Second Edition

ATHLETIC TRAINING
AND
SPORTS
MEDICINE

Second Edition

ATHLETIC TRAINING
AND
SPORTS
MEDICINE

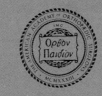

PUBLISHED BY THE

AMERICAN ACADEMY OF

ORTHOPAEDIC SURGEONS

Text Design: Angela Foote for The Book Department
Copyediting and Production: The Book Department, Inc., Boston
Medical and Technical Illustrations: Carol Binns, MA; Carol Capers, MSMI;
Heather Calehuff, ATC, PA-C; Sylvia Delk; Susan Banta; Laurel Cook; Sharon Ellis and Paul S. Foti
Photography: Steve Haywood; Yvonne Ehrhart; Dr. Edgardo Gonzalez-Ramirez and Katie Zernhelt
Cover Design: Hannus Design Associates
Cover Visuals: "Running Legs" by Vincent Perez;
background grid © UNIPHOTO/PICTOR INTERNATIONAL

SECOND EDITION

©1991 by the American Academy of Orthopaedic Surgeons

Telephone: 1-800-626-6726

ISBN 0-89203-044-5

Library of Congress Catalog Card Number 91-70295

10 9 8 7 6 5 4 3 2

Published and distributed by: American Academy of Orthopaedic Surgeons
6300 N. River Rd., Rosemont, IL 60018

Printed in the United States of America

Contents

Preface

In 1974, a workshop composed of representatives from the National Athletic Trainers Association (NATA), led by President Frank George, as well as members of the American Academy of Orthopaedic Surgeons (AAOS), met at Mount Hope Farm in Williamstown, Massachusetts. The purpose of the workshop was to devise educational programs to improve the training and health care of the athlete. Two major accomplishments resulted from this effort.

The first accomplishment, designed to increase the availability of skilled athletic trainers, was a proposed "alternative route" to becoming an athletic trainer that would permit interested faculty members to complete an approved training curriculum. Ultimately, these potential trainers would then be eligible to sit for the comprehensive certification exam. This alternative process was greatly aided by the contributions of Frank George, Lindsay McLean, and the late Sayers "Bud" Miller.

The second accomplishment was the development of a core curriculum. The impetus for this achievement came from Phillip B. Donley and William E. "Pinky" Newell. It was the strong recommendation of Phil Donley that a text be created for this educational program, and thus, the first edition of this text began to take shape. It was developed by editorial subgroups of NATA and members of the Sports Medicine Committee of AAOS.

Arthur Ellison, MD, the editor of the first edition of *Athletic Training and Sports Medicine*, stated in the Preface to that volume, "The reader is encouraged to consider this text to be in less than ultimate form. Sports medicine is dynamic and will continue to evolve. . . . It is the nature of Academy publications to grow and improve through revisions and subsequent editions. We hope this volume will be no exception, and that it will continue to evolve to better serve all of those who are concerned with and care for the athlete." As Dr. Ellison predicted, sports medicine has continued to evolve since the first edition was published, necessitating its revision.

For increased clarity, the second edition has been divided into eight sections:

Section One	Introduction
Section Two	Basic Concepts
Section Three	Diagnosis and Treatment of Specific Sports Injuries
Section Four	Medical Emergencies
Section Five	Preventing Injury
Section Six	Rehabilitation Techniques
Section Seven	Other Medical Issues
Section Eight	Selected Athletic Groups

Significant changes from the first edition include greatly expanded sections on the diagnosis and treatment of common injuries and medical problems seen in sport, updated chapters on medical emergency concerns, greater emphasis on the principles of conditioning and rehabilitation, and the inclusion of many more tables, charts, and figures to enhance readability.

It is hoped that the second edition of *Athletic Training and Sports Medicine* will continue to be not only a valuable textbook in athletic training and sports physical therapy curriculum programs, but also an important source of information for sports medicine physicians, exercise physiologists, and others involved in the care of athletes.

As this preface is written, the American Academy of Orthopaedic Surgeons is developing an Instructor's Manual to assist those who wish to use this edition as a course text. We feel this will be a significant supplement to the text.

My heartfelt thanks to all on the editorial board for the countless hours of work they contributed to the revision of this text. Their generosity in giving of both their time and expertise is greatly appreciated.

The editorial board wishes to express its appreciation to the members of NATA whose critiques were most helpful in the revision of this text: Dennis Aten, MS, PT, ATC; T. Ross Bailey, ATC; Gary Ball, ATC; Gerald Bell, EdD, PT, ATC; Marty Bradley, MS, ATC, EMT; Rod Compton, ATC; John Cottone, ATC; Michael Ferrara, ATC; Dan Foster, ATC; Suzanne Gewe, RN; Gordon Graham, PT, MS, ATC; Keith Handling, MS, PT, ATC; Peggy Houglum, RPT, ATC; Alexander Kalenak, MD; Kenneth Knight, PhD, ATC; Pete Koehneke, ATC; Roland LaRue, MA, PT, ATC; John Leard, MEd, PT, ATC; David Leigh, ATC; Brent Mangus, ATC; Dan Martin, ATC; Crayton Moss, MD, ATC; Robert Moss, ATC; Bobby Patton, EdD, ATC; John Powell, PhD, ATC; Carol Teitz, MD; Charles Vosler, ATC; and Don Zylks, PhD. Also thanks to The Coca-Cola Company and Southern Bell for contributing examples of their corporate wellness programs.

Special thanks to Leslie Neistadt for the many, many hours she spent on this project, both as an editorial board member and as a special assistant involved in the day-to-day organization of the manuscript. Also, many thanks to Carol Binns of the Hughston Sports Medicine Foundation for her valuable contribution in researching, selecting, and creating many of the medical illustrations in this edition. I'd also like to thank The Book Department, and in particular, Margaret Kearney, copyeditor, and Mary Day Fewlass, project manager. Their project management assisted us greatly in bringing this text to completion.

Finally, I wish to thank the staff of the American Academy of Orthopaedic Surgeons, particularly Sally King Jessee, publications manager, who served as project manager and oversaw the entire editorial and production process; and Kathy M. Brouillette, production editor, who worked on a daily basis for many months coordinating the production process and attending to the myriad details involved in a text of this magnitude. In addition, Mark W. Wieting, director of communications and publications, Marilyn L. Fox, PhD, assistant director, publications, and Keith Levine, marketing manager, all made valuable contributions to this text.

This second edition is an extension of the first, and its editorial board, Dr. Ellison; Arthur L. Boland, Jr., MD; Kenneth E. DeHaven, MD; Paul Grace, ATC; George Snook, MD; and Heather Calehuff, ATC, PA-C, should be recognized for having built a strong foundation with the first edition.

Letha Y. Hunter-Griffin, MD, PhD

Atlanta, Georgia

Acknowledgments

EDITORIAL BOARD

Chairman

Letha Y. Hunter-Griffin, MD, PhD
Peachtree Orthopaedic Clinic
Atlanta, Georgia

Members-at-Large

Tab Blackburn, PhD
Hughston Sports Medicine
  Foundation
Columbus, Georgia

Heather Calehuff, ATC, PA-C
Tuckahoe Orthopaedic Associates
Richmond, Virginia

Joe Gieck, EdD, ATC
Division of Sports Medicine and
  Athletic Training
University of Virginia
Charlottesville, Virginia

Paul Grace, ATC
Massachusetts Institute of
  Technology
Cambridge, Massachusetts

James Hill, MD
Northwestern Orthopaedic
  Associates
Chicago, Illinois

Stephen Hunter, MD
Hughston Sports Medicine
  Foundation
Columbus, Georgia

Terry Malone, EdD
Sports Medicine Center
Duke University
Durham, North Carolina

Leslie Neistadt, BA
Peachtree Orthopaedic Clinic
Atlanta, Georgia

CONTRIBUTORS

The Editorial Board of *Athletic Training and Sports Medicine* and the American Academy of Orthopaedic Surgeons wish to acknowledge the significant contributions made to this volume by the following individuals:

Julie Agel, MA, ATC
Seattle, Washington

David F. Apple, Jr., MD
Atlanta, Georgia

William D. Bandy, MA, PT, ATC,
  SCS
Conway, Arkansas

W. Daniel Caffrey, MD
Greensboro, North Carolina

John D. Cantwell, MD
Atlanta, Georgia

Bruce Cassidy, MD
Atlanta, Georgia

Rod Compton, MEd, ATC
Greenville, North Carolina

Patricia Darlington, ATC
Atlanta, Georgia

Craig Denegar, PhD
Slippery Rock, Pennsylvania

E. Randy Eichner, MD
Oklahoma City, Oklahoma

John P. Fulkerson, MD
Farmington, Connecticut

Robert Geller, MD
Atlanta, Georgia

J. Nicholas Gordon, MD
Atlanta, Georgia

Karl Kline, BMSc, PA-C
Atlanta, Georgia

Kenneth Knight, PhD, ATC
Terre Haute, Indiana

Wayne B. Leadbetter, MD
Rockville, Maryland

Laura Lodzinski, MEd
Atlanta, Georgia

Fred McGlynn, MD
Richmond, Virginia

Deborah Robinson MacLean, ATC
Atlanta, Georgia

John Marshall, BA, JD
Atlanta, Georgia

James Millhouse, PhD
Stone Mountain, Georgia

Lisa A. Nelson, ATC
Edmonds, Washington

Karen Nilson, MD
Seattle, Washington

Rebecca Oatts, MEd
Richmond, Virginia

JoAnn Patterson, PhD
Atlanta, Georgia

David Pawlowski, ATC
Richmond, Virginia

David Perrin, PhD
Charlottesville, Virginia

Larry Price, MA
Atlanta, Georgia

Stephen Rice, MD, PhD, MPH
Seattle, Washington

Robert Rotella, PhD
Charlottesville, Virginia

Cheryl Rubin, MD
Bridgewater, New Jersey

Ethan Saliba, MEd, ATC, PT
Charlottesville, Virginia

Anthony G. Smith, MEd, CSCS
Richmond, Virginia

The Editorial Board of *Athletic Training and Sports Medicine* and the American Academy of Orthopaedic Surgeons also recognize the contributions of the following individuals who served as editorial advisors:

Arthur L. Boland, Jr., MD
Boston, Massachusetts

Kenneth E. DeHaven, MD
Rochester, New York

John Feagin, MD
Durham, North Carolina

Keith L. Markey, MD
San Antonio, Texas

National Athletic Trainers' Association, Inc.

2952 STEMMONS • DALLAS, TX 75247 • (214) 637-6282 • FAX: (214) 637-2206

MARK J. SMAHA
PRESIDENT

ALAN A. SMITH, JR.
EXECUTIVE DIRECTOR

Dear Reader:

It is a pleasure to present to you the second edition of *Athletic Training and Sports Medicine*. The enthusiastic reception given the first edition has provided contributors with the impetus and encouragement to produce this text for our students of athletic medicine.

Since the beginning of the National Athletic Trainers Association in 1950, an important goal has been to upgrade educational standards within our profession. The publication of the second edition demonstrates a commitment to this concept and the opportunity for the physician and athletic trainer to work together in this endeavor.

On behalf of the members of the National Athletic Trainers Association, we thank the many contributors to the book and its many readers for their support.

Sincerely,

National Athletic Trainers Association

Mark J Smaha

Mark J. Smaha
President

INTRODUCTION

1

Emergence of Sports Medicine as a Discipline

CHAPTER OUTLINE

The Historical Development of
Sports Medicine
   The Early Sports Physicians and
   Trainers
   The Beginning of Physical
   Education in U.S. Schools
The Development of Athletic
Training and Sports Medicine
   Intercollegiate and Interscholastic
   Athletics

The Growing Need for Medical
   Care of Athletes
International Sports Medicine
Organizations
Sports Safety Organizations
Sports Organizations for the
Physically and Mentally Impaired

OBJECTIVES FOR CHAPTER 1

After reading this chapter, the student should be able to:
1. Discuss how the discipline of sports medicine evolved.
2. Identify various sports organizations whose development was closely
   linked to the development of sports medicine as a discipline and the
   sports medicine team.

INTRODUCTION

Throughout history, man's ability to survive has depended on physical capabilities. The speed, skill, and strength early man needed for survival were transformed into games of skill during times of peace. As civilization progressed and athletic contests became more organized, more highly trained and skilled athletes competed in teams. Maintaining fitness and recovering from injuries became increasingly important as the sophistication and popularity of athletic events grew. The need for physicians, trainers, and therapists knowledgeable in the care and rehabilitation of athletes grew simultaneously. Injury prevention through regulation of equipment and playing rules also became important.

Chapter 1 traces the evolution of the sports medicine team. The chapter begins with a brief history of early sports physicians and trainers. Next, the beginnings of physical education in the United States are described. The chapter goes on to describe the development of athletic training and sports medicine. Both disciplines were influenced by the emergence of intercollegiate and interscholastic organizations and the growing need for medical care as athletic participation increased. The last sections of Chapter 1 briefly mention international sports medicine organizations, sports safety organizations, and sports organizations for the physically and mentally impaired. ■

THE HISTORICAL DEVELOPMENT OF SPORTS MEDICINE

The historical development of any field is of interest, not only because it gives students familiarity with the people, places, and organizations that helped shape their area of interest, but also because it provides students with a sense of perspective—why did the field develop and how has it changed to meet the new demands of society?

The Early Sports Physicians and Trainers

The use of therapeutic exercises (medical gymnastics) was recorded as early as 800 to 1000 B.C. in the Atharva-Veda, a medical manuscript from India. Historians claim that the first sports physician was Herodicus. During the fifth century B.C., he treated athletes and other injured people in Athens with therapeutic exercises and diet.

Herodicus's colleagues criticized his approach as being harsh and radical. Yet, his fame spread, and other physicians came to observe and evaluate his techniques. His most famous pupil was Hippocrates, who later wrote of the value of exercise in treating many illnesses.

In the second century A.D., Galen was appointed physician to the gladiators and thus became the first physician known to occupy a position analogous to the team physician of today. Although he recognized the brutality and danger of some of the sporting events of his day, he taught and did an enormous amount of research in anatomy, physiology, and sports injuries. While he did not believe in excessive exercise, he did recommend exercise in moderation to maintain health and to treat many diseases.

In the fourth century A.D., Oribasius of

Pergamum claimed that the body's organs functioned better when they were physically stressed. He therefore endorsed an intensified form of exercise. In the fifth century A.D., the physician Aurelianus first recommended exercise during convalescence from surgery; he prescribed hydrotherapy and the use of weights and pulleys.

During the first five centuries of the Christian era, the invasions by the Barbarians, in combination with the medieval church's zealous destruction of Greek and, to some extent, Roman knowledge, led to the loss of many of the early medical texts. Fortunately, the Muslims, under the caliphate of al-Mansur and Harun al-Rashid, encouraged science and education. They ordered the earlier Greek, Roman, and Hebrew medical documents copied into Arabic. Thus, these works were preserved for later return to the Western world.

Hakim Avicenna (ibn-e-Sina), who lived from 980 to 1037 A.D., was probably the most famous Muslim writer. His standing in Islam was certainly equal to that of Galen in Rome. The Canon (Al-Qanun), his most famous medical book, describes prophylactic medical gymnastics and proposes rest, heat, massage, and exercise to aid recovery from illness and injury.

The Beginning of Physical Education in U.S. Schools

In the 15th century, Vittorino de Feltre and Maffeus Veginus reintroduced the Greek tradition of obligatory exercise and sports into the educational curriculum. This concept has influenced Western education ever since.

Physical education in the United States received its start at Amherst College in Amherst, Massachusetts, with the appointment in 1854 of Edward Hitchcock, Jr., as professor of physical education and hygiene. He developed a system of coordinated physical education for the college, incorporating the Swedish and German systems of gymnastics and running, as well as the American-style games of football, basket-

ball, and track. Dr. Hitchcock also served as the school physician for Amherst College. In this capacity, he instituted the study of anthropomorphic measurements of Amherst College students. He also kept systematic records of the incidence of disease and injury at Amherst College. His writings covered a broad range of subjects, such as "Athletics in American Colleges," "Basketball for Women," and "The Gymnastic Era and Athletic Era of Our Country." He is correctly identified as the founder of physical education in the United States; he was also the first team physician in America.

The American Alliance of Health, Physical Education, and Recreation (AAHPER) was founded in 1885 to promote the exchange of ideas and to stimulate research in exercise. It added Dance to its name in 1979 (AAHPERD), and has remained an active influence in health education, sports, and physical exercise. Its members include physical educators at all curriculum levels from elementary schools through colleges, as well as exercise physiologists, trainers, and physicians. This organization serves as the principal force for all physical education related activities in the United States.

AAHPERD developed the first standard fitness test for youth in 1958. This test, comprised of seven test items with results given in percentile scores, was adopted by the President's Council on Youth Fitness, the cabinet-level council formed by President Eisenhower. Physical education teachers gave the test in the fall and spring to grade school and high school students. Its intent was to measure and hence encourage the improvement of fitness during the school year.

The President's Council on Youth Fitness, whose name was changed to the President's Council on Physical Fitness under President Kennedy, continued to encourage the youth fitness program through national testing. In 1966, President Johnson began the President's Physical Fitness Awards Program, which gave awards to children who scored in the 85th percentile or higher on the fitness tests. Table 1.1 shows the

TABLE 1.1. Development of Government-Sponsored Fitness Programs for Youth

President	Organization	Comments
Eisenhower	President's Council on Youth Fitness	Developed as a cabinet-level position under the Secretary of the Interior
Kennedy	President's Council on Physical Fitness	Cabinet-level council under the Secretary of HEW
Johnson		Began physical fitness awards program
Nixon	President's Council on Physical Fitness in Sports	Abolition of the cabinet-level council; creation of a 15-member committee

development of government-sponsored fitness programs for youth.

Under President Nixon, the cabinet-level council was replaced by a 15-member committee renamed the President's Council on Physical Fitness in Sports. Advised by an appointed group of prominent sports persons, the council produced many publications emphasizing the development of lifetime sports activity.

In the 1980s, the President's Physical Fitness Awards Program was challenged by some physical educators who believed it focused too much on sports performance and athletic ability and too little on health-related fitness. In response, the AAHPERD developed the Lifetime Health-Related Fitness Test. Over the last decade, several other testing systems have been developed, not only to evaluate and record each child's fitness level, but also to use the scores to help each child establish an exercise program to improve his or her own fitness level. Table 1.2 compares these tests.

The American Medical Association's (AMA) Committee on Exercise and Physical Fitness was created in 1964 and continues to work closely with the President's Council on Physical Fitness in Sports, as well as with AAHPERD, for public education in this area and promotion of physical fitness for all ages. These organizations stress the need for the school system to be involved not only in providing classes for the development and measuring of youth fitness, but also in educating young people about the advantages of regular physical exercise.

THE DEVELOPMENT OF ATHLETIC TRAINING AND SPORTS MEDICINE

As competitive sports grew in the United States throughout the 20th century, individuals concerned with the safety of the athlete organized for mutual cooperation. Books were published on the prevention,

TABLE 1.2. Comparison of Youth Fitness Tests

AAHPERD Youth Fitness Test (modification from original 1958 test)	AAHPERD Health-Related Physical Fitness Test (1980)	President's Council on Physical Fitness in Sports Test (1986)
Sit-ups Pull-ups (boys) or flexed-arm hang (girls) Shuttle run 600-yard run walk 50-yard dash Standing broad jump	Sit-ups Mile run or 9-minute run Sit-and-reach flexibility test Sum of triceps and subscapular skinfolds	Curl-ups (bent-knee sit-ups) Pull-ups (boys) or flexed-arm hang (girls) Shuttle run Mile run/walk V-fit reach flexibility test

Source: *The Melpomene Journal*, vol. 7, no. 2 (Spring 1988).

recognition, and treatment of sports injuries. Perhaps some of the most outstanding of these early works were Sigren Weissbein's *Hygiene des Sports* in 1910, Byles and Osborne's *The Encyclopedia of Sports* in 1898, and Dr. S. E. Bilik's *Trainer's Bible* in 1916. In 1931, Walter Meanwell collaborated with Knute Rockne to produce the first American sports medicine work, which discussed the role of the athletic trainer and team physician in caring for the athlete.

In 1888, sports leaders interested in creating standards and guidelines for amateur athletics in the United States established the Amateur Athletic Union (AAU). Its original 15 member clubs have grown to several thousand clubs, which conduct local, state, regional, and national competitions in the United States and its territories. The AAU remains the largest U.S. nonprofit volunteer organization dedicated solely to the promotion and development of amateur sports and physical fitness programs. It sponsors the AAU/Junior Olympics and the AAU Senior Sports Program. It also provides awards to recognize fitness and sports achievements.

Intercollegiate and Interscholastic Athletics

In general, the development of athletic training and sports medicine in the United States is most closely tied to the development of intercollegiate and, to a lesser extent, interscholastic athletics. Hence, any discussion of the history of athletic training and sports medicine must include an understanding of the growth of organized competitive sports between and within our schools.

The National Collegiate Athletic Association (NCAA) was founded in 1906. Known initially as the Collegiate Athletic Association of the United States, it was formed by 62 representatives of 13 institutions. These individuals met at the urging of President Theodore Roosevelt, who was concerned over the number of injuries occurring in the poorly regulated sport of college football.

The NCAA initially functioned only as a discussion group and rule-making body, but it soon began to foster sports development in colleges and universities by sponsoring national championships, not only in football, but in many other sports as well. With its headquarters in Mission, Kansas, the NCAA remains a voluntary association devoted to the sound administration of intercollegiate athletics. Member colleges consider all athletic problems that cross regional or conference lines. Today the NCAA engages in the following activities:

▪ Develops, interprets, and enforces rules for sports safety.
▪ Conducts research on sports issues.
▪ Compiles sports statistics.
▪ Provides financial assistance to groups interested in promoting intercollegiate athletics.
▪ Answers questions on policies and other matters in intercollegiate athletics.
▪ Promotes participation in international sports programs.
▪ Administers insurance programs for member institutions and student athletes.
▪ Promotes community youth programs and administers national marketing programs.
▪ Promotes championship events and all other intercollegiate athletics through planned activities.

Any college or university may be elected to active membership in the NCAA if it is accredited by the recognized academic accrediting agency in its region, maintains at least four intercollegiate sports for men and four for women (one in each of the three traditional seasons), and complies with all NCAA legislation.

In 1920, the National Federation of State High School Associations (NFSHSA) was founded to promote the safe development of interscholastic activities. The National Federation believes such activities are a necessary part of the growth and development of young people.

Many college team physicians belong to

the sports medicine section of the American College Health Association (ACHA), an organization also founded in 1920. The ACHA offers a forum where representatives from college and university health centers, including physicians, nurses, pharmacists, trainers, and students, can work together to improve health care. The development of the sports medicine section within this organization has enabled college team physicians and trainers to cooperate in the exchange of ideas and information, which has led to improved medical supervision of both intercollegiate and intramural sports. The ACHA, in association with organizations such as the National Athletic Trainers Association (NATA) and the National Operating Committee on Standards for Athletic Equipment (NOCSAE), also participates in making recommendations regarding sports safety.

A number of basketball coaches from small colleges and universities throughout the country formed the National Association of Intercollegiate Basketball in 1940. Its initial function was the sponsorship of a small, invitational college tournament in basketball. In 1952 it changed its name to the National Association for Intercollegiate Athletics (NAIA) and expanded its role to include sponsorship of tournaments in a variety of sports, championing athletic opportunities for smaller schools. Members of the NAIA may also belong to the NCAA, and like the NCAA, the NAIA has been active in the promotion of sports safety.

The Growing Need for Medical Care of Athletes

Even though the NCAA, the NAIA, the ACHA, and the NFSHSA were interested in preserving the welfare of the athlete, their prime concern was the organization and promotion of sports competition. As the number of athletes participating in organized sports grew during the mid-1900s, a great demand for qualified persons to care for the medical needs of the athlete arose. Physicians interested in sports, many of

them former athletes themselves, were asked to provide emergency care of athletic injuries and to be available as medical consultants for this unique population of young, basically healthy individuals who demanded prompt, aggressive treatment of their injuries and as rapid a return to competition as safely possible.

Trainers were needed to assume the day-to-day responsibility for the medical care of the athlete. The trainer, serving as the link between physician and athlete and between athlete and coach, became responsible for preventing athletic injuries by instituting effective conditioning programs, by providing adequate protective equipment for the athlete (tape, pads, braces, bandages, etc.), and by advising the coach and the athlete on medical issues (proper hydration and other nutritional counseling, safety of the playing field, proper fit of equipment, etc.). When the physician was not present, the trainer assumed the responsibility of the initial evaluation and first-aid treatment of athletic injuries, making referrals to the team physician when needed. Rehabilitation of the injured athlete also fell into the trainer's domain.

As the demand on those in athletic training increased, they felt a need to organize on a national level to discuss issues of mutual concern such as ensuring the development of proper educational programs in the field of athletic training, establishing standards of care for athletic trainers, and exchanging ideas on injury management and prevention. Their first meeting was held in 1938 at the Drake Relays in Des Moines, Iowa. This meeting was organized primarily through the efforts of Bill Frey, trainer at the University of Iowa, and Charles Cramer, founder of the Cramer Chemical Company. Charles Cramer and his brother Frank did much to expand the knowledge of athletic training in the United States. Their company produced and distributed nationally a liniment to aid the healing of athletic injuries. The liniment was first developed by Charles himself to treat a sprained ankle. The Cramer Chemical Company not only produced one of the earliest newsletters in athletic training, *First Aider*, in 1936, but also was instrumental in contributing funds and ideas to the NATA.

At the Drake Relays meeting, Michael Chambers of Louisiana State University was appointed president of the NATA, and Bill Frey served as secretary-treasurer. The home office was designated as Iowa City. However, this early organization had difficulties gathering and maintaining support, and it was dissolved during the early war years of the 1940s.

Following the end of World War II, trainers in the various athletic conferences organized into associations for the purpose of exchanging ideas about athletic training. From these associations the desire to have a national body grew again. This time the local organizations were the instrumental force in recreating the NATA. Their first national meeting was held in 1950 at Kansas City, Missouri, and the following goals were established: to promote the exchange of ideas in athletic training, to develop athletic educational programs at the high school and college levels, to establish standards of performance for those in the field of athletic training, and to promote the overall development of athletics and fitness in the United States.

In 1956, the NATA began to publish *Athletic Training: Journal of the NATA*. Today, this journal remains a quarterly publication for the dissemination of recent developments in the field; it also provides a forum for the distribution of information of professional interest to the athletic trainer. The NATA established a code of ethics in 1957 to ensure the highest standards of conduct among its members. It has structured college curricula in athletic training and developed certification standards.

A group interested in furthering the development of sports research, both in the areas of basic science as well as in the clinically applied areas, and in promoting the interchange of knowledge among those in the various areas of sports medicine,

formed the American College of Sports Medicine in 1954. The membership of this organization consists of basic science physiologists, exercise physiologists, chemists, physicians, trainers, nutritionists, coaches, and others interested in fitness.

The American Medical Association in 1956 established the Committee for Sports Injuries to collect data on the prevalence and causes of injuries in sports and to make recommendations for injury prevention. Three years later this organization became known as the Committee on Medical Aspects of Sports. Through the committee's investigation, it became clear that a team approach, with the trainer and physician as the fundamental basis of the team, was necessary to provide proper medical care of the athlete and to decrease injuries. In 1966, the AMA House of Delegates endorsed a resolution recognizing the importance of qualified athletic trainers and encouraging their incorporation in all sports programs, further ensuring the necessary bond between trainer and physician as the core of the sports medicine team.

By the 1970s, the field of sports medicine was growing rapidly, mainly because more people were participating in both recreational and competitive athletics. Increasingly, orthopedic surgeons were asked to be present at sports events and to render care to the injured athlete. Family physicians, pediatricians, and internists also were asked to contribute to the athlete's care, but these professionals were more involved in preseason screening of athletes and in managing medical illnesses of the athletes than in treating their acute injuries.

A group of the first "Sports Orthopedists," spurred by such men as Jack Nicholas, Don O'Donoghue, and Jack Hughston, decided to form a smaller group within the larger American Academy of Orthopaedic Surgeons so that those primarily interested in treating athletic injuries could gather several times a year to discuss issues in sports medicine. Hence the American Orthopaedic Society for Sports Medicine (AOSSM) was created in 1972. Members of the AOSSM work to foster an awareness of the important relationship between the members of the sports medicine team through scholarship funds, scientific meetings, and educational publications and seminars. At their national meeting, they not only recognize outstanding leaders in sports orthopedics, but also present the Distinguished Service Trainer Award.

The trend toward specialization in sports medicine continued with the creation of the Sports Physical Therapy Section of the American Physical Therapy Association. Members of this group, which was founded in 1972, meet annually to exchange information on advances in sports therapy and to discuss common problems. The group sponsors research, as well as several educational conferences each year, which are open not only to members, but also to interested therapists, physicians, and trainers. Competency examinations in the area of sports physical therapy are recognized by the Board of Specialization of the American Physical Therapy Association.

Up-to-date listings of national sports organizations and sports medicine organizations, their date of founding, and their publications can be found in Table 1.3. The addresses of national sports medicine organizations, athletic trainers associations, high school and college organizations, and athletic injury data sources are listed at the end of the chapter.

INTERNATIONAL SPORTS MEDICINE ORGANIZATIONS

The development of sports medicine and athletic training paralleled the growth of organized sports competition, both in the United States and on the international level. The founding of the modern-day Olympics by Baron de Couberlin in 1896 probably marks the beginning of organized international competitive sports. The first Olympic Games were held in Athens, and 311 athletes representing 13 countries participated.

It was during the 1928 Second Winter Olympic Games in St. Moritz that Drs. F. Latarject of France and W. Knoll of Switzerland organized a meeting of 33 physicians, representing the 11 nations which attended

TABLE 1.3. National Sports Organizations

Organization	Date Founded	Publications
American Alliance for Health, Physical Education, Recreation, and Dance	1885	Journal of Physical Education Strategies Health Education Research Quarterly for Exercise and Sports
Amateur Athletic Union	1888	InfoAAU
National Collegiate Athletic Association	1906	NCAA General Information, 1987–88 NCAA News NCAA Sports Medicine Handbook
National Federation of State High School Associations	1920	National High School Sports Magazine 1987–1988 Handbook
United States Olympic Committee	1921	The USA in the Olympic Movement
National Athletic Trainers Association	1938	Injury Report: High School Reports Athletic Training: Journal of the NATA
National Association of Intercollegiate Athletics	1940	NAIA News
American College of Sports Medicine	1954	Medicine and Science in Sports and Exercise Exercise and Sport Science Reviews Sports Medicine (Bulletin)
National Federation of High School Athletic Coaches	1965	National Coach
American Orthopaedic Society for Sports Medicine	1972	American Journal of Sports Medicine
Sports Physical Therapy Section	1972	Journal of Orthopaedic and Sports Physical Therapy
National Strength and Conditioning Association	1978	NSCA Journal Journal of Applied Sport Science Research

the Games. This gathering might be considered the first meeting of the Federation Internationale Medico Sportiva (FIMS), also known as the International Federation for Sports Medicine. Still the leading international society for sports medicine, this organization is responsible for inaugurating sports-related research, promoting the study of medical problems in collaboration with various international sports federations, and organizing the International Congress of Sports Medicine, which is held simultaneously with the Olympic Games. The FIMS represents 78 national associations and serves as medical advisers to the International Olympic Committee.

Within the United States, the United States Olympic Committee (USOC), founded initially in 1921 as the American Olympic Association and renamed the USOC in 1961, is primarily responsible for the organization and development of U.S. team participation in the Olympic and Pan American Games. It coordinates amateur athletic activity relating to international competition and maintains the Olympic training centers in Colorado Springs, Colorado, Lake Placid, New York, and Marquette, Michigan, where athletes are sent to train after being chosen by the governing bodies of their various sports. In addition, the USOC also supports research in sports medicine, science, and safety.

SPORTS SAFETY ORGANIZATIONS

In any historical review, one should not forget to mention the contributions of organizations founded to ensure safety in sports through the safety testing of athletic equipment and the recording and analyzing of injury statistics.

The American Society for Testing and Materials (ASTM) has been developing standards for athletic equipment since 1898. The National Operating Committee for Standards in Athletic Equipment (NOCSAE), founded in 1969, conducts testing and research to develop standards in

and improve the quality of athletic equipment.

The U.S. Consumer Products Safety Commission sponsors the National Electronic Injury Surveillance System (NEISS), which monitors emergency room reports on injuries and accidents. This system began in 1972 and provides information to the commission and other agencies regarding the safety of consumer products.

The Injury Surveillance System of the NCAA was founded in 1982, initially to review football injuries and make recommendations to decrease their occurrence rate. It now monitors injury reports in all major sports. The NATA actively participates in collecting data for this system. The NCAA is also active in this area via the Committee on Competitive Safeguards and Medical Aspects of Sports, which recommends policies to promote the general health and well-being of the athlete.

The concern over catastrophic head and neck injuries in sports resulted in the establishment of committees that closely monitor the occurrence of such injuries and make recommendations to minimize their occurrence. The most active of these committees have been at the University of Pennsylvania and the University of North Carolina.

The NATA sponsors the National High School Injury Registry (NHSIR), a mechanism for gathering data relating to football, basketball, wrestling, and soccer injuries.

SPORTS ORGANIZATIONS FOR THE PHYSICALLY AND MENTALLY IMPAIRED

Concerns for the development of sports participation by the physically and mentally handicapped resulted in the founding of numerous organizations to further knowledge relating to the unique problems encountered by these athletes, as well as to develop sports participation opportunities for them. A discussion of these organizations and their activities is contained in Chapters 61 and 62.

IMPORTANT CONCEPTS

1. Historians identify Herodicus as the first sports physician.
2. President Eisenhower created the President's Council on Youth Fitness to upgrade physical education programs in U.S. schools.
3. The development of sports medicine in the United States is closely linked to the development of intercollegiate and interscholastic athletics.
4. As athletic participation increased, so did the demands on trainers and physicians to provide medical care for injured athletes.
5. The International Federation for Sports Medicine is the leading international society for sports medicine.
6. Sports safety organizations have played an important role in sports medicine through the safety testing of athletic equipment and the recording and analyzing of injury statistics.

SUGGESTED READINGS

Arnheim, D. D. *Modern Principles of Athletic Training: The Science of Sports Medicine: Injury Prevention, Causation, and Management*, 6th ed. St. Louis: Times Mirror/ Mosby College Publishing, 1985, pp. 1–75.

Beach, B. K., ed. *Journal of Physical Education, Recreation & Dance*, vol.56, no.4. Reston, Va.: American Alliance for Health, Physical Education, Recreation and Dance, 1985.

Bell, G. W., ed. *Professional Preparation in Athletic Training*. Champaign, Ill.: Human Kinetics, 1982.

Kulund, D. N., ed. *The Injured Athlete*, 2d ed. Philadelphia: J. B. Lippincott, 1988, pp. 1–48.

Larson, L. A., ed. *Encyclopedia of Sport Sciences and Medicine*. New York: Macmillan, 1971, pp. xxxiii–xlvii.

National Athletic Trainers Association. *Fundamentals of Athletic Training*, 2d ed. A Joint Project of the National Athletic Trainers Association, the Athletic Institute, and the Medical Aspects of Sports Committee of the American Medical Association. Chicago: The American Medical Association, 1971.

Nelson, A., ed. *Melpomene Journal*, vol. 7, no. 2. St. Paul, Minn.: Melpomene Institute for Women's Health Research, 1988.

O'Shea, M., ed. *A History of the National Athletic Trainers Association*. NATA, 1980.

Roy, S., and R. Irvin. *Sports Medicine: Prevention, Evaluation, Management, and Rehabilitation*. Englewood Cliffs, N.J.: Prentice-Hall, 1983, pp. 1–8.

Ryan, A. J., and F. L. Allman, Jr., eds. *Sports Medicine*. New York: Academic Press, 1974, pp. 3–55.

Williams, J. G. P., and P. N. Sperryn, eds. *Sports Medicine*, 2d ed. London: Edward Arnold, 1976, pp. 1–6.

SPORTS MEDICINE RESOURCES

NOTE: Many of the national organizations on this list have regional, state, or local chapters, with committees that deal with various aspects of sports medicine.

National Organizations

Amateur Athletic Union
3400 West 86th Street
P.O. Box 68207
Indianapolis, IN 46268
(317) 872-2900

American Academy of Family Physicians,
Sports Committee
8880 Ward Parkway
Kansas City, MO 64114
(816) 333-9700

The American Academy of Orthopaedic
Surgeons, Sports Medicine Committee
6300 N. River Road
Rosemont, IL 60018
(708) 823-7186

American Academy of Pediatrics, Sports
Committee
P.O. Box 927
Elk Grove Village, IL 60009
(708) 228-5005

American Academy of Pediatric Sports
Medicine
1729 Glastonberry Road
Potomac, MD 20854
(301) 424-7440

American Alliance of Health,
Physical Education, Recreation and Dance
1900 Association Drive
Reston, VA 22091
(703) 476-3400

American College of Sports Medicine
P.O. Box 1440
Indianapolis, IN 46206-1440
(317) 637-9200

American Medical Association
515 North State Street
Chicago, IL 60610
(312) 464-5000

American Orthopaedic Society for Sports
Medicine, Suite 115
2250 E. Devon Ave.
Des Plaines, IL 60018
(708) 803-8700

American Society for Testing and Materials
1916 Race Street
Philadelphia, PA 19103
(215) 299-5585

National Strength and Conditioning
Association
P.O. Box 81410
920 O Street
Lincoln, NE 68508
(402) 472-3000

Sports Physical Therapy Section of the
American Physical Therapy Association
2220 Grand View Drive, Suite 150
Fort Mitchell, KY 41017
(606) 341-6654

United States Olympic Committee
1750 East Boulder Street
Colorado Springs, CO 80909-5760
(719) 632-5551

Athletic Trainers Association

National Athletic Trainers' Association
2952 Stemmons Freeway, Suite 200
Dallas, TX 75247
(214) 637-6282

High School Organizations

National Federation of State High School
Associations
11724 Plaza Circle
P.O. Box 20626
Kansas City, MO 64195
(816) 464-5400

National High School Athletic Coaches
Association
P.O. Box 1808
Ocala, FL 32678
(904) 622-3660

College Organizations

National Association for Intercollegiate
Athletics
1221 Baltimore Ave.
Kansas City, MO 64105
(816) 842-5050

American College Health Association
P.O. Box 28937
Baltimore, MD 21240-8937
(410) 859-1500

National Collegiate Athletic Association
6201 College Blvd.
Overland Park, KS 66211-2422
(913) 339-1906

Athletic Injury Data Sources

National Athletic Head and Neck Injury
Registry
235 South 33rd Street
Weightman Hall
Philadelphia, PA 19104
(215) 662-4090

NEIS Data Highlights, 1988;
The Product Summary Report, 1989
National Electronic Injury Surveillance
System
U.S. Consumer Product Safety Commission,
Room 625
5401 Westbard Avenue
Washington, DC 20207

National Safety Council
1121 Spring Lake Drive
Itasca, IL 60143-3201
(708) 285-1121

New York State Public High School
Athletic Association
88 Delaware Avenue
Delmar, NY 12054
(518) 439-8872

NOCSAE Manual, 1987
National Operating Committee on
Standards for Athletic Equipment
11724 Plaza Circle
Kansas City, MO 64153
(816) 464-5470

Twenty Questions About ASTM
American Society for Testing and
Materials
1916 Race Street
Philadelphia, PA, 19103
(215) 299-5585

2

The Sports Medicine Team

OBJECTIVES FOR CHAPTER 2

After reading this chapter, the student should be able to:

1. Develop an active and assistive sports medicine team appropriate for a particular athletic situation.
2. Define the roles of the individual active team members according to the specific athletic situation.

INTRODUCTION

In some ways athletes are no different from nonathletic patients who sustain the same injuries and illnesses. However, athletes are different from the general population in that they impose higher functional demands on their cardiovascular, respiratory, and musculoskeletal systems. As do other healthy, highly motivated people, athletes want to recover maximum function. The primary goals of the sports medicine team are to prevent as many injuries and illnesses as possible, to treat injuries and illnesses when they do occur, and to arrange for complete rehabilitation so that injured athletes can return to their sports as quickly and as safely as possible.

Chapter 2 focuses on the sports medicine team. The chapter begins by describing the team approach—how a team consists of both active and assistive members and the key factors needed to develop a successful team. The rest of the chapter discusses the responsibilities of the active members of the team. ■

THE TEAM APPROACH

The special needs of today's athletes can best be provided through a team approach. Each team member has a role in ensuring that the athlete is competing safely and to full potential. The team member's role also includes trying to prevent injury or, once an injury occurs, trying to rehabilitate the athlete. Communication is essential between team members and is best achieved by defining roles and expectations of each member at the outset and making certain each team member understands his or her role and the role of others.

Active and Assistive Team Members

The sports medicine team should, in actuality, be two teams—an active team and an assistive team.

The **active team** in an intercollegiate sports program consists of the following individuals:

- Team physician
- Certified athletic trainer
- Coaches
- The athlete

- Parents of the athlete
- Athletic administrators/directors
- Family physician/pediatrician
- Student athletic trainers

Each member of the active team plays a vital role in the health, safety, and welfare of the athlete.

The **assistive team** in an intercollegiate setting is comprised of individuals who play important but secondary roles in the care of athletes. The assistive team consists of medical consultant specialists, allied medical personnel, and general consultants.

The following medical consultant specialists should be readily available for consultation to the team:

- Allergist
- Cardiologist
- Dermatologist
- Dentist/oral surgeon
- Gynecologist
- Internist
- Neurosurgeon
- Ophthalmologist
- Orthopedist (unless the same as the team physician)
- Otolaryngologist
- General surgeon
- Urologist
- Radiologist

Allied medical personnel who may be needed include the following:

- Physical therapist/sports therapist
- Emergency medical technician
- Laboratory technicians
- Nursing staff
- Optometrist
- Pharmacist
- Podiatrist
- Psychologist/mental health specialist
- Cardiac rehabilitation specialist

The general consultants whose involvement is advantageous to the team approach for the care of athletes include:

- Administrators
- Brace maker

- Orthotist
- Equipment manager
- Exercise physiologist
- Health educator
- Kinesiologist
- Lawyer
- Nutritionist
- Substance abuse personnel
- Strength coach

The interaction of the active medical team with these consulting groups enhances the success of the medical team's efforts to care for today's athletes adequately and properly.

Key Factors in Developing a Successful Team

The active medical team members are responsible for providing medical care for the athlete. The success of the program depends on the active team members' qualifications, interest, and abilities. Certainly, the knowledge, skills, and experience of the physician and trainer are key factors in developing a successful program, but communication between team members, role delineation, and respect for the medical team's capabilities are also vital.

Communication Between Team Members

The chain of command and lines of communication in a sports medicine team should be well established and followed. In a well-organized program, the team trainer is the liaison between all parties. Many programs utilize triplicate or four-page speed communication forms (Fig. 2.1). Using these forms helps the physician, athletic trainer, coach, athletes, and parents keep abreast of such issues as diagnosis, plan of action, restrictions, progress in rehabilitation, and expected date for return to action. If all team members are routinely appraised of this type of information, they can work together toward the athlete's safe return to play.

Sports Injury Clinic

Name_____Date_____

TO: Trainer_____

       Coach_____

       Parents_____

DIAGNOSIS_____

_____

_____

PLAN/COMMENTS_____

_____

_____

_____

_____

_____

STATUS _____Schedule a return visit

           _____Return to activity

           _____Return to full activity

Signed_____Date_____

ATHLETE'S COPY

OFFICE COPY

COACH'S COPY

ATHLETIC TRAINER'S COPY

FIGURE 2.1. A four-part speed communication form.

Delineation of Roles

The physician should communicate directly with parents regarding special or serious problems, particularly in a high school setting. By having a clear understanding of the injury and treatment plan, the parents can facilitate the athlete's recovery. Parents can monitor the athlete's activity outside the athletic arena and supervise an at-home rehabilitation program as directed.

The relationship between physician and trainer is most important for the smooth, efficient operation of the sports medicine program. These two individuals should be compatible, with mutual respect and confidence in each other's abilities. Possibly, the key ingredient in a successful physician-trainer relationship is understanding each other's roles.

Within the realm of the athlete-coach-trainer-physician interaction, it is paramount that all involved are in complete agreement as to who makes the medical decisions regarding who plays or practices. The final decision rests solely with the team physician, although input from the trainer, who has more day-to-day contact with the athlete, is vital.

Respect for the Medical Team

For the team approach to be effective, team members, athletes, and administrative personnel must have respect and confidence in the medical team's capabilities and techniques. The physician and trainer must keep the athlete's best interests in mind at all times and not yield to outside pressure. The coach can create the environment necessary for cooperation and proper care by acting intelligently and maturely, displaying trust and confidence in the trainer and medical team. Policies must ensure that everyone understands the process of deciding the availability of athletes for practice or competition. Strong administrative support is a must for the medical team's control of availability, as an administrator must be aware of these policies and be ready to control situations in which conflict might develop.

The ability to compromise on methodology without compromising oneself is also important for team members. The ability to plan ahead for problems and emergencies and then to act in tandem to detect common and unique problems and devise appropriate care results in efficient medical care.

Triage

Triage is usually much simpler in an athletic training room or on the playing field than in the hospital emergency department. Injuries that occur simultaneously among several team members are uncommon in sports. However, when they do occur, the team physician or trainer can rapidly assess the injuries, administer immediate first-aid treatment, and then refer and transport the injured athlete.

RESPONSIBILITIES OF ACTIVE TEAM MEMBERS

Each sports medicine "team" is going to vary according to the support staff available for the individual athletic situation. In the first portion of this chapter, we identified what would typically comprise a college-level team. Unfortunately, a majority of schools do not have access to all of the professionals described. Most often, specialized care is derived from community individuals who have a specific interest in sports medicine. Although several team members' roles are discussed in the following pages, these roles may need to be modified according to a specific setting (e.g., the athletic trainer in the college as opposed to the high school or the cardiac rehabilitation setting).

Role of the Team Physician

Supervision

The team physician is usually an orthopedic or sports medicine specialist whose role is to supervise the athletic trainer's care of athletic injuries and to advise on the overall conditioning program. The team physician is also responsible for performing or collecting and reviewing the data from the preparticipation physical evaluation and making the final determination of fitness for participation.

Medical Coverage

The team physician provides medical coverage for competitive events, especially contact sports, and is prepared to supply emergency evaluation, treatment, and triage of athletic injuries and illnesses. He or she also provides primary care of athletic injuries or arranges referrals to the family physician or specialist consultants as indicated. In addition, the team physician oversees or establishes the guidelines and procedures for trainer personnel to respond to emergencies and suggests emergency equipment needed for such situations.

Rehabilitation Plan

Following injury or illness, the team physician is responsible for setting up an appropriate rehabilitation plan, ensuring that the program is adequate, and assessing the athlete's readiness to return to activity.

Education

Finally, the team physician is responsible for educating coaches, trainers, administrators, athletes, and parents regarding the medical aspects of sports.

Role of the Athletic Trainer

Communication

The basic role of the athletic trainer is to stand at the "crossroads" between the physician, athlete, parent, and coach, making sure communication is adequate.

Record Keeping

The trainer has important record-keeping responsibilities, including preparticipation evaluations, communication forms, daily injury logs, and rehabilitation progress reports. Record keeping is not only important in assisting with communication, but also imperative for liability purposes.

Injury Prevention

The athletic trainer should be an adviser on basic conditioning programs and purchases and on the use of various types of exercise equipment. The athletic trainer, in conjunction with the equipment manager, coach, and athletic director, is also responsible for making sure playing conditions and equipment are safe prior to participation.

Injury Care

The athletic trainer's primary responsibility is to prevent injury, but when injuries do occur, it is important that the trainer be accessible so that proper first-aid care, referral, and transportation can be carried out. Injuries occur just as frequently at practices as they do in game play, and the athletic trainer is usually the key person in initial first-aid care. Athletic trainers who are unable to accompany their teams to away competitions should make arrangements with the home team's trainer to cover the team. When visiting teams arrive, athletic trainers should offer their sports medicine team's services to the visiting coach and/or trainer.

Rehabilitation

Once an injury does occur, the athletic trainer should work closely with the sports medicine team or supervising physician to implement the prescribed rehabilitation program. Intermittent testing and reevaluation of the injured athlete provide important quantitative information for both the physician and the coach in assessing readiness for return to activity.

Protective Taping and Bracing

The athletic trainer must be adept and knowledgeable in the techniques of taping, wrapping, and bracing and in the use of special padding and other protective equipment that may be used to supplement a rehabilitation program.

Care of the Training Room

Setting up and stocking the training room and sports training kits are additional duties of the athletic trainer. The kit should be stocked prior to games and practices. The trainer is also responsible for keeping the training room and therapeutic equipment clean and in good working condition.

Education

Finally, the athletic trainer should assist the physician in educating the coach, athlete, parents, and administrative personnel as to injury trends, injury potential, and prevention and care of injuries.

Role of the Coach

Education

The coach is responsible for teaching playing skills. As a member of the sports medicine team, he or she should impart a proper game philosophy and an overall safety awareness. Coaches can show their concern for safety by meeting with team members and perhaps parents to inform them of potential injuries and outlining means of prevention. The "win at all cost" syndrome can be dangerous and shows little regard for the safety of the athlete.

Safety Skills

Football coaches in particular should warn athletes of the potential for head and neck injuries and insist on blocking and tackling techniques that reduce the chance of injury. All coaches should recognize areas of physical hazards in their sports, inform athletes of injuries that might occur, and insist on skill techniques that minimize risk.

Conditioning

Teams should follow effective and safe conditioning programs, including off-season, preseason, and in-season programs that contain endurance, strength, flexibility, and agility components (see Chapter 45). Conditioning programs and practice schedules should be structured to prevent excessive fatigue and heat injuries.

First Aid in the Absence of an Athletic Trainer

The coach must also provide, or delegate to a competent aide, emergency care of athletic injuries and application of first aid in the absence of the trainer or team physician. At least one member of any coaching staff should have training in cardiopulmonary resuscitation and basic first aid. The coach should also communicate freely with the trainer and team physician regarding health and safety matters. When the coach is called on to carry out athletic training functions, there is a potential conflict of inter-est. For example, if a team is playing well and one of its members is injured, the coach can easily replace the injured athlete without jeopardizing the outcome of the game. If, however, the game is close and a key athlete is injured, the coach may unintentionally minimize the seriousness of the injury to avoid losing the game. The safety and well-being of the athlete must always have the highest priority.

Role of the Athlete

Conditioning

Athletes must play an active role in their own physical conditioning by participating in off-season, preseason, and in-season programs that contain endurance, strength, flexibility, and agility components.

Nutrition and Rest

Athletes should understand the importance of getting adequate nutrition and rest. A balanced diet provides the necessary raw material for the human body to create the energy needed to participate in any athletic event. The more balanced the diet, the more efficiently the body is able to break down and use the calories provided. Individual caloric requirements vary, based on basal metabolic rate, type of exercise, and body composition needed for the specific sport. The type of calories needed for efficient energy conversion is discussed more thoroughly in Chapter 42.

Adequate rest allows the body to perform more efficiently because excess energy is not expended on fighting fatigue. The mind is alert and more focused on the activity and task at hand.

Ingestion of Alcohol and Drugs

Athletes should refrain from ingestion of alcoholic beverages and drugs. In today's society, one would hope the athlete is aware of the detrimental effects narcotics and hallucinogenic drugs, steroids, and alcohol have on the body. Unfortunately, the transference of this information cannot be taken for granted. Coaches, trainers, physicians, and parents should take the time to educate the athlete in these areas. The athlete must understand how severely alcohol and drugs affect the mind and body, changes in reaction time, rational thinking, and the overall safety of both the athlete and his or her teammates—on and off the playing field.

Injury Reporting

Athletes should promptly report illnesses and injuries to the coach, trainer, or team physician and not attempt to hide medical problems, which may become more severe and create more disability and time lost.

Safety Skills

Athletes should become knowledgeable about injury and illness risks involved with their sports, and about safety and preventive measures that minimize those risks.

Proper Care and Fit of Equipment

Athletes are also responsible for the proper care and fit of their own equipment. Examining personal and borrowed equipment should be routine before and after each practice and competition. Repairs to broken straps, laces, and so forth should not be made during competition except in emergency situations. Repairs that are made during competition are usually temporary and may not be effective. Protective devices are discussed more fully in Chapter 44.

Role of the Parents

Nutrition and Rest

Parents should provide proper nutrition and encourage adequate rest for the athlete at home.

Psychological Support

Parents should encourage but not force their child into athletics. Parents also should help their child strike the all-important balance between education and sports.

Active Involvement

Parents should take an active role in ensuring that the proper coaching, equipment, and playing environment are provided to reduce the hazards of athletic participation. They should also be actively involved in booster organizations that help finance and support safe athletic programs.

Role of the Athletic Director

Organization

The athletic director is responsible for organizing athletic activities and taking steps to ensure that athletes are adequately protected and informed of potential risks. The athletic director should project the school's concern for injury prevention and care. This concern could be demonstrated to coaches by setting minimum standards of proficiency in cardiopulmonary resuscitation and first aid and by providing numerous opportunities for in-service training in injury prevention and care.

Medical Coverage

The athletic director should reflect the school's concern for the care of the athlete by providing adequate medical coverage. This coverage should include a medical insurance program, an athletic training program with adequate training room equipment and facilities, and, ideally, a certified athletic trainer to administer the program.

Safety Within the Program

The athletic director should provide supervision of the practice and playing environment as well as adequate and suitable maintenance of all athletic equipment. Additional responsibilities include providing the best possible officiating for competitive events, arranging for emergency transportation of injured athletes, and providing adequate security for both athletes and spectators.

Role of the Family Physician or Pediatrician

Continuity

The family physician provides important continuity of care and general counseling for the athlete.

Information Source

The family physician is often the primary source of preparticipation medical history and growth and development data.

Preparticipation Physical Evaluation

The family physician may also perform the preparticipation physical evaluation.

Role of the Student Trainer

Trainer Extender

The student trainer acts as an extension of the head athletic trainer. The actual role of the student trainer is not well defined, as it varies according to his or her maturity and experience. Whereas the student trainer at the high school level may be invaluable in helping to keep the training room neat and clean, keeping the training kits stocked, recording treatments and injuries, and so forth, the college-level student trainer may be an integral part of the taping team and actually cover sporting events.

Gradual Assumption of Trainer Responsibilities

At first, observing the program should be the student trainer's main activity. Once he or she becomes familiar and comfortable with procedures and skills, the student trainer can move on to easy duties and gradually progress to more involved responsibilities. It is important that student trainers be aware of and work within their limitations. They should also be encouraged to expand their knowledge and experience. In time, they can be an integral part of the work force for routine duties in practices and games.

Supervision and Education by Head Trainer and Team Physician

The head trainer and team physician should supervise the student trainers, advising and counseling them as necessary and requested. To make them more proficient, the head trainer and team physician should set up an in-service educational program that will provide student trainers with information and skills. It is advisable that student trainers take a basic first-aid and cardiopulmonary resuscitation (CPR) course. Several courses for student trainers at the high school level are taught throughout the country. At the college level most student trainers are interested in gaining knowledge and experience for future careers in a medically oriented specialty, such as premed, physical therapy, nursing, or athletic training. Specific athletic training programs and/or courses are often available at this level.

Role of the Assistive Team Member as a Primary Member of the Active Team

In specific situations, a specialist listed in an assistive role may act as a primary member of the active team. Examples include the physical therapist/sports therapist and the cardiac rehabilitation specialist.

Physical Therapist/Sports Therapist

The post-college-age athlete who has sustained an injury or undergone surgery may utilize the expertise of the physical therapist or the sports therapist. In the high school or college setting, specific testing equipment may not be available. Therefore, the physician may have to set up a program with the physical therapist for such tests, with supplemental rehabilitation from the athletic trainer.

Cardiac Rehabilitation Specialist

In this situation, the nursing staff, cardiologist, and cardiac rehabilitation specialist will play the major active roles.

IMPORTANT CONCEPTS

1. The three primary goals of the sports medicine team are to prevent injury and illness when possible, to treat injuries and illnesses promptly when they do occur, and to return injured athletes to play as quickly and safely as possible.
2. The active members of a sports medicine team are the team physician, athletic trainer, coaches, athletes, parents, athletic directors, family physician, and student trainers.
3. The assistive members of a sports medicine team are various medical consultant specialists, allied medical personnel, and general consultants.
4. The key factors in developing a successful sports medicine team are communication between team members, delineation of roles, and respect for the medical team.
5. The roles of the members of a sports medicine team vary and sometimes overlap, depending on the particular setting.

SUGGESTED READINGS

Arnheim, D. D. *Modern Principles of Athletic Training: The Science of Sports Medicine: Injury Prevention, Causation, and Management*, 6th ed. St. Louis: Times Mirror/ Mosby College Publishing, 1985, pp. 29–44.

Ehrlich, N. *The Athletic Trainer's Role in Drug Testing. NATA Journal* 21 (1986): 225–226.

Kuland, D. N., ed. *The Injured Athlete*. Philadelphia: J. B. Lippincott, 1982, pp. 1–4.

Magnus, B. "Sports Injuries to the Disabled Athlete and the Athletic Trainer." *NATA Journal* 22 (1987): 305–310.

Perrin, D., and S. Lephart. "The Role of the NATA Curriculum Director as a Clinician and Educator." *NATA Journal* 23 (1988): 41–43, 63.

Roy, S., and R. Irvin. *Sports Medicine: Prevention, Evaluation, Management, and Rehabilitation*. Englewood Cliffs, N.J.: Prentice-Hall, 1983, pp. 5–7.

3

Organization of a Sports Medicine Program

OBJECTIVES FOR CHAPTER 3

After reading this chapter, the student should be able to:

1. Describe the seven key elements of a sports medicine program.
2. List the seven standards for assessing the quality of a sports medicine program.
3. Identify the many features required in the construction, stocking, and operation of a central training room.
4. Explain and implement the various preventive, safety, and emergency standard procedures needed to operate an effective sports medicine program.
5. Discuss the educational needs in sports medicine/athletic training for athletic trainers, coaches, student trainers, and athletic administrators.
6. Explain and implement an evaluation monitoring system for the sports medicine program.

INTRODUCTION

Sports medicine programs exist in a variety of settings; the four most common are: a university/college or professional team, a high school, a recreational organization, and a health club/fitness center. This chapter directs its attention toward the university/college or professional team environment, although most aspects of a sports medicine program are applicable to each setting.

Chapter 3 presents the seven key elements of a sports medicine program: a needs assessment program, a well-equipped and organized central training room, standard procedures or protocols, a record-keeping system, the health care team, educational programs, and an evaluation system. Each of these elements is important to ensure a comprehensive and effective program. ■

A NEEDS ASSESSMENT PROGRAM

A thorough evaluation of current health and safety aspects of the sports program sets the stage for installation of a quality program. Defining standards of care and measuring where the program currently stands is a way to identify the program's strengths and weaknesses.

Standards of care have been established in many aspects of medicine. Seven such standards and methodology have now been developed for assessing the quality of a sports medicine program. These seven areas of assessment include staff training, athletic facilities, athletic equipment, emergency preparedness, central training room, provision of athletic health care and training services, and record keeping.

Staff training. An individual (or several individuals) who possesses current certification in cardiopulmonary resuscitation (CPR), current certification from the Red Cross in first aid, and athletic training skills shall be present at all sports practices and games.

Athletic facilities. The school is responsible for all athletic facilities and equipment utilized by its athletes. These facilities and the equipment must be maintained so as to minimize safety hazards and be appropri-ately organized so as to respond to emergencies resulting from athletic participation.

Athletic equipment. The school is responsible for selecting for the athlete protective equipment that is of high quality and meets the necessary protective functions of sports equipment. The school's responsibility includes proper fitting, inspection, maintenance, storage, cleaning, and establishment of appropriate standards for replacing old and defective equipment. All equipment shall protect the athlete as designed and not be a hazard to other athletes.

Emergency preparedness. The school shall be prepared to handle any medical emergencies that are associated with athletic participation.

Central training room. The school will provide a training room facility (or facilities) that will be the focus for the numerous services rendered to the athletes. This facility will be of adequate size; appropriately outfitted with the needed utilities, supplies, and equipment; and staffed by trained individuals so that all athletes in all sports can receive the attention and services they require.

Athletic health care and training services. The school is responsible for providing quality athletic health care services and athletic training services to athletes in all sports. These services include preventive measures (prehabilitation), the recognition and assessment of injuries, the administration of first aid, emergency measures, routine treatments, and rehabilitation following injuries.

Record keeping. Accurate, reliable record-keeping procedures shall exist to document all the health care services delivered to the athletes for injuries resulting from their athletic participation.

A CENTRAL TRAINING ROOM

The central training room, typically the prime focus of activity for the athletic trainer, is primarily a treatment facility; it may also serve as a rehabilitation room. Generally, the training room is not a weight-training or conditioning room.

The Physical Facility

The size and shape of the training room will help determine the usefulness of the facility. Depending on the number of athletes in the athletic program, the size and shape requirements will vary. Too often, not enough space is allocated for the training room. The location of the training room is also important. It must be as central as possible and provide equal access to male and female athletes.

The basic utilities needed in the training room are electricity, lighting, temperature control, ventilation, and plumbing. Each wall should have two electrical outlets. For the whirlpool, a ground fault detector/current interrupter is mandatory. The lighting should measure at least 30 foot candles at a height of 4 feet above the floor; if there are areas of varying illumination, make sure to use the brightest areas for the evaluation of athletes. Adequate ventilation is essential because of the presence of warm water in whirlpools and hydrocollators. Room temperature should ideally be between 68 and 70 degrees F (20 and 21 degrees C). Plumbing requirements include a deep sink with hot and cold running water, a whirlpool, and one or two floor drains.

Storage capabilities of the central training room should include a sufficient number of locked cabinets, lockers, and closets. Taping and treatment tables are also needed. There should be a desk, file cabinet, and telephone in the training room. A small table by the entrance to the room can hold the training room treatment log.

The layout of the training room will help establish proper traffic flow. Consider the constraints created by the shape of the room, the lighting and location of electrical outlets, telephone line, and plumbing. If the training room is small, set a bench outside or near the entrance so that athletes who are waiting for assistance can sit without getting in the way of the working trainers. Place those services used least often farthest from the entrance. Taping tables and the ice machine should be relatively close to the door (perhaps on either side of the entrance). The trainer's desk should be located where the trainer, while sitting at the desk, can observe all the activity in the room.

Supplies for the Training Room

Table 3.1 lists recommended supplies for a training room used to accommodate a school with an enrollment of 1,000 students and 17 to 20 varsity sports teams.

Money is frequently a limiting factor in supplying a training room. Some common money-saving techniques include the following:

- Use the bidding process when purchasing.
- Pool your bid with others in a consortium.
- Obtain free samples from athletic equipment vendors, athletic training supply vendors, local physicians, and pharmaceutical companies. Many

TABLE 3.1. Suggested Items for a Centralized Training Room

Item	Initial Ordering Quantity	Item	Initial Ordering Quantity
Ace wraps (4-inch)	2 dozen	dressings, nonstick sterile pads (Telfa, 3-by-4-inch)	100
Ace wraps (6-inch)	5 to 6 dozen	elastic tape, Elastikon or Conform (3-inch)	1 case
Ace wraps, double length (6-inch wide)	1 dozen	elastic tape, Elastikon or Conform (2-inch)	1 case
adhesive tape (1-1/2-inch)	35+ cases	elastic tape, Elastikon or Conform (1-inch)	1 case
alcohol, rubbing	8 pints	emergency kit: 25 cents (coins for pay telephone); emergency telephone numbers for nearest hospital, major trauma hospital/medical center, team physician, and 911; location of practice facility and vehicular gate; location of nearest telephone (plus key if the phone is in a locked maintenance shack); key to the vehicular gate (if it is locked); a map with inked-in route to nearest hospital and/or major trauma hospital/medical center; identification cards (the athlete's emergency information cards must be on hand at field or courtside for all practices and games)	2
alcohol dispenser	1		
antifungal powder/spray for athlete's foot/jock itch	6 1-ounce tubes		
antiseptic/antibiotic ointment	6 tubes, or 1 gross packet		
applicators, cotton-tipped swabs (6-inch length)	500, or 1 case		
applicator dispenser	1		
athletic training kits, empty	6		
Band-Aids (1-by-3-inch)	1,000, or 6 boxes		
Band-Aids, extra large (2-by-4-inch)	50		
Band-Aid dispenser	1		
basin, plastic, for holding wet Ace wraps in refrigerator	1		
blankets	3		
blister tape, Dermiclear (1/2-inch and 1-inch)	1 box		
bolt cutters for football	1		
broom and dust pan	1 each		
bulletin board and chalkboard	1 each	eyecup, sterile	2
butterfly closures or Steri-Strips	1 box, or 2 dozen packets	eye patches, sterile	1 box (36 patches)
cabinets or shelves for supplies	as needed	eyewash, sterile	12 bottles (1/2 ounce each)
callus trimmer, pumice stone, or emery board	2	felt for compression pads (1/4-inch and 1/2-inch-thick, 21-by-36-inch)	1 sheet
callus trimmer replacement blades	4	felt for horseshoes (1/4-inch and 1/2-inch-thick, 21-by-36-inch)	1 sheet
chairs for waiting athletes	2 or 3	first-aid cream	12 tubes
clock	1	flashlight or penlights (plus an extra light and batteries)	2
cloth ankle wraps (optional)	15		
combine roll dressing (Kerlix or Kling)	2 bags	foam padding (1/8-inch and 1/4-inch-thick, 40-by-40-inch)	2 each
collodion for cauliflower ear	1 pint	foam padding, adhesive backed (1/8-inch and 1/4-inch-thick sheets)	4 each
cotton, sterile	1 case		
cotton ball jar	1		
crutches (adjustable)	6 pairs		
cups, paper for drinking/ice massage (5- or 7-ounce)	5,000	gauze pads, sterile (4-by-4-inch)	1 case
disinfectant, spray or liquid, to clean training room	2 gallons	gauze pads, unsterile, for heel and lace pads in taping	2 cases

TABLE 3.1. (continued)

Item	Initial Ordering Quantity	Item	Initial Ordering Quantity
gauze pad dispenser	1	skin lubricant or petroleum jelly (Vaseline)	10 pounds
gauze rolls, for ankle and dressings (2-inch)	1 case	skin soap bars or liquid soap with wall dispenser	12 bars or 1 gallon
germicide or antiseptic, spray or liquid, for cleaning wounds	2 cases	slings or triangular bandages	12
heat balm (optional, not recommended but loved by athletes)	32 ounces	spine board (only for properly trained personnel)	1
heel cups for bruised heels	6	splints, air/vacuum, for stabilizing suspected fractures	3 sets
hydrocollator with 3 or 4 silica gel hotpacks	1	splints, finger	1 set
hydrocollator thick terry cloth towels (optional)	4	splints, "universal" type, knee corsets/immobilizer	4
hydrogen peroxide for cleaning wounds	12 bottles (8 ounces each)	splints, "universal" type, wrist immobilizer	6
ice chest	6	stretcher	2
ice machine	1	tables, taping (24-by-72-inch-long, 34- to 36-inch-high)	3 minimum
mirror	1	tables, treatment	1 minimum
moleskin and adhesive mesh	1 box each	tape adherent, spray	24 cans (10 ounces each)
nail clippers, large pliers type, for toes and fingernails	2 each	tape cutters	6
nasal sponges for treating bloody noses	3 dozen	tape cutter replacement blades	1 dozen
neck collars, foam (various sizes)	3	tape remover	1 gallon
neck collars, "Philadelphia" stiff type (various sizes)	3	thermometer, oral, or Tempadots	3 / 1 box (100/box)
oil, rubbing, for massage (optional)	1 gallon	tongue depressors	500 or 1 box
oral airway or oral screw (only for properly trained personnel)	1	tongue depressor dispenser	1
		towels	2 dozen
plastic bags, food storage size, for ice bags	2,000	tweezers and forceps	2 each
powder, cornstarch, for feet and body	12 (12-ounce cans)	underwrap (Prewrap or Prowrap)	4 cases
refrigerator with freezer	1	waste baskets, plastic (to fit foot for contrast therapy)	6
rubber gloves	2 boxes	waste baskets for waste (with 150 kitchen-sized plastic bags)	2
scale	1	water cooler or large jug/dispenser (5 gallon-sized)	1
scalpel blades, #11 and #15, disposable	6 each	weight charts	12
scissors for bandages and dressings	6 pairs	whirlpool	1
scissors, surgical	2 pairs	whirlpool cleaner/bathroom cleaner	1 gallon
sink, deep, with hot and cold water	1		
skin abrasion/burn dressing (Second Skin or Moreskin)	1 jar/pack		

pharmaceutical companies provide product teaching aids and anatomical models.

■ Obtain used equipment such as crutches and knee corset splints from a hospital emergency room, physical therapy department, or orthopedic clinic.

■ Split your order for supplies. Place a large order for the entire year to obtain the best price, but ask for the order to be delivered in several portions every few months to save costs as well as storage space and maintain fresh products in the training room.

An essential aspect of operating a successful training room is to adopt a central budgeting, ordering, and inventory process for supplies. (Samples of record sheets used for ordering are in Chapter 6.) Conduct an inventory to determine what is on hand. Review all purchases over the past few years to estimate the quantities of supplies consumed annually to avoid duplication in purchases and stockpiling by individual coaches of items that could be shared among many sports. Reviewing past purchases will also ensure that all athletes have access to the necessary medical and training supplies.

Staffing the Training Room

In planning staffing and hours of operation of the training room, one must consider not only the number of staff (athletic trainers, student trainers, etc.) but also the hours these staff people are available. Since the staff of the training room are generally the same individuals who cover sporting events and practices, the schedules of these events must be considered. Furthermore, the training room must be available to athletes during times that do not conflict with their sport or class schedules. Once a schedule of hours of operation and services provided during those hours is established, the schedule should be posted and made known to both athletes and coaches.

After consulting with the team physician, the trainer should establish a time for "sick call," when athletes with illness or injuries can report to be seen. Like the training room schedules, this time should not conflict with athletes' practice time or class schedules.

Sometimes, an after-hours "emergency" injury or illness evaluation needs to take place in the training room. A plan should specify the person or persons whom the ill or injured athlete should notify concerning the need for medical care and where the athlete should be seen and by whom.

Rules and Security in the Training Room

Establish proper decorum in the training room. Create a set of rules, display them prominently, and enforce them.

Security in the training room is important both for preventing the loss or theft of supplies and for ensuring the confidentiality of athletes' medical records. The training room staff should have a policy and forms available for issuing equipment and supplies to athletes. Cabinets, closets, desks, and file cabinets should be locked and access to the keys should be limited.

STANDARD PROCEDURES

Organizing a sports medicine program includes establishing written policies on standard procedures to expedite care of the athletes, prevent duplication of staff effort, and diminish chance for error. Guidelines for the preseason history, physical examination, and fitness screening are discussed in Chapter 5. Establishing policies on how athletes should access health care and supplies was considered in the previous section (see "A Central Training Room").

Policies regarding communicating with the parents of athletes, coaching staff, team physicians, and the press should be written, understood, and agreed upon by all members of the sports medicine team.

Policies for the payment of medical services rendered to athletes must be established and clearly communicated. For example, will the school pay all expenses incurred by the athlete for all medical services provided, or will the school be responsible only if the athlete is injured during practice or play or becomes ill or injured during a playing season? Are expenses for medical problems such as colds, sore throats, or urinary tract infections covered by the school, or are these expenses the responsibility of the athlete? If the athlete seeks medical care outside the care provided by the school, who will pay for that care? Clearly establishing policies such as these and making them known to the athletes at the beginning of the season will avoid confusion and conflict later.

Emergency care policies should include such things as a written checklist for stocking first-aid kits (Table 3.2), organizing sideline emergency equipment (Table 3.3),

and making sure an ambulance is present and an emergency facility is accessible during high-risk sporting events. Routine meetings should also be planned throughout the year to make certain that those staffing the training room, athletic games, and practices know where all emergency equipment and supplies are kept and are familiar with their use.

Instructions for routine situations such as the use of crutches, home management following a head injury, or return-to-play criteria following various injuries should be written so that all members of the sports medicine team agree on and understand the policies. Having these policies in writing will provide consistency throughout the program and diminish the chances for error and confusion.

Safety policies are also important, especially on such matters as when and how equipment, playing surfaces, and courts should be inspected and by whom. Faulty

TABLE 3.2. Suggested Supply List for First-Aid Kit

adhesive tape (1- to 1-1/2-inch rolls)	first-aid cream or ointment, antiseptic
airway	flashlight or penlight
alcohol or hydrogen peroxide	foam rubber
analgesic balm	
	gauze pads, sterile (3-by-3-inch)
Band-Aids (1-inch)	
bandage scissors and/or tape cutters	moleskin (6-by-10-inch)
butterfly bandages or Steri-Strips	
	pencil and paper
cloth ankle wraps, optional	plastic bags for ice or chemical ice
contact lens kit (mirror and wetting solution)	powder, talcum and/or foot powder
cotton balls	
cotton tip applicators, Q tips	rubber gloves
	skin lubricant (Vaseline)
disinfecting soap (pHisoHex, Cinder suds)	
	tape adherent, spray or tincture of benzoin
elastic tape (3-inch roll)	thermometer (or Tempadots)
elastic wraps, Ace (4-inch)	tongue depressors
elastic wraps, Ace (6-inch)	triangular bandage or sling
eyecup, sterile	tweezers
eye patches, sterile	
eyewash, sterile solution	underwrap (Prewrap or Prowrap), optional
	emergency information cards
felt (1/2-inch and 1/4-inch-thick, 6-by-6-inch)	
felt horseshoes	

TABLE 3.3. Suggested Items to Have on Hand at Athletic Events and Practices

emergency clipboard with the following infor-	crushed ice
mation:	plastic bags with ties
telephone numbers/location of nearest phone	6-inch elastic wrap bandages, wet and in ice
written directions to your location	drinking cups and drinking water*
map with written and marked routes to medical	towels
facilities	facial tissues
written emergency action plan	crutches
emergency transport vehicle	sling
keys to locked areas, as needed:	neck collars, foam
telephone	neck collar, rigid
storage areas	knee splint
offices	6-inch, double-length elastic wrap bandage
school building	felt pad with patella cutout for knee compression
training room	stretcher
gate keys, if gate is locked	air splints for extremities, assorted
coins for pay telephone	spine board (only for properly trained personnel)
identification cards with emergency information	bolt cutters†
first-aid kit (see Table 3.2)	screwdrivers: 1 regular and 1 Phillips†
ice chest	sharp pocket knife†

*Drinking water from a sanitary source should be of sufficient quantity for all athletes to drink 5 ounces every 20 to 30 minutes of activity.
†For use in removing face mask from football helmet.

equipment should be repaired and poor playing surfaces corrected. Hard objects in play areas should be padded. The athletes' personal sporting equipment, especially their protective equipment such as pads, helmets, mouth guards, and shields, should be inspected routinely. Any abnormalities found should be immediately reported to those with the authority and skill to correct them.

All written policies should be organized into a procedures manual that is readily available to all members of the sports medicine team. It should be mandatory for team members to review this manual at designated times, not only to ensure their knowledge of its content but also to make certain that policies are continually updated to reflect current standards.

A RECORD-KEEPING SYSTEM

Accurate, efficient record keeping is a vital component of a sports medicine program. The details of proper record keeping are discussed in Chapter 6.

THE HEALTH CARE TEAM

"People" are a key element of any program. Chapter 2 contains a complete discussion of the members of the health care team, including their roles and responsibilities.

EDUCATIONAL PROGRAMS

Obviously, knowledge about sports medicine and athletic training is essential in any sports medicine program. The National Athletic Trainers Association (NATA) has set educational requirements and testing procedures for certification in athletic training. The NATA provides sample curricula for programs (see Chapter 1) and sponsors continuing education programs for those involved in this area. The NATA's annual meeting provides an excellent arena for the presentation of new techniques and theories of treatment and the discussion of common problems.

Coaches should also be aware of sports medicine issues. In fact, many communities presently have requirements for coaches to participate in such classes as CPR, Red

Cross first aid, and some aspects of injury prevention and initial management.

If an athletic program is large enough to have student trainers, the head athletic trainer or a designee must assume the additional responsibility of providing an educational experience for these individuals. Although much of their learning is apprentice-style from other trainers, student trainers should attend formal classes on health issues, including classes on the prevention and early assessment of injuries and emergency procedures.

A library resource center should be accessible to the training room personnel, preferably within the training room itself. Posters and other educational materials should be on display. The budget for a sports medicine program should include an allotment for subscriptions to appropriate journals and books. If possible, the budget should provide money for continuing education courses for training room staff.

A PROGRAM EVALUATION SYSTEM

All seven elements in a sports medicine program should be evaluated periodically so improvements can be made.

Annual Needs Assessment

Although needs assessment is the initial step in organizing a sports medicine program, an annual informal assessment of needs, with a formal assessment every three to five years, ensures that new needs are being addressed by the program, and items or areas no longer important can be deleted.

Health Care Team and Education Element

Evaluation of the educational programs or materials can be done by testing before and after the program. Standardized tests can be used periodically to compare the educational level of those in the sports medicine program with established norms.

Standard Procedures

Monitoring whether standard procedures are followed is essential. Sideline safety and emergency preparedness can be measured by sideline observers. The checklist for recommended first-aid kit items in Table 3.2 can be used to determine if the kits are thoroughly and properly stocked. A system should be developed to monitor proper conditioning and stretching of the athletes as well as a program to check area safety, emergency equipment, water, emergency information/written action plan, and the availability of athletic trainers and coaches to care for athletes.

Records

Maintaining accurate and complete injury data is central to evaluating the effectiveness of an organized athletic sports medicine program. By tabulating the data, year-to-year trends in injuries can be tracked. By participating in a larger injury data bank, a school can compare its experience with the experience of other schools in the area and in the nation.

A Technique for Overall Program Evaluation

A good but complex method for evaluating the process of athletic health care provided to athletes is to use a case study technique. This method follows the quality of athletic health care services provided from the moment of injury, through first aid, diagnosis, treatment, rehabilitation, and return to play. An interview can be used to gather data about the injury from the athlete, coach, and athletic trainer. A brief one-page narrative is then prepared. Specific evaluation criteria are shared with the expert evaluators who will review each case. The areas of evaluation include:

1. Time frames
   a. Immediate crisis/moment of injury
   b. Later that day, prior to going home/to hospital

c. Next day until rehabilitation completed
d. Day of return to play
2. Categories of activities
    a. Injury recognition
    b. Transport
    c. Examination/assessment
    d. First aid and treatments
    e. Communication/advice
    f. Documentation/record keeping

The case study technique is very effective in identifying the strengths and weaknesses of any sports medicine program. This method provides a good overall evaluation of the health care available; it also incorporates the knowledge, preparedness, evaluation skills, record keeping, and advice provided by members of the sports medicine team (the athletic trainers, team doctors, student trainers, and coaches).

IMPORTANT CONCEPTS

1. The seven key elements of a sports medicine program are a needs assessment program, a well-equipped and organized central training room, standard procedures or protocols, a record-keeping system, the health care team, educational programs, and a program evaluation system.
2. The seven standards for assessing the quality of a sports medicine program are staff training, athletic facilities, athletic equipment, emergency preparedness, central training room, provision of athletic health care and training services, and record keeping.

3. An essential aspect of operating a successful central training room is to adopt a central budgeting, ordering, and inventory process for supplies.
4. Policies regarding issues such as communicating with parents, medical services, and safety of playing fields and equipment should be in writing and organized into a procedures manual.
5. A sports medicine program should budget time and money to be spent on continuing education and training for team members.

SUGGESTED READINGS

Arnheim, D. D. *Modern Principles of Athletic Training,* 7th ed. St. Louis: C. V. Mosby, 1989.
Rice, S. G. "Epidemiology and Mechanisms of Sports Injuries." In *Scientific Foundations of Sports Medicine,* edited by Carol C. Teitz, pp. 3–23. Toronto: B. C. Decker, 1989.
Rice, S. G., J. D. Schlotfeldt, and W. E. Foley. "The Athletic Health Care and Training Program: A Comprehensive Approach to the Prevention and Management of Athletic Injuries in High Schools." *The Western Journal of Medicine* 142 (1985): 352–357

FOR FURTHER INFORMATION

Athletic Health Care System
Division of Sports Medicine GB-15
Seattle, WA 98195
(206) 543-1550

National Athletic Trainers' Association
2952 Stemmons Freeway, Suite 200
Dallas, TX 75247
(214) 637-6282

National Interscholastic Athletic
Administrators Association
11724 Plaza Circle
P.O. Box 20626
Kansas City, MO 64195
(816) 464-5400

United States Sports Academy
One Academy Drive
Daphne, AL 36526
(205) 626-3303 or (800) 223-2668

4

Legal Responsibilities in Sports Medicine

OBJECTIVES FOR CHAPTER 4

After reading this chapter, the student should be able to:

1. Understand the relevance of torts in sports medicine, with special attention to the concepts of negligence, defenses to negligence, and liability for tortious acts.
2. Recognize liability issues involved in drug testing.
3. Comprehend the issue of contract claims in sports medicine.
4. Appreciate the need for protecting against liability suits.

INTRODUCTION

In the last 25 years, litigation involving schools and colleges has increased dramatically. Along with that increase has been a greater scrutiny of the activities of all of the employees of these institutions. The athletic trainer and team physician have not escaped this scrutiny. Thus, legal issues ranging from breach of contract and invasion of privacy to tort claims all can have a serious impact on the everyday activities of a sports medicine professional.

Chapter 4 begins with a brief definition of torts. The chapter then goes on to explain the doctrine of negligence and the defenses to negligence. The next section discusses the liability of the institution, the athletic trainer, and the team physician for tortious acts. Chapter 4 also mentions the liability issues involved in drug testing and drug treatment programs, and the use of contract claims in certain athletic injuries. The last section of Chapter 4 looks at ways sports medicine professionals can protect themselves against liability lawsuits. ▪

TORTS

There is no good definition of a *tort*. William L. Prosser (*Law of Torts*, 1971, p. 2) has described a tort as "a civil wrong, other than breach of contract, for which the court will provide a remedy in the form of an action for damages." This definition is obviously lacking in many respects, since it does not clearly define the type or nature of activity which will cause liability. It is easy to characterize torts as being either intentional or unintentional. Fortunately, there are very few intentional torts which would have a direct impact on the sports medicine professional, but the risk of claims for the unintentional tort (negligence) is great. However, the tort of battery, which is any unpermitted and intentional contact with another person, could be committed if medical treatment were undertaken without the consent of the patient. Other intentional torts such as libel and slander could also have an impact on the activities of the sports medicine professional.

NEGLIGENCE

If the conduct of an individual is unintentional but causes harm, then that conduct can be labeled **negligence**. A cause of action for negligence has four basic elements. First, there must be a duty that is recognized by law to conform one's conduct to a certain standard, called a **standard of care**. Thus, one must act reasonably in carrying out everyday activities, and a professional must exercise his or her professional activities with a reasonable degree of care and skill that is ordinarily employed by the profession generally. Statutory provisions would also constitute a duty, since all individuals who are regulated by statute are required to adhere to the provisions of that statute.

The second element of negligence is a breach of that duty. Thus, the failure to exercise reasonable care or the violation of a statute constitutes a breach of duty. The third element of negligence is that the breach of duty must be the "proximate cause" of a resulting injury. A substantial body of legal literature has been devoted to defining the concept of proximate cause. Generally, if the breach of duty is the substantial factor in bringing about the injury, then there will be liability for negligence. The concept of proximate cause is often discussed in terms of whether the injury was foreseeable if a particular duty was breached. The classic case in this area is

Palsgraf v. *Long Island Railroad Company.*[1] In that case a passenger was running to catch a train, and a train employee knocked a package from the passenger's arms. The package, which contained fireworks, fell on the tracks and exploded. The explosion turned over scales on the train platform, injuring the plaintiff. The court said there was no liability to this plaintiff, because negligence requires some relationship between the parties which must be based on the foreseeability of harm to the person who was actually injured. Thus, there usually is no duty owed to unforeseeable plaintiffs. However, there have been cases which have extended a duty to injured parties when the injury did not appear to be foreseeable. As a practical matter, courts will sometimes stretch the law in order to compensate an injured party.

The fourth and final element which is necessary for an action for negligence is that there must be some injury. The mere threat of harm is not sufficient to subject an individual to liability. The sports medicine professional has a duty to adhere to the recognized standard of care of the profession. For example, any guidelines developed by the American College of Sports Medicine would probably help to establish the standards of care. If these standards are breached and an injury results, then there would be liability for negligence.

DEFENSES TO NEGLIGENCE

The law has recognized that there are a number of situations in which certain activities will not generate liability for negligence. The following are several examples of generally recognized defenses to a negligence action.

Contributory and Comparative Negligence

If the individual who brings the lawsuit (the plaintiff) commits an act that causes his or

[1] 248 New York, 339 (1928)

her own injury, then there is no liability. For example, if an athlete is fitted improperly with a knee brace and later becomes angry and kicks a bench while wearing the brace and suffers a serious injury to the knee, the plaintiff's own act of kicking the bench would likely be **contributory negligence** and would bar any recovery against the individual who fitted the brace.

Some states recognize the theory of **comparative negligence**. Unlike contributory negligence, which bans all recovery by a plaintiff who is contributorily negligent, comparative negligence does as its name implies—it compares the negligence of the two parties. Thus, if an individual is speeding down the highway and another individual runs a stop sign and collides with the speeder, the speeder may be able to recover damages against the individual who ran the stop sign, but those damages will be reduced based on the jury's decision as to what percentage of the accident could be attributed to the speeder's own negligence due to his or her speeding. In sports activities where injuries often result due to a variety of factors, including behavior of the athlete, contributory and comparative negligence may be a viable defense.

Assumption of Risk

The law also recognizes that there are some risks inherent in all activities. It is assumed that an individual who participates in an activity and is injured as a result of the ordinary risk associated with the activity will not have an action for negligence. Thus, when a spectator attends a baseball game and is struck by a batted ball, that is one of the risks assumed in attending a baseball game. It can be argued that the risk of injury is inherent in many sports activities. In one case, a softball player at a college was chasing a foul ball and was injured when he stepped in a drainage ditch. He sued the college for negligence, but the court dismissed the case saying that the player assumed the dangers of the game, including falling in a clearly visible ditch.

Thus, an individual who has sued a sports medicine professional could well lose, based on an **assumption of risk** defense. However, if the sports medicine professional's own negligence contributed to that injury, then liability is still a possibility because the law does not require an individual to assume the risk of another's negligence.

Immunity

Two other types of defenses to a negligence action that can prevent any recovery for injury are sovereign and charitable immunity. The doctrine of **sovereign immunity** is an old doctrine based on the notion that the "king can do no wrong." Thus, it is a defense available only to a governmental entity. The defense of sovereign immunity is very specific to state law and has been in disfavor among many courts in the last few decades. Nevertheless, in some states it is still a viable defense to negligence.

The theory of **charitable immunity** is a doctrine based on the notion that a person who is carrying out a charitable function should not be held accountable for negligent acts. Thus, since many schools and colleges are considered to be charitable institutions, this defense is available if a state recognizes charitable immunity. The doctrine of charitable immunity has fallen into considerable disrepute and is not one that should be relied on under most circumstances. However, some states have passed statutes which would, in effect, grant charitable immunity to certain activities. For example, under Georgia law, volunteers for a sports program of a nonprofit association or any employees of such an association which conducts sports or safety programs are immune from liability for any acts or omissions committed in rendering services, if they were acting in good faith and unless their conduct amounted to willful and wanton misconduct or gross negligence. However, the statute also provides that this immunity is waived to the extent that there is any liability insurance for the claims which have been filed.

LIABILITY FOR TORTIOUS ACTS

Liability of the Institution

The law has long recognized that an employer can be held accountable for the wrongful acts of an employee that were committed in the scope of employment. This doctrine is often referred to as **vicarious liability** or **respondeat superior**; it means that the principal or employer must respond for the tortious conduct of the agent or employee.

Entities such as schools or colleges cannot act except through their employees or agents. Thus, for the institution to be liable for negligence, there must be some negligent action by an employee or agent of that institution. This negligence is then imputed to the employer so that the employer would be responsible to the plaintiff as a joint tortfeasor. That means that both the employer and the individual who committed the tortious act would be liable for any damages.

Athletic trainers and team physicians often are employed by institutions. However, many institutions will attempt to establish an independent contractor relationship between the physician and the trainer and the institution. If that independent contractor relationship is established, it is possible that liability for the institution might be avoided, because the tortious acts of an independent contractor are not imputed to the employer. However, an institution could still be liable for any injuries under a theory that it was negligent in selecting or supervising the trainer or physician.

If a sports medicine professional is acting as an independent contractor, then the insurance of the institution will not defend or protect the individual. It would be wise for the sports medicine professional to secure an indemnification agreement with the institution to assure that any claims made against that individual while acting on behalf of the institution would be covered out of the budget of that institution or by a special insurance policy. For example, in the case of *Hemphill* v. *Sayers*,[2] it was disclosed that Southern Illinois University provided such an indemnification agreement for the athletic director, the coach, and the athletic trainer. Such agreements also may be sufficient to provide an employee of a state institution with Eleventh Amendment immunity, which is a form of sovereign immunity that is available in federal court to states and their employees under certain circumstances.

The institution may also have liability if it fails to provide adequate health and medical care for its athletes. One frightening example is a case in which an individual had been deaf since birth and was a freshman on a college softball team. She was injured during a softball practice when a ball struck her in the right eye. The force of the ball striking her head could be heard from 80 to 100 yards away. Ice was applied, and she was told to go to her room and rest. The coach did not suggest that she go to see a doctor, although the school's medical clinic was across the street from the softball field. The next day the student had trouble with her vision and sought medical treatment. Unfortunately, the type of eye trauma she had suffered required prompt immobilization of the eye and absolute bed rest. Because this was not done, secondary hemorrhaging occurred, and she eventually lost sight in one eye. She filed suit against the institution and obtained a verdict of $800,000. The court said that the institution had a duty to ensure that medical assistance was available, and the coaches had a duty to evaluate the severity of an injury.[3] This case is the type that reinforces the need for trainers or other sports medicine professionals to be present at both practices and games, and they should ensure that follow-up medical treatment is obtained if an injury could be potentially serious.

The institution is responsible for providing competent medical care. Thus, a court in Illinois determined that a school district could be held liable, because the district was negligent in having an incompetent and untrained student provide medical care to an injured athlete. The injury resulted from an activity that took place away from school, but the injury was treated by a student assistant trainer for the football team before football practice.[4] In a recent case decided in Louisiana, the plaintiff attempted to establish that Louisiana State University had a duty to require club sport teams to have a "trainer/manager/coach" work with the rugby team to eliminate the dangerous conditions created by the lack of rest or conditioning. The court decided for the institution, because rugby was a club activity which was not controlled by the institution.[5] However, one could infer from the decision that a duty to have an athletic trainer could be imposed on an institution for sports which it controls and sponsors.

Liability of the Athletic Trainer

Although the professional competence of athletic trainers has improved as a result of national certification and state licensure, the risk of liability for negligence of trainers has also increased. There are now higher standards of care to which athletic trainers must adhere. The standards form a legal duty, the breach of which constitutes negligence if there is an injury. At a minimum, athletic trainers who work in states with licensure or certification requirements must conform to the standards of such licensure or certification. It is also likely that the national standards of care for athletic training would be applied to all certified trainers throughout the country.

---

[2]S.D. Ill. 1982, 552 F. Supp. 685 (1982)

[3]*Steinman* v. *Fontbonne College,* 664 F. 2d 1082 (8th Cir. 1981)

[4]*O'Brien* v. *Township High School District 214,* 415 N.E. 2d 1015 (Ill. 1980)

[5]*Fox* v. *Board of Supervisors of Louisiana State University and Agricultural and Mechanical College, et al.,* 559 So. 2d 850 (La. 1990)

It is not uncommon for an athletic trainer to be named in a lawsuit resulting from injury to an athlete. In one example, a student trainer for a college basketball team informed the team's treating physician that he had been "icing" the sprained ankle of a basketball player. The physician assumed that "icing" meant applying ice packs; instead, the trainer had used ice water immersion treatment for the ankle. The athlete slept overnight with the ankle submerged in a bucket of ice water and continued to immerse the foot for several days. After discovering that the basketball player was still using ice water immersion three days later, the trainer immediately called the physician, who instructed the trainer to stop the ice water treatment. Six days after the injury, the athlete visited the physician again and was diagnosed as having thrombophlebitis and frostbite of the fourth and fifth toes. Ultimately, muscle tissue in the foot had to be removed and one gangrenous toe had to be amputated. The athlete sued the college and the student trainer. The jury returned a verdict in favor of the institution, because the jury believed the athlete had been contributorily negligent in the situation and was responsible for his own injuries.[6] However, this case emphasizes the importance of clear communication between the physician and the athletic trainer. Fortunately, in this example, there was no liability for the sports medicine professionals, but there could easily have been a different result.

In another setting, a state university football player who sustained an injury to his cervical spine as a result of an allegedly defective football helmet sued not only the manufacturer of the helmet but also the athletic trainer. It was alleged that the trainer failed to warn the athlete of the dangers of the helmet.[7] Thus, it is possible that a

trainer could have a duty to warn an athlete of the inherent dangers of equipment which the athlete may use. If the trainer does not so warn the athlete, and the athlete is injured while using that equipment, then the trainer may be negligent.

It is incumbent on trainers to be aware of the standards of national organizations with regard to athletic activities. Trainers must not simply follow the practices that have always been used in the training room at their institution; they must also conform to the national standards of care for athletic trainers. Trainers must remain in close communication with the team physician about the treatment of injuries, and if they are unsure of the physician's orders, they should request written communication from the physician. Finally, if a state has a law requiring the licensure of athletic trainers, an institution must not hire a trainer who is not licensed. If some injury occurred as a result of the activities of such an individual, the plaintiff could argue that the violation of the athletic trainer licensing statute would be a breach of duty which could constitute negligence.

Liability of the Team Physician

The physician must practice with the level of reasonable skill and knowledge common for members of the medical profession in good standing. This obligation is really no different than that imposed on any physician practicing in a specialty area. A physician in general practice who treats a sports injury is expected to perform with the same degree of reasonable skill and knowledge that would be used by members of the profession in good standing. However, if the physician is practicing as a specialist in sports medicine, the standard of care is greater. The specialist will be held to a standard of care measured in terms of the specialty itself rather than the standard of the medical profession in general. Thus, the sports medicine practitioner would be required to perform with the same degree of

[6]*Gillespie* v. *Southern Utah State College,* 669 P. 2d 861 (Utah, 1983)

[7]*Hemphill* v. *Sayers,* 552 F. Supp. (S.D. Ill. 1982)

reasonable skill and knowledge that would be used by sports medicine experts across the country. In a situation in which the physician is unable to determine what "good medical practice" requires, it is appropriate to contact other members of the profession for aid in making that determination.

A physician is certainly not a guarantor of treatment procedures and will not be held liable for honest mistakes of judgment where proper treatment is open to reasonable doubt. Likewise, the physician should be cautious in making a prognosis. It is much more likely that an individual who is promised a successful recovery by a physician will sue the physician if such recovery does not take place, even if the physician has acted properly. A full explanation of the nature of the injuries and the possible consequences associated with that injury, both good and bad, should be explained to the patient. Once that is done, if the recovery is not as complete as hoped for, then the patient will at least have been aware of that possibility and will be less likely to believe that the physician is to blame. The general standard of care owed by a physician to any patient is not generally altered by the fact that the physician is not being compensated for his or her services. However, most states have a statutory provision which immunizes a physician or any other individual who renders emergency care at the scene of an accident, unless that person is compensated for such care. However, it is unlikely that a team physician could use such a statute to protect his or her actions in response to an emergency that was a part of the duties covered by the physician's agreement with an athletic program.

Once the treating physician accepts an athlete as a patient, the physician-patient relationship is established. Along with the establishment of such relationship comes the obligation to maintain, in confidence, medical information about the athlete. Thus, sports medicine physicians, as well as athletic trainers, should give no information about the athlete to outside individuals or teams without the specific consent of the athlete. Legitimate requests for information regarding prior injuries should normally be restricted to disclosure of the nature of the injury and the method of treatment.

The physician who is employed by an institution to treat the student athlete may be in a somewhat awkward position. The physician has a responsibility to the institution for which he or she works as well as to the athlete who is being treated. It is possible that the institution will have full access to the athlete's medical records, because the institution will have insisted that the athlete sign a consent form authorizing the release of such information to the institution. The physician may well be faced with pressure from the institution to certify that the athlete is ready to participate in athletic competition at the earliest possible opportunity. Obviously, the physician's greatest obligation is to the patient, regardless of the source of compensation for the medical treatment. The physician should never attempt to please the employing institution at the risk of the health of the athlete. In negotiating contracts with institutions for the treatment of athletes, the physician should insist that the decision regarding participation of an athlete in competition or practice should be left to either the athletic trainer or the physician. While assuming this responsibility may place a burden on the physician to make a determination whether a particular athlete is ready to resume competition, this approach is much safer than allowing nonmedical personnel to make such decisions. Certainly, if the physician does not meet the accepted medical standards of care for releasing an injured athlete for continued participation, then that physician could be liable for negligence if the athlete is injured. Nevertheless, the physician could also face liability if the injured athlete was not warned that he or she was not ready for participation if the institution has the authority to determine when an athlete can resume participation.

Under normal circumstances, a physician, before administering medical care, must obtain the consent of an adult patient. As discussed earlier in the chapter, failure to obtain such consent could result in liability for the physician for battery. The general rule for treatment of minors is that consent must be obtained from the parent or guardian, because a minor is deemed incapable of giving valid consent. Exceptions exist where minors can give valid consent in emergency situations when the parent or guardian is not available. The concept of **informed consent** varies from state to state. Generally, it is accepted that informed consent means the physician has "imparted some quantum of medical information relative to a proposed treatment which is sufficient to enable the patient to make an intelligent choice as to whether he or she should undergo such treatment." This definition typically includes a reasonable disclosure of alternatives, the danger of each, and the relative advantages and disadvantages of each. Some state laws do not require that a physician reveal the risk of failure of such treatment or the undesirable results which such treatment may produce. However, as discussed above, furnishing this information to the patient may prevent a patient from suing later should recovery be less than expected.

Physicians are often requested to do preparticipation physical evaluations of athletes. In so doing, the physician must act with the skill and knowledge that other members of the profession would use when acting under similar circumstances. The physician must be aware of the purpose of the evaluation, the nature of the conditions under which it was performed, the procedures generally used by other members of the profession in conducting such examinations, and the requirements of good medical practice in responding to the results of the examination. The physician should also detail, in writing, any concerns which he or she may have about the athlete's participation in an activity and should furnish a copy of this evaluation to the athlete, to the athlete's parents if the athlete is a minor,

and to the institution if the athlete consents to such communication.

LIABILITY ISSUES IN DRUG TESTING PROGRAMS

The National Collegiate Athletic Association (NCAA) has mandated drug testing in certain championship activities. As a result of this mandate, and in order to deal with a very real problem of drug abuse in this country, a number of colleges and universities have adopted drug testing and counseling programs for athletes. In fact, even some high schools have started to test their athletes for drugs.

The role of the athletic trainer and physician in these drug testing programs can be critical for two reasons. First, the physician may have prescribed drugs to an athlete which could result in a positive result on a drug test. The physician needs to communicate with the athletic trainer and the institution about any drugs an athlete may be taking. The physician also has to be certain that the use of such drugs will not endanger the health of the athlete if the drugs are used while in practice or in competition. Second, the physician and trainer will likely play a key role in the education and counseling of athletes who test positive for drugs.

Drug testing programs can raise a number of legal issues and questions such as invasion of privacy and the obligation of the physician when he or she obtains information from a patient/athlete that drugs are being used. In developing drug testing programs, the athletic trainer, the physician, and the institution's attorney should work in concert to define clearly the roles and expectations of all parties.

ATHLETIC INJURIES AND CONTRACT CLAIMS

When institutions cannot be held liable in a tort action for claims of negligence because of the principles of contributory negligence or charitable or sovereign immunity, plaintiffs' attorneys often will take a different approach in trying to obtain relief for their client. For example, an Ohio court stated that the University of Virginia could be liable for the cost of medical treatment for injuries received by an athlete while playing football. The court stated that a contract existed between the student and the college for the treatment of such injuries, and if the university breached that contract, it could be held liable for damages.[8] Similarly, a Georgia court, while denying relief to the athlete, stated that if the athlete had shown that his subsequent physical condition was the result of a prior football injury, then the college might have been contractually obligated to pay for all necessary medical treatment for the athlete several years after the injury.[9] Thus, an institution must carefully review the promises it makes to its athletes and realize that it could have a contractual duty to continue to provide medical care for those athletes based on such promises.

PROTECTING AGAINST LIABILITY SUITS

It is imperative that sports medicine professionals be aware that they are legally obligated to the standards established by their profession in carrying out their professional responsibilities. Failure to adhere to the standards of care may result in individual liability for the practitioner and liability for the employing institution. The sports medicine professional should be aware of the changes in sports medicine and conform his or her conduct accordingly. If the individual is not aware of such changes, he or she may be certain that if something happens, a jury will be made aware of the current standards of the profession and will hold the sports medicine professional accountable for adhering to the standards.

The sports medicine professional should seek out the advice of colleagues if there is any question about treatment for a particular condition. This action would be very helpful in the event of litigation to demonstrate that the practitioner took reasonable care to assure that the appropriate course of treatment was followed. Furthermore, it is important that the institution, the physician, and the athletic trainer maintain precise written records of treatment, physical conditioning of athletes, advice received from other professionals, and communications with athletes.

Because the cost of defending even a frivolous lawsuit can be substantial, all sports medicine practitioners should carry policies of liability insurance. Such policies will pay not only the cost of claims which might be awarded against the sports medicine professional, but also the costs of attorneys' fees and other expenses associated with litigation.

Sports medicine professionals must realize that their activities are subject to scrutiny because of the very visible nature of athletics in our society. With such scrutiny comes the possibility of litigation. However, adherence to the accepted norms of professional conduct will generally provide a complete defense should a lawsuit be filed.

[8]*Barile* v. *University of Virginia*, 441 N.E. 2d 608 (Ohio, 1981)

[9]*Eberhart* v. *Morris Brown College*, 352 S.E. 2d 832 (Ga. App. 1987)

IMPORTANT CONCEPTS

1. Conduct that is unintentional but causes harm is called negligence.
2. Defenses to negligence include contributory or comparative negligence, assumption of risk, and sovereign or charitable immunity.
3. For an institution to be liable for negligence, there must be negligent action on the part of an employee or agent of the institution.
4. Athletic trainers must conform to national standards of care for athletic training and to any state licensure or certification requirements to avoid liability for tortious acts.
5. A physician who is practicing as a specialist in sports medicine must conform to the same degree of reasonable skill and knowledge expected of sports medicine experts across the country to avoid liability for tortious acts.
6. The team physician and athletic trainer play key roles in drug testing programs.
7. Some injured athletes are bringing lawsuits against the institutions thought to be protected under charitable immunity defenses by claiming that the university breached the contract that existed between the athlete and the institution for the treatment of injuries.
8. Sports medicine professionals should be aware of current standards of the profession, document treatment and physical conditioning of athletes, and carry adequate liability insurance to protect themselves against the possibility of litigation.

TWO

BASIC CONCEPTS

5

The Preparticipation Physical Evaluation

OBJECTIVES FOR CHAPTER 5

After reading this chapter, the student should be able to:

1. Explain the underlying need for preparticipation physical evaluations.
2. Describe the techniques of preseason screening.
3. Describe disqualifying or restricting conditions for sports participation.
4. Become familiar with some additional areas of physical evaluation.

INTRODUCTION

The athlete's preparticipation evaluation is a vital part of all sports programs. It provides a thorough screening physical examination, as well as an evaluation of the athlete's fitness and performance potential. Chapter 5 begins by detailing the purposes of the preseason evaluation and suggesting the ideal setup for conducting the evaluation. After discussing how to organize the evaluation, the chapter explains how the ideal preseason physical evaluation is conducted. Then, any restrictions or disqualifying conditions that might be found are identified. The final section of Chapter 5 suggests additional tests that can be included in the physical evaluation or done at a later time. ■

PURPOSE OF THE EVALUATION

A preseason or preparticipation medical evaluation is required before any athlete can participate in an organized sport. This evaluation fulfills legal and insurance requirements. The preseason physical evaluation also yields a baseline of the athlete's fitness for participation. This baseline can be used as a record for later comparison should illness or injury occur during the course of the season and as an aid in setting criteria for return to play after injury.

The preparticipation physical evaluation may reveal deficiencies that place the athlete at higher risk for injury or disqualify the individual from participating in a specific sport altogether. Correctable or treatable physical conditions can be addressed early, thus decreasing the injury risk significantly during the actual playing season.

There are important considerations regarding the legality and scope of preseason assessment. First, parental or guardian consent should be obtained for permission to submit young people to this screening program. Second, the evaluation is a screening test—not a diagnosis and treatment session. When problems are found, athletes should be referred to specialists for definitive care and treatment.

THE IDEAL PRESEASON EVALUATION

The type of preseason evaluation will vary according to the requirements of the school or state, the availability of interested medical personnel, the space provided for evaluation, and the organization of the actual evaluation. The ideal evaluation is one with multiple specialty stations. This type of evaluation has the potential to provide the sports medicine team with the greatest amount of information about the athlete in the shortest period of time. The following description of an ideal circuit or station-type evaluation demonstrates the components of a comprehensive sports physical. While such an evaluation may be relatively easy to organize at the university or college level, specific constraints such as available space and personnel will require significant modifications at the junior high or high school level.

ORGANIZING THE EVALUATION

The evaluation circuit, ideally consisting of several specialty stations, should be set up well in advance in an area large enough to permit easy traffic flow and multiple evaluations. The examiner at each station should know the evaluation responsibilities of that particular station and make sure that ample supplies are easily accessible.

The coaching staff should advise athletes of the physical's starting time, which may be staggered according to last name (A–K 3:00, K–P 4:00, etc.), sport, or other delineation. The coach should also request that athletes arrive in loose-fitting shorts and shirts or gym suits.

Prior to arriving at the evaluation, athletes should fill out medical history and immunization forms. For junior high and high school physicals, a parent's or guardian's signature is necessary to allow athletes to participate in the examination. Permission must also be given for them to compete in the school's athletic program, travel with the team, and receive emergency treatment when the parent cannot be reached.

Some parents may not automatically grant permission to treat their son or daughter in an emergency situation because of their religious beliefs. These circumstances must be addressed on an individual basis, and an amenable agreement must be reached prior to allowing participation. Insurance coverage should also be verified, particularly if medical coverage is the responsibility of the athlete's family. The review of the athlete's medical history during the preparticipation examination provides an opportunity to verify that all these forms have been signed.

Figure 5.1 is an example of a form that can be used for data collection. Some preseason evaluations also include assessment of an athlete's level of fitness and conditioning. Basic tests for flexibility, strength, power, cardiovascular endurance, and body fat percentage can provide the coaching and training staffs with vital information about an athlete's performance, potential, and injury risk.

Athletes who return annually for evaluation may not have to repeat the entire screening because some portions are likely to remain unchanged from year to year—for example, ophthalmologic, otologic, and orthopedic examinations. A thorough oral history each year can indicate areas where new illnesses or injuries require further evaluation.

CONDUCTING THE EVALUATION

Basically, the preparticipation physical evaluation consists of a review of the athlete's medical history, a general physical, and an orthopedic examination.

Review of Athlete's Medical History

The athletic or student trainer, nurse, or coach should review for completeness the medical history form that the athlete brings to the exam. Significant past illnesses and injuries, allergies, and medications should be circled or highlighted, making the circuit move more quickly. A computer at this station is a helpful tool for collating this information with required permission forms, the athlete's insurance coverage, and parents' or guardians' home and work telephone numbers in case of an emergency. The following equipment is needed: table, extra pens, and a computer (optional).

General Physical

Height/Weight

The coach, assistant coach, or an interested parent can take this information. A height/weight scale is needed for this part of the physical exam.

Urinalysis

A urinalysis is a test for abnormal glucose and protein levels; it should be performed by the training staff or a nurse using Clinix Stix, Combistix, or a comparable product. Protein levels are frequently elevated to trace or 1+ in the adolescent and should not necessarily be considered abnormal. However, elevated protein levels should be investigated further to rule out any underlying pathology. Elevated glucose levels also require closer evaluation. The following equipment is needed for a urinalysis: a bathroom facility, urinalysis reagent strips, disposable gloves, paper cups with a place for the athlete's name, a pen, a plastic-lined garbage can, and a table.

Blood Pressure/Pulse

These measurements should be taken in a quiet area by the athletic trainer or student trainer, a nurse, or a paramedic. The blood pressure of young children between the ages of 6 and 11 should not exceed 130/80

Exam Number: _____

ATHLETIC EXAMINATION FORM

Name: _____ *(Circle One)* Sex: **M** or **F** Race: **B W** or **O**

School Name _____ School No. _____ Birthdate _____ Dominant Hand **R** or **L**

Sport(s) _____

AGE/GRADE	YEAR ( )	YEAR ( )	YEAR ( )	YEAR ( )	COMMENTS/INTERIM CHANGES	

HISTORY

Illness						
Injuries						
Operations						
Medications						
Allergies						
Other						
(Initial)						

PHYSICAL

H.E.E.N.T.						
Heart						
Lung						
Abdomen						
Skin						
Other						
(Initial)						
Height/Weight						
BP						
Pulse						
Lab: UA/						
Dental						

FIGURE 5.1. A preparticipation physical evaluation form.

	YEAR ( )		YEAR ( )		YEAR ( )		YEAR ( )		COMMENTS/INTERIM CHANGES	
ORTHOPAEDICS	L	R	L	R	L	R	L	R		
Shoulder										
Elbow										
Hip										
Knee										
Ankle										
Spine										
Other										
(Initial)										
FLEXIBILITY	L	R	L	R	L	R	L	R		
Heelcords										
Hamstrings										
Other										
STRENGTH	L	R	L	R	L	R	L	R		
Hip Flexor										
Shoulder										
Thigh Girth										
Other										
(Initial)										
FITNESS										
Body Fat %										
	L	R	L	R	L	R	L	R		
Reaction										
	L	R	L	R	L	R	L	R		
Grip Strength										
Pull or Hang										
Run										
Reach/Jump										
Put										
Sit Ups										
Other										
CHECK OUT								CONDITIONS/REASONS		
Pass										
Fail										

TABLE 5.1A. Detecting Cardiac Risks in School Examinations: Key Physical Findings of Cardiac Evaluation by School Physician

1. Heart rate over 120 beats/min
   a. If repeated tests on second occasion are high, suggest monitoring and recording of pulse at home by a trained parent or nurse friend.
   b. Pulse recovery tests after jumping or hopping exercises are useless routines except for multiple extrasystoles or arrhythmias.

2. Multiple extrasystoles or arrhythmias. Check after jumping or hopping 20 times to ascertain if arrhythmias appear or disappear.

3. Resting blood pressure over 130/80 mm Hg for students aged 6 to 11 years, over 140/90 mm Hg for students aged 12 to 18 years.
   a. For validity, be certain that the pressure cuff covers at least two thirds of the upper arm, from elbow to shoulder (Adult cuff = 30 x 13 cm; pediatric cuff = 22 x 10 cm; obese cuff = 39 x 15 cm).
   b. If high, repeat test three times and take average.

4. All systolic murmurs grade 3 to 6 or louder at any location; all diastolic murmurs of any intensity at any location; or any continuous murmur. Heart should be auscultated at four chest locations:
   a. Pulmonic area (second intercostal space at left sternal border).
   b. Aortic area (second intercostal space at right sternal border).
   c. Tricuspid area (fourth intercostal space at left sternal border).
   d. Mitral area (fourth intercostal space at left midclavicular line).

5. Routinely palpate femoral and brachial pulses. Note if absent or if large discrepancy exists between them.

mm Hg; for youths between 12 and 18 years, the blood pressure should not exceed 140/90 mm Hg. Individuals with recorded high blood pressure should be tested again on two separate occasions. Referral to a physician is appropriate if the blood pressure remains high. A resting pulse rate should not exceed 100 beats per minute. The following equipment is needed: a table, two chairs, a watch with a second hand, a stethoscope, and a sphygmomanometer (blood pressure cuff).

Eye Examination

A Snellen Vision Chart or Titmus machine is commonly used to perform the visual examination. The examiner should note if the athlete wears contact lenses or glasses, and the test should be administered with the athlete wearing them. Visual fields should be checked for blind spots. Eyeglass lenses should be protective in nature. If possible, athletes who wear contacts or glasses should carry an extra pair in case of loss or damage. The following equipment is needed for performing eye examinations: a measuring tape, an appropriate eye chart, and a 3-by-5-inch card to cover the eye.

Skin/Mouth/Nose/Ears/Throat/Neck

A physician should examine these areas of the athlete and note any abnormalities. An athlete who has a contagious skin rash should be restricted from play until the infection is under control. The following equipment is needed: tongue depressors, ophthalmoscope, and gloves.

Chest: Heart/Lungs

A physician should examine an athlete's heart and lungs. (The information in Tables 5.1A, B, and C will be helpful in screening cardiac abnormalities and determining contraindications to sports participation.) For an asthmatic athlete, the physician must make certain that the condition is well controlled prior to clearing the individual for sports participation. The asthmatic's medication must be labeled and readily available in the team's training kit. The following equipment is needed for this part of the physical exam: stethoscope, examination table, and curtain or dividers.

Lymphatic, Genitalia, Abdomen

A physician can detect an enlarged liver and spleen, solitary paired organ, or hernias in this portion of the evaluation. The following equipment is needed: gloves, examination table, and curtain or dividers.

Dental

A dentist should examine the athlete's mouth and teeth for soft tissue lesions and decayed, broken, or abscessed teeth. Abnormalities of the teeth and gums due to the use of smokeless tobacco are increasing in younger people. The need for a custom-

TABLE 5.1B. Contraindications to Sports Participation by Patients with Disqualifying Cardiac Conditions

	Contraindication	
	---	---
Condition	Strenuous Sports	Nonstrenuous Sports
1. Severe mitral stenosis or insufficiency	Absolute	Relative
2. Aortic stenosis or insufficiency	Absolute	Relative
3. Idiopathic hypertrophic subaortic stenosis	Absolute	Relative
4. Active myocarditis	Absolute	Absolute
5. Systemic hypertension	Relative	Relative
6. Pulmonary hypertension	Absolute	Relative
7. Significant arrhythmias (atrioventricular and tachycardias)	Absolute	Relative
8. Cyanotic heart disease (postoperative)	Relative	Relative
9. All other congenital heart disease (postoperative)	Relative	Relative

TABLE 5.1C. Detecting Cardiac Risks in School Examinations: Key Historic Facts Obtained from Students, Parents, and School Health Records

1. Cyanotic heart disease early in life
2. Murmur early in life based on anatomic diagnosis of
   a. Left-to-right shunt
   b. Pulmonic or aortic stenosis
3. Rheumatic heart disease
4. Fainting spells (syncope)
5. Chest or abdominal pains (not otherwise diagnosed)
6. Dyspnea on exertion
7. Cardiac surgery
8. Enlarged heart
9. Cardiac rhythm disturbances
10. Familial heart disease* or rhythm disturbances
11. Functional or innocent murmur of four or more years' duration

*Hypertension, early stroke (under 50 years), or early coronary (under 50 years) in close relatives.

Source: Tables 5.1A, B, and C from Schell, N.B. "Cardiac Evaluation of School Sports Participants: Guidelines Approved by the Medical Society of the State of New York." *NY State J Med* 1978; 78: 942–943. Reprinted by permission from the New York State Journal of Medicine, copyright by the Medical Society of the State of New York.

fitted mouthpiece for athletes who have braces should also be determined at this examination. The following equipment is needed for the dental exam: tongue depressors, flashlight, and gloves.

Orthopedic Examination

An orthopedic surgeon should evaluate any prior injuries sustained by the athlete, or any problem areas noted in the past. Orthopedic disqualifications are sport-specific. Existing conditions should be evaluated to determine if the conditions could be improved adequately with rehabilitation, bracing, medication, padding, rest, or surgery. The following equipment is needed: examination table and a curtain or dividers.

DISQUALIFYING OR RESTRICTING CONDITIONS

After the physical evaluation, the athletic trainer, in consultation with the team physician, reviews the physical forms and makes decisions to pass or fail athletes, with or without restrictions (Table 5.2). In the event of any restrictions, suggestions for rehabilitation, areas that need rechecking, or recommendations for further evaluation, the athletic trainer informs parents and coaches.

If additional testing is recommended, clearance to participate is withheld until the problem is proved to be of no consequence. Examples of these problems include diastolic blood pressure above 90 mm

---

TABLE 5.2. Conditions of Passing or Failing Evaluation

A. PASSED
   Unconditional
   No reservations
   Cleared for all sports and all levels of exertion
   No preexisting or current medical problems
   No contraindications for collision or contact sports

B. PASSED with conditions
   Has a medical problem needing follow-up
   1. Can participate in sports at present
   2. Follow-up must be prior to sports activities

C. PASSED with reservations
   1. No collision sports (hockey, rugby, lacrosse)
   2. No contact sports (football, basketball, wrestling)

D. FAILED with reservations
   Not cleared for REQUESTED sport (other sports will be considered)
   1. Collision not permitted, contact to be limited
   2. Contact not permitted, noncontact sports allowed

E. FAILED with conditions
   Can be reconsidered when medical problem is addressed

F. FAILED
   Unconditional
   No reservations
   Cannot be cleared for any sport or any level of competition

---

Hg, elevated levels of glucose or protein in the urine, acute or chronic infection, skin rash, inguinal hernia, undescended testicle, or scoliosis. Limited participation may be permitted with certain disqualifying abnormalities, noted on the history or physical evaluation, until the abnormality is corrected. Specific sports in which the athlete may participate should be listed. Copies of the evaluation should be kept on file, sent to the family physician, and sent to the athlete's parents or guardians.

Disqualifying conditions vary according to the sport in which the athlete desires to participate.[1] Table 5.3 identifies the condition with the type of sport. The following disqualifying conditions are identified in greater detail.

[1]Disqualifying conditions are also listed in the *Medical Evaluation of the Athlete: A Guide*, rev. ed. (Chicago: American Medical Association, 1976).

Head Trauma/Repeated Concussions

The severity of head trauma and the frequency of injury are important factors for a physician to consider before permitting an athlete with a prior history of head injury to participate in collision or contact sports. Some athletes may demonstrate emotional disturbances following head trauma; they should not be allowed to play until a neurologist evaluates them.

A general rule many team physicians use is the "1-2-3 rule": One concussion and the athlete is out of the game; two concussions and the player is out for the season; three concussions and the athlete should no longer play. See Chapter 30 for a more detailed discussion of head injuries.

Loss of Vision

An athlete who has lost an eye or has loss of vision in one eye, severe myopia, or previous retinal detachment should be advised of the dangers of participating in a contact or collision sport. Today, equipment that is available will offer protection for the athlete with such conditions. Protective eye guards have been developed for a number of sports, including football. Face shields have been developed to allow participation in sports that require helmets. Even though these protective devices are available, it is the athletic trainer's and physician's duty to explain the dangers of competing in certain sports to the athlete and the parents if the athlete is a minor. It is also advisable to have an ophthalmologist examine the athlete's eyes prior to participation.

One Kidney

Most physicians agree that the risk of injury for an athlete with one kidney far outweighs the benefits of granting the athlete permission to participate in collision or contact sports. Although the injury rate is low, the kidney area is difficult to protect. Injury to a single kidney could lead to dependence on dialysis or even require organ transplantation for survival.

TABLE 5.3. Conditions Disqualifying an Athlete for Sports Participation*

Condition	Type of Sport			
	Collision[a]	Contact[b]	Endurance[c]	Other[d]
General				
Acute infection	X	X	X	X
Physical immaturity	X	X		
Hemorrhagic disease	X	X	X	
Diabetes (inadequately controlled)	X	X	X	X
Jaundice	X	X	X	X
Eyes				
Absence of an eye	X	X		
Severe myopia or field cuts	X	X		
Ears				
Deafness	X			
Respiratory tract infection	X	X	X	X
Symptomatic TB	X	X	X	X
Pulmonary insufficiency	X	X	X	X
Cardiovascular system				
Mitral or arterial stenosis, coarctation of aorta	X	X	X	X
Cardiac	X	X	X	X
Cyanotic CHD	X	X	X	X
Hypertension[e]	X	X		
Arrhythmia[e]	X	X		
Previous heart surgery[e]	X	X		
Abdomen				
Hepatomegaly	X	X		
Splenomegaly	X	X		
Genitourinary system				
Absence of a kidney	X	X		
Renal disease[e]	X	X	X	X
Hernia	X	X	X	
Absence of a testicle[f]	X	X		
Musculoskeletal system				
Chronic or unhealed injuries[e]	X	X	X	X
Functional inadequacy incompatible with contact or skill demands of sport	X	X	X	
Head and nervous system				
History of signs of previous serious head trauma	X	X		
Convulsive disorder, not controlled on medicines[e]	X	X	X	
Controlled convulsive disorder[e]	X			
Previous surgery on head	X	X		
Skin				
Boils, impetigo, or herpes simplex	X	X		

*Based on recommendations of the American Medical Association Committee on Medical Aspects of Sports
[a]Football, rugby, and hockey.
[b]Lacrosse, baseball, soccer, basketball, wrestling, and so forth.
[c]Cross country, track, tennis, crew, swimming, and so forth.
[d]Bowling, golf, archery, field events, etc.
[e]Each patient should be judged on an individual basis, but it is probably better to encourage a young boy or girl to participate in a noncontact sport rather than a contact sport.
[f]The Committee approves the concept of participation in sports for youths with only one testicle or with an undescended testicle except in specific cases, such as an inguinal canal undescended testicle, following appropriate medical evaluation to rule out unusual risk of injury.
Source: Portions adapted with permission from *Pediatrics,* May 1988; 81:5. Copyright © 1988 American Academy of Pediatrics.

One Testicle

The athlete who has only one testicle should be advised to participate in noncontact sports rather than strenuous or violent contact sports. The use of scrotal cups has lessened the chance of significant injury for the athlete who, along with his family, chooses to assume the risk.

Marfan's Syndrome

Marfan's syndrome, a disease affecting the collagen system, has recently gained notoriety because of its association with sudden death in athletes. This inherited condition presents with ocular, cardiac, and musculoskeletal abnormalities. Ocular abnormalities often include an upward displacement of the lens of the eye, caused by lack of connective tissue. Cardiac abnormalities, such as aortic dilation, present with abnormal heart sounds. Skeletal abnormalities are easier to screen in a general physical evaluation. Kyphoscoliosis and pigeon or convex chest are often seen (Fig. 5.2). An athlete with Marfan's syndrome will frequently have an arm span longer than his or her height. Another orthopedic sign can be detected by having the athlete adduct his or her thumb across the palm, wrapping the fingers around it. If the thumb sticks out beyond the fifth finger, it could indicate the presence of this condition (Fig. 5.3). An additional test is to have the athlete encircle his or her wrist with the thumb and fifth finger of the opposite hand. If the thumb and finger overlap, a further workup should be considered (Fig. 5.4). A family history of Marfan's syndrome should alert the physician to the need for further evaluation.

ADDITIONAL AREAS OF PHYSICAL EVALUATION

Testing an athlete's flexibility, strength, power, cardiovascular endurance, and body fat percentage can yield important information regarding potential problems. Such testing can be done during the preparticipation physical evaluation or at a later time.

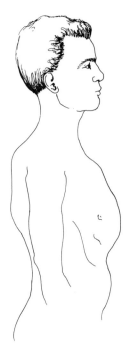

FIGURE 5.2. Pigeon chest is a skeletal abnormality associated with Marfan's syndrome.

Testing Flexibility

A few simple tests will determine where an athlete's flexibility falls on the spectrum of muscle tightness. The sit-and-reach test indicates low back and hamstring tightness (Fig. 5.5). The athlete sits with legs straight, places both feet against a box, and reaches the fingertips of both hands over a ruler attached to the box. The measurement is read in inches, either plus or minus, depending on the tightness found. Most athletes should strive to achieve either zero or plus scores. Minus scores indicate muscle tightness, and that particular athlete may have to work harder than average on joint flexibility.

For a test of upper-extremity flexibility at the shoulder, the athlete stands with arms flexed at 90 degrees, elbows fully extended. The athlete externally rotates both arms as far as possible. Athletes who can rotate their palms beyond horizontal, making the hypothenar eminence higher than the thenar eminence, are considered "loose."

A simple test of active dorsiflexion at the ankle measured with a goniometer can as-

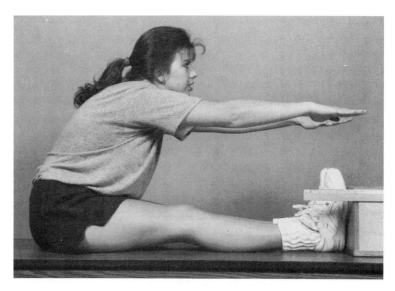

FIGURE 5.5. The sit-and-reach test indicates low back and hamstring tightness.

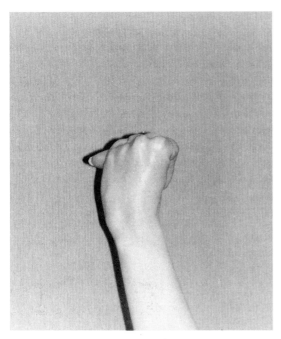

FIGURE 5.3. The athlete's thumb extends beyond the fifth finger, indicating the possible presence of Marfan's syndrome.

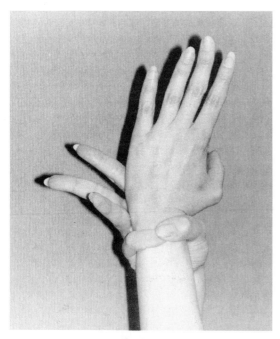

FIGURE 5.4. Another orthopedic sign of Marfan's syndrome is seen in this photo where the thumb overlaps the fifth finger as the athlete encircles the opposite wrist.

sess tightness and its possible relation to present and future athletic conditions. Athletes should be able to achieve at least 15 degrees of active dorsiflexion as a guard against athletic injury.

To test hip flexor tightness the athlete lies supine and pulls one knee completely to the chest with both arms, while extending the opposite leg onto the floor or table. Athletes should be able to extend the leg fully. The degrees of hip flexion of the extended leg indicate the extent of iliopsoas tightness on the same side. The test is reversed for the opposite hip.

All of these tests determine tightness or looseness for individual athletes. Flexibility testing is described further in Chapter 45. Any athlete found to have a specific deficit should be placed both on a specialized stretching program that addresses the particular problem and on a general program designed by the coach and trainer.

Testing Strength

Baseline muscular strength is established during the orthopedic examination by manual muscle testing that compares the extremities. The athletic training staff and coaches can obtain further strength measures in a variety of ways. For example, dynamometers have been developed to measure grip strength and strength of the shoulder abductors and adductors. Another common way to test muscular strength is through isotonic weight testing. Baseline measures of strength are determined using the best score among three trials of a one-repetition maximum lift of an isotonic weight. After each attempt, a rest period is allowed. The athlete continues until he or she has lifted the maximum weight possible. Many conditioning and strengthening programs are based on percentages of this maximum lift.

Testing Power

Baseline power measurements can be obtained in a variety of ways. The most common power test is the vertical jump test. The athlete stands near a wall or measuring device and reaches as high as possible. From a stand-still position, the athlete attempts to jump straight up, marking the highest point. The measurement consists of the difference between the two markings. Another power test is the Margaria stair-climb test. The athlete runs up a set of stairs and is timed between the third and ninth steps. Power is calculated by dividing the product of the athlete's body weight and the height his or her body displaces in running up the stairs by the time required to travel from the third to ninth steps. The following formula applies:

$$\text{Power kg m/sec} = \frac{w\,(\text{kg}) \times D\,(\text{m})}{t\,(\text{sec})}$$

The results of an athlete's power scores are usually compared to generalized norms.

Isokinetic devices such as the Cybex (Lumex, Ronkonkema, NY), Kincom (Chattrex, Chattanooga, TN), and Biodex (Biodex Corp., Shirley, NY), are more accurate in measuring strength and power. These machines accommodate resistance and are safe for testing a recovering injured extremity. Power and endurance testing is as important as strength testing following an injury and should be used to compare the injured extremity to the noninjured extremity.

Testing Cardiovascular Endurance

The 12-minute run test correlates well with tests that measure maximum oxygen consumption. Most coaches and trainers hope their athletes have been working on their aerobic conditioning program for 2 to 3 months prior to the first day of practice. They hope testing on opening day will show that athletes can cover at least 1.75 miles in 12 minutes and are therefore in superb condition. Most good college athletes can run 1.5 miles in 8.15 minutes.

Testing Body Fat Percentage

Measurement of body fat percentage is important in preseason screening for two reasons. First, it allows the athletic trainer to monitor how much fat weight, as opposed to lean muscle weight, the athlete can safely lose during the year. Second, it allows the sports medicine staff to differentiate between athletes who have large frames due to large muscle mass and those who truly carry excess fat and could be healthier, less of an injury risk, and more efficient if they were to lose weight. Underwater weighing is probably the most accurate technique for testing body fat percentage, but it requires special equipment, trained personnel who do this type of testing frequently, and an abundance of time.

Caliper testing is potentially easier and less time-consuming than underwater weighing. Measurements of subcutaneous fat are believed to be directly related to internal fat percentage. Measurements are taken by pinching the subcutaneous fat folds between the thumb and forefinger, pulling it away from the muscle mass. The skinfold thickness calipers are placed beside the finger and thumb, with millimeters recorded from the calipers. Generally, three measurements each are taken at six sites on the body, with the average measurement used for calculations. The six sites commonly used are the mid-triceps, subscapu-

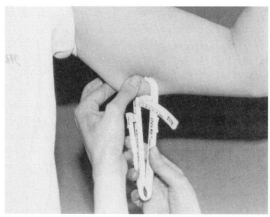

FIGURE 5.6. Caliper skin-fold test for measuring body fat percentage. The triceps is measured half-way between the top of the shoulder to the elbow in the midline of the triceps.

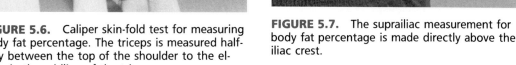

FIGURE 5.7. The suprailiac measurement for body fat percentage is made directly above the iliac crest.

lar, suprailiac, abdominal, upper part of the thigh, and mid-axillary.

Body fat percentage can be calculated in several ways.[2] In the following formula for women, the triceps and suprailiac measurements are used:

Body density (gm/cc) = 1.0764
$$- (0.00088 \times \text{tricep})$$
$$- (0.00081 \times \text{suprailiac})$$

Percentage body fat (%) =
$$(4.570/\text{body density} - 4.142) \times 100$$

The triceps is measured halfway between the tip of the shoulder to elbow in the midline of the triceps (Fig. 5.6). The suprailiac measurement is made directly above the iliac crest (Fig. 5.7).

The formula for men utilizes subscapular and thigh measurements.

Body density (gm/cc) = 1.1043
$$- (0.00131 \times \text{subscapular})$$
$$- (0.001327 \times \text{thigh})$$

Percentage body fat (%) =
$$(4.570/\text{body density} - 4.142) \times 100$$

[2]The formulas for calculating body fat are reprinted with permission of Macmillan Publishing Company from *Physical Fitness*, 3rd edition by Bud Getchell. Copyright © 1983.

The subscapular measurement is taken obliquely, just below the tip of the scapula (Fig. 5.8). The thigh is measured along the inside of the proximal third (Fig. 5.9).

It is very important to measure each site on the same side of the body. Age is also a factor in the calculation and the comparison of measures to normative data. Table 5.4 shows body fat norms for young adults age 16 to 25. The percentage of body fat for men and women increases slightly with age.

By using hand-held calipers or a computerized calculating system, age and caliper measurements are calculated automatically, making this task extremely easy.

TABLE 5.4. Body Fat Norms for Young Adults

Category	Women	Men
Very low fat	14.0–16.9	7.0–9.9
Low fat:trim	17.0–19.9	10.0–12.9
Average	20.0–23.9	13.0–16.9
Above normal	24.0–26.9	17.0–19.9
Very high fat	27.0–29.9	20.0–24.9
Obese	30.0+	25.0+

Source: Reprinted with permission of Macmillan Publishing Company from *Physical Fitness*, 3rd edition by Bud Getchell. Copyright © 1983.

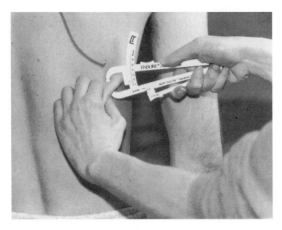

FIGURE 5.8. The subscapular measurement for body fat percentage is taken just below the tip of the scapula.

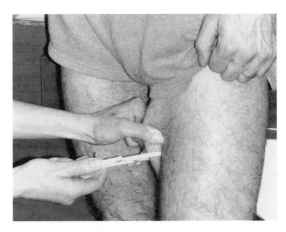

FIGURE 5.9. The thigh is measured for body fat percentage along the proximal third, along the inside of the thigh.

IMPORTANT CONCEPTS

1. A preparticipation physical evaluation fulfills legal and insurance requirements, reveals deficiencies that may disqualify or restrict an athlete from participating in a particular sport, and gives a baseline of the athlete's fitness, which can be used for later comparison should an injury occur.
2. The ideal preseason evaluation is a circuit evaluation, whereby multiple specialty stations are set up in an area large enough to permit easy traffic flow and multiple evaluations.
3. The basic preseason evaluation includes (1) a history of prior medical problems or injury, (2) a complete general physical evaluation that includes eye and dental exams, and (3) an orthopedic examination.
4. Disqualifying or restricting conditions that result from a preseason evaluation include elevated protein and glucose levels, high blood pressure, prior head trauma, having a single paired organ, and Marfan's syndrome.
5. Additional tests of flexibility, strength, power, cardiovascular endurance, and body fat percentage can be performed during the preseason evaluation or later to gain further information on potential physical problems.

SUGGESTED READINGS

Abdenour, Thomas E., and Nancy J. Weir. "Medical Assessment of the Prospective Student Athlete." *Athletic Training* 21 (1986): 122–123, 186.

American Medical Association. *Medical Evaluation of the Athlete: A Guide*, rev. ed. Chicago: American Medical Association, 1976.

Brown, Eugene W., and Crystal F. Branta, eds. *Competitive Sports for Children and Youth: An Overview of Research and Issues.* Champaign, Ill.: Human Kinetics, 1988.

Caine, Dennis J., and Jan Broekhoff. "Maturity Assessment: A Viable Preventive Measure Against Physical and Psychological Insult to the Young Athlete?" *The Physician and Sportsmedicine* 15 (March 1987): 67–80.

Cantwell, J. D. "Marfan's Syndrome: Detection and Management." *The Physician and Sportsmedicine* 14 (July 1986): 51–55.

Committee on Sports Medicine, American Academy of Pediatrics. *Sports Medicine: Health Care for Young Athletes.* Evanston, Ill.: American Academy of Pediatrics, 1983.

Dorsen, P. J. "Should Athletes with One Eye, Kidney, or Testicle Play Contact Sports?" *The Physician and Sportsmedicine* 14 (July 1986): 130–138.

DuRant, R. H., C. Seymore, C. W. Linder, and S. Jay. "The Preparticipation Examination of Athletes: Comparison of Single and Multiple Examiners." *American Journal of Diseases of Children* 139 (1985): 657–661.

Feinstein, Ronald A., Earl J. Soileau, and William A. Daniel, Jr. "A National Survey of Preparticipation Physical Examination Requirements." *The Physician and Sportsmedicine* 16 (May 1988): 51–59.

Galioto, Frank M., Jr. "Identification and Assessment of the Child for Sports Participation: A Cardiovascular Approach." *Clinics in Sports Medicine* 1 (1982): 383–396.

Garrick, J. G., and N. J. Smith. "Pre-Participation Sports Assessment." *Pediatrics* 66 (1980): 803–806.

Goldberg, B., A. Saraniti, P. Witman, et al. "Pre-participation Sports Assessment—An Objective Evaluation." *Pediatrics* 66 (1980): 736–745.

Harvey, Jack. "The Preparticipation Examination of the Child Athlete." *Clinics in Sports Medicine* 1 (1982): 353–369.

Hunter, S. C. "Screening High School Athletes." *Journal of the Medical Association of Georgia* 74 (1985): 482–484.

Hunter, Stephen C., William C. Etchison, and Brian C. Halpern. "Standards and Norms of Fitness and Flexibility in the High School Athlete." *Athletic Training* 20 (1985): 210–212.

Jones, R. "The Preparticipation, Sport-Specific Athletic Profile Examination." *Seminars in Adolescent Medicine* 3 (1987): 169–175.

Komadel, L. "The Identification of Performance Potential." In *The Olympic Book of Sports Medicine* (vol. 1, *Encyclopaedia of Sports Medicine*), edited by A. Dirix, H. G. Knuttgen, and K. Tittel, pp. 275–285. Oxford: Blackwell Scientific, 1988.

Kreipe, R. E., and H. L. Gewanter. "Physical Maturity Screening for Participation in Sports." *Pediatrics* 75 (1985): 1076–1080.

Leach, R. "Medical Examination of Athletes." In *The Olympic Book of Sports Medicine* (vol. 1, *Encyclopaedia of Sports Medicine*), edited by A. Dirix, H. G. Knuttgen, and K. Tittel, pp. 572–582]. Oxford: Blackwell Scientific, 1988.

Linder, C. W., R. H. DuRant, R. M. Seklecki, et al. "Preparticipation Health Screening of Young Athletes: Results of 1268 Examinations." *American Journal of Sports Medicine* 9 (1981): 187–193.

Livingston, Samuel, and Wulfred Berman. "Participation of the Epileptic Child in Contact Sports." *Journal of Sports Medicine* 2 (1974): 170–174.

Lysens, R., A. Steverlynck, Y. van den Auweele, J. Lefevre, L. Renson, A. Claessens, and M. Ostyn, "The Predictability of Sports Injuries." *Sports Medicine* 1 (1984): 6–10.

McKeag, D. B. "Preseason Physical Examination for the Prevention of Sports Injuries." *Sports Medicine* 2 (1985): 413–431.

Micheli, Lyle J., and Kevin R. Stone. "The Pre-Sports Physical: Only the First Step." *Journal of Musculoskeletal Medicine* 1 (1984): 56–60.

Micheli, Lyle J., and John G. Yost. "Preparticipation Evaluation and First Aid for Sport." In *Pediatric and Adolescent Sports Medicine*, edited by Lyle J. Micheli, pp. 30–48. Boston: Little, Brown, 1984.

Myers, G. C., and James G. Garrick. "The Preseason Examination of School and College Athletes." In *Sports Medicine*, edited by Richard H. Strauss, pp. 237–249. Philadelphia: W. B. Saunders, 1984.

Rooks, D. S., and L. J. Micheli. "Musculoskeletal Assessment and Training: The Young Athlete." *Clinics in Sports Medicine* 7 (1988): 641–677.

Rose, K. D. "Which Cardiovascular 'Problems' Should Disqualify Athletes?" *Physician and Sportsmedicine* 3 (June 1975): 62–68.

Roy, S., and R. Irvin. "The Preparticipation Physical Examination." In *Sports Medicine: Prevention, Evaluation, Management, and Rehabilitation*, pp. 11–27. Englewood Cliffs, N.J.: Prentice-Hall, 1983.

Runyan, D. K. "The Pre-participation Examination of the Young Athlete: Defining the Essentials." *Clinical Pediatrics* 22 (1983): 674–679.

Salem, D. N., and J. M. Isner. "Cardiac Screening for Athletes." *Orthopedic Clinics of North America* 11 (1980): 687–695.

Shaffer, T. E. "The Health Examination for Participation in Sports." *Pediatric Annals* 7 (October 1978): 666–675.

Shephard, Roy J. *Physical Activity and Growth*. Chicago: Year Book Medical Publishers, 1982.

Smith, Nathan J., and Carl L. Stanitski. "The Preparticipation Health Evaluation for the Scholastic and Collegiate Athlete." In *Sports Medicine, A Practical Guide*. Philadelphia: W. B. Saunders, 1987, pp. 1–15.

Spack, Norman P. "Medical Problems of the Exercising Child: Asthma, Diabetes, and Epilepsy." In *Pediatric and Adolescent Sports Medicine*, edited by Lyle J. Micheli, pp. 24–133. Boston: Little, Brown, 1984.

Strong, W. B., and Charles W. Linder. "Preparticipation Health Evaluation for Competitive Sports." *Pediatrics in Review* 4 (1982): 113–121.

Strong, W. B., and D. Steed. "Cardiovascular Evaluation of the Young Athlete." *Pediatric Clinics of North America* 29 (1982): 1325–1339.

Tennant, F. S., Jr., K. Sorenson, and C. M. Day. "Benefits of Preparticipation Sports Examinations." *Journal of Family Practice* 13 (1981): 287–288.

Tucker, J. B., and J. T. Marron. "The Qualification/Disqualification Process in Athletics." *American Family Physician* 29 (1984): 149–154.

6

Record Keeping

OBJECTIVES FOR CHAPTER 6

After reading this chapter, the student should be able to:

1. Describe the types of forms for which the athletic trainer is often responsible.
2. Review the information contained in each type of form.
3. Discuss the utilization of these forms in an athletic training situation.

INTRODUCTION

Paperwork is one of the "chores" of the athletic trainer. Most athletic trainers are more comfortable working with people and find that the long hours and intense level of activity involved with athletic training do not allow much time or enthusiasm for record keeping. However, the athletic trainer has to devote a certain amount of time to records, especially when one considers that many athletes work out year-round and the number of athletic activities is increasing. Trying to remember all events specific to an athlete's activity certainly is not easy for today's athletic trainer.

Chapter 6 begins with a discussion of successful record keeping. The remainder of the chapter focuses on the following commonly kept records: administrative forms, preseason forms, injury forms, annual reports, and national registries. All of these forms may be amended to suit the individual needs of the athletic program for which they are to be used. ■

SUCCESSFUL RECORD KEEPING

Records should not be kept simply for the sake of record keeping or out of fear of lawsuits. Records are kept as a log or journal of the athlete's injuries, treatment, observations, and recovery. The information must be accurate and available for study or review. The athletic trainer, team physician, and athletic administrator should determine which records to keep and how to do so with utmost accuracy.

Self-discipline and organization are the keys to successful record keeping. Good records are an athletic trainer's means of accountability to peers, coaches, administrators, and physicians. Having a secretary, student, or clerical assistant help with record keeping will allow a trainer to perform other necessary tasks. An athletic trainer who is poorly organized will have a difficult time with both accuracy and information, making any records virtually useless. In such cases, the responsibility of record keeping should be given to another staff member.

Sometimes records are kept in a college or university health center. In such situations, the records may not have to be duplicated by the athletic trainer. In the case of the high school athlete, the athletic trainer is usually the primary record keeper, and he or she must be especially diligent in record keeping.

Time should be set aside daily or several times a week for updating and recording athletic medical records. Failure to do so results in either forgotten or distorted information. If lack of time is a problem in record keeping, then a priority system should be implemented so that documentation of serious injury, unsafe practices, and equipment takes precedence over other data. The trainer can use a daily diary to record major happenings. All records become legal documents and are extremely important in instances of legal action.

Athletic health care cannot be compromised because of record keeping. Some trainers may become so involved in record keeping that they have limited time for interacting with the athletes.

Equipment for Record Keeping

Equipment for record keeping may range from a log book and file cabinet in a desk to an extensive computer system (Fig. 6.1). Increasingly, computers are becoming popular in athletic training rooms because they are coming down in price and are capable of storing large amounts of easily accessible information.

A computer can be programmed to keep all essential records. When necessary, the computer's printer can produce the hard copies needed, thus saving additional turn-around time previously necessary when a secretary typed records for the athletic trainer. At year's end, in just a matter of minutes the computer can tabulate all injuries, all of a particular type of injury, the number of types of treatment, the number of treatments per athlete, the number of injuries per sport, or a variety of other combinations of data requested by the sports medicine staff. When this efficiency is contrasted with the laborious time spent with handwritten records and their tabulations, it is evident that computers are becoming a must for the successful and organized athletic trainer.

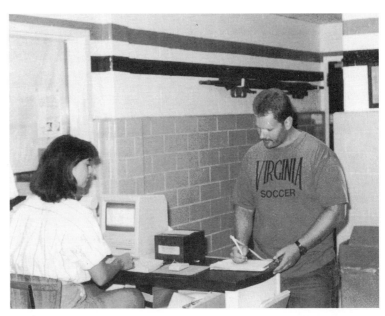

FIGURE 6.1. Computers are increasingly used by athletic trainers because they are coming down in price and are capable of storing large amounts of easily accessible information.

Storage of Records

Records kept by the athletic trainer should be safely stored and kept confidential from those other than the sports medicine staff. The athlete, however, should be allowed access to his or her own records at any time. How long records are stored varies, depending on the athletic organization and the state in which it operates. Most records should probably be kept two years or more after the statute of limitations has run out in the respective state. For the athlete who is a minor, the statute of limitations applying to legal action will not begin until he or she reaches the legal age limit, usually 18 years old. Records kept in hospitals and other health care centers will be maintained as required by those institutions.

ADMINISTRATIVE FORMS
Equipment Check-Out Forms

Equipment check-out forms are important to keep down costs of reusable items (Fig. 6.2). These items are issued during the season and checked in after their use or at the end of the competitive season or school year. Examples include crutches, braces, elastic wraps, and protective pads.

Inventory Forms

A running inventory needs to be kept to ensure a constant monitoring of supplies. Figure 6.3 illustrates a yearly record of supplies on hand that were ordered at the beginning of the school year, and supplies on hand that remain at the end of the year. Some athletic trainers prefer to do a semi-annual inventory. Figure 6.3 may be modified for this purpose.

Health Insurance Forms

The job description of the athletic trainer often includes the processing of health insurance information. Figure 6.4 contains the kind of information that the athletic trainer or the trainer's assistant needs to process insurance claims as efficiently as possible.

Equipment Check-Out

Name	Sport	Address / Phone	Date Out	Date In

FIGURE 6.2. An equipment check-out form.

YEAR _____					YEAR _____			
Item	Stocked	Ordered	On hand 5/30	Used	Stocked	Ordered	On hand 5/30	Used

FIGURE 6.3. An inventory supply form.

Student-Athlete Medical Insurance Information
(Please type or use ballpoint pen and print.)

Sport _____   Social Security Number _____

Student-Athlete

Complete Full Name _____
   (No Initials)   Last   First   Middle

Date of Birth _____   Year in School _____

Primary Insurance Information

Insurance Company Name _____

Address _____

_____

Insurance Company's Telephone Number: (___) _____

Employer's Name _____

Address _____

_____

Employer's Telephone Number: (___) _____

Policyholder's Name _____

Relationship _____   Social Security Number _____

Policy Number _____   Effective Date _____

Authorization to Release Benefits to Medical Center and Appropriate Physician

Date _____   Signed _____
                  Student-Athlete (or parent, if minor)

Authorization to Pay Insurance Benefits to Medical Center/M.D.

Date _____   Signed _____
                  Insured

FIGURE 6.4. A medical insurance form.

Student Athletic Trainer Time Sheet

Name	Time In	Time Out	Total Time	Nature of Work

FIGURE 6.5. A student athletic trainer's time sheet for logging trainer hours for certification.

Student Athletic Trainer Time Sheets

Student athletic trainers are required to have a certain number of hours of athletic training experience, depending on their program of certification. Figure 6.5 illustrates one method in which these student trainer hours may be logged in an accurate manner.

Medications Forms

Dispensing medications is the responsibility of the team physician. Figure 6.6 shows one way of keeping an accurate record of medications dispensed. Information from this kind of record may be later transferred to the athlete's individual file.

PRESEASON FORMS

Preseason forms should be completed before the athlete is allowed to check out equipment or begin the first team practice session.

Physical Examination Forms

A copy of the physical examination form illustrated in Figure 6.7 should be kept with the athletic trainer. The athletic trainer should review each form for information that would indicate potential problems for the athlete. This information should be transferred to the individual's file.

Pre- and Postseason Screening Examination Forms

Screening of the athlete for musculoskeletal weaknesses should be performed both preseason and postseason to determine strength and flexibility deficits, as well as to record body fat and physical fitness indexes. Figure 6.8 illustrates one such screening form.

Permission-for-Treatment Forms

A necessary form, especially for athletes under 18 years of age, is the permission-to-treat form. The one shown in Figure 6.9 incorporates with the form an explanation of who the certified athletic trainer is and an invitation to parents to meet and discuss any concerns they may have with the trainer. At this time, the parent receives an introduction to the training room environment and the types of treatments and rehabilitation that are provided.

Medication Check-Out

Date	Name	Sport	Physician	Diagnosis	Medication	Dosage

FIGURE 6.6.   A medication check-out form.

Intercollegiate Athlete Interim History and Physical Examination

Student's Interim Medical History
(To be completed by student or parents yearly)

Name of Student _____ Age _____

Address _____ Phone _____

Sport _____

1. List illnesses or injuries requiring medical attention, including hospitalization and/or surgical procedures in the past 12 months _____

_____

2. Are you currently under a physician's care and if so, for what condition? _____

_____

3. List medications currently taken _____

_____

4. List current allergies (e.g., food, insect, medication) _____

_____

5. Have you ever had mononucleosis? If yes, when? _____

_____

Physician's Certificate
(To be filled in and signed by the examining physician)

Name of Student _____
                         (Please Print)

Age _____ Height _____ Weight _____ Blood Pressure _____

Significant Past Illness or Injury _____

_____

Respiratory _____

Cardiovascular _____

Liver _____ Spleen _____ Hernia _____

Musculoskeletal _____ Skin _____

Neurological _____ Genitalia _____

Laboratory: Urinalysis _____ Differential _____

Comments _____

Completed Immunizations: Tetanus _____ Other _____
                                            Date   Date

I certify that I have on this date examined this student and find him/her physically able to compete in the supervised activities *not crossed out below.*

BASEBALL	FIELD HOCKEY	SOCCER	TRACK
BASKETBALL	FOOTBALL	SOFTBALL	VOLLEYBALL
CHEERLEADER	GOLF	SWIMMING	WRESTLING
CROSS COUNTRY	LACROSSE	TENNIS	OTHER _____

Date of Examination _____ Signed _____ , M.D.

Physician's Address _____ Phone _____

FIGURE 6.7. A preseason physical examination form.

Name ______________________ Sport ______________________

	Date														
	Height														
	Weight														
STRENGTH	Caliper														
	Orthotron 60°/sec Left														
	Right														
	Shoulder	R	L	R	L	R	L	R	L	R	L	R	L	R	L
	Abduction														
	Adduction														
FLEXIBILITY	Ankle														
	Back														
	Hamstrings														
	Hip Flexors														
	Hip (External Rotation)														
	Time - 40														
	Vertical Jump														
	Injuries														

FIGURE 6.8. A flexibility test form.

Release Forms for Athletes with Increased Risks

Some injuries are unavoidable in athletics—a reality that athletes and parents alike must accept. Figure 6.10 is an example of a form for the athlete who is permitted to participate despite a high risk of injury. The information on this form is important not only from an educational perspective but also from one of liability should legal action be initiated at a later date due to injury to the athlete.

Standard Release-for-Football Forms

Figure 6.11 is a standard release form for the sport of football. Similar forms should be used for athletes in all sports. This failure to warn is currently being used in litigation when an athlete is injured.

Drug-Screening Forms

When drug screening is part of the athletic training program, the athlete has to provide a document that indicates he or she under-

---

Permission for Treatment

As many of you know, we have employed a certified athletic trainer, Miss DeDe Jackson, to help provide the best athletic health care for your son or daughter. We would like to invite you to stop by the school to meet her or contact her about any athletic health care problems that may occur during the season. In addition, Miss Jackson will be available by appointment during teacher-parent conference or at parent-teacher night. Our first parent-teacher night will be September 10, at which time we invite you to visit Miss Jackson in our training room at the entrance to the gymnasium.

Should a medical emergency occur, we will make every effort to contact you about treatment for your son or daughter. In the event you cannot be reached, we ask that you give us permission to provide emergency medical treatment and any follow-up care by a licensed physician.

_____

In the event I cannot be reached by telephone, I grant permission to the Fluid School System to provide emergency treatment for _____ (son or daughter) and follow-up care by a licensed physician of the Commonwealth of Virginia.

Name _____

Address_____

Phone numbers and time of day at each number I may be contacted:

_____

Signed _____ Date _____

FIGURE 6.9. A permission-to-treat form.

Release Form for Athletes with Increased Risks

Release:

I understand that football is a hazardous sport. It has been explained to me, and I understand that there is a risk of injury to my eyes in participating in the sport. I also understand that as I only have functional sight in my right eye, there is risk that I could be permanently blinded should I have my sight impaired through injury to my left eye.

I accept this risk and agree not to hold responsible any individuals employed by the Fluid School System should I sustain any such injury resulting in sight impairment as a result of injury to my eye(s) through athletic competition in football.

Signed _____   _____
                    (Student)   (Parent)

Date _____   Date _____

FIGURE 6.10. A standard athletic release-of-liability form.

Standard Release for Football

Name _____
(Please Print)

This is to certify that I have carefully read and fully understand the warning label(s) attached inside and/or outside of the football helmet I have checked out from the University of Virginia Athletic Department. The label reads:

WARNING — NO HELMET CAN PREVENT ALL HEAD OR NECK INJURIES A PLAYER MIGHT RECEIVE WHILE PARTICIPATING IN FOOTBALL. Do not use this helmet to butt, ram, or spear an opposing player. This is in violation of the football rules, and such use can result in severe head or neck injuries; paralysis or death to you; and possible injury to your opponent.

On some of our helmets, the label reads:

WARNING: Do not use this helmet to butt, ram, or spear an opposing player. This is in violation of the football rules, and can result in severe head, brain, or neck injury; paralysis or death to you; and possible injury to your opponent.
There is a risk these injuries may also occur as a result of accidental contact without intent to butt, ram, or spear.

I also understand that football is a potentially injurious sport and agree to accept the risk of injury associated with competition in the sport.
No helmet can prevent all such injuries.

Player Signature _____ Date _____

NOTE: One copy of this form is to be given to the player, and one copy is to remain on file in the equipment room.

FIGURE 6.11. A standard release-for-football form.

stands the policies and procedures and is willing to submit to drug testing. Figure 6.12 is an example of this kind of form.

INJURY FORMS

Written injury reports enable all personnel to contribute to the well-being of the athlete in that the record becomes a teaching implement for undergraduate and graduate student athletic trainers. An organized, sequential, and systematic approach to record keeping can only sharpen the clinical skills of the athletic trainer. Filling out injury report forms disciplines the trainer to think logically and express precisely the whole progression of the condition of the athlete.

Individual Athlete's Record

The individual athlete's record should contain injury, treatment, and rehabilitation progress, as well as information deemed important to the individual's personal situation. The athletic record should be well organized and complete. The information should be systematic in its logic and continuity so that other athletic training personnel can easily interpret the information. Other personnel reading the individual athlete's record can find out such things as how the injury occurred, when it occurred, and what kind of treatment was applied. This communication with other personnel illustrates the reasons why treatments are carried out.

Consent to Testing of Urine Sample and Authorization for Release of Information

I hereby acknowledge receipt of a copy of the University of _____ Intercollegiate Athletics Drug Policy. I further acknowledge that I have read this policy and fully understand its provisions.

It is my understanding that signing this consent form and returning it is a prerequisite to becoming a member of the intercollegiate team at the University of _____ . I further understand that I may refuse to sign this consent form, but as a consequence, I must forego participation in intercollegiate sports at the University.

I am aware that I am expected to abide by team rules, that such rules are subject to change, and that I may be dismissed from the team and/or deprived of my grant-in-aid or scholarship for failure to abide by such rules. I acknowledge my understanding that the use or abuse of drugs not prescribed by a physician for a specific medical condition is a violation of team rules.

I hereby consent to have samples of my urine collected and tested for the presence of certain drugs or substances in accordance with the provisions of the University of _____ Intercollegiate Athletics Drug Policy.

I further authorize the head athletic trainer at the University of _____ to make a confidential release to the head coach of any intercollegiate sports in which I am a team member; the athletic director at the University of _____ ; physicians at the Student Health Office, and my parent(s) or legal guardian(s) (if a minor) of all information and records, including test results, you may have relating to the screening or testing of my urine sample(s) in accordance with the provisions of the University of _____ Intercollegiate Athletics Drug Policy, which is applicable to all intercollegiate athletes at the University of _____ . To the extent set forth in this document, I waive any privilege I may have in connection with such information. I further agree that, in the event the results of my drug-screening test are positive, I will follow the procedures enumerated in the section of the policy entitled "Effect of Positive Test Results."

The University of _____ , its Board of Visitors, its officers, employees, and agents are hereby released from legal responsibility or liability for the release of such information and records as authorized by this form.

Signature _____   Print Full Name _____

Date _____   Intercollegiate Sport _____

FIGURE 6.12.   A standard drug-testing consent form.

Notes to the athlete's record that are added during the course of the year or the season should be brief and to the point. It has been remarked that the length of the note is inversely proportional to its value. An example of an individual record form is shown in Figure 6.13.

Use of SOAP or SOP Notes

Some clinical athletic trainers like to use SOAP or SOP notes. These forms are a variation of the athlete's record. The acronyms are based on the following phrases:

*S*ubjective statements by the athlete that include the athlete's current or chief complaints and a history of injury, including description and mechanism, date of injury, functional impairments, pain, and discomfort.

*O*bjective record of what the athletic trainer observes, measures, and palpates, such as strength, range of motion, instability, and atrophy. The motor and sensory nervous system, both peripheral and central, may need evaluation, as may the musculoskeletal, cardiac, vascular, and dermatologic

---

Individual Athlete Record

Name _____   Age _____

Address _____   Sport _____

Parent's Name _____

Address / Phone(s) _____

Allergies (drug, insect) _____

Permanent Medical Information (prior injuries, illnesses) _____

Injuries, illnesses _____

Date	Injury / Illness	Treatment / Comments

FIGURE 6.13.   An athlete's record form.

systems. Functional assessments such as posture, endurance, and gait should also be noted. Other objective assessments would include edema, ecchymosis, and gait analysis, such as limping, use of a cane, crutches, or bracing.

*A*ssessment of the athlete's problem is next—that is, the trainer's professional judgment as to what is happening, how the athlete is reacting to the treatment—in short, what the trainer thinks.

*P*lan is the final step of what the trainer does with the above information to continue or change treatment, to consult with other specialties, educate the athlete, and so forth.

*S*ubjective as in the SOAP note.
*O*bjective as in the SOAP note.
*P*rogram for the treatment and rehabilitation of the athlete. For example, whirlpool, hamstring stretching, and straight leg raising with a 1-pound weight might be appropriate for the athlete with patellar tracking problems. Modalities, sets, and repetitions of strength, range of motion, and endurance programs, as well as home instructions, are included.

The athletic trainer in the training room usually finds the SOP note more appropriate. The SOP note could be implemented when filling out an initial injury report (Fig. 6.14).

Within this program, both long- and short-term goal setting for the athlete begins. Short-term goals are emphasized, especially for the athlete who will require long-term rehabilitation. The findings in the subjective and objective categories are used to project these goals.

Progress notes within the SOP system are added only as change occurs in any of the three areas. In this way, a lot of unnecessary

Name _____   Date/Time: 9/8/90 4:00 P.M.

Sport _____

S — Athlete indicated he/she was hit on the lateral left knee as he/she was running during a
     football game 9/8/90, at approximately 3:00 P.M. Chief complaint is pain, swelling, loss of
     range of motion, and function.
O — Slight edema; pain with valgus stress; no instability; minus 5 degrees extension, plus 100
     degrees flexion; gait tentative; athlete is hesitant about weight bearing.
P — Wrapped knee with elastic bandage, elevated leg, iced knee for 20 minutes. Gave crutches
     and instructed athlete in crutch walking. Referred athlete to Dr. Smith.

Athletic Trainer Signature _____   Date_____

FIGURE 6.14. A SOP note.

writing is eliminated. In both the SOAP and SOP systems, the stress is on functional activity. Using the information on a SOAP or SOP note, another athletic trainer can determine where the athlete is in the program to return to competition.

Regular Review of Records

A review of records should be a regular process in record keeping. In the case of SOAP or SOP notes, the records should be assessed for completeness, reliability, sound analytical sense, and efficiency.

When checking for completeness, the trainer should ask these questions: Are all problems identified? Is the plan of action for all problems dealt with?

When checking for reliability, these questions should be asked: Are the records up-to-date? Accurate? Have the plans been carried out? Have the most recent or appropriate techniques been used?

In assessing whether the records make sound analytical sense, these are questions to be asked: Are valid judgments demonstrated to manage the problems? Do the data support the plan implemented? Is the plan consistent with current therapy?

Finally, efficiency is judged by asking the following questions: Has the problem been solved in a reasonable amount of time? If not, why not? What alternatives have been

used, and have they been timely and applied as quickly as possible?

This review of records—often done at the end of a season, semiannually, or at least yearly—gives the athletic trainer an opportunity to judge whether his or her records are logical, the techniques are scientifically sound, and the information is properly prioritized. Changes in record keeping may be in order following this review. Any changes should be written and distributed to the other athletic training personnel.

Individual Injury Report Forms

Figure 6.15 is a sample injury report form that may be filled out and placed in an athlete's file. This type of report can be filled out daily and filed as the athletic trainer or administrative personnel has time. Individual injury report forms are good time-savers because the athletic trainer does not have to go constantly to the athlete's personal file to record information. The athletic trainer can carry a daily diary or log to record short notes that will be transcribed later.

Injury Report to Parents

Another important form for the secondary school athletic training program is the report to parents (Fig. 6.16), which allows the

Injury Report Form

Name _____

Date / Time _____   Sport _____

Injury and Description of Injury _____

_____

Athlete's Complaint(s) _____

_____

Evaluative Findings _____

_____

Treatment and/or Triage _____

Athletic Trainer Signature _____

FIGURE 6.15. An injury report form.

Secondary School Athletic Injury Home Report

TO: Mr. & Mrs. Jim James
FROM: Jack Smith, ATC
RE: Billy James

Injury: Billy has received an injury to his left ankle. Our impression is that it is a moderate sprain.

Treatment: We suggest that you have him elevate the ankle and apply an elastic wrap and ice for 20 minutes each hour before bedtime.

Follow-up: I would like him to report to the training room tomorrow morning before school for further evaluation.

If you have any questions, please contact me at school (555-1289) or at home (555-8708).

FIGURE 6.16. An injury-report-to-parents form.

Treatment Record

Date / Time	Sport	Name	Initial–A.T.	Injury	Treatment	Comments

FIGURE 6.17. A treatment record form.

trainer to report the injury, its treatment, and suggested follow-up procedures to the parent in written rather than verbal form. This approach not only enables the trainer to show concern in a professional manner, but also avoids any confusion and misunderstanding that might result if the parent's only report of the injury and its treatment came from the athlete.

Treatment Records

Treatment records indicate the athlete's compliance to recommended treatment;

but more important, they show that the athlete is receiving proper care. Figure 6.17 is an example of a record that can easily be kept by hand or on a computer for fast individual recall of the record. A space for comments by the athletic trainer is important so that the trainer can note changes in the condition of the athlete's injury.

Referral Forms

A referral form (Fig. 6.18) is especially useful when a number of different physicians are involved, as is the case with the high school athletic trainer. Often, what the player communicates to the physician is not exactly what the athletic trainer has told the student, and what the student passes on to the athletic trainer from the physician may also be inaccurate. Most physicians feel more comfortable with referral forms, especially when the athlete will not be under the physician's direct supervision. The use of referral forms by a trainer also indicates to the physician the trainer's interest in carrying out the physician's instructions and the trainer's concern for the athlete. Referral forms should also be kept with the individual's file.

Coach's Injury Report Forms

Finally, the athletic trainer should complete the coach's injury report (Fig. 6.19). This report should be updated daily and given to the coach at the beginning of each day so that the coach can plan to eliminate any players listed on the injury report from the practice schedule.

OTHER REPORTS

Annual Reports

An annual report may be compiled and submitted to the athletic department of the athletic training program. This report should include monies allocated at the beginning of the school year and monies actually spent over the course of the year. At this time, an analysis of the program may be included with recommendations for the next year's budget and reasons for the recommendations. The number of athletes treated and a breakdown of injuries sustained may be useful information to report when planning the budget for the following year.

It is important for an athletic trainer to establish priorities and goals for future athletic training programs. A three- to five-year plan that encompasses budget, supplies, equipment, staff, and facilities should be prepared.

Referral Form

TO: Dr. Jones
FROM: DeDe Jackson, ATC

_____ is being referred for evaluation
(Name) and treatment. Please indicate below your impression and follow-up treatment.

Diagnosis _____

Your Treatment _____

Check or note treatment by athletic trainer:

Modality
ice   electrical stimulation
heat   therapeutic exercise
  hot packs   strength
  whirlpool   range of motion
  contrast   endurance
ultrasound   other
traction

Date of functional participation

No contact _____

Limited contact _____

Limited running _____

Other _____

Full practice _____

Special pads/support _____

Date of next appointment _____

FIGURE 6.18. A referral form.

National Registries

National registries record athletic injuries by age, gender, and sport (see Chapter 1). The athletic trainer may be responsible for reporting athletic injuries to one or more national registries. Data from the national registries are used to recognize injury patterns so that sports may be made safer through changes in rules and equipment.

Coach's Injury Report

Date _____

Sport _____

Name	Injury	Practice Limitation

FIGURE 6.19. A coach's injury report form.

IMPORTANT CONCEPTS

1. Administrative forms, while not medically pertinent, are important for keeping track of supplies, medical costs, and student trainer hours.

2. Preseason forms must be completed before the athlete begins practice.

3. Injury forms must be kept up-to-date, describing in detail the aspects of the athlete's record of injury, the prescribed treatment, and the rehabilitation plan. Other injury forms pertain to physician referral, parental injury information, and the coach's injury reports.

4. Annual reports and national registries allow the athletic trainer an opportunity to analyze budget, treatment, and injury patterns to plan more effectively for the next season.

SUGGESTED READINGS

Feitelberg, S. B. *The Problem Oriented Record in Physical Therapy*. Burlington: University of Vermont, 1975.

Hill, J. R. *The Problem-Oriented Approach to Physical Therapy Care*. Washington, D.C.: American Physical Therapy Association, 1977.

7

Introduction to Biomechanics

OBJECTIVES FOR CHAPTER 7

After reading this chapter, the student should be able to:
1. Understand the effects of force on a body.
2. Recognize the three types of energy (potential, kinetic, and work) and their interrelationships.
3. Define the principles of strength, stress, strain, stiffness, and elasticity.
4. Understand the biomechanical basis of musculoskeletal injuries.

INTRODUCTION

The relationship of force to motion, or biomechanics, is important in understanding not only the mechanism of athletic injury, but also the principles of rehabilitation. The athlete, in performing intense activity, uses large muscular forces that place significant biomechanical loads on the bones, joints, ligaments, tendons, capsules, and muscles. Whether or not these body parts are injured depends on such factors as strength, elasticity, and the amount of deformation they can undergo before failure.

Chapter 7 begins with an explanation of the effects of force and the concepts of potential, kinetic, and work energy. How force and energy impact on bone strength and stiffness is discussed next, followed by the effects of loading on the soft tissues and repetitive loading on the bones. The last section of Chapter 7 describes how kinematic data are used to analyze motion in a joint, specifically the knee. ▪

EFFECTS OF FORCE

External and Internal Effects

When force is applied to a body, it has two effects: the first is external and causes the body to accelerate; the second is internal and produces a **deformation**, or state of mechanical strain in the body. For example, when a tennis racket hits a tennis ball, the two effects are easily seen under high-speed photography. The external effect accelerates the tennis ball, which goes over the net into the opposite court. The internal effect, or the deformation, changes the ball's shape when the racket's strings flatten one surface of the ball. These two effects occur whenever forces are applied to bodies. In the case of a boxer struck by a heavy blow, the external effect of the force is easily seen as the boxer is knocked down and accelerated to the mat. Not so apparent is the internal effect or change in shape of the boxer's face as the glove strikes it.

Linear Acceleration

Acceleration and internal deformation are caused by forces. A **force** is an action that changes the state or motion of a body to which it is applied. **Linear acceleration** is the change in an object's speed in a straight direction.

Moments of Torque and Inertia

Most of our actions involve forces that act through a lever arm, producing a moment of torque. A **moment of torque** is a force that acts through a distance, or more precisely defined, the perpendicular distance from the line of force application to the center of motion or fulcrum of the structure. Forces are defined in terms of pounds of force or in metric terms, newtons. Moments of torques are defined in terms of foot-pounds or newton-meters. **Moment of inertia** is defined as a measure of resistance to change.

Determining Joint Forces

The relationship between force and motion is summed up in two mathematical relationships:

$$F = ma,$$

reads as "force (F) equals mass (m) times acceleration (a)."

$$T = Ia,$$

reads as "torque (T) equals moment of inertia (I) times acceleration (a)."

By finding the linear acceleration in the case of forces, or the angular acceleration in the case of torques, the forces about a human joint during various athletic activities can be found. For example, when someone punts a football, stroboscopic or motion pictures can help reveal acceleration. Once the moment of inertia is known, the torque can be calculated from the formula:

$$T = Ia,$$

where T is the torque expressed in foot-pounds (ft-lbs) or newton-meters (N-m); I is the mass moment of inertia, in newton-meters times seconds squared (N-m·sec²); and a is the angular acceleration, in radians per seconds squared (r/sec²).

The torque is a product not only of the mass moment of inertia and the angular acceleration of the body part, but also of the main muscle forces accelerating the body part and the perpendicular distance of the force from the instant center of the joint (lever arm). Thus:

$$T = Fd,$$

where F is force expressed in pounds or newtons and d is the perpendicular distance expressed in feet or meters.

Since T is known and d can be measured on the body part from the line application of the force to the instant center of the joint, the equation can be solved for F. When F has been calculated, the remaining problem can be solved like a static problem using simplified techniques from biomechanics to determine the minimum magnitude of the joint reaction force acting on the joint at a certain instant in time.

An example illustrates the use of dynamic analysis to calculate the joint reaction force on the tibiofemoral joint at a particular instant in time during dynamic activity —that of kicking a football. A stroboscopic film of the knee and lower leg shows that the maximal angular acceleration occurred at the instant the foot struck the ball; the lower leg was almost vertical at this instant. From the film the maximal angular acceleration was computed to be 453 radians per seconds squared. From anthropometric data tables, the mass moment of inertia for the lower leg was determined to be 0.35 newton-meter times seconds squared. The torque about the tibiofemoral joint was calculated according to the equation, torque equals mass moment of inertia times angular acceleration ($T = Ia$):

$$(0.35 \text{ N-m} \cdot \text{sec}^2) \times (453 \text{ r/sec}^2)$$
$$= 158.5 \text{ N-m}$$

After the torque was determined to be 158.5 newton-meters and the perpendicular distance from the patellar tendon to the instant center for the tibiofemoral joint was found to be 0.05 meter, the muscle force acting on the joint via the patellar tendon was calculated using the equation, torque equals force times distance ($T = Fd$):

$$158.5 \text{ N-m} = F \cdot 0.05 \text{ m}$$

$$F = \frac{158.5 \text{ N-m}}{0.05 \text{ m}}$$

$$F = 3{,}170 \text{ N}$$

The maximal force exerted by the quadriceps muscle during the kicking motion was 3,170 newtons. Thus, very large forces are produced during athletic activities.

During walking and running, the knee, hip, and ankle joints experience very high loads. **Load** is defined as any force or combination of forces, applied to the outside of a structure, and therefore sustained or carried by the matter in the structure. In level walking, the forces on the hip, knee, and ankle joints are three to five times body weight. With running and more rigorous activities, the forces may rise. The hip joint has a characteristic force pattern during normal gait, with a high force at heel strike and at toe-off. Even during stance phase, the forces are at least body weight.

ENERGY

Defining Potential, Kinetic, and Work Energy

Another concept of great interest to the athletic trainer is that of energy. There are three types of energy: potential, kinetic, and work. **Potential energy (PE)** is the energy stored in a body by virtue of its position in space and is equal to the mass times the vertical height (*h*): $PE = mh$. **Kinetic energy (KE)** is the energy of a moving body, and it equals one-half of the mass times the velocity (*v*) squared: $KE = \frac{1}{2}mv^2$. **Work energy (WE)** is the energy stored in a structure under deformation and is defined as the force times the distance a body is deformed: $WE = Fd$.

Interrelationships of Potential, Kinetic, and Work Energy

During athletic activity there is a constant conversion from potential energy to kinetic energy to work energy back to kinetic or potential energy. For instance, a skier standing on top of a hill has very large amounts of potential energy. He starts to come down the hill by converting his potential energy into kinetic energy. As he increases in speed, he may feel uncomfortable and turn up into the hill again, converting some of the kinetic energy back into potential energy as he goes upward on the hill. Alternatively, he converts some kinetic en-

ergy into work energy by deforming his skis and deforming the snow.

Much more energy is involved in athletic and other activities than is required to break a single bone. For instance, it requires only 80 kilogram-centimeters (kg-cm) of energy to fracture a tibia, although a skier going 30 kilometers per hour possesses 2,000 kg-cm of energy. Large, fast athletes performing at high levels of intensity must be able to dissipate large amounts of kinetic energy without injury.

BONE STRENGTH AND STIFFNESS

Viscoelastic and Anisotropic Properties

All biological materials are **viscoelastic**—that is, their deformation behavior is time dependent. They are also **anisotropic**—that is, their properties are specific to the direction of force application. In the case of bones, this means that the strength of the material depends on the rate that it is loaded and the direction of loading.

Strength and Stiffness

Strength and stiffness are the important mechanical properties of bone. These properties can best be understood for bone or any other material by examining the material under loading. When a load in a known direction is placed on a structure, the deformation of that structure can be measured and plotted on a load-deformation curve, and the strength and stiffness of the structure can be determined.

The Load-Deformation Curve

Interpreting the Graph

A hypothetical **load-deformation curve** for a somewhat pliable material is shown in Figure 7.1. When a load is applied within the elastic region of the curve (A-B area in Fig. 7.1) and is then released, the structure returns to its original shape—that is, no permanent deformation occurs. If loading

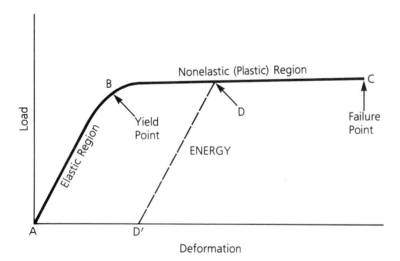

FIGURE 7.1. Load-deformation curve for a somewhat pliable material. The amount of permanent deformation that occurs if the structure is loaded to point D and then unloaded is represented by the distance between A and D. B represents the yield point at which deformation occurs. (From V. H. Frankel and M. Nordin. *Basic Biomechanics of the Skeletal System*, 2d ed. Philadelphia: Lea & Febiger, 1989.)

continues, some regions of the material begin to yield permanently (B-C area in Fig. 7.1). If loading continues past this yield point and into the nonelastic region of the curve, permanent deformation results. If loading in the nonelastic region continues, an ultimate failure point is reached.

Determining Structural Strength

The load-deformation curve shows three parameters for determining the strength of a structure:

- The load the structure can sustain before failure.
- The deformation it can sustain before failure.
- The energy it can store before failure.

On the curve, the ultimate failure point indicates the strength in terms of load and deformation. The size of the area under the entire curve indicates strength in terms of energy storage. In addition, the slope of the curve in the elastic region indicates the stiffness of the structure.

Computing Mechanical Behavior of Different Materials

The load-deformation curve is useful for determining the strength and stiffness of whole structures of various sizes, shapes, and material compositions. To examine the mechanical behavior of the material that composes a structure and to compare the mechanical behavior of different materials, test specimens and testing conditions must be standardized. When samples of standardized size and shape are tested, the load per unit area and the amount of deformation in terms of length can be determined. The curve that is generated is called the **stress-strain curve**.

Stress and Strain

Stress is the load per unit area which develops on a plane surface within a structure in response to externally applied loads. It is expressed in force units per area. The three

units most commonly used for measuring stress in bone samples are newtons per centimeter squared (N/cm²); newtons per meter squared, or pascals (N/m²; Pa); and mega-newtons per meter squared, or megapascals (MN/m²; MPa). Pounds per square inch (psi) is also used.

Strain is the deformation at a point in a structure under loading. Two basic types of strain exist: *normal strain*, which is a change in length, and *shear strain*, which is a change in angle. Normal strain is the amount of deformation (lengthening or shortening divided by the structure's original length). It is a nondimensional parameter expressed as a percentage (for example, centimeter per centimeter). Shear strain, under conditions of torque loading, is the amount of angular deformation in a structure—that is, the amount that the original angle of the structure changes. It is expressed in radians (one radian equals approximately 57.3 degrees).

Developing a Stress-Strain Curve

Stress and strain values can be obtained for bone by placing a standard specimen of bone tissue in a testing jig and loading it to failure (Fig. 7.2). The strain that results can be illustrated in a stress-strain curve (Fig. 7.3). The regions of the stress-strain curve are similar to those of the load-deformation curve. Loads in the elastic region do not cause permanent deformation or strain. Once the yield point is exceeded, however, permanent deformation occurs.

Stiffness and strength. The stiffness of the material is represented by the slope of the curve in the elastic region. The strength in terms of energy storage is represented by the area under the entire curve, and this is called the toughness of the material.

Stress-strain curves for metal, glass, and bone illustrate the differences in mechanical behavior among these materials (Fig. 7.4). Variations in stiffness are reflected by differences in the slope of the curve in the elastic region. Metal has the steepest slope and is thus the stiffest material. A value for

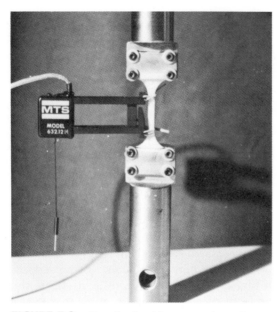

FIGURE 7.2. Standardized bone specimen in a testing machine. The strain between the two gauge arms is measured with a strain gauge. The stress is calculated from the total load measure. (From V. H. Frankel and M. Nordin. *Basic Biomechanics of the Skeletal System*, 2d ed. Courtesy of Dennis R. Carter, Ph.D. Philadelphia: Lea & Febiger, 1989.)

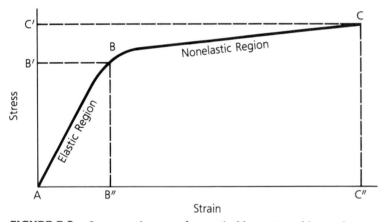

FIGURE 7.3. Stress-strain curve for cortical bone tested in tension. Yield point (B)—point past which some permanent deformation of the bone occurs.
Yield stress (B′)—load per unit area that the bone sample sustained before nonelastic deformation.
Yield strain (B″)—amount of deformation that the sample sustained before nonelastic deformation. The strain at any point in the elastic region of the curve is proportional to the stress at this point.
Ultimate failure point (C)—the point past which the sample failed.
Ultimate stress (C′)—load per unit area that the sample sustained before failure.
Ultimate strain (C″)—amount of deformation that the sample sustained before failure. (From V. H. Frankel and M. Nordin. *Basic Biomechanics of the Skeletal System*, 2d ed. Philadelphia: Lea & Febiger, 1989.)

stiffness is found by dividing the stress anywhere in the elastic portion of the curve by the strain at that point. This value is called the **modulus of elasticity** (Young's modulus). Stiffer materials have higher moduli.

The elastic region of the curve. The elastic portion of the stress-strain curve for metal is a straight line, indicating linearly elastic behavior. Precise testing has shown that the elastic portion of the curve for bone is not straight but curves slightly, indicating that bone is not linearly elastic in its behavior. Some yielding may occur when the bone is loaded in the elastic region. The difference in nonelastic behavior for the two materials is due to differences in micromechanical events during mechanical yielding. Yielding in bone (tested in tension) is caused by debonding of the osteons and microfracture and the role of the organic components. Yielding in metal (tested in tension) is caused by plastic flow and formation of slip lines. Slip lines are formed when the planes of atoms of the atomic lattice structure dislocate relative to one another.

Defining Brittle and Ductile

Materials are classified as brittle or ductile, depending on the amount of deformation they undergo before failure. Glass, a typical brittle material, deforms little before failure, as indicated by the absence of a nonelastic (plastic) region on the stress-strain curve (see Fig. 7.4). Soft metal, a typical ductile material, deforms extensively before failure, as indicated by a long, nonelastic (plastic) region on the curve (see Fig. 7.4). The fracture surfaces of the two materials reflect this difference in amount of deformation (Fig. 7.5). A ductile material pieced together after fracture will not conform to its original shape, but brittle material will.

SOFT TISSUES UNDER LOADING

The soft tissues that make up ligaments, tendons, and capsules exhibit a specific type of behavior under loading. When a liga-

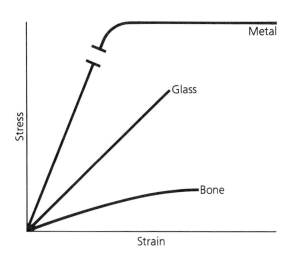

FIGURE 7.4. Stress-strain curves for three materials: metal, glass, and bone. The elastic portion of the graph for bone is slightly curved, indicating that bone is not linearly elastic in its behavior. Soft metal is a ductile material and therefore has no plastic region.   (From V. H. Frankel and M. Nordin. *Biomechanics of the Skeletal System,* 2d ed. Philadelphia: Lea & Febiger, 1989.)

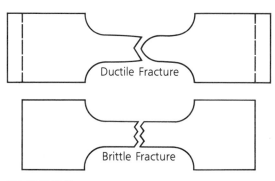

FIGURE 7.5. Fracture surfaces of a ductile and brittle material. The dotted lines on the ductile material indicate the original length of the structure, before deformation. The brittle material deformed very little before fracture.   (From V. H. Frankel and M. Nordin. *Basic Biomechanics of the Skeletal System,* 2d ed. Philadelphia: Lea & Febiger, 1989.)

ment is subjected to loading, microfailure takes place even before the yield point is reached. When the yield point is exceeded, the ligament begins to undergo gross failure, and simultaneously the joint begins to displace abnormally. Because failure of a ligament leads to a large joint displacement, the surrounding structures such as the joint capsule and other ligaments may also be damaged. In a clinical test, the anterior drawer test, force was applied to a cadaver knee up to the point of anterior cruciate ligament failure and a ligament-bone preparation was tested. Figure 7.6 depicts the progressive failure of this ligament and displacement of the joint. At maximum load the joint had displaced several millimeters. The ligament was still in continuity even though it had undergone extensive macro- and microfailure and extensive elongation. The force-elongation curve generated during this experiment indicates where microfailure of the ligament begins.

The results of this in-vitro test can be correlated with clinical findings. In Figure 7.7, the curve for the experimental study is divided into three regions. The first region corresponds to the amount of load placed on a ligament during clinical tests of joint stability. The second region corresponds to the amount of load placed on the ligament during physiologic activity. The third region corresponds to the amount of load imposed on the ligament from the beginning of microfailure to complete rupture.

Ligament Injuries

Ligament injuries fall into three categories, depending on their severity. Injuries in the first category result in pain but no joint instability on clinical examination. However, microfailure of the collagen fibers may have occurred.

Injuries in the second category produce severe pain and some degree of joint instability clinically. Progressive failure of the collagen fibers has taken place, producing partial ligament rupture. The strength and stiffness of the ligament may be decreased by 50 percent or more. Often, the joint instability produced by a partial rupture of a ligament is masked by muscle activity, and thus the clinical test for joint stability is often performed under anesthesia.

Injuries in the third category produce severe pain during the course of trauma,

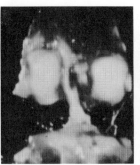
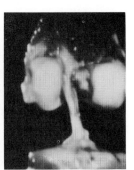
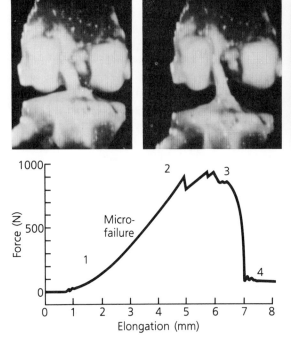

FIGURE 7.6. Progressive failure of the anterior cruciate ligament. Almost 8 mm of joint displacement took place before the ligament reached complete failure. (From V. H. Frankel and M. Nordin. *Basic Biomechanics of the Skeletal System*, 2d ed. Philadelphia: Lea & Febiger, 1989. Courtesy of Frank R. Noyes, M.D., and Edward S. Grood, Ph.D.)

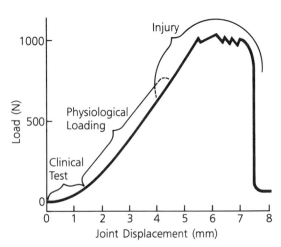

FIGURE 7.7. The curve in Figure 7.6 converted to a load-displacement curve and divided into three regions that correlate with clinical findings. (From V. H. Frankel and M. Nordin. *Basic Biomechanics of the Skeletal System*, 2d ed. Philadelphia: Lea & Febiger, 1989.)

with less pain after injury. Clinically, the joint is found to be completely unstable. Most collagen fibers have ruptured, but a few may still be intact, giving the ligament the appearance of continuity, although it is unable to support any loads.

Loading of a joint that is unstable due to ligament or joint capsule rupture produces abnormally high stresses on the joint cartilage. This abnormal type of loading of the cartilage in the knee has been correlated with osteoarthritis in humans and animals.

Muscles Under Loading

The strength of bone is influenced not only by the loading rate and loading direction, but also by muscle activity. When bone is loaded in vivo, contraction of the muscles attached to the bone substantially alters the magnitude and type of stress within the bone. This muscle contraction can decrease or eliminate tensile stress in the bone by producing compressive stresses that partially or totally neutralize the tensile stresses.

The effect of muscle contraction can be illustrated in a tibia subjected to three-point bending. Figure 7.8a shows the leg of a skier who is falling forward, subjecting his tibia to a bending moment. High tensile stress is produced on the posterior aspect of this tibia, and high compressive stress acts on the anterior aspect. Contraction of the triceps surae muscles produces a high compressive stress on the posterior aspect (Fig. 7.8b), neutralizing the high tensile stress and thereby protecting the tibia from fail-

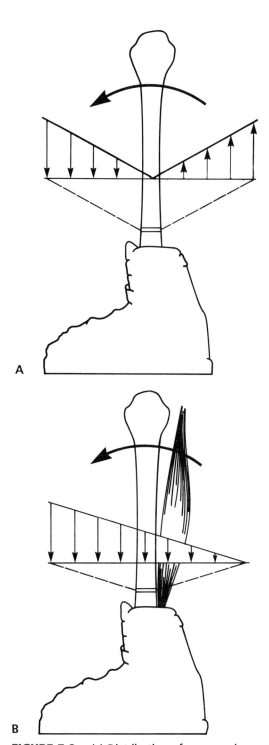

FIGURE 7.8. (a) Distribution of compressive and tensile stresses in a tibia subjected to three-point bending. (b) Contraction of the triceps surae muscles produces high compressive stress on the posterior aspect, neutralizing the high tensile stress. (From V. H. Frankel and M. Nordin. *Basic Biomechanics of the Skeletal System*, 2d ed. Philadelphia: Lea & Febiger, 1989.)

ure in tension. This muscle contraction may result in a higher compressive stress on the anterior surface of the tibia. Adult bone can usually withstand this stress, but immature bone, which is weaker, may fail in compression.

Muscle contraction produces a similar effect on the hip joint (Fig. 7.9). During locomotion, bending moments are applied to the femoral neck, and tensile stress is produced on the superior cortex. Contraction of the gluteus medius muscle produces compressive stress that neutralizes this tensile stress, with the net result that neither compressive nor tensile stress acts on the superior cortex. Thus, the muscle contraction allows the femoral neck to sustain higher loads than otherwise possible.

FRACTURE OF BONE UNDER REPETITIVE LOADING

Mechanism of Fatigue Fracture

Bone fracture that occurs after many loading cycles is called a **fatigue fracture**. Fatigue fractures occur when terrain, footwear, or exercise regimen changes. To understand fatigue fractures one must understand the interrelationships of the mechanical properties of bone, the properties of muscle, the effect of muscle activity on loading of bones, and the cyclic properties of loading. Under excessive compression loading, bone fails because many small microcracks are produced. Under excessive tensile load of the bone, the osteons are debonded at the cement lines. Either tension failure of bone, compression failure, or combinations of these will take place.

Fractures can be produced by a single load or the repeated application of a smaller load. A fatigue fracture is typically produced by either a few high loads or many small or normal loads.

The Fatigue Curve

The interplay of the load and repetition for all materials can be plotted on a fatigue

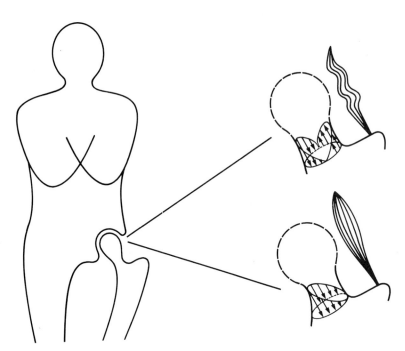

FIGURE 7.9. Stress distribution in a femoral neck subjected to bending. (From V. H. Frankel and M. Nordin. *Basic Biomechanics of the Skeletal System*, 2d ed. Philadelphia: Lea & Febiger, 1989.)

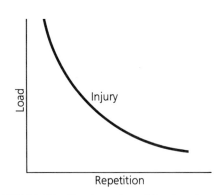

FIGURE 7.10. The interplay of load and repetition represented on a fatigue curve. (From V. H. Frankel and M. Nordin. *Basic Biomechanics of the Skeletal System*, 2d ed. Philadelphia: Lea & Febiger, 1989.)

curve (Fig. 7.10). For some materials (some metals, for example), the fatigue curve is asymptotic, indicating that if the load is kept below a certain level, the material will remain intact, no matter how many repetitions. For bone tested in vitro, the curve may not be asymptotic. Fatigue microfractures may be created in bone subjected to low repetitive loads.

Yield Strength

Testing of bone in vitro also reveals that bone fatigues rapidly when load or deformation approaches the yield strength of the bone; that is, the number of repetitions that are needed to produce a fracture greatly diminishes.

Effect of Frequency of Loading

In repetitive loading of living bone, the amount of load and the number of repetitions affect the fatigue process, as does the frequency of loading. Since living bone is self-repairing, a fatigue fracture only results when the remodeling process is outpaced by the fatigue process—that is, when the frequency of loading precludes the remodeling that is necessary to prevent bone failure.

Fatigue fractures are usually sustained during continuous, strenuous physical activity. Such activity causes the muscles to lose their tone or become fatigued. When muscles "fatigue," their ability to contract is reduced; as a result, they are less able to store energy and thus to neutralize the stress imposed on the bone. The resulting alteration of the stress distribution in the bone causes abnormally high loads to be imposed on the bone, and a fatigue fracture may occur.

Failure may occur on the tensile side, the compressive side, or both sides of the bone. Failure on the tensile side results in a transverse crack, and the bone may proceed rapidly to complete fracture. Fatigue fracture on the compressive side appears to occur more slowly; the remodeling is less easily outpaced by the fatigue process, and the bone may not proceed to complete fracture. A schema for effective exercise of bone fatigue is shown in Figure 7.11.

KINEMATICS

Kinematic data are used to analyze motion in a joint. Internal joint function can be determined with an instant center analysis. For more complex joints a complex rotation or a screw axis must also be determined. The instant center technique permits the center of motion to be determined for a joint in any range of motion. For example, in the knee, surface joint motion occurs between the tibial and femoral condyles and also between the femoral condyles and the patella.

The instant center locations for the range of knee motion for 0 to 90 degrees have been determined. Tangential sliding at the joint surface was found in all cases. An investigation of the instant center pathway for the tibiofemoral joint in knees with internal derangements found that in all cases the instant center was displaced from the normal position during some portion of the motion examined.

The abnormal instant center pathway for one subject, a 35-year-old man with a bucket-handle derangement, is shown in Figure 7.12. If the knee is extended and flexed about a displaced instant center, the tibiofemoral joint surfaces do not slide (tangentially) throughout the range of motion but become either distracted or compressed (Figs. 7.13a, b). Such a knee is analogous to a door with a bent hinge, which no longer fits into the doorjamb.

If the knee is continually forced to move about a displaced instant center, it will gradually adjust to this situation by either stretching the ligament and supporting structures of the joint or exerting abnormally high forces on the articular surfaces.

Internal derangements of the tibiofemoral joint may interfere with the so-called screw-home mechanism, a combination of knee extension and external rotation of the tibia (Fig. 7.14). The tibiofemoral joint is not a simple hinge joint but has spiral, or helical, motion. The spiral motion

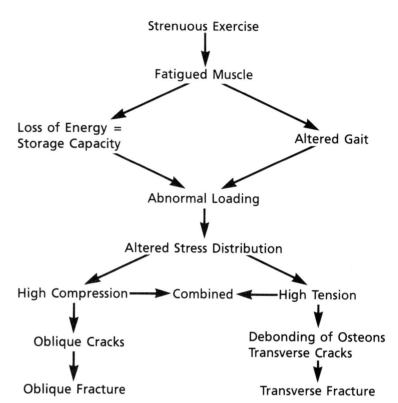

FIGURE 7.11.   Schema for effective exercise of bone fatigue.   (From V. H. Frankel and M. Nordin. *Basic Biomechanics of the Skeletal System,* 2d ed. Philadelphia: Lea & Febiger, 1989.)

of the tibia about the femur during flexion and extension results from the anatomic configuration of the medial femoral condyle.

In a normal knee the medial femoral condyle is approximately 1.7 centimeters longer than the lateral femoral condyle. As the tibia slides under the femur from the fully flexed to the fully extended position, it ascends and then descends the curve of the medial femoral condyle and simultaneously rotates externally. This motion is reversed as the tibia moves back into the fully flexed position. The screw-home mechanism gives more stability to the knee in any position than would be possible if the tibiofemoral joint were a just simple hinge joint.

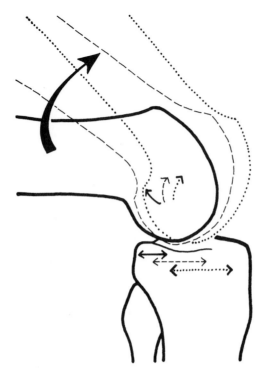

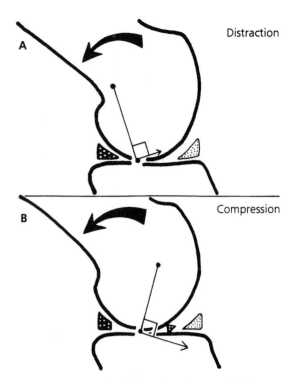

FIGURE 7.12. In this bucket-handle derangement, the abnormal center jumps at full extension of the knee. (From V. H. Frankel and M. Nordin. *Basic Biomechanics of the Skeletal System,* 2d ed. Philadelphia: Lea & Febiger, 1989. Adapted from Frankel et al., *J. Bone Joint Surg.,* 53A: 945–962, 1971.)

FIGURE 7.13. Surface motion in two tibiofemoral joints with displaced instant centers. The right-angle lines indicate the direction of displacement of the contact points. (a) With further flexion, the tibiofemoral joint is distracted (arrow). (b) With further flexion, the joint is compressed (arrow). (From V. H. Frankel and M. Nordin. *Basic Biomechanics of the Skeletal System,* 2d ed. Philadelphia: Lea & Febiger, 1989.)

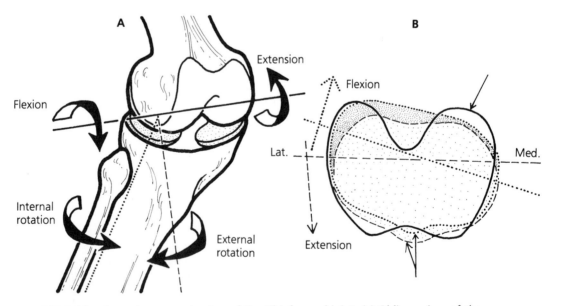

FIGURE 7.14. Screw-home mechanism of the tibiofemoral joint. (a) Oblique view of the femur and tibia. Shaded area indicates the tibial plateau. (b) Top view showing the position of the tibial plateau on the femoral condyles in knee flexion and extension. The light shaded area indicates the position of the plateau in knee flexion; the dark shaded area shows its position during knee extension. (From V. H. Frankel and M. Nordin. *Basic Biomechanics of the Skeletal System,* 2d ed. Philadelphia: Lea & Febiger, 1989. Adapted from Helfet: *Disorders of the Knee.* Philadelphia: J. B. Lippincott, 1974.)

IMPORTANT CONCEPTS

1. A force is an action that changes the state or motion of a body to which it is applied.
2. The three types of energy are potential, kinetic, and work energy.
3. A load-deformation curve measures and plots the deformation of a structure from a load placed on it in a known direction.
4. Stress is the load per unit area which develops on a plane surface within a structure in response to externally applied loads, and strain is the deformation of a point in a structure under loading.
5. Failure of a ligament from loading leads to simultaneous joint displacement.
6. A fatigue fracture occurs when the bone fails because of many small microcracks that occur from overloading.
7. Kinematic data are used to analyze motion in a joint.

SUGGESTED READINGS

D'Ambrosia, R. D., and D. Drez, Jr., eds. *Prevention and Treatment of Running Injuries*, 2d ed. Thorofare, N.J.: Slack Incorporated, 1989.

Teitz, C. C., ed. *Scientific Foundations of Sports Medicine*. Toronto: B. C. Decker, 1989.

Woo, S. L-Y., and J. A. Buckwalter, eds. *Injury and Repair of the Musculoskeletal Soft Tissues*. Park Ridge, Ill.: American Academy of Orthopaedic Surgeons, 1988.

8

Physiology of Tissue Repair

CHAPTER OUTLINE

OBJECTIVES FOR CHAPTER 8

After reading this chapter, the student should be able to:

1. Understand the basic structure and function of the tissues that are commonly injured in sports trauma.
2. Recognize the role of transition in load or use as an initiator of injury and breakdown.
3. Be familiar with the initiating mechanisms, mediators, and cellular events in the process of sports-induced inflammation and injury repair.
4. Define the terms *regeneration, repair,* and *degeneration.*
5. Describe the site of action and potential benefits of commonly prescribed therapeutic drugs and modalities.
6. Be able to characterize specific responses in tissues commonly injured in sports.
7. Define pain in the context of sports injury.
8. Explain the rationale and limitations of current grading concepts for soft tissue injury in sports trauma.
9. List examples of sports-induced injury that are not classically inflammatory.

INTRODUCTION

When a sports injury occurs, any of a number of tissue responses can take place. Some of these responses are predictable, but others are unexpected. Although the predictability of wound healing and repair forms the basis of present-day therapy, those who treat injured athletes soon become aware of the vast number of variables that defeat the textbook application of such logic to any single case. In addition, it is not clear whether the stages of wound healing seen after an acute sports injury occur in exactly the same manner as in cases of chronic, or overuse, sports injury. The goal of sports medicine therapy is to minimize the adverse effects of traumatic inflammatory responses while promoting tissue repair, thereby expediting a safe return to performance.

Chapter 8 begins by describing the structure and function of connective tissue (tendons, muscles, ligaments, cartilage, and bone), synovium, and nerves. Tissue response to physical injury is discussed next, followed by a description of tissue-specific injury response patterns. The last section of Chapter 8 discusses clinical grading systems. ■

STRUCTURE AND FUNCTION OF INJURED TISSUES

The individual cell holds the key to the regulation of the body's trauma response. Sports medicine therapy is increasingly challenged to understand and anticipate these cellular responses in predicting the recovery from injury or to justify the value of any therapeutic measure. Thus, this discussion is an invitation to "think like a cell" and to see that the body's cellular response to sports trauma takes place in the context of a changing biochemical environment, constantly influenced by such factors as oxygen tension, nutrition, genetic endowment, and aging, and modified by physical forces that initiate communication to and between cells. The result is the maintenance of structural integrity during use and tissue renewal after injury.

Connective Tissue

Tendon, muscle, ligament, cartilage, and bone are known as the **connective tissues**. That sprains are the most common acute sports injury underscores the vulnerability of these "connecting" tissues. Chronic overuse sports injuries most often involve the muscles, tendons, and their attachments. The following discussion focuses on those aspects of connective tissue structure and function that aid in understanding the events involved in inflammation, healing, and repair of such structures.

Composition

Connective tissues are composed of two basic elements, cells and extracellular matrix. Cell composition varies greatly in normal connective tissues. Because tendon, ligament, and cartilage have relatively few cells, the response to injury in these tissues relies on the migration of reparative cells—neutrophils, histiocytes, fibroblasts, or macrophages—to the damaged area. In contrast, two of the most actively repairing tissues, bone and muscle, are characterized by abundant pluripotential cells—osteoblasts in bone and myoblasts in muscle—which are readily available to begin the repair process.

To a great extent, the form and function of connective tissues are distinguished by their extracellular matrix composition. Once considered an inert, amorphous ground substance, the **matrix** is now known to be a vital, responsive, biochemical, saline gel that contains many important types of important macromolecules, including collagen, proteoglycans, hyaluronic acid, elastin, and fibronectin. There is growing evidence that the matrix may be the modulating medium that prompts cells to change their patterns of protein synthesis in re-

TABLE 8.1. Types and Properties of Collagen

Type	Chains	Macromolecular Association	Aggregate Form	Localization
I	α 1(I), α 2(I)			Most abundant collagen: Ubiquitous—Bone, Tendon, Capsules, Muscle, etc.
II	α 1(II)			Major cartilage collagen: Cartilage, Nucleus pulposus, Vitreous humor.
III	α 1(III)			Found in pliable tissues: Blood vessels, Muscle, Uterus, etc.

Source: Adapted from W. B. Leadbetter, J. A. Buckwalter, and S. L. Gordon. *Sports-Induced Inflammation: Clinical and Basic Science Concepts.* Park Ridge, Ill.: American Academy of Orthopaedic Surgeons, 1990.

sponse to load or use. For example, cartilage cells remain in a differentiated state only so long as they are in contact with Type II collagen and surrounding matrix.

Of the many macromolecules found in the extracellular matrix, collagen and proteoglycans are the most abundant. **Collagen**, a family of stiff, helical, insoluble protein macromolecules, provides the scaffold for tensile strength in fibrous tissue and, with additional mineralization, for rigidity in bone. Seventy to 90 percent of the dry weight of ligament and tendon is collagen; in bone it is 90 percent. A function of the fibroblast, collagen synthesis begins inside the cell and leads to the secretion of a three-peptide chain procollagen molecule (Fig. 8.1). Enzymatic cleavage of the low molecular weight ends of the procollagen molecule produces the tropocollagen form that self-assembles extracellularly into the collagen fibril (fibrillogenesis). Of the types of collagen, Types I–III are important in musculoskeletal tissue (Table 8.1).

Type I collagen, the normal fabric of tendon, ligament, muscle, and bone, derives its strength from the 2 to 3 covalent intermolecular bonds, or cross-linking, found in each collagen molecule (Fig. 8.2). This cross-linking is tissue specific, with strong trivalent bonding associated with high tensile demands, as in the Achilles tendon or the anterior cruciate ligament. Under increasing load, these cross-links give way, leading to fibril failure and eventual tendon rupture. Failure begins at 8 to 10 percent strain (change in length/length).

Type II collagen is the principal collagen of articular cartilage. Type III collagen has smaller fibrils and fewer cross-links. During repair, increased quantities of Type III collagen are often deposited, resulting in long-term structural weakening and delayed recovery. In time, Type III collagen is gradually replaced by Type I collagen.

In bone, osteoblasts synthesize an organic matrix called *osteoid*, of which 70 percent is Type I collagen. During mineralization, collagen fibers provide sites for the deposit of the hydroxyapatite crystals that give bone its hardness and rigidity.

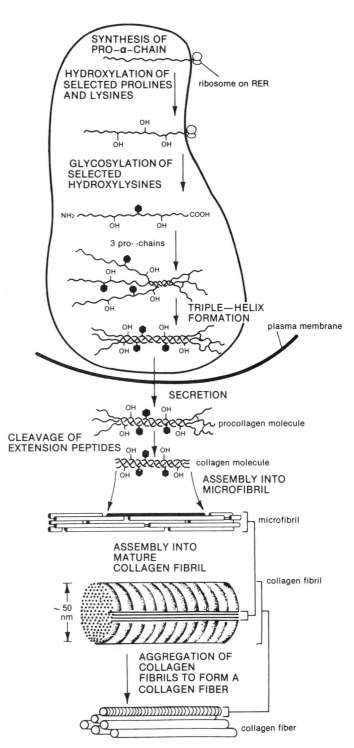

FIGURE 8.1. Intracellular and extracellular events of collagen synthesis and fibrillogenesis. (From J. G. Gamble. *The Musculoskeletal System—Physiological Basics.* New York: Raven Press, 1988, p. 63.)

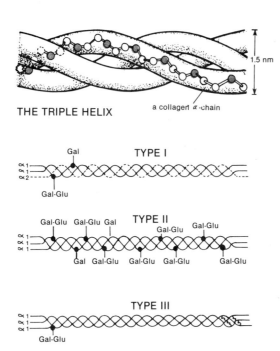

THE TRIPLE HELIX

a collagen α-chain

1.5 nm

TYPE I

Gal

Gal-Glu

TYPE II

Gal-Glu Gal-Glu Gal   Gal-Glu   Gal-Glu

Gal   Gal-Glu   Gal-Glu Gal-Glu   Gal-Glu

TYPE III

Gal-Glu

FIGURE 8.2. Under the triple helix structure are schematic drawings of three types of musculoskeletal collagen (gal = galactose, glu = glucose). Type III collagen, the weakest form, is deposited in increased quantities during tissue repair. (From J. G. Gamble, *The Musculoskeletal System—Physiological Basics.* New York: Raven Press, 1988, p. 61.)

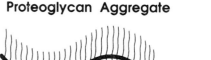

Proteoglycan Aggregate

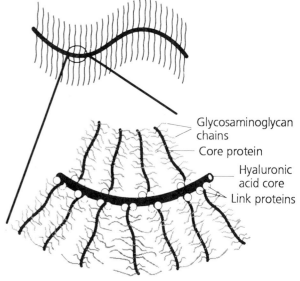

Glycosaminoglycan chains
Core protein
Hyaluronic acid core
Link proteins

FIGURE 8.3. Schema of a typical cartilage proteoglycan aggregate. Attachment of the individual proteoglycans to the central chain of hyaluronic acid is mediated by the link proteins. (Adapted from Leadbetter, W. B., Buckwalter, J. A., Gordon, S. L. *Sports-Induced Inflammation: Clinical and Basic Science Concepts.* Park Ridge, Ill.: American Academy of Orthopaedic Surgeons, 1990.)

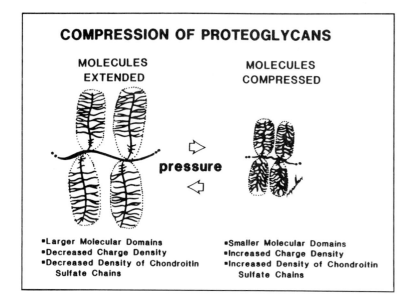

COMPRESSION OF PROTEOGLYCANS

MOLECULES EXTENDED

MOLECULES COMPRESSED

pressure

- Larger Molecular Domains
- Decreased Charge Density
- Decreased Density of Chondroitin Sulfate Chains

- Smaller Molecular Domains
- Increased Charge Density
- Increased Density of Chondroitin Sulfate Chains

FIGURE 8.4. Changes in load alter the shape and electrostatic properties of the proteoglycan molecular aggregate. (From Simon, S. R., Riggins, R. S., Wirth, C. R., Fox, M. L. *Orthopaedic Science: A Resource and Self-Study Guide for the Practitioner, Syllabus.* Park Ridge, Ill.: American Academy of Orthopaedic Surgeons, 1986.)

Proteoglycans, the other principal group of matrix macromolecules, possess great water-binding capacity. Proteoglycans vary in composition according to tissue type and, linked with hyaluronic acid, form the largest molecular aggregates in the body. They function as enormous electrostatic sponges to give articular cartilage its compression resistance and viscoelastic properties (Figs. 8.3 and 8.4).

Vascular Supply

Blood supply in connective tissue varies both in availability and pattern. Inflammation has been defined as the local reaction of vascular connective tissues to injury; therefore a blood supply is needed to generate a classic inflammatory response. Blood vessels carry the polymorphonuclear leukocytes that initiate wound débridement and activate reparative cells. Because articular cartilage is avascular, as well as alymphatic and aneural, it is not surprising that pure cartilage lesions have no inflammatory healing response. Tendon vascular sources are variable and often segmental. The blood supply to such structures as the rotator cuff and Achilles tendon is tenuous. As a result, intermittent ischemia caused by excessive compression, torsion, traction, or bony impingement produces a reduction in blood supply that can cause an accumulative diminishment in oxygen and nutrition. This deprivation leads to degenerative cellular change and chronic, insufficient healing.

Unlike tendon and cartilage, muscle and bone are highly vascular. Ten percent of cardiac output goes to bone. Both tissues demonstrate prominent but different repair patterns. Bone is repaired by complete regeneration, muscle by a combination of scar formation and regeneration.

Regulation of Connective Tissue Metabolism

No single central control mechanism regulates the metabolism of connective tissue. Instead, the diverse cell types that make up connective tissue exert a high degree of interrelated homeostatic control.

Mediators are protein messengers that allow cell-to-cell self-regulation. Cell-synthesized mediators include such platelet-synthesized growth factors as histamine, complement factor, prostaglandin, interleukin-1, bradykinin, and leukotrienes. In all, over 300 cell-synthesized mediators have been identified.

The breakdown products of connective tissue matrix molecules can also act to modify cell activity. In this open system, a given mediator can have multiple actions, depending on its matrix context, its interaction with other mediators, its concentration, and, importantly, the timing of its arrival at the site of activity. These variable functions have caused confusion, and several mediators have been "rediscovered" and given different names. Target cell protein synthesis or lack of synthesis is signaled by such cues as the three-dimensional molecular configuration and electrical charge of the

mediator interacting with cell wall receptor sites. When a target cell receives such cues, it is said to be "activated."

Mediators should be understood as the normal requirements of connective tissue homeostasis, which under unusual conditions, such as injury, inflammation, atrophy, or degeneration, can cause mediators to act pathologically. For example, certain prostaglandins that protect gastric lining from hyperacidity can also be injurious and require suppression by anti-inflammatory drugs in sports injury.

Morphostasis is the process by which tissues renew their cell populations and their matrix content. As previously noted, cell-matrix interaction is governed by precisely timed stimulating (anabolic) or inhibiting (catabolic) factors. In connective tissue, morphostasis is responsible for a continual turnover of collagen. Although difficult to quantify, collagen turnover is most rapid in bone and is very slow in articular cartilage.

Load and use are the primary mechanisms of connective tissue change in response to sports activity. **Load** represents mechanical force, and **use** refers to both repeated movement and the accumulation of load over time. As such, repetition, as seen in endurance sports, can take the form of both cyclic loading and overuse. Cells may be seen as the transducers of load in this process. Cells respond to load by changing shape or composition, protein synthesis, growth rate, mitochondrial density, and collagen turnover rate. Extremes of overload or immobilization increase their synthesis of matrix degradative enzymes, called *breakdown*. In theory, a "physiologic window of stress" response defines the synthetic, homeostatic, and degradation cell behavior for any of a given athlete's tissues (Fig. 8.5). The effect of load on tissues is described by strain and stress. **Strain** implies deformation whereas **stress** is the internal molecular energy resistance to strain. Research suggests that both strain and stress may promote cellular or matrix biologic responses (Fig. 8.6).

Transition is a common cause of sports injury. As previously defined by Lead-

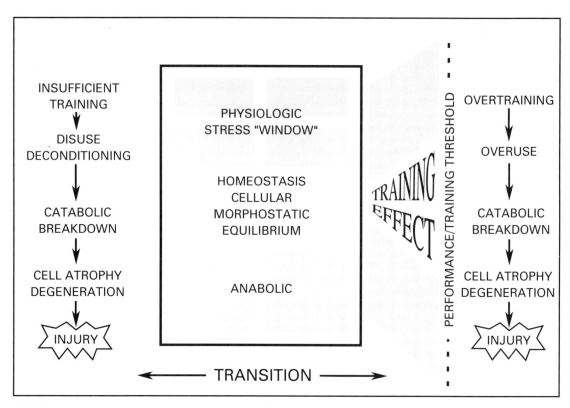

FIGURE 8.5. Hypothetical physiological stress "window" of cell response to level of activity. As previously defined by Leadbetter, transition, or change in activity level, is rate sensitive; that is, a more rapid transition produces a more drastic response.

better, the **principle of transition** states that sports injury is likely to occur when the athlete incurs any change in load or use of the involved part. Examples include increases in performance level; improper

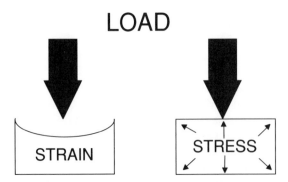

FIGURE 8.6. Load effect on tissues: strain is a measure of deformation under load; stress is the internal molecular resistance to deformation under load. Either can induce a cell response.

training; changes in equipment; environmental changes, such as new surfaces or a different training altitude; alterations in frequency, intensity, or duration of training; attempts at mastering new techniques; and even body growth itself. The transitional theory emphasizes that adaptation to physical demand is a time-dependent cellular process, and that any sudden, ill-timed activity change, whether in training or during recovery from injury, can result in an undesired breakdown response that exceeds the tissue's ability to repair itself. Transitionally induced injuries can usually be avoided by proper coaching and training supervision.

Aging and genetic factors can influence an athlete's capacity to adapt to transitions in load or use. In aging, there is a decrease in basal functional capacity and a reduced ability to adapt and recover from environmental stress. For example, given equal resting pulse rates, the maximal increase with exercise becomes smaller with age, and the time required for return to normal heart rate is extended. Aging collagen undergoes a process of *maturational stabilization*, in which the reducible cross-linkages gradually become more molecularly bound. This results in a less compliant, less tension-resistant tissue. The loss of water content that accompanies aging brings a loss of resilience and tolerance to deformation. In general, after injury the young heal faster.

Genetic predisposition to injury has received little attention, but familial patterns have been documented in such conditions as the occurrence of rotator cuff complaints, lumbar disc degeneration, and Achilles tendon ruptures. The term **mesenchymal syndrome** describes a group at risk for connective tissue breakdown in the face of relatively benign load or use. Such athletes may be plagued by multiple complaints, including cervical or lumbar disc degeneration, rotator cuff tendinitis, lateral or medial elbow tendinitis, carpal tunnel syndrome, patellar tendinitis, Achilles tendinitis, and plantar fasciitis. In this group, the association of several of these diagnoses in one individual is striking and cannot be explained. Although the sites of injury are the same as would be seen in other populations of injured athletes, this subgroup has an inflammatory or degenerative reaction that is more severe than expected. Because of increased susceptibility, the affected athlete must be counseled to train properly, avoid abusive techniques, and be aware of transitional risks.

Other Tissues Involved in Sports Injury

Synovium

The synovial tissue that lines joints, bursae, tendons, and ligaments is complex, highly permeable, and well supplied by blood vessels. The synovium is not a continuous barrier; instead, it admits to the joint a filtrate of serum. This serum, or **synovial fluid**, lacks fibrinogen, meaning it does not clot. Synovial fluid is a source of lubrication and nutrients for joint chondrocytes and has a high concentration of hyaluronic acid. It also contains lymphocytes and other cells that react strongly to injury, which means that synovium is capable of an explosive inflammatory response. The quantities of synovial fluid produced in response to trauma contain a high concentration of lysosomal enzymes. These enzymes degrade hyaluronic acid and decrease the protective viscosity of the synovial fluid.

Nerves

Peripheral nerves are groupings of nerve fibers, called *axons*. Afferent axons carry nerve impulses to the spinal column; efferent axons carry impulses from the spinal column distally, to the outer parts of the body. The axons are arranged in bundles, called **fascicles**, that are covered by a tough outer layer, called the *perineurium*. Connective tissue septa and special cells called *Schwann cells* surround the axons. In case of injury, these cells provide a source of fibroblastic activity and mediator release to trigger an inflammatory reaction. A well-developed network of lymphatic and blood vessels provides nutrition and takes part in the inflammatory response to trauma.

TISSUE RESPONSE TO PHYSICAL INJURY

Definition of Sports Injury

From the athlete's point of view, an athletic injury is any painful problem that prevents or hampers usual sports performance. To the sports medicine professional, this imprecise definition is especially prone to inaccuracy in soft tissue diagnosis. Epidemiologic research uses such variables as duration of disability, need for medical attention, and degree of structural tissue damage to define injury. Tissue damage is further defined as functional and structural defects resulting from traumatically induced biochemical, ultrastructural, microscopic, and macroscopic changes.

Injuries are classified as acute or chronic. **Acute injury** is characterized by a rapid onset, macrotraumatic event, with a clearly identifiable initiating cause or moment of onset. Such injuries are typified by a sudden crisis, followed by a fairly predictable, though often lengthy, resolution to healing. Lateral collateral ligament sprain of the ankle and fracture of the distal radius are examples of acute injuries.

Chronic injury is characterized by a slow, insidious onset, implying a gradual development of structural damage that leads to a threshold episode, most often heralded by pain and/or signs of inflammation. Chronic injury lasts months or even years and is characterized by persistence of the symptoms. Tendinitis, bursitis, and fasciitis are typical chronic complaints. The period between acute and chronic injury is termed the **subacute stage**, occurring approximately 4 to 6 weeks after the initial trauma.

The Inflammation–Repair Process

Sports-induced inflammation (L. *inflammatio; inflammari*—to set on fire) is a localized tissue response initiated by the injury or destruction of vascularized tissues exposed to excessive mechanical load. It is a time-dependent, evolving process, characterized by vascular, chemical, and cellular events and leading to tissue repair, regeneration, or scar formation. Sports-induced inflammation can lead to spontaneous resolution, fibroproductive healing, regeneration, or chronic inflammatory response.

Historically, the four signs of inflammation were heat (*calor*), redness (*rubor*), swelling (*tumor*), and pain (*dolor*). To these was added a fifth sign: loss of function (*functio laesa*). Pain, which as tenderness is a local sign, is also a symptom, which limits its use in quantifying the extent of inflammation. It is also difficult, based on pain alone, to determine the site of a structural injury in a multistructured area, such as the shoulder, low back, or knee. Yet, modern-day clinicians still tend to refer to any painful site as inflamed. This generalization is probably incorrect, because there are relatively painless inflammations (for example, the subtle effusion that may be associated with early joint trauma) and there are also painful noninflammations (for example, some forms of tendonopathy and myofascial trigger points). Growing evidence suggests that in addition to true inflammatory responses, characterized by initial vascular disruption, there are also other injury responses caused by alterations in cell matrix. These various tissue responses may represent different stages in the overall spectrum of response to a given athletic injury (Fig. 8.7).

If sufficient damage has occurred, inflammation is a required step in the activation of wound repair. Tissue cell necrosis, result-

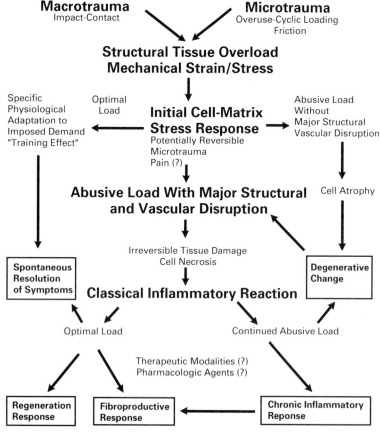

FIGURE 8.7. Pathways in tissue response to sports trauma. (From Leadbetter, W. B., Buckwalter, J. A., Gordon, S. L. *Sports Induced Inflammation: Clinical and Basic Science Concepts.* Park Ridge, Ill.: American Academy of Orthopaedic Surgeons, 1990.)

ing from damage and hypoxia at the injury site, initiates the inflammatory process. This nonspecific response to physical trauma resembles the body's response to infection, chemical injury, or thermal injury. In inflammation, the body attempts to limit the extent of injury, to remove devitalized tissue from the wound, and to initiate repairs. Inflammation is not necessarily dose-related. Severe local inflammation can result from a relatively minor injury. In sports, the sudden swelling of a bursa or tendon is a prime example of disproportionate inflammatory reactions. This inability to finely regulate the inflammatory process may further tissue damage. In sports trauma, a heightened reaction of this sort can further damage local tissue.

Regeneration and repair are necessary for the survival of all living organisms. In **regeneration**, new matrices and cells that are identical in structure and function to those they replace are formed. In phylogenetically advanced organisms, the regenerative process becomes increasingly complex. Amphibians are the most advanced animals able to regenerate a lost extremity. For the human who has suffered sports trauma, only limited regeneration of epithelium, endothelium, and components of connective tissue is possible. In **repair**, damaged or lost cells and matrices are replaced by new cells and matrices that are not necessarily identical in structure and function to normal tissue. Repair is often accomplished by fibrous scar, the common patching material for wound healing. Inflammation and repair responses vary considerably in different sports-injured tissues.

There are three phases in the normal **inflammation–repair process** of sports-induced soft tissue or bone injury: acute vascular inflammatory response, repair–regeneration, and remodeling–maturation (Fig. 8.8).

Phase I: Acute Vascular Inflammatory Response

The first phase, the acute vascular inflammatory response to injury, is essentially similar in both soft tissue and bone. The initial reaction to trauma is fostered by a complex series of vascular, humoral, and cellular events that are controlled at all stages by chemical mediators. Many of these mediators are produced at the injury site by cells brought to the site as part of the vascular response to the injury. Also known as the *reaction phase*, the first phase is characterized by inflammatory cell mobilization, aided by an acute vascular response that begins within moments of injury and lasts for a few minutes to several days.

Alterations in the anatomy and function of microvasculature are among the earliest responses to injury. An acute vasoconstriction lasts a few minutes and is followed by vasodilatation, primarily of precapillary arterioles that bring increased blood flow to the injured area, causing swelling. Blood from the disrupted vessels collects locally and, with cellular debris and early necrotic tissue, forms a **hematoma**. The extent of the initial hematoma and the area of devitalized tissue define the **zone of primary injury**. A **humoral response** is nearly coincident with neurovascular events and centers on

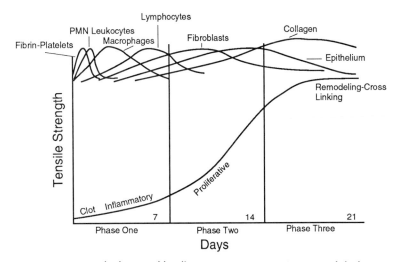

FIGURE 8.8.   Ideal wound-healing response curve. In sports injuries, reinjury on return to play can alter the curve. Tensile strength of injured ligaments may reach only 50 to 70 percent of normal after one year.   (Adapted from Gamble, J. G. *The Musculoskeletal System—Physiological Basics.* New York: Raven Press, 1988, p. 173.)

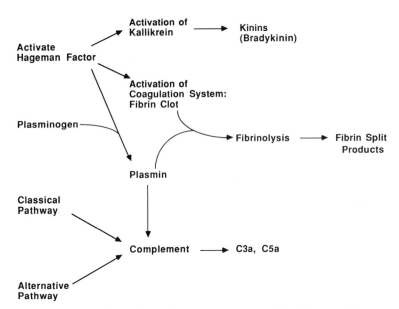

FIGURE 8.9. Plasma-derived mediators, activated by injury, initiate enzymatic production of the pain stimulator bradykinin. Two pathways produce complement-derived C3a and C5a, which modulate the immune function. (From Leadbetter, W. B., Buckwalter, J. A., Gordon, S. L. *Sports-Induced Inflammation: Clinical and Basic Science Concepts.* Park Ridge, Ill.: American Academy of Orthopaedic Surgeons, 1990.)

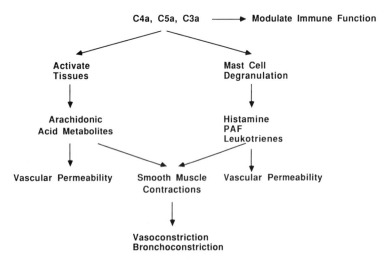

FIGURE 8.10. Arachidonic acid production and complement activation of mast cell degranulation cause both edema and vasoconstriction. This sequence is seen in allergic reactions as well as in muscle strains. (From Leadbetter, W. B., Buckwalter, J. A., Gordon, S. L. *Sports-Induced Inflammation: Clinical and Basic Science Concepts.* Park Ridge, Ill.: American Academy of Orthopaedic Surgeons, 1990.)

the activation of Hageman factor (clotting factor XII) in the plasma, resulting in four subsystems of mediator production that have the following functions:

1. The coagulation systems reduce blood loss by local clot formation, a process activated in part by collagen exposed in the walls of damaged blood vessels.
2. Fibrinolysis discourages widespread blood clotting by fibrin degradation.
3. Kallikrein produces the strong vasodilator bradykinin which increases capillary permeability and edema.
4. Complement activation produces anaphylatoxin, which activates chemotaxis —the attraction of inflammatory cells and the activation of phagocytosis and wound débridement (Fig. 8.9).

Stimulated by the complement system, mast cells and basophils release histamine. Platelets, in addition to providing clot formation, are the primary source of serotonin. Histamine and serotonin work to increase vascular permeability (Figs. 8.10 and 8.11).

Cellular response is associated with vascular changes that occur at the postcapillary venule. The lining of the venules develops gaps in response to the vasoactive mediators, such as complement-derived C5a, histamines, serotonin, bradykinin, leukotrienes, and prostaglandins, released from both plasma and cellular sources (Fig. 8.12). Common initiating mechanisms for mediator release range from local ischemia produced by extrinsic pressure (such as seen in shoulder impingement syndromes) to major traumatic disruption of blood vessels and tissue structure (such as seen in severe tendon or muscle strains). These changes in vascular permeability cause a flow of fluids into the interstitial tissues, referred to as **edema**.

At the same time, leukocytes (white blood cells), which have been drawn to the walls of blood vessels near the injury site by changes in electrostatic charge, immigrate through the vascular walls and migrate unidirectionally (chemotaxis) toward increasing concentrations of chemotactic media-

Ag + IgE ⟶ Mast Cell/Basophil ⟶ Histamine, PAF, LTC_4, D_4, E_4

Thrombin, Collagen ⟶ Platelet ⟶ Histamine, Serotonin

Phagocytic Chemotactic ⟶ Leukocytes ⟶ PAF, Leukotrienes,
Stimulus   Prostaglandins

FIGURE 8.11. Cell-derived vasoactive mediators. Leukotrienes (LTC4, D4, E4) are derived from leukocytes and are also produced by mast cells. Together with platelet-activating factor (PAF), histamine, serotonin, and prostaglandins, they produce chemotactic, vascular, and smooth muscle effects. Similar mediator release occurs in allergic reactions with the stimulus of antigen (Ag) and immunoglobulin E (IgE). (From Leadbetter, W. B., Buckwalter, J. A., Gordon, S. L. *Sports-Induced Inflammation: Clinical and Basic Science Concepts.* Park Ridge, Ill.: American Academy of Orthopaedic Surgeons, 1990.)

tors at the site of injury (Fig. 8.13). Leukocytes produce platelet-activating factor, prostaglandins, and leukotrienes, which further increase vascular permeability. Leukocytes and phagocytic macrophages act at the injury site to remove damaged cell material. Granules within the leukocytes release hydrolytic enzymes, which hydrolyze cell membrane phospholipids, producing arachidonic acid. The resulting *arachidonic acid cascade* (Fig. 8.14) is an enzymatically driven sequence, leading to the production of prostaglandins, thromboxanes, leukotrienes, eicosanoids, and slowly reacting substance of anaphylaxis (SRS-A). Collectively, these polypeptide proteins activate further inflammatory cellular behavior. For this reason, they are the targets of modern-day, anti-inflammatory drug therapy. The intense chemical activity and exudation of this phase produce the initial clinical signs of inflammation, edema, and hypoxia, and create the **zone of secondary injury** (Fig. 8.15).

Phase II: Repair–Regeneration

Repair–regeneration of soft tissue. Beginning at 48 hours and lasting up to 6 to 8 weeks, a second wave of cells composed of fibroblasts begins the process of wound repair and collagen synthesis. At the same time, a process of vascular proliferation and ingrowth, *angiogenesis*, occurs; tiny blood

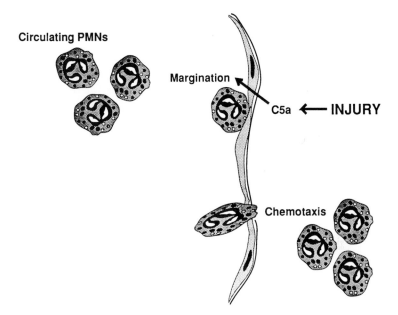

FIGURE 8.12. Polymorphonuclear cells (PMNs) respond to injury first by adhering to the vascular walls (margination). They then move to the injury site through gaps in the endothelial cell lining, a process called diapedesis. (From Leadbetter, W. B., Buckwalter, J. A., Gordon, S. L. *Sports-Induced Inflammation: Clinical and Basic Science Concepts.* Park Ridge, Ill.: American Academy of Orthopaedic Surgeons, 1990.)

vessels grow and anastomose with each other to form a new capillary bed. Granulation tissue is the visible evidence of this process. Various growth factors that promote this activity, including macrophage, fibroblast, nerve, and platelet-derived growth factors, have been identified. Hypoxia (reduced oxygen supply) also stimulates vascular ingrowth and collagen synthesis.

Chemoattractant	Target	Recruit
C_{5A}, platelet factor 4 Elastin peptides F-Met peptides	Inflammatory cells Neutrophils Monocytes	Phagocytes
PDGF, fibronectin Lymphokines, monokines Complement peptides	Connective tissue cells Fibroblast Smooth muscle cells	Matrix producing cells
Fibronectin, laminin Monokines	Endothelial cells	Vascular system

FIGURE 8.13. **Chemoattractants in wound repair.** (From Simon, S. R., Riggins, R. S., Wirth, C. R., Fox, M. L. *Orthopaedic Science: A Resource and Self-Study Guide for the Practitioner, Syllabus.* Park Ridge, Ill.: American Academy of Orthopaedic Surgeons, 1986.)

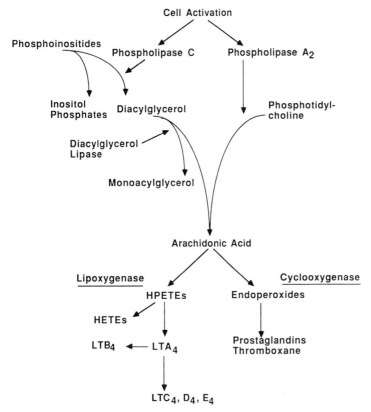

FIGURE 8.14. Generation of arachidonic acid metabolites. Cell membrane phospholipids and fatty acids are broken down into arachidonic acid, which is further broken down into HETEs (hydroxyeicosatetranoic acids), HPETEs (hydroperoxyeicosatetranoic acid compounds), and leukotrienes (LTB4, LTA4, LTC4, D4, and E4). (From Leadbetter, W. B., Buckwalter, J. A., Gordon, S. L. *Sports-Induced Inflammation: Clinical and Basic Science Concepts.* Park Ridge, Ill.: American Academy of Orthopaedic Surgeons, 1990.)

The new collagen, which begins to appear in wounds about 4 days after injury, is predominantly Type III. This hastily produced collagen is described as immature. At first it is soluble because it lacks cross-links between tropocollagen molecules, which makes it more susceptible to enzymatic degradation. As the wound matures and cross-linking becomes established, collagen degradation decreases and the wound's tensile strength increases. During this phase, myofibroblast cells cause the wound to contract, or shrink, which accounts for some of the decrease in ligament laxity and muscular flexibility after injury.

Repair–regeneration of bone. Special cells, called *osteoclasts*, perform functions analogous to those carried out in soft tissue by macrophages and leukocytes and débride fractured bone surfaces, removing damaged bone. Mesenchymal cells from periosteal blood vessels and bone periosteum proliferate and differentiate into collagen-forming and cartilage-forming cells. Capillaries grow among these cells, forming a fibrovascular tissue known as *callus* that bridges the gap between bone ends. This process is known as **enchondral bone healing.** The new bone so produced is relatively weak and is converted to lamellar or mature bone during later remodeling. Another kind of bone repair, **direct bone healing**, occurs when the broken bone ends are immobilized and are in contact, which allows direct deposit of woven bone without the intermediate step of callus formation. Fractures not fixed by metal plates, screen, or rods usually heal by the enchondral process. Arbitrarily, the stage at which a fracture has healed sufficiently to allow activity approaching normal function marks the end of this phase in hard tissue.

Phase III: Remodeling-Maturation

The remodeling–maturation phase is characterized by a trend toward decreased cellularity and an accompanying decrease in synthetic activity; increased organization of extracellular matrix; and a more normal biochemical profile. There is a shift from Type III collagen to Type I collagen, with collagen turnover approaching normal levels. A summary of the cellular and chemical events leading up to Phase III is presented in Figure 8.16.

Maturation, the final stage of remodeling, is sometimes considered a separate, fourth phase of the injury–repair cycle. Such a distinction seems arbitrary. Maturation is quite variable in duration and end point. The factors that influence maturation are animal model and tissue specific.

In bone remodeling, maturation implies the restoration of the original cortex. New bone is organized along lines of stress and mechanical forces; it is a process that may continue for many years after fracture.

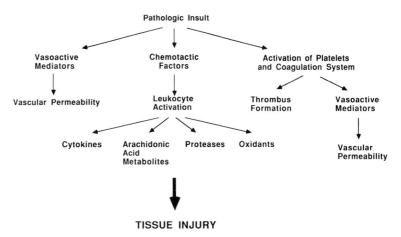

FIGURE 8.15. Factors contributing to the zone of secondary injury after an inflammatory response. (From Leadbetter, W. B., Buckwalter, J. A., Gordon, S. L. *Sports-Induced Inflammation: Clinical and Basic Science Concepts.* Park Ridge, Ill.: American Academy of Orthopaedic Surgeons, 1990.)

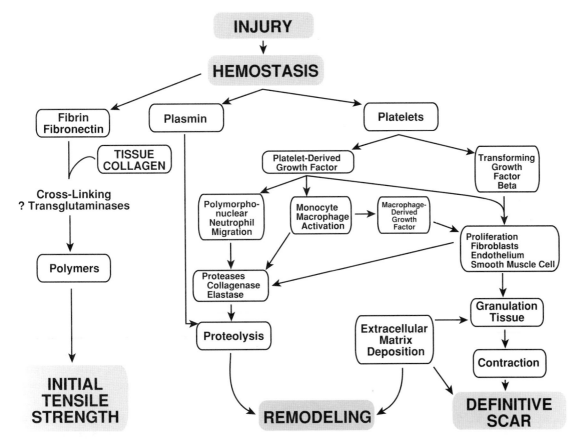

FIGURE 8.16. Summary of events in injury-healing response. Interactions among components of hemostasis, growth factors, platelet-derived growth factor (PDGF), transforming growth factor beta (TGFB), macrophase-derived growth factor (MDGF), extracellular matrix (ECM), and cells during the repair reaction. The actual interactions taking place in an individual injury determine the outcome of healing. (From Leadbetter, W. B., Buckwalter, J. A., Gordon, S. L. *Sports-Induced Inflammation: Clinical and Basic Science Concepts.* Park Ridge, Ill.: American Academy of Orthopaedic Surgeons, 1990.)

Remodeling–maturation of soft tissue. Starting about 3 weeks after injury, and continuing for a year or more, collagen remodeling proceeds under the influence of activity-induced load, as collagen fibers reorient themselves along the lines of tensile force. Electric fields may also play a part in the orientation of collagen fibers. This theory is the basis for electrobiological stimulation of healing. During Phase III, immature, Type III collagen is converted to the stronger Type I form. However, the ultimate tensile strength of the scar can be as much as 30 percent less than that of the original tissue.

Remodeling–maturation of bone. The remodeling–maturation process in bone is

also affected by mechanical load and resulting piezoelectric effects. In a long-bone fracture, bone-forming osteoblasts are directed by bioelectrical triggering to the concave, compression, electronegative aspect of the fracture, where observed bone deposition will be greatest. Bone-removing osteoclasts digest bone on the convex, tension, electropositive side of the fracture. The remodeling phase of bone healing is essentially a more rapid form of normal bone turnover, culminating in the restoration of sufficient shape and/or strength.

Alternative Injury Responses

Not all sports injuries generate an inflammation–repair reaction. In some cases of chronic injury of collagen in tendon, ligament, or fascia, infiltration of leukocytes and macrophages does not occur. Theoretically, a cell atrophy–degeneration cycle may explain these observations.

Atrophy–Degeneration Cycle

In **atrophy**, a cell's size and function decrease in response to an environmental signal. Protein synthesis decreases, along with such activities as energy production, replication, storage, and contractility. Immobilization is one cause of cell atrophy. Other causes include an inadequate oxygen supply, decreased nutrition, a drop in endocrine hormones, chronic inflammation, and aging (Fig. 8.17).

In **degeneration**, a tissue changes from a higher to a lower or less functionally active form. Degeneration weakens structures, making them more vulnerable to sudden dynamic overload or cyclic overloading, which can lead to fatigue and failure. Traumatic disruption can cause vascular injury and initiate a renewed inflammation–repair process. Although rest can allow an atrophied cell to recover, a lack of physical stimulation can prevent a sufficient healing response. Under such circumstances, the athlete, upon returning to sports activity, would not have substantially changed or

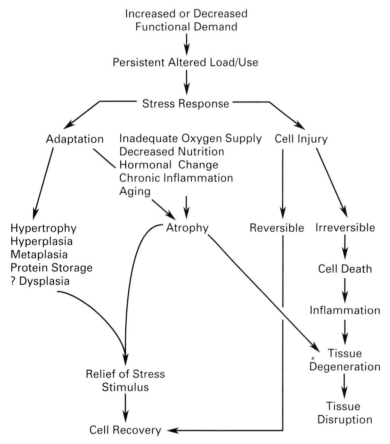

FIGURE 8.17. Cell stress responses to altered load or use. (From Rubin, E., and Farber, J. L. *Pathology.* Philadelphia: Lippincott Co., 1988.)

improved tissue integrity. For this reason, protected activity or therapeutic exercise is usually a better treatment than complete rest.

Chronic Inflammatory Response

After an acute injury, the replacement of leukocytes by macrophages, plasma cells, and lymphocytes in a highly vascularized and innervated loose connective tissue milieu defines a chronic inflammatory condition. Such tissue is seen in chronic sports injuries. Lateral epicondylar injury of the elbow, commonly known as tennis elbow, is an example. However, not all chronic sports injury complaints involve a chronic inflammatory response. The mechanisms that convert acute inflammation to a chronic inflammatory process are not understood, but overuse or overload, combined with possible cumulative microtrauma, is a contributing factor. Chronic inflammatory response can accompany atrophy and degeneration at the site of injury.

Inflammation–Repair Modifiers

Modifiers of sports-induced inflammation may be employed to decrease pain, allowing rehabilitation to begin. Modifiers are also used to avoid the risk of atrophy, neurological discoordination, and altered muscle function. As a part of rehabilitative therapy, a modifier can minimize such effects of immobilization as adhesions, joint stiffness, and cartilage degeneration. Modifiers decrease inflammation in freshly healed tissues during retraining and reconditioning and control the symptoms of inflammation in overuse injuries, especially chronic symptoms related to earlier injuries. Modifiers can also help limit the zone of soft tissue necrosis following acute trauma and limit the dysfunctional behavior caused by pain.

Drug Modifiers

Nonsteroidal, anti-inflammatory drugs (NSAIDs) are commonly given to athletes after an injury or surgery, but the effectiveness of NSAIDs in treating chronic overuse injury has been questioned. NSAIDs are analgesics and antipyretics—that is, they relieve pain and reduce fever. NSAIDs block the breakdown of arachidonic acid to prostaglandin. The toxicity of NSAIDs is related to their capacity to inhibit prostaglandins (Fig. 8.18), and the risks involved must be carefully weighed in view of their recently reported toxicity to the liver and kidneys. Fortunately, NSAIDs have not been shown to slow the normal healing process. At present, oral anti-inflammatory agents are used primarily to relieve pain. Acetaminophen, a commonly prescribed neutral compound, does not concentrate in inflammatory sites or in inflammatory cells and works solely as a pain reliever.

Steroids also affect the arachidonic acid cascade sequence, and their use (both orally and by injection) in sports trauma is even more controversial. To date, research on the effects of steroids has two limitations. First, because there is no good overuse animal model, normal tendons have been used or inflammation has been artificially induced. Second, most animal models do not react to these substances in the same way that humans react. Because there is controversy regarding the suppression of collagen synthesis during repair phases of the inflammation–repair response, current clinical practice avoids injecting steroid preparations directly into tendons. Local injection into a synovial cavity, bursa, or tendon synovial sheath is currently the most accepted application of steroid use in sports trauma.

Some researchers have advised injecting corticosteroids after muscular strain or other acute macrotrauma in order to reduce the acute inflammatory zone of secondary injury, but the effectiveness of this treatment has not been substantiated by controlled study. If used, steroid injection should be limited to no more than two to three treatments to any one anatomic area, and treatments should be spaced over several weeks. A mandatory rest period of 2 to 4

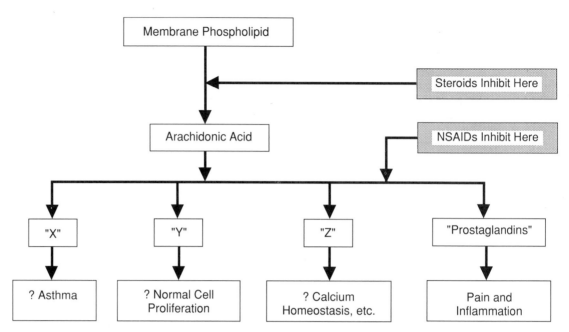

FIGURE 8.18. Scheme for arachidonic acid metabolism showing how the sites of action of corticosteroids differ from those of nonsteroidal anti-inflammatory drugs. Because corticosteroids suppress other pathways in addition to pain and inflammation, their potential side effects are **greater.** (From Goodwin, J. S. "Mechanism of Action of Corticosteroids." In *Mediguide to Inflammatory Diseases.* New York: Lawrence Delacorte Publishers, 1987, vol. 6:1.)

weeks is advised to avoid potential suppression of the healing-repair process. The relief of pain is not a measure of recovery of structural integrity. The best use for anti-inflammatory medication is to make it easier for the athlete to cooperate with more effective therapy, such as rehabilitative and reconditioning exercises.

Modalities

The physical modalities include cryotherapy (cold), thermotherapy (heat), ultrasound (high-frequency sound waves), and galvanic stimulation (electric current). Animal modeling is essentially impossible for chronic overuse injuries, and with only limited laboratory testing, there has been much debate about the effectiveness of these physical techniques and when and how they should be used. Clinical experience suggests that their use during the first phase of the inflammatory process can reduce pain, ede-

ma, and muscle spasm, allowing early mobilization of the injured part and shortening the period of disability.

Cryotherapy decreases some of the effects of inflammation, particularly edema. In the acute animal injury model, researchers have seen faster resolution of hematoma, increased vascular ingrowth at the site of injury, quicker regeneration of injured tissue, and more rapid recovery of tensile strength. Paradoxically, cold has actually been found to aggravate prostaglandin mediated inflammation. Compression adds measurably to the penetration of cooling and the efficacy of cryotherapy.

Thermotherapy reduces muscle spasm and stiffness, and eases motion at joints and between fascial planes. The molecular basis remains poorly understood; what is known is that increased temperature reduces resistance to flow of viscous hyaluronate solutions and influences collagen's physical state. Application of heat also heightens synovial cell metabolism and the formation of hyaluronate in synovial fluid.

Ultrasound has long been used to treat inflammatory conditions, but its benefits and the mechanisms involved have not been verified by research. Higher intensities, because they create heat, have limited use. Lower intensities do not create heat, and are gaining wider use in the promotion of wound healing. The lower-intensity sound waves increase the flow of ions and metabolites over cellular membranes and intracellular structures and also alter membrane permeability—changes that are believed to increase cell nutrition. Ultrasound is claimed to reduce edema and ease the pain of muscle spasms. By enhancing the degranulation of mast cells by increasing the transport of calcium ions, ultrasound releases chemotactic agents that draw cellular components to the site of inflammation. These components act to expedite repair, improve the attraction of macrophages, increase collagen production, promote wound contraction, and enhance vascular ingrowth.

High-voltage, pulsatile **galvanic stimulation** provides an external electrical stimulation of more than 100 volts with a pulsatile wave form that is between 5 and 100 microseconds in duration. Electrical chemical effects are claimed to occur at both cellular and tissue levels. In the absence of control studies, the effect of galvanic treatment on inflammation is conjectural, but clinical observation suggests that it may modulate pain, facilitate resolution of edema, and enhance local circulation.

Therapeutic Exercise

Rehabilitative therapeutic exercise has the strongest rationale for use in the treatment of sports-induced inflammation and injury. Cellular and biomechanical responses to exercise documented in tendon, ligament, and muscle include changes in collagen turnover rate; changes in collagen cross-linking at the intramolecular and intermolecular level; alteration in tissue water and electrolyte content; and changes in the ar-

rangement, number, and thickness of collagen fibrils. Under the effects of load, collagen fibers may transmit physical signals, inducing changes in cellular metabolism and synthesis of proteoglycans and matrix. Both tension and pressure have been shown to modify cell synthesis in tendon and articular cartilage, and these changes can hasten the return of structural integrity.

TISSUE-SPECIFIC INJURY RESPONSE PATTERNS

Muscle Injury

Muscle injuries can be caused by strain or by a direct blow. Although muscle cells are permanent cells and have no proliferative capacity, reserve cells that lie in the basement membrane of the muscle fiber are able to proliferate and differentiate, forming new skeletal muscle. Thus, the regeneration of muscle fibers and even complete muscle tissue is possible. When muscle tissue is completely disrupted, scar tissue forms. Scar tissue prevents the muscle from regenerating and creates adhesions that restrict function. Healed muscle can lose up to 50 percent of its strength.

Muscle strain can be caused by excessive stretching or by violent contracture. There are three types of response to injury: delayed onset muscle soreness, acute muscle soreness, and injury-related soreness.

Delayed onset muscle soreness (DOMS) appears 12 to 48 hours after an exercise session and is characterized by tenderness on palpation, by increased muscle stiffness, and by a reduction in range of motion. DOMS is probably not inflammatory. Research has found that few macrophage cells are present at such injury sites, and classic inflammatory changes are not predominant. In the absence of inflammation, the pain is probably caused by noxious neuropeptide proteins, such as substance P, or by reduced blood flow and lack of oxygen in the injured area.

Acute muscle soreness is also caused by a reduction in blood flow under conditions of

TABLE 8.2. Terminology of Tendon Injury Classification

New	Old	Definition	Histological Findings	Clinical Signs and Symptoms
Paratenonitis	Tenosynovitis Tenovaginitis Peritendinitis	An inflammation of only the paratenon, either lined by synovium or not	Inflammatory cells in paratenon or peritendinous areolar tissue.	Cardinal inflammatory signs: swelling, pain, crepitus, local tenderness, warmth, dysfunction.
Paratenonitis with tendinosis	Tendinitis	Paratenon inflammation associated with intra-tendinosis degeneration	Same as I, with loss of tendon collagen fiber disorientation, scattered vascular ingrowth but no prominent intra-tendinous inflammation.	Same as I, with often palpable tendon nodule, swelling and inflammatory signs.
Tendinosis	Tendinitis	Intratendinous degeneration due to atrophy (aging, microtrauma, vascular compromise, etc.)	Noninflammatory intratendinous collagen degeneration with fiber disorientation, hypocellularity, scattered vascular ingrowth, occasional local necrosis or calcification.	Often palpable tendon nodule that is *asymptomatic*. Swelling of tendon sheath is absent.

Tendinitis	Tendon strain or tear	Symptomatic degeneration of the tendon with vascular disruption and inflammatory repair response	Three recognized subgroups: each display variable histology from purely inflammation with acute hemorrhage and tear to inflammation superimposed upon pre-existing degeneration, calcification and tendinosis changes in chronic conditions.
			1. Acute
			2. Subacute
			3. Chronic
			  a. Interstitial microinjury
			  b. Central tendon necrosis
			  c. Frank partial rupture
			  d. Acute complete rupture
				Symptoms are inflammatory and proportional to vascular disruption, hematoma or atrophy-related cell necrosis. Symptom duration defines each subgroup:
				
				Less than 2 weeks
				4-6 weeks
				Over 6 weeks.

isometric contracture. This raises the levels of lactic acid and potassium and stimulates the nerve nociceptors, which receive and pass on the pain signal. Rapid onset of pain sensation within a minute of contracture, with relief of the pain within 2 or 3 minutes after relaxation and restored circulation, is characteristic. The burning sensation associated with weight lifting is an example of acute muscle soreness.

Injury-related muscle soreness results from a discoordination of antagonist and agonist functions about a joint during rapid movement. Tendon and muscular strains can cause significant muscle fiber disruption, producing hemorrhage and initiating a true inflammatory response.

Myositis ossificans, a bony deposit within the muscle, is associated with severe or repeated injury-related blood clots within the muscle. Symptoms include prominent local swelling, tenderness, and loss of adjacent joint motion. Inflammation associated with trauma can set off a complex series of biochemical changes that trigger bone formation within the muscle. Histologically, an early inflammatory cell reaction leads to the active proliferation of various cells,

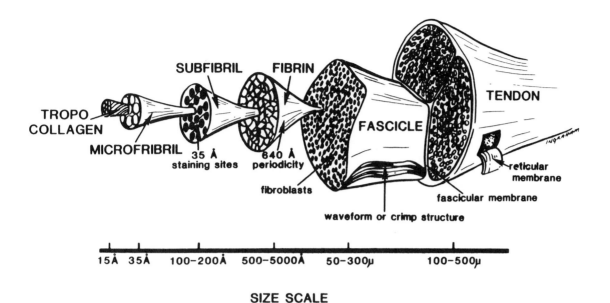

FIGURE 8.19. Microanatomy of muscle tendon. Structural failure starts at the tropocollagen level. (From Simon, S. R., Riggins, R. S., Wirth, C. R., Fox, M. L. *Orthopaedic Science: A Resource and Self-Study Guide for the Practitioner, Syllabus.* Park Ridge, Ill.: American Academy of Orthopaedic Surgeons, 1986.)

eventually creating a mass with a rim of bone surrounding a zone of dense fibrous tissue. These bony deposits occur in 13 to 20 percent of quadriceps contusions.

Myofascial pain syndrome is a painful musculoskeletal response that can follow muscle trauma. Myofascial trigger points are small cordlike or nodular sites that are associated with local muscle spasms and are acutely painful. **Fibrositis** is a diffuse, multiple-site complaint that is not associated with muscle spasm or weakness and that most often affects women between the ages of 40 and 60. It is not caused by trauma and is associated with emotional disturbances. One of its symptoms is generalized soreness. Both myofascial pain syndrome and fibrositis may be of neurogenic origin at the central or spinal level. Neither condition is inflammatory.

Tendon, Tendon Insertion, and Fascia Injury

Because of their prevalence in sports, injuries to tendons and tendon insertions have received considerable attention. There are many types of tendon and fascia injuries. **Enthesopathy** is an injury in which tendon fibers are torn directly off their insertion. The **tendinosis lesion** is an asymptomatic tendon degeneration caused either by aging or by cumulative microtrauma without inflammation. **Peritendinitis** involves tenosynovitis of the tendon sheath (Table 8.2) and is marked by pain, swelling, and, occasionally, local crepitus.

In **tendinitis**, there is injury to the tendon proper and, if partial tearing is involved, there will be vascular injury and intratendinous inflammation. Normal tendon has a tensile strength that measures 45 to 98 N/mm, but at 8 to 10 percent strain, tendon begins to fail (Figs. 8.19 and 8.20). The stage at which this failure causes pain and the mechanisms involved in healing of this type of injury are matters of conjecture. It is not clear whether inflammation leads to degeneration, or if inflammation is the result of mechanical failure. Present evidence from biopsy suggests that inflammation follows tendon tears.

Fascial injuries and tendon injuries are similar, in that inflammation is secondary to tears. In some sites, including the plantar fascia, chronic repetitive microtears can

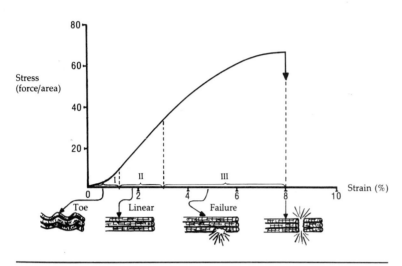

FIGURE 8.20. Stress-strain curve for tendon failure caused by cross-link fractures, the breaking of molecular bonds between tropocollagen molecules. (From Curwin, S., and Stanish, W. D. *Tendinitis: Its Etiology and Treatment.* Lexington, Mass.: Collamore Press, 1984.)

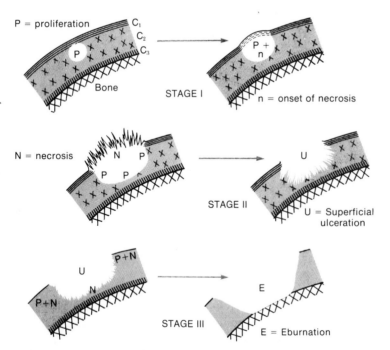

FIGURE 8.21. Stages of articular cartilage degeneration in response to load. (From Ficat, R. P., and Hungerford, D. S. *Disorders of the Patellofemoral Joint.* Baltimore, Md.: The Williams & Wilkins Co., 1977.)

cause formation of periosteal new bone, or **spurs**.

In injury to both tendon attachment and fascia, granulation tissue that is characterized by capillary ingrowth, scattered nerve endings, and occasional macrophages can form. Damaged tendon or fascia often has a dull look. Under a microscope, a loss of the normal wavy, crimped collagen fiber array and normal cellularity is noted—a change termed **mucoid degeneration**. Inflammation is not usually present unless tearing has occurred.

Cartilage Injury

Because of the lack of blood vessels, lymphatics, and nerves, partial thickness cartilage injuries do not repair. In cartilage lesions, an inflammatory response is generated only if the subchondral bone is also injured, because this type of injury allows inflammatory cells to enter the wounded area from the marrow. Healing of full-thickness osteochondral lesions takes place by fibrocartilaginous replacement. When normal cartilage is exposed to excessive pressure or shear, isolated chondrocyte necrosis can occur. Resultant softening of the articular surface is called **chondromalacia**. When chondrocytes in the intermediate zones of the articular surface are subjected to load, a blistering of the surface occurs, followed by cellular necrosis and fatigue rupture of the fiber network of the matrix. This leads to further degeneration, loss of proteoglycan content, and continued softening. Eventual total loss of the articular covering exposes the underlying subchondral bone. This process is known as **eburnation** (Fig. 8.21). The inflammatory symptoms associated with cartilage injury may be caused by shedding of enzymatically produced matrix breakdown products and secondary stimulation of the synovium.

Ligament Injury

Healing of sprained ligament tissue is analogous to healing in other vascularized tissues. Disruption of a ligament is followed by hematoma and soft tissue inflammatory repair. Full recovery may take more than a year, and ultimately tensile strength can be reduced by 30 to 50 percent. Most newly synthesized collagen in the ligament scar is Type III, which reverts over time to Type I. Immobilization after injury causes cell atrophy, increases the risk of rupture under load, and decreases the rate of healing. Controlled exposure to load can speed ligament healing. Although ligament is similar to tendon in that both tissues have few reparative cells and a high ratio of matrix to cell content, no ligament lesion analogous to the tendinosis lesion has been documented. Recent evidence suggests that ligaments differ from tendons at the cellular level and that individual ligaments may differ from each other in the same way. Cell structure, rates of maturation, and metabolic activity may differ from ligament to ligament. Tendons and ligaments share the structural property of **crimp**, a regular, wavy undulation of cells and matrix that is seen under a microscope. This crimp acts as a buffer or shock absorber that allows the ligament to avoid damage during elongation. Under load, the crimp pattern slowly straightens out (Fig. 8.22). Ligaments also seem to soften at higher temperatures, which may explain why heat is of benefit in mobilizing joints.

Synovial Injury

Synovial tissue is found in bursa, common tendon sheath linings, and joints. Synovial Type A macrophagelike cells make up 20 to 30 percent of the synovial lining. These cells are active in phagocytosis and the degradation of particulate matter from the cavities they surround, and they demonstrate pronounced immunologic and inflammatory potential. Bursitis and synovitis are accurate descriptions of histopathology. Vascular endothelial cells in the synovium maintain nutrition and also participate in inflammatory reactions to trauma. Afferent neurons in the synovium and joint capsule contain Substance P, a neuropeptide that is a primary source of

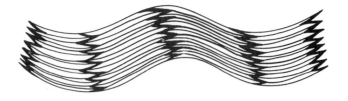

FIGURE 8.22. Crimp pattern of relaxed collagen typical of ligament and tendon tissues. Collagen fibers straighten completely at about 4 percent elongation. Beyond this limit, tropocollagen molecular stress occurs. (From Curwin, S., and Stanish, W. D. *Tendinitis: Its Etiology and Treatment.* Lexington, Mass.: Collamore Press, 1984.)

pain after injury. Both connective tissue fibroblasts and macrophages would appear to assume the structure and function of synovial lining cells under conditions as yet to be precisely defined. A special synovial cell has been identified to interdigitate with immune T-lymphocytes, a cell known to mediate chronic inflammatory processes. The synovial membrane contains freely available, unsaturated phospholipids—a ready source of prostaglandin production through the arachidonic acid cascade. Synovial lining cells have been noted to bind antigen antibody complex, present antigen to T-lymphocytes, produce cytokines that promote the activation and proliferation of T-lymphocytes, and respond to signals from mononuclear cells.

Explosive bursal swellings, such as are seen in the olecranon bursa of the dart thrower or the prepatellar bursa of the wrestler, and the marked peritendinitis reactions brought on by overuse seem to be triggered by conditions of use as well as friction. Trauma to a bursa or joint, with vascular injury and bleeding, rapidly triggers this inflammatory process. Lysosomal enzymes are released into the bursal or joint space, and damage to exposed articular surfaces and tendons is often evidenced by loss of matrix and proteoglycans. Medication to reduce inflammation is used to treat inflammatory conditions of synovium through direct suppression of the arachidonic acid cascade.

Frozen shoulder describes the restricted movement of the shoulder joint that occurs after acute trauma or periarticular biceps or rotator cuff injury. Hypertrophic inflammatory synovitis is associated with intra-articular and pericapsular adhesions, which are referred to as **adhesive capsulitis.** These joint contractures appear to result from recurrent traumatic insults, inflammation, and proliferative scar formation with contracture.

Bone Injury

The acute response to injury of bone has been described. A subtle stress reaction of bone is that caused by chronic overuse. In applying the training principle of specific adaptation to imposed demand, Wolff stated the often quoted law, "Every change in the form and function of a bone or in its function alone is followed by a certain definite change in its external conformation." Abrupt shifts in load or chronic cyclic accumulations of load can cause bone fatigue and eventual partial or complete fracture. If normal cortical bone remodeling is accelerated, resorption can occur too rapidly, weakening the bone cortex and leading to microfracture. When this occurs, the old bone must then be rebuilt anew (Fig. 8.23). During this transition, which takes time, the athlete is vulnerable to injury. The lower extremities account for 95 percent of all stress fractures in athletes, which reflects the mechanical nature of the process. Although pain is present, this process is not inflammatory. Effective treatment emphasizes a reduction in load and allows protected activity to allow the bone to react by producing a stronger and more durable structure.

Stress reactions are a symptom of abusive training or overload, often caused by mechanical vulnerabilities such as leg-length discrepancy or hyperpronation of the foot.

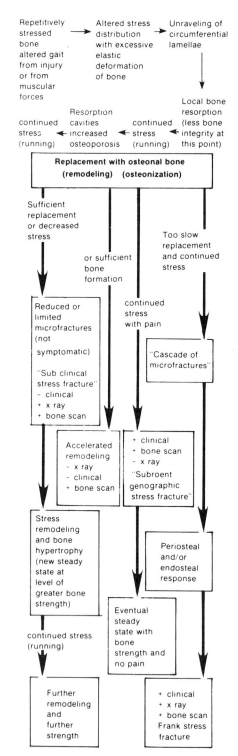

FIGURE 8.23. Theoretical flow pattern of stress reaction of bone. (From McBryde, A. M., Jr. "Stress Fractures in Runners." In *Prevention and Treatment of Running Injuries,* ed. D'Ambrosia, R., and Drez, D. Thorofare, N.J.: Slack, Inc., 1982.)

In the tibia and in the fifth metatarsal, stress reactions can persist despite proper care and can require bone grafting. Not much is known about the histology of **osteoperiostitis** because biopsy material is rarely obtained in cases of chronic overuse. The inflammation is probably caused by separation of the periosteum by the tension overload of muscle attachments, or by a direct blow, causing bleeding under the periosteum. In **shin splints**, or **posterior tibial stress syndrome**, the site of cyclic overuse injury is at the posterior tibial and soleus muscular attachments and origins on the tibia. Resistant cases treated surgically have shown chronic periosteal inflammation at these sites.

Nerve Injury

Sports-related nerve injuries are most often caused by compression or traction. External pressure equal to 20 to 30 mm Hg can compromise microcirculation, and shear stresses at the compression site cause additional microvascular injury and ischemia. The earliest sign of injury to a nerve is the accumulation of fluid in the tissue surrounding the nerve. Pressure levels of 30 to 50 mm Hg can block nerve conduction as a result of depletion of oxygen. With traction, or stretching, of human nerve tissue, gradual structural and mechanical failure begins to occur at strain levels between 11 and 17 percent, and disruption occurs at 15 to 23 percent. The tough connective tissues around them protect peripheral nerves from such trauma. Nerve roots, because they lack these covering tissues, have less elasticity and tensile strength, which helps to explain the vulnerability to stretching of the brachial plexus or cervical nerve roots.

Partial damage to nerves, affecting only the outer protective layers, or leaving those layers and affecting only the nerve tissue itself, triggers neural growth factors and initiates nerve regrowth. Total disruption of the nerve, called **neurotmesis**, can occur with a cut or violent traction, and without surgical repair, only random regrowth can occur, resulting in a **neuroma**, or nerve

tumor. Neuromas can also result from external nerve pressure, as is seen in Morton's neuroma of the digital nerves of the foot. Nerve regrowth must compete with the scar formation secondary to inflammation, which, after a period of several months, will stop further nerve regrowth. Axon regrowth to the site of injury occurs at a rate of almost 1 mm per day or 2.5 cm per month. In motor nerves, end-organ degeneration of the muscle motor plate synapse may occur before reinnervation, limiting recovery. **Neuralgia** is a paroxysmal pain felt along the course of one or more nerves due to some irritation or inflammation.

CLINICAL GRADING SYSTEMS IN SPORTS TRAUMA

Systems for grading the severity of sports-induced soft tissue inflammation and the progress of healing are used to recognize the severity of injury, to judge its resolution, and to make recommendations on level of activity and return to competition. Such staging concepts for sports trauma, which have been applied to both acute and chronic injuries, attempt to describe subjective or qualitative symptoms or behaviors in quantitative terms. An early example, the traditional American Medical Association classification of ligament injury, set up three grades: Grade I, mild stretching; Grade II, partial tear; and Grade III, severe complete tear. These grading systems are based on the assumption that (1) there is a measurable response to soft tissue injury; (2) the duration and subjective appreciation of severity and type of pain correlate directly with the degree of tissue injury; and (3) a given level of pain correlates with a specific quality of tissue pathology.

Although these assumptions have been substantiated in many cases, they have not been scientifically documented and there are exceptions. A weak point in such grading systems is the middle grade, which often shares signs and symptoms of both lesser and higher grades of injury. Despite their shortcomings, these systems can be

TABLE 8.3. The Clinical Grading of Sports-Induced Soft Tissue Inflammations

Grade	Subjective Pain Pattern	Physical Signs	Tissue Damage	Healing Potential	Relevant Therapeutic Measures	
I	Pain after activity only. Duration of symptoms less than two weeks. Spontaneous relief within 24 hours.	Nonlocalized pain.	Micro Injury	Potential spontaneous resolution	Proper warmup and conditioning. Avoidance of abrupt transition in activity level.	Training, coaching and self-help measures often effective.
II	Pain during and after activity, but no significant functional disability. Duration of symptoms greater than two weeks, less than 6 weeks.	Localized pain. Minimal or no other signs of inflammation.			Analysis of technique and efficiency. Decrease transitional abuse and improve training.	
III	Pain during and after sport lasting for several days despite rest with rapid return upon activity. Significant functional disability. Duration of pain greater than 6 weeks. Night pain may occur.	Intense point tenderness with prominent inflammation (edema, effusion, erythema, crepitus, etc.).	Macro Injury	Permanent scar and residual tissue damage more likely	Medical assessment of structural vulnerability (e.g. flat feet, inflexibility, muscle weakness, etc.). Protected activity (e.g. bracing). Modification or substitution of different sports exercise to avoid excessive load on injured part.	Medical diagnosis and opinion valuable.
IV	Continuous pain with sport and daily activity. Total inability to train or compete. Night pain common.	Grade III symptoms plus tissue breakdown, atrophy, etc. Impending or actual tissue failure.			Surgical treatment often indicated to stimulate fibrous scar and repair or create structural alteration such as releases or decompression, potential permanent withdrawal from activity (e.g. deg. joint disease).	

Source: Adapted from Leadbetter, W. B., Buckwalter, J. A., and Gordon, S. L. *Sports-Induced Inflammation: Clinical and Basic Science Concepts.* Park Ridge, Ill.: American Academy of Orthopaedic Surgeons, 1990.

used as guidelines to grade severity of injury, the stages of healing, the phases of rehabilitation and therapy, and the timing of return to active participation.

These staging systems must distinguish between the symptom of pain and the presence of inflammation. To the degree that there are multiple pathways for the origin of pain, as well as modifications of its appreciation at the level of the brain, attention is again called to the role of load and heretofore undiscovered mechanically and biochemically mediated effects on cell and matrix. A unified grading scheme based on the present sports medicine literature is shown in Table 8.3. Because accurate diagnosis can be difficult, those responsible for diagnosing and treating sports-related soft tissue injury often find such grading systems very helpful. Their use also draws attention to the cycle of inflammation and repair which can suggest preventive and self-adjustment measures to the injured athlete.

IMPORTANT CONCEPTS

1. Sports injuries produce both predictable and unpredictable tissue responses. Variables affecting such response include severity, mode of onset, age, genetics, and the individual demands of a given sport.
2. Successful sports medicine treatment demands an understanding of the body's cellular responses and the ability to modify cellular activity.
3. Tendon, muscle, ligament, cartilage, and bone are known as the connective tissues. Extracellular matrix composition most distinguishes the form and function of all connective tissue. There is great variability in cell population, vascularity and innervation of connective tissues.
4. There is no single central control mechanism for the regulation of connective tissue metabolism; mediators are protein messengers that allow cell to cell regulation of all trauma responses.
5. Synovium is a highly differentiated connective tissue with marked capability for immunologic and inflammatory response.
6. Sports-induced inflammation is a localized tissue response initiated by the injury or destruction of vascularized tissues exposed to excessive mechanical load. It is a time dependent evolving process characterized by vascular, chemical and cellular events leading to spontaneous resolution, fibroproductive heal-

ing (tissue repair), tissue regeneration, or chronic inflammatory response.
7. The four "cardinal signs" of classical inflammation are: heat, redness, swelling, and pain. To these was added the so-called fifth sign: loss of function.
8. In regeneration, new matrices and cells that are identical in structure and function to those that they replace are formed; sports trauma most often results in a less efficient form of healing known as repair, in which damaged or lost cells and matrices are replaced by new cells and matrices that are not necessarily identical in structure or function to the normal tissue.
9. *Load* represents mechanical force, and *use* refers to both repeated movement and the accumulation of load over time.
10. *Strain* implies deformation of a structure, and *stress* is the internal molecular energy resistance to strain.
11. The principle of transition states that sports injury is most likely to occur when the athlete experiences any change in load or use of the involved part.
12. In *atrophy*, a cell's size and function decrease in response to an environmental signal.
13. The three phases of the inflammation–repair process are acute vascular inflammatory response, repair–regeneration, and remodeling mat-

uration. These phases are characterized by vascular, cellular, and humoral responses.

14. In degeneration, a tissue changes from a higher to a lower or less functionally active form.

ACKNOWLEDGMENT

Portions of this chapter are based on material and discussions from "Inflammation and Healing of Sports-Induced Soft-Tissue Injuries," a workshop jointly sponsored by the Foundation for Sports Medicine Education and Research, an affiliate of the American Orthopaedic Society for Sports Medicine, and the National Institute of Arthritis and Musculoskeletal and Skin Diseases. Proceedings of the workshop were published in *Sports-Induced Inflammation: Clinical and Basic Science Concepts*, edited by Wayne B. Leadbetter, MD; Joseph A. Buckwalter, MD; and Stephen L. Gordon, PhD, Park Ridge, IL 1990, American Academy of Orthopaedic Surgeons.

SUGGESTED READINGS

Bryant, W. M. "Wound Healing." *CIBA Clinical Symposia* 29 (1977): 1–36.

Cailliet, R. *Soft Tissue Pain and Disability*. Philadelphia: F. A. Davis, 1977.

Castor, C. W. "Regulation of Connective Tissue Metabolism." In *Arthritis and Allied Conditions: A Textbook of Rheumatology*, 11th ed., edited by D. J. McCarty, pp. 256–272. Philadelphia: Lea & Febiger, 1989.

Clancy, W. G., Jr. "Tendinitis and Plantar Fasciitis in Runners." In *Prevention and Treatment of Running Injuries*, edited by R. D'Ambrosia and D. Drez, Jr., pp. 77–87. Thorofare, N.J.: Charles B. Slack, 1982.

Colosimo, A. J., and F. H. Bassett, III. "Jumper's Knee: Diagnosis and Treatment." *Orthopaedic Review* 19 (1990): 139–149.

Cox, J. S. "Current Concepts in the Role of Steroids in the Treatment of Sprains and Strains." *Medicine and Science in Sports and Exercise* 16 (1984): 216–218.

Curwin, S., and W. D. Stanish. *Tendinitis: Its Etiology and Treatment*. Lexington, Mass.: Collamore Press, 1984.

Estwanik, J. J., and J. A. McAlister. "Contusions and the Formation of Myositis Ossificans." *The Physician and Sportsmedicine* 18 (April 1990): 53–64.

Ficat, R. P., and D. S. Hungerford. *Disorders of the Patello-femoral Joint*. Baltimore: Williams & Wilkins, 1977.

Fox, R. J., M. Lotz, and D. A. Carson. "Structures and Function of Synoviocytes." In *Arthritis and Allied Conditions: A Textbook of Rheumatology*, 11th ed., edited by D. J. McCarty, pp. 273–287. Philadelphia: Lea & Febiger, 1989.

Frank, C., D. Amiel, S. L.-Y. Woo, et al. "Normal Ligament Properties and Ligament Healing." *Clinical Orthopaedics and Related Research* 196 (1985): 15–25.

Gallin, J. I., I. M. Goldstein, and R. Snyderman, eds. *Inflammation: Basic Principles and Clinical Correlates*. New York: Raven Press, 1988.

Gamble, J. G. *The Musculoskeletal System: Physiological Basics*. New York: Raven Press, 1988.

Hunt, T. K., and J. E. Dunphy, eds. *Fundamentals of Wound Management*. New York: Appleton-Century-Crofts, 1979.

Hunter-Griffin, L. Y., ed. *Clinics in Sports Medicine*, vol. 6, no. 2. Philadelphia: W. B. Saunders, 1987.

Kellett, J. "Acute Soft Tissue Injuries—A Review of the Literature." *Medicine and Science in Sports and Exercise* 18 (1986): 489–500.

Knight, K. L. *Cryotherapy: Theory, Technique and Physiology*. Chattanooga, Tenn.: Chattanooga Corporation, Education Division, 1985.

Lachmann, S. *Soft Tissue Injuries in Sport*. Oxford: Blackwell Scientific Publications, 1988.

Leadbetter, W. B., J. A. Buckwalter, and S. L. Gordon, eds. *Sports-Induced Inflammation: Clinical and Basic Science Concepts*. Park Ridge, Ill.: American Academy of Orthopaedic Surgeons, 1990.

Majno, G. *The Healing Hand: Man and Wound in the Ancient World*. Cambridge, Mass.: Harvard University Press, 1975.

McBryde, A. M., Jr. "Stress Fractures in Runners." In *Prevention and Treatment of Running Injuries*, edited by R. D'Ambrosia and D. Drez, Jr., pp. 21–42. Thorofare, N.J.: Charles B. Slack, 1982.

Menard, D., and W. D. Stanish. "The Aging Athlete." *American Journal of Sports Medicine* 17 (1989): 187-196.

Parker, R. D., A. I. Froimson, D. D. Winsberg, et al. "Frozen Shoulder. Part I: Chronology, Pathogenesis, Clinical Picture, and Treatment." *Orthopedics* 12 (1989): 869–873.

Peacock, E. E., Jr. *Wound Repair*, 3rd ed. Philadelphia: W. B. Saunders, 1984.

Pérez-Tamayo, Ruy. *Mechanisms of Disease: An Introduction to Pathology*, 2nd ed. Chicago: Year Book Medical Publishers, 1985, p. 182.

Puzas, J. E., M. D. Miller, and R. N. Rosier. "Pathologic Bone Formation." *Clinical Orthopaedics and Related Research* 245 (August 1989): 269–281.

Robinson, D. R. "Physiology and Pharmacology of Anti-Inflammatory Drugs." *Contemporary Orthopaedics* 2 (1980): 242–245.

Rogers, E. J., and R. Rogers. "Fibromyalgia and Myofascial Pain: Either, Neither, or Both?" *Orthopaedic Review* 18 (November 1989): 1217–1224.

Rubin, E., and J. L. Farber, eds. *Pathology*. Philadelphia: J. B. Lippincott, 1988.

Simon S. R., R. S. Riggins, C. R. Wirth, and M. L. Fox, eds. *Orthopaedic Science: A Resource and Self-Study for the Practitioner: Syllabus*. Park Ridge, Ill.: American Academy of Orthopaedic Surgeons, 1986.

Solomonow, M., and R. D'Ambrosia. "Biomechanics of Muscle Overuse Injuries: A Theoretical Approach." *Clinics in Sports Medicine* 6 (1987): 241–257.

Sporn, M. B., and A. B. Roberts. "Transforming Growth Factor-β: Multiple Actions and Potential Clinical Applications." *Journal of the American Medical Association* 262 (1989): 938–941.

Stauber, W. T., V. K. Fritz, D. W. Vogelbach, et al. "Characterization of Muscles Injured by Forced Lengthening: I. Cellular Infiltrates." *Medicine and Science in Sports and Exercise* 20 (1988): 345–353.

Teitz, C. C., ed. *Scientific Foundations of Sports Medicine*. Toronto: B. C. Decker, 1989.

van der Meulen, J. C. "Present State of Knowledge on Processes of Healing in Collagen Structures." *International Journal of Sports Medicine* (supplement 1) 3 (1982): 4–8.

Weiler, J. M., J. P. Albright, and J. A. Buckwalter. "Nonsteroidal Anti-Inflammatory Drugs in Sports Medicine." In *Nonsteroidal Anti-Inflammatory Drugs: Mechanisms and Clinical Use*, edited by A. J. Lewis and D. E. Furst. New York: Marcel Dekker, pp. 71–88, 1987.

Woo, S. L.-Y, and J. A. Buckwalter, eds. *Injury and Repair of the Musculoskeletal Soft Tissues*. Park Ridge, Ill.: American Academy of Orthopaedic Surgeons, 1988.

9

Topographic Anatomy

CHAPTER OUTLINE

OBJECTIVES FOR CHAPTER 9

After reading this chapter, the student should be able to:

1. Understand the terminology used to describe topographic anatomy.
2. Recognize the topographic anatomy of specific body regions.
3. Describe the sensory dermatome scheme.

INTRODUCTION

An understanding of the topographic anatomy of the body enables the athletic trainer to assess an athlete's injury quickly and to convey accurate information regarding the injury to other medical personnel. Chapter 9 discusses the terminology used, the topographic anatomy of specific body regions, and the skin dermatome scheme. ■

OVERVIEW OF TOPOGRAPHIC ANATOMY

Importance of Landmarks

The surface of the body has many definite features. These landmarks are guides to structures that lie beneath them, giving clues to the anatomy of the body through its external features, or its **topography**. A knowledge of the superficial landmarks of the body, or the **topographic anatomy**, allows the well-trained athletic trainer to evaluate the seriousness of an injury quickly and to anticipate complications.

Terminology of Topographic Anatomy

All athletic trainers should be familiar with the language of topographic anatomy so they can relate specific information with the least possible confusion.

The Anatomic Position

Picture the body in the standard position, which is always standing erect, facing the trainer, with the arms at the sides, palms forward. When the terms "right" and "left" are used, they refer to the athlete's right and left. The principal regions of the body are the head, neck, thorax (chest), abdomen, and extremities (arms and legs).

An anatomic or injured part may be described as being in a certain plane or section of the body. Because the human body is three-dimensional, planes can be used as points of reference. The three planes most commonly referred are the **coronal** (frontal), **sagittal** (vertical), and **transverse** (horizontal) **planes** (Fig. 9.1).

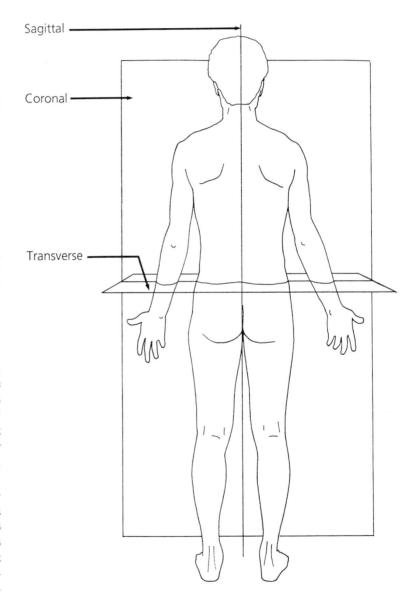

FIGURE 9.1. Three planes of the human body.

Specific Location Terms

The surface of the front of the body, facing the trainer, is the **anterior surface**. The surface of the body away from the trainer is the **posterior surface**. An imaginary vertical line drawn from the middle of the forehead through the nose and the umbilicus (navel) to the floor is termed the **midline**. Areas that lie away from this line are termed **lateral**, and areas that lie toward it are termed **medial**; we speak, for example, of the medial and lateral surfaces of the knee, elbow, or ankle. The **superior portion** of the body is that portion nearer the head or cephalad end; the **inferior portion** is that portion nearer the feet or caudad end. The

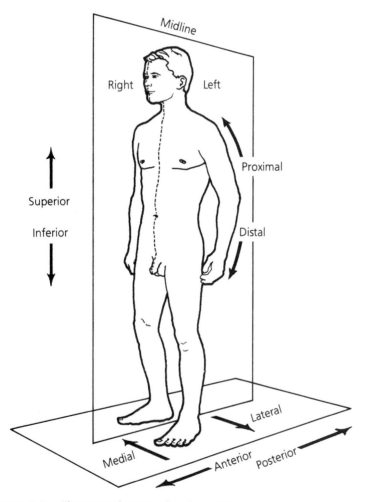

FIGURE 9.2. The general terms of topographic anatomy are used to describe the location of wounds and injuries.

nose, for example, is superior to the mouth, while the umbilicus is inferior to the chest.

Proximal refers to a location on an extremity that is nearer to the trunk, and to any location on the trunk that is nearer to the midline or to the point of reference named. **Distal** is the opposite of proximal and refers to a location on an extremity nearer to the free end—the end not attached to the trunk. Similarly, distal refers to any location on the trunk that is farther from the midline or from the point of reference named. For example, the elbow is distal to the shoulder but proximal to the wrist and hand (Fig. 9.2).

In general, the arms and legs refer to the upper and lower extremities. Specifically, the upper portion of the lower extremity from the hip joint to the knee is the thigh. The lower portion from the knee to the ankle is the leg. The upper portion of the upper extremity from the shoulder to the elbow is the arm. The lower portion from the elbow to the wrist is the forearm.

By using these terms and recalling the description of the standard anatomic position, the trainer can describe the location of an injury so that another trainer or emergency response personnel will know immediately where to look and what to expect.

Role of Topographic Anatomy in Inspection of Injuries

Inspection is the simplest component of the primary and secondary surveys of injured persons (see Chapter 11). Inspection requires no special dexterity or strength on the part of the trainer; nor does it cause the athlete pain or risk of further injury. Because thorough inspection yields much information regarding the extent of injury, its importance cannot be overemphasized; more facts are missed by not examining an athlete thoroughly than by not knowing a specific anatomic relation.

Trainers can develop their own method for inspecting the athlete, but any method should be systematic, thorough, and performed in exactly the same sequence for all athletes. Developing a routine will help the trainer avoid overlooking a critical but perhaps subtle sign. The examination should begin at the head and proceed through the neck, thorax, abdomen, pelvis, and the extremities. It is especially crucial to compare a given injured region with the corresponding uninjured region on the opposite side.

TOPOGRAPHIC ANATOMY OF SPECIFIC BODY REGIONS

Head

The head is divided into the cranium and the face. An imaginary horizontal plane that passes across the top of the ears and eyes separates the superior (top) and inferior (bottom) portions of the head.

Cranium

The area above the imaginary horizontal plane is called the **cranium**. It contains the brain, which connects with the spinal cord through a large opening at the base of the skull (the **foramen magnum**) and in the center of the upper part of the neck. The most posterior portion of the cranium (the back of the head) is the **occiput**. On each side, the lateral and most anterior portions of the cranium are called the **temples** or **temporal regions**; more posteriorly are the **parietal regions** (Fig. 9.3). The pulse of the temporal artery can be felt just anterior to the ear.

Face

Just below the imaginary horizontal plane lie the ears, eyes, nose, mouth, cheeks, and jowls that make up the face. Gross injuries of these structures are not difficult to recognize. The orbital rim of the **maxilla** is prominent below the eye, while the **zygomatic bone** (cheekbone) is also obvious (see Fig. 9.3).

By viewing the face from the side, one can observe the eyeball recessed in the **orbit**, which is composed of the frontal bone of the skull, the maxilla, and the zygomatic bone (see Fig. 9.3). The bony ridges of the

frontal bone and maxilla protect the eye superiorly and inferiorly. The zygomatic bone protects the eye laterally; the maxilla protects the eye medially. These ridges protect the eye and obviously receive the greatest force of any impact. A bruise, laceration, or abrasion in these locations must always be viewed, therefore, as a possible sign of a major underlying fracture. Frequently, a fracture of the maxilla will trap one or more of the muscles that control motion of the eye. In this situation, the affected eye will often look down and its motion in other directions will be limited. This type of fracture is called a "blow-out" fracture of the floor of the orbit.

Only the proximal third of the nose, the **bridge**, is formed by bone; the remainder is a cartilaginous framework. Any injury of the proximal third is therefore cause to suspect an underlying fracture, while an

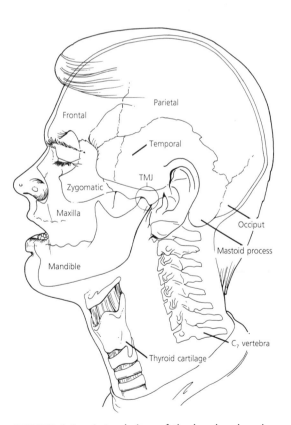

FIGURE 9.3. Lateral view of the head and neck showing the bone structure and regions of the head.

abrasion on the tip of the nose usually is a minor lesion. Bleeding or discharge from the nose after a head injury should always be investigated further. A nasal discharge of clear cerebrospinal fluid is an indication of a fracture of the anterior portion of the skull. A bloody discharge or leaking of clear fluid from the ear suggests a fracture of the skull involving its base.

Unlike the nose, the exposed portion of the ear, or the **pinna**, is composed entirely of cartilage covered by skin, and injuries are usually obvious. Immediately anterior to the notch at the middle of the anterior border of the exposed ear is the easily palpable temporal artery. If you hold a finger gently on the temporal artery at this site and then open your mouth, you will immediately appreciate that the articulation of the mandible with the undersurface of the skull, the **temporomandibular joint** (TMJ), lies at this site. The **tragus**, or small, rounded, fleshy protuberance immediately at the front of the ear canal, lies over the area where the temporal artery may be palpated. The lobes are the dependent fleshy portions at the bottom of each ear.

The prominent, hard, bony mass at the base of the skull, about 1/2 inch posterior to the tip of the lobe of the ear, is called the **mastoid process**. In athletes who have suffered a serious skull fracture involving the base, an ecchymosis (a purplish-blue bruise) may appear in this region some hours after the injury. This finding is subtle and is often overlooked or misdiagnosed as a simple bruise.

Neck

The neck contains many structures, including the cervical or upper **esophagus** and the **trachea** (windpipe). The first seven vertebrae (bony segments of the spinal column) form the **cervical spine**, which lies in the neck. The carotid arteries may be found at either side of the trachea, together with the jugular veins and several nerves (Fig. 9.4).

Several useful landmarks are present in the neck. Most obvious is the firm, prominent **thyroid cartilage** in the center of the

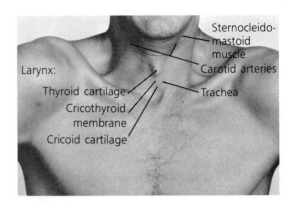

FIGURE 9.4. Anterior view of the neck.

anterior surface commonly known as the "**Adam's apple**"; it is more prominent in men than women. Approximately 3/4 inch inferior to the upper border of this prominence is a marked soft tissue depression about 1/4 inch wide that separates the thyroid cartilage from a second, somewhat less noticeable, cartilage—the **cricoid cartilage**. The cricoid cartilage is palpable as a firm ridge 1/8 to 1/4 inch thick. The thyroid and cricoid cartilages form the framework of the **larynx** (voice box). The soft tissue depression represents the area of the **cricothyroid membrane**, which is a substantial sheet of fascia (connective tissue) connecting the two cartilages. The cricothyroid membrane is covered at this point only by skin.

Inferiorly from the larynx, several additional firm ridges are palpable in the trachea. These ridges are the cartilages of the trachea. The trachea connects the larynx with the main **bronchi** (airways) of the lungs. On either side of the lower larynx and the upper trachea lies the **thyroid gland**. Unless it is enlarged, this gland is usually not palpable.

Pulsations of the carotid arteries are easily palpable about 1/2 to 3/4 inch lateral to the larynx. Lying immediately adjacent to these arteries are the internal jugular veins and important nerves. Obviously, injuries that involve these areas of the neck may cause rapid, fatal bleeding.

Posteriorly, the **spinous processes** of the cervical vertebrae are palpable prominences in the midline of the neck; they become

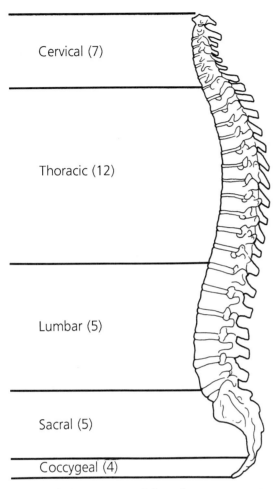

FIGURE 9.5. Regions of the spine.

Cervical (7)

Thoracic (12)

Lumbar (5)

Sacral (5)

Coccygeal (4)

The **spine** is essentially the central structure of the body on which all of the extremities and ribs articulate. The spine also serves as the protective canal for the neural **spinal cord** that extends from the brain to the body and extremities.

Vertebrae of the Spinal Column

Approximately 33 vertebrae form the spinal column. Most of the spine is formed of separate vertebrae, but in the lower section the segments are fused together.

The spinal column is divided into five major regions. The **cervical spine** consists of the 7 vertebrae that support the skull. The next 12 vertebrae compose the **thoracic spine** and have attached **ribs**. The **lumbar spine** consists of 5 vertebrae. The **sacrum** also has 5 vertebrae which are fused in a solid bony mass. The last 4 vertebrae form the **coccyx** or distal tip of the spine.

Anatomy of the Vertebrae

A typical vertebra has a solid **body**, an encircling **neural arch**, and posterior and lateral spinous processes (Fig. 9.6). The vertebral bodies are stacked on each other much like building blocks. The **fibrocartilaginous discs** act as spacers and shock absorbers between each vertebral body. The neural arch behind each body encompasses

more obvious as they progress down the spine. They are most easily palpable when the neck is in extreme flexion. At the base of the neck posteriorly, the spinous process of the seventh cervical vertebra is usually the most prominent. Ordinarily, the larynx lies just anterior to the fifth and sixth cervical vertebrae.

Spine

The **spinal column** consists of a series of interconnecting bones (**vertebrae**) that extend from the base of the skull to the tip of the coccyx (Fig. 9.5). Each spinal bone articulates with the next one and has interposing fibrocartilaginous discs that act as spacers and cushions for the spine.

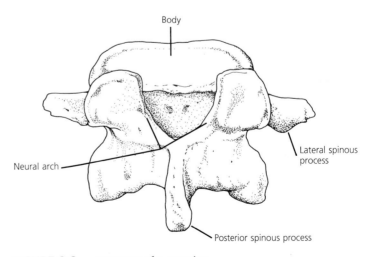

FIGURE 9.6. Anatomy of a vertebra.

and protects the spinal cord as it passes the length of the spine. Openings in the arches called **foramina** allow paired branches of nerves to exit the spinal cord at each vertebral level.

The sets of joint articulations above and below each neural arch allow limited motion between the vertebrae. The fusion of the sacrum eliminates these joints and discs at this level. The paired **transverse processes** and single **posterior process** allow for the attachment of strong intervertebral ligaments that support the spine and also provide anchors for muscles attached to the spinal column.

The cervical vertebrae are modified to allow mobility of the head. The first vertebra beneath the skull is the **atlas** and has no body. Its special articulations with the base of the skull and the second vertebra, or **axis**, allow most of the rotatory motion of the head. The remaining 5 cervical vertebrae are designed to provide flexion and extension of the head and neck. The 12 thoracic vertebrae allow little motion for the spine. Articulation with the ribs creates stability in the thoracic spine. The 5 lumbar vertebrae are more massive in structure than the cervical vertebrae, thus allowing them to tolerate greater load bearing. Their joint articulations allow moderate flexion and extension of the lumbar spine. Because of the increased weight load in the lower spine, a greater risk of disc and bone injuries exists in this area from the overload stresses. The sacrum is modified to be the supporting base of the spinal column and to articulate with the pelvic bones. The coccyx plays no role in the spinal column in weight bearing or neural protection.

Thorax

The **thorax** (chest) is the cavity that contains the heart, lungs, esophagus, and the great vessels (the aorta and the two venae cavae). It is formed by the 12 thoracic vertebrae and 12 pairs of ribs. The **clavicle** (collarbone) overlies its upper boundaries in front and articulates with the **scapula** (shoulder blade), which lies in the muscular

tissue of the thoracic wall posteriorly. **Pleura** (smooth, glistening tissue) lines the chest cavity, arches high in a dome behind each clavicle superiorly, and inferiorly covers the upper surface of the diaphragm, the lower boundary of the thorax (Figs. 9.7a, b). The dimensions of the thorax are defined by the bony rib cage and its attachments.

Anteriorly, in the midline of the chest, is the **sternum** (breastbone). The superior border of the sternum forms the easily palpable **jugular notch**. The inferior end of the sternum forms a narrow cartilaginous tip called the **xiphoid process**.

In the midline of the upper back, the spinous processes of the 12 thoracic vertebrae can be palpated. Ten of these vertebrae are connected anteriorly to the sternum or to the costal arch by the first through the tenth ribs. The eleventh and twelfth ribs do not connect to the sternum or the arch and are therefore called **floating ribs**. An interposed costal cartilage forms the articulation between the ribs and the sternum or the arch. Inferiorly, the cartilages themselves become longer and form the palpable **costal arch**, which is the definite boundary of the lower border of the thorax and the upper border of the abdomen. The arch itself is made up of the fused costal cartilages of the sixth through the tenth ribs. The jugular notch of the sternum lies at the level of the second thoracic vertebra. The xiphoid tip lies approximately at the level of the ninth thoracic vertebra.

The major palpable landmarks in the chest are obviously the ribs, most of which can be easily felt. The first rib is not palpable on either side, since it is hidden under and behind the clavicle, which joins the sternum. Both the clavicle and sternum are easily felt. Just inferior to the junction of the clavicle and sternum is a prominence on the breastbone, called the **angle of Louis**. This prominence always lies opposite the space between the second and third ribs (second intercostal space). Orientation for counting ribs can be from this prominence and the palpable interspace opposite it.

On the male chest the nipples lie at the level of the interspace between the fourth

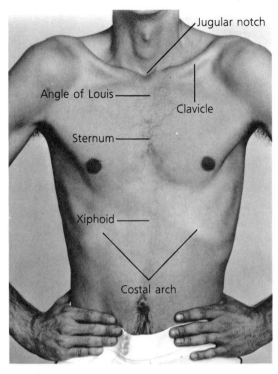

FIGURE 9.7a. Anterior aspect of the chest wall.

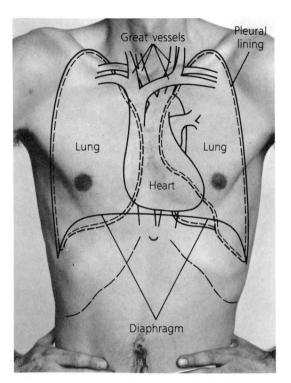

FIGURE 9.7b. Anterior aspect of the chest with the positions of the important chest organs.

and fifth ribs. In the female, breasts vary in size, and consequently nipple position may vary. The center of the breast, however, still lies at the interspace between the fourth and fifth ribs.

Posteriorly, the scapula overlies the thoracic wall and is contained within heavy muscles. When the athlete is standing, the two scapulae should lie at approximately the same level, with their inferior tips at about the seventh thoracic vertebra. If one scapula lies noticeably higher than the other, it may be an indication of neuromuscular or bony injury.

The **diaphragm** is a muscular dome forming the undersurface of the thorax, separating the chest and abdominal cavities. Anteriorly, it is attached to the costal arch. Posteriorly, it is attached to the lumbar vertebrae. It moves up and down with normal breathing for a distance of one or two intercostal spaces. Injuries of the lower portion of the lung and the diaphragm from penetrating wounds obviously depend on

the position of the diaphragm at the time of injury. Similarly, injuries of the lower chest may easily involve the diaphragm.

Within the thoracic cage, the most prominent structures are the heart and lungs. The **heart** lies within the pericardial sac immediately under the sternum and immediately above the midportion of the diaphragm. It extends from the second to the sixth ribs anteriorly and from the fifth to the eighth thoracic vertebrae posteriorly. Ordinarily it lies from the midline to the left midclavicular line in the fifth intercostal space. Diseased hearts may be larger or smaller.

The major blood vessels traveling to and from the heart lie deep within the chest. On the right side of the spinal column the superior and inferior venae cavae carry blood to the heart. Just beneath the upper third of the sternum, the arch of the aorta and the pulmonary artery rise to distribute blood to the body and to the lungs, respectively. The arch of the aorta passes to the left and lies alongside the left side of the spinal column as it descends deep within the chest and into the abdomen. The esophagus lies behind the trachea and directly on the spinal column as it passes through the chest into the abdomen.

All the space within the chest not occupied by the heart, the great vessels, and the esophagus is occupied by the **lungs**. Anteriorly, the lungs extend down to the surface of the diaphragm at the level of the xiphoid process. Posteriorly, the lungs continue in contact with the surface of the diaphragm down to the level of the twelfth thoracic vertebra.

Abdomen

The **abdomen** is the second major body cavity. It is bounded superiorly by the diaphragm, inferiorly by a plane extending from the pubic symphysis through the sacrum, anteriorly by the anterior abdominal wall, and posteriorly by the posterior abdominal wall. It contains the major organs of digestion and excretion.

The Four Abdominal Quadrants

Although there are several methods of referring to the various portions of the abdomen, the simplest and most common uses abdominal quadrants. In this method, the abdomen is divided into four equal parts by two lines that intersect at right angles at the umbilicus. The quadrants thus formed are right upper, right lower, left upper, and left lower (Fig. 9.8), where "right" and "left" are the athlete's right and left, not the observer's. Pain or injury in a given quadrant usually arises from or involves the organs in that quadrant. Specifying a particular quadrant allows the organs that are injured or diseased or that may require emergency attention to be identified quickly and clearly.

In the **upper right quadrant**, the major organs are the **liver**, **gallbladder**, and a portion of the **colon** (Fig. 9.9). The greater portion of the liver lies in this quadrant

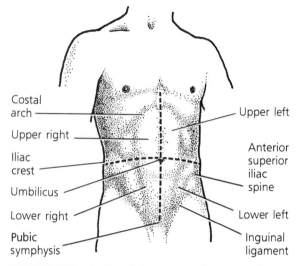

FIGURE 9.8. In the abdomen, quadrants are the easiest system for identifying areas. Major bony landmarks are also shown.

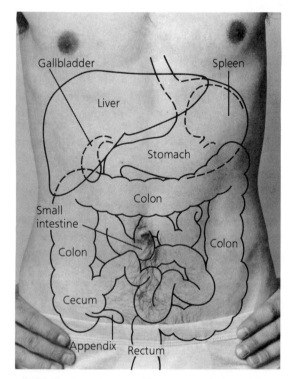

FIGURE 9.9. Anterior view of the abdomen with the position of the major abdominal organs outlined.

almost entirely under the protection of the eighth to twelfth ribs. It extends through the entire anteroposterior depth of the abdomen. Injuries in this quadrant are frequently associated with injuries of the liver. Tenderness without injury in the right upper quadrant is usually due to gallbladder disease.

In the **left upper quadrant**, the principal organs are the **stomach**, the **spleen**, a portion of the **transverse** and **descending colon**, and a small portion of the liver. The stomach and the spleen are almost entirely protected by the left rib cage. The spleen lies lateral and posterior in this quadrant, under the diaphragm and immediately beneath the ninth to eleventh ribs. This organ is frequently injured, especially in association with fracture of these ribs. Tenderness or pain in the left upper quadrant often indicates a ruptured spleen.

In the **right lower quadrant**, the principal organs are two portions of the large intestine: the **cecum** and the **ascending colon**. The **appendix** is a small tubular structure attached to the lower border of the cecum. Appendicitis is the most frequent cause of tenderness and pain in this region.

In the **left lower quadrant** the principal organs are the **descending colon** and the **rectosigmoid colon**. The pain of diverticulitis (inflammation of a diverticulum) often localizes to the left lower quadrant.

Many organs lie in one or more quadrants (Fig. 9.10). The **small bowel**, for instance, encircles the umbilicus, and parts of the small bowel occupy all four quadrants. The **large bowel** arises laterally in the right lower quadrant and completely encircles the abdomen in one sweep, coming to lie in all four quadrants also. The **urinary bladder** lies just behind the junction of the pubic bones at the middle of the abdomen; therefore, it lies in both lower quadrants. The **pancreas** lies transversely on the posterior body wall behind the abdominal cavity and therefore is in both upper quadrants. The **kidneys** lie in the same plane as the pancreas, behind the abdominal cavity. They lie completely above the level of the umbilicus,

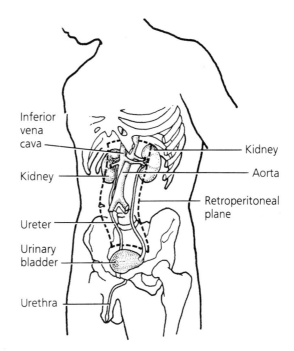

FIGURE 9.10.   Several organs lie in more than one quadrant.

extending from the eleventh thoracic vertebra to the third lumbar vertebra. They are approximately 4 to 6 inches long and lie in an angle formed by the spinal column and the lower ribs, the **costovertebral angle**. They are each attached to the bladder by tubular structures called **ureters**, which lie in the same plane behind the abdominal cavity. These tubes pass on either side of the spinal column along the posterior wall of the abdomen into the pelvis to enter the bladder.

Posterior Landmarks of the Abdomen

Posteriorly, one does not usually refer to quadrants. The posterior portions of the iliac crest and the midline spines of the five lumbar vertebrae are the predominant landmarks of reference.

The Pelvic Cavity

Properly speaking, organs that lie in the lowest portions of the abdominal cavity are in the **pelvic cavity**. This cavity is bounded

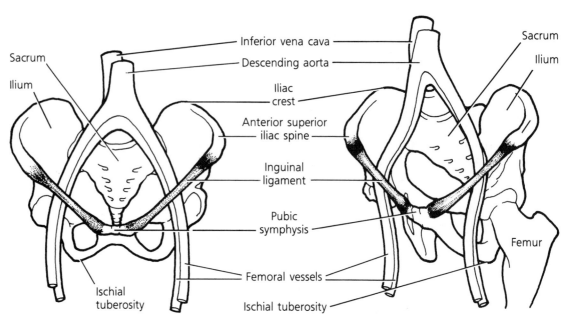

FIGURE 9.11. The pelvis is composed of several separate elements and bears the sockets for the hip joints. The inguinal ligament lies just above the femoral vessels and helps protect them.

by the sacrum behind and the pubis in front. It lies between the most inferior portions of the pelvic bone. The female reproductive organs (the **uterus, ovaries,** and **fallopian tubes**) and the **rectum** and **urinary bladder** are situated in this cavity, which is continuous with the abdominal cavity above.

Topographic Landmarks of the Abdomen

In the abdomen the chief topographic landmarks are the costal arch, the umbilicus, the anterior superior iliac spines, the iliac crests, and the pubic symphysis. The **costal arch** is the fused cartilages of the sixth through the tenth ribs. It forms the superior arching boundary of the abdomen. The **umbilicus**, a constant structure, is in the same horizontal plane as the fourth lumbar vertebra and the superior edge of the **iliac crest**, the outer, uppermost rim of the pelvic bone. The umbilicus overlies the division of the aorta into the two common iliac arteries. The **anterior superior iliac spines** are the

hard bony prominences at the front on each side of the lower abdomen just below the plane of the umbilicus. At the center of the lowermost portion of the abdomen, another hard bony prominence, the **pubic symphysis**, can be felt. The **bladder** lies just behind this bone. Injuries of the bladder frequently accompany fractures of the pelvis.

Pelvis

The **pelvis** is a closed bony ring consisting of the sacrum in the midline posteriorly, two iliac bones laterally, two ischial bones inferiorly, and two pubic bones anteriorly. The latter three bones—the **ilium**, the **ischium**, and the **pubis**—fuse to form a single bone, called the **innominate bone** (Fig. 9.11). Gentle pressure on each anterior superior iliac spine or on the iliac crests in an athlete with a pelvic fracture usually causes pain at the fracture site. On each side of the pelvis are deep sockets. They receive each **femoral head** and form the **hip joints**.

Posteriorly, the pelvis presents a flattened appearance, mainly because of the configuration of the sacrum. In the sitting position, a bony prominence is easily felt in the middle of each buttock. These prominences are the **ischial tuberosities**. The **sciatic nerve** carrying major motor and sensory innervation to the foot and leg passes lateral to the tuberosity as it enters the thigh (Fig. 9.12). With fractures of the pelvis in this region or a posterior hip dislocation, pressure on this nerve results in pain or paralysis.

Other Pelvic Structures

Located between the pubic symphysis and the anterior superior iliac spine on each side of the lower abdomen is a palpable, tough band of tissue, the **inguinal ligament** (Fig. 9.13). Deep to this ligament pass the femoral nerve, artery, and vein, and muscles to the lower extremity. The femoral artery is easily palpable just distal to the midpoint of the ligament. The femoral nerve lies immediately lateral to the artery, and the femoral vein lies just medial to it.

Lower Extremity

The lower extremity consists of the hip, thigh, knee, leg, ankle, and foot.

Hip

Strictly speaking, the hip is a joint articulating the **femur** (the main supporting bone of the thigh) with the innominate bone (the bone formed by the fusion of the ilium, ischium, and pubic bones). Just distal and posterolateral to this joint is a bony prominence present on each femur called the **greater trochanter** (Fig. 9.14). In examination, the position of this prominence should always be compared with that on the opposite side. Changes in the relative positions of these prominences may indicate underlying hip fractures or dislocations. The hip joint itself is superior and medial to the greater trochanter and about 1 inch lateral and 1 inch inferior to the pulsations of the femoral artery at the inguinal ligament (Fig. 9.15).

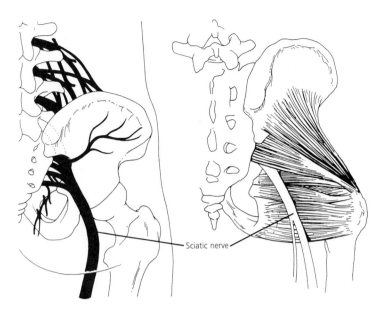

FIGURE 9.12. Posterior views of sciatic nerve as it enters the thigh.

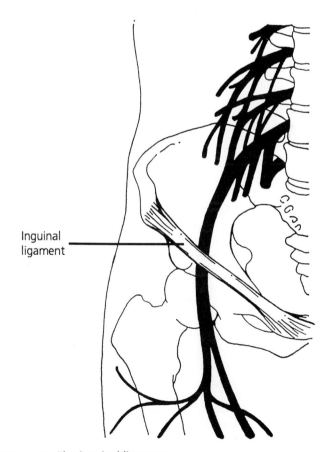

FIGURE 9.13. The inguinal ligament.

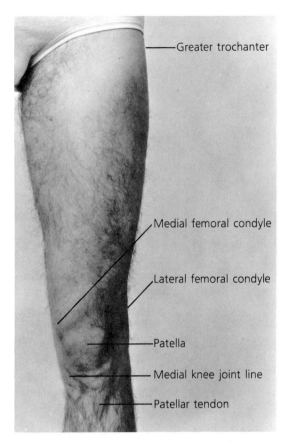

FIGURE 9.14. Anterior view of the thigh and knee.

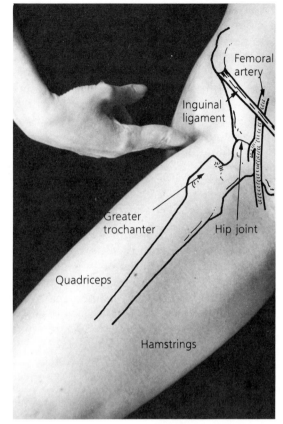

FIGURE 9.15. Anatomy of the hip.

Thigh

The thigh extends from the hip joint to the knee. The underlying femur has few landmarks, except the greater trochanter and the distal femoral condyles, but fractures of this large bone, when displaced or angulated, can be localized without great difficulty. The powerful muscles which attach to the femur can drive fractured segments of bone through the skin after an injury. The examination of a suspected femoral fracture must be done carefully to avoid converting a closed fracture into an open one.

Knee

The knee is a compound joint. Its patellofemoral articulations aid the **quadriceps** in its function as a decelerator of the body and a dynamic stabilizer of the knee (Fig. 9.16).

The **tibiofemoral joint** is a polycentric hinge joint that bears the body's weight during locomotion. The major ligamentous support structures of the knee include the **tibial collateral ligament**, which extends from the medial condyle of the femur to the medial condyle of the tibia and its shaft, and the **fibular collateral ligament**, which attaches to the lateral condyle of the femur and the lateral surface of the head of the fibula. Deeper to these structures lie the shorter capsular ligaments that extend from the femur to the meniscus and from the meniscus to the tibia. The **meniscus** itself acts as a gasket and an encircling band to stabilize the knee. The connection between the capsular ligaments and the meniscus adds significant stability to the knee joint.

Two major intra-articular ligaments provide additional static stability to the knee.

The **anterior cruciate ligament** passes from the lateral intercondylar notch to attach anteriorly on the articular surface of the tibia and serves primarily to prevent anterior translation of the tibia. The **posterior cruciate ligament** passes from the medial intercondylar notch of the femur and attaches on the posterior aspect of the tibia to its articular surface. It prevents posterior translation of the knee, and its attachment on the femur overlies the polycentric axis of flexion and extension of the knee (Fig. 9.17). The rotatory axis of the knee also lies in the plane of the posterior cruciate ligament.

The **patella** (kneecap) lies anteriorly to the knee joint, within the **quadriceps femoris tendon**, and thus is an important part of the extensor mechanism of the knee (see Fig. 9.16). A fracture of the patella will frequently interrupt this tendon, and the athlete will be unable to extend the leg at the knee. A gap in the patella itself may also be palpated in these cases. Normally, the patella rides smoothly in a groove on the anterior surface of the distal femur. This groove lies between the rounded condyles that make up the distal end of the femur and the articular surface of the knee joint. When the patella is dislocated, it is usually displaced laterally from the groove beyond the lateral condyle. In such cases, the leg is fixed in flexion at the knee, and the pain is extreme. The actual joint line of the knee is usually 1 inch inferior to the lower margin of the patella, and it can be easily felt by palpating on either side of the patellar tendon with the knee flexed at 90 degrees.

Leg

The leg is the portion of the lower extremity extending from the knee joint to the ankle joint (Fig. 9.18). The bones of the leg are the **tibia**, the familiar shinbone, and the **fibula**. The broad **tibial plateau** forms the lower surface of the knee joint. The entire extent of the tibia can be palpated just under the skin on the medial surface.

The head of the fibula lies at the posterolateral corner of the knee. The fibula is most

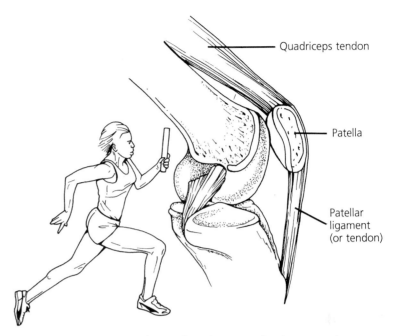

FIGURE 9.16.   The quadriceps functions as a decelerator and stabilizer.

easily palpated with the knee flexed to 90 degrees. Passing immediately distally around this bony prominence is the **peroneal nerve**, which controls movement at the ankle and sensation over the top of the foot. Injury of the fibula in this region should always prompt comparison of the function of the nerve with that on the opposite side of the athlete's body.

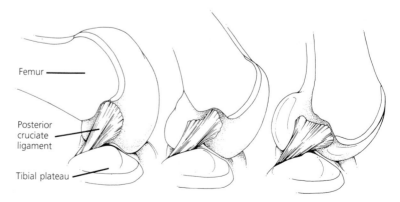

FIGURE 9.17.   The attachment of the posterior cruciate ligament overlies the polycentric axis of flexion and extension of the knee.

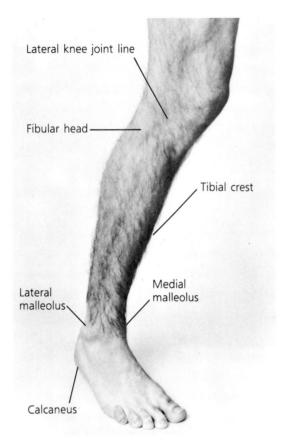

FIGURE 9.18. Anterolateral view of the leg and foot, showing the bony prominences.

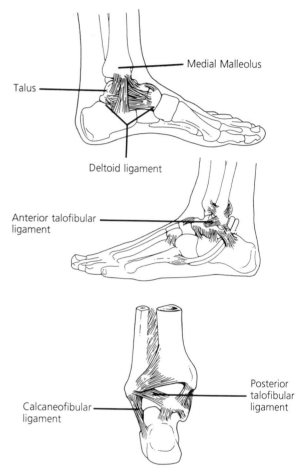

FIGURE 9.19. Major support ligaments of the ankle.

Ankle

The ankle is easily located by identifying the prominent distal ends of both the tibia and the fibula (see Fig. 9.18). Usually visible even in individuals with large or fat legs, these knobs are called, respectively, the **medial malleolus** and the **lateral malleolus**, and they form the socket of the ankle joint. Within the socket sits the **talus** (anklebone), which in turn articulates with the **calcaneus** (heelbone or **os calcis**) inferiorly.

The major support ligaments of the ankle are the **deltoid ligament**, medially, and a three-part **lateral ligament structure** (Fig. 9.19). The deltoid ligament derives its name from its fan shape as it originates on the medial malleolus and spreads to attach to the medial border of the talus. The three lateral ligaments of the ankle are the **ante-** rior talofibular ligament, the elongated **calcaneofibular ligament**, and the **posterior talofibular ligament**.

Ankle ligament injuries usually involve the lateral structures, most often the anterior talofibular ligament and the calcaneofibular ligament. The shorter bony strut of the medial malleolus on the inside of the ankle cannot prevent the ankle from turning in when forced. Excessive forces can stretch and tear the lateral ligaments causing inversion injuries.

Foot

The calcaneus (heelbone) is palpable through the skin of the heel. The extremity is completed by the **tarsal bones**, 5 **metatar-**

sal bones, which form the substance of the foot, and 5 toes formed of 14 **phalanges**.

Inspection of the Lower Extremity

Inspection of the lower extremity can give many clues to an injury, particularly fractures and dislocations. Noting the relative position of bilateral structures helps diagnose other injuries from the hip joint to more distal areas in the extremity. In assessing injuries in the lower extremity, if the patellae are at the same level on either side, the injury is probably below the knee. If they are not, the injury may be above the knee. Most people with hip fractures have a shortened, externally rotated leg. In these individuals, the patella may be above the patella on the opposite side, facing outward. A dislocated hip may cause the extremity to shorten, flex, and internally rotate, in which case the patella may face its neighbor. Careful inspection allows the trainer to make all these observations.

Upper Extremity

The upper extremity extends from the shoulder to the fingertips. It is composed of the shoulder, arm, elbow, forearm, wrist, and hand.

Shoulder

The shoulder girdle (Fig. 9.20) is composed of the clavicle anteriorly, scapula posteriorly, and the humeral head laterally. Injury of these structures may present as "pain in the shoulder."

The **clavicle** is attached medially to the sternum at the **sternoclavicular joint**. It is palpable throughout its entire length, from the sternum to its attachment to the scapula at the **acromioclavicular joint**. Acromioclavicular dislocations or separations can be easily palpated. Fractures of the clavicle are not only easily palpable but also usually visible.

The **scapula** is a broad, flat bone overlying the posterior wall of the thorax and articulating with the clavicle and humerus. Injury

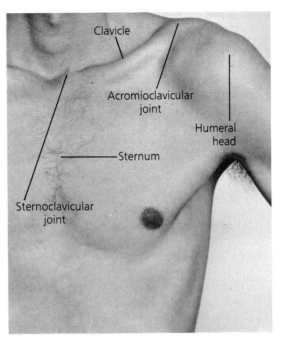

FIGURE 9.20.   The rounded prominence of the shoulder girdle laterally is created by the humeral head, covered by muscle.

of this bone is rare because of its protected situation. It ordinarily is palpable, especially the transverse ridge or spine running across the upper portion of each scapula.

The external appearance of the shoulder as a unit is that of a gently rounded area without major noticeable prominences. The very top of the shoulder corresponds to the acromioclavicular joint. This joint lies about 1¼ inches from the lateral surface of the arm. The most lateral structure of the shoulder is the rounded head of the humerus, the bone of the arm, which accounts for the rounded appearance of the shoulder in general. If the humeral head is dislocated from its articulation with the scapula, it is no longer laterally located, and the configuration of the shoulder may change from a rounded to a more angular appearance. Injuries that do not involve the joint itself fail to produce this change.

Arm

The arm extends from the shoulder to the elbow, and the supporting bone is the

humerus. The arm offers few specific landmarks. Displaced or angulated fractures of the humerus are generally easy to diagnose. The **radial nerve**, carrying sensation to the greater portion of the back of the hand and motor function that controls extension of the hand at the wrist, wraps very closely around the shaft of the humerus in its midportion. Fractures in this region demand careful testing of the function of this nerve.

Elbow

The elbow presents several bony landmarks (Fig. 9.21). The **medial** and **lateral condyles** of the humerus form the medial and lateral borders of the upper surface of the elbow joint. They are easy to palpate at the distal end of the elbow joint and at the distal end of the humerus with the elbow flexed. A third prominence is the most posterior portion of the elbow at its apex, called the **olecranon process** of the ulna. Fractures about the elbow usually result in distortion of the normal alignment of these three prominences.

Immediately posterior to the medial condyle of the humerus is a groove in which the **ulnar nerve** passes. This groove can be easily felt by extending the elbow fully. The ulnar nerve is extremely important, as it controls sensation over the fourth and fifth fingers and most of the muscular function of the hand. The ulnar nerve is easily damaged in elbow injuries. Contusions to this nerve at the elbow produce tingling in the fourth and fifth fingers, an event referred to as injuring the "funny bone."

The **median nerve** may also be injured about the elbow. This nerve lies near the anterior surface of the elbow, approximately in the midline. It is more protected in this area by adjacent muscles than is the ulnar nerve.

Forearm

The forearm is composed of two bones, the **ulna** and the **radius**. The ulna is larger in the proximal part of the forearm, and the radius is larger in the distal part. The entire **ulnar shaft** from the tip of the olecranon process distally can be palpated, as it lies just under the skin on the posterior surface of the forearm (Fig. 9.22). The radius is covered by muscles and cannot be palpated except in the lower third of the forearm where it enlarges to form a major portion of the wrist joint.

Wrist

Just as the two bones of the leg form a socket for the ankle joint, there are bony prominences on the ends of the radius and ulna to form the socket for the wrist joint (see Fig. 9.22). Here they are called **styloid processes.** Both the **radial styloid** and the **ulnar styloid** are easily palpable. The radial styloid is on the thumb side of the wrist, and the ulnar styloid is on the little finger side. Simultaneous palpation of these two processes will reveal that the radial styloid

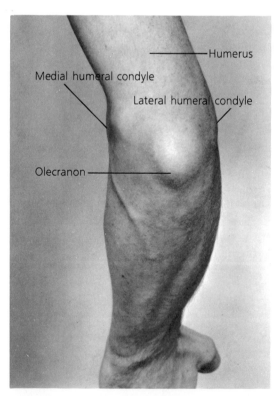

FIGURE 9.21. Posterior view of the elbow, showing the three bony prominences.

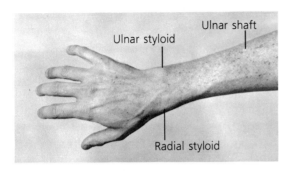

FIGURE 9.22. Dorsal view of the forearm and wrist.

process usually lies about half an inch distal to that of the ulna. With displaced wrist fractures, this relationship may be reversed, or the processes may lie at the same level.

Hand

The hand articulates with the forearm through the 8 **carpal bones**. The palm of the hand is formed by 5 **metacarpal bones** and the thumb and fingers by the 14 phalanges.

Arterial Pulse Points

At any point where an artery passes over a bony prominence or lies close to the skin, it can be palpated and the arterial pulse taken. These points are called **arterial pressure points** because it was initially believed that compression at one of these points would help control hemorrhage distal to it. Although this principle is sound and applies to any artery in the body, pressure over any single artery rarely stops circulation distal to that point completely, because more than one artery is always supplying blood to an injury site. Therefore, local pressure on the wound remains the best method to control hemorrhage.

At major arterial pulse points (Fig. 9.23) it is usually easy to find the arterial pulse and to ascertain correctly the presence of cardiac activity or the absence of a proximal arterial injury.

Anterior to the upper portion of the ear, just over the temporomandibular joints, lie the **superficial temporal arteries** that supply

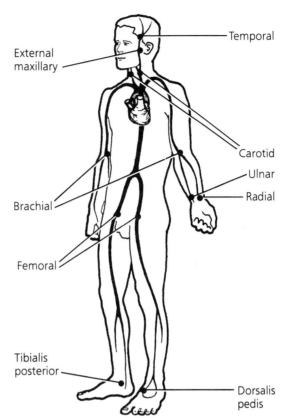

FIGURE 9.23. Major arterial pulse points.

the scalp. Anterior to the angle of the mandible, on the inner surface of the lower jaw on either side, one may palpate the **external maxillary arteries**, which contribute much of the blood supply to the face. The **carotid arteries** may be compressed anteriorly against the transverse processes of the sixth cervical vertebra just behind the artery. At the inner surface of the arm, the **brachial artery** may be palpated approximately 1½ inches above the elbow. Arterial pulsation may be felt in both the **radial** and **ulnar** arteries at the wrist and at the bases of the thumb and little finger, respectively.

The **femoral artery** may be palpated as it issues from beneath the inguinal ligament in the groin. Just posterior to the medial malleolus is the **posterior tibial artery**. On the anterior surface of the foot just lateral to the major extensor tendon of the great toe is the **dorsalis pedis artery**. This artery is not as constantly present as the posterior

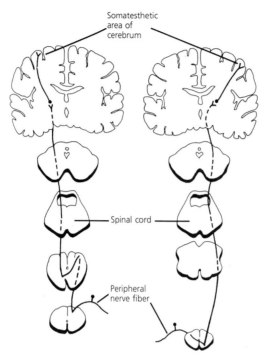

FIGURE 9.24. The left side of the brain receives sensory input from the right side of the body and vice versa.

tibial artery, but when present, its pulsations may be felt easily.

SKIN DERMATOMES

Sensations of touch, pain, temperature, and position follow similar neurological patterns from the stimulus site to the brain. Peripheral nerve fibers pass to the spinal cord and cross to the opposite side before reaching the brain. They terminate through synapses in the somatesthetic area of the cerebrum. Thus, the left side of the brain receives these sensory inputs from the right side of the body and vice versa (Fig. 9.24).

The sensory patterns on the skin follow a distinct scheme, which is related to the paired nerve roots emanating from the spinal cord. The cranial nerves receive sensation from the face. This pattern of innervation of the skin is called a **sensory dermatome scheme** (Fig. 9.25).

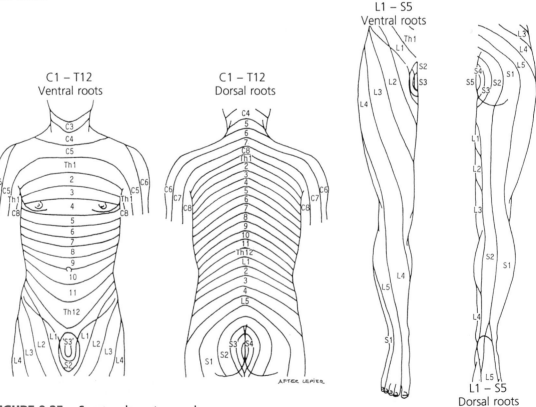

FIGURE 9.25. Sensory dermatome scheme.

IMPORTANT CONCEPTS

1. Knowledge of topographic anatomy is essential for conducting a thorough inspection of the injured athlete.
2. Use of correct terminology enables the athletic trainer to convey much useful information quickly and accurately.
3. The head consists of the cranium and face.
4. The neck contains the upper portion of the esophagus, the trachea, and the first seven vertebrae.
5. The spine serves as a protective canal for the spinal cord and is the central structure of the body on which all extremities and ribs articulate to form the complete skeleton.
6. The thorax contains the heart, lungs, esophagus, diaphragm, and great vessels (the aorta and two venae cavae).
7. The abdomen contains the major organs of digestion and excretion; the lower portion of the abdomen, referred to as the pelvic cavity, contains the organs of reproduction, the rectum, and the urinary bladder.
8. The pelvis is a closed bony ring, consisting of the sacrum and the innominate bone that connects the trunk to the lower extremities.
9. The lower extremity consists of the hip, thigh, knee, leg, ankle, and foot.
10. The upper extremity consists of the shoulder, arm, elbow, forearm, wrist, and hand.
11. The shoulder girdle is composed of the clavicle, scapula, and humeral head.
12. Arterial pressure points are places where an artery passes over a bony prominence or lies close to the skin; there the artery can be palpated and the arterial pulse taken.
13. Sensations of touch, pain, temperature, and position follow similar neurological patterns of innervation called a sensory dermatome scheme.

SUGGESTED READINGS

Backhouse, Kenneth M., and Ralph T. Hutchings. *Color Atlas of Surface Anatomy: Clinical and Applied.* Baltimore: Williams & Wilkins, 1986.

Clemente, Carmine D. *Anatomy, A Regional Atlas of the Human Body,* 3rd ed. Baltimore: Urban & Schwarzenberg, 1987.

Gray, Henry. *Anatomy of the Human Body,* 30th American ed. Philadelphia: Lea & Febiger, 1985.

McMinn, R. M. H., and R. T. Hutchings. *Color Atlas of Human Anatomy,* 2nd ed. Chicago: Year Book Medical Publishers, 1988.

Netter, Frank H., et al. *The CIBA Collection of Medical Illustrations.* Vol. 8, *Musculoskeletal System.* Part I, *Anatomy, Physiology, and Metabolic Disorders.* Summit, N.J.: CIBA-Geigy, 1987.

Sobotta, Johannes. *Atlas of Human Anatomy,* 10th English ed., vol. 1: "Head, Neck, Upper Extremities;" vol. 2: "Thorax, Abdomen, Pelvis, Lower Extremities, Skin". Baltimore: Urban & Schwarzenberg, 1983.

Warfel, John H. *The Extremities: Muscles and Motor Points,* 5th ed. Philadelphia: Lea & Febiger, 1985.

————. *The Head, Neck, and Trunk,* 5th ed. Philadelphia: Lea & Febiger, 1985.

10

Evaluation of the Ill and Injured Athlete

CHAPTER OUTLINE

Role of the Athletic Trainer
The Clinical Evaluation Process
   The Medical History
   Physical Testing of the Injured
   Athlete
     Stress Testing
     Manual and Mechanical Muscle
     Testing

Range-of-Motion and
Goniometry Testing
Motor and Sensory Function
Testing
Functional Assessment

OBJECTIVES FOR CHAPTER 10

After reading this chapter, the student should be able to:
1. Describe the role of the athletic trainer in evaluation of the ill and injured athlete.
2. Describe the nine steps in obtaining a medical history.
3. Define and describe the physical evaluation of an injured athlete.

INTRODUCTION

Most injuries and illnesses suffered by athletes do not require emergency care. When emergency care is not required, the athletic trainer must decide whether the athlete should be treated in the training room, referred to a physician or hospital, or referred to other medical and allied health professionals such as a dentist or counselor. Chapter 10 describes the evaluation process that the athletic trainer must carry out in order to make these decisions. The chapter describes the nine steps involved in obtaining a medical history and the tests that are performed during a physical examination of the injured athlete. ■

ROLE OF THE ATHLETIC TRAINER

When an athlete's injury or illness does not require emergency care, the athletic trainer is often required to perform a thorough clinical evaluation to determine the nature of the injury or illness, the need for referral to the team physician for further examination and treatment, or the practicality of treating the athlete according to routine standing orders from the team physician. Once a diagnosis is made, a treatment program can be designed to return the athlete to competition. However, treatment other than initial first aid should not begin until a diagnosis is made.

Athletes will consult the athletic trainer for assistance in a variety of circumstances, ranging from acute injuries sustained in a game or in a practice to overuse injuries and chronic injuries that are affecting their performance, as well as medical concerns that are unrelated to an athletic injury. Because each situation is different, only general guidelines can be provided regarding the chronology and content of the evaluation process.

THE CLINICAL EVALUATION PROCESS

The Medical History

The initial, and probably most important, step in the clinical evaluation process is the medical history. A complete history is obtained when the right questions are asked.

The process of obtaining a history requires a great deal of practice and experience before the athletic trainer develops a comfortable and effective style. In many instances, the medical history alone describes the illness or the injury sustained, and the physical evaluation only substantiates the athletic trainer's assessment.

The process of taking a medical history varies, depending on individual circumstances. An athlete who has provided a detailed preseason history and who is well known to the athletic trainer will be managed differently from an athlete whom the trainer has never met. Whichever is the case, the athletic trainer must be certain to have all of the necessary medical information before continuing the evaluation with physical testing. The results of the evaluation should be recorded in the SOAP notes as discussed in Chapter 6.

The medical history consists of the following nine steps. Individual circumstances will make some steps more or less important and may affect the order in which they are addressed.

1. *Look at the athlete.* Does the athlete appear anxious? Is his or her posture normal? Does he or she walk and move freely or limp or guard the injury?

2. *Identify the athlete.* The athletic trainer should note the athlete's name, age, and gender, and identify what sport and position the person plays.

3. *Identify the chief complaint.* Specifically, why is the athlete seeking medical assistance at this time?

4. *Review the athlete's medical history and pertinent previous traumatic events.* The trainer must determine if the current problem is recurrent or chronic. Has the athlete ever suffered a similar injury or illness? Has the athlete ever sustained an injury, or had surgery on the injured or opposite extremity? If there is a history of a recurrent or chronic condition, the trainer should find out how the problem was treated and if the treatment was thought to be successful.

5. *Review the symptoms.* The trainer determines if the athlete has a fever, nausea, or dizziness, or has swelling or numbness. What is the athlete's interpretation of the injury or illness? In asking about the athlete's pain, the trainer will find the PQRST mnemonic helpful:

- *Provocation*—What caused or causes the pain? Is it acute, subacute, or chronic? For example, the athlete may state, "It hurts when I throw a curve ball," "The pain in my wrist started when I fell during practice last Friday," or "My shoulder has been giving me trouble since last season."
- *Quality*—Is the pain sharp, aching, burning, dull, etc.?
- *Region and/or radiation*—Where does it hurt? Does the pain radiate? For example, in an athlete complaining of back pain, does the pain radiate down the legs?
- *Severity*—How intense is the pain? Does it affect sleeping or studying?
- *Timing*—When does it hurt, for how long, and what makes the pain better or worse?

6. *Review the athlete's social history and personal health habits.* Occasionally, questions regarding the athlete's social and personal life (sexual activity, drug use, eating habits, etc.) are necessary. While the athletic trainer is usually concerned with musculoskeletal injuries, he or she is often viewed by the athlete as a knowledgeable allied health care provider who can be consulted about other health concerns. The athletic trainer should always maintain the confidentiality of the athlete's medical history, especially with regard to social and personal habits.

The athletic trainer will encounter athletes who are pregnant and athletes who have sexually transmitted diseases, serious eating disorders, and problems with substance abuse and depression. Most athletic trainers have minimal experience and expertise in these areas. Therefore, a variety of medical specialists should be included in the sports medicine team on a formal or informal basis and a mechanism for confidential referral should be developed by the team physician and athletic trainer before a crisis arises.

7. *Review the athlete's family history.* In addition to an athlete's social and personal history, the athlete's family history may provide important information about the athlete's current condition. Anxiety over family crises and health issues may be manifested as physical and psychological concerns on the part of the athlete. By discussing the athlete's family history, the athletic trainer and team physician are better prepared to provide the medical and social support the athlete needs.

8. *Define the problem or complaint.* The trainer should review the features of the medical history that appear to be related to the chief complaint of the athlete. This process assures that the athletic trainer has understood the athlete correctly and allows the athlete an opportunity to add additional information.

9. *Palpation.* Palpation means to examine by touch. It may be considered a separate step in the clinical evaluation, but is included as part of the medical history because it is a logical extension of the process of identifying the location and cause of the athlete's symptoms. In general, palpation should be conducted at the end of the medical history to avoid the tendency

to touch, push, and pry without listening to the athlete. Frequently, the athlete can define the problem, and therefore, unnecessary and sometimes painful palpation can be avoided. The athletic trainer should identify the areas of swelling, local tenderness, heat, deformity, and crepitus or grating as the injury or painful area is being palpated.

There is a corollary to the nine steps in the medical history: think anatomically! The athletic trainer should review the regional anatomy and function of structures in the area identified by the athlete's chief complaint.

The medical history usually provides a working diagnosis that can be confirmed by physical examination and special tests such as x-rays. Occasionally, the medical history does not provide a working diagnosis or the physical examination fails to confirm the athletic trainer's suspicions. Despite that possibility, there is no substitute for obtaining a complete medical history in the clinical evaluation.

Physical Testing of the Injured Athlete

Several procedures are useful in the clinical evaluation to confirm the working diagnosis obtained from the medical history, to document the athlete's status, or to chart the athlete's progress through treatment and rehabilitation. These procedures include the following:

- Stress testing of the ligaments that are supporting joints to determine the severity of a sprain.
- Manual muscle testing to determine the force generated by a particular muscle group.
- Range-of-motion assessment through goniometry to document the degree of restricted motion.
- Sensory nerve assessment.
- Assessment of the athlete's functional performance in tasks specific to the demands of the sport.

This section provides an introduction to these various tests. More extensive information may be found in the references listed at the end of the chapter. Other testing, such as taking the athlete's temperature, may also be appropriate but are not addressed in this chapter (see Chapter 11).

Stress Testing

Stress testing involves placing a stress on the ligaments supporting a joint. Generally, the uninjured extremity is tested first to determine the normal ligamentous stability and to permit the athlete to experience the maneuver on a pain-free joint. It is important to note previous injuries to the uninvolved side so that a joint with residual instability is not considered normal.

The medical history usually suggests that certain structures have been injured. These structures are examined last because stress testing may cause pain and guarding that will limit further testing. All of the structures of an injured joint should be stress tested—not just those the athletic trainer suspects have been injured.

In general, a painful stress test with minimal joint laxity and a firm end point indicates a first-degree sprain. A second-degree sprain demonstrates a marked degree of laxity with a firm end point and pain with stress testing. A third-degree sprain results in extreme laxity and a very soft end point, which usually indicates that soft tissues other than the stressed ligament are resisting the force applied. Frequently, the athlete experiences little or no pain when a third-degree sprain is stressed because the ligament is completely torn, and therefore is not stressed during testing. (Stress testing of the major ligaments of the elbow, knee, and ankle is outlined in Chapters 17, 21, and 23, respectively.)

Manual and Mechanical Muscle Testing

Manual muscle testing involves resisting the active contraction of a muscle group for the purpose of comparing the muscle func-

MUSCLE EXAMINATION

Patient's Name _____ Chart No. _____

Date of Birth _____ Name of Institution_____

LEFT   RIGHT

				Examiner's Initials				
				Date					
				NECK Flexors — Sternocleidomastoid					
				Extensor Group					
				TRUNK Flexors — Rectus abdominis					
				R. Ext. abd. obl. ⎱ Rotators ⎰ L. Ext. abd. obl. L. Int. abd. obl. ⎰ ⎱ R. Int. abd. obl.					
				Extensors ⎰ Thoracic group ⎱ Lumbar group					
				Pelvic elev. — Quadratus lumb.					
				HIP Flexors ⎰ Iliopsoas ⎱ Sartorius					
				Extensors — Gluteus maximus					
				Abductors ⎰ Gluteus medius ⎱ Tensor fascia lata					
				Adductor group					
				Lateral rotator group					
				Medial rotator group					
				KNEE Flexors ⎰ Biceps femoris ⎱ Inner hamstrings					
				Extensors — Quadriceps femoris					
				ANKLE Plantar flexors ⎰ Gastrocnemius ⎱ Soleus					
				FOOT Invertors ⎰ Tibialis anterior ⎱ Tibialis posterior					
				Evertors ⎰ Peroneus brevis ⎱ Peroneus longus					
				TOES M. P. flexors — Lumbricals					
				I. P. flexors (Prox.) — Flex. digit. br.					
				I. P. flexors (Distal) — Flex. digit. l.					
				M. P. extensors ⎰ Ext. digit. l. ⎱ Ext. digit. br.					
				HALLUX M. P. flexor — Flex. hall. br.					
				I. P. flexor — Flex. hall. l.					
				M. P. extensor — Ext. hall. br.					
				I. P. extensor — Ext. hall. l.					
				GAIT:					

GRADING SYSTEM

Completes range of motion against gravity	*Completes range of motion*	*No range of motion*
N Normal —with full resistance at end of range	F Fair —against gravity	T Trace —slight contraction
G Good —with some resistance at end of range	P Poor —with gravity decreased	0 Zero —no contraction

FIGURE 10.1. Manual muscle exam. (From Daniels, Lucille, M.A., and Catherine Worthingham, Ph.D., D.SC. *Muscle Testing: Techniques of Manual Examination,* 5th edition. Philadelphia: W. B. Saunders Company, 1986, pp. 9–10.)

MUSCLE EXAMINATION

LEFT   RIGHT

				Examiner's Initials							
				Date							
				SCAPULA	Abductor	Serratus anterior					
					Elevator	Trapezius (superior)					
					Depressor	Trapezius (inferior)					
					Adductors	{ Trapezius middle) { Rhomboid maj. & min.					
				SHOULDER	Flexor	Deltoid (anterior)					
					Extensors	{ Latissimus dorsi { Teres major					
					Abductor	Deltoid (middle)					
					Horiz. abd.	Deltoid (posterior)					
					Horiz. add.	Pectoralis major					
					Lateral rotator group						
					Medial rotator group						
				ELBOW	Flexors	{ Biceps brachii { Brachialis { Brachioradialis					
					Extensor	Triceps brachii					
				FOREARM	Supinator group						
					Pronator group						
				WRIST	Flexors	{ Flex. carpi rad. { Flex. carpi uln.					
					Extensors	{ Ext. carpi rad. l. & br. { Ext. carpi uln.					
				FINGERS	M. P. flexors	Lumbricals					
					I. P. flexors (Prox.)	Flex. digit. sup.					
					I. P. flexors (Distal)	Flex. digit. prof.					
					M. P. extensor	Ext. digit. com.					
					Adductors	Palmar interossei					
					Abductors	Dorsal interossei					
					Abductor digiti minimi						
					Opponens digiti minimi						
				THUMB	M. P. flexor	Flex. poll. br.					
					I. P. flexor	Flex. poll. l.					
					M. P. extensor	Ext. poll. br.					
					I. P. extensor	Ext. poll. l.					
					Abductors	{ Abd. poll. br. { Abd. poll. l.					
					Adductor pollicis						
					Opponens pollicis						
				FACE:							

Additional data:

149

tion with the opposite extremity or an expected level. Manual muscle testing is useful in determining the severity of a strain, in evaluating strength losses following joint injury or surgery, and in deciding if an injury to the nervous system has resulted in a motor deficit.

Generally, the athlete's muscle is stressed throughout the functional range of motion. Manual testing of each muscle group should be done as part of the preseason screening examination. These results can be recorded in chart form (Fig. 10.1, on pages 148–149) and kept in the athlete's file, along with Cybex testing scores, flexibility scores, joint range-of-motion and laxity assessment, and other baseline data.

Following an injury, manual muscle testing in the area of injury is done, and scores are compared to those of the preseason screening. Flexibility scores and joint range-of-motion and laxity assessment are also performed and compared with the preseason determination during the injury assessment process.

The force of the muscle contraction is graded in a standardized manner familiar to physicians, athletic trainers, and physical therapists (Table 10.1). Manual muscle testing does not attempt to quantify precisely the force generated by a muscle group. However, the procedure is very useful in the clinical evaluation of musculoskeletal

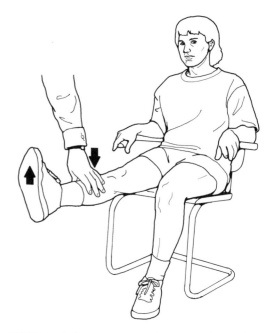

FIGURE 10.2. Knee extension manual muscle test.

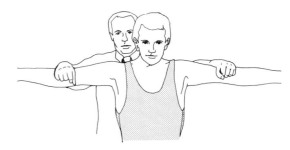

FIGURE 10.3. Shoulder abduction manual muscle test.

injuries. Figures 10.2 and 10.3 illustrate manual muscle testing of the knee extensors and shoulder abductors.

Mechanical computerized muscle testing can be performed on dynamometers such as the Cybex (Lumex Inc., Ronkonkomo, New York) or Kin Com (Chatex, Chattanooga, Tennessee). These devices offer more precise quantification of muscle function and are very useful in charting the athlete's recovery and providing motivation during rehabilitation. However, they are expensive and do not replace manual muscle testing in the initial examination.

TABLE 10.1. Manual Muscle Strength Grading

Muscle Strength	(%)	Concentration	Grade
Complete range of motion (ROM) against gravity, with full resistance	100	Normal	5
Complete ROM against gravity, with some resistance	75	Good	4
Complete ROM against gravity, with no resistance	50	Fair	3
Complete ROM, with gravity omitted	25	Poor	2
Evidence of slight contractility, with no joint motion	10	Trace	1
No evidence of muscle contractility	0	Zero	0

Range-of-Motion and Goniometry Testing

The active range of motion of the joints of an injured extremity should be measured and quantified with a standard goniometer (a protractor used to measure joint range of motion). If the range of motion is restricted, then the athlete's progress in regaining motion can be easily documented. Assessing the range of motion is especially important in the postoperative course of joint reconstructive surgery following fractures and dislocations. Goniometry is also used during the preparticipation physical evaluation. Standard goniometric measurements of the shoulder, elbow, hip, knee, and ankle are illustrated in Figures 10.4 through 10.20.

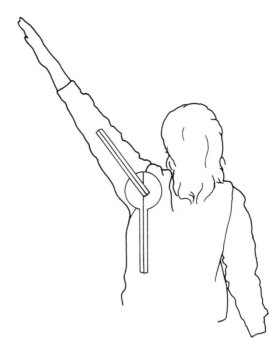

FIGURE 10.6.   Recording shoulder abduction.

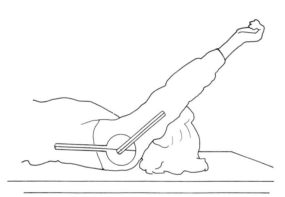

FIGURE 10.4.   Recording shoulder forward flexion.

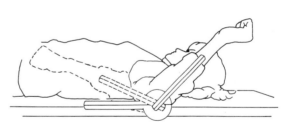

FIGURE 10.7.   Recording shoulder internal rotation.

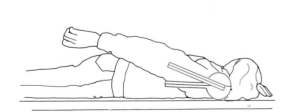

FIGURE 10.5.   Recording shoulder backward extension.

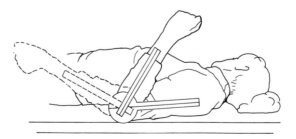

FIGURE 10.8.   Recording elbow extension.

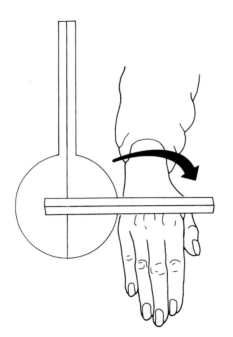

FIGURE 10.9. Recording forearm pronation.

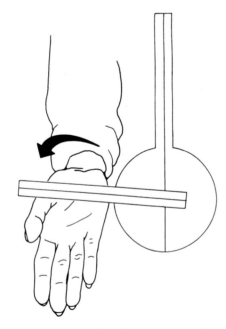

FIGURE 10.10. Recording forearm supination.

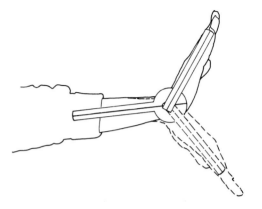

FIGURE 10.11. Recording wrist flexion.

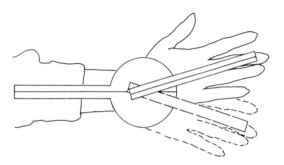

FIGURE 10.12. Recording wrist ulnar deviation.

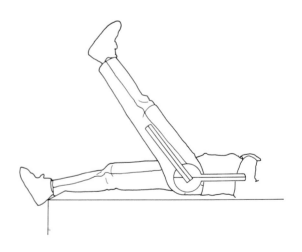

FIGURE 10.13. Recording hip flexion.

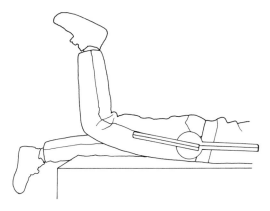

FIGURE 10.14. Recording hip extension.

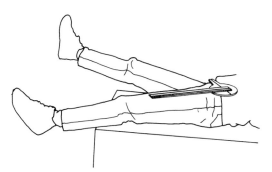

FIGURE 10.15. Recording hip abduction.

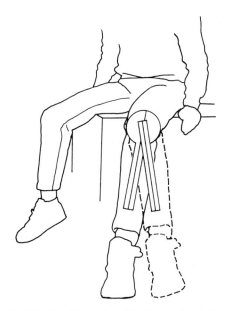

FIGURE 10.16. Recording hip internal rotation.

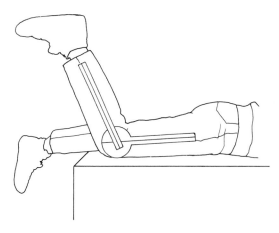

FIGURE 10.17. Recording knee flexion.

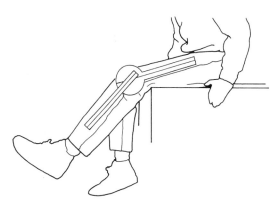

FIGURE 10.18. Recording knee extension.

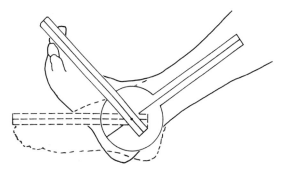

FIGURE 10.19. Recording ankle plantar flexion.

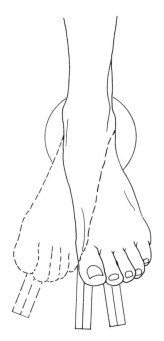

FIGURE 10.20. Recording ankle inversion.

Motor and Sensory Function Testing

Injuries to the central and peripheral nervous systems can result in motor and sensory deficits. The athletic trainer must be familiar with the motor and sensory distribution of the peripheral and spinal nerves. Motor and sensory function should be assessed following head and neck trauma, whenever fractures and/or dislocations are suspected, and any time the athlete complains of altered sensation.

Functional Assessment

A final clinical evaluation should be undertaken before the injured athlete is given permission to return to practice and competition. When the athlete demonstrates adequate joint stability, normal nervous system function, unrestricted range of motion, and 85 to 90 percent muscle strength, a functional assessment should be performed before the athlete returns to play.

The functional assessment should be tailored to the athlete's sport and position. The trainer should have the athlete perform the tasks required by his or her sport using normal movement patterns in a pain-free manner. Unfortunately, a functional assessment is often not conducted because of the inconvenience of taking athletes to the gym or practice field and watching them run, cut, jump, back pedal, throw, and catch. Many athletes are returned to practice solely on their report of pain-free activities of daily living and normal range of motion and strength. Some of these athletes have not, in fact, fully recovered the timing and the specific movement patterns necessary for their sport, and these deficits may predispose them to reinjury.

Athletes should advance from individual to team drills as their progress permits. The athletic trainer, team physician, strength and conditioning coach, and the team coach must work to help athletes regain their sport-specific skills before full practice and competition are allowed.

IMPORTANT CONCEPTS

1. The athletic trainer performs a thorough evaluation to determine the nature of the illness or injury, the need for referral to the team physician for further examination and treatment, or the practicality of treating the athlete according to routine standing orders from the team physician.
2. The medical history, probably the most important step in the clinical evaluation process, provides a working diagnosis that can be confirmed by physical examination and special tests such as x-rays.
3. Stress testing, manual muscle testing, range-of-motion assessment, sensory nerve assessment, and assessment of functional performance confirm the working diagnosis from the medical history.

SUGGESTED READINGS

Hoppenfeld, S. *Physical Examination of the Spine and Extremities.* New York: Appleton-Century-Crofts, 1976.

Kendall, F. P., and E. K. McCreary. *Muscles: Testing and Function,* 3d ed. Baltimore: Williams & Wilkins, 1983.

Magee, D. J. *Orthopedic Physical Assessment.* Philadelphia: W. B. Saunders, 1987.

Norker, C. C., and J. J. White. *Measurements of Joint Motion: A Guide to Goniometry.* Philadelphia: F. A. Davis, 1985.

11

Emergency Assessment of the Injured Athlete

CHAPTER OUTLINE

OBJECTIVES FOR CHAPTER 11

After reading this chapter, the student should be able to:
1. Explain the difference between a sign and a symptom.
2. List the body's nine diagnostic signs and normal measurements/responses for each.
3. Describe how changes in any of the diagnostic signs, along with symptoms, can assist the athletic trainer in the initial assessment of the injured athlete.
4. Explain the process of conducting a primary and secondary survey on the injured athlete.
5. List and describe the conditions and injuries requiring priority for management and triage.

INTRODUCTION

Accurate, efficient assessment of the athlete by the athletic trainer at the scene of injury is essential for proper emergency care of the athlete. By adopting a standardized approach, the trainer does not overlook important details and knows how to respond to any situation that may arise, including situations involving several injured people where triage is required.

Chapter 11 begins by detailing the nine diagnostic signs that the trainer observes during the emergency assessment of the injured athlete. The chapter then describes the primary and secondary surveys that the trainer conducts to observe and evaluate the injured athlete's medical problems. The last section of Chapter 11 explains how triage is carried out. ▪

THE NINE DIAGNOSTIC SIGNS

Part of the physical examination of any injured or ill athlete is noting certain **signs** that are manifestations of changes in body function apparent to the athletic trainer, and hence, different from **symptoms**, which are evidence of changes in body function apparent to the athlete and expressed to the athletic trainer as subjective complaints. The nine essential diagnostic signs—pulse, respiration, blood pressure, body temperature, color of the skin, status of pupils, state of consciousness, ability to move, and reaction to pain—can be observed rapidly during examination. Together with question-ing about symptoms and the physical examination, they form the basis for diagnosis or further evaluation.

Pulse

Normal Pulse Rate

The **pulse** is the pressure wave, traveling along the arteries, caused by the contraction of the heart. The usual pulse rate in adults is 60 to 100 beats per minute (40 to 60 beats per minute in most well-trained athletes); in children the usual rate is 80 to

100 beats per minute. The pulse can be palpated (felt by touch) at any site on the body where an artery passes over a bony prominence or is close to the skin.

Palpation of the Pulse

Commonly, the place to palpate the pulse is in the wrist. The fingertip is placed over the palmar surface of the wrist where the radial artery is fairly superficial (Fig. 11.1a). However, palpation of the radial pulse may be difficult in an emergency and not always accurate. Instead, the carotid artery in the neck is the preferred site to palpate the pulse, although the pulse can be felt in other major arteries. For example, the athlete's pulse can be taken under the anterior border of the sternocleidomastoid muscle (Fig. 11.1b). The athlete must always be lying down or sitting, and the pulse taker must palpate gently. If no pulse is detected, an unconscious athlete should be considered pulseless and without effective circulation of the blood to the organs of the body. Cardiopulmonary resuscitation (see Chapter 37, "Basic Life Support") should be instituted immediately.

Changes in Pulse Rate and Volume

Changes in the rate and volume of the pulse are important findings in emergency medical care. The pulse rate is easily checked and reflects the rapidity of the heart contractions. The pulse volume describes the sensation the contraction gives to the palpating finger. Normally, the pulse is a strong, easily felt impulse reflecting a full blood volume. A rapid, weak pulse can result from dehydration or shock from loss of blood; a rapid, bounding pulse is present in fright or hypertension. The absence of a pulse means the specific artery is blocked or injured, the heart has stopped functioning (cardiac arrest), or death has occurred. Changes in the pulse directly reflect changes in heart rate in response to injury or alarm, changes in circulating blood volume, or changes in the vascular bed.

The pulse should be taken immediately and then periodically during emergency

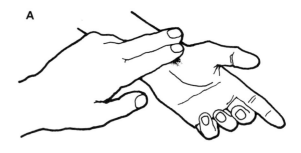

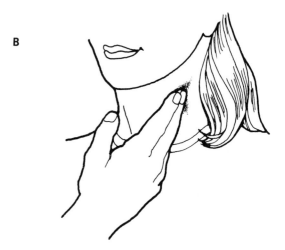

FIGURE 11.1. (a) Radial and (b) carotid pulses are usually easily palpated.

treatment to note any changes. The pulse rates should be written down as they are taken, along with the character of the pulse (whether it is weak or strong). Keep in mind that following a severe injury, initial vital signs may be normal, but they can change rapidly and the athlete's condition may deteriorate quickly. Pulse measurement and skin color (discussed later in the chapter) are the two most common indicators of blood flow during initial assessment of an injured athlete.

Respiration

Normal Breathing

Normal breathing is easy, without pain or effort. The rate of respiration can vary widely, although it is usually between 12 and 20 breaths per minute. Well-trained athletes may breathe only 6 to 8 times a minute. In most individuals the resting respiratory rate rarely exceeds 20 breaths per minute.

Changes in Breathing

Following an injury, a record should be made of the initial rate and character of respiration when the athlete is first evaluated. Then, any changes that occur during assessment should be noted. Rapid, shallow respirations are seen in shock. Deep, gasping, or labored breathing may indicate partial airway obstruction or pulmonary disease. In respiratory arrest, there is no movement of the chest and abdomen. Severe metabolic disturbances which produce a chemical **acidosis** or **alkalosis** may cause an altered respiratory rate. By decreasing the breathing rate, one retains carbon dioxide and can neutralize a metabolic acidosis. By increasing the breathing rate, one increases the amount of carbon dioxide expired, and hence can neutralize a metabolic alkalosis. If no metabolic abnormality exists, **hyperventilation**, or an increase in breathing rate, will result in the athlete rapidly breathing off carbon dioxide, and can quickly cause a temporary metabolic alkalosis manifested by numbness, tingling, and a feeling of light-headedness. Hyperventilation may occur as a response to metabolic disturbances and decreased tissue oxygen, the latter frequently occurring in the unconditioned athlete. Hyperventilation is also a common manifestation of fear. Breathing into a paper bag—that is rebreathing one's own air—rapidly reverses this alkalosis. Increased athletic activity, especially in unconditioned athletes, may result in an increase in breathing rate.

Frothy Sputum

An injured athlete who starts to cough up frothy sputum, with blood at the nose and mouth, probably has an injury to the lung, as can occur when the lung is perforated by a fractured rib. Frothy pink or bloody sputum may also be a manifestation of pulmonary edema, which can accompany acute cardiac failure or severe lung contusion.

Breath Odor

Occasionally, one can learn much from the smell of an athlete's breath. The breath of an intoxicated athlete typically smells like alcohol. The breath of an athlete in severe diabetic acidosis may have a sweet or fruity odor. Any particularly obvious odor should be noted and recorded.

Blood Pressure

Blood pressure is the pressure of the circulating blood against the walls of the arteries. In the normal person the arterial system is a closed system, attached to a pump (the heart), and completely filled with blood. Any changes in the pressure indicate changes in the volume of the blood, in the capacity of the vessels, or in the ability of the heart to pump. Changes in blood pressure, like those in the pulse, can occur rapidly.

Systolic and Diastolic Pressure

Blood pressure is recorded at systolic and diastolic levels. **Systolic pressure** is the level present during contraction of the heart muscle. **Diastolic pressure** is the level present during relaxation of the heart muscle. Systolic pressure is the maximum pressure to which the arteries are subjected, and diastolic pressure is the minimum pressure constantly present in the arteries. Usually, these pressures change in a parallel fashion —that is, they both rise or they both fall. Brain damage in an athlete with a head injury sometimes causes a rise in the systolic pressure, with a stable or falling diastolic pressure. Systolic and diastolic pressures that approach each other—that is, as the systolic pressure falls the diastolic pressure rises—occur in cardiac tamponade, a condition in which the balloonlike covering of the heart fills with blood.

Blood pressure is measured with a sphygmomanometer and a stethoscope (Fig. 11.2). The pressure reading is in millimeters of mercury (mm Hg) and is recorded in

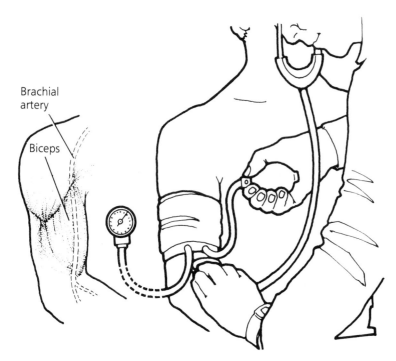

Brachial
artery

Biceps

FIGURE 11.2. The proper location for and application of the sphygmomanometer and stethoscope.

the form systolic/diastolic. The cuff of the sphygmomanometer is fastened about either arm above the elbow and is inflated with a rubber bulb until the mercury column or the needle of the dial stops moving with the pulse. This point, usually between 150 and 200 mm Hg on the scale, should be 50 mm Hg higher than uppermost pressure so as not to miss very high blood pressures. The blood pressure cuff should be periodically recalibrated to ensure the accuracy of readings taken.

The stethoscope bell is placed over the brachial artery at the front of the elbow. Air is slowly released from the bulb as the gauge returns to zero. The point at which the first sounds of the pulse are heard through the stethoscope is the systolic pressure. The point at which the sounds disappear is the diastolic pressure.

At times no pressures can be heard. The athletic trainer must rely on watching for movement in the gauge at the moment of systolic pressure and seeing such move-

ment stop at the diastolic level. Then the athletic trainer should try to obtain the systolic pressure by the palpation method. With this technique, the athlete's radial pulse is palpated, and then the sphygmomanometer cuff is inflated. The pulse will disappear when the cuff pressure exceeds the systolic blood pressure. The cuff pressure is increased approximately 50 mm Hg above the point at which the pulse disappears. The cuff is then deflated gradually. When the palpating fingertip first feels a return of the radial pulse, the pressure recording on the gauge equals the systolic blood pressure.

Normal Blood Pressure

Blood pressure levels vary with age and sex. A useful rule of thumb for normal systolic pressure in the male is 100 plus the age of the athlete, up to a level of 140 to 150 mm Hg. Normal diastolic pressure in the male is 65 to 90 mm Hg. Both pressures are about 10 mm Hg lower in the female.

Changes in Blood Pressure

Blood pressure can fall markedly in states of shock, after severe bleeding, or following a heart attack. Lowered blood pressure means that there is insufficient volume or cardiac output in the arterial system to supply blood to all of the organs of the body. Some of these organs are at great risk of being severely damaged if they are deprived of an adequate blood supply for even a short period of time. The causes of low blood pressure must be rapidly ascertained and treated.

If blood pressure is abnormally high, the vessels in the arterial circuit may be damaged or blocked. It is equally important that the causes of this state be ascertained and treated.

Blood pressure can change rapidly during transport of an injured athlete to the hospital. Emergency department personnel must know the status of the blood pressure as early as possible, and any changes before arrival at the hospital. Therefore, during emergency medical care of the athlete, the athletic trainer should check and record the pressure at intervals as necessary, together with the time each reading was taken. If the athlete's pressure cannot be heard on one extremity, the trainer should always try the opposite extremity, as conditions such as occlusions in major arteries to the limb in which the flow can be blocked or diminished unilaterally do occur.

Exercise should only mildly increase the blood pressure, pulse, and respiratory rate in the fit athlete. However, the anxiety associated with an athletic competition may result in an increase in blood pressure in individuals with essential or labile hypertension. To identify those athletes with labile blood pressure, multiple determinations should be made in varying emotional situations. These athletes should be referred for further medical evaluation and counseling. Severely overweight, recreational athletes with mild hypertension frequently can return their pressures to normal with weight reduction and salt restriction.

Body Temperature

Normal Body Temperature

Normal body temperature is 98.6 degrees Fahrenheit (37 degrees Centigrade). When basal body temperature rises, blood is shunted to the peripheral circulation and sweating increases. When the sweat begins to evaporate, body temperature falls. If basal body temperature drops, blood is shunted away from the skin to the core to preserve heat. Also, the shivering reflex is initiated to raise body heat.

Body temperature is usually measured by placing the bulb of a thermometer beneath a person's tongue. The thermometer should be left in place with the mouth closed for approximately 3 minutes. With a child or uncooperative adult, the thermometer can be placed in the axilla (armpit), and the arm kept at the side. Axillary temperatures are notoriously inaccurate, take a long time to

register accurately (10 minutes), and should be used only if an oral temperature cannot be taken. Rectal temperature is very accurate and is usually taken, if necessary, in the emergency department. Rectal temperature is routinely 1/2 to 1 degree above oral temperature and is taken with a special rectal thermometer left in place for 1 minute. Rectal temperatures should be used to obtain core temperature in evaluating heat or cold injuries.

Changes in Body Temperature

Illness or injury produces changes in temperature. A cool, clammy (damp) skin indicates a general response of the sympathetic nervous system to body insult, such as blood loss (shock) or heat exhaustion (water loss). As a result of nervous stimulation, sweat glands become hyperactive and skin blood vessels contract, resulting in cold, pale, wet, or clammy skin. These signs are often the first indication of shock and must be recognized as such. Exposure to cold produces a cool, dry skin. A dry, hot skin may be caused by fever or by exposure to excessive heat, with profound water loss, as in heatstroke.

The exercising athlete might experience mild elevation of temperature, regardless of the weather conditions. However, any and all temperature elevations or depressions (in cold weather) should be assumed to be abnormal and investigated further by the team physician.

Skin Color

Normal Skin Color

In lightly pigmented people, skin color depends primarily on the presence of circulating blood in the subcutaneous blood vessels. In deeply pigmented people, skin color depends primarily on the pigment.

Changes in Skin Color

Pigment may hide skin color changes resulting from illness or injury. In athletes with deeply pigmented skin, the athletic trainer may need to look for changes in the fingernail beds, in the sclera (the white portion of the eye), or under the tongue. In lightly pigmented athletes where changes may be seen more easily, the colors of medical importance are red, white, and blue.

A red skin color may accompany high blood pressure, certain stages of carbon monoxide poisoning, and heatstroke. The athlete who has severe high blood pressure may sometimes be plethoric (dark, reddish-purple skin color). An athlete with carbon monoxide poisoning is usually cherry red, as is the heatstroke patient.

A pale, white, ashen, or grayish skin indicates insufficient circulation. It is most often seen in shock, acute heart attack, or certain stages of fright.

A bluish skin color, referred to as cyanosis, indicates poor oxygenation of the circulating blood. Poorly oxygenated blood is very dark and causes the overlying tissue to appear blue. Cyanosis may result from respiratory insufficiency due to airway obstruction or inadequate lung function. It is usually first seen in the fingertips and around the mouth.

Skin color changes also occur in certain systemic diseases. In diseases of the liver, for example, bilirubin, a normal reddish-yellow pigment of the biliary system, may increase and be deposited in the skin, turning it yellow.

Exercise normally increases skin blood flow and perspiration, producing reddish, clammy skin. Exposure to winter conditions may cause frostbite or freezing of the skin, accompanied by a characteristic whitish color.

Eye Pupils

Normal Eye Pupil Size

The pupils, when normal, are regular in outline and usually the same size. Anyone examining the pupils must remember to check for the presence of contact lenses or prostheses (glass eyes).

Constricted pupil

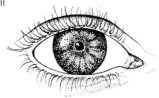

Dilated pupil

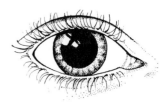

FIGURE 11.3.   Normal pupillary diameter is 2 to 3 mm.

Changes in Eye Pupil Size

Changes and variation in the size of one or both pupils are important signs in emergency medical care. Constricted pupils (Fig. 11.3) are often present in a drug addict or in an athlete who is suffering from a central nervous system disease or injury. Dilated pupils indicate a relaxed or unconscious state. Such dilation usually occurs rapidly —for example, within 30 seconds after cardiac arrest. Head injury or prior drug use, however, may cause the pupils to remain constricted, even in athletes who are in cardiac arrest.

A small percentage of normal persons have anisocoria (unequal pupil size). This finding should be highlighted on the athlete's preparticipation physical evaluation because it is an important piece of information if the athlete is unconscious or has sustained a head injury. If a history is unavailable, always assume that inequality of pupil size following an injury is a manifestation of head trauma and demands immediate physician evaluation.

Pupils ordinarily constrict promptly when light shines into the eye. This is the eye's normal protective reaction. The pupils fail to constrict when a light shines into the eye in cases of disease, poisoning, drug overdose, and injury. In death, the pupils are widely dilated and fail to respond to light. With exercise, the pupils will sometimes dilate due to the excitement; more often they remain normal in size.

State of Consciousness

Normal State of Consciousness

Under normal conditions, a person is alert, oriented (knows time, place, and what day it is), and responsive to vocal or physical stimuli (Fig. 11.4).

Changes in State of Consciousness

Any change from a normal, alert, and oriented state is indicative of illness or injury. Changes may vary from mild confusion to deep coma. Recording such changes is very important in emergency medical care.

Changes in mental status should be recorded periodically following injury while awaiting and during transport to a medical facility. On arrival at the emergency room, these changes should be relayed to emergency room personnel.

Ability to Move

The inability of a conscious person to move voluntarily is known as **paralysis**. Paralysis of both arms and legs indicates a high cervical spine injury. Paralysis of one side of the body (hemiplegia) may be caused by bleeding within the brain, a clot in a vessel (stroke), or a partial high cervical spine injury. Ability to move the arms but inability to move the legs after an accident generally indicates injury to the spinal cord somewhere below the neck.

All paralyzed individuals need immediate transport, with special precautions given to stabilization of the spine to avoid increased injury (see Chapter 32).

Reaction to Pain

Normal Reaction to Pain

Reaction by vocal response or body movement to painful physical stimulation such

NEUROLOGICAL CHECKLIST				
Time				
Talks	yes / no	yes / no	yes / no	yes / no
Follows commands	yes / no	yes / no	yes / no	yes / no
Pupil diameter	L R mm mm	L R mm mm	L R mm mm	L R mm mm

FIGURE 11.4. The neurological checklist used to record periodic observations of the athlete's level of consciousness.

as deep pressure to the sternum or pinching the Achilles tendon is a normal response of the body. Loss of this sensation following an injury or drug overdose reflects a lowering of the normal state of consciousness of the individual.

Changes in Reaction to Pain

The loss of voluntary movement of the extremities after an injury may be accompanied by loss of sensation in these extremities. Occasionally, movement is retained, and the athlete complains only of numbness or tingling in the extremities. This sensation can occur with spinal cord injury or with stretching or compression of the peripheral nerve supplying the extremity. Severe pain in the extremity, with loss of skin sensation, may be the result of the extremity's main artery being blocked (occlusion). In such a case the pulse in the extremity is absent. The athlete can usually move the extremity but often holds it immobile because of pain. All athletes who complain of loss or altered sensation in an extremity following an injury should be evaluated immediately by a physician. They should be assumed to have a spinal cord injury until proven otherwise, and thus they should be immobilized for transport immediately, in accordance with the precautions for transporting individuals with suspected spinal cord injuries.

CONDUCTING PRIMARY AND SECONDARY SURVEYS

Primary Survey

The **primary survey** (Fig. 11.5) is designed to discover and correct any immediate life-threatening problems. It begins as soon as the trainer reaches the injured player. During the primary survey, the athletic trainer needs only to talk, feel, and observe. No diagnostic equipment is needed. Inquiries should be brief and pertinent, with no detailed questioning at this time. Four diagnostic signs—state of consciousness, respiration, skin color, and pulse—should be observed.

During the primary survey, the athletic trainer must follow a definitive, step-by-step outline of action in observing the diagnostic signs. A disorganized or unplanned approach will result in lost time, inhibit emergency care, and create confusion at the scene. The trainer must remain calm no matter what the situation may be. A calm attitude instills confidence in the athlete. A record of initial observations should be started.

Secondary Survey

Upon completing the primary survey and controlling any immediate life-threatening problems, the athletic trainer should begin the **secondary survey**, which involves a more thorough examination of the athlete and, if necessary, preparation for transporting the athlete from the field to an emergency facility (see Fig. 11.5).

The athletic trainer should question the conscious athlete to determine symptoms and then note and record all of the athlete's complaints. Questioning is the best way to identify an underlying disease or injury process. The athletic trainer should be familiar with any important medical history and, if not, ask the athlete whether any similar episodes have occurred previously. Allowing the athlete to talk is very helpful, but at times the athletic trainer must direct the conversation so as to focus on the medical history.

Having obtained as much pertinent medical information as possible, the athletic trainer should thoroughly examine the area of injury. The examination should be conducted in a standard fashion. The effective secondary survey requires inspection, palpation, listening, and even, occasionally, the sense of smell to identify all abnormalities. The athletic trainer should become proficient enough to complete the examination within a few minutes. Except in life-threatening emergencies, this secondary survey should be completed before beginning stabilization and transport.

When the athlete is unconscious, the athletic trainer should first attend to life-threatening situations, and then evaluate the diagnostic signs. Immediate observers, such as other players, officials, or coaches, may provide important information and should be consulted. Ambulance assistance for stabilization and transport should be called for immediately. The telephone numbers of the rescue squad, hospital emergency department, team physicians, and consultants (home and office) should always be attached to the athletic training room phones and be present in the "on the field" trainer kit.

TRIAGE

Triage, or the assignment of treatment priorities, is required when injuries occur to more than one athlete at one time—for example, a team bus accident, lightning, or heat injury. Athletes with certain conditions or injuries have a priority for treatment and transportation.

Triage is generally divided into three categories: highest priority, second priority, and lowest priority. Highest-priority patients must be treated first at the scene and transported immediately. The following injuries or medical problems constitute the highest-priority category:

- Airway and breathing difficulties.
- Cardiac arrest.
- Uncontrolled or suspected severe internal bleeding.

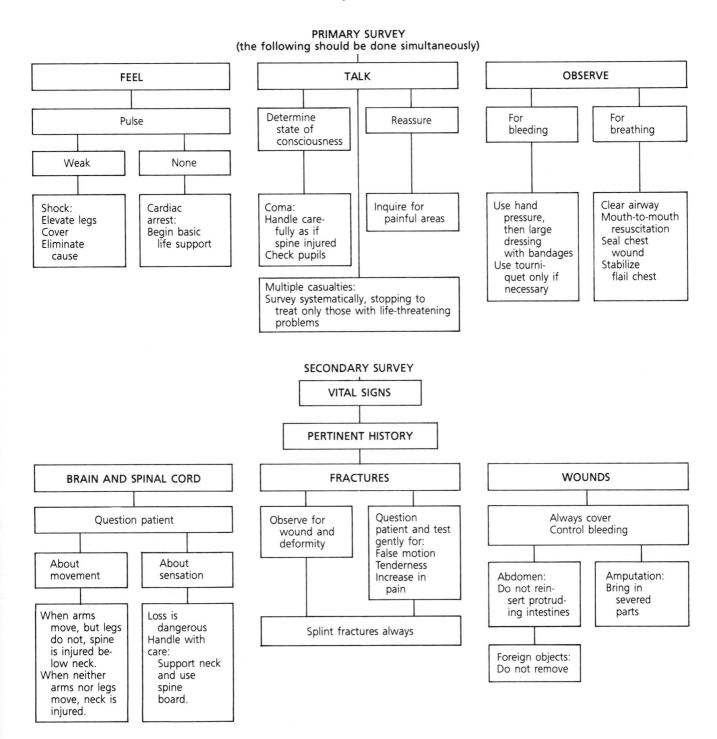

FIGURE 11.5. Primary and secondary surveys for patient assessment.

- Open chest or abdominal wounds.
- Severe head injuries with evidence of brain damage, however slight.
- Several medical problems: diabetes with complications, cardiac disease with failure.
- Dislocations associated with lost pulses.

Second-priority patients are treated at the scene and transported if necessary after the highest-priority patients have been transported. The following injuries constitute the second-priority category:

- Major or multiple fractures.
- Back injuries with or without spinal damage.

Lowest-priority patients are handled last. These patients are beyond help because they have died, or their injuries are minor fractures, scrapes, or contusions.

Leadership is paramount during triage. Someone must be in command to guide the sorting of injured people into treatment categories and to use help efficiently and effectively as it arrives. This duty falls to the most highly trained medical person.

IMPORTANT CONCEPTS

1. A sign is an objective change in body function apparent to the trainer, while a symptom is a subjective change in body function apparent to the athlete and expressed to the athletic trainer.
2. The nine diagnostic signs are pulse, respiration, blood pressure, body temperature, skin color, pupil size, state of consciousness, ability to move, and reaction to pain.
3. The goal of the primary survey is to discover and correct any immediate, life-threatening problems.
4. The goal of the secondary survey is to examine the athlete more thoroughly in preparation for transport from the field.

SUGGESTED READINGS

American Academy of Orthopaedic Surgeons. *Emergency Care and Transportation of the Sick and Injured*, 4th ed. Park Ridge, Ill.: American Academy of Orthopaedic Surgeons, 1987.

———. *Workbook for Emergency Care and Transportation of the Sick and Injured*, 4th ed. Park Ridge, Ill.: American Academy of Orthopaedic Surgeons, 1987.

12

Sports Psychology and the Injured Athlete

CHAPTER OUTLINE

INTRODUCTION

In recent years, athletic trainers have given increased attention to the psychological component involved in the rehabilitation of athletic injuries. As athletic trainers have become increasingly aware of the psychological aspect of injury and its relationship to physical rehabilitation, new information has become available for helping athletes reshape their perception of their injury and make the transition back into practice and competition smoother.

Chapter 12 begins by discussing how important a relationship built on mutual trust and respect is to the psychological well-being of the injured athlete. The chapter then describes the athlete's typical psychological reactions to injury: denial, anger, depression, and acceptance. Several of the psychological strategies that will enhance the rehabilitation process are presented in the next section. The last two sections of Chapter 12 describe the injury-prone athlete and several types of problem athletes. ■

DEVELOPING A RELATIONSHIP BETWEEN ATHLETE AND TRAINER

The development of a relationship built on trust and mutual respect between the athletic trainer and the injured athlete is essential to the athlete's psychological well-being and eventual return to the athletic field. Such a relationship is fostered, in part, by the trainer being a good listener and knowing what to say to the athlete at the right time. Effective trainers must, in addition, be adept at motivating injured athletes through encouragement and by providing feedback promoting a positive attitude toward rehabilitation. To be effective motivators and encouragers, athletic trainers must become skilled at viewing and interpreting injuries from each athlete's perspective in order to meet a particular athlete's individual needs.

The relationship that develops between athlete and trainer determines the trainer's ability to promote the athlete's psychological well-being. The trainer's expertise, dress, speech, organization, professional membership, and training-room manner all communicate the preparedness and capability to provide quality care and influence the trust that can develop between trainer and athlete. While effective use of a good sense of humor is appropriate and helpful, it is best to avoid sarcastic attempts at humor. The trainer must become skillful at listening attentively with trust, care, and concern to athletes' comments.

One of the complexities in the athletic environment is that often several individuals are concerned with the performance of a team or individual. A close, cooperative relationship must be fostered if the organization is to work effectively. When players voice dissatisfaction, the best approach may be to make constructive suggestions or simply to listen without comment. But athletic trainers should not use players as counselors to help deal with their own complaints. Coaches, athletes, and physicians should view the trainer as a team member who is willing and eager to fulfill the role of trainer and is not engaged in second guessing or criticizing colleagues.

Communication Based on Trust

Optimal communication between athlete and trainer cannot occur without complete trust. In this context, trust is a perception by an athlete that the trainer would never do anything that was not in the athlete's best interest or vice versa. Trust is not something that is given automatically; it must be earned. In the ideal situation, trust becomes a two-way street, with trainer and athlete having complete trust in each other.

A good athletic trainer realizes that trust does not mean that there will always be agreement over decisions. But when decisions are made, the best interests and goals of the athlete are considered first and foremost. Good trainers constantly ask themselves these questions:

- Is this decision in the best interest of the athlete?
- Will the athlete perceive this decision as being in his or her best interest? If not, why not?

- How can I help the athlete to understand that this decision is in his or her long-term best interest despite the athlete's inability to see it as such at the present time?
- Should I be trusted?
- Do my athletes all behave as though they trust me?
- How can I continue to be trusted?
- Am I always honest with athletes and am I always there to help them when they need me?

The majority of athletes behave up to the level to which they are trusted or act down to the level to which they are distrusted. There are, of course, exceptions. An athletic trainer must have confidence in his or her ability to develop trust and should respond with understanding if this trust is violated. If repeated violations occur, it may be necessary to sit down with individual athletes and discuss the importance of trust and the potential consequences of repeated violations of trust. A trainer must realize that many athletes have probably had an abundance of past experiences with trainers and others who have not reinforced the development of trust.

The Importance of Effective Listening

Communicating with athletes should be a regular part of any trainer's responsibility. It should not occur only when athletes are injured. Communication is a two-way process of speaking to and listening to others. Some trainers may mistakenly believe that they are always supposed to do the speaking and their athletes should always do the listening. Not true; effective trainers learn not only when and how to speak to athletes but also when and how to listen to athletes.

When a trainer and an athlete are interacting, the athlete often telegraphs needs and sources of motivation. Effective listening requires that the trainer examine every statement of substance made by each athlete. When the trainer is engaged in an emotionally charged discussion—for example, an athlete is demanding to participate despite a potentially serious injury—it is best for the trainer not to disagree, argue, or try to convince the athlete that he or she is wrong and the trainer is right. The trainer must recognize that such a strategy will either end the conversation or cause it to become more emotionally charged and less productive. Instead, the trainer should rephrase the athlete's comments and repeat them to the athlete in an understanding and empathetic tone of voice. This simple strategy, if not made too obvious, will provide a release for the athlete's passion. Once the emotion is removed, effective communication and progress can begin.

Obstacles to Effective Listening

There are several ways in which trainers can learn to improve their listening skills (it is a good idea to teach athletes how to listen also). The first step is to recognize the obstacles to effective listening. The most typical problems occur in the following situations:

- The trainer concentrates mainly on what to say next rather than on what the athlete is saying now.
- The trainer allows certain statements the athlete makes to trigger distractions so that the rest of what the athlete says goes unheard.
- The trainer interrupts the athlete's statement.
- The trainer feels threatened by the athlete's comments and begins to prepare a defense rather than continuing to listen to the athlete.
- The trainer nods at the wrong time or otherwise shows signs of merely pretending to be interested in the athlete's statements.
- The trainer gives the impression that listening to the athlete is being done out of a sense of duty rather than from a true desire to understand the person.

Trainers must learn to listen for ideas rather than just words. If an athlete says

something important or stimulating that is best not forgotten, the trainer should make a written note and return immediately to listening. A quick note will keep the trainer from being distracted by trying to remember the important point and will allow listening to continue. The important point can be discussed later in the conversation. As trainers become more successful at active listening, their ability to communicate with athletes will improve and they will gain confidence in their communication skills. Trainers who listen effectively are capable of effective communication.

Effective Listening as a Method of Effective Counseling

One of the most important methods of effective counseling is listening attentively for the message of the athlete. Trainers are sometimes thinking about what the athlete will say next and thus miss what the athlete is really saying. Trainers have to learn to keep personal troubles to themselves and not play down the importance of what the athlete believes is a problem. The trainer must show genuine concern about any problem the athlete discloses and avoid criticizing the athlete who expresses fear or discomfort.

Often people are uncomfortable because they view their feelings as not normal when, in fact, their feelings are quite typical in such situations. By "normalizing" the behavior—that is, telling the athlete that other people feel the same way and that so and so was able to solve the problem in such and such a fashion—the trainer can often move the athlete from worrying to problem solving.

If the athlete's statements or conclusions do not seem true, the trainer can suggest that "from my perspective" things look a little different. Athletes often are too self-critical or pessimistic. If the trainer reinterprets their situation more favorably, much of their discomfort may disappear.

Athletes tend to become discouraged when problems seem insurmountable and progress seems too slow. Focusing on goals and progress rather than on errors and shortcomings may help. The trainer should assist the athlete in setting a series of objectives that lead toward a goal. Marking progress along the way will enhance the athlete's performance and satisfaction.

Athletes can experience psychological difficulties in their personal lives or professional environments. The stress of competition may also aggravate a nonathletic problem. These difficulties make athletes uncomfortable and can detract from their performance. Because the coaches decide who plays, athletes may hide personal problems from them. Athletes are often more willing to discuss their concerns with the trainer, and they need a trainer who has the patience and concern to listen to these personal problems. Athletic trainers must avoid becoming so "busy" with specific athletic training work that they don't have time to listen to these problems. Not saving any time for listening to personal problems is as serious a mistake for the trainer as spending every minute of time listening to athletes' problems.

Referral for Professional Help

Athletes may express their psychological discomfort by frequent physical complaints or by showing undue concern over minor injuries. A trainer can help in these situations by assisting the athlete with minor problems and referring more serious problems to psychiatrists or psychologists who have expertise in treating athletes. If the disturbance is mild but persistent, and does not improve with the assistance of trainers and coaches, then it is advisable to seek additional help. Referral should be mandatory if psychological stress is intense or persistent or if there is any suggestion of suicide or loss of contact with reality. The team physician and trainer should together ensure that any athlete with serious psychological problems receives professional treatment. Determining the availability of sport psychologists or psychiatrists in the area in advance of any problem is a wise precaution.

Some of the conversation between a trainer and an athlete may relate to the athlete's personal condition, and some may be social, but some of the athlete's comments may express worries, concerns, fears, or other psychological states. The trainer should be alert for such expressions. In many instances, a good listener is all that the athlete wants or requires. In other cases, the athlete is signaling that there is a problem and it might be serious enough to require professional help.

The Importance of Encouragement

Effective trainers have mastered the science and art of motivating people through the process of encouragement. Since the early writings of the well-known psychologists, Alfred Adler and Robert White, it has been recognized that personal growth does not occur without encouragement. Encouragement, the first step in any change process, is a significant process that all trainers must understand and master so that they may effectively use it to their advantage.

It is unlikely that anyone in the athletic training profession has the luxury of working exclusively with "turned-on," enthusiastic athletes. To the contrary, most teams have some athletes who are "turned-off" and quite lacking in enthusiasm. To be as successful as possible, trainers have to be able to excite these athletes, as well as continue to stimulate enthusiasm in athletes who are already enthusiastic and encourage those athletes who begin at a neutral point.

Developing Perceptual Alternatives

Athletic trainers who are good at encouraging people have learned the importance of developing **perceptual alternatives**—that is, viewing and interpreting the same situation in many different ways. The more ways trainers can observe an athlete's behavior, the greater the likelihood that trainers will understand all of their athletes and be capable of helping individuals with problems.

As trainers learn to develop perceptual alternatives, they must understand the differences between (1) athletes who ask and/or expect the trainer to be flexible and encouraging and (2) athletes who take advantage of the situation so they can justify being lazy or irresponsible. Some athletes will unknowingly fail to develop their potential fully if their trainer is too understanding. Effective trainers learn to realize when to bend to meet an athlete's needs and when the athlete needs to bend to the trainer's wishes in order to rehabilitate optimally. The openness that these trainers display causes their athletes to model their behavior and be more receptive to suggestions themselves.

Unfortunately, some trainers never learn to develop perceptual alternatives and remain rigid and closed to new and perhaps better ideas. Often, they have lost their enthusiasm and desire to give their time and energy to their athletes. This situation is particularly unfortunate when the trainer is young and has little or no experience. Trainers who function in this manner will not reach their potential. Often, these trainers feel threatened and attempt to protect themselves by defending their beliefs, no matter how illogical they sound. These trainers have stagnated at an early age and denied themselves the opportunity to grow and improve. Such growth can happen only by questioning beliefs and values.

Open-minded trainers who constantly strive to improve throughout their careers may still respond in old, stereotypical ways in certain situations. But they do so because they have studied other responses and decided the old way is the better way. They are not, however, afraid to risk finding out that their old way may have been wrong. It is this attitude that allows open-minded trainers to reduce their weaknesses and maximize their strengths.

Most athletic trainers need to work at developing perceptual alternatives. Trainers who are interested in self-improvement will find the following exercises useful:

Exercise 1. Think for a moment of two different athletes: one you really enjoy working with and one you find difficult because he or she tries your patience. Write down five to seven qualities or characteristics that accurately describe them—first the athlete that you enjoy and then the one you dislike.

Now look carefully at the lists you have developed. Did you tend to see positive qualities in the athlete you don't enjoy? Chances are that if you are seeing only negative qualities in the athlete, you have not been very encouraging to this athlete. It is probably reflected in how often you smile, respond enthusiastically, and provide confidence-provoking statements to this athlete. Most likely, you are discouraging this athlete. Try to focus on some positive qualities in this person and express them in your interactions with him or her. Continue with this strategy and watch what happens to the communication between the two of you and to the athlete's attitudes and behaviors during the rehabilitation process.

Exercise 2. Constantly look for other ways in which you have possibly helped to discourage athletes. See if you can do something different that can encourage them. Decide that you will make at least one encouraging comment to an athlete you have tended to discourage each day for the next 2 weeks and study the response you get.

Exercise 3. Identify an athlete to whom you do not tend to give very much feedback. Perhaps it is a bottomline player. Maybe it is even a regular. Try to determine if there is a good reason for this athlete to get a reduced quantity and quality of feedback from you. If not, commit yourself to change.

Exercise 4. Imagine that you are one of the best athletes at your school. Now, from that athlete's perspective, write a paragraph describing what you see, think, and feel about the trainer.

Exercise 5. Imagine that you are one of the poorest players at your school. Now, from that athlete's perspective, write a paragraph describing what you see, think, and feel about the trainer.

Exercise 6. Some time in the near future take an opportunity to sit down individually with the athletes you identified in exercises 4 and 5 and ask them the same questions to which you responded. Were your responses similar? Were you afraid to find out? Are you willing to realize that you may not view yourself the same way as athletes view you?

Exercise 7. Begin to develop perceptual alternatives. Try to recall the last time that you had a disagreement with an athlete or a coach. Remember that person's position on the issue. Put yourself in that person's position, which may be quite different from yours. Try to recall when you were in that person's perspective. You are developing perceptual alternatives if you are beginning to understand the other person's point of view. You need not agree with someone else's point of view, but if you can understand different perspectives, you perhaps will be patient enough to be a more encouraging athletic trainer.

It is far easier for trainers to view the world from a self-oriented perspective and to spend great amounts of energy convincing themselves and others that their view is correct. On the other hand, scientists studying perception often marvel at the tendency of injured athletes to see most rehabilitation problems as stemming from poor trainers. A few years later the same athletes become trainers and view the same problems as being caused by athlete-centered problems such as a poor attitude. Effective trainers remember how they and other athletes viewed the sports world when they were players and use this knowledge to work in a more effective manner.

Just the opposite interaction typically occurs when athletic trainers focus mainly on the negative qualities of athletes who have very different beliefs, values, and behaviors. Typically, these athletes get far more negative feedback from their trainers. Such athletes begin to feel uncomfortable and lose confidence in the trainer. Trainers often respond by discouraging these athletes even more, emphasizing their shortcomings on a daily basis. Their perception of the athletes is that they are not "fitting the mold."

Focusing on the Athletes' Positive Qualities

Trainers must realize that it is difficult to be an encouraging leader while focusing primarily on the negative qualities of athletes. Trainers can improve their coaching skills to a great extent by focusing on the positive qualities in athletes.

It has been well documented that a self-fulfilling prophecy occurs when trainers focus on the positive aspects of their athletes. Trainers tend to give a greater quality and quantity of feedback when they view athletes in this positive perspective. Athletes who are viewed by their trainers as being capable of successful rehabilitation in time come to view themselves in a similar manner. Because of their enhanced self-perception, these athletes develop increased motivation and are likely to follow the trainer's suggestions.

Effective trainers recognize the importance of encouragement and use it to their advantage with as many athletes as possible. Only trainers who have developed perceptual alternatives will be capable of behaving in this manner.

Fostering a Positive Attitude Toward Rehabilitation

Clearly, feedback from the trainer to the athlete is a factor in the way an athlete thinks, feels, and behaves in the training room. Successful trainers are not only honest and direct but also able to foster a positive attitude toward rehabilitation. The following are some basic guidelines for giving feedback that will enable a trainer to help the athlete build a positive attitude and self-confidence.

1. Learn to give compliments—pay attention to the kind of feedback you usually give and become comfortable about giving compliments. Discard the myth that complimenting an athlete will lead to laziness and/or poor compliance.

2. Be direct with compliments—some trainers are very direct with criticism but give compliments in indirect ways. Give compliments directly to an athlete and at least occasionally in front of the athlete's teammates.

3. Be as specific as possible with compliments by pinpointing behaviors, attitudes, and situations.

4. Be consistent with compliments by making praise a regular form of feedback. The more consistently praise is received from a trainer, the easier it will be for an athlete to listen to, accept, and learn from criticism.

5. Use constructive criticism as opposed to destructive criticism, which typically focuses on what the athlete did wrong or failed to do ("you missed a treatment" or "you were late"). The danger of destructive criticism is that the athlete tends to replay these negative thoughts over and over again in his or her mind and in essence mentally starts practicing the mistake. Constructive criticism, on the other hand, focuses on what the athlete should have done instead of the error. Tell athletes what to do correctly next time rather than what they did wrong this time.

6. Criticize behaviors only. It is crucial to save criticism for specific, unacceptable behaviors rather than for some aspect of the person's character or personality.

ATHLETES' PSYCHOLOGICAL REACTIONS TO INJURY

The treatment of any injury requires attending to both physical and psychological needs. Athletes depend on the ability of their bodies to perform at or near optimal levels. Failure to perform optimally is little more than an irritant to the nonathlete or recreational athlete. To the competitive athlete, however, performance can be the cornerstone of social and economic success and important to self-esteem. Thus, caring for the psychological needs of the injured athlete is a major challenge.

From the perspective of a competitive athlete, an injury is any physical problem that interferes with performance. The aches and pains that follow a contact sport that many nonathletes would consider injuries do not fall into the category of injuries by competitive athletes. Yet a sprain, which would merely be an inconvenience to the nonathlete, could seriously incapacitate the competitive athlete. Thus, the psychological reactions of competitive athletes depend on their perceptions of the injury's severity —not as a threat to life or source of unbearable pain, but as an interference with peak performance.

While emotional reactions to injuries are partially caused by pain associated with tissue damage, they also are caused by the significance and the amount of attention focused on an injury. Competitive athletes' self-esteem is frequently tied closely to their capacities to excel physically. Their social roles are often based on their ability to perform, and they spend a large amount of time attending to their bodies. Athletes are likely to react emotionally if they perceive that an injury might threaten their capacity to perform. The amount and type of reaction vary considerably from athlete to athlete, which complicates the assessment and treatment of injuries.

The focus here is on non-life-threatening injuries and other injuries that do not require immediate hospitalization. With such injuries the athlete's psychological needs become a key consideration. In dealing with these needs, trainers should first become familiar with an athlete's typical reaction to pain. Even though some athletes frequently overreact to slight injuries, the trainer should always assume an injury is serious until it has been thoroughly evaluated. During and after evaluation, the trainer can help control the athlete's discomfort and emotional reaction by using a reassuring manner when speaking and by directing the athlete's attention away from the injury. By maintaining eye contact and voice contact with the athlete, the trainer is helping the athlete to concentrate on something other than the injury. The athlete who has developed confidence in the trainer before the injury will find the trainer's presence very reassuring. Hearing from the trainer that the condition can be treated will lessen the athlete's anxiety and help control pain. The trainer should never lie, but neither should the trainer make any unnecessary statements regarding potential complications.

Psychological Phases Following Injury

Injured athletes typically go through four psychological phases: denial, anger, depression, and acceptance. These phases occur in differing sequences and with varying degrees of intensity. In some cases, one or more of the phases may even be omitted.

Denial Phase

In the denial phase, the athlete says nothing is really wrong and he or she will be ready to play on Friday: "This can't happen to me, only to others." It is not up to the trainer to convince the athlete otherwise. A physician makes the diagnosis and outlines the necessary treatment. However, the athletic trainer often interprets the medical diagnosis for the athlete and helps the athlete reshape his or her perception of the injury. At this point, most athletes leave the denial phase. Others seek second and third opinions, thus prolonging this phase.

Anger Phase

Once athletes can no longer deny an injury, they often become angry at themselves, those around them, and everything in general. Now is the time for the athletic trainer to back off. Challenging anger only makes matters worse. Things get said that are not meant to be said, thus damaging the athlete-trainer relationship. Once the athlete has more self-control, the trainer can begin reasoning with the individual.

Depression Phase

Depression begins after anger subsides, and it is often the longest phase. The athlete believes his or her season or career is over. Often the athlete's life's goals are related to sport, and now these goals may no longer be achievable. In cases of an athlete's first injury, depression may be especially severe. Dealing with this phase takes a great amount of patience. In fact, during all three of these phases, the trainer must constantly repeat goals and reinforce exercises and routines, often daily, because the athlete is not listening very well to what is being said. Trainers often say an athlete's frustration is more difficult to deal with than the actual injury.

Acceptance Phase

In the final, or acceptance, phase, maximum effort is applied to rehabilitation. Hopefully, the athlete reaches this phase in a short time. The skill of the athletic trainer in helping the athlete achieve this phase can influence the length of rehabilitation.

Athletes Who Deny Pain or Loss of Function

Some athletes are able to ignore pain signals or deny loss of function from injuries. They can tolerate high levels of pain and apparently believe it is to their advantage not to acknowledge discomfort. Trainers should watch athletes during and after competition to try to detect signs of injury, paying particular attention to those who have had hidden injuries in the past. Coaches often are the ones who see injuries occur or note performance deficits. Their help is important in identifying injuries and convincing athletes that possible injuries require evaluation. The welfare of the athletes and the team is best served by rapid evaluation and subsequent treatment of any injuries.

Athletes Who View Injury as a Source of Relief

While some athletes will deny discomfort from an injury if their opportunity to play is threatened, other athletes consider injury a source of relief rather than a threat. Competition is not just an opportunity to triumph; it also holds the risk of failure. When others expect the athlete to succeed but circumstances such as intense competition make the athlete less confident, the threat of failure and the pressure to succeed can produce great psychological discomfort. An injury—even a small injury—can provide a socially acceptable reason to avoid the pressure.

When the athletic trainer notices that an overreaction to an injury is threatening an athlete's ability to compete, and when the athlete is showing less than expected psychological discomfort, it would be worthwhile for the trainer to discuss the athlete's perception of the situation and reaction to pressure. Trainers can help these athletes perceive the competitive situation as less of a threat and more of an opportunity. It is senseless to suggest that an athlete will perform above his or her potential or succeed without further effort. Urging such athletes to focus on possible success, and not on possible failure, will help them to perceive competition more positively and reduce the need to escape.

Dealing with an Athlete's Perception of Injury

Athletes perceive injuries in different ways. Some perceive an injury as a disaster; others view an injury as an opportunity to show courage; and yet others find an injury a welcome relief from the embarrassment of poor performance, lack of playing time, or a losing season. Injured athletes may wonder whether they will completely recover. They must be prepared for the end of participation but remain positive and enthusiastic about the prospect of total recovery. For some athletes an injury means an attack on their self-image and a lost opportunity to display prowess. If an injury should end their athletic career, these athletes may suffer an "identity crisis."

With some injured athletes, emotional and irrational thinking sometimes takes over. These athletes become lost in "the

work of worry," excuse their own mistakes and responsibilities, and are overwhelmed by anxiety. Such self-defeating thought patterns may interfere with the rehabilitation process.

Athletes who are thinking irrationally often exaggerate the meaning of an event, disregard important aspects of a situation, oversimplify events as good or bad or right or wrong, overgeneralize from a single event, or draw unwarranted conclusions, even though evidence is lacking or contradictory. They may, for example, decide that the trainer is giving preferential treatment to "major-sport" athletes over "minor-sport" ones. They may exaggerate the meaning of getting injured, thinking the injury has ended their athletic career. They may disregard important aspects of a situation and become terribly discouraged after, for example, 10 days of therapy, even though they were told it would take at least 2 or 3 weeks to complete the therapy. An example of an injured athlete who oversimplifies events or overgeneralizes from a single event is the athlete who knows of another athlete who had a similar injury and failed to recover despite intensive rehabilitation. Therefore, the irrational-thinking athlete decides that there is no hope of recovery. Then there are the athletes who once injured decide they are "injury prone." They become more and more anxious, and as a result do in fact begin to experience frequent injuries.

Effective Psychological Responses for the Athlete

When injury occurs, athletes should be encouraged to view the injury in a rational, self-enhancing way rather than from a self-defeating perspective. They should understand that when an injury blocks the attainment of important goals, it is reasonable and appropriate to think of the injury as unfortunate, untimely, and inconvenient and to feel irritated, frustrated, and sad. It is unreasonable, however, for athletes to convince themselves that the situation is hopeless, that the injury should be hidden from their coach or trainer, that the season or their career has ended, and that they will never again be able to perform effectively.

Athletes with emotional self-control will be able to cope with their injury by responding rationally to it and not being overwhelmed by it. They can best exert self-control if they have knowledge of their injury and the rehabilitation process. Athletes cannot be positive and relaxed if they are uninformed, anxious, and left wondering about the outcome. Much of the anxiety experienced by injured athletes results from uncertainty, misconceptions, or inaccurate information. If uncertainty persists, they may have trouble getting through the denial, anger, and depression phases. Honest and accurate information, along with hope, helps them move into the acceptance phase. Furthermore, athletes who understand what they are doing in rehabilitation and why are more likely to work hard and be able to provide useful information to the trainer about their progress.

What athletes say to themselves and imagine after an injury has occurred helps to determine their behavior. They can learn coping skills to control their thoughts and what they say to themselves. Athletes who notice faulty or self-defeating internal dialogues should know how to use their coping strategies to change their thinking. They may use an intervention strategy such as thought stoppage. **Thought stoppage** is a technique whereby the athlete, upon recognizing faulty thinking, says "stop" and then repeats self-enhancing thoughts. An effective sports psychologist can help athletes recognize faulty thought patterns and anticipate destructive thoughts; the sports psychologist can then "inoculate" the athlete with coping strategies. Team physicians and athletic trainers can also learn to teach these coping strategies. Good coping strategies may shorten the time injured athletes need to progress from denial to acceptance to productive rehabilitation, and ultimately to a safe, successful return to competition.

In addition to coping with faulty thinking, injured athletes sometimes have to cope with the conditions of the hospital and training room and the stress of special treatment procedures. They should be encouraged to express their feelings, establish rapport with hospital and training room personnel, and balance the expectation of receiving help from others with retaining independence.

PSYCHOLOGY OF ENHANCING REHABILITATION

Athletic trainers can help shape athletes' perceptions in a positive way by encouraging them to view their injury in a rational, self-enhancing way rather than from a self-defeating point of view. A number of coping techniques are available to help athletes control their thoughts and perceptions about their injury. It is also important that athletic trainers encourage their injured athletes to be cooperative and patient. Cooperation and patience are essential because of the time injured athletes must dedicate, the effort they must exert, and the pain they must sometimes endure while undergoing rehabilitation.

Recent years have witnessed rapid advancement in the development of psychological strategies for enhancing the effectiveness of rehabilitation for injured athletes. Athletic trainers will find it helpful to have at least a basic understanding of these strategies.

Building Cooperation and Patience

During treatment, pain and fear are no longer major psychological factors, but depression and impatience may decrease athletes' contribution to rehabilitation. The cooperation of athletes is essential for successful rehabilitation because they are the ones who must dedicate the time, exert the effort, and endure the pain usually involved. Trainers can improve cooperation during rehabilitation by giving clear explanations, outlining procedures used in treatment, and making reasonable predictions of athletes' expected return to competition.

Setting Attainable Goals

By offering an optimistic expectation, measuring progress daily, and breaking programs into small subgoals so that improvement is more visible, athletic trainers can alleviate some of their athletes' emotional discomfort. Discussing the feasibility of returning to the previous level of performance or regaining the previous position on the team and making reasonable and appropriate estimates for achieving these goals are good ways to maintain morale.

Encouraging Participation in Rehabilitation

One way to encourage athletes' participation in rehabilitation is to involve them in planning treatment schedules and setting goals along the route to complete recovery. If athletes understand the relationship between a procedure and the eventual return of function and ability to compete, their motivation to follow the treatment will increase. Setting goals and measuring improvement are also ways to help convince athletes that their injured part has recovered and can be used with confidence when they return to play. Athletes can lose confidence in their ability to perform at previous levels, even when their injury is totally rehabilitated. Therefore, treatment requires rehabilitating an athlete's state of mind as well as his or her body.

Maintaining Association With the Team

With prolonged recovery, athletes' social status and rewards often dramatically decrease. Friendships based on team membership become threatened. Trainers should try to keep injured athletes involved with the team, either with light workouts or with suggestions to coaches that injured players assist with coaching or managerial tasks. Maintaining a team association can keep injured athletes' motivation to return to play from fading.

Using Visual Imagery as a Coping Skill

The imagination of athletes can greatly influence their response to an injury. Often they imagine the worst thing that could happen—"I'll never play again." Athletes can be taught to control their visual images and to direct them productively to reduce anxiety and to aid in rehabilitation. Visual imagery strategies include emotive imagery, body rehearsal, mastery rehearsal, and coping rehearsal.

Emotive Imagery

In **emotive imagery**—a technique that helps athletes feel secure and confident that their rehabilitation will be successful—scenes are imagined that produce positive, self-enhancing feelings, such as enthusiasm, self-pride, and confidence. Some athletes, for example, will recall successful recovery from an earlier injury and their return to competition. Others may envision the admiration they will receive from their coach, teammates, and friends for overcoming the injury. Basically, athletes are instructed to think of other athletes who have overcome the same injury and to generate other scenes that produce positive feelings.

Body Rehearsal

In **body rehearsal**—a mental rehearsal technique now being investigated—the athlete is given a detailed explanation of his or her injury. Whenever possible, colored pictures are used to help the person develop a mental picture of the injury. Then the healing process and the purpose of the rehabilitation techniques are carefully explained so that the athlete can envision what is happening internally to the injured part during the rehabilitation process. After clearly visualizing the healing process, the athlete is asked to imagine the process in color during treatments and at intervals throughout the day. Body rehearsal shows promise for becoming a way to influence healing.

Mastery Rehearsal and Coping Rehearsal

Mastery rehearsal involves mentally practicing a desired outcome in an enthusiastic and positive way; **coping rehearsal** involves mentally practicing solutions to difficult situations, with an emphasis placed on effective responses. Mastery rehearsal and coping rehearsal are used to prepare athletes for difficult situations and to help them achieve important goals. For example, mastery rehearsal for knee surgery might go like this:

> I'm looking forward to surgery and feel great about the upcoming operation and rehabilitation. I'm glad I'll no longer be bothered by my knee. I have a qualified surgeon who'll perform the operation successfully. I'll begin rehabilitation shortly afterward with a caring, talented athletic trainer. Rehabilitation will be short and successful. Each day, I'll make progress. In a few weeks, I'll be training again. I'll feel good and be excited. I know I'll be successful.

Coping rehearsal for knee surgery might go like this:

> I'm looking forward to surgery, but I'm anxious. I'm likely to become even more anxious as the day of surgery approaches. Whenever I realize that my mind is running wild with anxiety, I'll "stop" and replace these thoughts with helpful thoughts and "let go" and relax.
>
> Rehabilitation will be long and demanding, challenging my self-discipline and willpower. If I want to reach the goals I've outlined, I can't let the injury stand in my way. I must have confidence in my ability to overcome this challenge.
>
> What must I do? I'll work out a plan that will prepare me for successful rehabilitation. I must keep cool and not respond emotionally. If I find myself responding emotionally, I'll relax and become more aware of my self-state-

ments. If I'm thinking self-defeating thoughts, I'll "stop" them and repeat helpful thoughts to myself. If I become discouraged, I'll think of athletes who have overcome far worse injuries than mine. An injury such as mine has ruined some athletes' careers, but successful athletes realize that successful management of injuries and rehabilitation is part of becoming a successful athlete.

> There will be many excuses for not going to therapy: "I can't find time." "I'm too busy." "I have a test tomorrow." "The training room hours are ridiculous." I will make sure that I'm ready to deal with these excuses because I realize that they will only work against me. I will always find a way to get my treatments.

> There will be days when I'll see little or no progress in therapy. I will also probably experience pain that is likely to make me tense, irritable, and frustrated. When this occurs, I must remember to stay calm and positive and to keep my sense of humor. Then the trainer will enjoy helping me more, and I'll feel better about myself. Think how good I'll feel when my rehabilitation is successful.

Enhancing Self-Control of Pain

Pain is influenced by motivational and cognitive factors. Athletes can be taught non-imagery and imagery strategies to control or eliminate pain. They must be careful, of course, not to block out completely pain signals that could be warnings of danger.

Pain has three dimensions: sensory-discriminative, motivational-affective, and cognitive-evaluative. Each dimension needs different coping skills.

The Sensory-Discriminative Dimension of Pain

For the sensory-discriminative dimension, relaxation techniques can control the sensory input of pain and reduce the tension that otherwise magnifies the pain intensity. Other strategies include attention diversion, somatization, imaginative inattention, transformation of context, and relaxation.

Attention diversion. Athletes can exclude the sensation of pain by diverting their attention to other stimuli in the external environment. They can, for example, do mental arithmetic, count ceiling tiles, or plan their daily schedule.

Somatization. Another nonimagery strategy is **somatization**. Athletes focus directly on the pain at the injured area and ignore other sensations. If, for example, they have to immerse their foot into ice water, they focus on a feeling of pleasant dampness and numbness.

Imaginative inattention. Imaginative inattention requires athletes to imagine "goal-directed fantasies" that are pleasant and allow them to ignore the pain. They become totally absorbed in the guided fantasy, such as a perfect performance in an upcoming contest. They may also imagine the injured or painful part to be numb or minimize the pain as being insignificant or unreal.

Transformation of context. Athletes may also imaginatively transform the context in which they are feeling the pain. They acknowledge the pain and include it in a fantasy, transferring the context or the setting in which the pain occurs. They may, for instance, imagine themselves to be a spy who has been shot and is now in a car that is being chased down a winding mountain road by enemy agents. The car chase should require more attention than the pain.

Relaxation. Relaxation can also reduce the sensation of pain. Athletes imagine that it is a summer day and they are relaxing in a rowboat on a calm pond, or that their injured part is warm and heavy.

The Motivational-Affective Dimension of Pain

A second dimension of pain is the motivational-affective dimension. Negative feelings of anxiety and helplessness may increase the perception of pain, whereas positive feelings of confidence and control decrease it. Thought-stoppage techniques and positive self-statements may help.

The Cognitive-Evaluative Dimension of Pain

The third dimension is the cognitive-evaluative dimension. How intense athletes expect the pain to be will usually influence how much pain they report. Thought stoppage and self-instruction statements are valuable.

Biofeedback is another way to gain control over pain. Athletes' awareness is raised and their self-control is improved by monitoring various measurements of psychophysiologic processes. Biofeedback may also be used to show athletes the effectiveness of their self-control strategies.

Systematic Desensitization

Despite the great advances in physically preparing athletes for a return to sport after an injury or surgery, little use has been made of systematic psychological rehabilitation. As a result, psychological scars may be overlooked. These "scars" may be rational or irrational anxieties that cause athletes to lose their ability to concentrate and may lead to reinjury or to injury of another area. It also may take a long time for athletes to regain their confidence for peak performance.

Systematic desensitization may be used to rehabilitate injured athletes psychologically. Desensitization helps athletes handle anxiety by combining relaxation training and visual imagery. When possible, systematic desensitization should be supplemented by biofeedback training.

At the onset of rehabilitation, the sports psychologist encourages athletes to talk about their anxieties concerning the injury and their return to competition. Athletes are then introduced to relaxation training techniques. They practice them by using a tape recording each day at home or in a private room next to the training room. Once athletes become skilled at relaxing on cue, they are ready to start desensitization procedures.

Systematic desensitization lasts for 20 to 30 minutes a day. It is timed so that psychological rehabilitation is completed when the athlete is physically ready to return to play. A fear hierarchy that applies specifically to the athlete's fears or anticipated fears should be established. This hierarchy is a list of 5 to 10 situations that elicit a progressive increase in anxiety.

Desensitization starts with step one on the fear hierarchy. In imagining the first step, the athlete tries to remain as relaxed as possible. Electromyography or thermal biofeedback may be used to measure muscle tension and relaxation. If this equipment is not available, the athlete should indicate the degree of relaxation on a scale of 1 through 10 (1 = very tense; 10 = very relaxed). The therapist calls off the numbers 1 through 10, and the athlete raises an index finger at the appropriate number. The athlete may proceed to the next step after indicating deep relaxation and confidence while imagining the previous step on the fear hierarchy. The process is repeated until the athlete can relax on cue and stay relaxed while imaging each step on the fear hierarchy. After successfully completing the fear hierarchy, the athlete should be ready mentally to return to athletics. In addition to going through mental desensitization, the athlete should go through each step of the fear hierarchy physically before returning to competition.

The following steps represent the football running back's fear hierarchy for a shoulder injury.

1. You are told by the trainer that you are ready to return to practice.
2. You're in the huddle for the first time after return to practice, and you must block.
3. You're in the huddle for the first time after return to practice, and you must carry the ball on a sweep play.
4. You're in the huddle for the first time after return to practice, and you must carry the ball on a dive play.
5. You must jump high in the air to catch a pass with a defender about to tackle you on the side of the injured shoulder.
6. You must jump high in the air to catch a pass with a defender about to tackle you on the side opposite the injured shoulder, and you are about to land on the injured shoulder on a turf field.
7. You are successfully running the ball on various plays and avoiding or breaking tackles. (This was the state of the athlete's mental process before the injury.)

Here is a basketball player's fear hierarchy for an ankle sprain.

1. You are going on the basketball court to practice.
2. You begin practice by running wind-sprints.
3. You are now in a "wave" drill, and you practice your defensive step slide.
4. You practice shooting with no defense.
5. You are running lay-ups in practice.
6. You are in a scrimmage, and you shoot over a defensive player.
7. You shoot over a defensive player, and you are fouled.
8. You are in practice and will rebound a ball to start a fast break, and there is no defense.
9. You rebound a ball during a scrimmage and turn to give an outlet pass.
10. In a scrimmage, you jump high to rebound a basketball; when you come down, you land on another player's foot, but you still turn and throw an outlet pass.

THE "INJURY-PRONE" ATHLETE

Physical Causative Factors

Some athletes are more prone to injury than others, perhaps because of physical reasons such as limb malalignment, joints that are too loose or too tight, poor strength, or strength imbalance. Such athletes might not be fully fit; their poor endurance leads to fatigue, a slower reaction time, and reduced coordination. In addition, they may not be warming up correctly.

Emotional Causative Factors

Athletes may also be tense, depressed, or preoccupied with problems in school, social problems, or problems at home. The mental changes may be subtle, but the team physician, trainer, or sports psychologist can often tell that something is wrong. These athletes may uncharacteristically jump the gun, start fights, miss foul shots, or otherwise not be concentrating on the task. They may have trouble sleeping, show a changed behavior pattern, and have mood changes. Talking with these athletes will sometimes uncover the source of the problem, and the difficulty can then be dealt with.

Predisposing Attitudes: The False Image of Invulnerability

In addition to predisposing personality factors, there are also potentially predisposing attitudes that have been fostered by many coaches. These attitudes usually "sound good," and athletes who accept them typically "look tough" and appear to have "great attitudes." Unfortunately, when taken too far, as is often the case for many highly motivated and coachable athletes, these well-learned attitudes become counterproductive and predispose athletes to injury.

The Myth of Giving 100 Percent

Often coaches systematically teach their athletes that mental toughness and giving 100 percent effort all of the time are necessary for success in sport. Athletes must be taught that "trying your hardest" is not the same as "doing your best" and that giving 100 percent all of the time will simply guarantee mental weakness rather than mental toughness. The reality is that giving 100 percent all of the time is impossible to

do. A full acceptance of the false attitudes or an extreme reaction to these attitudes may increase the likelihood of injury and failure.

Playing Through Pain

Many highly motivated athletes learn to "play through" almost any kind of pain. Developing such an ability may result in an often-injured athlete who seldom, if ever, performs in a fully healthy state. Such athletes usually have short-lived athletic careers and lives filled with pain and suffering from masked injuries that they were tough enough to play through.

Rewards for "Tough" Players

Unfortunately, in sports—especially in contact sports—athletes who accept these predisposing attitudes receive an abundance of rewards. The promise of such rewards often leads athletes to an extreme psychological reaction of wishing to win the admiration and respect of coaches, trainers, teammates, and fans. The more these athletes enjoy the rewards for displaying these attitudes, the more they are willing to do whatever is necessary to earn them.

Bodies and Minds Left Vulnerable to Injury

Gradually, the well-intentioned appearance of mental toughness and dedication evolves into the projection of a false image of invulnerability. As athletes strive to live up to this impossible image, problems begin to appear. Gradually, players and coaches alike accept as fact that "tough" athletes never need a rest, never miss a play, never go to the training room, and never let a "minor" injury keep them from playing. Failure to live up to this image of invulnerability is considered a sign of weakness. Unfortunately, for athletes with this belief system their self-pride is attached to never missing a practice or game. Their bodies are therefore left extremely vulnerable to injury. Their minds are left unprepared for the incapacitating injury or lifelong pain that may follow.

Ensuring a Healthy Adaptation to Injury and Life

A major change in attitude is required to ensure a healthy adaptation to injury and life after athletics. Without this change, athletes who hold predisposing attitudes will not accept the reality that they are vulnerable and can get hurt physically and scared psychologically. This change of attitude is crucial if athletes are to accept injuries as a natural occurrence in sport and be capable of responding positively to them. Such acceptance will enable athletes to develop to their fullest ability and allow coaches, athletic trainers, and physicians to fulfill their respective roles effectively. The hazards of holding mistaken attitudes must be realized before the specific psychological strategies presented can be most fully utilized.

Care and Concern of Sports Leaders

Some sports leaders mistakenly believe that the best way to foster a rapid recovery from injury is to make injured athletes feel unimportant as long as they are injured. Leaders who hold this view clearly communicate to their athletes that they care for them only as performers. Such leaders communicate this message by isolating injured athletes from healthy team members. Some leaders go so far as to refuse any form of verbal communication while using body language to suggest that injured athletes should feel guilty for not helping the team win. Others of this persuasion suggest that their injured athletes are malingerers, lack mental toughness and desire, or are not fully committed to the success of the team.

Sports leaders must realize that the time during which athletes are recovering from injury is crucial for either developing or destroying trust. It is during this time that leaders have a chance to demonstrate care and concern and show that they are as committed to their injured athletes as they ask these athletes to be to them.

Trust in Sports Leaders

Successful sports leaders must help athletes realize that attitudes such as desire, pride, and commitment are beneficial at the right time and place, but that these attitudes may also be hazardous to present and future health if they are taken to the extreme. The key is for leaders to do what is in the best interest of injured athletes. When this approach is followed, athletes, coaches, trainers, and teams alike will have the best possible chance of attaining their fullest potential. When this approach is not followed, there is still a chance that the athletes themselves will put sport in proper perspective. They will do so, however, out of distrust rather than trust, and perhaps in the end decide that athletics are unimportant and a means for personal abuse rather than an opportunity for positive growth and fulfillment.

PROBLEM ATHLETES

All sports medicine specialists must recognize that certain athletes are particularly difficult. Five of the most typical problem types are categorized as (1) dependent, attention-loving athletes, (2) resistant athletes, (3) childlike athletes, (4) angry athletes, and (5) unmotivated athletes.

Successful rehabilitation of problem athletes requires a positive relationship between the parties involved. Staff members must at all times remain professional, helpful, and friendly, and at the same time not allow such closeness to interfere with effective feedback and treatment. When the relationship becomes too close, objectivity in assessment and treatment is lost. At the same time, understanding and empathy are crucial. Furthermore, experiencing an array of human emotions does not make a relationship ineffective. Such shared emotions are normal and often allow for the empathy necessary for the ideal relationship. Some practical ideas of communicating with these five types of problem athletes are suggested in the following sections.

Dependent, Attention-Loving Athletes

Athletes who need attention and who enjoy being dependent on others make constant and extreme demands on the training room staff. They make others feel responsible for them and their health. Their behavior breeds dependency. The normal services other athletes receive on a day-to-day basis are never good enough for them; dependent, attention-loving athletes always want more attention, time, and help.

In general, athletes of this type refuse to accept the responsibility of taking care of themselves. They want others to take care of them and, because of their athletic abilities, have often been able to find people quite willing to do so. These athletes develop innocent and devious behaviors for at-· taching themselves to giving people in the helping professions. Training room staff members often find out after the fact that they have been taken advantage of by such athletes.

Athletic trainers must set reasonable time limits for themselves when caring for dependent, attention-loving athletes; otherwise, these athletes will overwork them. And the trainer who does set such limits must not allow the unhappy athlete to take over another staff member.

Some athletes will respond to limits being set with frustration, hostility, and hurt feelings. In the past these responses have commonly helped them get the attention they desire. In some cases athletes with such needs will not be content to live within the stated boundaries. Sports medicine specialists must be willing to continue to work with these athletes.

Resistant Athletes

Athletes who resist treatment make the training room staff's job most difficult. Whereas it is common for the dependent type to make the staff feel needed and respected, resistant athletes are perceived as showing no respect or appreciation for the rehabilitation skills of the staff. Although there are various reasons for the resistant behaviors of such athletes, it is usually best to avoid psychological interpretations unless guided by a trained psychologist. For most athletes of this type, the staff should not take personal offense at the attitudes of these athletes. Many athletes will change their attitudes and behaviors when the staff's responses are combined with humor.

After trying a strategy of mixing humor with advice and not getting satisfactory results, the staff should employ a more straightforward approach. Sometimes it is best simply to tell these athletes that the decision is theirs: live with your injury, suffer through an extremely slow recovery, or follow the recommended rehabilitation regimen. The training room staff makes it clear that they can live with the injury and the lack of treatment if the athlete is able to do so. Leaving the decision in the athlete's hands often leads the athlete to make a commitment to rehabilitation. Too often training room staff members are hesitant to allow their athletes to make this kind of decision for fear they might choose to refuse treatment. This lack of confidence on the part of the staff will not encourage the development of self-responsibility so necessary for athletes. Staff members who become impatient with resistant athletes may show signs of fatigue, overwork, or burnout. Some resistant athletes need to be referred to a different staff member who might communicate more effectively with this type of problem athlete.

Childlike Athletes

It is not uncommon for even the toughest and most mature athletes to regress to a more childlike state when they are injured. This reality makes sense, particularly for athletes with disabling injuries that require a prolonged rehabilitation period, when it is understood that, as with young children, many everyday activities require help from another adult. Depending on the athlete's personality, a variety of behavior patterns will occur. Some athletes like being waited on, some withdraw and become quiet and shy, some lose their tempers, and some whine and get lost in self-pity.

When childlike behaviors occur, training room staff members should recognize and accept such behavior and at the same time help these athletes to anticipate what is happening. It is then appropriate to give the athletes control and self-responsibility over their rehabilitation to foster more mature behavior.

Angry Athletes

Obviously, no training room staff member enjoys being verbally attacked or ridiculed by athletes receiving treatment. Although an athlete's normal response to injury is easy to understand, displays of prolonged or persistent anger, particularly when directed at the training room staff members, should not be tolerated. Anger is best responded to immediately and directly. Rather than attempting to explain the anger, it is best for training room staff members to show empathy and firmness while asking questions of the athlete intended to facilitate an understanding of the response in question.

The major goal in working with an angry athlete is to establish a workable relationship between the parties involved. To do so, the staff member involved must stay calm while establishing the necessary boundaries. Staff members who respond to angry athletes by shouting back and acting irrationally will only ensure that there will be no resolution. Likewise, displaying bitterness toward an angry athlete will further hinder the desired relationship. In any case the sooner a calm and objective relationship

is established, the sooner rehabilitation goals can be achieved.

Unmotivated Athletes

Injured athletes display a lack of motivation for many reasons. Some athletes arrive in the training room for treatment with an extremely negative attitude, which hinders progress. Others are injured for the first time and know of friends who, despite efforts to rehabilitate themselves, did not make a healthy return to competition. As a result, these athletes assume that there is no reason to be motivated. Still others are despondent about their injury and have developed a counterproductive habit of complaining and questioning everything they are asked to do.

In all cases the underlying problem must be addressed. Athletes cannot be forced to have a great attitude; they can, however, be helped to develop a positive outlook toward their treatment. The training room staff can cite numerous examples of athletes with similar injuries who, as a result of a positively motivated attitude, successfully recovered. A variety of strategies are useful, including motivational tapes, stories, or videos that help inspire athletes to think about how good they will feel upon their return to competition.

Training room staff members must accept the fact that while they may be able to inspire athletes for a short time, they cannot force athletes to accept something they do not want. However, unmotivated athletes can be taught how motivated athletes think when they are going through rehabilitation. Once unmotivated athletes understand such thinking patterns, they will be able to motivate themselves. When all other attempts fail, the training room staff must remember the importance of maintaining an enthusiastic, optimistic attitude so as to serve as effective role models.

IMPORTANT CONCEPTS

1. A relationship built on trust and mutual respect between the athletic trainer and the injured athlete is essential to the athlete's psychological well-being and eventual return to play.
2. Effective listening is the key to effective communication.
3. The athletic trainer must learn to distinguish minor emotional problems that can be dealt with from severe psychological stress that requires referral of the athlete for professional help.
4. Successful athletic trainers have learned the importance of developing perceptual alternatives as a way of motivating athletes through the process of encouragement.
5. Successful athletic trainers are able to foster a positive attitude toward rehabilitation in their injured athletes.
6. The four phases an injured athlete typically goes through are denial, anger, depression, and acceptance.
7. Some athletes deny pain or loss of function following an injury.
8. Some athletes view injury as a source of relief from the pressure to succeed.
9. An athlete's perception of injury may lead to anxiety and irrational thinking.
10. Athletic trainers can help athletes to view their injuries in a rational, self-enhancing way rather than from a self-defeating perspective.
11. Psychological strategies for enhancing the effectiveness of rehabilitation for injured athletes include building cooperation and patience, using visual imagery as a coping skill, enhancing self-control of pain, and systematic desensitization.
12. Some athletes are injury prone for physical and emotional reasons.
13. Five categories of problem athletes that have been recognized by sports psychologists are attention-loving athletes, resistant athletes, childlike athletes, angry athletes, and unmotivated athletes.

SUGGESTED READINGS

Averill, J. "Personal Control over Aversive Stimuli and Its Relationship to Stress." *Psychology Bulletin* 80 (1973): 286–303.

Bean, K. L. "Desensitization, Behavioral Rehearsal, the Reality: A Preliminary Report on a New Procedure." *Behavioral Therapy* 1 (1970): 525–545.

Beck, A. "A Cognitive Therapy: Nature and Relation to Behavior Therapy." *Behavioral Therapy* 2 (1970): 194–200.

Blitz, B., and A. J. Dinrstein. "The Role of Attentional Focus in Pain Perception: Manipulation of Response to Noxious Stimulation by Instructions." *Journal of Abnormal Psychology* 77 (1971): 42–45.

Bramwell, S. T., M. Masuda, N. N. Wagner, and T. H. Holmes. "Psychosocial Factors in Athletic Injuries: Development and Application of the Social and Athletic Readjustment Rating Scale (SARRS)." *Journal of Human Stress* 1 (1975): 6–20.

Burns, D. D, ed. *Cekcs Depression Inventory. Feeling Good: The New Mood Therapy.* New York: Signet, 1978.

Chaves, J. F., and T. X. Barber. "Cognitive Strategies, Experimental Modeling, and Expectation in the Attenuation of Pain." *Journal of Abnormal Psychology* 83 (1974): 356–363.

Coddington, R. D., and J. R. Troxell. "The Effect of Emotional Factors on Football Injury Rates: A Pilot Study." *Journal of Human Stress* 6 (1980): 3–5.

Cohen, F. "Personality, Stress and the Development of Physical Illness." In *Health Psychology: A Handbook: Theories, Applications, and Challenges of a Psychological Approach to the Health Care System.* Edited by Stone, G. C., F. Cohen, N. E. Adler, et al. San Francisco: Jossey-Bass, 1979.

Curtian, L. A. F. "Evaluation of the Injury Prone Athlete: A Multidimensional Approach." Master's thesis, University of Virginia, 1988.

Dinkmeyer, D., and R. Dreikurs. *Encouraging Children to Learn: The Encouragement Process.* Englewood Cliffs, N.J.: Prentice-Hall, 1963.

Evans, M. B., and G. L. Paul. "Effects of Hypnotically Suggested Analgesia on Physiological and Subjective Responses to Cold Stress." *Journal of Consulting and Clinical Psychology* 35 (1970): 362–371.

Foreyt, J. P., and D. P. Rathjen, eds. *Cognitive Behavior Therapy: Research and Application.* New York: Plenum Press, 1978.

Gordon, S. "Sport Psychology and the Injured Athlete: A Cognitive-Behavioral Approach to Injury Response and Injury Rehabilitation." *Sports Science Periodical on Research and Sport* (March 1986): 1–10.

Green, R., and J. Reyhner. "Pain Tolerance in Hypnotic Analgesia and Imagination States." *Journal of Abnormal Psychology* 77 (1977): 42–45.

Hamburg, D., and J. E. Adams. "A Perspective on Coping Behavior." *Archives of General Psychiatry* 17 (1987): 277–284.

Jacobson, E. *You Must Relax.* New York: McGraw-Hill, 1934.

Jacobson, E. *Progressive Relaxation: A Physiological and Clinical Investigation of Muscular States and Their Significance in Psychology and Medical Practice,* 2d ed. Chicago: University of Chicago Press, 1938.

Jacobson, E. *Anxiety and Tension Control: A Physiologic Approach.* Philadelphia: J. B. Lippincott, 1964.

Janis, I. L. *Psychological Stress: Psychoanalytic and Behavioral Studies of Surgical Patients.* New York: John Wiley & Sons, 1958.

Johnson, R. "Suggestions for Pain Reduction and Response to Cold-Induced Pain." *Psychology Reports* 18 (1966): 79–85.

Kavanaugh, R. E. *Facing Death.* Los Angeles: Nash Publishing, 1972.

Kübler-Ross, E. *On Death and Dying.* New York: Macmillan, 1969.

Kulund, D. N., ed. *The Injured Athlete,* 2d ed. Philadelphia: J. B. Lippincott, 1988.

Lazarus, R. S. "Psychological Stress and Coping in Adaptation and Illness." *International Journal of Psychiatry Medicine* 5 (1974): 321–333.

Lindemann, E. "Symptomatology and Management of Acute Grief." *American Journal of Psychiatry* 101 (1944): 141–148.

Lipowski, Z. J. "Physical Illness, the Individual and the Coping Processes." *Psychiatry in Medicine* 1 (1970): 91–102.

Lynch, G. A. (1988). "Athletic Injuries and the Practicing Sport Psychologist: Practical Guidelines for Assisting Athletes." *The Sport Psychologist* 2 (1988): 161–167.

Lysens, R., Y. Vanden Auweele, and M. Ostyn. "The Relationship between Psychosocial Factors and Sports Injuries." *Journal of Sports Medicine and Physical Fitness* 26 (1986): 77–84.

Mahoney, M. J. *Cognition and Behavior Modification.* Cambridge, Mass.: Ballinger, 1974.

Meichenbaum, D. *Cognitive-Behavior Modification: An Integrative Approach.* New York: Plenum Press, 1977.

———. *Cognitive Behavior Modification*. Morristown, N.J.: General Learning Press, 1978.

Melzack, R., and K. L. Casey. "Sensory, Motivational, and Central Control Determinants of Pain: A New Conceptual Model." In *The Skin Senses*, edited by D. R. Kenshalo, pp. 423-443. Springfield, Ill.: Charles C Thomas, 1968.

Melzack, R., and P. D. Wall. "Pain Mechanisms: A New Theory." *Science* 150 (1965): 971-979.

Moss, R. H. *The Crisis of Physical Illness: An Overview in Coping with Physical Illness*. New York: Plenum Medical Book Co., 1979.

Pate, R. R., B. McClenaghan, and R. Rotella. *Scientific Foundations of Coaching*. Philadelphia: Saunders College Publishing, 1984.

Reeves, J. "EMG—Biofeedback Reduction of Tension Headache: A Cognitive Skills Training Approach." *Biofeedback and Self Regulation* 1 (1976): 217–225.

Rotella, R. J. "Systematic Desensitization: Psychological Rehabilitation of Injured Athletes." In *Sport Psychology: From Theory to Practice*, edited by L. Bunker and R. Rotella. Charlottesville: University of Virginia, Department of Health and Physical Education, 1979.

Rotella, R. J., and S. R. Heyman. "Stress, Injury, and the Psychological Rehabilitation of Athletes." In *Applied Sport Psychology: Personal Growth to Peak Performance*, edited by J. M. Williams. Palo Alto, Calif.: Mayfield Publishing, 1986.

Samples, P. "Mind Over Muscle: Returning the Injured Athlete to Play." *The Physician and Sportsmedicine* 15 (October 1987): 172-180.

Selye, H. *The Stress of Life*. New York: McGraw-Hill, 1956.

Smith, R. E., F. L. Smoll, and N. J. Smith. "Stress Psychological Assets, and Reduction of Athletic Injuries." Research conducted for Washington Interscholastic Activities Association, University of Washington, 1987.

Sternbach, R. A. *Pain: A Psychophysiological Analysis*. New York: Academic Press, 1968.

Stout, C. L. "The Physiological and Psychological Aspects of Depression Resulting from Injury." Unpublished manuscript, 1977.

———. "The Interrelationship of Stress, Injury, and Depression and the Influence of Exercise." Unpublished manuscript, 1979.

Suls, J., and B. Mullen. "Life Events, Perceived Control and Illness: The Role of Uncertainty." *Journal of Human Stress* 7 (1981): 30–34.

Vanderpool, J. P. "Stressful Patient Relationships and the Difficult Patient." In *Rehabilitation Psychology: A Comprehensive Textbook*, edited by D. W. Krueger, pp. 167-174. Rockville, Md.: Aspen Systems, 1984.

Weiss, M. R., and R. R. Troxel. "Psychology of the Injured Athlete." *Athletic Training* 21 (1986): 104–109.

THREE

DIAGNOSIS AND TREATMENT OF SPECIFIC SPORTS INJURIES

THE MUSCULOSKELETAL
SYSTEM AND SKIN

13

The Musculoskeletal System

CHAPTER OUTLINE

Bones
  Anatomic Areas
  Histology
  Bone Growth and Remodeling
Joints
  Functional Anatomy

Joint Motion
  Histology and Physiology
Muscles
  Skeletal Muscle
  Special Muscles

OBJECTIVES FOR CHAPTER 13

After reading this chapter, the student should be able to:
1. Understand the organization and functional concepts of the musculoskeletal system.
2. Describe the functional anatomy, histology, and physiology of bones, joints, and muscles.

INTRODUCTION

The musculoskeletal system protects the vital organs of the body but is itself at risk of injury. Musculoskeletal injuries are common among athletes, and trainers who have an appreciation of how the musculoskeletal system is organized will be better prepared to handle these injuries. Chapter 13 presents the functional anatomy, histology, and physiology of the bones, joints, and muscles that compose the musculoskeletal system. ■

BONES

The **skeleton** forms the supporting framework of the human body (Fig. 13.1). Normally, it is composed of 206 bones that give form to the body and, with the joints, allow bodily motion. The skeleton also protects vital internal organs by shielding them: the brain lies within the skull; the heart, lungs, and great vessels are within the thorax; much of the liver and spleen are protected by the lowermost ribs; and the spinal cord is contained within and protected by the bony spinal column formed by the vertebrae.

Bones of the skeleton come into contact with one another at **joints**, where they are moved by the action of **muscles**. The skeleton thus is a rigid framework for the attachment of muscles and protection of organs and a flexible framework to allow the parts of the body to move by muscular contraction. The skeletal framework allows an erect posture against the pull of gravity and gives recognizable form to the body.

Bones must be rigid and unyielding to fulfill their function, but they must also grow and adapt as the human being grows. As a rule, bone growth is complete by late teens. Unless some abnormality is present, there is usually little outward skeletal change after this period. Because bones in young children are more flexible than bones in the adult, they are less likely to sustain displaced fractures but more likely to sustain a greenstick or buckle (torus) fracture.

Depending on shape and function, parts of a bone may be designated by specific names. The **head** of a bone is the rounded end that allows joint rotation. The region below the head is frequently called the neck. The **shaft** is the long, straight, cylindrical midportion of a bone.

The **condyles** (called malleoli at the ankle and styloid processes at the wrist) are prominences at one or both ends of the bone that usually serve as points of ligament attachment. **Tuberosities** and **trochanters** are prominences on the bone where tendons insert. The **epiphyseal plate** is a transverse cartilage plate near the end of a child's bone; it is responsible for growth in bone length.

Each bone is composed of a protein framework that allows its growth and remodeling. Calcium and phosphorus are deposited into this framework to make the bone hard and strong. Throughout a person's lifetime, calcium and phosphorus are constantly being deposited in bone and withdrawn from it under the control of a very complex metabolic system. This ability to grow as well as to repair by forming new bone is a phenomenon unique to bone tissue.

Bones are just as much living tissue as muscle and skin. A rich blood supply constantly provides the oxygen and nutrients that bones require. Each bone also has an extensive nerve supply, primarily from the periosteum. Thus, bone fracture produces severe pain from irritation of its nerves as well as heavy bleeding from damage to its blood vessels.

Anatomic Areas

For descriptive purposes, bones can be divided by the gross structures into long bones such as the tibia or humerus, short bones such as the metatarsal and metacarpal bones, and flat bones such as the scapula and clavicle. Long bones can further be divided into the **diaphysis**, or straight part of a long bone; the **epiphysis**, or end of a long bone; and the **metaphysis**, or flared area joining the diaphysis to the epiphysis (Fig. 13.2).

In growing bone, the growth plate, or **physis** (also termed the epiphyseal plate), separates the metaphysis from the epiphysis (see Fig. 13.2). The physis is the transverse plate of cartilage cells responsible for the longitudinal growth of bone (see section on bone growth and remodeling which follows). Furthermore, each bone is composed of a dense outer layer of bone called **cortical bone** (or the bone's cortex) and a less dense, more trabecular layer of bone called **cancellous bone**. The central open area of the bone is termed its **medullary canal** or **cavity**.

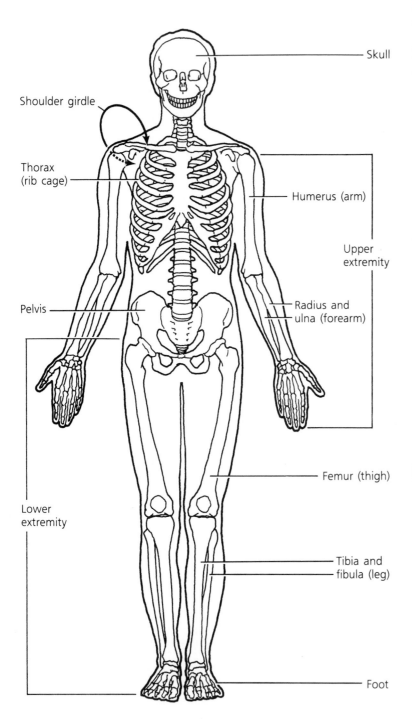

FIGURE 13.1. The human skeleton forms the frame of the body.

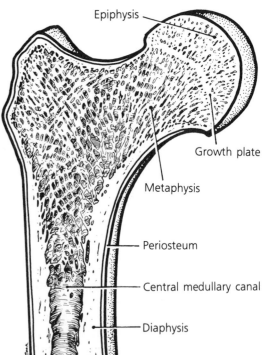

FIGURE 13.2. Anatomy of a bone.

Cortical bone predominates in the diaphyseal region of long bones, whereas cancellous bone predominates in the epiphyseal and metaphyseal regions.

The outer covering of bone, the **periosteum**, is formed by a dense layer of connective tissue which has osteogenic potential. **Endosteum** refers to a similar tissue which forms the inner layer of long bones.

Histology

Bone may be divided into **nonlamellar bone**, or **woven bone**, which is an immature bone, and mature **lamellar bone**, which is arranged in layers. Lamellar bone may be further divided into nonhaversian and haversian bone. *Haversian bone* consists of lamellar bone arranged around a central canal (Fig. 13.3). This arrangement of a central canal with surrounding layers of lamellar bone is called a *haversian system* or *osteon*. The haversian bone may be primary haversian, which is bone formed in place of connective tissue, or secondary haversian, formed in place of preexisting bone.

Bone cells consist of **osteoblasts**, which lay down new bone; **osteocytes**, which maintain mature bone; and **osteoclasts**, which resorb bone (Fig. 13.4). The fine channels extending through the bone and connecting the osteocytes are called *canaliculi*. They contain extracellular fluid that can transport nutrients to the osteocytes; they also provide a large area for the exchange of minerals. The osteoblast initially deposits unmineralized bone tissue (osteoid), which over an interval of approximately 15 days becomes mineralized. The osteoclast is present in depressions that are called *Howship's lacunae* along calcified resorbing bone.

Bone is composed of one-third organic matrix and two-thirds mineral. The mineral in bone is a form of amorphous tricalcium phosphate and hydroxyapatite, or $Ca_{10}(PO_4)_6(OH_2)$. The matrix is composed of 95 percent collagen, 1 percent glycosaminoglycans, 2 percent water, and 2 per-

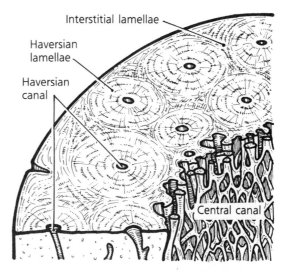

FIGURE 13.3. Histologic cross section of bone showing Haversian bone and lamellar bone around a central canal.

cent bone cells. Bone does not grow interstitially but by apposition and resorption on its surface. Less than 5 percent of the adult bone surfaces are being formed or resorbed at any one time.

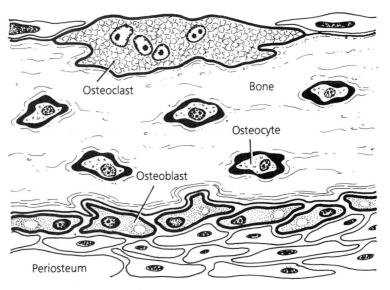

FIGURE 13.4. Bone cells.

Bone Growth and Remodeling

Bone formation and resorption occur along vertical tunnels in the bone. Most bones are formed by remodeling of a cartilage model. This is termed **enchondral ossification**. The longitudinal growth of a long bone is an example. The physis grows by interstitial deposition of cartilage beneath the metaphysis. The cartilage cells die, and the cartilage is invaded by blood vessels. New bone is deposited on the cartilage model, and the cartilage is reabsorbed. Bone grows in width by apposition of new bone on the periosteal surface and remodeling of the metaphysis, a process called **funnelization**.

Bone may be formed without preexisting cartilage in a growth process called **intramembranous ossification**. The bones of the vault of the skull are formed by intramembranous ossification. Centers of ossification are places where bone begins to be laid down. The primary center of ossification of a long bone is in the diaphysis and is present by the end of the fourth month of gestation. The secondary centers of ossification are formed in the epiphysis of the long bone. Each bone has a characteristic time of appearance of the secondary centers of ossification.

Bone growth and remodeling are affected by many factors, including hormones (such as parathyroid), adequacy of minerals (such as calcium and phosphorus), adequacy of vitamins (such as vitamin D), protein supply, and activity level. Bone responds to physical stresses or the lack of them. Bone is deposited on areas subjected to stress and reabsorbed from areas where little stress is present. This phenomenon is termed **Wolff's law**. A bone subjected to prolonged immobilization, such as when a cast is worn, is protected from use and becomes thinner. This loss of bone substance is called **osteoporosis of disuse**.

JOINTS

Wherever two bones come into contact, they form a **joint articulation**. Some joints allow motion—for example, the knee, hip, or elbow—whereas other bones fuse with one another at joints, producing a solid, immobile bony structure. The skull is composed of several different bones that fuse as the person grows into adulthood. The infant, whose bones are not yet fused, has soft spots called **fontanelles** between the skull bones. Many joints of the body are named by combining the names of the two bones forming that joint—for example, the sternoclavicular joint is the articulation between the sternum and the clavicle.

Functional Anatomy

Inside some joints, most notably the knee, cartilaginous cushions reduce the space between the bones and aid in the joint's gliding motion. Such a cushion is called a **meniscus** or sometimes simply a **cartilage**. When injured and torn from its attachment, the meniscus can produce symptoms of locking or catching in the joint.

In joints that allow motion, the bone ends are held together by a fibrous tissue capsule. At certain points around the joint, the capsule is lax and thin to allow motion in a certain plane, while in other areas it is thick and resists stretching or bending. These bands of tough, thick capsule are called **ligaments**. A joint that is virtually surrounded by tough, thick ligaments, such as the sacroiliac, has little motion, whereas a joint with few ligaments, such as the shoulder, is free to move in almost any direction (and is, as a result, more prone to dislocation).

Joint Motion

The degree of freedom of motion at a joint is determined by the extent to which the ligaments hold the bone ends together and by the configuration of the bone ends themselves. The hip joint is a ball-and-socket joint that allows internal and external rotation as well as bending. The finger joints are typical hinge joints, with motion restricted to one plane. They can bend (flex) and straighten (extend). Rotation is not possible because of the shape of the joint surfaces, and bending to the right or left is prevented by the strong ligaments on either side. Thus, while the amount of motion varies from joint to joint, all joints have a definite limit beyond which motion cannot occur. When a joint is forced beyond this limit, some structures are inevitably damaged. The bones forming the joint may break, or the supporting capsule and ligaments may be disrupted.

Motion of a joint is produced by the action of muscles. Muscles of the extremities are attached through their tendons to two bones (Fig. 13.5a). The muscle originates from one bone, and its other end inserts into the second bone. When the muscle shortens (contracts) (Fig. 13.5b), the ends of the bones will be brought closer together, with motion at the intervening joint. Muscles on the opposite side of the limb will relax (lengthen) to allow this motion. When motion in the opposite direction is desired, the second group of muscles contract and the first relax, rotating the joint back to its original position (Fig. 13.5c).

Histology and Physiology

The ends of bones that articulate with each other to form a moving joint are covered with a smooth, shiny surface called **articular cartilage**. The articular cartilage consists of four distinct cell zones: a superficial tangential or gliding zone, a transitional or intermediate zone, a radial zone, and a calcified zone (Fig. 13.6). A thin line called the **tidemark** lies between the radial and the calcified zone. Adult hyaline (articular) cartilage contains fewer cells than most other adult tissues. Mature cartilage is avascular, aneural, and alymphatic. Collagen fibers in the matrix provide stiffness to the articular

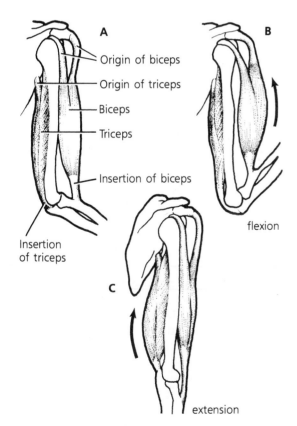

FIGURE 13.5. (a) The mechanism of joint motion powered by two opposing muscles. (b) Biceps contraction flexes the elbow and (c) triceps contraction extends the elbow.

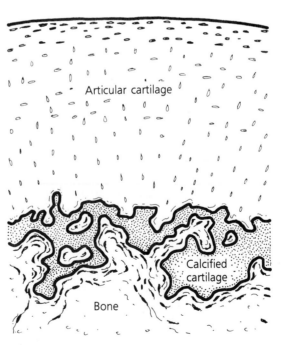

FIGURE 13.6. Histologic cross section through a gliding surface.

cartilage. Under normal adult conditions, articular cartilage cells do not undergo mitosis (cell division for new growth). Even in the presence of injury, the articular cartilage repair response is severely limited.

Articular cartilage has a high content of water (between 65 and 80 percent) present in the form of a gel. Collagen makes up 90 percent of the protein content. The cartilage contains complex large molecules called *mucopolysaccharides*, such as chondroitin sulfate. Also present are macromolecules called *protein polysaccharides*, consisting of a protein core with large chains of sulfated polysaccharides. The protein polysaccharides are highly charged molecules and are important in providing resiliency to the cartilage.

The inner surface of the joint capsule (the **synovium**) produces a fluid that nourishes and lubricates the articular cartilage—**synovial fluid**. Normally, only a few cubic centimeters of synovial fluid are present in a joint. The fluid is a source of nutrition for the hyaline cartilage and a lubricant for the joint. With injury or disease, more fluid is produced to protect the joint, resulting in swelling inside the capsule, as in the condition called "water on the knee."

Nutrients are diffused from the synovial fluid through the matrix of the articular cartilage. Very little nutrition passes from the vascular bone into the cartilage. The metabolic rate of articular cartilage, however, is high, and the anaerobic metabolic pathway is well developed.

MUSCLES

Almost all body systems and most organs have some muscular elements. Muscles may be classified as skeletal or special.

Skeletal Muscle

Skeletal muscle forms the major muscle mass of the body. It is called *skeletal* because it attaches to the bones of the skeleton. It is also called *voluntary muscle* because all skeletal muscle is under direct

voluntary control of the brain and can be contracted or relaxed at will. It is frequently also called **striated muscle** because it has characteristic stripes, or striations, under the microscope. All bodily movement is a result of skeletal contraction or relaxation. Most often a given motion is the result of several muscles working together, contracting or relaxing simultaneously.

Muscles function as agonists when they cause body movement. An antagonist causes motion opposite to the agonist muscle. An example is the biceps brachii and the triceps. Muscles must function in a coordinated manner, with synergistic muscles contracting as agonists contract and antagonists relax. Skeletal muscles cause movement by acting on bone, which functions as a lever, and across a joint, which acts as a fulcrum.

Skeletal muscles are under the direct control of the nervous system and respond to a willed command, as in the movement of an arm or leg. Nerves pass directly from the spinal cord to all skeletal muscles. Movements are voluntarily initiated and involuntarily coordinated. When the normal nerve supply is lost, a voluntary muscle can be neither contracted nor relaxed and becomes limp and useless.

Most of these skeletal muscles attach directly to bones by **tendons**—tough, rope-like cords of fibrous tissue. Usually these attachments are at two definite points. A muscle and its tendon pass between two bony attachments called the **origin** of the muscle and the **insertion** of the muscle (Fig. 13.7). When a muscle contracts, a line of force or pull is created between the origin and the insertion—that is, between the two bones to which the muscle is connected. Most voluntary muscles pass over or across joints. Movement can take place because of these joints.

An **aponeurosis** is a broad, fibrous sheet attaching a muscle to another muscle. **Ligaments**, or fibrous bands, attach bones to bones. Overexertion or excessive stretching may produce an injury in which the muscle, its tendon, or its aponeurosis is torn. Mus-

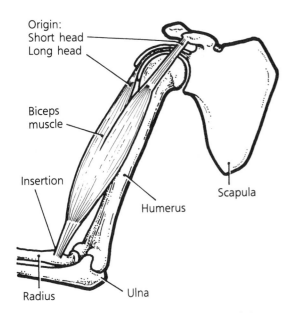
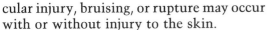

FIGURE 13.7. The origin and insertion of the biceps. Contraction of the biceps flexes the elbow.

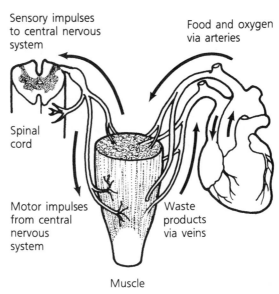

FIGURE 13.8. Arterial blood carries nutrients and oxygen to skeletal muscles, and venous blood removes metabolic waste.

cular injury, bruising, or rupture may occur with or without injury to the skin.

All skeletal muscles are supplied with arteries, veins, and nerves (Fig. 13.8). Blood brings oxygen and nutrients to muscles and carries away the waste produced by muscle contractions. Muscles cannot function without a continuous supply of nutrients and continuous removal of waste. Cramps may result when insufficient oxygen or nutrients are available or when acidic waste products accumulate.

Muscle contraction requires an energy source, **adenosine triphosphate (ATP)**, as well as magnesium and calcium ions. ATP is a high-energy, phosphate-containing compound. A complex series of metabolic pathways exist for the synthesis of ATP. As ATP and oxygen are depleted and anaerobic glycolysis occurs, lactic acid is produced and an oxygen debt is created. Once exertion is finished, extra oxygen is consumed and the lactic acid is removed. The oxygen debt may be as much as six times the basal oxygen consumption. Trained athletes contract smaller oxygen debts than do untrained persons.

A muscle may contract fully or partially. A contraction may result in a change in length, tension, or both. Each individual muscle fiber contracts maximally or not at all. Increasing a muscle's force of contraction results from recruiting additional muscle fibers. A single motor neuron innervates multiple muscle fibers and constitutes a functional unit, the motor unit. Recruitment of several motor units increases the force of contraction. A single action potential causes a muscle twitch.

Both the tension that a muscle develops when stimulated and the passive tension vary with the length of the muscle fiber. The greatest contractile force develops when the muscle is at its resting length. If the muscle is passively stretched beyond its resting length, the passive tension in the muscle increases, but the active tension that the muscle can develop decreases.

There are two major types of muscle fibers: Type I and Type II. Whole muscles are composed of Type I (red) and Type II (white) fibers of varied properties. **Type I muscle fibers** are rich in oxidative metabolic enzymes and myoglobin, whereas **Type II**

muscle fibers have high concentrations of enzymes for anaerobic glycolysis and less myoglobin. Myoglobin acts as a storage site for oxygen and is believed to speed the inward diffusion of oxygen into the muscle fiber. Type I fibers have slow contraction times and are predominantly used for sustained work. Type II fibers have rapid, short contraction times and fewer fibers per motor unit. Type II fibers are specialized for fine-skilled movements. Some of these differences between Type I and Type II fibers are related to neural innervation. Experimentally, reversal of the innervation can alter the properties of a muscle fiber, changing the fiber type. The different quantities of Type I and Type II muscle fibers may explain individual differences in athletic ability, such as the sprinter versus the marathon runner.

Special Muscles

The special muscles of the body are not part of the skeletal muscular system and are noted here only for completeness. The **involuntary muscles** carry out much of the automatic work of the body. This type of muscle is called **smooth muscle**. It forms the bulk of the gastrointestinal system, the bladder, and the ureters. It is found in nearly all the vessels and in bronchi. It is under involuntary nervous control and responds to stimuli such as heat or fright, or the need to relieve waste or to dilate or constrict vessels. No voluntary control is exerted over this type of muscle. Involuntary muscles are discussed in chapters dealing with the systems they serve.

The **diaphragm** is both an involuntary and a voluntary muscle. It is attached to the costal arch and the lumbar vertebrae. When a breath is taken, the diaphragm flattens, and its center part moves down. The volume of the chest cavity is increased, and inspiration can take place. Breathing is an automatic function that continues when a person sleeps and at all other times. Automatic control of breathing can, however, be temporarily overridden by conscious will, and a person can breathe faster or slower, or hold his or her breath. However, in the end, automatic control of breathing resumes. Hence, although the diaphragm looks like voluntary, skeletal muscle and is attached to the skeleton, it behaves like involuntary muscle most of the time.

The heart, or **cardiac muscle**, is a large muscle which is responsible for pumping blood to the tissues. It must function continuously from birth to death. It is a specially adapted involuntary muscle with a particularly good blood supply and its own regulatory system. It can tolerate interruption of its blood supply only for a few minutes before severe chest pain and the signs of a heart attack develop. Like all other involuntary muscles, it is under the automatic control of the autonomic nervous system.

IMPORTANT CONCEPTS

1. Bones come in contact with one another at joints, where they are moved by the action of muscles.
2. Bones can be long (tibia, humerus), short (metatarsals, metacarpals), or flat (scapula, clavicle).
3. Bone is composed of cells called osteoblasts (which lay down new bone), osteocytes (which maintain mature bone), and osteoclasts (which resorb bone).
4. Factors that affect bone growth and remodeling are hormones (parathyroid), min-erals (calcium, phosphorus), vitamins (vitamin D), protein supply, and activity level.
5. Joints that are surrounded by tough, thick ligaments have little motion, whereas joints surrounded by few ligaments are free to move in almost any direction.
6. Tendons attach muscle to bone, aponeuroses attach muscle to muscle, and liga-ments attach bone to bone.
7. Skeletal muscle, which forms the major muscle mass of the body, attaches to the bones of the skeleton.

SUGGESTED READINGS

Albright, James A., and Richard A. Brand, eds. *The Scientific Basis of Orthopaedics,* 2d ed. Norwalk, Conn.: Appleton & Lange, 1987.

Alho, A., T. Husby, and A. Høiseth. "Bone Mineral Content and Mechanical Strength: An ex Vivo Study on Human Femora at Autopsy." *Clinical Orthopaedics and Related Research* 227 (1988): 292–297.

Baldwin, K. M. "Muscle Development: Neonatal to Adult." *Exercise and Sport Sciences Reviews* 12 (1984): 1–19.

Benjamin, M., E. J. Evans, L. Copp. "The Histology of Tendon Attachments to Bone in Man." *Journal of Anatomy* 149 (1986): 89–100.

Brighton, C. T. "Longitudinal Bone Growth: The Growth Plate and Its Dysfunctions." In *Instructional Course Lectures,* vol. 36, edited by P. P. Griffin, pp. 3–25. Park Ridge, Ill.: American Academy of Orthopaedic Surgeons, 1987.

Chapman, A. E. "The Mechanical Properties of Human Muscle." *Exercise and Sport Sciences Reviews* 13 (1985): 443–501.

Cruess, Richard L., ed. *The Musculoskeletal System: Embryology, Biochemistry, and Physiology.* New York: Churchill Livingstone, 1982.

Currey, J. D. "Strain Rate and Mineral Content in Fracture Models of Bone." *Journal of Orthopaedic Research* 6 (1988): 32–38.

Fiore, Mariano S. H. di. *Atlas of Normal Histology,* 6th ed. Edited by Victor P. Eroschenko. Philadelphia: Lea & Febiger, 1989.

Fulkerson, John P. "Structure and Function of Joints." In *Scientific Foundations of Sports Medicine,* edited by Carol C. Teitz, pp. 261–270. Toronto: B. C. Decker, 1989.

Garrett, William E., and Pamela W. Duncan. "Basic Science of Musculotendinous Structure." *Sports Injury Management* 1 (1988): 1–42.

Gladden, L. Bruce. "Lactate Uptake by Skeletal Muscle." *Exercise and Sport Sciences Reviews* 17 (1989): 115–155.

Gollnick, P. D., and D. R. Hodgson. "The Identification of Fiber Types in Skeletal Muscle: A Continual Dilemma." *Exercise and Sport Sciences Reviews* 14 (1986): 81–104.

Gollnick, Philip D., and Bengt Saltin. "Skeletal Muscle Physiology." In *Scientific Foundations of Sports Medicine*, edited by Carol C. Teitz, pp. 185–241. Toronto: B. C. Decker, 1989.

Haines, Duane E. *Neuroanatomy: An Atlas of Structures, Sections, and Systems*, 2d ed. Baltimore: Urban & Schwarzenberg, 1987.

Hensinger, Robert N. *Standards in Pediatric Orthopedics: Tables, Charts, and Graphs Illustrating Growth*. New York: Raven Press, 1986.

Jones, Norman L., Neil McCartney, and Alan J. McComas, eds. *Human Muscle Power*. Champaign, Ill.: Human Kinetics, 1986.

Junqueira, Luiz C., José Carneiro, Robert O. Kelley. *Basic Histology*, 6th ed. Norwalk, Conn.: Appleton & Lange, 1989.

Kelly, Douglas E., et al. *Bailey's Textbook of Microscopic Anatomy*, 19th ed., edited by D. E. Kelly, R. L. Wood, and A. C. Anders. Baltimore: Williams & Wilkins, 1989.

Komi, P. V. "Physiological and Biomechanical Correlates of Muscle Function: Effects of Muscle Structure and Stretch-Shortening Cycle on Force and Speed." *Exercise and Sport Sciences Reviews* 12 (1984): 81–121.

Laughlin, M. H., and R. B. Armstrong. "Muscle Blood Flow during Locomotory Exercise." *Exercise and Sport Sciences Reviews* 13 (1985): 95–136.

Loeb, G. E. "The Control and Responses of Mammalian Muscle Spindles during Normally Executed Motor Tasks." *Exercise and Sport Sciences Reviews* 12 (1984): 157–204.

Marcus, Robert, and Dennis R. Carter. "The Role of Physical Activity in Bone Mass Regulation." *Advances in Sports Medicine and Fitness* 1 (1988): 63–82.

Mayne, Richard, and Michael H. Irwin. "Collagen Types in Cartilage." In *Articular Cartilage Biochemistry*, edited by Klaus E. Kuettner, Rudolf Schleyerbach, and Vincent C. Hascall, pp. 23–38. New York: Raven Press, 1986.

Nelson, C. L. "Blood Supply to Bone and Proximal Femur: A Synopsis." In *Instructional Course Lectures*, vol. 37, edited by F. H. Bassett, III, pp. 27–31. Park Ridge, Ill.: American Academy of Orthopaedic Surgeons, 1988.

Otten, E. "Concepts and Models of Functional Architecture in Skeletal Muscle." *Exercise and Sport Sciences Reviews* 16 (1988): 89–137.

Perugia, Lamberto, Franco Postacchini, and Ernesto Ippolito. *The Tendon: Biology—Pathology—Clinical Aspects*. Milano: Kurtis, 1986.

Puzas, J. E., M. D. Miller, and R. N. Rosier. "Pathologic Bone Formation." *Clinical Orthopaedics and Related Research* 245 (1989): 269–281.

Rall, J. A. "Energetic Aspects of Skeletal Muscle Contraction: Implications of Fiber Types." *Exercise and Sport Sciences Reviews* 13(1985): 33–74.

Ratzin, Jackson, G. Catherine, and Arthur L. Dickinson. "Adaptations of Skeletal Muscle to Strength or Endurance Training." *Advances in Sports Medicine and Fitness* 1 (1988): 45–59.

Roesler, H. "The History of Some Fundamental Concepts in Bone Biomechanics." *Journal of Biomechanics* 20 (1987): 1025–1034.

Schenk, Robert K., Peter S. Eggli, and Ernst B. Hunziker. "Articular Cartilage Morphology." In *Articular Cartilage Biochemistry*, edited by Klaus E. Kuettner, Rudolf Schleyerbach, and Vincent C. Hascall, pp. 3–22. New York: Raven Press, 1986.

Schoutens, A., E. Laurent, and J. R. Poortmans. "Effects of Inactivity and Exercise on Bone." *Sports Medicine* 7 (1989): 71–81.

Stauber, W. T. "Eccentric Action of Muscles: Physiology, Injury, and Adaptation." *Exercise and Sport Sciences Reviews* 17 (1989): 157–185.

Williams, I. F. "Cellular and Biochemical Composition of Healing Tendon." In *Ligament Injuries and Their Treatment*, edited by D.H.R. Jenkins, pp. 43–57. Rockville, Md.: Aspen Systems, 1985.

Woo, Savio L-Y., and Joseph A. Buckwalter, eds. *Injury and Repair of the Musculoskeletal Soft Tissues*. Park Ridge, Ill.: American Academy of Orthopaedic Surgeons, 1988.

14

Acute Soft Tissue and Musculoskeletal Injuries

CHAPTER OUTLINE

OBJECTIVES FOR CHAPTER 14

After reading this chapter, the student should be able to:

1. Describe the physical examination of the athlete with an acute musculoskeletal injury.
2. Discuss the mechanisms and management of soft tissue injuries.
3. Assess and provide emergency treatment for the athlete with a fracture, dislocation, or sprain.
4. Develop a plan for injury management.

INTRODUCTION

Athletic injuries can be classified as acute or overuse injuries. Acute injuries, such as lacerations, abrasions, sprains, dislocations, and traumatic fractures, occur suddenly, with a single application of force. Overuse injuries, such as tendinitis and stress fractures, occur from repeated stresses or microtrauma (see Chapter 15). Much can be learned about the nature of an injury when the mechanism through which it occurred is established.

Chapter 14 introduces some basic concepts regarding the mechanisms of acute injuries to the skin and musculoskeletal system. The chapter begins with a description of how the trainer examines athletes with injured limbs. Then the chapter presents the mechanisms and management of soft tissue injuries, fractures, and dislocations. The last section of Chapter 14 focuses on the importance of forming an injury management plan. ■

EXAMINATION OF ACUTE MUSCULOSKELETAL INJURIES

The following three steps are essential in the examination of *all* athletes with acute musculoskeletal injuries:

- Perform a general assessment of the athlete.
- Conduct an examination of the injured limb and evaluate distal neurovascular function.
- Keep the athlete calm.

General Assessment of the Athlete

The trainer must first perform a general, primary assessment of the injured athlete before treating an injured limb. Even when multiple injuries have occurred, the athlete's general condition must first be assessed and stabilized.

Examination of the Injured Limb

The trainer can examine and evaluate the injured limb using the following five steps.

Step 1: *Look at the injury.* The clothing should be gently and carefully removed from the injured limb to allow a thorough inspection. The trainer should be looking for the following problems:

- An open fracture or dislocation.
- Deformity (determined by comparing with the opposite limb).
- Swelling and ecchymosis.

Step 2: *Question the athlete.* The trainer should ask the conscious athlete about the mechanism of injury and what he or she heard and felt. The athlete can usually describe the injury and localize the point of maximal discomfort. If even the slightest motion increases the pain, no further motion should be attempted. The trainer should eliminate this step if the athlete complains of neck or back pain, because even slight motion might permanently damage the spinal cord.

Step 3: *Feel the limb.* The trainer gently palpates the injured extremity to identify point tenderness, which is the best indicator of an underlying fracture, dislocation, or sprain.

Step 4: *Assess limb function.* The trainer asks the athlete to move the injured limb carefully if no crepitus (a grating, grinding sensation from fractured bone ends rubbing against each other) or deformity has been noted.

Step 5: *Evaluate neurovascular parameters.* An equally important step in assessing musculoskeletal injury is a critical evaluation of the neurovascular function of the limb. Many important vessels and nerves lie close to the bone, especially around the major joints. Any fracture or dislocation may have associated vessel or nerve injury. The trainer must carry out neurovascular evaluation initially and repeat the evaluation every 30 minutes until the athlete is transported to a hospital. It is also imperative that the trainer recheck the athlete's neurovascular status after any manipulation of the limb, such as splinting, because movement may cause a bone fragment to press against or impale an important nerve or vessel. A pulseless limb will die if circulation is not restored, and an athlete with this problem must receive high priority for emergency care.

The trainer should evaluate and record the following neurovascular parameters for each injured limb.

- *Pulse.* Palpate the pulse distally to the point of injury.
- *Capillary filling.* Note the skin color, identifying any pallor or cyanosis. The capillary bed is best judged in the finger or toe under the nail. Firm pressure on the tip of the nail causes this bed to blanch or turn white. Upon release of the pressure, the normal pink color should return by the time it takes to say "capillary filling." If the color does not return in this 2-second interval, capillary filling is considered delayed, indicating impaired circulation.
- *Sensation.* The athlete's ability to perceive light touch in the fingers or toes distal to a fracture site is a good indication that the nerve supply is intact. In the hand, check and record touch sensation on the pulp of the index and little fingers. In the foot, check and record feeling on the pulp of the great toe and on the dorsum of the foot laterally.
- *Motor function.* When an injury is proximal to the hand or to the foot, estimate muscular activity. Test each muscle group and grade as indicated in Table 10.1 on page 150. If such testing produces pain in the athlete, do not persist with this part of the examination.

In the unconscious athlete, some of the neurovascular parameters cannot be evaluated because they require the athlete's cooperation. After the primary assessment is completed and vital functions are stabilized, any limb deformity, swelling, ecchymosis, or false motion should be considered evidence of a fracture and treated as such. The distal pulses and capillary filling can still be monitored in the unconscious, injured athlete. Any unconscious, injured athlete should be assumed to have suffered a spinal injury that requires spine board immobilization.

Keeping the Athlete Calm

As always, when an athlete sustains an acute injury or experiences a sudden illness, keeping the athlete calm is of paramount importance. The reassuring manner of the skilled athletic trainer instills confidence in the athlete, allowing the trainer to proceed with evaluation and institution of emergency care.

SOFT TISSUE INJURIES

Injuries to the soft tissues surrounding the skeletal system—muscles and their tendons, ligaments, nerves, blood vessels, and the skin—are common in athletics. The injured athlete needs to be evaluated as soon as an injury occurs. Early recognition and immediate care can minimize the severity of the injury and often prevent serious complications and disability.

Most injuries involve some soft tissue, skin, skeletal muscle, or fascia (the fibrous tissue that encloses muscles). An injury may be closed or open. In **closed injuries**, soft tissue damage occurs beneath the skin with no break in the surface involved. In **open injuries**, the surface of the skin or the mucous membrane that lines the major body orifices (mouth, nose, anus, and vagina) is broken.

Bruises and Contusions

Mechanism of Injury

A blunt object that strikes against the body with sufficient force crushes the tissue beneath the skin. Within this tissue, a **contusion** (bruise) develops (Fig. 14.1). Subsurface damage may extend for varying depths beneath the skin. Small blood vessels in the tissues usually tear, and varying amounts of blood and plasma leak into the wound and produce swelling and pain. The blood in the tissues gradually migrates toward the skin and causes an **ecchymosis** (a black-and-blue discoloration).

When considerable amounts of tissue are damaged or torn, or when large blood ves-

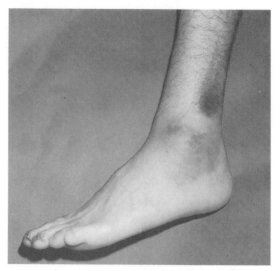

FIGURE 14.1. A contusion, characterized by swelling and ecchymosis, has developed in this closed soft tissue injury to the ankle.

sels are disrupted at the site of the contusion, a lump may develop rather rapidly from a pool of blood collecting within the damaged tissue. This condition is called a **hematoma**, or literally, a blood tumor. In all fractures, a hematoma collects around the broken ends of the bones. With the fracture of a large bone such as the femur or pelvis, more than a liter of blood can be lost from injured vessels that are leaking into the tissues.

Management of Bruises and Contusions

Small bruises require no special emergency medical care. With severe, closed soft tissue injuries, extensive swelling and bleeding beneath the skin may cause shock. Applying local padding and a soft roller bandage for counterpressure can partially control this bleeding in the extremities. Elevating the extremity and applying ice locally to the area are also helpful in decreasing bleeding of injured tissue and preventing initial tissue swelling. If the athlete has suffered extensive soft tissue damage, the athletic trainer should suspect that underlying fractures are involved.

Open Wounds

Open wounds cause obvious bleeding and are subject to direct contamination and thus infection.

Mechanism of Injury

There are four major causes of open soft tissue injury: abrasions, lacerations, avulsions, and puncture wounds.

An **abrasion** is a loss of a portion of the epidermis and part of the dermis from having been rubbed or scraped across a hard surface (Fig. 14.2a). It is extremely painful, and blood may ooze from injured capillary vessels at the surface. However, the wound does not penetrate completely through the skin.

A **laceration** is a cut produced by any object that leaves a smooth or jagged wound through the skin, damaging the subcutaneous tissue, underlying muscles, nerves, and blood vessels (Fig. 14.2b).

An **avulsion** is an injury in which a piece of skin with varying portions of subcutaneous tissue or muscle is either torn loose completely or left hanging as a flap (Fig. 14.2c).

A **puncture wound** results from a splinter, cleat, or other pointed object (Fig. 14.2d). External bleeding is usually not severe because the wound is small, but puncture wounds are difficult to cleanse and are prone to infection. A deep wound may injure major vessels within body cavities and require an exploratory operation in the chest, abdomen, or involved extremity. Extensive damage should always be suspected. The trainer should *never* attempt to remove an impaled object.

Management of Open Wounds

Abrasions generally do not bleed extensively. Small abrasions may be cleansed with soap and water and covered with a sterile dressing that does not adhere to the wound, such as a Telfa bandage. Sterile analgesic preparations or antibiotic ointments may be used but are not substitutes for thorough

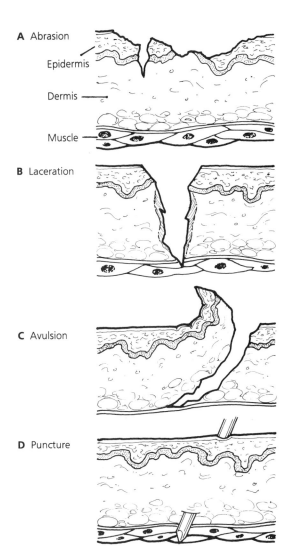

FIGURE 14.2. The four general types of open soft tissue injuries: (a) Abrasions involve loss of variable depths of the dermis and epidermis. (b) Lacerations are cuts produced by sharp objects. (c) Avulsions raise flaps of tissue, usually along normal tissue planes. (d) Puncture wounds may penetrate to any depth.

cleansing of the wound. Extensive abrasions, such as the "road rash" bicyclists can get from high-speed falls, are very painful. A physician's assistance may be needed to control pain during cleansing and dressing of these wounds.

Treatment of small lacerations can often be managed by the athletic trainer. Bleeding from these wounds should be controlled with direct pressure. After bleeding is controlled, the wound should be cleansed with soap and water. An antiseptic solution such as Betadine may also be applied. The wound is closed by pulling the edges of the wound together with adhesive strips such as Steri-Strips. Tincture of benzoin may be applied to the skin around the wound to improve the adhesion of the strips.

Larger lacerations and avulsions require evaluation and treatment by a physician. The athletic trainer should quickly assess the severity of the bleeding and the amount of blood lost and then work to control the bleeding and immobilize the injured part, prevent further wound contamination, and keep the athlete calm. The trainer should not do anything to clean these wounds beyond removing surface particles. Topical analgesics and antiseptics should not be applied because they can make the wound more difficult to clean and suture. When in doubt regarding the need for suturing or wound care, the trainer should control the bleeding, prevent further wound contamination, and refer the athlete to a physician.

Ordinarily, avulsed tissues separate at normal anatomic planes—for example, between muscle and subcutaneous tissue. Occasionally, avulsed tissue will be torn completely free and will be lying apart from the athlete. All avulsed tissue should be retrieved and transported to the hospital with the athlete because reattachment may be possible. Avulsions of fingers or extremities can separate portions of tissue. Any pieces should be wrapped in sterile gauze, placed in a plastic bag, and then put in a cooled container. The tissue should not be allowed to freeze.

Minor puncture wounds are treated in the same manner as abrasions. Because the surface of puncture wounds is not as exposed as the surface affected by abrasions, these wounds are difficult to clean and prone to infection. The trainer should refer athletes with puncture wounds that contain debris to a physician for treatment. The trainer should also check the athlete's record of tetanus inoculation as a part of the treatment of all open wounds.

Evaluating puncture wounds involves evaluating the intactness of nerves, vessels, and muscles in the area of the wound. Large puncture wounds may bleed extensively and require control of bleeding by applying direct pressure and dressing and bandaging the wound. The trainer then must refer the athlete to a physician for further evaluation and treatment.

Occasionally, an object such as a splinter of wood or a piece of glass is the cause of a puncture wound and is known as an **impaled foreign object**. In addition to local control of bleeding, there are three rules to apply when treating an athlete with an impaled foreign object:

- *Do not remove the object* (Fig. 14.3a). Removing the object may cause hemorrhage or damage nearby nerves or muscles. Try to stop any bleeding from the entrance wound by direct pressure, but do not exert any force on the impaled object itself or on tissue directly adjacent to its cutting edge to avoid further tissue damage (Fig. 14.3b).
- *Use a bulky dressing to stabilize the object.* The impaled foreign body itself should be incorporated within the dressing to reduce its motion after the bandage is applied (Figs. 14.3c, d).
- *Transport the athlete promptly to the emergency department with the object still in place.* Ordinarily, surgery is necessary to remove the object, so the tissues immediately around the object will be directly examined and treated.

Sometimes, a very long impaled object must be shortened to allow transport. Because even the slightest movement may cause severe additional pain, hemorrhage, or damage of the tissue around the object, the object must be made very secure, before it is cut, and any motion transmitted to the athlete must be kept to a minimum. Pain,

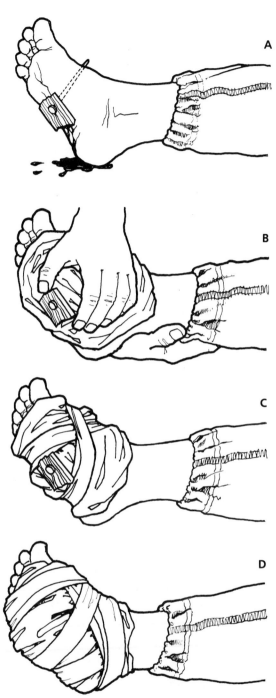

FIGURE 14.3.   Treating an athlete with an impaled foreign object: (a) Leave the impaled object in place. (b) Control bleeding with pressure. (c) Apply a bandage about the object to stabilize it and to maintain pressure. (d) Use a bulky final dressing to protect the athlete during transportation.

because it may aggravate shock in the athlete who has undergone severe hemorrhage, must be avoided whenever possible.

Muscle Strains

Mechanism of Injury

Sudden overload of a musculotendinous unit can cause the fibers of the muscle and tendon to tear, a condition called a **strain** (Fig. 14.4). The signs and symptoms of muscle strain include pain over the site of injury, muscle spasm, and loss of strength. It is often difficult to differentiate between mild and moderate strains. Knowing the extent of the pain, spasm, and weakness is

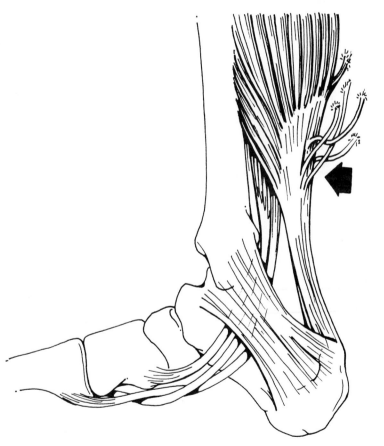

FIGURE 14.4.   A strain occurs when a sudden overload of a musculotendinous unit causes the fibers of the muscle and tendon to tear.

useful in estimating the extent of the injury and the time lost from athletic activity.

Severe strains often result in palpable deformities and the absence of function. The trainer must be careful not to misinterpret the actions of synergistic muscles in the examination of severe strains. For example, the posterior tibialis and peroneal muscles assist the triceps surae with plantar flexion. Following rupture of the Achilles tendon, some ability to plantar flex the unweighted foot will remain due to the actions of the muscles.

Management of Muscle Strains

Following the initial physical examination, muscle strains should be managed with rest, ice, compression, and elevation. This

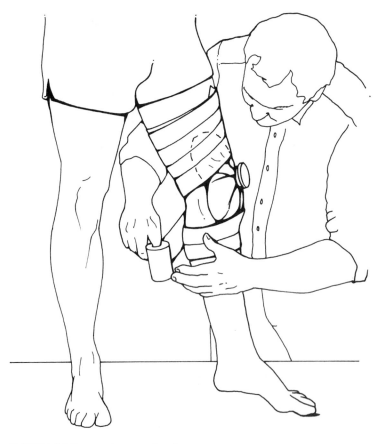

FIGURE 14.5. Ice bag application.

treatment reduces tissue damage from bleeding and swelling. Crushed ice in a plastic bag, held in place with an elastic bandage (Fig. 14.5), may be applied for 20 to 30 minutes every 1½ to 2 hours. The athletic trainer should be aware that a very small percentage of athletes may experience adverse reactions to ice application such as frostbite and nerve damage. Therefore, any application of ice should be monitored. Extra caution should be taken when ice is placed directly over subcutaneous nerves (e.g., the ulnar nerve behind the elbow and the peroneal nerve behind the knee) to prevent damage to these structures by cold exposure.

Strains that are too painful for normal walking or that cause pain when the athlete moves the injured part should be protected and rested. Crutches, slings, and commercial ankle, knee, and wrist splints should be available in the athletic training room.

Definitive treatment of strains will depend on the extent of the injury and the athlete's sport and position. Timely examination of all but very minor strains by a physician is essential, so that a treatment and rehabilitation plan can be established.

Ligament Sprains

Mechanism of Injury

Although **sprain** has been used in a very general sense to refer to an injury to a joint where ligaments are stretched or torn but the joint is not completely dislocated (i.e., an ankle sprain), it more specifically refers to the injury to the ligament itself—that is, a sprain of the anterior fibular talar ligament of the ankle. As such, ligament sprains are graded according to the following classification.

- *Grade I (mild).* The ligament is stretched, but there is no loss of continuity of its fiber.
- *Grade II (moderate).* The ligament is partially torn, resulting in some increased laxity to the joint.

- *Grade III (severe)*. The ligament is completely torn, resulting in laxity (instability) of the joint which it stabilizes.

Ligament tears can be seen with deep lacerations, but more commonly they occur when a joint is forced beyond its normal range of motion. The following are signs of a ligament sprain:

- *Tenderness*. Point tenderness can be elicited over the injured ligament.
- *Swelling and ecchymosis*. There is typically swelling and ecchymosis at the point of ligament laxity.
- *Instability*. Gently stressing the injured ligament will increase pain and demonstrates an increased abnormal range of motion in Grade II and III ligament sprains. It is important to compare the findings on the injured limb to the opposite limb (or to records of ligament instability as noted on the preseason screening exam) before deciding that there is a loss of stability.
- *Inability to use the extremity*. Because of the pain of the injury, the athlete may not be able to use the limb normally.

Management of Ligament Sprains

The management of a ligament sprain depends on the degree of injury. A first-degree sprain is treated with rest, ice, compression, and elevation until the acute symptoms subside. A rehabilitation program to strengthen the area will prepare the athlete for return to activity. A second-degree sprain is treated similarly, but may in addition require immobilization of the injured area. Depending on the location and severity of the injury, a third-degree sprain may require either immobilization or surgical intervention to restore continuity of the ligament. Some severe ligamentous injuries can be managed successfully on a conservative program.

Nerve Injuries

The human nervous system is highly complex. It is divided into a **central nervous system**, consisting of the brain and spinal cord, and a **peripheral nervous system**, which includes the nerves innervating the muscles (the **motor nerves**) and the nerves sending sensory information from the skin, muscles, and joints to the brain (the **sensory nerves**).

Mechanism of Injury

The nerves of both the central and peripheral nervous systems can be damaged in athletic injuries. Fractures and dislocations of the vertebrae, especially in the cervical region, can damage the spinal cord and result in permanent disability. Peripheral nerve injuries are usually associated with lacerations, dislocations, and fractures. However, injuries such as a brachial plexus stretch (shoulder "burner") may be limited to the peripheral nerves.

Unfortunately, potentially catastrophic injuries to the cervical spine are difficult to evaluate and usually require x-ray examination. The potential for damage to the spinal cord should be recognized when the mechanism of injury could have resulted in injury to the cervical spine. An athlete suffering a head injury should be evaluated for injury to the cervical spine, and an athlete rendered unconscious from trauma should always be treated as if a cervical spine injury has been sustained.

Management of Nerve Injuries

The function of the peripheral nervous system should be assessed following sprains, dislocations, suspected fractures, and deep lacerations of the skin. The nerve function can be easily assessed by checking motor function and sensation distal to the injury. The extent and location of loss of motor function or sensation should be noted, and the athlete should be promptly referred to a physician.

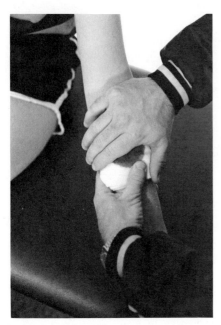 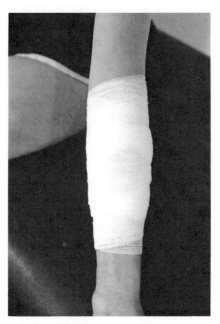 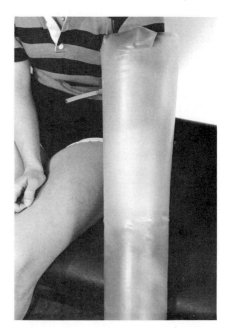

14.6a. Direct pressure applied by hand using a sterile dressing.

14.6b. Direct pressure applied by a pressure bandage.

14.6c. Direct pressure applied by an air splint.

Blood Vessel Injuries

Mechanism of Injury

Damage to the large arteries and veins is not common in athletic injuries. However, deep skin wounds can lacerate these vessels and present a life-threatening emergency. Bright red, spurting blood from a wound indicates bleeding from an artery. Arterial bleeding can result in the loss of a large volume of blood and produce life-threatening **hemorrhagic shock**.

Fractures and dislocations can lacerate large vessels or press down on them, occluding blood flow. The absence of a pulse or poor capillary refill distal to the site of injury indicates that the vessels have been compromised. Prompt medical attention is required to prevent additional injury due to limited blood flow to the area.

Management of Blood Vessel Injuries

External bleeding should be controlled. Suspected fractures and dislocations should be carefully splinted to prevent injury to the nervous and vascular systems during transport of the athlete. The trainer should always check neurovascular function after applying a splint to be sure that the splint is not causing complications.

Dressings and Bandages

Soft tissue injuries must be bandaged and sometimes splinted. (Splinting is discussed later in the chapter.)

Functions

Dressings and bandages have three main functions: to control bleeding, to protect a wound from further damage, and to prevent further contamination and possible infection. The initial step in controlling bleeding is the application of direct pressure. Pressure may be applied with a sterile dressing by the hand (Fig. 14.6a), by a pressure bandage (Fig. 14.6b), or by an air splint (Fig. 14.6c). Care should be taken to avoid putting heavy pressure over possible fractures, especially at the skull. Wounded extremities should be elevated, if a fracture can be ruled out. Only rarely, pressure-point control or a tourniquet is necessary to control severe arterial bleeding. (See Chapter 39 for information on these techniques.)

Frequently, splinting the extremity can help control bleeding from soft tissue wounds, whether or not they are associated with a fracture. An air splint exerts a considerable amount of gentle pressure throughout the entire length of the extremity and may control bleeding more readily than a local pressure dressing. When bleeding is associated with a soft tissue wound accompanying a fracture, splinting is absolutely necessary for adequate control of soft tissue bleeding. Further, splinting an extremity with severe soft tissue injury immobilizes the injury and allows the athlete to be moved more readily and comfortably without sustaining further damage.

Wound contamination and resultant secondary infection are less likely if sterile materials are used for the initial dressing. Every effort should be made to keep foreign matter out of the wound. Hair, clothing, dirt, and fluids all increase the danger of secondary infection. However, in initial treatment, the trainer should not try to remove material embedded in the wound. Only the foreign matter on the surface around the wound should be removed. A physician should perform the final, definitive cleaning of the wound. Much time can be lost in a fruitless attempt to clean a wound that requires surgery.

Any clothing that is covering a wound must be removed. It is often better to tear or cut clothing away from the wound than to remove it as one would normally, since any motion may be painful and cause additional tissue damage and contamination. Even a minor movement may cause excruciating pain for the athlete.

Dressings should never interfere with circulation. After applying a dressing, the trainer should always check the distal limb for signs of impaired circulation or loss of skin sensation.

Types of Dressings

Several different materials can be used to apply the four most commonly used dressings: universal, stabilizing, occlusive, and pressure dressings.

Universal dressings. A **universal dressing** is made of thick, absorbent material; it measures 9 by 36 inches and is packed folded into a compact size. Although universal dressings are available commercially, they can be made at a reasonable cost. Bandage material is available in 9-inch-wide, 20-yard rolls. When cut in a 36-inch-long piece and folded on itself three times, from each end, each length becomes a compact dressing that fits conveniently into a number 2 paper bag. The end of the bag can be folded and stapled. The package can be sterilized by local hospital personnel and placed in a protective plastic bag with a soft roller bandage. It is an efficient, reasonably priced dressing for wounds or burns and can serve as padding for splints.

Stabilizing dressings. Dressings must remain in place during transport. Soft roller, self-adherent bandages, rolls of gauze, triangular bandages, or adhesive tape can be used as **stabilizing dressings**. Soft roller bandages are probably the easiest to use because they are slightly elastic, the layers adhere to one another, and the end of the roll can be tucked back into the layers. Triangular bandages can hold a dressing in place if the ends of the bandage can be tied together. Adhesive tape can hold small bandages in place and help secure other dressings. Remember, however, that some people are allergic to ordinary adhesive tape. Elastic bandages should not be used to secure dressings, because they may distribute pressure unevenly and produce complications.

Occlusive dressings. **Occlusive dressings** are used for sucking chest wounds and abdominal eviscerations. These wounds must be sealed so that air does not pass through.

With sucking chest wounds a large enough dressing must be used so that the dressing itself is not sucked into the chest cavity. Sterile aluminum foil is a satisfactory, nonadherent, occlusive dressing for both sucking chest wounds and abdominal eviscerating wounds. The entire roll of foil can be sterilized in its package, and the remainder resterilized after each use. Adhesive tape may be needed to secure the bandage.

Pressure dressings. A **pressure dressing** is recommended to control bleeding from a wound. The pressure applied must exceed the pressure in the bleeding vessels. The universal dressing is a perfect initial layer for a pressure dressing because it can be folded or opened to adapt to most wound sizes. After the dressing is in place, hand pressure is applied on the wound through the dressing until the bleeding has slowed or stopped. Continued pressure can be maintained by firmly applying a roller bandage to the injured part. If bleeding continues or recurs, the original dressing and bandages should be left in place, and another large dressing should be applied and secured with another roller bandage.

FRACTURES AND DISLOCATIONS

Because musculoskeletal injuries occur so frequently, the trainer must be able to evaluate them properly and master the skills necessary for their initial emergency care. Appropriate emergency care of fractures and dislocations not only decreases immediate pain and reduces the possibility of shock, but also improves the athlete's chances for a rapid recovery and early return to normal activity.

Fractures

A **fracture** is any break in the continuity of a bone, ranging in severity from a simple crack to more severe shattering of the bone with multiple fracture fragments. There is no difference between a fractured or broken bone; both terms describe the same injury.

Classification of Fractures

In the initial evaluation of a fracture, the most important factor to identify is the integrity of the overlying skin and soft tissues. Thus, fractures are always classified as open (compound) or closed.

In an **open fracture**, or **compound fracture**, the overlying skin has been lacerated by the sharp bone ends protruding through the skin or by a direct blow that breaks the skin at the time of fracture. The bone may or may not be visible in the wound. The wound may be only a small puncture, or a gaping hole exposing much bone and soft tissue. In a **closed fracture**, the bone ends have not penetrated the skin, and no wound exists near the fracture.

It is extremely important to determine at once whether the fracture is open or closed. Open fractures are often more serious than closed fractures because they may be associated with greater blood loss; also, because the bone is contaminated by exposure to the outside environment, the wound may become infected. For these reasons, all fractures should be described to emergency department personnel as open or closed, so that the proper treatment can be undertaken as soon as the athlete arrives at the hospital.

Fractures are also described by the degree of displacement of the fragments. **Nondisplaced fractures** may be difficult to diagnose without x-ray films. The fracture may be thought to be only a bruise or sprain. A high index of suspicion is necessary when a trainer evaluates an injured athlete who is complaining of extremity pain. An athlete exhibiting any of the signs or symptoms of fracture must be treated as if he or she has a fracture.

A **displaced fracture** produces deformity of the limb. The deformity is slight if the displacement is minimal, or extreme with gross displacement of the fragments. Many different deformities may occur. Angulation and rotation of the limb distal to the fracture site are common displacements. In addition, the limb may be shortened if the fracture fragments are displaced and their

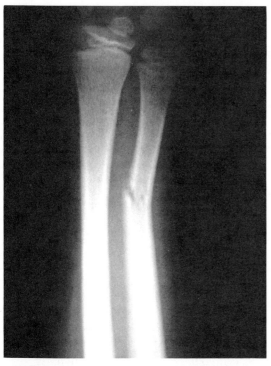

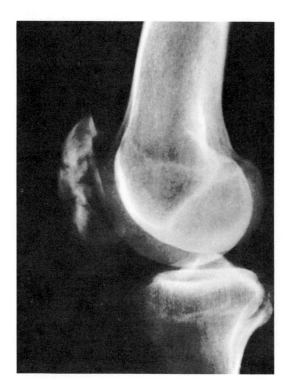

FIGURE 14.7.   An incomplete, or greenstick, fracture.

ends overlap. Particular types of fractures may be described as follows:

- A **greenstick fracture** occurs only in children and is an incomplete fracture that passes only part way through the shaft of a bone (Fig. 14.7).
- A **comminuted fracture** occurs when the bone is broken into more than two fragments (Fig. 14.8).
- A **pathologic fracture** occurs through weak or diseased bone and is produced by minimal force.
- A **stress** or **fatigue fracture** occurs when the bone is subjected to frequent, repeated stresses such as from running or marching long distances, much as a paper clip can be broken by repeated bending back and forth.
- An **epiphyseal fracture** occurs in growing children and involves injury to the growth plate of a long bone (Fig. 14.9). This fracture may lead to an arrest of bone growth. Proper treatment reduces this risk.

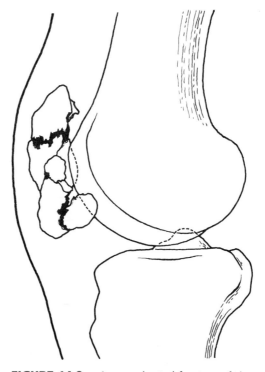

FIGURE 14.8.   A comminuted fracture of the patella: (top) x-ray; (bottom) line drawing.

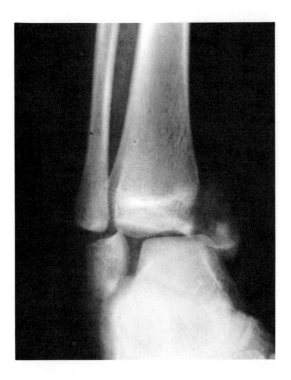

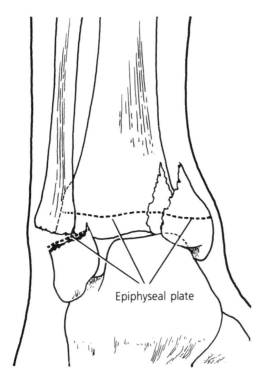

Epiphyseal plate

FIGURE 14.9. Transverse fracture through the growth plate of the distal fibular epiphysis and a vertical fracture through the tibial epiphysis: (top) x-ray; (bottom) line drawing.

Signs and Symptoms of Fractures

Any athlete who complains of musculoskeletal pain must be suspected of having a fracture. While bone ends that are protruding through the skin or gross deformity of a limb makes recognition of fractures easy, many fractures are less obvious. The athletic trainer must know the seven signs of fractures that follow. The presence of any one of these signs should arouse suspicion of a fracture, and proper emergency treatment should be instituted.

- *Deformity.* The limb may lie in an unnatural position—shortened, angulated, or rotated at a point where no joint exists. If the deformity is unclear, the opposite limb provides a mirror image for comparison. Always compare the injured limb to the uninjured opposite limb when checking for deformity.
- *Tenderness.* Tenderness is usually sharply localized at the site of the break. The sensitive spot can be located by gently pressing along the bone with one fingertip. This sign, called **point tenderness**, is the most reliable indication of an underlying fracture.
- *Inability to use the extremity* (**guarding**). An athlete with a fracture or serious injury usually "guards" the injured part and refuses to use it because motion increases pain. One might say that athletes attempt to splint their own fractures to minimize pain. Occasionally, nondisplaced fractures are not very painful, and some athletes may continue to use a painful limb even when it is fractured.
- *Swelling and ecchymosis.* Fractures are virtually always associated with swelling and bruising of the surrounding soft tissues. These signs are present following almost any injury and are not specific for fractures. However, rapid swelling immediately after a fracture is usually due to bleeding into the soft tissues from damaged blood vessels. Indeed, the swelling

may mask a limb deformity produced by the broken bones. Generalized edema of the limb also occurs 12 or more hours after the fracture.

- *Exposed fragments.* In an open fracture, bone ends may protrude through the skin or be seen in the depths of the wound itself. When the limb is manipulated, two additional signs of fracture may appear.
- *Crepitus (grating).* A grating or grinding sensation called **crepitus** can be felt and sometimes even heard when bone ends impinge or move on one another.
- *False motion.* Motion at a point in the limb where it usually does not occur is indicative of bone fracture. (See Chapter 10 for a discussion of evaluation of joint range of motion.)

The first five signs of fracture need to be evaluated to diagnose a fracture in the field. Crepitus and false motion are extremely painful, and the limb should not be manipulated to elicit these signs if other signs of a fracture are present. If a fracture is suspected, appropriate splinting and referral for an x-ray examination should be implemented.

Dislocations

Dislocation means disruption of a joint so that the bone ends are no longer in contact (Fig. 14.10). Frequently, the stabilizing ligaments of the joint are torn at the time the joint dislocates. A **fracture-dislocation** is a combined injury in which the joint is dislocated and a part of the bone near the joint is fractured as well (Fig. 14.11).

With dislocation of a joint, injury to the stabilizing ligaments and capsule is so severe that the joint surfaces are completely displaced from one another. The bone ends are locked in the displaced position, making any attempted joint motion very difficult and very painful. The joints most susceptible to dislocation are the shoulder, elbow, hip, ankle, and the small joints of the fingers.

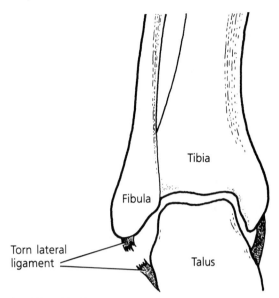

FIGURE 14.10.   A dislocated ankle joint; the bone ends are no longer in contact.

The following are signs and symptoms of a dislocated joint:

- Marked deformity of the joint.
- Swelling of the joint.
- Pain at the joint, aggravated by any attempt at movement.
- Marked loss of normal joint motion (a "locked" joint).

Management of Fractures and Dislocations

Emergency management of fractures, dislocations, and sprains occurs after the injured athlete's vital functions have been assessed and stabilized. All open wounds should be covered completely with a dry, sterile dressing, and local pressure should be applied to control bleeding. The open fracture should then be managed in the same way as a closed fracture. Emergency department personnel should be notified of all open wounds so dressed and splinted.

All fractures and dislocations should be splinted before the athlete is moved, unless the athlete's life is immediately threatened. Splinting, in addition to facilitating the

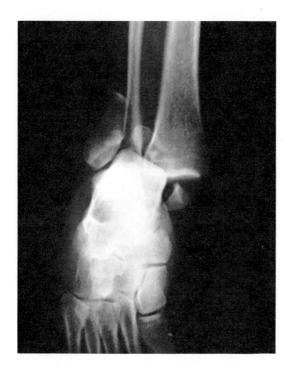

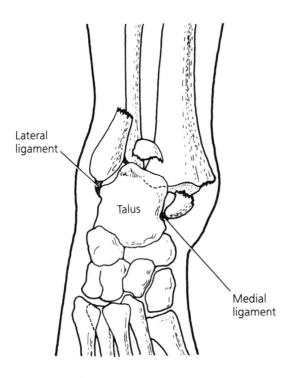

FIGURE 14.11. Fracture-dislocation of the ankle joint. X-ray shows the talus dislocated from the distal tibia with fracture of both the medial and lateral malleoli.

transfer and transportation of the athlete, has the following advantages:

- Prevents movement of fracture fragments or a dislocated joint.
- Reduces pain.
- Prevents laceration of the skin by the broken bones, which converts a closed fracture into an open one.
- Prevents the restriction of distal blood flow resulting from pressure of the bone ends on blood vessels.
- Controls excessive bleeding into the tissues at the fracture site.

Common Splints and Their Application

A **splint**, which is a device that prevents an injured part from moving, can be fashioned from many materials. If no splinting materials are available, the arm can be bound to the chest, and the injured leg can be splinted to the uninjured leg to provide at least temporary stability. However, an adequate supply of standard commercial splints should be on hand (Fig. 14.12), and improvisation should be necessary only occasionally. There are three basic types of splints: rigid, soft, and traction.

Rigid splints. **Rigid splints** are made from firm material and are applied to the sides, front, or back of an injured extremity to prevent motion at the injury site. Common examples include padded board splints, molded plastic and metal splints, padded wire ladder splints, and folded cardboard splints.

Two athletic trainers should follow these steps to apply rigid splints.

1. First trainer: gently support the limb and apply steady traction until the splint is completely applied.
2. Second trainer: place the rigid splint under or alongside the limb and continue the application.
3. Place padding to ensure even pressure and even contact between the limb and the splint, with particular attention to bony prominences.

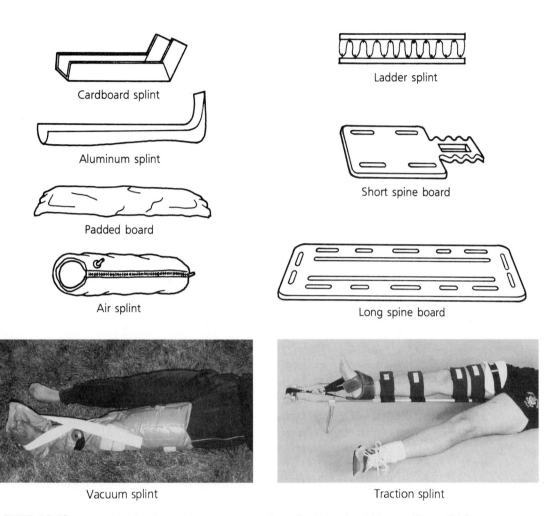

Cardboard splint

Aluminum splint

Padded board

Air splint

Ladder splint

Short spine board

Long spine board

Vacuum splint

Traction splint

FIGURE 14.12. A good selection and adequate number of splints should be readily available.

4. Apply bindings to hold the splint securely to the limb.
5. After application, check and record distal neurovascular function.

With severe deformities, as seen with most dislocations, or when gentle traction produces resistance or pain, the deformed limb must be splinted in the position of deformity. This can be done efficiently by applying padded board splints to each side of the limb and securing them with soft roller bandages, or by applying a vacuum-type splint.

Soft splints. A commonly used soft splint is the precontoured, inflatable, clear plastic **air splint**. These splints are available in a variety of sizes and shapes, with or without a zipper that runs the length of the splint. After application, the splint is inflated by mouth—*never* with a pump. The air splint is comfortable to the athlete, provides uniform contact, and has the added advantage of applying gentle pressure on a bleeding wound.

The air splint does have some disadvantages. One problem is that the pressure tends to straighten deformities. Also, the zipper can become stuck, become clogged with dirt, or freeze in cold weather. With extreme temperature changes, the air pressure in the splint varies, decreasing with cold and increasing with warmth.

Before one applies an air splint, the wound should first be covered with a dry, sterile dressing. The method of applying an air splint depends on whether it has a zipper. With zipper splints, the trainer holds the injured limb slightly off the ground with gentle traction; places the open, deflated splint around the limb; zips it up; and inflates it by mouth.

With the nonzipper or partial zipper type, two trainers should follow these steps.

1. First trainer: put your arm through the splint and then grasp the hand or foot of the injured limb.
2. Second trainer: support the athlete's injured limb.
3. First trainer: apply gentle traction to the hand or foot while sliding the splint onto the injured limb. (Always include the hand or foot of the limb in the splint.)
4. First trainer: inflate the splint by mouth.

With either type of air splint, the pressure in the splint should be tested after application. With proper inflation, a firm pinch between the thumb and index finger near the edge of the splint should just compress the walls of the splint together. As with any splint, distal neurovascular function must be checked and recorded after application.

Other soft splints such as **pillow splints** and the **sling and swathe** are widely used.

A recently developed splinting technique uses a vacuum created by suction to expand synthetic beads, creating a rigid splint. **Vacuum splints** are not temperature sensitive and form around deformities. They are secured around the limb with Velcro strips rather than being pulled up the length of the limb. They do not need to be removed for x-ray evaluation.

Traction splints. A **traction splint** holds a lower extremity fracture or dislocation immobile and exerts steady longitudinal pull on the extremity. Most commercial traction splints can be used on either lower extremity. A traction splint should not be used on an upper extremity fracture because the major nerves and blood vessels in the axilla cannot tolerate countertraction. Countertraction is essential to the proper function of the traction splint and occurs when traction is applied to the foot through the ankle hitch. The padded half-ring, which seats against the ischial tuberosity of the athlete's pelvis, applies countertraction. The ischium and the groin must be well padded and excessive pressure avoided, especially on external genitalia. Commercial padded ankle hitches are readily available and must be used rather than pieces of rope, cord, or tape. Such improvised hitches are painful and can obstruct circulation in the foot.

Traction splints are used to secure fractures of the shaft of the femur. Fractures of the tibial shaft and about the hip or knee can also be effectively splinted with this device if gentle traction on the limb does not decrease the distal pulse or produce pain as the limb is aligned.

Commercial traction splints are fairly expensive and require practice for effective application. Unless a traction splint is on hand and the trainers are proficient in its application, the trainer should identify a fracture requiring traction splinting and request assistance from a rescue squad.

The Rules of Splinting

A trainer about to apply a splint should follow these 12 general rules of splinting:

1. Remove clothing from the area of any suspected fracture or dislocation.
2. Note and record the circulatory and neurologic (motion and sensation) status distally to the site of injury before and after splinting.
3. When splinting a fracture, make sure the splint immobilizes the joints above and below the injured bone.
4. When splinting a dislocation or sprain, make sure the splint immobilizes the bones above and below the injured joint.
5. During splint application, move the limb as little as possible.
6. Straighten a severely deformed limb with constant, gentle, manual traction

only if necessary to incorporate the limb into a splint.

7. If gentle traction increases the athlete's pain substantially or if the limb resists alignment, splint the limb in the position of deformity.

8. In all suspected neck and spine injuries, correct the deformity only as necessary to eliminate airway obstruction and to allow effective application of a splint.

9. Cover all wounds with a dry, sterile dressing before applying a splint.

10. Pad the splint to prevent local pressure.

11. Do not move or transport athletes before splinting the injured extremity.

12. When in doubt, *splint.*

Rules 6 and 7 refer to the use of traction in managing musculoskeletal injury. **Traction** is defined as the action of drawing or pulling on an object. Traction, especially if excessive, can be harmful to an injured limb. When applied correctly, however, traction stabilizes the bone fragments and improves overall alignment. The trainer should not attempt to reduce the fracture or force all of the fragments back into anatomic alignment. This task is the physician's responsibility. In the field, the goals of traction are to stabilize the fracture fragments to prevent excessive movement and align the limb sufficiently to allow it to be placed in a splint.

Transporting Limb-Injured Athletes

After the injured limb has been adequately splinted, the athlete is ready to be transferred to a litter and transported to the hospital. The best position for the athlete depends on the type of injury. With most isolated upper extremity fractures, the athlete is most comfortable in a semi-seated position, rather than lying flat. Either position, however, is acceptable. With lower extremity injuries, the athlete should lie supine with the limb elevated slightly, about 6 inches, to minimize swelling. In all cases, the injured limb must not flop about or dangle off the edge of the litter.

The trainer can minimize swelling to some degree by applying cold packs, if readily available, to the injury site. Care should be taken to avoid placing the cold pack directly on the skin or other tissues.

Very few, if any, musculoskeletal injuries require rapid ambulance transportation. Once dressed and splinted, the limb is stable, and orderly transportation can be undertaken. If the hospital is only a few minutes away, reckless speeding to the emergency department makes little or no difference in the athlete's eventual outcome. If the treatment facility is an hour or more away, or if the athlete's limb is pulseless, evacuation of the athlete via helicopter or rapid ground transportation should be given a high priority.

FORMING A MANAGEMENT PLAN

The team physician and athletic trainer must plan for injury management. The supplies for managing most injuries, such as splints and bandages, should be available at the site of the event. Occasionally, special equipment, such as a traction splint, or additional help in protecting a suspected spinal injury is necessary. An ambulance service or rescue squad is sometimes required to transport injured athletes.

Planning for injury management should not be relegated to a trivial formality. A system for ensuring that specific supplies are available in the designated place and are in working order prevents confusion and mismanagement when an injury does occur. The local emergency medical service should be contacted before each season, taken on a tour of the various athletic facilities, and included in the emergency plan.

In the emergency plan, physicians, trainers, coaches, and administrators—all members of the sports medicine team—should be familiar with and able to practice their responsibilities in an emergency. A telephone should be available at all events. Coins should be on hand if a pay phone must be used. Emergency phone numbers and instructions to the caller should be posted near the telephone. Locked gates and doors should be opened (the person with the key must be on hand) to allow easy access for emergency medical personnel.

Each acute injury must be evaluated and managed on an individual basis, but well-established injury management and emergency plans will assist the athletic trainer in providing prompt, effective care to the athlete. Communication, organization, and practice prevent the confusion and chaos that can hinder the quality of care rendered to an injured athlete.

IMPORTANT CONCEPTS

1. Three steps essential in the examination of athletes with acute musculoskeletal injuries are performing a general assessment of the athlete, conducting an examination of the injured limb and evaluating distal neurovascular function, and keeping the athlete calm.

2. In soft tissue injuries, small blood vessels in the tissues tear, and varying amounts of blood and plasma leak into the wound and produce swelling and pain.

3. The four major causes of open wounds are abrasions, lacerations, avulsions, and puncture wounds.

4. Muscle strain, caused by the fibers of a muscle or its tendon tearing, is managed with rest, ice, compression, and elevation.

5. The signs and symptoms of a ligament sprain include point tenderness, swelling, instability, and inability to use the extremity.

6. The function of the peripheral nervous system should be assessed following sprains, dislocations, fractures, and deep lacerations of the skin.

7. Arterial bleeding from a wound is life-threatening and requires prompt, medical attention.

8. The most commonly used dressings are universal (for burns, wounds, padding for splints), stabilizing (for keeping dressings in place during transport), occlusive (for keeping air out of sucking chest wounds and abdominal eviscerating wounds), and pressure dressings (for control of bleeding).

9. The signs and symptoms of a fracture include deformity, point tenderness, guarding, swelling and ecchymosis, exposed fragments, crepitus, and false motion.

10. A dislocation occurs when the bone ends forming a joint are displaced.

11. All suspected fractures and dislocations should be splinted before the athlete is moved.

12. Proper splinting prevents movement of the injured limb, reduces pain, prevents laceration of the skin by broken bones, prevents restriction of distal flow resulting from pressure on the bone ends on blood vessels, and controls bleeding.

13. A coordinated plan for managing an emergency should be established and practiced.

SUGGESTED READINGS

American Academy of Orthopaedic Surgeons. *Emergency Care and Transportation of the Sick and Injured*, 4th ed. Park Ridge, Ill.: American Academy of Orthopaedic Surgeons, 1987.

Bergeron, J. D. *First Responder*, 2d ed. Englewood Cliffs, N.J.: Prentice-Hall, 1987.

Fahey, T. D. *Athletic Training: Principles and Practice.* Palo Alto, Calif.: Mayfield Publishing, 1986.

Hollinshead, W. H., and C. Rosse. *Textbook of Anatomy*, 4th ed. Philadelphia: Harper & Row, 1985.

McArdle, W. D., F. I. Katch, and V. L. Katch. *Exercise Physiology: Energy, Nutrition, and Human Performance*, 2d ed. Philadelphia: Lea & Febiger, 1986.

McMinn, R. M. H., and R. T. Hutchings. *Color Atlas of Human Anatomy*, 2d ed. Chicago: Year Book Medical Publishers, 1988.

15

Overuse Injuries of the Musculoskeletal System

CHAPTER OUTLINE

Mechanisms of Injury	Management of Overuse Injuries
Causative Factors	Diagnosis
Intrinsic Factors	History
Extrinsic Factors	Physical Exam
Inflammation	Diagnostic Studies
Tissues Prone to Overuse Injuries	Treatment
Muscles	Rest
Tendons	Anti-inflammatory Medications
Bursae	Modalities
Cartilage	Rehabilitation
Bones	Causative Factors
Nerves	

OBJECTIVES FOR CHAPTER 15

After reading this chapter, the student should be able to:

1. Distinguish between acute and overuse injuries.
2. Define intrinsic and extrinsic causes of overuse injuries and give examples of each.
3. Explain the role of inflammation in overuse injuries.
4. List the tissues that can be affected by overuse injuries and explain the mechanisms by which each is injured.
5. Describe the steps in diagnosing overuse injuries.
6. Describe the goals of treatment and the steps used in the treatment of overuse injuries.

INTRODUCTION

Injuries to the musculoskeletal system can be classified as either acute or overuse. Overuse injuries, in contrast to acute injuries, are not the result of a single incident or force, but instead result from a series of repetitive forces that overwhelm the tissue's ability to repair itself. Overuse injuries constitute a significant portion of the injuries related to sports.

Chapter 15 presents a general overview of the mechanisms and management of overuse injuries. The chapter begins with a brief explanation of the difference between causative extrinsic and intrinsic factors. Next, the process of inflammation is described, followed by a discussion of the tissues that are prone to overuse injuries. The second half of Chapter 15 focuses on the steps of diagnosis and the types of treatment for overuse injuries. ■

MECHANISMS OF INJURY

Causative Factors

Factors that lead to overuse injuries can be divided into two categories: intrinsic and extrinsic.

Intrinsic Factors

Those factors associated with anatomy, biomechanics, and physiology of the injured athlete are called *intrinsic factors*. Common intrinsic factors include leg-length difference, poor flexibility, muscle weakness or imbalance, and abnormal alignment.

Often, other injuries can cause or exacerbate intrinsic problems. For example, an injured limb that is not properly rehabilitated may result in residual muscle weakness or pain, which then causes a change in the forces that are normally applied to that or another body part during activity. Weakness itself may lead to the inability of that part to withstand even the same force and number of repetitions that were easily tolerated prior to the injury.

Extrinsic Factors

Extrinsic factors include training errors, such as too much distance, too much intensity, running up hills, running on hard or uneven surfaces (Fig. 15.1), inadequate equipment (Fig. 15.2), or improper technique. Because of the great number of repe-

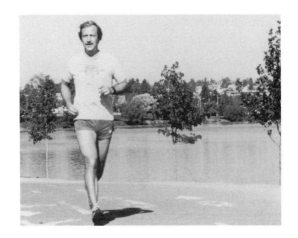

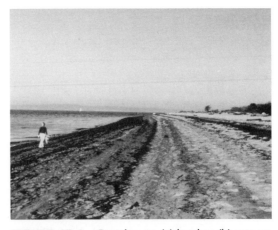

FIGURE 15.1. Running on (a) hard or (b) uneven surfaces is an example of an extrinsic factor that could lead to overuse injury.

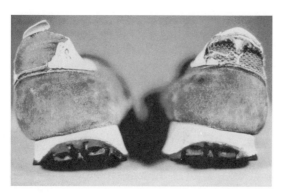

FIGURE 15.2. Shoes should be inspected for signs of excessive or unusual wear.

titions of movements required to train for and compete in sports, especially endurance sports, any of these intrinsic or extrinsic factors, alone or in combination, can add to the stresses already imposed on the tissues and thus create overload, which leads to injury.

Inflammation

A process common to all injury and especially important in the development of overuse injuries is **inflammation**, or the localized heat, redness, swelling, and pain that accompany musculoskeletal injuries. Inflammation, which can occur in a variety of forms, is an extremely complex and not well-understood series of steps that involves many different types of cells, enzymes, and other physiologically active substances.

In overuse injuries, the additive effects of repetitive forces lead to **microtrauma**, or the destruction of a small number of cells. The breakdown products of these destroyed cells probably trigger the inflammatory process. The first step is a short period of vasoconstriction to help control bleeding. Within minutes, the local capillaries dilate, and the pressure within them increases, causing leakage of fluid and cells into the area. Many types of white blood cells are also attracted to the area by *chemotactic factors*. The cells are active in the cleanup of damaged tissue, but because of the en-

zymes that are contained in them, they can destroy normal surrounding tissue. Other cells that migrate to the area form new capillaries and connective tissue.

Although inflammation is a necessary part of the healing process, it can become self-perpetuating and lead to chronic inflammation and the destruction of normal surrounding tissue.

Tissues Prone to Overuse Injuries

Muscles

Muscle injuries resulting from overuse commonly result in delayed muscle soreness. This soreness is the result of mechanical damage to the muscles and surrounding connective tissue. It usually occurs 12 to 48 hours after exercise and persists for 4 to 12 days. It produces tenderness to palpation, stiffness, and pain with movement.

Tendons

Tendons commonly become inflamed as the result of overuse, leading to **tendinitis**. Tendons are composed of dense connective tissue arranged in parallel and interspersed with mucopolysaccharide. They are very strong and can usually withstand the distractive forces placed on them when the muscle contracts. They can fatigue with repetitive loading, however, as is seen in overuse injuries. Fatigue occurs most frequently where the tendon attaches to bone because the blood supply is especially poor at this point.

Tendons are surrounded by either a loose connective tissue called the *peritendon* or a sheath called the *synovial sheath*. These structures are susceptible to repeated pressure or friction, which leads to inflammation and eventually **peritendinitis** or **tenosynovitis**.

Bursae

Bursae are sacs formed by two layers of synovial (joint lining) tissue. They are located at sites where there is friction between tendon and bone, or skin and bone. They normally contain a thin layer of joint fluid. They can become inflamed, however, from repetitive friction from the overlying tendon or external pressure. The inflammation, called **bursitis**, causes swelling from an increase in fluid in the bursa. If the inflammation is prolonged, the bursae walls may thicken, and sometimes the adjacent tendon degenerates or becomes calcified, causing a chemical bursitis.

Cartilage

Cartilage is made up of collagen, a proteoglycan gel, a few cells, and 60 to 80 percent water. It is located at the ends of bones where they meet other bones. Although cartilage is metabolically active, it has no blood or lymphatic supply. It therefore has little ability to repair itself. Cartilage is protected from injury by a thin layer of fluid that lubricates the opposing surfaces and keeps them apart. The cancellous or spongy bone beneath the cartilage is also able to deform and protect the cartilage from injury. These protective mechanisms may fail, however, and lead to wearing and damage of the cartilage. This damage occurs most frequently because of poor alignment and resulting abnormal forces on the cartilage. Once damaged, the hyaline cartilage that lines the ends of bones cannot be repaired. It is replaced instead by fibrocartilage, which is not as strong or as durable as hyaline cartilage.

Bones

Bone, in contrast to cartilage, has great power to repair itself. In fact, the strength of bone is dependent on the forces placed on it, and the size and the shape of the bone are a result of a complex series of forces, or **loads**, including tension, compression, shear, bending, and torsion. Bone remodels as the result of these forces.

The first step in bone remodeling is **resorption**, or taking away bone. Then new bone is laid down. Bone fractures when the load placed on it is sufficient to overcome its mechanical strength. Fracture can occur as the result of a single large force or a repetitive series of smaller ones. The ability of the bone to withstand the repetitive forces of sports depends on the amount of load, the number of repetitions, and the frequency of repetitions. When the resorption of bone outpaces bone formation, **stress fractures** can result.

Nerves

Nerve tissue is very susceptible to compression and to decreases in oxygen supply and, therefore, is susceptible to overuse trauma by a variety of mechanisms. Direct pressure on a nerve, either repetitively or for a prolonged period of time, may cause injury.

Activities that lead to swelling or to muscle hypertrophy can also cause injury to nerves by putting pressure on them as they pass through areas where they have limited space. Nerves can also be damaged by repetitive stretching as the result of abnormal joint function.

MANAGEMENT OF OVERUSE INJURIES

Management of overuse injuries, as well as other injuries and illnesses, follows a logical sequence of steps, starting with diagnosis and ending, hopefully, with return to play. Specific injuries and their treatment are covered in other chapters. This section outlines the general steps that the trainer should follow in the management of overuse problems.

Diagnosis

History

The first step in diagnosis is taking a complete and accurate history. In overuse problems it is important to determine the onset of symptoms and their progression. Commonly, the symptoms may be minor at first, sometimes noted initially during activity and sometimes only after activity. As the symptoms progress, they may become more and more noticeable, either during activity or at rest. The history must include the specific activities that cause pain, either at the time of activity or after cessation. It is also important to determine any changes in external factors that may have led to the symptoms. For example, training errors commonly contribute to overuse problems, so asking the athlete whether the duration or intensity of training has changed or if new equipment or a new technique has been introduced may give clues to the etiology of the problem.

Physical Exam

Examination of the athlete should start with inspection. The trainer should look for any signs of redness, swelling, or discoloration. The trainer should also observe alignment of the limb.

Palpation for tenderness can frequently pinpoint the anatomic site of the problem and the structure that is injured. Careful attention to detail, keeping in mind the anatomic landmarks, is essential. Palpation can also detect minimal swelling that is not obvious from observation alone. A determi-

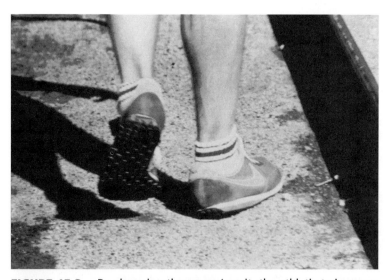

FIGURE 15.3. By observing the runner's gait, the athletic trainer can perform a functional assessment to determine if any intrinsic factors should be considered during diagnosis and treatment.

nation should also be made regarding the size of the area that is affected. Is there point tenderness or a more diffuse area of soreness?

Range-of-motion, both active and passive, and strength determinations should be made and compared with the uninjured side. The trainer can also do a functional assessment by watching the athlete perform routine movement such as walking, squatting, throwing, and so forth, depending on the injury (Fig. 15.3). This step is important not only in helping to make the diagnosis, but also in helping to determine if any biomechanical or intrinsic factors are present and should be dealt with during treatment and rehabilitation.

The trainer should also evaluate the vascular and nervous systems in the body part that is being assessed. Noting the pulse in an extremity, as well as skin color and speed of capillary filling after mild pressure is applied, is helpful in determining if there is any compromise in blood supply.

Any numbness or decreased or increased sensation should be carefully mapped to determine distribution. These observations, along with the presence or absence of any specific muscle weakness or the absence of deep tendon reflexes, can be used to determine nerve involvement.

Diagnostic Studies

Sometimes an accurate diagnosis requires further diagnostic studies to confirm the clinical impression and to rule out other possible causes of the symptoms. **X-rays** are helpful in evaluating bone, but sometimes a **bone scan** (a nuclear imaging technique) is required to confirm or deny the suspicion of a stress fracture. The reason is that stress fractures occur at a microscopic level, and x-ray findings usually only show evidence of the healing process, which may not be apparent for three weeks or more, if at all.

Special x-rays called **tomograms**, which take multiple views at varying depths through the thickness of bone, can also be helpful in some instances. **Magnetic reso-**

nance imaging (MRI), or computer-assisted imaging produced by placing an individual in the core of a magnet, is a relatively new technique which has been helpful in diagnosing soft tissue abnormalities such as tumors, cysts, and herniated intervertebral discs.

Occasionally, surgery is required to make an accurate diagnosis. **Arthroscopic surgery**, in which the interior of a joint is visualized through a scope attached to a camera, has been an important advancement in the diagnosis and treatment of sports-related injuries. Overuse injuries of the knee, shoulder, and elbow occasionally require this technique.

Electrodiagnostic studies, such as electromyographic (EMG) tests and nerve conduction studies, are also useful for assessing nerve damage due to overuse.

Treatment

The goals of treatment in overuse injuries are (1) to reduce pain and inflammation and promote healing and (2) to rehabilitate the injured part in order to prevent recurrence of that injury or the development of another related injury. Rest, anti-inflammatory medications, and treatment modalities all have the purpose of reducing pain and inflammation and promoting the body's healing process.

Rest

Rest can be accomplished in a variety of ways, depending on the nature and extent of the problem. Intended to make the person symptom-free, rest can range from merely altering or stopping the activity to using protective devices like crutches, splints, or casts.

The benefits of rest must always be weighed against the problems that arise with disuse—for example, muscle atrophy and decreased flexibility. The goal of treatment is to use the minimum amount of immobilization necessary to allow proper healing to occur.

Anti-inflammatory Medications

Anti-inflammatory drugs reduce inflammation by blocking the synthesis of prostaglandins, a group of substances that have widely varying effects on different tissues. Prostaglandins are important mediators of inflammation, causing vasodilation and potentiating edema as well as sensitizing the tissues to painful stimuli. Medical professionals, therefore, frequently prescribe anti-inflammatory drugs (usually nonsteroidal anti-inflammatories such as aspirin or ibuprofen) to reduce pain and quiet the inflammatory response.

Modalities

Ice, heat, electrical stimulation, and massage often are used in treating overuse injuries. They are important components in a total treatment plan and can be used alone or in combination to help reduce pain, swelling, muscle spasm, and stiffness and to hasten healing and rehabilitation. They are covered in more depth in Chapter 50.

Rehabilitation

Probably the most important aspect of treatment of overuse injuries is rehabilitation. The goal is to correct problems in strength, flexibility, or proprioception (sensory awareness of position in space). These problems could have been a cause of the injury, sometimes resulting from another injury such as an acute ankle sprain, or they could be the result of the current injury. In either case, it is imperative to correct these problems before the athlete returns to full activity because failure to do so will very likely result in recurrence of the same injury or in development of a new overuse problem. Techniques of rehabilitation are discussed in Chapter 49.

Causative Factors

While rehabilitation is proceeding, treatment of the injured athlete should address possible causative factors. Sometimes a single factor such as a training error can be

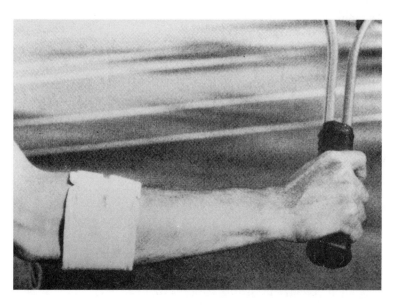

FIGURE 15.4. An arm brace will alter the distribution of forces to an injured area.

identified; more frequently, however, a combination of factors are additive and lead to the development of the injury.

Extrinsic causes should be identified and alleviated, a process that often requires the cooperation of both the athlete and the coach. A careful evaluation of technique, equipment, and training schedule will often yield valuable information and lead to appropriate recommendations to help prevent further injury.

Intrinsic factors related to strength, flexibility, and proprioception can be addressed in the rehabilitation program. Other intrinsic factors that cannot be corrected with rehabilitation can sometimes by addressed by appliances such as braces or orthotics (Fig. 15.4). Occasionally, surgery may be required to correct anatomic or biomechanical problems.

IMPORTANT CONCEPTS

1. Overuse injuries result from a series of repetitive forces which overwhelm the body's ability to repair itself.
2. Causative factors can be divided into intrinsic factors (those associated with anatomy, physiology, and biomechanics) and extrinsic factors (those that are external to the person experiencing the injury).
3. Inflammation can be an important perpetuating factor in overuse problems.
4. Many tissues, including tendons, bursae, muscles, cartilage, bones, and nerves, can be affected by overuse.
5. Accurate diagnosis is important in the management of overuse injuries and includes obtaining an accurate history, a physical exam, and sometimes diagnostic studies.
6. The goals of treatment include reducing pain and inflammation to promote healing and rehabilitating the injured part.

SUGGESTED READINGS

Arnheim, D. D. *Modern Principles of Athletic Training: The Science of Sports Medicine: Injury Prevention, Causation, and Management,* 6th ed. St. Louis: Times Mirror/Mosby College Publishing, 1985.

Curwin, S., and W. D. Stanish. *Tendinitis: Its Etiology and Treatment.* Lexington, Mass.: Collamore Press, 1984.

Frankel, V. H., and M. Nordin, eds. *Basic Biomechanics of the Skeletal System.* Philadelphia: Lea & Febiger, 1980.

Hunter-Griffin, L. Y., ed. *Clinics in Sports Medicine,* vol. 6, no. 2. Philadelphia: W. B. Saunders, 1987.

16

The Shoulder

CHAPTER OUTLINE

OBJECTIVES FOR CHAPTER 16

After reading this chapter, the student should be able to:

1. Describe the anatomy and basic functions of the joints of the shoulder girdle.
2. Evaluate injuries to the shoulder girdle.
3. Describe appropriate treatment for major injuries to the shoulder girdle.
4. Describe rehabilitation programs for injuries to the shoulder girdle, with ideas on progression to return to activity.

INTRODUCTION

In athletics, injuries to the shoulder from acute trauma or overuse are common. Chapter 16 begins with a discussion of the anatomy and biomechanics of the shoulder, followed by a description of the mechanisms of shoulder injury. The chapter next stresses the importance of performing an initial assessment, administering first aid following an acute shoulder injury, and evaluating the painful shoulder which results from an overuse injury. The evaluation and treatment of common shoulder injuries (e.g., dislocations, fractures, and rotator cuff injuries) are discussed, and examples of rehabilitation exercises are presented. ■

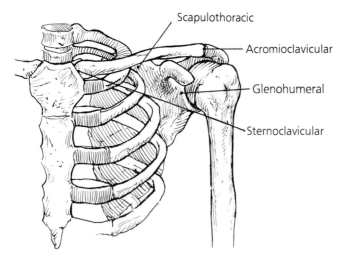

FIGURE 16.1. The four shoulder articulations.

Scapulothoracic

Acromioclavicular

Glenohumeral

Sternoclavicular

ANATOMY OF THE SHOULDER

The shoulder is a complex structure that comprises four separate joints: glenohumeral, acromioclavicular, sternoclavicular, and scapulothoracic (Fig. 16.1). Motion of the arm on the trunk involves coordinated movements of all of these joints. An understanding of the topical anatomy of the shoulder, as presented in Chapter 9 and reviewed in Figure 16.2, is important in evaluating shoulder injuries, since much of the anatomy is easily palpable beneath the skin.

Bones and Joints

The shoulder girdle is composed of three bones: the **scapula**, **humerus**, and **clavicle**.

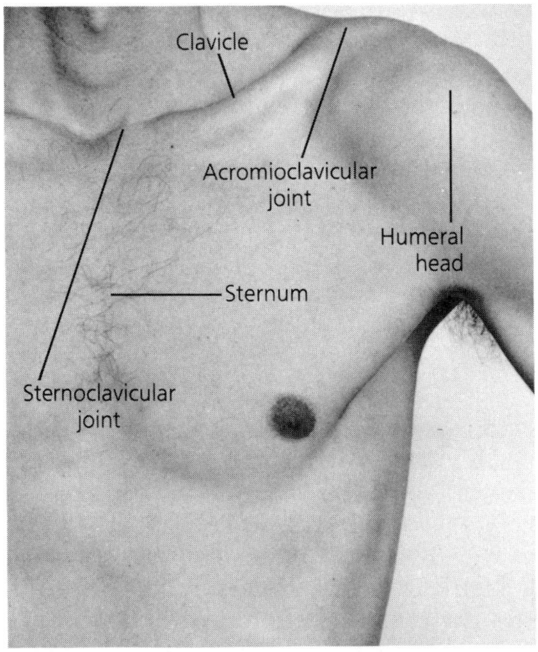

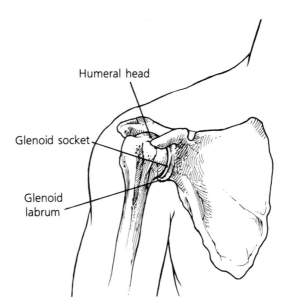

FIGURE 16.2. Surface anatomy of the shoulder girdle.

FIGURE 16.3. The glenohumeral joint.

Among these three bones, two joints exist: the **glenohumeral joint** and the **acromioclavicular joint**. The bones of the shoulder girdle are attached to the trunk through two other articulations: the **scapulothoracic joint**, in which the scapula is suspended from the posterior thoracic wall through muscular attachments to the ribs and spine, and the **sternoclavicular joint**, which lies between the clavicle and the sternum.

The glenohumeral joint (which many refer to as "the shoulder joint proper") is a relatively unstable joint. It consists of a large humeral head which lies in the shallow socket of the glenoid fossa of the scapula (Fig. 16.3). This arrangement, although it permits a remarkable range of motion—an advantage for throwing and other upper extremity activities—puts the glenohumeral joint at a greater risk for acute and overuse injuries. Glenohumeral joint stability is increased somewhat by the **glenoid labrum**, a fibrocartilaginous rim around the glenoid that slightly widens and deepens the socket (Fig. 16.4), and by the capsule

and the **rotator cuff**, a musculotendinous cuff that reinforces the capsule. The acromial process of the scapula forms a roof over the glenohumeral joint, creating the subacromial space in which lies the **subacromial bursa** and rotator cuff. The bursa acts as the "protective" tissue between the cuff and the bony acromion. Its purpose is to cushion the cuff below from repetitive trauma of the bony acromion above. This bursa is frequently irritated and inflamed with repetitive overhead activities. The **coracoac-**

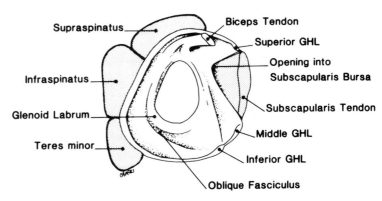

FIGURE 16.4. The glenoid labrum slightly widens and deepens the glenoid fossa, increasing glenohumeral joint stability.

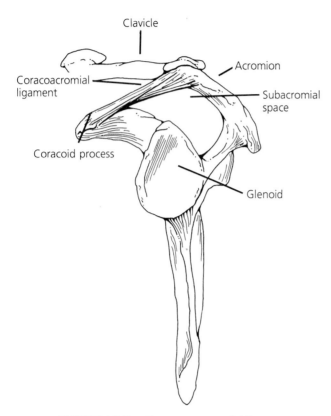

FIGURE 16.5. The coracoacromial ligament defines and narrows the subacromial space.

romial ligament, which lies anteromedially and superior to the glenohumeral joint, further defines (and narrows) the subacromial space (Fig. 16.5).

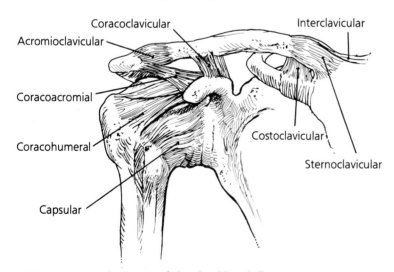

FIGURE 16.6. Ligaments of the shoulder girdle.

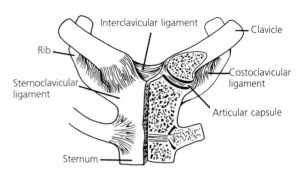

FIGURE 16.7. The sternoclavicular joint.

The acromioclavicular joint is capable of small rotatory movements. The joint capsule is reinforced by strong stabilizers, the **coracoclavicular ligaments** (the conoid and trapezial ligaments), which join the coracoid process to the outer, inferior surface of the clavicle and the acromioclavicular ligament, which runs transversely across the joint (Fig. 16.6). The trapezius and deltoid muscles overlie the joint.

The sternoclavicular joint is the only true joint between the upper extremity and the trunk, since the scapula does not articulate with the posterior thoracic wall as a true joint. The sternoclavicular joint has motion in all planes, but with limited excursion. Its stability is maintained by the capsule, which is reinforced by ligaments between the medial aspect of the clavicle, the sternum, and the first rib (Fig. 16.7).

Although not a true joint since there are no bony articulations, the scapulothoracic junction functions as a joint in shoulder motion. The scapula glides on the posterior thoracic rib cage, where it is stabilized by muscular attachments.

Muscles

The muscles of the shoulder girdle can be thought of in terms of "layers." The muscles of the most superficial layer are the **pectoralis major**, the **deltoid**, and the **trapezius**. The pectoralis major and deltoid lie anteriorly; superiorly and laterally is the deltoid; and posteriorly are the trapezius and deltoid (Fig. 16.8).

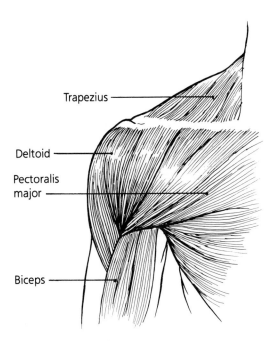

FIGURE 16.8.   The major shoulder muscles.

Four muscles comprise the deeper muscular layer called the *rotator cuff of the
shoulder* (Fig. 16.9). The **subscapularis** arises from the ventral surface of the scapula
and inserts on the lesser tuberosity. The
supraspinatus, infraspinatus, and **teres minor** arise from the dorsal surface of the
scapula and insert on the greater tuberosity.
The supraspinatus is the most superior of
these muscles, and the teres minor is the
most inferior (Fig. 16.10).

The **biceps brachii** is a deep anterior muscle of the shoulder. It has two heads of
origin: the long head arises from the superi-
or rim of the glenoid and then passes
through the shoulder joint under the rotator cuff lying in the bicipital groove between the proximal tuberosities of the humerus (see Fig. 16.8). The short head arises
from the coracoid process and joins the long
head in the arm. Both heads insert on the
radial tuberosity.

The **serratus anterior** and the **rhomboids,
levator scapulae,** and **latissimus dorsi** are
muscles of the trunk that help to stabilize
and maneuver the shoulder girdle (Fig.
16.11).

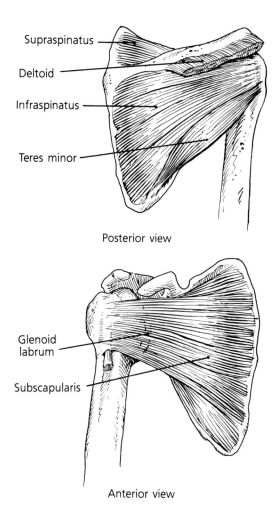

FIGURE 16.9.   Posterior and anterior views of
the rotator cuff muscles and insertions.

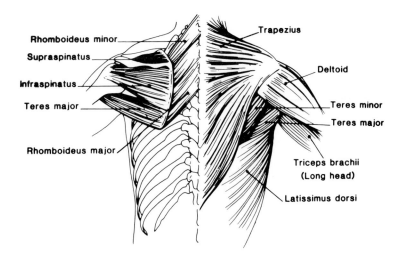

FIGURE 16.10.   Posterior view of the shoulder and trunk.

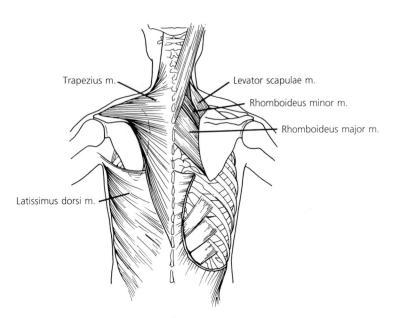

FIGURE 16.11. Muscles of the trunk help to stabilize and maneuver the shoulder girdle.

Range of Motion

Motion of the upper extremity involves movement in all four joints of the shoulder girdle. The movements of the shoulder are illustrated in Figure 16.12 and can be described as follows:

- *Flexion*, in which the arm starts at the side and elevates in the sagittal plane of the body anteriorly.
- *Extension*, in which the arm starts at the side and elevates in the sagittal plane of the body posteriorly.
- *Adduction*, in which the arm moves toward the midline of the body. *Abduction*, in which the arm moves away from the midline of the body.
- *Internal rotation*, in which the arm rotates medially, inward toward the body.
- *External rotation*, in which the arm rotates laterally, or outward, from the body.

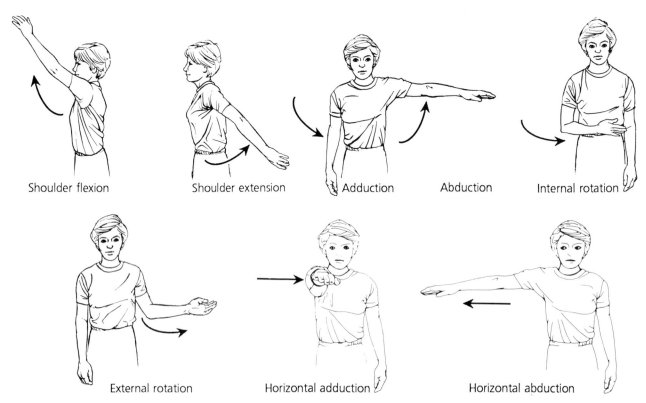

FIGURE 16.12. Movements of the shoulder.

- *Horizontal adduction* (horizontal flexion), in which the arm starts at 90 degrees of abduction and adducts forward and medially toward the center of the body.
- *Horizontal abduction* (horizontal extension), in which the arm starts at 90 degrees of abduction and moves outward, away from the body.

The deltoid muscle is the primary abductor of the arm, with assistance from the supraspinatus muscle. However, all of the rotator cuff muscles are essential for effective abduction of the arm, as they must stabilize the humeral head in the glenoid during abduction.

The infraspinatus, teres minor, and posterior deltoid muscles are the prime external rotators of the shoulder. External rotation of almost 90 degrees is necessary to prevent impingement of the greater tuberosity on the acromion during abduction. Elevation of the lateral aspect of the scapula is necessary for full forward flexion and abduction. This range of motion is accomplished by the upper part of the trapezius muscle and the underlying serratus anterior muscle. Forward flexion is mainly accomplished by the clavicular portion of the deltoid, part of the pectoralis major, and the biceps brachii muscles. Extension is primarily the function of the posterior deltoid and latissimus dorsi muscles.

Adduction is accomplished primarily by the pectoralis major and latissimus dorsi muscles. Internal rotation is primarily a function of the subscapularis muscle, with assistance from the pectoralis major and latissimus dorsi muscles as they adduct, flex, or extend.

The function of the various muscles of the shoulder changes, depending on the position of the shoulder itself. For example, in the act of throwing, when the arm is brought into abduction, extension, and external rotation, the primary internal rotators of the shoulder change from the subscapularis to the pectoralis major and latissimus dorsi muscles.

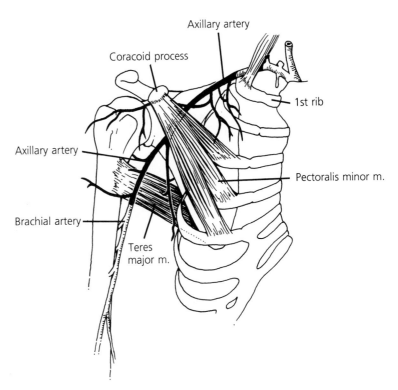

FIGURE 16.13.   The axillary artery.

The Neurovascular Supply of the Shoulder Girdle

The axillary artery traverses the axilla. It extends from the outer border of the first rib to the lower border of the teres minor muscle, at which point it becomes the brachial artery. The axillary artery lies deep to the pectoralis muscle but is crossed in its midregion by the pectoralis minor tendon, just before the tendon inserts into the coracoid process (Fig. 16.13). The axillary vein traverses with the axillary artery. Branches from the axillary artery supply most of the shoulder girdle.

A few other arteries contribute to the vascular supply of the shoulder. For example, the suprascapular artery, a branch off the thyrocervical trunk of the subclavian artery, joins the suprascapular nerve as it arises quite early off the brachial plexus. Together, they traverse the superior border of the scapula to supply the supraspinatus muscle; then they travel around the lateral

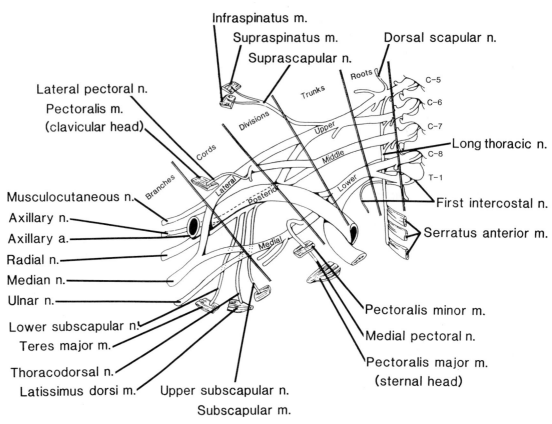

FIGURE 16.14. The brachial plexus.

border of the scapular spine to supply the infraspinatus and teres minor, as well as contributing to the teres major muscle. Impingement of the suprascapular nerve as it courses around the scapular spine can occur in throwing athletes.

The *brachial plexus* is the name given to the complex mingling of nerves from the ventral rami of the fifth through the eighth cervical nerves and the first thoracic nerve (Fig. 16.14). These nerve roots ramify and divide, forming trunks which ramify and divide again into cords. The cords then ramify to form the peripheral nerves that supply the upper extremity. This network of nerve fibers begins with the joining of the ventral rami proximally in the neck and continues anteriorly and distally, crossing into the axillary region obliquely under the clavicle at about the junctional area of the distal one-third and proximal two-thirds of the clavicle. Clavicular fractures in this area

carry the potential of damaging the plexus. The plexus lies inferiorly to the coracoid process. At the level of the coracoid process, the brachial plexus cords are forming the peripheral nerves which continue down the arm.

The muscles of the shoulder girdle are supplied by the nerves that arise at all levels of the plexus. For example, the axillary nerve supplying the deltoid arises from the posterior cord. The suprascapular nerve, as just indicated, arises quite early from the plexus and innervates the subscapularis, teres major, and latissimus dorsi muscles.

The neurovascular anatomy of the shoulder is quite complex. Those caring for athletes with injuries to this area are encouraged to refer to texts as needed when neurovascular problems arise. It is important, however, to keep in mind that the neurovascular supply to the shoulder girdle crosses underneath the lateral clavicle; traveling obliquely, it courses inferior to the coracoid process and crosses over into the axillary region to enter the upper extremity at about the level of the humeral neck. Moreover, the neurovascular supply to the shoulder is not only from the axillary artery and nerves in the axilla; neurovascular contributions to the shoulder girdle also arise more proximally for the neurovascular bundle as it goes beneath the clavicle on its way to the axilla.

BIOMECHANICS

Normal Biomechanics

When the arm is at the side, the deltoid muscle exerts an upward and outward force. The rotator cuff muscles exert a downward and inward force. Acting together, the vertical forces cancel each other and combine to stabilize the humeral head in the glenoid. The slight horizontal force of the deltoid acts below the center of rotation of the humeral head. This force is opposite in direction to the horizontal force of the rotator cuff, which is applied above the center of rotation. Forces such as these act synergistically to effect smooth abduction and are known as a *force couple*.

Altered Biomechanics

Examples of altered biomechanics are present in a variety of pathologic conditions. When abduction is attempted with a rotator cuff tear, the greater tuberosity of the humeral head tends to rise and impinge on the undersurface of the acromion. Abduction is laborious up to a point of 90 degrees. Conversely, in axillary nerve lesions where innervation of the deltoid muscle is impaired, abduction is difficult or impossible to initiate or sustain. Thus, the dominant muscle in the shoulder region for abduction is clearly the deltoid; in the absence of the rotator cuff muscle, however, the effectiveness of the deltoid is markedly diminished.

If the scapula is restrained from movement, the humerus can abduct only to 120 degrees. Moreover, full abduction depends on the posterior deltoid, teres minor, and infraspinatus muscles also externally rotating the humerus to allow the greater tuberosity to lie posteriorly to the acromion. The simultaneous movement of both the scapula and the humerus, which produces a smooth, rhythmic motion, is called *scapulohumeral rhythm*. For every 30 degrees of abduction, 20 degrees of motion occurs at the glenohumeral joint, and 10 degrees is due to the scapula's rotating on the thorax (2 to 1 ratio).

Motion of the humerus in the glenoid can be described in terms of the center of rotation, or the pivot shift point about which the humerus appears to rotate. Using x-ray and graphic analysis, one can determine the instant center of rotation for any movement. As long as the rotator cuff exerts a compression force, the glenohumeral joint is stable and the humeral head rotates on a fixed center of rotation. Excessive movement of the humeral head in a vertical or horizontal direction results in varying instant centers of rotation. This variance occurs if the conformity of the joint is disturbed, as when the labrum is torn with a shoulder dislocation. Among other factors causing this variance is an imbalance of forces between the deltoid and the rotator cuff. In a rotator cuff tear, for example, severe pain disturbs the muscle coordination of the scapulohumeral rhythm; or perhaps a single rotator cuff muscle is weak compared to the others, as in the case of entrapment of the suprascapular nerve in baseball pitchers.

Throwing Mechanism

Any overhead throwing act, whether it be hitting a tennis ball, throwing a ball, or throwing the javelin, represents a very complex activity. The throwing act places great stress on the anterior and posterior structures of the shoulder; hence, overuse injuries commonly occur.

To understand the injuries associated with the throwing athlete, one must appreciate the complex mechanics of throwing. There are five phases of the throwing act:

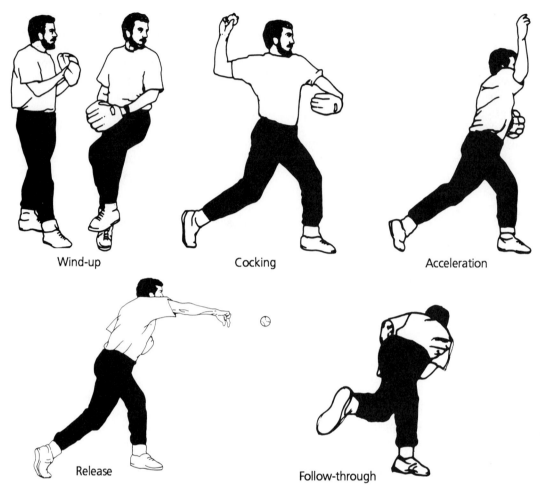

Wind-up

Cocking

Acceleration

Release

Follow-through

FIGURE 16.15. The throwing act: (a) wind-up, (b) cocking, (c) acceleration, (d) release, (e) follow-through.

wind-up, cocking, acceleration, release, and follow-through (Fig. 16.15).

To throw a baseball in an overhead position, the pitcher begins wind-up from either a full position or a stretch position. The wind-up phase initiates the rhythm and coordination of the throwing act, as the pitcher generates the forces necessary to propel the ball toward the plate. The cocking phase begins when the ball and glove separate, and it ends when the shoulder is at the extreme of external rotation. At this point, the pitcher's hips are rotated, and the lower extremities are beginning to rotate forward as the body begins to move forward. A synchronous chain of events occurs during cocking, beginning with the lower

extremity and progressing to the upper extremity. The rotator cuff muscles and deltoid are responsible for bringing the arm into the externally rotated abductive position. As a general rule, the shoulder is positioned at approximately 90 degrees of abduction, as much as 135 to 165 degrees of external rotation, and 15 degrees of horizontal abduction. Whether the pitcher throws from an overhead position, three-quarters position, or side-arm position, the angle at the shoulder stays the same. It is the lean of the body that will determine the pitcher's type of delivery.

In the acceleration phase, the anterior muscles horizontally adduct and internally rotate the humerus, as does the momentum of the derotation of the rest of the body, as the arm is brought forward for ball release. The rotator cuff is relatively quiet during this stage; the triceps works to extend the elbow from 90 degrees to about 30 degrees.

Ball release occurs in just a few milliseconds; remember, the hand is moving as fast as the ball is at this point. Once ball release occurs, the follow-through phase takes place. Tremendous deceleration by the muscles of the rotator cuff stops horizontal adduction and internal rotation of the humerus and stabilizes the humerus in the glenoid. Concurrently, the biceps brachii muscle acts to stop elbow extension by pulling anteriorly across the shoulder. The rotator cuff is under its greatest strain in this eccentric maneuver.

Throwing sport activities, such as throwing a football, serving a tennis ball, or making overhead racquetball shots, are merely variations of this basic theme. All of the motions have different mechanics but can be analyzed from this example. In the crawl stroke in swimming, for example, the humerus abducts above neutral, and irritation to the rotator cuff from impingement can occur if the rotator cuff muscles are not strong enough to hold the humeral head firmly in the glenoid fossa. In tennis, impingement can occur when the player abducts the humerus above 90 degrees during a serve or with overhead strokes.

MECHANISMS OF INJURY

Shoulder injuries can be caused by acute trauma or by movements repeated over time.

Acute Trauma From Direct Force

Strictly differentiating between direct and indirect forces in a specific injury may be difficult but is informative in understanding the mechanism of injury. For example, acromioclavicular joint dislocations classically result from falling directly on the tip of the acromion. The clavicle is driven superiorly by the force of the fall, resulting in

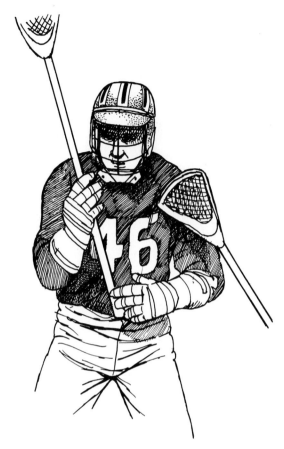

FIGURE 16.16.   A posterior glenohumeral joint dislocation is more likely to result from a direct blow to the anterior aspect of the shoulder when the arm is held in internal rotation.

disruption of the stabilizing ligament of this joint. Posterior glenohumeral dislocations are most likely to occur from direct blows to the anterior aspect of the shoulder, when the arm is held in internal rotation (Fig. 16.16); the humeral head is forced posteriorly out of its shallow glenoid. Direct blows are also the cause of fractures of the scapular body and the clavicle.

Acute Trauma From Indirect Force

Indirect forces are classically involved in the anterior shoulder dislocation. The humeral head is levered anteriorly, as the arm is brought into extremes of abduction, extension, and external rotation. This injury

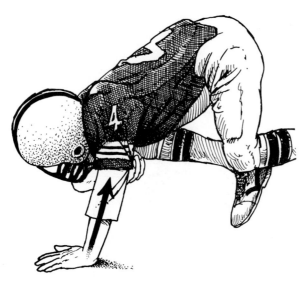

FIGURE 16.17. A fracture of the humeral head region may occur with a fall on the outstretched arm.

sometimes occurs during arm tackle in football. Another example of indirect injury to the shoulder is a fall on the outstretched hand, which can result in a fracture of the humeral head region (Fig. 16.17).

Chronic Repetitive Movements

Any injury caused by repetitive submaximal stress to a tissue which overwhelms the body's natural repair processes is termed an **overuse injury.** For example, the impingement syndrome can result from repetitive abduction and internal rotation of the humerus, causing swelling and scarring in the rotator cuff and the subacromial bursa. Once swollen, this thickened, edematous tissue can more easily be further impinged under the anterior rim of the acromion and the coracoacromial ligament. Such repetitive trauma may eventually lead to actual tears in the cuff.

INITIAL ASSESSMENT AND FIRST AID

An assessment of the shoulder should take place immediately following injury. After obtaining a brief history of the mechanism

of injury, the athletic trainer should conduct a cursory vascular assessment of the upper extremity prior to removing the athlete's clothing and protective equipment. The radial and ulnar arterial pulses should be palpated and assessed, and a sensory examination of the entire upper extremity done, especially in obvious glenohumeral dislocations. Following sensory examination, the trainer should assess motor function. (With any evidence of neurovascular compromise of the upper extremity, the athlete should be transported immediately to a medical facility.) Once the athlete's clothing and protective equipment have been removed, the trainer can perform a more thorough neurovascular examination.

After assessing neurovascular status, the athletic trainer should observe the shoulder area for any obvious deformity, lacerations, abrasions, hemorrhage, or swelling. These signs indicate the location of damaged underlying structures. The trainer then palpates the area of injury to determine the location of tenderness and the presence of any obvious bony deformity that might indicate fracture or dislocation. If possible, the trainer should try to move the shoulder passively through a complete range of motion. If successful, the trainer should then ask the athlete to move the shoulder actively through its entire range. Of course, pain may prevent active motion, and any limitation of motion or movement because of pain should be noted. If the athlete experiences significant pain, the trainer should immobilize the shoulder in a sling and swathe for protection pending more thorough evaluation off the field. Ice can be applied to the injured area to decrease pain and swelling.

EVALUATION OF A PAINFUL SHOULDER

Steps of Evaluation

Often an athlete complains of a shoulder that has been painful for several hours or weeks. The examination on this occasion differs from the evaluation of an acute injury on the field. Steps in the evaluation consist of taking a history, inspecting the shoulder, palpating the painful area, assessing both active and passive range of motion and strength, and conducting stress tests.

History

A detailed history of the onset of symptoms, the relationship of symptoms to sport performance, and activities of daily living should be obtained, as well as a history of any prior injury or shoulder pain. The athlete should be asked to state the location of pain and if the location varies with the time of day or the activity. A description of the pain should also be obtained. For example, is the pain throbbing, aching, sharp, stabbing, or burning? The duration of symptoms should be noted. Have symptoms progressed during this time? Are there associated symptoms to the pain—for example, tingling, weakness, snapping, radiation, catching? What factors aggravate the pain? What relieves it?

Inspection for Deformity

When inspecting the shoulder, the athletic trainer should look at the relationship of the acromion to the clavicle at the acromioclavicular joint. Is there any chronic separation? Is there scapular winging from a long thoracic nerve palsy? Is there any atrophy of the deltoid, supraspinatus, or infraspinatus muscles?

Palpation

The acromioclavicular joint and glenohumeral joint should be palpated. Both of these joints should be assessed for laxity and put through a range of motion. Note should be made of any clicks, such as that which occurs with abduction (external rotation of the shoulder as the humeral head rolls over an irregular glenoid rim). On palpation, one can frequently locate the area of maximal tenderness. The biceps tendon should be palpated for congruity and for localized tenderness in this area. Both the long head and the indirect head of the coracoid can be

felt. The subacromial bursa should be palpated to assess whether there is fluid present in it. Palpation of the clavicle can assess any irregularities that are secondary to an old fracture.

Assessing Range of Motion

Both active and passive range of motion should be noted, as well as the degree of motion and the coordination of motion. That is, does the scapulothoracic motion follow smoothly with the glenohumeral motion or is the abduction motion of the shoulder coming only from abduction of the glenohumeral joint without participation of the scapulothoracic junction?

Assessing Strength

In assessing strength, the athletic trainer should test all muscles about the athlete's shoulder as in a routine muscle assessment examination.

Conducting Stress Tests

When assessing a painful shoulder, the athletic trainer can apply various stress tests, among them the apprehension test, the sulcus sign, the relocation test, the Yergason test, the clunk test, the posterior shoulder stability test, the glenohumeral translation test, and the impingement test.

Apprehension test. The apprehension test is used for determining glenohumeral instability. Generally, if there is anterior shoulder laxity, the athlete will become apprehensive if the shoulder is abducted and externally rotated. This maneuver mimics the position of dislocation, causing reflexive guarding on the part of the athlete.

Sulcus sign. The acromioclavicular distraction test, or sulcus sign, is used for determining whether there is a lax capsule. With the athlete sitting, with his or her arm at the side, a distraction force is applied along the humerus. If there is a lax capsule, one would expect to see a hollowing out just distal to the joint.

Relocation test. The relocation test is another test for shoulder instability. If the athlete's pain and apprehension with external rotation and abduction increase when a forward force, an anterior translation force, is put on the humeral head, as opposed to decreasing when a posterior translation force is put on the humeral head, the athlete is likely to have some anterior instability in the glenohumeral joint.

Yergason test. The Yergason test, used to evaluate biceps tendon stability, is done with the athlete standing or sitting. The elbow is flexed to 90 degrees, and the forearm is pronated. The examiner holds the athlete's wrist, while the athlete actively supinates against the examiner's resistance. If this maneuver produces pain localized to the bicipital groove, it suggests disease in the long head of the biceps tendon.

Clunk test. The clunk test is used to determine glenoid labrum tears. The athlete lies supine. The examiner externally rotates and abducts the arm, using gentle pressure at the elbow while keeping his or her other hand on the anterior surface of the glenohumeral joint. The arm can be internally and externally rotated in the abducted position. As it is put through this range of motion, one can occasionally feel the humeral head clicking or popping or clunking over an irritated glenoid.

Posterior shoulder stability test. To test posterior shoulder stability, the examiner stands with his or her elbow extended; the athlete is supine, and the glenohumeral joint is maximally relaxed. The examiner grasps the humeral head with one hand, and while controlling the arm with his or her opposite hand at the athlete's elbow, the examiner tries not only to bring the shoulder anteriorly to note anterior shoulder laxity, but also to force the shoulder posteriorly to test the stability of the posterior structures.

Glenohumeral translation test. With the athlete sitting or supine, the examiner uses one hand to stabilize the scapula; with his or her opposite hand, the examiner grasps the humeral head and applies first an anterior and then a posterior force to note the degree of glenohumeral translation in both the anterior and posterior planes.

Impingement test. The impingement test is used to define the degree of subacromial irritability. The glenohumeral joint is abducted, flexed forward, and internally rotated, causing impingement of the supraspinatus tendon underneath the anterior process of the acromion and the coracoacromial ligament. If the tendon or the bursa above it is inflamed, this maneuver reproduces the athlete's pain.

Referred Pain

When evaluating a painful shoulder, the trainer should remember that pain in the shoulder can be referred from other areas. For example, cardiac problems can present with left shoulder pain. The pain from cervical disc disease or cervical vertebral facet disease is frequently referred to the posterior shoulder (primarily the trapezius muscle). Unlike primary shoulder pain, the pain of cervical disease will radiate from the trapezius down into the shoulder rather than primarily emanating from the shoulder. Stretching of the brachial plexus in the thoracic outlet can also present as shoulder pain (see Chapter 32).

Apical lesions in the lung can present as either anterior or posterior shoulder pain. In this particular instance, the pain typically worsens with time, despite conservative care. One should be suspicious of a pulmonary lesion that produces shoulder pain if the pain is felt deep within the shoulder and the painful area cannot easily be palpated or reproduced on reexamination of the athlete's shoulder.

Abdominal injuries, such as injuries to the spleen and gallbladder, can conceivably result in shoulder pain, but these intra-abdominal problems more typically result in complaints of pain in the posterior thoracic region.

EVALUATION AND TREATMENT OF SPECIFIC INJURIES

When the upper extremity is subjected to abnormal forces, the resulting injuries may be bony or soft tissue, depending primarily on three elements: the direction of the force, the magnitude of the force, and the rapidity with which it is applied. In general, the bony shoulder girdle has a rich blood supply that enables rapid healing; bony injuries may heal even in the face of some movement at the fracture site. Ligaments and tendons of the shoulder are not as well vascularized; therefore, their healing time may be prolonged.

Sternoclavicular Dislocation

In the skeletally mature athlete, there is generally no associated fracture when the sternoclavicular joint is injured. The injury is to the soft tissue and consists of a tear of the sternoclavicular joint capsule. The injury may range from a mildly symptomatic sprain to a complete **sternoclavicular dislocation**, with disruption of the entire anterior capsule and its restraining ligaments.

Anterior Sternoclavicular Dislocation

The most common type of sternoclavicular dislocation is the **anterior sternoclavicular dislocation**. This dislocation is easily recognized clinically by the anterior prominence of the proximal clavicle on the involved side. Radiographic documentation of an anterior sternoclavicular joint dislocation is difficult but can be confirmed by special views.

While dislocation of the anterior sternoclavicular joint may cause considerable distress initially, the symptoms usually subside rapidly, with no functional loss to the shoulder. A variety of surgical and nonsurgical approaches to treat acute anterior sternoclavicular dislocations have been advocated. Surgical procedures may result in significant complications. For example, functional motion for rotation and eleva-

tion of the clavicle at the sternoclavicular joint might be lost, which would hinder normal movement of the glenohumeral joint. Since there is little evidence to suggest that surgery improves the functional results of this injury, nonsurgical treatment is most frequently recommended. Closed treatment modalities vary from a sling alone to attempts at closed reduction. While closed reduction can be successful initially, it is difficult to maintain. Sometimes, the "popping" sternoclavicular joint may be more of a nuisance than a functional problem.

Posterior Sternoclavicular Dislocation

In contrast to the anterior dislocation of the sternoclavicular joint, **posterior sternoclavicular dislocation**, although much less common, has a higher morbidity, with potential injury to the great vessels, the esophagus, and the trachea (Fig. 16.18). Presenting symptoms vary from mild to moderate pain in the sternoclavicular joint region to hoarseness, difficulty in swallowing, or severe respiratory distress. Subcutaneous emphysema from tracheal injury may be seen. Special radiographic views confirm the dislocation.

In most instances, particularly when performed early, closed reduction of a posteri-

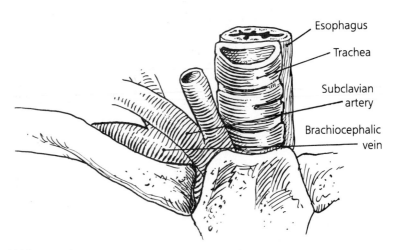

FIGURE 16.18. A posterior sternoclavicular joint dislocation may result in injury to adjacent soft tissue structures.

or dislocation is successful and stable. To achieve reduction, a pillow is placed under the upper back of the supine athlete and gentle traction is applied, with the shoulder held in 90 degrees of abduction and in maximum extension. Occasionally, open reduction or surgical manipulation under general anesthesia is required.

Epiphyseal Fracture of the Distal Clavicle

In athletes under 25 years of age, sternoclavicular injuries may not result in true dislocations, but rather in fractures through the growth center of the proximal aspect of the clavicle. **Clavicular epiphyseal fractures** may appear clinically as dislocations, especially if some displacement is present, and they can be treated conservatively. They are typically not associated with growth deformities. Reduction of the fracture is not usually required unless the displacement is severe. Symptomatic treatment until the athlete is pain free is all that is required. A Kenny Howard splint used to treat acromioclavicular joint dislocation may be used if there is significant displacement. Remodeling occurs readily.

Occasionally, a youngster who fell on the shoulder will complain several weeks later about an enlarging mass at the sternoclavicular joint. The mass is generally firm and may be slightly tender, depending on the time that has elapsed since injury. This mass most likely represents the healing callus of a clavicular epiphyseal fracture. Radiographs will confirm the diagnosis.

Rehabilitation of Sternoclavicular Injuries

While the athlete is in the immobilization device, simple activities can be performed to maintain strength in the upper extremity. Isometrics for external and internal rotation, abduction and adduction, and extension and flexion can be done many times throughout the day. A ball of putty or grip apparatus can be utilized to maintain grip.

Once the athlete has healed sufficiently to allow range of motion and strengthening, an exercise routine can be started (see pp. 258–263). Emphasis should be on gaining full range of motion in all directions. For strengthening, the various motions of the shoulder should be strengthened against gravity, working up to 5 sets of 10 repetitions, two to three times a day, working initially to 5 pounds. Once range of motion and strength approach the preinjury level, then functional activities can be emphasized as the athlete prepares to return to sport participation. When the athlete returns to play, generally no special braces, splints, or pads are necessary.

Clavicular Fractures

Despite the proximity of vital structures, **clavicular fractures** which occur during sport participation are rarely associated with arterial or nerve damage. Accompanying soft tissue pathology is also uncommon. Midclavicular fractures account for 80 percent of clavicular fractures (Fig. 16.19); distal fractures, 15 percent; and proximal fractures, 5 percent. Most fractures of the shaft of the clavicle heal uneventfully.

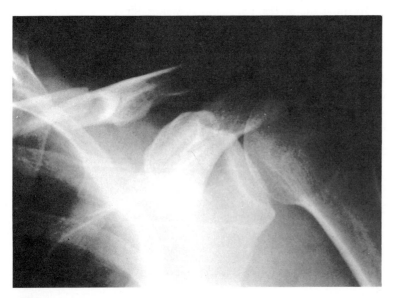

FIGURE 16.19. Radiographic appearance of a midclavicular fracture.

The potential for a rare but serious neurovascular complication, such as a tear of the subclavian artery or injury to the brachial plexus, must be kept in mind when evaluating and treating clavicular fractures; as with sternoclavicular dislocations, a neurovascular exam on initial evaluation is very important. Pulses in the distal part of the upper extremity, strength, and sensation should all be evaluated carefully.

Because the clavicle is a single, bony structure that fixes the shoulder girdle to the thorax, a fracture through it causes the shoulder to sag downward and forward. The pull of the sternocleidomastoid muscle displaces the proximal fragment superiorly. In the older child or the adult, the size of the bone and the muscular development hinder the initial reduction and maintenance of reduction. In addition, distal fractures of the clavicle, more common in older age groups, may involve tears of the coracoclavicular ligament. Such a tear allows the proximal clavicle to ride up superiorly, mimicking an acromioclavicular dislocation. Delayed union in this type of fracture is far greater than with other clavicular fractures.

Mid- and proximal clavicular fractures in all age groups are usually treated with figure-eight strapping, tightened periodically to maintain good shoulder position. Athletes should be instructed that the strap is a reminder not to allow their shoulder to sag forward. The strap should not be applied so tightly that it puts significant pressure on the axilla. In the first few days following injury, a sling on the affected side may also be used to support the extremity. In distal clavicular fractures, an acromioclavicular joint splint such as the Kenny Howard splint to depress the clavicle may effect a better reduction than a figure-eight sling.

Once the clavicular fracture has healed, range-of-motion and strengthening exercises should be performed. Athletes should not be allowed to return to play until achieving their preinjury shoulder strength. Generally, no special braces or pads are utilized when the athlete returns to play.

Acromioclavicular Joint Injuries

Acromioclavicular separations or **sprains** vary in severity, depending on the extent of injury to the stabilizing ligaments and capsule. If the blow producing the injury is mild, usually only a partial tear of the acromioclavicular ligament occurs, producing a first-degree injury. When the acromioclavicular ligament is completely torn but the coracoclavicular ligament remains intact, a second-degree injury that involves subluxation or partial displacement results. The subluxation is not always obvious on physical examination, but the diagnosis can be confirmed by an x-ray of the shoulder with the shoulder girdle weighted (see the following paragraph). When the force is severe enough to tear the coracoclavicular ligament as well as the acromioclavicular ligament and capsule, a third-degree injury occurs. The resulting displacement of the joint is often obvious on observation and can be confirmed by a shoulder radiograph.

For the weighted shoulder x-ray, 10-pound weights are attached to both of the athlete's wrists rather than held in the athlete's hands. When the weights are held in the hands, the increased muscular effort required to hold them may mask the degree of separation (Fig. 16.20). An anteroposteri-

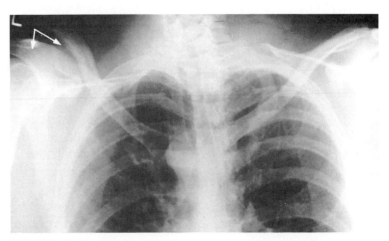

FIGURE 16.20. A third-degree acromioclavicular sprain seen on a weighted x-ray. Note the increased coracoclavicular space on the right.

or x-ray of the entire upper thorax allows the vertical distance between the coracoid and the clavicle on both the involved and uninvolved sides to be compared. An increase in this distance on a "nonweighted" radiograph indicates incompetence of coracoclavicular ligaments and categorizes the injury as a third-degree separation.

The athlete who has sustained an acromioclavicular joint injury will typically leave the field holding his or her arm close to the side. The examiner should review the mechanism of injury with the athlete, observing whether the athlete fell on the outstretched arm or received a heavy blow to the acromial area. A blow to the acromial area would demonstrate pain and soreness in the area, whether there was a sprain or just a contusion. When checking for looseness of the acromioclavicular joint, the examiner is advised to manipulate the clavicle at midshaft rather than at the acromioclavicular joint to rule out pain from the contusion to the area. Occasionally, there is an obvious deformity or easily detected motion at the acromioclavicular joint, which makes it easy to diagnose the injury. The more difficult injury to determine is the mild injury. To aid in this evaluation, the athlete puts the hand of his or her affected arm on the opposite shoulder (if possible), and then the examiner gently applies a downward pressure at the athlete's affected elbow, noting if such a maneuver elicits pain at the acromioclavicular joint.

Management of acromioclavicular joint injuries depends on their severity. First- and second-degree sprains of the joint frequently can be successfully managed with a sling alone until discomfort dissipates, usually within 2 to 4 weeks, followed by a rehabilitation program to restore normal range of motion and strength to the upper extremity.

The treatment of third-degree sprains or complete dislocations varies. Some physicians advocate open reduction. Others believe that third-degree sprains should be treated nonsurgically, since many athletes can and do function well with complete dislocation of the acromioclavicular joint. Surgery, when performed, is generally directed at reconstruction of the conoid and trapezoid ligaments (the coracoclavicular ligaments).

Nonsurgical treatment can either be with a sling for comfort or can involve the use of an acromioclavicular sling to try to achieve reduction of the dislocation. The athlete on whom this device is used must be followed carefully to make certain that the pressure applied by the sling to the distal clavicle is sufficient to afford reduction but not great enough to cause compromise of the skin. Ice and other modalities are utilized to decrease initial soreness in an acute acromioclavicular joint injury. The athlete's pain initially limits range-of-motion and strengthening exercises. The athlete's progress is determined by his or her ability to achieve full range of motion activity, a process carried out gently and gradually. Isotonic strengthening exercises then follow, although isometric exercises can be done earlier when range of motion is still limited.

Before an athlete can return to play with a mild injury, he or she should have full range of nonpainful motion and no tenderness upon direct palpation of the acromioclavicular joint or pain when manual traction is applied to it.

Rotator Cuff Injuries

Rotator Cuff Impingement

When the detailed anatomy of the shoulder region and the mechanics of the overhead throw are considered, the prevalence of injuries to the rotator cuff becomes understandable. With prolonged, repetitive overhead activities, such as pitching, serving in tennis, or swimming the crawl, the rotator cuff may impinge on the acromion and the overlying coracoacromial ligament. **Rotator cuff impingement** causes microtrauma to the cuff, resulting in local inflammation, edema, cuff softening, pain, and poor function of the cuff. These problems precipitate even greater impingement, producing a "cycle of injury" (Fig. 16.21). High stress on the rotator cuff, as in eccentric deceleration during throwing, can also cause intrinsic rotator cuff tendon injury. Blood supply to this tendon is precarious, diminishing the capacity for healing.

Physical Examination

The athlete with an impingement syndrome will generally show increased pain on external rotation and abduction. Generally, weakness and pain in the rotator cuff are evident when manual muscle testing is done. Muscle testing should be done with the shoulder in abduction in the "empty-can position" (Fig. 16.22), as well as horizontal abduction and external rotation with the humerus at 90 degrees and at 0 degrees.

Passively, when the arm is taken into a position of horizontal adduction, flexion, and internal rotation, the athlete will experience discomfort. This maneuver will also elicit pain in an athlete with acromial joint dysfunction, but in this latter instance, palpation of the acromioclavicular joint also results in discomfort, differentiating acromioclavicular joint dysfunction from impingement phenomenon.

Differentiation From Chronic Cuff Tears

Frequently, it is difficult to differentiate the pain that results from the impingement phenomenon from pain that is secondary to a partial or full thickness tear of the rotator cuff (see Chronic Rotator Cuff Tears, page 250). Unlike acute tears of the rotator cuff, chronic rotator cuff tears may present insidiously, with slowly increasing symptoms. In some instances, this pathology may represent an extension of the impingement phenomenon—that is, repetitive impingement causes thinning of the cuff, which then goes on to sustain a degenerative tear.

Radiographic evaluation of the shoulder with an arthrogram or magnetic resonance imaging (MRI) study may be useful in diagnosing chronic rotator cuff tears in the

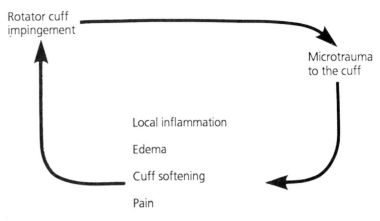

FIGURE 16.21. Rotator cuff impingement "cycle of injury."

athlete who has signs and symptoms of chronic impingement, but does not improve on a conservative treatment program for same.

If there is a tear of the rotator cuff and arthrographic dye is injected into the glenohumeral joint, the dye will leak into the subacromial space. If a partial-thickness tear is present, pooling of the dye in the partial cuff tear will be evident on a radiograph. The MRI study is useful for visualizing the cuff tissue itself.

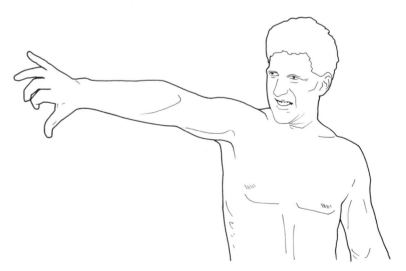

FIGURE 16.22. Muscle testing with the shoulder abducted in the "empty can" position.

Treatment

Conservative treatment of shoulder impingement consists of oral anti-inflammatories and modalities such as heat and cold, iontophoresis or phonophoresis, and microelectric nerve stimulation. The latter modalities will help decrease inflammation and therefore promote healing. Conservative treatment for impingement must also include an exercise program to strengthen the rotator cuff, as it is only with restoration of normal function of the cuff tissue that the glenohumeral mechanics will be improved and the impingement phenomenon will no longer be present.

Steroid injections into the rotator cuff are rarely done. Steroids, if injected directly into the tendinous cuff, can cause softening or weakening of the cuff itself and perhaps predispose it to tear.

Activity modification is frequently recommended, especially in the acutely symptomatic athlete. Decreasing repetitive overhead activities while maintaining the conditioned state is also recommended.

Surgical correction for impingement is done only after prolonged conservative treatment (6 months to a year) fails to yield significant improvement. Special radiographic views can be taken of the subacromial space to see whether spurs exist on the undersurface of the acromion. Spurs can cause a mechanical narrowing of the subacromial space. If the subacromial space is narrow, releasing the coracoacromial ligament, combined with shaving the undersurface of the acromion (partial acromionectomy), may result in relief of symptoms. This procedure can be done arthroscopically, although some surgeons still prefer an open approach. With arthroscopic débridement of the subacromial space, the athlete frequently has less postoperative morbidity and can begin a return-to-throwing program in 6 to 8 weeks. Following any surgical procedure, range of motion is achieved before strengthening exercises are started. The exercises used are similar to those of a conservative strengthening program.

Chronic Rotator Cuff Tears

Chronic rotator cuff tears typically result from degeneration within the rotator cuff tendon. It has been theorized that the poor blood supply to the tendon promotes early degeneration. Repetitive activity, especially in the athlete with a restricted subacromial space, may also be a contributing factor. A minor traumatic event—for example, a fall on the outstretched arm that causes the humeral head to be impacted against the acromion—may cause a full-thickness tear in the athlete with mild or moderate tendon degeneration.

The athlete with a chronic rotator cuff tear may describe a gradual loss of strength in abduction and external rotation, with increasingly persistent pain in this range. Night pain is common, as well as pain with overhead activity. The pain is difficult to locate but is usually described as being deep in the shoulder.

If the rotator cuff tear is small, a prolonged period of rest (4 to 9 months) may result in healing. Range-of-motion exercises are also recommended, unless they cause significant discomfort. When cuff exercises cause pain, they should be discontinued for several weeks and replaced by range-of-motion exercises.

If prolonged rest or rest with controlled exercise does not improve the athlete's symptoms, surgical repair of the tear is recommended. The thin, degenerated tissue of a chronic rotator cuff tear makes surgical repair more difficult than repair of an acute rotator cuff tear. Subacromial decompression to increase the subacromial space may be done during cuff repair, especially if the subacromial space is diminished by spurs noted radiographically.

Rehabilitating the shoulder following rotator cuff repair requires 6 months to a year of gradually increasing exercises until full function returns. The program selected will vary, depending on the extent of the tear and the type of repair performed. Generally, initially following repair, isometric exercises only are done. The athlete then progresses to shoulder shrugs; elbow, hand, and grip strengthening; and pendulum exercises. At 4 weeks, progressive abduction and external rotation in the supine position on the table or floor can usually begin. At 6 weeks, the athlete may be able to begin some gentle, active strengthening exercises against gravity for flexion, abduction, prone horizontal abduction, and external rotation side lying (athlete lying on unaffected side and gradually flexing to 90 degrees). The goals are to bring the athlete to the point at which he or she can perform 5 sets of 10 repetitions, twice a day, with 5 pounds, in all of the different exercise positions, and to obtain functional range of motion.

Tennis players, throwers, and swimmers in the competitive high school, college, and professional age groups may sustain partial rotator cuff tears merely from repetitive overhead activity. In the conservative treatment of this injury, emphasis on prone horizontal abduction and prone external rotation is important to try to restore strength to the cuff, and hence, restore normal shoulder mechanics. External rotation stretching in three positions also seems to be a stimulus to healing of the posterior rotator cuff by providing stress lines for the orderly arrangement of collagen tissue and by stimulating blood flow to the area. If a 6-week conservative program of exercise, followed by a gradual return to activity, does not result in steady improvement, further diagnostic evaluation with an arthrogram, MRI study, or arthroscopic evaluation of the cuff may be recommended. Arthroscopic débridement of abnormal cuff tissue may promote healing in athletes with partial-thickness posttraumatic tears.

Following débridement, the athlete immediately begins range-of-motion and strengthening exercises. When the athlete can externally rotate at 2 to 3 pounds pain-free, a return-to-throwing program can be started (see Interval Throwing Program on p. 258). It typically requires 6 to 12 months for a throwing athlete to return to sport following arthroscopic débridement of a partial thickness rotator cuff tear.

Glenoid Labrum Injuries

The glenoid labrum is the soft tissue rim around the glenoid fossa that "deepens" the socket and provides stability for the humeral head. A mixture of cartilage and ligamentous connective tissue, it is intimately connected with the surrounding capsule.

Glenoid labrum tears can occur from repetitive shoulder motion or from acute trauma. In the athlete with repeated anterior subluxation of the shoulder, tears of the middle and inferior portion of the glenoid labrum can occur. The tear enhances anterior instability. Glenoid labrum tears may also result from anterior instability during the acceleration phase of throwing or during the deceleration phase of the throwing act, from the biceps pulling on the anterior labrum.

Athletes who are weight training may develop a glenoid labrum tear with repetitive bench pressing and overhead pressing. Weakness in the posterior rotator cuff can aggravate this pathology. Glenoid labrum tears can occur from acute trauma, such as falling on an outstretched arm; they can also occur in the leading shoulder of batters or golfers who ground their bats or clubs.

An athlete with a glenoid labrum injury may describe the pain as pain that interrupts the smooth functioning of the shoulder in the performance of the activity. On examination, the athlete may have discomfort on forced external rotation at 90 degrees of abduction; this discomfort typically does not increase as the arm goes into further abduction. Frequently, a glenoid labrum disruption can be felt as a "pop" or "click" on a forced external rotation of the torn labrum. The athlete may also experience discomfort on forced horizontal adduction of the shoulder. Manual muscle testing may show associated weakness in the rotator cuff.

With more recent advances in soft tissue visualization using such instruments as the MRI and CT (computed tomography) scan following injection of contrast dye into the shoulder joint, labrum injuries may be detected at an early date. Radiographic confirmation of suspected glenoid labrum defects can be done using either MRI or CT.

If conservative range-of-motion exercise and gradual return to activity are not successful, arthroscopic intervention may be performed for débridement of the labrum. At the time of arthroscopy, care must be taken not to débride the inferior labrum, as doing so may increase anterior shoulder instability and, hence, increase the risk of anterior shoulder dislocation. Range-of-motion exercises progressing to 25 repetitions and strengthening exercises progressing to 5 sets of 10, twice a day, progressing to 5 pounds, typically begin immediately after surgery. The athlete who has débridement of a small superior or middle glenoid labrum tear may frequently progress into a throwing program 2 to 3 weeks after surgery and be ready to throw in a game within 3 months (see Interval Throwing Program on p. 258).

Bicipital Tendinitis

The long head of the biceps muscle extends intra-articularly under the acromion through the rotator cuff to its insertion at the top of the glenoid. The same mechanism that initiates the impingement syndrome symptoms in rotator cuff injuries can inflame the tendon in its subacromial location, producing **bicipital tendinitis**. Bicipital tendinitis may also result from subluxation of the tendon out of its groove in the proximal humerus (the bicipital groove, Fig. 16.23). This condition occurs with rupture of the transverse ligament.

The symptoms of bicipital tendinitis, whether due to impingement or tendon subluxation, are essentially the same. Pain is localized to the proximal humerus and the shoulder joint. Resistive supination of the forearm aggravates pain, since the biceps' primary function is supination. Pain may also occur on manual muscle testing of the elbow flexors and on palpation of the tendon itself. The Yergason test (see p. 244)

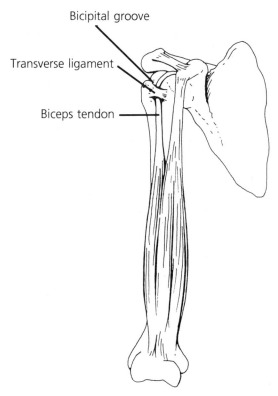

FIGURE 16.23. The biceps tendon lies within the bicipital groove.

is used to test for instability of the long head of the biceps in its groove.

If bicipital tendinitis is associated with the shoulder impingement syndrome, therapy directed to the impingement syndrome may result in spontaneous resolution of the bicipital tendinitis. If subluxation of the tendon within its groove is the cause of irritation, conservative treatment includes modalities, followed by restriction of activities initially, with slow resumption of activity after a period of rest. Strengthening muscles which assist the biceps in elbow flexion and forearm supination may also be helpful. Steroid injections are hazardous because they may promote tendon degeneration. If symptoms are persistent, tenodesis of the biceps tendon directly into bone or transplantation of the long head into the short head of the biceps may be considered in the older athlete. Unfortunately, recovery from such a procedure is difficult; it is doubtful that a highly competitive athlete would be able to return to peak performance following this procedure.

Bursitis of the Shoulder

Bursitis of the shoulder refers to inflammation of the subacromial bursa. Inflammation of the bursa is generally secondary to shoulder impingement, and hence, the signs and symptoms are similar, as is the treatment.

Rotator cuff strengthening and stretching exercises may reduce the symptoms. With return of the cuff's normal function (depressing the humeral head and stabilizing the glenohumeral joint), there is greater room under the acromial arch, and, therefore, less impingement and irritation.

Scapular Fractures

Scapular fractures may be divided into three groups: those involving the glenoid joint, those of the spine and acromion process, and those of the body. Those involving the glenohumeral joint are most frequent, and those of the body are least common. Fractures of the glenoid usually involve the rim and are associated with dislocation or subluxation of the shoulder. They are usually minimally displaced, and treatment is dictated by the shoulder subluxation, not by the scapular fracture.

Fractures of the acromion may occur in connection with acromioclavicular separations. These minimally displaced fractures are likewise treated as the acromioclavicular separation. Occasionally, a markedly displaced acromial fracture with substantial acromioclavicular disruption requires surgical treatment. Any time severe trauma occurs to the shoulder or when crepitus or acute tenderness is localized over the scapula, an x-ray of the scapula may be needed. Referral of this athlete to the team physician for evaluation is appropriate.

Fractures of the body and spine of the scapula can be treated in the same manner as the surrounding soft tissue—that is, by

cold applications for the first 48 hours to minimize bleeding, followed by heat and early mobilization. Considerable displacement is not incompatible with a good result and can be accepted. Once the fracture is stabilized, the athlete should begin range of motion exercises and strengthening of the muscles of the shoulder girdle in order to be able to return to his or her previous level of activity.

Shoulder Dislocation (Glenohumeral Dislocation)

The glenohumeral joint is notable for its mobility but not for its stability. Bony articular contact is minimal, and the capsular ligaments are lax in all but the extremes of shoulder motion. Consequently, control of the joint is provided primarily by the dynamic action of muscles. When the forces driving the glenohumeral joint toward the limits of its normal range of motion exceed the restraining strength of the shoulder muscles and capsular ligaments, the humeral head may displace from the joint. This injury is called **glenohumeral dislocation** or, more commonly, **shoulder dislocation**. The majority of glenohumeral dislocations and subluxations are anterior and inferior to the glenoid rim.

Anterior Glenohumeral Dislocation

Anterior glenohumeral dislocation occurs when external rotation/abduction force on the humerus or a direct posterior or posterolateral blow on the shoulder is great enough to displace the humeral head, and the anterior capsule is either stretched or torn within its substance or torn from its attachment to the anterior glenoid (Fig. 16.24). The head may be displaced into the subcoracoid, subglenoid, subclavicular, or intrathoracic position.

Two gross pathological lesions are typical (Fig. 16.25). One is the **Bankart lesion**, an anterior capsule injury associated with a tear of the glenoid labrum. The other is an indentation or compression fracture of the

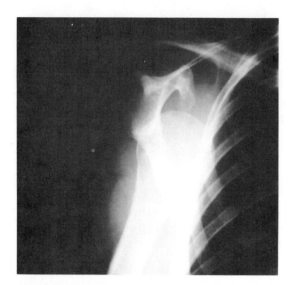

FIGURE 16.24. Anterior glenohumeral dislocation seen on x-ray.

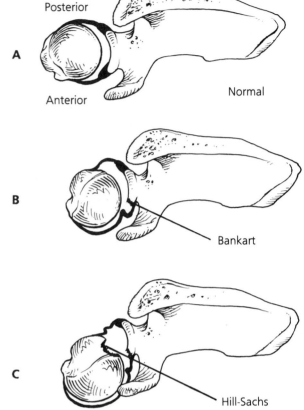

FIGURE 16.25. Normal appearance of the anterior glenohumeral joint and two gross pathological lesions: (a) normal appearance, (b) Bankart lesion, (c) Hill-Sachs lesion.

articular surface of the humeral head that is created by the sharp edge of the anterior glenoid as the humeral head dislocates over it. This is termed the **Hill-Sachs lesion**. Both lesions predispose to recurrent dislocations as they result in a compromise of the mechanical stability of the glenohumeral joint when the arm is placed in abduction and external rotation.

Two other associated injuries occur with some frequency in the young athlete. One is avulsion of the greater tuberosity from the humerus caused by traction from the rotator cuff. The second is an injury to the axillary nerve, which supplies the deltoid muscle and skin over the proximal lateral area of the arm. This nerve may be contused, stretched, or torn during an anterior dislocation. Its function may be temporarily or permanently lost, resulting in denervation of a portion of the deltoid muscle, and hence, its loss of function as well as the loss of sensation on the proximal lateral area of the arm. In the majority of cases, the nerve is stretched or contused, and hence, recovers, resulting in return of deltoid function and return of sensation to the upper outer arm. It is possible for persistent axillary nerve palsy to occur after shoulder reduction, either because the axillary nerve

has been stretched to a point beyond which it cannot recover or because it has been torn. The function of this nerve should always be tested at examination before and after reduction.

Athletes who have just sustained a shoulder dislocation will typically try to support their injured extremity by holding their forearm with their opposite hand. They generally know that their shoulder is dislocated and will say so. On physical examination of the athlete with an anterior-inferior dislocation, the examiner will note a space underneath the acromion where the humeral head should lie and a palpable mass representing the humeral head in the anterior axilla.

Anterior glenohumeral dislocation is a common injury in athletics. Because recurrent dislocations are not uncommon, one needs to distinguish between athletes who have sustained an acute dislocation and those who have sustained a recurrent dislocation. The athlete with an initial dislocation typically has sustained considerable trauma. The possibility of associated fractures and nerve injuries is high. The exception to this rule is the rare athlete who has significant congenital laxity of the glenohumeral joint. Athletes who have had a prior glenohumeral joint dislocation or who have congenital laxity of the joint have compromised shoulder stability. Therefore, they can sustain a recurrent dislocation from minimal trauma. Hence, associated injuries are less frequently seen in this population. Furthermore, reduction of their dislocation may be accomplished with minimal effort. Attempted reduction of a recurrent dislocation or of a dislocation in a congenitally lax athlete is reasonable. If the shoulder does not easily reduce, however, the arm should be placed in a sling and the athlete transferred to a medical facility for complete evaluation, including radiographs.

Anterior glenohumeral dislocations can be reduced by several techniques. Longitudinal traction can be exerted on the affected arm with slight external movement, followed by internal movement of the arm. The athlete should be counterbalanced by a sheet or towel in the axilla (Fig. 16.26). Care should be taken to avoid direct pressure on neurovascular structures in the axilla injury or fracture. In another technique, the athlete lies between two tables, with the head resting on one table and the body on the other. The affected arm is between the tables, with a 5- to 10-pound weight tied to it. A variation of this position is to have the athlete lie prone on a table, with the arm hanging off the side of the table, with a weight affixed to it. As the musculature about the shoulder relaxes from the force of the weight, spontaneous reduction takes place. Although the Kocher maneuver (a procedure in which the elbow is flexed and the arm is externally rotated with traction

applied at the elbow) is an acceptable method of reduction, it can, if done improperly, cause increased forces on the humeral neck, resulting in a fracture. Caution must be taken to place adequate traction on the arm before external rotation is attempted.

Following the initial dislocation, it is usually advisable to immobilize the shoulder in internal rotation for 3 to 6 weeks. The athlete will probably not return to competition before 6 weeks and healing may take longer. Prior to return to play, the athlete should regain normal strength without pain and have normal range of motion. All muscles of the shoulder should be strengthened. Emphasis should be placed on strengthening the rotator cuff, since one of its main functions is to stabilize the humeral head in the glenoid fossa. Upon return to routine weight-training activities, the athlete should avoid wide grips on the bench press and deep shoulder dips. Any activity that causes increased stress on the anterior capsule should be modified. With recurrent shoulder dislocations, minimal immobilization until pain subsides is generally recommended. Range-of-motion and strengthening exercises are then begun.

Multiple restraining devices are available to prevent recurrent dislocations. These devices attempt to keep the arm from going into abduction, extension, and external rotation. These devices can be effective, but they do restrict the athlete's shoulder motion, which is a disadvantage in certain

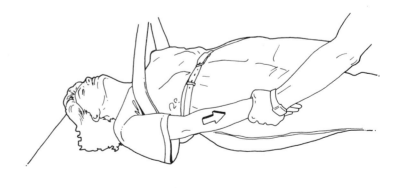

FIGURE 16.26. Reduction of an anterior glenohumeral dislocation using longitudinal traction.

sports, especially if the affected extremity is the dominant extremity. If the athlete has sustained multiple dislocations, surgical reconstruction of the shoulder joint may be advisable, but only after all factors such as the number of dislocations, the circumstances of each dislocation, and whether the dominant arm is involved are considered.

The orthopedic literature presents a wide variety of shoulder repairs; which the recurrence rate for many of the more common repairs is approximately the same. Most procedures involve repair of the glenoid defect and tightening of the anterior capsule and ligamentous structures through an anterior incision. Alternatively, especially in throwing athletes, a block of bone can be transferred surgically from the coracoid process to the anterior glenoid rim to "deepen" the socket in order to prevent future dislocations. Shoulder repairs in which only the torn glenoid labrum needs to be repaired can be done arthroscopically, a procedure associated with less initial postoperative morbidity than open repair.

For most surgical procedures, aggressive range-of-motion exercises are not started until approximately 3 weeks postoperatively. The athlete's goal is to try and gain full abduction and 90 degrees of external rotation. Procedures that employ bony block (if the block is securely fixed by screw or staple) may allow earlier range-of-motion activities. In some cases, external rotation and abduction may begin as early as 10 days postoperatively. The strengthening routine for these athletes can also begin utilizing the antigravity positions earlier than they are used following soft tissue repairs. By 12 weeks athletes who have progressed well with their initial program can begin a variety of weight-training activities. Again, emphasis on avoiding exercises that stress the anterior capsule is recommended.

Posterior Glenohumeral Dislocation

Although **posterior glenohumeral dislocation** results from a different set of forces than that of anterior dislocation, in many

ways the pathology is similar. The posterior capsule is either stretched, torn, or disrupted from the posterior glenoid. A reverse Hill-Sachs lesion is created on the anterior articular surface by the posterior lip of the glenoid. With an anterior glenohumeral dislocation, the rotator cuff or its bony attachment at the greater tuberosity may be injured by stretching; with a posterior dislocation, the subscapularis or its insertion on the lesser tuberosity may be injured.

The posterior glenohumeral dislocation may be difficult to diagnose. In contrast to anterior shoulder dislocation, where the deformity is easily visible and the position of the arm is extreme, an athlete who has sustained a posterior dislocation may present with a normal anterior contour to his or her shoulder. Chest muscles appear intact, and in the well-developed individual with a large deltoid, it is difficult to see that the shoulder is depressed. A cardinal sign of a posterior shoulder dislocation is prominence of the humeral head posteriorly in the shoulder; again, this prominence can be masked by heavy deltoid musculature. What cannot be masked, however, is that the shoulder is held in internal rotation and cannot be externally rotated.

All shoulder injuries sustained on the playing field should first be evaluated by observation, by gentle palpation, and by attempts at bringing the joint carefully and gently through a full range of motion. Restriction of the joint motion is an indication for transfer to a medical facility and radiographic examination. Even with the aid of standard radiographs, posterior dislocations may go unrecognized. Thus, if the shoulder's inability to rotate externally is noted during a careful physical exam, the athlete may need additional radiographs to document the humeral head's position in the glenoid.

A posterior dislocation of the glenohumeral joint is reduced by applying traction in the line of the adducted deformity and concomitant direct anterior pressure on the humeral head. If the maneuver is done gently after total body relaxation, reduction should be atraumatic.

For an initial dislocation, immobilization for 3 to 6 weeks is warranted. The recurrent dislocation should be treated symptomatically, and surgical treatment considered.

Shoulder Subluxation: Anterior and Posterior

Some athletes will have laxity in either the posterior or anterior capsule. They may never have had a frank dislocation. These loose-jointed individuals often develop a painful shoulder, especially if rotator cuff strength decreases. They may develop fatigue fracture of the glenoid labrum or inflammation of the rotator cuff because of the stress put on the cuff as it tries to stabilize the humeral head during the activity. On occasion, various surgical procedures may be performed to stabilize this individual. Generally, this type of athlete will do well with a rotator cuff strengthening program.

The **dead arm syndrome** is the name used to describe a condition that occurs in throwing athletes who during a contest are suddenly unable to throw and state that after ball release their arm goes numb and is extremely weak. Their symptoms may be vague. Many of these athletes have some anterior shoulder laxity on a congenital basis or from prior injury, either acute or repetitive stress. The dead arm syndrome may also occur in football players who are hit on the anterior portion of their glenohumeral joint and sustain a posterior subluxation that stretches their neurovascular structures in the anterior part of their shoulder.

In the thrower with the dead arm syndrome, physical evaluation may reveal a positive impingement sign, weakness in the rotator cuff, and frequently, laxity in the anterior capsule. Neurological evaluation may be normal. These athletes should initially rest and then strengthen the muscles about the shoulder. A progressive return to throwing is then started in hopes of returning these athletes to sport without recurrence of their symptoms. If an athlete fails to improve in the above program, operative correction of the anterior shoulder laxity may be necessary.

For football players with posterior subluxation, the signs and symptoms will generally disappear within 15 to 30 minutes. Athletes who have no residual neurological problems and who have full strength may return to play. Learning how to block and tackle may help prevent this injury.

Fractures of the Proximal Humerus

Fractures of the proximal humerus, although they occur infrequently in sports, may create one or more fragments in the following locations: the joint surface and anatomical neck; the greater tuberosity (the attachment site for the rotator cuff); the lesser tuberosity (the attachment site for the subscapularis); and the shaft and the surgical neck area.

As previously mentioned in the section on glenohumeral dislocation, occasionally fractures (especially those of the articular surface or greater tuberosity) are associated with dislocation of the humerus in the glenoid; the injury is then termed a *fracture-dislocation of the shoulder.* Healing of these injuries depends on the number of fragments, the degree of displacement of the fragments, and the extent of disruption of the blood supply to the fragments. In the young athlete, epiphyseal (growth plate) injuries to the proximal humerus can occur. The separate growth centers of the articular surface, the greater and lesser tuberosities, coalesce into a single center by age 7. The remaining growth plate does not close until 20 or 22 years of age. Fracture separations of this area can occur at any age until the growth plate closes. Fractures in this area usually do not arrest growth.

In the mature athlete, primary healing of proximal humeral fractures with conservative treatment (sling or sling and swathe) is usually the rule unless the fracture fragments are significantly displaced. Stiffness, even in young people, remains a threat following these injuries because the soft tissues that envelope the shoulder joint lose their range of excursion with injury and immobilization. Pendulum exercises can be done early in the course of healing of these injuries to avoid postinjury stiffness if possible. When healing progresses, active and then passive range-of-motion exercises are started later and are coupled with strengthening exercises for all the shoulder girdle muscles (see pp. 260-263).

Adhesive Capsulitis (Frozen Shoulder)

Adhesive capsulitis, often called **frozen shoulder**, is a clinical entity that begins with any type of inflammatory process about the shoulder (e.g., rotator cuff tendinitis). The inflammation leads to a progressive limitation in the range of motion of the shoulder joint, primarily in the joint capsule. The disease as classically described moves through three phases.

The first, or active, phase begins with the production of capsular scar tissue that progressively matures. The athlete is uncomfortable, primarily at night, and shoulder motion becomes progressively limited. Range-of-motion activities for external rotation and abduction will help decrease the loss of motion and time of dysfunction.

The second phase occurs when the shoulder has essentially undergone a fibrous arthrodesis. The shoulder motion is markedly limited. Pain progressively diminishes as the shoulder becomes stiffer.

During the third phase, the resolution phase, the shoulder becomes progressively supple and gradually returns to normal; symptoms are minimal. The overall time from onset to resolution varies, but may be as long as 18 to 24 months.

Diagnosis in the early phases of adhesive capsulitis is often difficult. Clinical signs include inability to bring the arm up the back to the same level as the opposite, normal shoulder. Examination of the shoulder with the arm abducted to 90 degrees shows varying degrees of loss of internal and external rotation, but especially external rotation. Similar findings may be noted when the adducted arm is examined.

Radiographic confirmation of adhesive capsulitis can be done by arthrography, which will demonstrate marked reduction in the capacity of the joint. Often the affected shoulder will not take more than 2 to 3 ml of dye, although normal shoulder capacity is approximately 12 ml.

Treatment modalities vary, but most athletes can be managed conservatively with modalities and progressive range-of-motion activities. Early, aggressive range-of-motion exercises are encouraged. More rarely, surgical manipulation under general anesthesia may be warranted. Adhesive capsulitis is most frequently seen in the older, recreational athlete. It is also common in nonathletic people, particularly females in their 30s and 40s. No inciting factor may be identifiable in this population, and many factors relating to the pathology of this lesion are still unknown.

REHABILITATION EXERCISES

For most shoulder pathology, high-repetition, low-weight exercise will restore range of motion and strength. The athlete should begin with a basic program and advance slowly to heavier training.

Most range-of-motion activities are done with at least 25 repetitions, three times a day or more, and strengthening activities are done with 5 sets of 10 repetitions, two to three times a day, working from 0 to 5 pounds. Even though unable to complete a full range of motion, the athlete should at least begin working without weight against gravity to develop strength in the motion he or she has. The athlete will thus progress much more quickly than if he or she waited to achieve full range of motion before beginning any strengthening exercises.

Interval Throwing Program

The **interval throwing program** is designed to allow the athlete to get a light workout several times a day at a submaximal level, never trying to fatigue the arm. The arm will gradually become stronger and more conditioned to the throwing act. The program should begin with a thorough stretching of the throwing extremity and application of moist heat, followed by ice, if appropriate. Even though the athlete could throw at a more intense level, that is not the idea of this program. It is the slow buildup and conditioning of the arm that will allow the athlete to progress and not be reinjured. The regimen is to throw 2 days and rest 1 day. One interval is one long toss and one short toss. The goal is to increase the number of intervals per session gradually.

Each throwing session begins with several minutes of 10-foot tossing to get the arm warm for long tossing. The athlete may gradually work to his or her long-toss distance. It is not necessary to start at the set distance. The long toss may start with throws that will just roll to the athlete's partner and will graduate to one hop and then the fly. The long-toss and short-toss intervals may progress independently of each other.

Progress may not be in a straight line upward. Advances and regressions will occur, and some soreness is expected. Athletes should ease off when they hurt. They should not advance to the next phase until they are completely comfortable at the present phase. The phases of an interval throwing program are outlined in Table 16.1.

TABLE 16.1. Phases of an Interval Throwing Program

Phase	Long Toss		Short Toss	
Phase I	feet	(90)	feet	(30)
Interval/day (2)	minutes	(5)	minutes	(5)
Rest between (15–30)	throws	(25)	throws	(50)
	intensity	(to tolerance)	intensity	(work to ½ speed)
Phase II	feet	(120)	feet	(60)
Interval/day (2)	minutes	(5)	minutes	(5)
Rest between (15–30)	throws	(25)	throws	(50)
	intensity	(to tolerance)	intensity	(work to ½ speed)
Phase III	feet	(150)	feet	(60)
Interval/day (2)	minutes	(5)	minutes	(5)
Rest between (15–30)	throws	(25)	throws	(50)
	intensity	(to tolerance)	intensity	(work to ¾ speed)
Phase IV	feet	(180)	feet	(60)
Interval/day (2)	minutes	(5)	minutes	(5)
Rest between (15–30)	throws	(25)	throws	(50)
	intensity	(to tolerance)	intensity	(work to ¾ speed, mound)
Phase V	feet	(210)	feet	(60)
Interval/day (2)	minutes	(5)	minutes	(5)
Rest between (15–30)	throws	(25)	throws	(50)
	intensity	(to tolerance)	intensity	(½ to ¾ speed, mound, breaking ball)
Phase VI	feet	(250)	feet	(60+)
Interval/day (2)	minutes	(5)	minutes	(5)
Rest between (15–30)	throws	(25)	throws	(50)
	intensity	(to tolerance)	intensity	(¾ full speed, mound, breaking ball)

Shoulder Program

Circumduction

Position: leaning over, with opposite arm on table and chest parallel to floor; involved arm hanging straight down, body totally relaxed

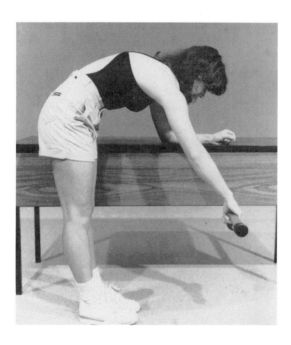

Procedure: Move body and let arm swing clockwise, counterclockwise, forward and backward, and side to side. Perform _____ times, _____ times daily. Progress to _____ times, _____ times daily.

Supine Flexion

Position: lying on back

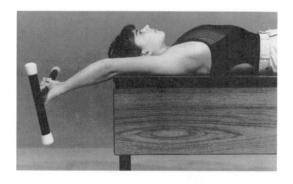

Procedure: Grip stick with hands together and elbows straight and move both arms over the head as far as possible and hold for a count of _____. Relax and repeat _____ times, _____ times per day. Progress to _____ times, _____ times daily.

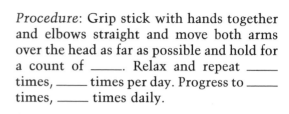

Supine External Rotation

Position: lying on back, with involved arm out to the side at 90 degrees and elbow at 90 degrees

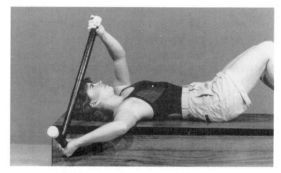

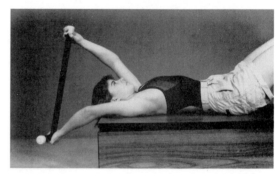

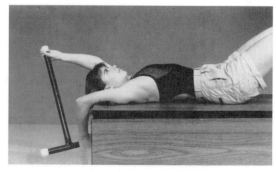

Procedure: Use stick to push the arm straight back into external rotation. Hold for a count of _____. Relax and repeat _____ times, _____ times daily. Repeat this at 135 degrees (about halfway to the ear) and full abduction (next to the ear). Progress to _____ times, _____ times daily.

Supine Internal Rotation

Position: lying on back, with involved arm out to the side at 90 degrees and elbow at 90 degrees

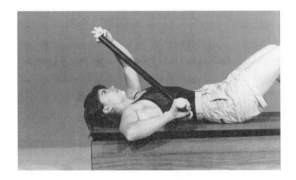

Procedure: Use stick to push arm straight into internal rotation. Hold for a count of _____. Relax and repeat _____ times, _____ times daily. Progress to _____ times, _____ times daily. The athlete may find it helpful to have someone hold his or her shoulder down.

Supine Abduction

Position: lying on back, with involved arm on the surface, as high toward the ear as possible, with palm up

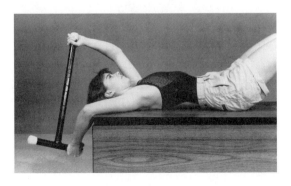

Procedure: Slide arm along surface toward the ear. Use stick or opposite hand to help pull. Hold for a count of _____. Relax and repeat _____ times, _____ times daily. Progress to _____ times, _____ times daily.

Horizontal Adduction Stretch

Position: sitting, standing, or supine

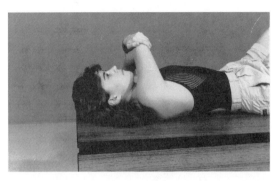

Procedure: Grasp elbow of involved arm with opposite hand and pull arm across front of chest. Hold for _____ counts. Relax. Repeat _____ times, _____ times daily. Progress to _____ times, _____ times daily.

Shoulder Shrugs

Position: standing, arms by side, _____-pound weight in hand

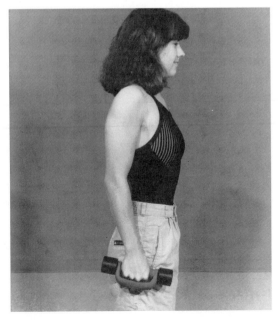

Procedure: Lift shoulders straight up to your ears for a ____ count; then pull shoulders back and pinch shoulder blades for a ____ count. Relax and repeat ____ times, ____ times daily. Progress to ____ pounds, ____ times, ____ times daily.

Shoulder Flexion

Position: standing, with ____-pound weight in hand

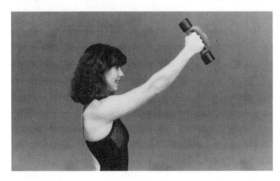

Procedure: Raise arm out to the front of body with thumb up as high as possible. Hold for a ____ count. Relax and repeat ____ times, ____ times daily. Progress to ____ pounds, ____ times, ____ times daily.

Supraspinatus

Position: standing, with ____-pound weight in hand

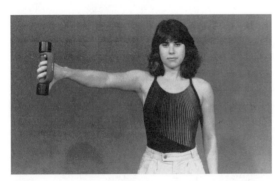

Procedure: Turn the hand so the thumb points at a spot 2 inches in front of the side seam of the pant leg. Raise arm out to the side to eye level. Hold for a ____ count. Relax and repeat ____ times, ____ times daily. Progress to ____ pounds, ____ times, ____ times daily.

Shoulder Abduction

Position: standing, with ____-pound weight in hand

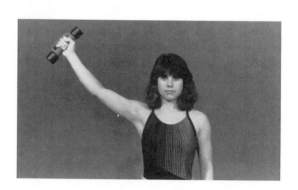

Procedure: Raise arm out to the side of body as high as possible while rotating arm externally with palm up. Hold for a ____ count. Relax and repeat ____ times, ____ times daily. Progress to ____ pounds, ____ times, ____ times daily. You may be asked to hold weight with thumb pointed straight ahead and to raise arm only to shoulder level.

Prone Horizontal Abduction

Position: lying on table or bed, on stomach, with involved arm hanging straight to the floor

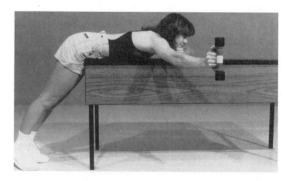

Procedure: With ____-pound weight in hand, raise arm out to the side, with thumb up and hand at eye level. Hold for a ____ count. Relax and repeat ____ times, ____ times daily. Progress to ____ pounds, ____ times, ____ times daily.

Shoulder Extension

Position: lying on stomach, with arm hanging off table, thumb pointing out as far as possible

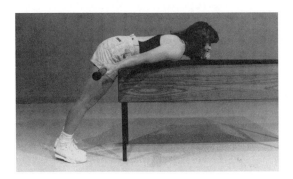

Procedure: With _____-pound weight in hand, lift arm into extension. Hold for a _____ count. Relax and repeat _____ times, _____ times daily. Progress to _____ pounds, _____ times, _____ times daily.

External Rotation—Prone

Position: lying on stomach, elbow level with shoulder, and arm supported at the elbow

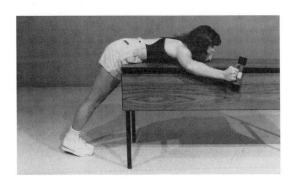

Procedure: Use a _____-pound weight in hand and lift hand up into external rotation level with table. Hold for a _____ count. Relax and repeat. Perform _____ times, _____ times daily. Progress to _____ pounds, _____ times, _____ times daily.

External Rotation—Side Lying

Position: lying on noninjured side, elbow of injured arm at side and flexed to 90 degrees, allowing hand to lie across stomach

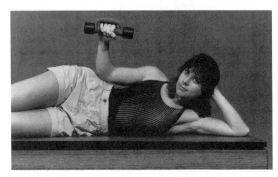

Procedure: With _____-pound weight in your hand, lift hand upward as high as possible. Hold for a _____ count. Relax and repeat _____ times, _____ times daily. Progress to _____ pounds, _____ times, _____ times daily.

Internal Rotation—Side Lying

Position: lying on injured side, elbow of injured arm flexed to 90 degrees

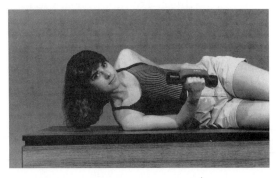

Procedure: With _____-pound weight in hand, lift hand toward stomach. Hold for a _____ count. Relax and repeat. Perform _____ times, _____ times daily. Progress to _____ pounds, _____ times, _____ times daily.

IMPORTANT CONCEPTS

1. The bones of the shoulder are the scapula, humerus, and clavicle.
2. The joints of the shoulder are the glenohumeral, acromioclavicular, scapulothoracic, and sternoclavicular.
3. The rotator cuff of the shoulder is formed by four muscles: the subscapularis, supraspinatus, infraspinatus, and teres minor.
4. Acute trauma from direct force is classically responsible for acromioclavicular and glenohumeral dislocations and scapular and clavicular fractures.
5. Chronic repetitive movements can result in overuse injuries that cause rotator cuff problems and problems with posterior shoulder structures.
6. The trainer should assess neurovascular status in the initial examination of the injured shoulder.
7. Generally, in the skeletally mature athlete, there is no associated fracture with a sternoclavicular joint injury.
8. Midclavicular breaks account for 80 percent of clavicular fractures.
9. Acromioclavicular separations are classified as first-degree (a partial tear of the acromioclavicular ligament only), second-degree (the acromioclavicular ligament is completely torn but the coracoclavicular ligament remains intact), or third-degree (both the acromioclavicular ligament and the coracoclavicular ligament are torn and the joint is displaced).
10. With repetitive overhead activities, the rotator cuff impinges on the coracoacromial ligament, resulting in local inflammation, edema, softening, and pain.
11. Glenoid labrum injuries can occur from overuse or acute trauma.
12. Bicipital tendinitis is usually a secondary finding to a primary cause, such as an impingement syndrome or biceps tendon subluxation.
13. Glenohumeral joint dislocation (shoulder dislocation) occurs when forces driving the glenohumeral joint toward the limits of its normal range exceed the restraining strength of the shoulder muscles and capsular ligaments, and the humeral head tears out of the joint and lodges outside.
14. Fracture of the proximal humerus may create fragments in the joint surface and anatomical neck, the greater tuberosity, the lesser tuberosity, and the shaft and surgical neck.
15. Adhesive capsulitis begins with inflammation about the shoulder, which leads to progressive limitation in the range of motion of the shoulder joint, primarily in the joint capsule.
16. For most shoulder pathology, high-repetition, low-weight exercise will restore range of motion and strengthen the upper extremity.

SUGGESTED READINGS

Alderink, G. J., and D. J. Kuck. "Isokinetic Shoulder Strength of High School and College-Aged Pitchers." *The Journal of Orthopaedic and Sports Physical Therapy* 7 (1986): 163–172.

Blackburn, T. "Throwing: Mechanics, Pathomechanics, Evaluation, and Treatment." Paper presented at the 63rd Annual APTA National Convention, San Antonio, Texas, June 28, 1987.

Brunet, M. E., R. J. Haddad, Jr., and E. B. Porche. "Rotator Cuff Impingement Syndrome in Sports." *The Physician and Sportsmedicine* 10 (December 1982): 86–94.

Cailliet, R. *Shoulder Pain*. Philadelphia: F. A. Davis, 1966.

———— *Shoulder Pain*, 2d ed. Philadelphia: F. A. Davis, 1981, pp. 11–44.

Cybex, Division of Lumex, Inc. *Cybex Data Reduction Computer: A Handbook for Using the Cybex Data Reduction Computer*. Ronkonkoma, N.Y.: Cybex, 1983.

———— *Isolated Joint Testing and Exercise: A Handbook for Using the Cybex II and the U.B.X.T.* Ronkonkoma, N.Y.: Cybex, 1983.

Davies, G. J. *A Compendium of Isokinetics in Clinical Usage*. LaCrosse, Wis.: S. & S. Publishers, 1984.

Davies, G. J., J. A. Gould, and R. L. Larson. "Functional Examination of the Shoulder Girdle." *The Physician and Sportsmedicine* 9 (June 1981): 82–104.

Donatelli, R. "Mobilization of the Shoulder." In *Physical Therapy of the Shoulder*, edited by R. Donatelli, pp. 241–262. New York: Churchill Livingstone, 1987.

Durnin, J. V., and M. M. Rahaman. "The Assessment of the Amount of Fat in the Human Body from Measurements of Skinfold Thickness." *British Journal of Nutrition* 21 (1967): 681–689.

Duvall, E. N. "Critical Analysis of Divergent Views of Movement at the Shoulder Joint." *Archives of Physical Medicine and Rehabilitation* 36 (1955): 149–154.

Einhorn, A. R., D. W. Jackson. "Rehabilitation of the Shoulder." In *Shoulder Surgery in the Athlete*, edited by D. W. Jackson, pp. 103-118. Rockville, Md.: Aspen Systems, 1985.

Freedman, L., and R. R. Munro. "Abduction of the Arm in the Scapular Plane: Scapular and Glenohumeral Movements: A Roentgenographic Study." *Journal of Bone and Joint Surgery* 48A (1966): 1503–1510.

Halbach, J., and R. Tank. "The Shoulder." In *Orthopaedic and Sports Physical Therapy*, edited by J. A. Gould III, and G. J. Davies, pp. 497–517. St. Louis: C. V. Mosby, 1985.

Hoppenfeld, S. *Physical Examination of the Spine and Extremities*. New York: Appleton-Century-Crofts, 1976, pp. 1–34.

Inman, V. T., J. B. de C. M. Saunders, and L. C. Abbott. "Observations on the Function of the Shoulder Joint." *Journal of Bone and Joint Surgery* 26 (1944): 1–30.

Ivey, F. M., Jr., J. H. Calhoun, K. Rusche, and J. Bierschenk. "Isokinetic Testing of Shoulder Strength: Normal Values." *Archives of Physical Medicine and Rehabilitation* 66 (1985): 384–386.

Jackson, D. W., and B. K. Graf. "Decompression of the Coracoacromial Arch." In *Shoulder Surgery in the Athlete*, edited by D. W. Jackson, pp. 51–63. Rockville, Md.: Apsen Systems, 1985.

Jobe, F. W., and C. M. Jobe. "Painful Athletic Injuries of the Shoulder." *Clinical Orthopaedics and Related Research* 173 (1983): 117–124.

Jobe, F. W., D. R. Moynes, J. E. Tibone, et al. "An EMG Analysis of the Shoulder in Pitching: A Second Report." *American Journal of Sports Medicine* 12 (1984): 218–220.

Kapandji, I. A. *The Physiology of the Joints: Annotated Diagrams of the Mechanics of the Human Joints*, 2d. ed. Vol. 1: "Upper Limb." Edinburgh: Churchill Livingstone, 1982.

Kaput, M. "Anatomy and Biomechanics of the Shoulder." In *Physical Therapy of the Shoulder*, edited by R. Donatelli, pp. 1–16. New York: Churchill Livingstone, 1987.

Kegerreis, S. "Shoulder Impingement Syndrome: Conservative Management Based on Applied Anatomy and Biomechanics." Paper presented at the APTA State Chapter Meeting, Little Rock, Arkansas, October 8, 1986.

Kendall, F. "Functional Manual Muscle Testing and Evaluation." Presented at Arkansas PTA State Chapter Meeting, Little Rock, Arkansas, October 7, 1986.

Kendall, H.O., and F. P. Kendall. "Developing and Maintaining Good Posture." *Physical Therapy* 48 (1968): 319–336.

Lucas, D. B. "Biomechanics of the Shoulder Joint." *Archives of Surgery* 107 (1973): 425–432.

McLeod, W. D., and J. R. Andrews. "Mechanisms of Shoulder Injuries." *Physical Therapy* 66 (1986): 1901–1904.

Moffroid, M., R. Whipple, J. Hofkosh, et al. "A Study of Isokinetic Exercise." *Physical Therapy* 49 (1969): 735–747.

Murphy, T. "Shoulder Pain in Swimmers: Mechanics, Pathomechanics, Evaluation, and Treatment." Paper presented at the 63rd Annual ATPA National Convention, San Antonio, Texas, June 28, 1987.

———— "External and Internal Shoulder Rotation Strength and Endurance in Swimmers: Relation to Swimmer's Shoulder Pain." Paper presented at the 7th Annual Combined Physician-Therapist Conference, Williamsburg, Virginia, December 4, 1986.

Murray, M. P., D. R. Gore, G. M. Gardner, et al. "Shoulder Motion and Muscle Strength of Normal Men and Women in Two Age Groups." *Clinical Orthopaedics and Related Research* 192 (1985): 268–273.

Neer, C. S. II. "Impingement Lesions." *Clinical Orthopaedics and Related Research* 173 (1983): 70–77.

Nitz, A. J. "Physical Therapy Management of the Shoulder." *Physical Therapy* 66 (1986): 1912–1919.

Peat, M. "Functional Anatomy of the Shoulder Complex." *Physical Therapy* 66 (1986): 1855–1865.

Poppen, N. K., and P. S. Walker. "Normal and Abnormal Motion of the Shoulder." *Journal of Bone and Joint Surgery* 58A (1976): 195–201.

Rathbun, J. B., and I. Macnab. "The Microvascular Pattern of the Rotator Cuff." *Journal of Bone and Joint Surgery* 52B (1970): 540–553.

Saha, A. K. "Dynamic Stability of the Glenohumeral Joint." *Acta Orthopaedica Scandinavica* 42 (1971): 491–505.

Scagnelli, P. "Management of Myofascial Dysfunction of the Shoulder." In *Physical Therapy of the Shoulder*, edited by R. Donatelli, pp. 263–284. New York: Churchill Livingstone, 1987.

Soderberg, G. L. *Kinesiology: Application to Pathological Motion.* Baltimore: Williams & Wilkins, 1986, p. 110.

17

Arm, Elbow, and Forearm

CHAPTER OUTLINE

Anatomy
  Osseous Structures
  Ligaments
  Muscles
  Nerves, Vessels, and Bursae
Injuries to the Arm
  Contusions
  Injuries to the Radial Nerve
  Fractures of the Humerus
Injuries to the Elbow
  Contusions
  Injuries to the Ulnar Nerve
  Olecranon Bursitis

Strains
Epicondylitis
Sprains
Dislocation
Fractures
Valgus Extension Overload
Injuries to the Forearm
  Contusions
  Acute Tenosynovitis
  Nerve Injuries
  Fractures
Rehabilitation Exercises

OBJECTIVES FOR CHAPTER 17

After reading this chapter, the student should be able to:

1. Describe the anatomy of the arm, elbow, and forearm.
2. Recognize the various types of injuries which may be sustained by the arm, elbow, and forearm, and describe the appropriate treatment for each injury.
3. Instruct the athlete in strengthening exercises for the arm, elbow, and forearm.

INTRODUCTION

Upper extremity injuries caused by acute trauma or recurrent overuse are common in the athletic population. The function of the arm, elbow, and forearm depends on musculotendinous units which originate proximal to the shoulder joint and insert distally near the wrist and hand. An appreciation of the anatomy of these adjacent regions is essential to a complete understanding of extremity problems.

Chapter 17 begins with the anatomy of the arm, elbow, and forearm— the bones, ligaments, muscles, nerves, vessels, and bursae. The chapter next discusses the evaluation and management of common arm, elbow, and forearm injuries. The last section of Chapter 17 presents strengthening exercises to aid in the rehabilitation of the arm, elbow, and forearm.

■

ANATOMY

Osseous Structures

The **humerus**, distal to the humeral head, is cylindrical in its proximal and midportion and then becomes flattened in the antero-posterior direction just proximal to its distal articulating surface (Fig. 17.1). At the elbow, the humerus has two articulating areas: the convex capitellum laterally, and the trochlea medially, which has a spool-shaped depression articulating with the ulna. Extending proximally from these humeral condyles are the medial and lateral epicondylar ridges, to which the forearm flexor pronator muscles attach medially, and the extensor supinator muscles, laterally. The medial epicondyle is more prominent than the lateral and has a cartilaginous apophyseal growth plate that does not close until 16 or 17 years of age.

The **ulna** is a large bone proximally but becomes narrower as it extends distally toward the wrist. The proximal part of the ulna has a deep, semilunar notch that articulates with the trochlea of the humerus as a hinged joint. This articulation is very stable, allowing flexion and extension only. The olecranon process of the ulna extends posteriorly, preventing hyperextension of the elbow, and the coronoid process of the ulna extends anteriorly, preventing hyperflexion. The oblique inclination of the trochlear articulation with the ulna pro-

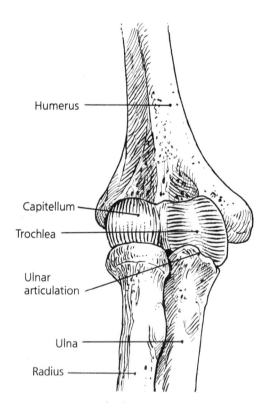

FIGURE 17.1. The humerus.

duces a valgus-carrying angle of 5 to 20 degrees.

The **radius** is much larger distally at the wrist and narrows as it extends proximally to the radial neck and the radial head. The radial head is a round, concave disc that articulates with the convex capitellum of the humerus. The radius rotates over the ulna, allowing pronation and supination of the forearm. A strong ligament extends around the head and neck of the radius, allowing motion along the longitudinal axis but restricting anteroposterior motion. The radius is closely approximated to the ulna distally and proximally. However, it has a radial bow in its midportion, separating it from the ulna. An interosseous membrane connects the two bones in the forearm and separates the anterior flexor compartment from the posterior extensor group.

Ligaments

The **medial collateral ligament** of the elbow consists of anterior, posterior, and oblique components (Fig. 17.2). A portion of the anterior fibers is tight throughout the range of motion of the elbow. The more anterior fibers are tight in extension, whereas the posterior portion is tight in flexion. This anterior band extends from the medial epicondyle to the medial aspect of the coronoid process. The posterior fibers of the medial collateral ligament are fan-shaped and thin compared with the anterior fibers. They are tight only beyond 90 degrees of flexion. They originate on the medial epicondyle and extend down to the medial side of the olecranon. The oblique portion of the medial collateral ligament is less important clinically and extends from the medial side of the olecranon to the medial side of the coronoid process.

The **lateral collateral ligament** consists of a capsular thickening, extending from the lateral epicondyle to the annular ligament.

Muscles

The **biceps muscle** extends from its two origins, one in the superior region of the glenoid and the other on the coracoid process, distally to attach into the tuberosity of the radius. The **brachial muscle** originates on the humerus, extends anteriorly across the elbow joint, and attaches to the ulna.

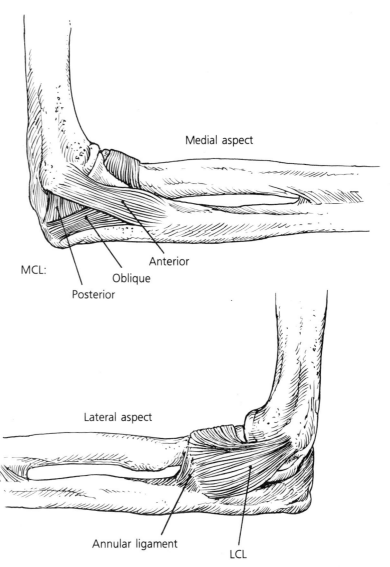

FIGURE 17.2. Medial and lateral aspects of the collateral ligaments.

The extensor muscle, the **triceps**, originates from both the inferior-posterior aspect of the glenoid and the posterolateral aspect of the humerus and extends into its attachment on the olecranon.

The **flexor pronator muscle group** of the forearm and wrist originates on the medial epicondyle and then extends along the epicondylar ridge. These muscles extend down the forearm anteriorly into their attachments at the wrist and fingers. The **extensor supinator muscle group** originates on the lateral epicondyle and extends down the forearm dorsally into the wrist and hand.

Nerves, Vessels, and Bursae

The **brachial artery** and **median nerve** course medially down the arm and across the anterior aspect of the elbow joint. The median nerve crosses the anterior aspect of the elbow and descends into the forearm between the two heads of the pronator teres muscle. It then courses toward the wrist between the flexor sublimis and profundus muscles, entering the palm of the hand from beneath the transverse carpal ligament. The **radial nerve** begins superiorly and medially in the upper arm and winds around the humeral shaft, covered by the triceps, and then extends over the lateral epicondylar ridge, across the anterior aspect of the elbow joint. A major terminal branch of the nerve, the **posterior interosseus nerve**, winds around the radius to the dorsal side of the forearm under the supinator muscle. The **ulnar nerve** passes behind the medial epicondyle at the elbow and extends into the forearm between the two heads of the ulnar flexor muscle of the wrist. At the wrist, the nerve passes laterally to the pisiform bone. The **radial** and **ulnar arteries** accompany their respective nerves along the distal half of the forearm (Fig. 17.3). Knowing the relationships of these vessels and nerves is important in assessing possible neurovascular complications of upper extremity injuries.

The **olecranon bursa** of the elbow separates the skin from the underlying ulna. It allows the soft tissue to glide smoothly over this bony prominence. The **radial humeral bursa** is located anteriorly between the radial head and the lateral epicondyle.

INJURIES TO THE ARM

Contusions

Contusions to the arm are common in contact sports. Direct blows sustained while tackling and blocking can produce bleeding within muscle groups and subperiosteally

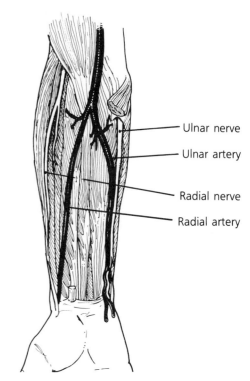

FIGURE 17.3. Arteries and nerves of the forearm.

Ulnar nerve
Ulnar artery
Radial nerve
Radial artery

along the humerus. Contusions within the muscles, particularly the triceps, biceps, and brachial muscles, can be painful and result in restricted motion and disability of the arm.

A common site of contusion in the arm is over the lateral aspect of the humerus, just distal to the attachment of the deltoid and lateral to the biceps muscle. Here, either a severe single blow or repeated injuries from blocking and tackling can cause subperiosteal hematoma formation, with subsequent calcification within the hematoma that eventually matures to bony trabeculae and is called **myositis ossificans** or **tackler's exostosis**. The lower edge of a poorly fitted shoulder pad can contribute to trauma in this area.

The clinical symptoms of contusions of the arm are pain, stiffness, and associated weakness within the involved muscle groups. On examination, the tenderness and swelling must be localized carefully, and any neurological impairment must be noted. Hematoma formation within the muscle groups can lead to calcification and permanent restriction of motion and function. Consequently, careful diagnosis and prompt treatment are important. The typical tackler's exostosis does not involve the adjacent muscle group but presents as a painful, firm mass just distal to the deltoid insertion.

Depending on the severity of the injury, ice applications, compression bandages, and immobilization, either singly or all together, can be used. A sling or a posterior splint may be necessary to restrict motion and relieve pain for the first 48 hours. A compressive bandage of sheet wadding and elastic bandages, extending from the fingertips to the axilla, is often helpful. A constricting bandage around the elbow is to be avoided, since venous return may be obstructed by such a dressing.

Ice applications are generally continued for 48 to 72 hours, or at least until the inflammatory response and swelling appear to be controlled. Thereafter, gentle, active range-of-motion exercises are initiated. Heat may be helpful as part of later treatment plans.

Strengthening exercises to rehabilitate the injured area should be done within the pain-free arc of motion. Active stretching is pursued, but passive stretching should be avoided initially since overstretching an injured muscle could damage it further. A vigorous rehabilitation program for strengthening the triceps and biceps muscle groups should wait until a painless, full range of motion is achieved. Protective padding can be used when the athlete returns to contact sports.

Injuries to the Radial Nerve

The radial nerve winds around the posterolateral aspect of the humerus, protected by the triceps muscle. It then extends over the lateral epicondyle, where it is more subcutaneous and vulnerable to injury. Contusions in this region of the arm may injure the radial nerve.

One of the clinical symptoms of radial nerve injury is pain in the arm, extending down the forearm toward the wrist. Numbness and tingling may also be noted in the dorsum of the wrist. The first dorsum web space of the hand may be numb and the wrist extensors weak, producing the characteristic wrist drop.

Initial treatment consists of immobilization in a cock-up splint in dorsiflexion and a sling. Ice can be used to relieve the swelling, although the ice should not be placed directly over the nerve, as nerve injury from application of ice has been reported. Although many of these lesions are self-limiting and recover spontaneously, others may result in serious hemorrhage within the nerve sheath, resulting in permanent loss of function. A physician should see athletes with radial nerve injury promptly in order to assess the neurological status and to initiate appropriate care.

Fractures of the Humerus

Humeral shaft fractures in the athletic population result from direct force as well as from indirect rotatory torque. A fall on a flexed elbow can result in a humeral shaft fracture. A sudden, severe rotatory force extending through a fixed forearm and elbow, such as in arm wrestling, can produce a spiral fracture of the humeral shaft.

The clinical symptoms of humeral shaft fractures are pain and weakness in the upper extremity, which may extend along the entire course of the upper extremity. Clinical examination often shows swelling and tenderness along the shaft of the humerus. The athlete's ability to flex or extend the elbow does not rule out a fractured humerus. Again, because of the proximity of the radial nerve to the humeral shaft, neurological assessment must be carried out to be certain the nerve is not injured (Fig. 17.4).

Initial treatment of humeral fractures consists of splinting. A sling and a swathe can be used effectively if the individual is not comfortable wearing a posterior splint out of plaster. The athlete must be referred

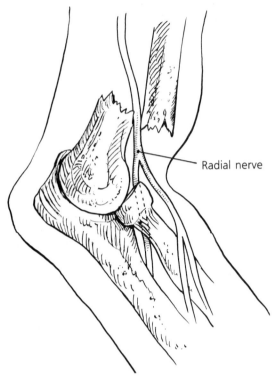

Radial nerve

FIGURE 17.4. The radial nerve is subject to injury in a humeral shaft fracture.

to a physician for definitive treatment. Closed reduction and a plaster cast are usually required.

INJURIES TO THE ELBOW

Contusions

Contusions about the elbow resulting from falls or direct blows are common. The olecranon and epicondylar ridges are particularly vulnerable to direct trauma. The medial epicondyle is more protected than the lateral. The lateral epicondyle is often contused and remains painful if not appropriately treated.

Treatment of these contusions is similar to that described for the arm. Applications of ice and compression bandages for 24 to 48 hours help to reduce swelling and pain. The ice should not be applied directly over the ulnar nerve. A sling may be used when motion at the elbow joint is painful. When the acute inflammatory response has subsided, heat may aid the rehabilitation program. Appropriate protection can help avoid recurrent injuries. Both hard and soft pads can be utilized and should be sport specific.

Injuries to the Ulnar Nerve

The ulnar nerve runs subcutaneously in a groove in the posteromedial aspect of the medial epicondyle. Consequently, it is vulnerable to a direct blow in this area. Such a blow may produce numbness and tingling in the forearm and hand, as when the so-called funny bone is hit. A fascial sheath holds the ulnar nerve within its groove. Occasionally, this sheath is injured, causing subluxation of the nerve from the groove. Flexion and extension of the elbow with valgus force may irritate the nerve as it subluxes in its groove.

The symptoms of ulnar nerve contusions are pain and numbness extending into the fourth and fifth fingers of the hand. Weakness of the interossei muscles of the hand may be present, as well as weakness of tip flexion of the fourth and fifth digits. On clinical exam, the ulnar groove is often tender directly over the nerve. Pressure in this area may produce symptoms extending down into the hand. Sensation along the fourth and fifth fingers, as well as strength of the muscles, particularly the adductor of the little finger and abductor of the index finger, should be carefully assessed.

The initial treatment for contusions of the ulnar nerve consists of rest and application of cold packs to the area. The elbow may be immobilized with a sling. If a nerve injury is suspected, the athlete must be referred to a physician for further evaluation. Many of these lesions are incomplete tears and will subside spontaneously. However, more severe injuries result in hemorrhage within the nerve fibers and sheath. Such hemorrhaging can produce permanent scarring with loss of nerve function and can require surgical decompression and anterior transposition of the nerve.

Olecranon Bursitis

The olecranon bursa of the elbow is equally traumatized by multiple small blows to the olecranon area or by a single traumatic event, such as a fall on the flexed elbow, or by recurrent irritation from repetitive flexion-extension activity of the elbow, allowing the skin to slide repetitively over the bursa and irritate it. Swelling and hemorrhage develop within the bursal sac, producing sensations of pain and stiffness posteriorly. The clinical exam will show local swelling and tenderness over the olecranon bursa (Fig. 17.5). The examiner should inspect for erythema, which may indicate an infectious bursitis rather than a traumatic one. One should also be concerned about infection as a cause of the bursitis if the athlete's pain is very severe and there is no history of trauma.

Initial treatment of olecranon bursitis consists of compression and ice application to reduce the swelling and inflammation. Immobilization with a splint or sling may be indicated. When swelling is marked, aspiration of the fluid within the bursa can be helpful. When aspiration is done, it should be performed with great caution, using all the principles of sterile technique. Because of the poor blood supply to this area, infections may easily occur. When athletes with olecranon bursitis return to competition, this area should be protected with padding. Individuals with chronic or recurrent olecranon bursitis may require surgical excision of the bursa.

Strains

Strains of the musculotendinous units of the upper extremity vary from mild, first-degree injuries to severe, third-degree muscle tears. An elbow forced into extension produces a load on the contracting biceps and brachial muscles that can result in partial or complete disruptions of these musculotendinous units. Similarly, a flexion force against the contracting triceps can result in its avulsion from the olecranon or

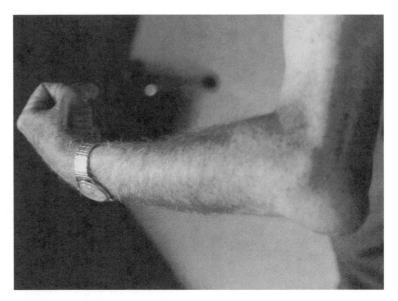

FIGURE 17.5.   Swelling over the olecranon bursa indicates bursitis.

in an avulsion fracture of the olecranon itself. These musculotendinous units can be injured not only from violent forces but also from repeated microtrauma, such as that which occurs in throwers or rowers.

Symptoms from such chronic trauma, including pain, stiffness, and restricted motion, are gradual in onset but can be equally disabling. On clinical examination, swelling and tenderness should be carefully localized. Although most of these injuries are partial tears, a complete tear with avulsion of the biceps or brachial muscles from their attachments on the radius and ulna, respectively, is possible. Careful palpation and comparison with the normal side help to determine the presence of a complete tear. Each major muscle should be examined individually. Referral to a physician for clinical evaluation and radiographs of the injured elbow may be indicated, as frequently there are associated avulsion fractures. The neurological status of an athlete with a presumed acute muscle strain must also be carefully assessed.

Initial treatment of a strain includes application of ice, compression bandages, and immobilization. In mild first- and second-degree injuries, the ice and immobilization can generally be discontinued after the first 48 hours. Heat treatment with whirlpools or hydrocollator packs may be helpful after the inflammatory response and swelling subside. Stretching exercises, resistive exercises, or massage are generally avoided in the acute injury stage. Rest is essential until a pain-free range of motion is achieved. Exercising these musculotendinous units prematurely may result in calcification within the muscle mass (myositis ossificans), which may lead to permanent restriction of the elbow motion. The athlete who returns to competition may benefit from protective taping to prevent hyperextension forces at the elbow.

An athlete with a third-degree muscle injury should be referred promptly to a physician. Avulsion of the biceps from the radial tuberosity and complete avulsion of the triceps from the olecranon both require surgical reattachment of the tendon. A prolonged period of disability follows surgical repair of these injuries. At least several months are required to regain strength and range of motion.

Epicondylitis

Epicondylitis is an inflammatory response to overuse of either a flexor or an extensor muscle group attaching into the medial and the lateral epicondyle of the humerus, respectively. **Tennis elbow**, or lateral epicondylitis, is perhaps the most common of these injuries. Medial epicondylitis is a frequent occurrence in athletes participating in the throwing sports. Repeated overload of these musculotendinous units attaching into the epicondyle is usually the cause of these conditions.

Although tennis elbow is frequently associated with weekend tennis players, golfers, and bowlers, it occurs regularly in experienced players, too. Factors influencing this condition include faulty techniques, particularly with the backhand in tennis, excessive pronation, and inadequate sport equipment (racket, ball, club, etc.). Relative weakness of the extensor muscle group compared with the flexors has also been incriminated.

Athletes such as baseball pitchers and tennis players with a vigorous overhead motion may have symptoms along the medial epicondyle as a result of valgus forces through the elbow joint. The ulnar nerve must be examined to rule out subluxation or entrapment of that nerve in the groove behind the medial epicondyle.

The typical lateral epicondylitis produces pain localized to the lateral epicondyle. The pain may radiate down the forearm extensor muscle group or up into the brachial radialis muscle. The pain is intensified by resistive extension of the wrist and fingers as well as by shaking hands. Pressure over the lateral epicondyle is painful. In medial epicondylitis, pain is present with palpation over the medial epicondyle and is intensified by forceful wrist flexion.

The initial treatment of epicondylitis, whether medial or lateral, is rest, ice, and nonsteroidal anti-inflammatory medications. Injections of soluble corticosteroids into acute lesions often help, but the extremity should be rested for several weeks following an injection. Steroid injections into muscle or tendon may cause necrosis of tissue that must heal before the athlete can participate in vigorous activities. Heat prior to activity may be helpful once the acute inflammatory response subsides. A rehabilitation program to strengthen the extensor muscle groups is indicated once pain has subsided sufficiently. Injuries to these structures can decrease flexibility, so stretching must be part of rehabilitation. Because faulty technique may cause the injury to recur, the athletic trainer should view the athlete's serve or delivery with the coach to correct any biomechanical faults. Although most cases of epicondylitis subside with conservative programs over a 6- to 12-month period, some become chronic and disabling. In these cases, surgical intervention may be indicated to release the aponeurotic attachments of the involved muscle group at the epicondylar level.

Sprains

Falls on the outstretched hand produce hyperextension or varus/valgus forces that injure the ligamentous structures of the elbow as well as the musculotendinous unit. Partial or complete tears to medial ligamentous structures of the elbow can also occur from large valgus-extension forces generated during the act of throwing. With injuries to the medial side of the elbow, the ulnar nerve should be carefully examined to rule out possible subluxation or contusion to the nerve.

Athletes with sprains may complain of pain diffusely above the elbow. They often are unable to throw or grasp because of pain. Physical examination shows local tenderness over the medial collateral ligament. Possible injury to the muscular attachments of the flexor muscle groups must also be carefully assessed. Since the elbow is stable in extension, the elbow should be stressed at 20 to 30 degrees of valgus flexion to determine whether the ligament is completely disrupted (Fig. 17.6). Avulsion injuries through the physis of the medial epicondyle in adolescents are not uncommon with this mechanism of injury. These athletes have localized pain at the medial epicondyle, and usually the avulsed fragment can be felt under the skin. Radiographic evaluation is needed in order to confirm the diagnosis.

A first- or second-degree partial sprain of the medial collateral ligament should be treated with ice, compressive bandaging, and immobilization in a sling or posterior splint. Ice is cautiously applied to the medial aspect of the elbow to avoid cold injury to the ulnar nerve. Complete disruption of the medial stabilizing structures or an avulsion fracture of the medial epicondyle requires surgical correction.

Dislocation

Dislocation at the elbow is a severe, traumatic injury that can be caused most commonly by either a fall on the fully extended elbow or a sudden, violent, unidirectional

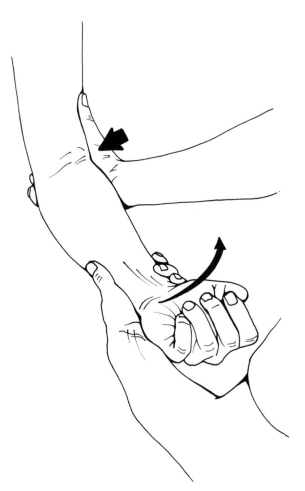

FIGURE 17.6.   In evaluating a possible elbow sprain, the athletic trainer stresses the elbow at 20 to 30 degrees of valgus flexion to determine whether the ligament is completely disrupted.

blow to the elbow. The pain is immediate and severe, with total loss of function in the elbow and obvious deformity (Fig. 17.7). Numbness, especially along the ulnar nerve, is often present, indicating injury to this structure. Frequently, there are associated fractures of either the forearm bones or the radial head or coronoid process of the ulna. Hence, immediate transportation to a medical facility for x-ray films and further evaluation is mandatory. Closed reduction typically requires regional or general anesthesia. The elbow should be carefully splinted for protection during transport.

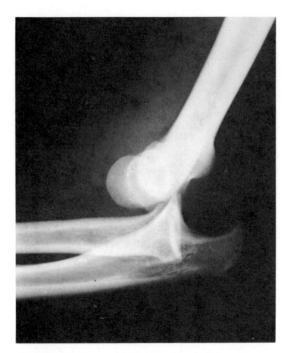

FIGURE 17.7. X-ray film of elbow dislocation.

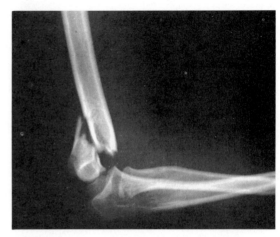

FIGURE 17.8. X-ray film of a supracondylar fracture.

Fractures

Elbow fractures are some of the most severe problems an athlete can encounter. Stiffness, limitation of motion, angular deformities, growth disturbances, and neurovascular problems frequently result. Except for undisplaced fractures, surgical intervention is often necessary.

Supracondylar fractures of the humerus are usually caused by falls on the outstretched arm. Diagnosis is easy in the displaced fracture because of the severe pain and deformity (Fig. 17.8). Neurovascular status of the hand and forearm should be assessed. Immediate referral to a medical facility for further treatment is mandatory.

Fractures of the olecranon are usually the result of direct trauma. If displaced, these fractures generally do not respond to conservative treatment because the pull of the triceps further distracts the fragments, and surgical treatment is indicated.

Undisplaced fractures of the radial head generally respond to conservative care with pain and swelling controlled by ice, sling, and a short period of splinting, followed by gentle, active exercise until the fracture is healed. Displaced fractures of the radial head require surgical intervention.

Fractures in children's elbows are complicated by the concern of growth deformity

Dislocations of the radial head may occur with and without associated ulnar fractures. If the displacement is severe, incarceration of the ruptured annular ligament of the radius within the joint may block closed reduction, necessitating surgery.

Following an elbow dislocation, many months of physical therapy are needed to restore full function. If the elbow is stable following reduction (and it generally is), the elbow is splinted for only several weeks until the acute pain subsides. Then early active range of motion is begun. Close monitoring by the trainer as the athlete proceeds with rehabilitation is needed to ensure steady progress in regaining range of motion and then strength. The athlete may be able to return to play within 4 to 6 months but can be out of the sport for up to 12 months or more.

Recovery from fracture-dislocations at the elbow is even more difficult, since the fracture not only may disrupt the joint surface but also may necessitate stabilization in a splint, thus preventing initiating early motion.

resulting from malalignment of the reduction or injury to the growth center. Open reduction with pin fixation is usually required with displaced fractures.

One of the most serious complications in supracondylar fractures is ischemic necrosis of the forearm muscles, known as **Volkmann's contracture** (Fig. 17.9). It is caused by compression or damage to the vascular supply to the forearm, either from the initial injury or from swelling of tissues following injury. Because the muscles of the forearm are enclosed in tight fascial compartments, their expansion is limited by these fascial sheaths. A cast or compressive dressing used to treat an elbow or forearm fracture can be responsible for further compression. Signs of an impending compartment syndrome are coldness, stiffness, and numbness of the fingers. The symptom of severe increasing pain in the forearm is a warning that treatment must be instituted immediately. The presence of a radial pulse is not a reliable indicator of adequate circulation to the forearm muscles, as the terminal arterioles and capillaries are the first to close with increasing tissue pressure, not the major arterial supply. The diagnosis of a true compartment syndrome is confirmed by using tissue manometers to measure compartment pressures.

Frequently, if the athlete with early signs of increasing tissue pressure (pain, coldness, and decreased motion) is treated by removal of all compressive dressings (casts, Ace bandage, etc.) and the extremity is elevated, swelling will decrease and the athlete will recover without the need for surgical release of fascial compartments. Close monitoring during this initial period is needed, however, to make certain that swelling is decreasing and that the extremity is recovering.

Valgus Extension Overload

During the acceleration phase of the throwing act, a valgus force is produced across the medial side of the elbow. This force stresses the medial flexor muscle mass and the me-

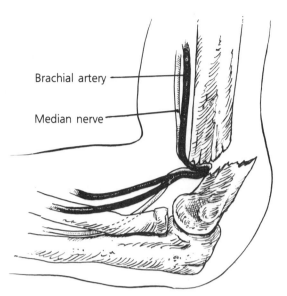

Brachial artery

Median nerve

FIGURE 17.9. Volkmann's contracture, or ischemic necrosis of the forearm muscles, is a complication of a supracondylar fracture.

dial elbow joint ligaments. There may actually be a stretching of the medial ligaments in either acute disruption or a repetitive overload situation. When the medial joint becomes unstable, stress is put on the ulnar nerve, the radius-capitellum joint, and the olecranon fossa. Avascular necrosis of the capitellum and olecranon spurs may develop, and the athlete may lose full extension of the elbow.

This syndrome may develop slowly. Initially, the athlete will only have vague pain along the medial aspect of the elbow and ache following practice or play. By continuing to play without proper treatment, the athlete will most likely develop increasing pain, clicking, and frequently, an elbow effusion.

Conservative care involves an initial period of rest, followed by a range-of-motion and strengthening program, as outlined in the exercises on page 279–281, especially for the medial stabilizers of the elbow. Taping the elbow for support and closely examining the throwing technique may be helpful. Sometimes, in severe cases, up to a year off from throwing is required. Surgeons consider arthroscopic débridement of the elbow an option if all conservative treatment fails to improve symptoms.

INJURIES TO THE FOREARM

Contusions

Contusions of the forearm are common during athletic competition. These injuries should be treated with ice, rest, and elevation in a sling. Fractures must be carefully ruled out, and the complication of compartment syndromes must be avoided. Myositis ossificans is not common following forearm injuries.

Acute Tenosynovitis

Acute tenosynovitis involving the extensor and flexor tendons of the wrist is seen in certain athletic activities. Particularly with rowers, repeated dorsiflexion of the wrist while feathering the oar leads to extensor tenosynovitis. Similarly, a prolonged tight grip on the oar may result in flexor tendinitis, not only in the forearm but often extending down into the fingers. Examination reveals tenderness, swelling, and crepitus over the involved tendons.

Treatment includes rest, ice, and nonsteroidal anti-inflammatory drugs. Additional physical therapy modalities may help to decrease inflammation. Referral to a physician for an injection of cortisone may be needed in recalcitrant cases, but the cortisone must be injected into the tendon sheath and not the tendon itself. A period of immobilization should follow such an injection. Since this is a self-limiting condition, it is best to treat the tendinitis conservatively and avoid injections if possible. Following resolution of acute symptoms, strengthening of the forearm muscles should be instituted to prevent reinjury. The athlete's technique should always be reviewed prior to resumption of activity to make certain inadequate technique does not result in recurrence of symptoms.

Nerve Injuries

In athletes, most nerve injuries are the result of direct trauma, associated with either a contusion or a fracture. However, repeated muscular activity may result in nerve entrapment.

The median nerve may be compressed by hypertrophy of the pronator teres through which it passes. Pain may be felt in the forearm, but numbness and weakness may extend distally into the hand. This condition occurs in tennis players from overuse or an abnormal gripping of the racquet. The median nerve may also be compressed at the wrist (**carpal tunnel syndrome**) and produce similar symptoms in the hand and forearm.

On examination, tenderness proximally in the forearm suggests the pronator teres syndrome. Weakness in the thenar muscle group and numbness in the median nerve distribution of the hand are present in both of these conditions. Electromyography and nerve conduction studies help to localize the site of nerve entrapment.

Treatment consists of ice, rest, and nonsteroidal anti-inflammatory drugs. Occasionally, a persistent nerve compression requires surgical decompression. In those cases related to an abnormal grip, the coach, trainer, and player should carefully assess techniques and equipment.

Fractures

Children frequently break the forearm bones (the radius and ulna) during athletic practice and competition. The mechanism of injury is usually a fall on the outstretched arm or a direct blow. One or both bones may be fractured, or one bone may fracture and the other dislocate at the adjacent elbow joint. A **Monteggia fracture** is a dislocation of the radial head in association with an ulnar fracture; a dislocated ulna with a fractured radius is called a **Galeazzi fracture**. These are serious injuries that require prompt treatment by a physician.

A fracture must be suspected whenever the forearm is severely injured. Initial inspection may reveal an obvious deformity, particularly when the middle or distal third of the forearm is fractured. The bones must be gently palpated, for tenderness and crepitus. Neurovascular status must be observed and recorded before applying a splint to immobilize the fracture. It is essential that the physician who will evaluate the athlete later and who may find neurovascular compromise be told if the nerves and vessels were damaged by the initial injury or by subsequent swelling.

REHABILITATION EXERCISES

Though it is difficult to isolate every muscle in the forearm with a certain exercise, the following exercises will enhance the majority of those muscles. As always, stretching *and* strengthening are encouraged.

Grip

Position: standing or sitting

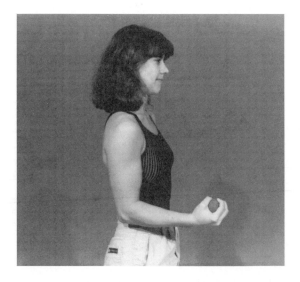

Procedure: Grip apparatus, putty, small rubber ball, etc. Perform this gripping exercise as much as possible, all day long.

Stretch Flexors

Position: elbow completely straight

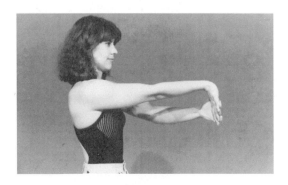

Procedure: With palm facing up, grasp the middle of the hand and thumb. Pull wrist down as far as possible. Hold for _____ counts. Relax and repeat _____ times, _____ times daily. This can be done isometrically by holding the wrist in neutral and pulling against the opposite hand into flexion for _____ counts. Perform _____ times, _____ times daily.

Stretch Extensors

Position: elbow completely straight

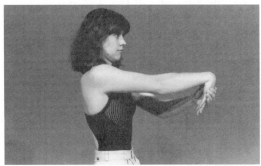

Procedure: With palm facing down, grasp the back of the hand and pull wrist down as far as possible. Hold for a _____ count. Relax and repeat _____ times, _____ times daily. This exercise can be done isometrically by holding the wrist in neutral and pulling against the opposite hand into extension for counts. Perform _____ times, _____ times daily. Progress to _____ times, _____ times daily.

Wrist Curls

Position: forearm supported on a table, with hand off edge; palm facing upward

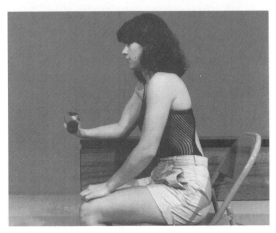

Procedure: Using ____-pound weight, lower the hand as far as possible and then curl it up as high as possible. Hold for a ____ count. Relax and repeat ____ times, ____ times daily. Progress to ____ pounds, ____ times, ____ times daily.

Wrist Reverse Curls

Position: forearm supported on a table, with hand off edge, palm facing downward

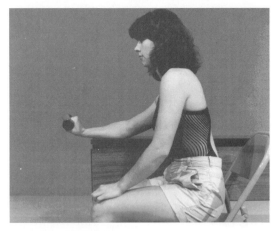

Procedure: Using ____-pound weight, lower the hand as far as possible and then curl it up as high as possible. Hold for a ____ count. Relax and repeat ____ times, ____ times daily. Progress to ____ pounds, ____ times, ____ times daily.

Pronation

Position: forearm supported on a table, with wrist in a neutral position

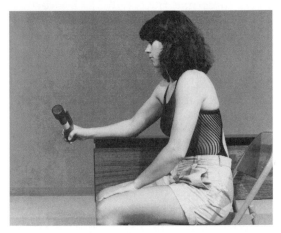

Procedure: Using a ____-pound weight held in a "hammering" position, roll wrist into pronation as far as possible. Relax and hold for a ____ count. Raise back to starting position. Relax and repeat ____ times, ____ times daily. Progress to ____ pounds, ____ times, ____ times daily.

Supination

Position: forearm supported on a table, with wrist in a neutral position

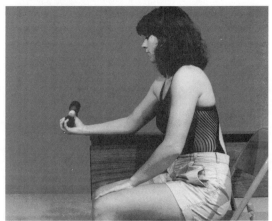

Procedure: Using a ____-pound weight held in a hammering position, roll wrist into full supination. Hold for a ____ count. Raise to starting position. Repeat ____ times, ____ times daily. Progress to ____ pounds, ____ times, ____ times daily.

Biceps Curl

Position: sitting or standing with arm hanging down

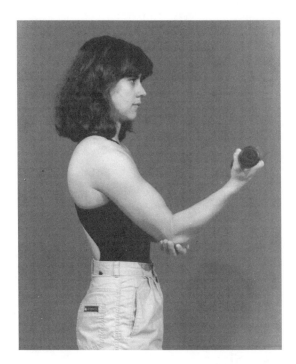

Procedure: Support arm at elbow with your opposite hand. Using a ____-pound weight, bend elbow to full flexion, hold for a ____ count, then straighten arm completely. Relax and repeat ____ times, ____ times daily. Progress to ____ pounds, ____ times, ____ times daily.

French Curl

Position: arm raised overhead; opposite hand giving support at elbow

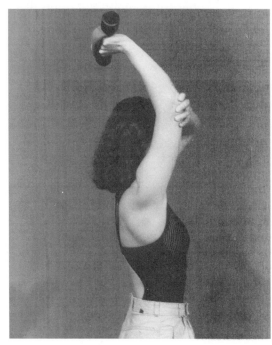

Procedure: Using a ____-pound weight, straighten elbow over head, hold for a ____ count. Relax and repeat ____ times, ____ times daily. Progress to ____ pounds, ____ times, ____ times daily.

(Important Concepts appear on next page.)

IMPORTANT CONCEPTS

1. The bones of the arm, elbow, and forearm are the humerus, the ulna, and the radius.
2. Knowing the relationships of the vessels and nerves of the arm, elbow, and forearm is important in assessing possible neurovascular complications of upper extremity injuries.
3. Most injuries of the arm, elbow, and forearm can be treated with ice, rest, elevation, and nonsteroidal anti-inflammatory drugs.
4. A hematoma formation that calcifies and eventually matures to bony trabeculae is called myositis ossificans or "tackler's" exostosis.
5. Tennis elbow is an inflammatory response to overuse of the extensor muscle group that attaches into the lateral epicondyle of the humerus.
6. A serious complication of a supracondylar fracture is ischemic necrosis of the forearm muscles, known as Volkmann's contracture.
7. Dislocation at the elbow is a severe, traumatic injury that causes immediate pain, total loss of function, and obvious deformity.
8. A Monteggia fracture is a dislocation of the radial head in association with an ulnar fracture, and a Galeazzi fracture is a dislocation of the ulna with a fractured radius.

SUGGESTED READINGS

Bennett, G. E. "Shoulder and Elbow Lesions of the Professional Baseball Pitcher." *Journal of the American Medical Association* 117 (1941): 510–514.

Berg, K. "Prevention of Tennis Elbow through Conditioning." *The Physician and Sportsmedicine* 5 (1977): 110.

DeHaven, K. E., and C. M. Evarts. "Throwing Injuries of the Elbow in Athletes." *Orthopedic Clinics of North America* 4 (1973): 801–808.

Jobe, F. W., H. Stark, and S. J. Lombardo. "Reconstruction of the Ulnar Collateral Ligament in Athletes." *Journal of Bone and Joint Surgery* 68A (1986): 1158–1163.

Larson, R. L., and R. O. McMahan. "The Epiphyses and the Childhood Athlete." *Journal of the American Medical Association* 196 (1966): 607–612.

Norwood, L. A., J. A. Shook, and J. R. Andrews. "Acute Medial Elbow Ruptures." *American Journal of Sports Medicine* 9 (1981): 16–19.

Tivnon, M. C., S. H. Anzel, and T. R. Waugh. "Surgical Management of Osteochondritis Dissecans of the Capitellum." *American Journal of Sports Medicine* 4 (1976): 121–128.

Wilson, F. D., J. R. Andrews, T. A. Blackburn, et al. "Valgus Extension Overload in the Pitching Elbow." *American Journal of Sports Medicine* 11 (1983): 83–88.

18

Hand and Wrist

CHAPTER OUTLINE

OBJECTIVES FOR CHAPTER 18

After reading this chapter, the student should be able to:

1. Understand the anatomy of the hand and wrist.
2. Recognize the various types of finger, hand, and wrist injuries which can occur and the recommended treatment for each.
3. Describe the rehabilitation of hand and wrist injuries.

INTRODUCTION

In the course of their work, athletic trainers will encounter many hand and wrist injuries. "Baseball finger," "jersey finger," "coach's finger," and "gamekeeper's thumb" are some of the more common sprains, fractures, and muscle-tendon injuries seen, but many other injuries to the bones, tendons, and ligaments of the wrist and hand are also possible. Chapter 18 presents the anatomy of the region, followed by a discussion of the diagnosis, management, and rehabilitation of common hand and wrist injuries. ■

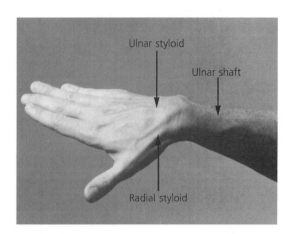

FIGURE 18.1. Posterior view of the forearm, wrist, and hand.

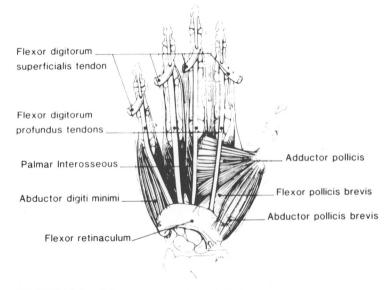

FIGURE 18.2. Palmar cross-section of the hand.

ANATOMY

Bones, Tendons, and Ligaments

The distal ulna and radius form the base for the wrist joint. The **ulnar styloid** and **radial styloid** are the most prominent ends of the bones, which are easily palpable at the wrist (Fig. 18.1). Eight **carpal bones** form the wrist. The carpals are interconnected themselves by a complex system of joint capsules and ligaments, and are joined by ligaments to the radius and ulna proximally and the metacarpals distally. The five **metacarpals** lying distal to the carpals form the palm of the hand. Finally, the **phalanges** make up the finger bones (three in each finger and two in the thumb).

Each bone, except the carpals, is joined by tendons that flex or extend the joints on the dorsal and palmar surfaces (Fig. 18.2). At the proximal levels, intrinsic muscles of the hand also produce motion to either side. The same possibilities for motion are provided at the wrist, with muscles and tendons that produce flexion, extension, abduction, adduction, rotation, or combinations thereof. The thumb, in addition, has the power of opposition. This entire unit is the most versatile, functional unit that has evolved in animals.

Neurovascular Supply

A network of the branches of the radial and ulnar arteries and their accompanying veins supply blood to the hand. After entering the hand, the radial and ulnar arteries divide into two branches that form the superficial and deep volar arches, which anastomose and send common branches to the fingers. The nerve supply to the hand is through the radial, ulnar, and median nerves, which innervate the muscles and provide a sensory distribution to the hand in a fairly regular pattern, subject to some variations (Fig. 18.3). The **ulnar nerve** innervates the little finger and ulnar side of the ring finger on the dorsal and volar surfaces; the **median nerve** innervates the remainder of the volar surface of the hand and fingers; and the **radial nerve** innervates the dorsum of the hand (see Fig. 18.3). The radial nerve supplies the muscles that extend the fingers at the knuckles or metacarpophalangeal (MCP) joints. The median nerve controls the muscles that oppose the thumb to the fingers and control flexion of the thumb, and middle fingers at the distal interphalangeal (DIP) and proximal interphalangeal (PIP) joints. The ulnar nerve supplies the intrinsic muscles that move the fingers apart (abduct) or together (adduct) when they are held in full extension as well as flexion of the DIP joint of the ring and little fingers. The radial and ulnar nerves control extension of the wrist, and the median and ulnar nerves control flexion.

Nomenclature

When describing injuries of the hand, nomenclature can be confusing. The problem arises because the first finger rests on the second metacarpal. To avoid confusion, it is best to describe metacarpal injuries by their numbers—that is, first, second, third, fourth, and fifth metacarpal—and digital injuries by their names—that is, thumb, index, middle or long, ring, and little finger.

FINGER, HAND, AND WRIST INJURIES

In general, injuries to the fingers that require immobilization should be splinted, with the interphalangeal joints held in full extension. The few injuries that require immobilization in flexion must be closely supervised to prevent the development of

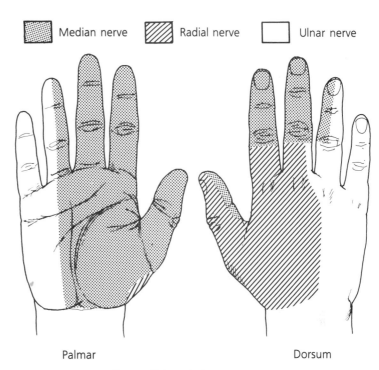

Median nerve   Radial nerve   Ulnar nerve

FIGURE 18.3.   Median, radial, and ulnar nerve distribution to the hand.

flexion contractures. The ligaments of the interphalangeal joints are tightest in extension and more relaxed when the joint is flexed. Because of this, a joint that has been fixed in a fully straight position for several weeks is usually easy to mobilize, whereas a finger joint that has been held in flexion for a prolonged period may be very difficult to straighten.

Fingertip Injuries

The most common injuries to the fingertips are direct contusions from a thrown object impaling the finger or from the finger being jammed against or crushed by an object. **Subungual hematomas**, a collection of blood beneath the nail, often result from such injuries. Treatment for subungual hematoma consists of soaking the finger in ice water for 10 to 15 minutes to decrease bleeding and swelling. It will also provide temporary analgesia (pain relief). Radiographs are usually required to rule out accompanying fracture of the distal phalanx. If no fracture exists, the hematoma may be drained by carefully melting a hole through the nail with a disposable electrocautery unit, if available, or with the end of a paper clip heated to cherry red in a flame (cigarette lighter or alcohol lamp). If an underlying fracture is present, the trainer may elect not to drain the hematoma because doing so converts a closed fracture into an open one, increasing the risk of infection.

An athlete's fingernail may be avulsed by being caught in an object or in an opponent's clothing. A partially avulsed nail can be restored to near anatomic position by manipulation and held in place by clear tape. This treatment affords a protective layer to a very sensitive nail bed. The nail should be removed only if absolutely necessary. If the nail is completely avulsed, the trainer should apply a protective dressing of fine-mesh gauze and petroleum jelly to the bed and change it regularly to keep the bed clean. A plastic "cage" over the affected fingertip provides additional protection and often allows the athlete to play. Disruption of the nail bed, by either laceration or crush injury, should be brought to the immediate attention of the physician.

A **paronychia** is an infection along the edge of the nail that can cause purulent drainage. Treatment consists of warm water soaks; protection with a dry, sterile dressing; and referral to a physician for possible drainage or antibiotics.

A **felon** is an infection of the pulp of the fingertip and may follow a puncture wound of the fingertip from a needle or even a severe contusion. As a closed space infection it causes extreme tenderness and firmness of the fingertip. If treatment is delayed, infection may spread to the adjacent area, and serious complications may arise. Prompt referral to a physician is advised.

The **mallet** or **baseball finger** is caused by a sudden flexion force on the DIP joint while the finger is actively extended, such as when the player is poised to catch a ball (Fig. 18.4). Such a mechanism results in a rupture of the extensor tendon at or near its insertion on the terminal phalanx. The ath-

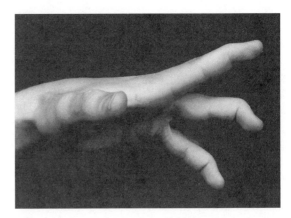

FIGURE 18.4. Mallet finger injury. Distal phalanx is no longer able to extend in long finger.

lete can no longer actively extend the terminal joint. The terminal phalanx is usually held in partial flexion but may be extended passively by the examiner. Athletes with mallet injuries should have an x-ray of their finger to note if a fracture of the distal phalanx is present and if it is associated with any subluxation of the joint. Initial treatment is ice and elevation, followed by splinting of the DIP joint in full extension. Surgery is usually not required unless a large fracture of the joint has significant displacement or subluxation.

The counterpart of the mallet finger, the **jersey finger**, is caused by a sudden, forceful extension of the DIP joint while held in flexion, typically when a tightly held jersey is torn out of the grasp of a would-be tackler. An avulsion of the long flexor tendon from its attachment to the distal joint can result. On examination, the athlete cannot flex this joint, although the joint can be passively flexed. The jersey finger injury must be recognized early and the athlete referred for immediate physician evaluation, as delay in treatment may compromise repair and result in the athlete's needing a tendon graft rather than primary repair of the injured tendon.

Proximal Finger Joint Injuries

Injuries of the proximal finger joint can occur as described for the fingertips. In addition, forceful twisting injuries may result from grabbing or being grabbed, or catching fingers on opponents' clothing or equipment.

Hyperextension Injury

One of the most common injuries of the PIP joint is the hyperextension injury, where the finger is bent forcibly backward, stretching or rupturing the volar plate on the palmar side of the joint. In more severe injuries, dorsal dislocations, rupture of the collateral ligaments, or fractures may occur. Often, with a simple hyperextension injury in which no structures are torn, the joint will swell, in a fashion similar to the swelling seen with a direct blow to the fingertip—that is, a direct compression injury to the PIP joint. With hyperextension injuries, the palmar side of the joint is tender on examination, and attempts to hyperextend the joint cause pain. Evaluation should include a stress examination of the collateral ligaments to be certain they are intact. Finger hyperextension injuries associated with either significant pain or swelling will need to be referred for radiographic evaluation to make certain there is not an associated fracture.

Initial treatment of hyperextension injuries is ice, elevation, and splinting with avulsion fractures of the volar surface of either the DIP or the PIP joint. Splinting in slight flexion for 10 to 14 days is generally preferred. Then the affected finger is buddy taped to the adjacent finger to encourage range-of-motion exercise to achieve full extension and flexion. Failure to splint and supervise these injuries satisfactorily until they are completely healed may result in a painful, stiff finger with a fixed flexion deformity of the joint, frequently termed the **coach's finger**. Surgery is rarely required in these injuries unless fractures involving the joints, subluxation, or marked instability of the collateral ligaments exist.

Dislocations

In dislocations of the PIP joint, the athlete's middle phalanx usually dislocates dorsally on the proximal phalanx. The cause is most often a hyperextension force, and the dislocation is an extension of the simple hyperextension injury. Ordinarily, the finger is foreshortened with obvious swelling and deformity.

In athletes, many of these dislocations are treated at the sidelines, with simple, longitudinal distraction that produces successful and prompt reduction. Nevertheless, a physician should evaluate the integrity of the collateral ligaments and obtain x-ray films to check for associated fractures and to ensure that the reduction is satisfactory. The finger may be splinted with the PIP and DIP joints in extension for several weeks prior to beginning active motion. In fact, to prevent stiffness, the athlete may be encouraged to perform range-of-motion exercises of the finger out of the splint early in the postinjury period. Surgery is rarely required, except for serious fracture of the joint surface or persistent subluxation.

Collateral Ligament Tears

Hyperextension injuries can also cause tears of the collateral ligaments, even though collateral ligament tears are more commonly associated with a force applied to the sides of the fingers. Swelling of the joint is common, but obvious deformity is rare. To assess the integrity of the collateral ligaments, the trainer should apply a lateral force to the joint, first fully extended and then flexed approximately 30 degrees. Minor tears may produce joint laxity up to 10 degrees, and a definite end point is felt. With complete ruptures, greater laxity is apparent. Stress after an acute injury may be too painful for the athlete to tolerate, and the examination may be compromised because of guarding on the part of the athlete. On careful examination, tenderness is usually localized to the side of the ligament rupture.

Most ligament tears can be treated by splinting, with the joint extended, or by taping the injured finger to the adjacent finger. More severe or complete ruptures may require surgical repair.

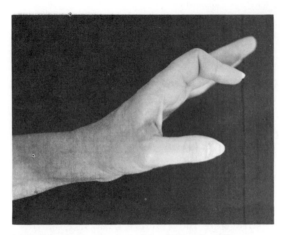

FIGURE 18.5. Boutonnière deformity. The proximal joint flexes while the distal joint hyperextends.

Boutonnière Deformity

The **boutonnière deformity** is caused by rapid, forceful flexion at the PIP joint (Fig. 18.5). The central slip of the extensor tendon of the middle phalanx ruptures with associated separation and palmar displacement of the lateral band. This injury leaves no effective, active extensor mechanism of the middle joint. As a result, the proximal joint flexes, and the distal joint tends to hyperextend, producing the deformity.

Initial treatment is splinting the finger in full extension. Occasionally, surgical repair is required to regain full function. For this reason, early evaluation by a physician is recommended. As with other finger injuries, radiographs to detect associated fractures are recommended.

Finger Fractures

In general, fractures of the hand require physical assessment and radiographic evaluation. Treatment is often complex, and the functional result may depend on the expertise of the person managing these injuries. The clinical diagnosis is obvious if there is gross deformity. However, in many occult, or nondisplaced, fractures, clinical diagnosis may be difficult. The most reliable sign of injury is localized tenderness, but this does not specifically localize the injury to soft tissue or bone. The safest course is to refer the athlete to a physician for radiographic evaluation whenever a fracture is suspected. The old adages of "It's not broken if you can move it" or "if it doesn't swell" are unreliable.

The four fingers must move as a unit. Failure to maintain the longitudinal and rotational alignments severely hampers grasping or manipulating small objects within the palm. The most difficult alignment to evaluate and maintain is rotation. Failure to correct a malrotation causes one finger to overlap the other when a fist is made. The easiest way to assess rotation is to flex all the fingers, bringing them as close together as possible, remembering that the fifth finger should point toward the middle of the wrist. If in doubt, the trainer should compare the alignment with the unaffected hand, or his or her own hand.

Thumb Injuries

The thumb is a unique digit because it has only two phalanges and one interphalangeal joint. Generally, all of the injuries described for the fingers can also affect the thumb, with the exception of the boutonnière deformity.

Because the MCP joint of the thumb is more exposed than its counterparts in the fingers, it is subject to a rupture of the ulnar collateral ligament—an injury peculiar to this joint and more commonly known as the **gamekeeper's thumb** (Fig. 18.6). While originally described in gamekeepers because they chronically stressed this ligament when wringing the necks of rabbits, it is seen in many contact sports such as football and wrestling as well as in skiing. It is caused by forceful abduction of the thumb away from the hand, with the MCP joint in extension. On examination, there is usually local tenderness on the ulnar side of the MCP joint. Diagnosis is confirmed by stressing the joint laterally in extension and then in 30 degrees of flexion, looking for laxity of the joint on the ulnar side. With partial ligament tears, a definite end point is felt, and only modest lateral laxity is noted. In the more severe, or complete, tears, laxity of 45 degrees or more is noted, and no discrete end point is felt. In all cases, the laxity of the involved thumb must be compared with the uninvolved thumb to determine what is normal for that athlete.

Stability of the ulnar collateral ligament is critical to normal hand function, particularly fine pinching, such as in grasping a key, between the thumb and index finger. Therefore, a physician should evaluate all cases of collateral ligament injuries in the thumb. A radiograph should be obtained to reveal fractures or volar subluxation of the joint. Incomplete tears are generally treated with immobilization in a thumb spica cast for 4 to 6 weeks. However, complete disruption of the ligament typically requires surgical repair to gain an effective result. Generally, undisplaced avulsion fractures of the thumb at the site of injury heal with cast immobilization.

Palmar and Dorsal Hand Injuries

Mid-Hand Contusions

Simple contusions of the hand produce a soft, painful, bluish discoloration of the dorsum of the hand, and must be differentiated from metacarpal fractures. Treatment is ice, compression, and elevation of the hand. Disability seldom lasts longer than 2 or 3 days.

Thenar and Hypothenar Eminence Contusions

Contusions of the thenar and hypothenar eminences are seen most often in baseball, hockey, and handball players. These contusions follow trauma and appear as tender, painful swelling of the fleshy areas at the base of the thumb or the little finger. They can be confused with a tendon sheath infection or a carpal or metacarpal fracture. Treatment is ice, compression, elevation, and protective padding, such as a sponge

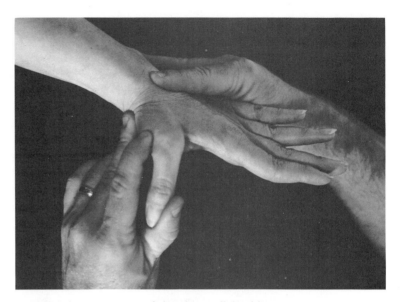

FIGURE 18.6.   Rupture of the ulnar collateral ligament (gamekeeper's thumb) can be exhibited by laxity when stressing the metacarpophalangeal joint laterally.

rubber doughnut. Splinting to rest the injured muscles may be needed, and disability may last 4 days or longer if the injury is severe.

Dislocation of the MCP Joints

MCP joint dislocations usually follow hyperextension injuries, with the proximal phalanx dislocating dorsally in respect to the metacarpal head (Fig. 18.7). The joint

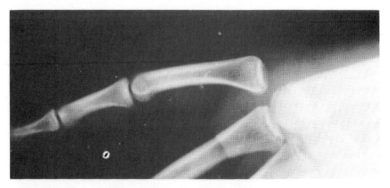

FIGURE 18.7.   Dislocated metacarpophalangeal joint. (From Paul M. Weeks. *Acute Bone and Joint Injuries of the Hand and Wrist.* St. Louis: C. V. Mosby, 1981.)

remains hyperextended and foreshortened, with obvious deformity. Simple injuries may be reduced by closed means. Occasionally, a dimple may be apparent on the skin of the palm, which indicates a "complex" or irreducible dislocation. This dislocation will not respond to closed manipulation because the metacarpal head is entrapped by the surrounding soft tissues of the volar plate, which is interposed within the joint. These injuries ordinarily require open surgical reduction. A physician should evaluate all dislocations of the MCP joints.

Rupture of the Transverse Metacarpal Ligament

Rupture of the transverse metacarpal ligament is an unusual injury caused by a spreading force to the fingers, such as a faulty catch, that forces the fingers apart and spreads the interior metacarpal joints. The intrinsic muscle attachments can also be ruptured. On physical examination, the athlete's hand is tender and swollen over the area where the ligament attaches. Stress testing reveals a loss of stability. Treatment includes rest in a splint, progressing to buddy taping and early range-of-motion exercises, with frequent checks to make sure stability is being maintained.

Metacarpal Fractures

Metacarpal fractures, particularly of the neck of the fifth metacarpal, are relatively common. The latter is caused by a direct blow to the MCP joint with a clenched fist, as when striking a hard object. Ordinarily, the MCP joint is depressed, and there is tenderness, swelling, and angulation on the back of the hand. A referral to a physician for further evaluation, including radiographs, is important. Axial compression, twisting stress, or direct blows can also cause metacarpal fractures. In general, the metacarpal shafts are splinted to one another and are more stable when fractured than are the phalanges. Shortening and rotation can occur, however, necessitating surgical fixation to restore alignment and length.

Oblique fractures through the joint of the first metacarpal are usually unstable and result in a dissociated dislocation of the carpometacarpal joint. They typically require surgical correction and pin fixation to maintain their reduced position. Fractures through the base of the first metacarpal, as long as the fracture does not go through the joint surface, may usually be treated with closed reduction and cast immobilization for 4 to 6 weeks or until the fracture is healed. Some angular deformity but no rotational deformity can be accepted in these injuries.

Wrist Injuries

Injuries to the wrist that present pitfalls in diagnosis are considered here. These injuries may result in chronic pain and disability, and the seriousness of the injury may be easily overlooked initially.

Carpal Scaphoid Fractures

Fractures of the carpal scaphoid may occur following falls on the outstretched hand. Initially they may be difficult to see radiographically. Therefore, if the athlete has significant pain and/or swelling in the snuffbox on evaluation following trauma to the wrist, splint immobilization (using a thumb spica) is recommended. Radiographs should be repeated in 10 to 14 days when bone absorption at the fracture site makes the injury more apparent radiographically. If a definitive diagnosis is needed sooner than 10 days, a bone scan can be done. It will show increased uptake of tracer at the navicular if a fracture is present.

The scaphoid distal pole has a tenuous blood supply, and therefore, fracture nonunions of this area are a complication of fractures to the mid- and distal poles of this bone. Close monitoring of this injury is needed. Operative correction is generally recommended for displaced scaphoid fractures, and many physicians recommend operative stabilization of the nondisplaced unstable fracture.

Base of Second and Third Metacarpal Fractures

Although other metacarpal fractures were discussed with injuries to the hand, fractures of the base of the second and third metacarpals are considered with the wrist, as symptoms are closely involved with wrist function. These fractures are often associated with subluxation of the carpometacarpal joint and result in tenderness in this area. This fracture typically occurs from a fall on the volar-flexed wrist. X-ray films may or may not show a small flake of bone just dorsal to the base of the metacarpal. Tomography may be needed to localize fractures and detect any subluxation. Reduction of the subluxed metacarpal is necessary for future function.

Rotatory Dislocation of the Radioulnar Joint

Rotatory dislocation of the radioulnar joint is a hyperpronation injury whose only signs may be pain and disability on movement of the wrist and a shift of the ulnar styloid to the center of the bone on an anteroposterior x-ray view of the wrist. There may be a click on supination of the wrist. Cast immobilization in supination for about 4 weeks is generally recommended. The dislocation will stay reduced in this position.

Hamate Hook Fractures

Hamate hook fractures occur with a strong, twisting force or from a direct blow (Fig. 18.8). The athlete presents with tenderness over the hypothenar eminence and an inability to perform twisting motions, such as a golf swing. A radiograph of the wrist (carpel tunnel view) discloses this disabling fracture.

Radiocarpal Joint Injuries

The radiocarpal joint can be sprained, but it is rarely dislocated except at the distal radioulnar joint (see above). If the force applied, often from a fall on the outstretched arm with hand extended, is severe, the

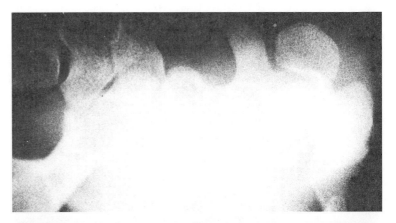
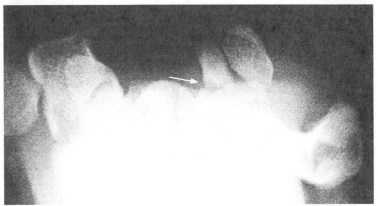

FIGURE 18.8.   Hamate hook: normal (top) and fracture (bottom).

radius usually fractures, frequently with the tip of the ulna as well, resulting in the so-called **Colles' fracture** (Fig. 18.9). As previously noted, this same mechanism may produce other injuries in the upper extremity. In the growing child, the epiphyseal plate can be injured. These injuries must be diagnosed and treated, or growth or angular deformity may result. A sudden twisting injury to the wrist may also tear the articular disc of the wrist. This small, fibrocartilaginous structure, called the **triangular fibrocartilaginous complex** (TFCC), located between the distal end of the ulna and the carpals, results in point tenderness just distal to the ulna and pain on wrist motion. Routine radiographs are normal, and an arthrogram is necessary for diagnosis. The

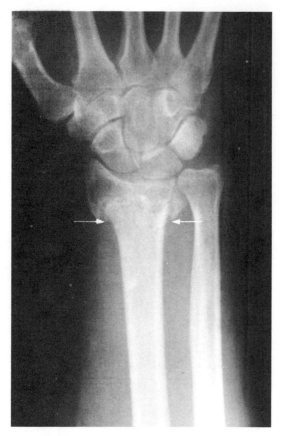

FIGURE 18.9. Colles' fracture.

athlete should be referred to a physician if a TFCC injury is suspected.

Injuries to the Skin: Lacerations and Abrasions

Hand abrasions should be completely cleaned and all foreign matter removed. The entire hand should be scrubbed with surgical soap for at least 10 minutes and the abrasion washed with a prepared iodine solution. All imbedded foreign matter should be removed from the abrasion. Often this can be accomplished by scrubbing with one of the prepackaged sterile brushes impregnated with water-soluble iodine compounds. The abrasion should be dressed with a nonadherent dressing and inspected daily for signs of infection. Soak-

ing wounds in hydrogen peroxide may help to clean abrasions.

Superficial lacerations of the fingers and the back of the fingers and hand may be treated with careful scrubbing, removal of debris, and then loosely closing the area with butterfly tapes. If the laceration crosses a joint on the dorsal surface, it may spread with motion, and splinting of the joint may be required during the first few days of healing. All deep lacerations, particularly those of the palm of the hand, should be referred to a physician promptly.

Evaluating the extent of the laceration, including nerve status, vascular status, and tendon injury, is essential. Evaluation should include sensory testing using a pin on each side of the digits distal to the laceration to determine whether the palmar and digital nerves are intact. In most cases, evaluation using touch only is deceptive, as the athlete thinks he or she feels touch when the sense is actually transmitted through proprioceptive elements within the joints. Therefore, evaluation with a sterile pin is recommended. As previously noted, sensory innervation of the hand may vary slightly. The examiner should be aware of these variations.

To assess the integrity of the tendons, the examiner observes the hand in the resting position. Normally, all fingers flex slightly at rest. With loss of a flexor tendon, one or more fingers remain extended. To test for continuity of the long flexors of the thumb or fingers (profundus), the examiner holds the proximal joints straight and asks the athlete to bend the distal joints (Fig. 18.10). The athlete can do this only if the long flexor tendon is intact. To check for the short flexor tendons (flexor sublimis), the athlete holds all fingers extended except for the finger being examined. When the athlete is asked to flex this digit, the long flexors will remain tethered, and only the flexor sublimis of the finger being examined will be able to cause flexion of the PIP joint. Each of the four fingers must be assessed separately.

Puncture wounds may on superficial evaluation appear trivial, but a small puncture

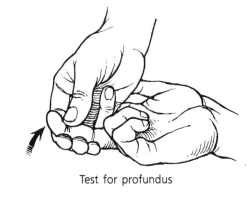

Test for profundus

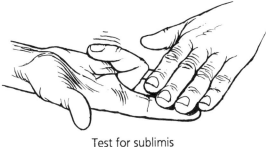

Test for sublimis

FIGURE 18.10.   Test for integrity of tendons of the fingers.

wound of the skin may be associated with more serious injury to deeper structures. Furthermore, puncture wounds have a high incidence of infection. When evaluating the athlete with this injury, the examiner must carefully check for disturbance of nerve and tendon function, particularly if the puncture wound is to the palm. Treatment is thorough cleaning with soaks in warm water and appropriate germicidal agents, followed by a sterile dressing and referral to a physician. A tetanus toxoid booster is needed if the athlete's tetanus immunization is not current. Puncture wounds of the fingertip can produce a felon, a fingertip injury discussed earlier in the chapter.

Human bites most commonly occur on the knuckle, when a closed fist strikes a human tooth. The severity of human bites must be recognized, as the human mouth harbors many organisms resulting in significant wound contamination. These wounds require special and intensive treatment.

They should be thoroughly cleaned, and antibiotics are frequently prescribed. These wounds should always be left open. Bite injuries must be examined to make certain that the extensor tendon of the MCP joint has not also been injured.

REHABILITATION OF HAND AND WRIST INJURIES

Rehabilitation of the injured hand is important to achieve a good functional outcome following injury. In complex injuries, failure to follow through with rehabilitation may lead to stiffness and limited function despite perfect primary care.

In general, the goals of rehabilitation are to minimize swelling and mobilize the hand as soon as the injured parts permit. Initially, simple active motion is begun while protecting the area of injury from stress. Thereafter, resistance and strengthening exercises are added progressively. A specific exercise routine lasting only 5 to 10 minutes is prepared for each athlete to be performed two to three times per day. In many cases, a splint may be removed for these exercise periods and replaced when completed. Short periods of active motion permit early return of function without resulting in swelling or further injury.

In some injuries, protective splinting and padding may allow the athlete to return early yet safely to sport participation. For example, fractured metacarpals, especially the third and fourth, frequently can be taped together and protective sponge rubber or Styrofoam padding used.

Fractures of the second and fifth metacarpals are less stable, and this form of treatment is not as effective. The phalanges may be taped to their adjacent fingers and splinted with Styrofoam or rubber protective splints, and the thumb may be fitted with an adhesive tape checkrein to protect a gamekeeper's thumb after initial healing has occurred. (See Chapters 43 and 44 for taping techniques and the use of protective devices.)

IMPORTANT CONCEPTS

1. Eight carpal bones form the wrist, 5 metacarpals form the palm of the hand, and 14 metacarpals make up the fingers and thumb.
2. The radial and ulnar nerves control extension of the wrist, and the median and ulnar nerves control flexion.
3. A subungual hematoma, a collection of blood beneath the nail, often results from contusion to the fingertip.
4. Hyperextension injury of the PIP joint occurs when the finger is bent forcibly backward, stretching or rupturing the volar plate on the palmar side of the joint.
5. The MCP joint of the thumb is more exposed than its counterparts in the fingers and is subject to rupture of the ulnar collateral ligament, an injury known as the gamekeeper's thumb.
6. Metacarpal fractures, particularly of the neck of the fifth metacarpal, are relatively common and treatment generally consists of splinting the metacarpal shafts to one another.
7. Fractures of the base of the second and third metacarpals are closely involved with wrist function and often associated with subluxation of the carpometacarpal joint.
8. Puncture wounds of the hand may be associated with more serious injury to the deeper structures (nerves and tendons, for example) and have a high incidence of infection.
9. The goals of rehabilitation of hand and wrist injuries are to minimize swelling and mobilize the hand as soon as the injured parts permit.

SUGGESTED READINGS

Black, S. A. "Blistered and Torn Hands Disrupt Gymnast Training." *First Aider* 118 (1979): 10–11.

Blazina, M. E., and C. Lane. "Rupture of the Insertion of the Flexor Digitorum Profundus Tendon in Student Athletes." *Journal of the American College Health Association* 14 (1966): 248–249.

Browne, E. Z., Jr., H. K. Dunn, and C. C. Snyder. "Ski Pole Thumb Injury." *Plastic and Reconstructive Surgery* 58 (1976): 17–23.

Burton, R. I., and R. G. Eaton. "Common Hand Injuries in the Athlete." *Orthopedic Clinics of North America* 4 (1973): 809–838.

Gieck, J. H., and F. C. McCue, III. "Splinting of Finger Injuries." *Athletic Training* 17 (1982): 215.

Green, David P., ed. *Operative Hand Surgery*, 2d ed. New York: Churchill-Livingstone, 1988.

Lichtman, David M., ed. *The Wrist and Its Disorders*. Philadelphia: W. B. Saunders, 1988.

McCue, F. C., III, W. H. Baugher, D. N. Kulund, et al. "Hand and Wrist Injuries in the Athlete." *American Journal of Sports Medicine* 7 (1979): 275–286.

Spinner, Morton, ed. *Kaplan's Functional and Surgical Anatomy of the Hand*, 3d ed. Philadelphia: J. B. Lippincott, 1984.

19

The Pelvis

OBJECTIVES FOR CHAPTER 19

After reading this chapter, the student should be able to:

1. Understand the anatomy and function of the pelvis.
2. Recognize minor injuries of the pelvis and their treatment.
3. Recognize major injuries of the pelvis and realize the importance of providing emergency treatment prior to transport to the hospital.

INTRODUCTION

Pelvic injuries are not a common entity in sports; however, they can range from functional aggravation to life-threatening emergencies. An understanding of the anatomy of the pelvis and its potential injuries is important to the athletic trainer, who may be the first to assess and manage these problems. Chapter 19 describes the structural anatomy of the pelvis and reviews the minor and major pelvic injuries that can occur during sports activities. ■

ANATOMY

The **pelvis** is composed of several large flattened bones that form a ring which functions as a major support structure of the human skeleton (Fig. 19.1). It has adapted to allow man's upright posture and gait.

The **sacrum**, which is a flattened fusion of bones from the spinal column, forms the posterior aspect of the **pelvic ring** and is the base support of the upright spinal column. The **coccyx**, or terminal portion of the spinal column, consists of three to five vertical segments attached below the sacrum. The two **innominate bones** form a fibrous articulation with the sacrum and curve anterior-

ly to unite and form an anterior fibrous joint called the **symphysis pubis** or **pubic symphysis**. Each innominate bone is a fusion of three bones: the **ilium**, **ischium**, and **pubis**. The ring formed by the pelvis supports abdominal contents, contains the birth canal in women, and allows passage of the excretory canals. The **iliac crest** is the outer, uppermost margin of the ilium. The four **iliac spines** are sharp points of muscular attachments: the anterior superior, anterior inferior, posterior superior, and posterior inferior iliac spines. The ilium has attachment points for paraspinous and abdominal muscles as well as major muscle groups from the thigh. The **ischial tuberosity,** or **prominence**, serves as the attachment for the **hamstring muscles** and is the major weight-bearing structure for sitting. The **adductor muscles** of the thigh have major attachments to the pubic bone.

At the junction of the ilium, ischium, and pubic bones, the innominate bone is modified to form the **acetabulum**, the socket that acts as the receptacle for the hip joint.

MINOR PELVIC INJURIES

Sacroiliac Strain

Because the pelvis withstands significant functional forces, it is at risk of stress injuries.

The **sacroiliac joint** is an irregularly contoured fibrous joint that normally has no active motion. Acute trauma or repetitive stresses can create irritation in this joint and result in low back pain. Rest, therapy modalities, and specific rehabilitative exer-

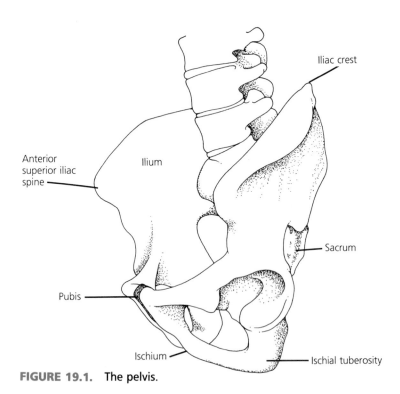

FIGURE 19.1. The pelvis.

cises often are necessary to relieve sacroiliac dysfunction.

Avulsions

Multiple avulsion injuries can occur about the pelvis. The **rectus femoris muscle**, the anterior thigh muscle of the quadriceps group, can pull from its direct attachment to the anterior superior iliac spine, causing a painful injury that is localized and disabling (Fig. 19.2). Point tenderness is easily noted at the injury site. Sometimes the reflected head of the rectus femoris pulls from the anterior inferior iliac spine, causing a deep disabling pain in the groin area.

Immediate treatment for rectus femoris avulsion injuries includes rest, icing to decrease pain and swelling, and analgesic medications for relief of pain. After the acute phase of the injury, the athlete should be maintained on crutches for continued rest of the injured site. Slow progression to motion is begun, and eventually strengthening exercises, such as leg lifts in the sitting and prone positions, are instituted. When the athlete is able to sprint and run free of pain, return to sports activities is possible. Flexibility exercises for the rectus femoris are important to prevent reinjury.

Hamstring strains or **tears** from the ischium are usually acute and dramatic (see Fig. 19.2). Adolescents may actually have a portion of bone avulsed from the ischium that can be detected radiographically. These injuries are very disabling and require a long period of rest and rehabilitation.

Avulsion injuries of the hamstrings usually require 3 to 4 months to resolve completely. Initially, these injuries are treated with rest, icing (if indicated), and analgesic medications. Crutches may be necessary to allow the athlete to ambulate without excessive pain or stress on the injured site. After acute symptoms have abated, the athlete can begin active rehabilitation of the hamstrings with curl exercises against gravity and then progress to heavier resistance exercises. Recovery is slow because the hamstrings are such a dynamic muscle group in the act of running. Once the ath-

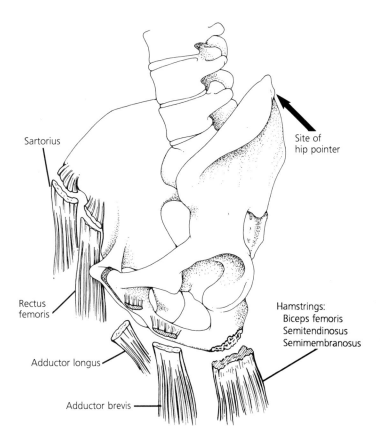

FIGURE 19.2.   Sites of avulsion injuries.

lete is pain free, sports activities can be resumed gradually. Continued flexibility exercises are important to prevent reinjury.

Avulsions of the adductor muscles from the pubis are less common but can also be very disabling (see Fig. 19.2). Bone fragments from the pubis can be detected radiographically. Rarely, these bony attachments have to be reattached surgically.

Hip Pointer

Contusions over the prominence of the iliac crest can irritate the attachments of the abdominal and thigh muscles, causing a very painful problem called a **hip pointer** (see Fig. 19.2). Treatment is rest, anti-inflammatory medications, and topical modalities such as heat. Athletes who continue sports activities with a hip pointer injury will have persistent pain and limited function, and recovery can be prolonged.

Coccygodynia

A fall on the buttock area can cause contusion or even fracture of the coccyx. This injury, called **coccygodynia**, can be very painful but is not permanently disabling. Initial treatment consists of ice and heat modalities with pain medications. A soft cushion is often necessary for sitting. Coccygodynia symptoms can become chronic but usually resolve in a few weeks.

Osteitis Pubis

Osteitis pubis is an arthritic condition resulting from continued stress on the pubic symphysis, a fibrous joint. A chronic strain of the pubic symphysis can result from repetitive stress activities such as long-distance running. Localized pain and difficulty during running activities are usually the clinical symptoms. Treatment is rest, heat, and anti-inflammatory medication.

MAJOR PELVIC INJURIES

Pelvic Fractures

The pelvis can be fractured from direct compression—that is, it can be literally crushed by a heavy impact (Fig. 19.3). This kind of impact can occur during falls from heights or from motor vehicle accidents. An indirect force such as the knee striking a wall can drive the femoral head into the pelvis and also cause a fracture.

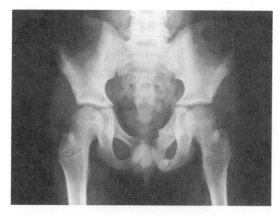

FIGURE 19.3. X-ray of pelvic fracture.

Signs and Symptoms

The athlete usually complains of pain in the pelvic region. Topographic deformity is rare, but there may be some soft tissue swelling at the injury site. There may also be a contusion or abrasion over the iliac crest if the fracture resulted from a direct blow. The most important signs in diagnosing pelvic fractures are pain that is felt when the iliac crests are compressed together or tenderness on palpation at the pubic symphysis or sacroiliac joints.

Associated Injuries of the Genitourinary System

Injuries of the genitourinary system, such as rupture of the bladder or a laceration of the urethra, are frequently associated with pelvic fractures and must be suspected. In an athlete with a suspected or known pelvic fracture, the trainer must always check for abdominal pain and tenderness, as well as hematuria (blood in the urine or blood around the urethral opening).

Blood Loss

Fracture of the pelvis may be associated with blood loss severe enough to cause hypovolemic shock and death. The trainer should keep in mind the possibility of shock as a result of the fracture and take steps to combat it. Open fracture of the pelvis with obvious external bleeding is uncommon because heavy musculature surrounds the pelvis. The extent of blood loss in a closed pelvic fracture may not be apparent because the hemorrhage occurs within the pelvic cavity and into the retroperitoneal space and thus is not visible. The athlete's vital signs must be evaluated as soon as possible and carefully monitored during stabilization and transport.

Immobilization

An athlete with a suspected pelvic fracture should be immobilized on a long spine board before being transported to the hospital. The foot of the spine board should be elevated 6 to 12 inches to reduce the pooling of blood or fluids in the athlete's lower extremities.

Treatment of Major Pelvic Injuries

Major pelvic injuries are an orthopedic emergency and should be left to the care of a physician. Acute treatment may include fluid and blood replacement for shock conditions. The athlete should be maintained on bed rest and close observation during the acute phase of the injury.

The physician will decide if the fracture can be treated conservatively with rest to allow healing of the fracture. Certain pelvic fractures are grossly unstable and require surgical intervention to reduce and stabilize the bones in a functional position. Recovery from these major injuries can be slow; it may take up to a year before the athlete completes rehabilitation and can return to sports activities. A significant portion of the athlete's rehabilitation should consist of general conditioning because of the prolonged activity associated with serious pelvic injuries.

IMPORTANT CONCEPTS

1. The pelvis is composed of multiple flat bones (sacrum and innominate) that form a fused interior ring for maximum strength and support of the human skeleton.
2. The sacrum is the base of support for the spinal column and upper body.
3. Innominate bone forms hip joint articulations for the lower extremity.
4. Muscle attachments for the upper body are on the iliac crest and pubis and for the lower body, on the ilium, ischium, and pubis.
5. The fibrous sacroiliac joint can be injured acutely or with stress overload.
6. Avulsion injuries of the pelvis can include avulsion of the rectus femoris, hamstring, and adductor muscles.
7. The pelvis can be fractured from direct compression or from an indirect force such as the knee striking a wall and driving the femoral head into the pelvis.
8. Athletes with suspected pelvic fractures must be immobilized on a long spine board, with the foot of the board elevated 6 to 12 inches to prevent pooling of liquids in the lower extremities.

SUGGESTED READINGS

Ekberg, O., N. H. Persson, P.-A. Abrahamsson, et al. "Longstanding Groin Pain in Athletes: A Multidisciplinary Approach." *Sports Medicine* 6 (1988): 56–61.
Koch, R. A., and D. W. Jackson. "Pubic Symphysitis in Runners: A Report of Two Cases." *American Journal of Sports Medicine* 9 (1981): 62–63.
Lachmann, Sylvia. *Soft Tissue Injuries in Sport*. Oxford: Blackwell Scientific Publications, 1988.

Liebert, P. L., J. A. Lombardo, and G. H. Belhobek. "Acute Posttraumatic Pubic Symphysis Instability in an Athlete." *The Physician and Sportsmedicine* 16 (April 1988): 87–90.

Lloyd-Smith, R., D. B. Clement, D. C. McKenzie, and J. E. Taunton. "A Survey of Overuse and Traumatic Hip and Pelvic Injuries in Athletes." *The Physician and Sportsmedicine* 13 (October 1985): 131–141.

Metzmaker, J. N., and A. M. Pappas. "Avulsion Fractures of the Pelvis." *American Journal of Sports Medicine* 13 (1985): 349–358.

Noakes, T. D., J. A. Smith, G. Lindenberg, et al. "Pelvic Stress Fractures in Long Distance Runners." *American Journal of Sports Medicine* 13 (1985): 120–123.

Pearson, R. L. "Osteitis Pubis in a Basketball Player." *The Physician and Sportsmedicine* 16 (July 1988): 69–72.

Renström, P., and L. Peterson. "Groin Injuries in Athletes." *British Journal of Sports Medicine* 14 (1980): 30–36.

Sim, F. H., and S. G. Scott. "Injuries of the Pelvis and Hip in Athletes: Anatomy and Function." In *The Lower Extremity and Spine in Sports Medicine*, vol. 2, edited by James A. Nicholas and Elliott B. Hershman, pp. 1119–1169. St. Louis: C. V. Mosby, 1986.

Smodlaka, V. N. "Groin Pain in Soccer Players." *The Physician and Sportsmedicine* 8 (August 1980): 57–61.

Waters, P. M., and M. B. Millis. "Hip and Pelvic Injuries in the Young Athlete." *Clinics in Sports Medicine* 7 (1988): 513–526.

Wiley, J. J. "Traumatic Osteitis Pubis: The Gracilis Syndrome." *American Journal of Sports Medicine* 11 (1983): 360–363.

20

Hip and Thigh

OBJECTIVES FOR CHAPTER 20

After reading this chapter, the student should be able to:
1. Understand the functional anatomy of the hip and thigh.
2. Recognize, assess, and manage sports injuries to the hip and thigh.
3. Describe rehabilitation exercises for the hip and thigh.

INTRODUCTION

The hip is the articulation of the lower extremity with the body. Like the shoulder, it is a ball-and-socket joint, but it has far more structural stability in its design. The thigh extends the length of the femur and contains the great muscles that power bipedal locomotion. Chapter 20 reviews the structural anatomy of the hip and thigh and details the most common sports injuries as well as other major injuries of the hip and thigh. The last section of Chapter 20 contains several rehabilitation exercises. ▪

ANATOMY

Hip Joint

The articulation of the femur with the pelvis forms the **hip joint**, a ball-and-socket joint (Fig. 20.1). The ball is the **femoral head**. Below the head, the femur narrows into the **femoral neck**. Just distal to the neck, the bone widens into two large prominences, the **lesser trochanter** (medial) and the **greater trochanter** (lateral). The **acetabulum**, or socket of the joint, is deepened and reinforced by a fibrocartilaginous rim, the **labrum acetabulare**. The joint is encased in a

tough fibrous capsule lined by synovial tissue that nourishes the joint. Three extremely strong ligaments, the **iliofemoral**, **pubofemoral**, and **ischiofemoral**, surround the joint anteriorly and posteriorly and reinforce the capsule.

Bursae of Hip

Of numerous bursae about the hip joint, the two most important are the **trochanteric bursa**, located just behind the greater trochanter and deep to the gluteus maximus and tensor fascia lata muscle, and the **iliopsoas bursa**, located between the capsule and the iliopsoas muscle anteriorly (Fig. 20.2).

Hip Muscles

Motion of the hip joint includes flexion, extension, abduction, adduction, circumduction, and rotation. The primary flexors of the hip are the iliopsoas, sartorius, rectus femoris, and adductor muscles. The primary extensors of the hip are the gluteus maximus and hamstrings. Adduction is primarily from the adductors and medial hamstrings. The primary abductors are the tensor fascia lata and gluteus minimus and medius muscles. The internal rotators are the gluteus medius and minimus, tensor fascia lata, adductors, and iliopsoas muscles. The external rotators include the glu-

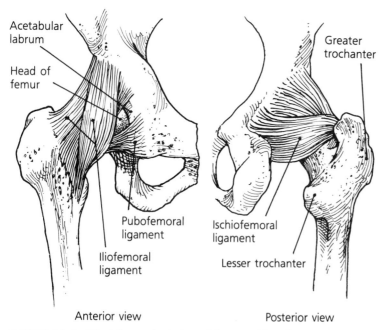

Acetabular labrum

Head of femur

Greater trochanter

Pubofemoral ligament

Ischiofemoral ligament

Iliofemoral ligament

Lesser trochanter

Anterior view

Posterior view

FIGURE 20.1. Hip joint: articulation of femur with pelvis.

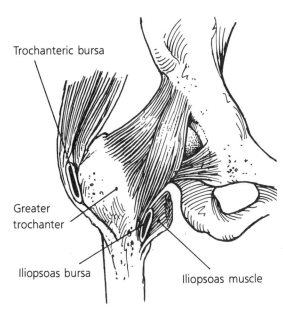

FIGURE 20.2. Trochanteric and iliopsoas bursae.

teus maximus, piriformis, obturator, and gemellus muscles (Fig. 20.3).

Thigh Bone

The **femur** is the largest, longest, and strongest bone in the body and is almost perfectly cylindrical in shape. The shaft is bowed slightly outward and forward to accommodate the stress of locomotion and weight bearing.

Thigh Muscles

There are four major groups of muscles in the thigh: flexors, extensors, abductors, and adductors. The strongest group are the knee extensors (**quadriceps**) on the anterior aspect. The quadriceps consist of the rectus femoris, vastus intermedius, vastus medialis, and the vastus lateralis. The rectus femoris originates on the anterior superior and the posterior superior iliac spines; the others arise from the shaft of the femur. They all converge to form the **quadriceps tendon**, inserting into the patella and extending on as the patellar tendon to the

tibial tuberosity. In addition, the rectus femoris acts as a hip flexor.

The **hamstrings** are strong flexors of the knee and major extensors of the hip. The hamstrings on the posterior aspect of the thigh are composed of the biceps femoris, semitendinosus, and semimembranosus muscles (Fig. 20.4). All three muscles originate on the tuberosity of the ischium. The biceps has two heads: the long head arises from the medial aspect of the ischial tuberosity; the short head arises from the linea aspera of the femur. It inserts on the head of the fibula and lateral condyle of the tibia. The biceps courses along the lateral side of the posterior thigh, while the semitendinosus and semimembranosus muscles course along the medial aspect of the femur. The gracilis and sartorius muscles, while not technically hamstring muscles, contribute to the medial hamstrings through a conjoined tendon called the **pes**

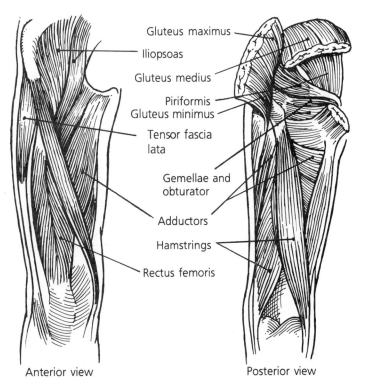

Gluteus maximus
Iliopsoas
Gluteus medius
Piriformis
Gluteus minimus
Tensor fascia lata
Gemellae and obturator
Adductors
Hamstrings
Rectus femoris

Anterior view   Posterior view

FIGURE 20.3. Hip muscles.

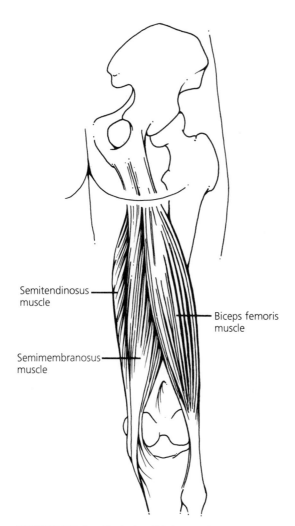

Semitendinosus muscle

Biceps femoris muscle

Semimembranosus muscle

FIGURE 20.4. Posterior thigh muscles.

anserinus (goose foot), which inserts onto the upper medial aspect of the tibia.

The adductor muscles consist of the adductor magnus, brevis, and longus muscles; the pectineus; and the gracilis. The adductors arise from the pubic ramus and insert along the medial aspect of the distal femur. The gracilis attaches to the tibia through the pes anserinus tendons. They adduct the hip and help in hip and knee flexion.

The hip abductors consist of the tensor fascia lata and gluteus medius and minimus muscles. They originate along the crest of the ilium. The gluteus medius and minimus insert on the greater trochanter, and

the tensor fascia lata courses along the outer aspect of the thigh as the iliotibial band, inserting on the lateral aspect of the femoral condyle and tibia.

The extensor muscles of the thigh are supplied by the femoral artery and nerve, which course from the inguinal area down the adductor canal. Branches from the artery and nerve supply the extensor muscles. The hamstrings are innervated by the sciatic nerve, which runs from the pelvic sciatic notch through the short external rotators and down the posterior thigh deep to the hamstring musculature. The hamstrings are nourished by the femoral artery. The adductors are supplied by the obturator nerve, which begins in the obturator foramen of the pelvis and branches to innervate the adductor musculature. The thigh muscles are covered and divided into groups by a heavy, fibrous sheath, the **fascia**.

OVERUSE INJURIES OF THE HIP

Bursitis

The trochanteric and iliopsoas bursae may become inflamed (**bursitis**) from overuse, such as occurs in jogging. If the trochanteric bursa is involved, there is usually aching and pain after running. The discomfort is localized laterally over the greater trochanter and can be elicited by palpation in this area. In running, the repetitive movement of the iliotibial tract over the greater trochanter irritates the bursa and can cause inflammation. If the iliopsoas muscles are involved, the pain is more medial and anterior in the groin. The site of tenderness is not readily palpated, but discomfort can be elicited by passive rotatory motion of the hip. This irritation can be caused by the repetitive motion of the iliopsoas tendon against the hip capsule during running.

Treatment includes rest of the hip joint, daily use of ice packs or ice massage, and nonsteroidal anti-inflammatories. The trainer should also observe the athlete carefully for any biomechanical problems, such as leg length discrepancy or muscle contracture that could predispose to the bursitis.

Synovitis

Synovitis of the hip is a generalized, nonspecific inflammation of the lining of the hip joint. It may be caused by direct injury, such as a blow or twisting, or by overuse. Bacterial infections can also cause synovitis. Hip joint pain sometimes radiates down the medial aspect of the thigh to the knee via the obturator nerve. On observation, the athlete often rests with the hip slightly flexed and externally rotated to relieve the painful pressure in the hip joint caused by the synovitis. Any type of motion usually causes pain, and the athlete has an antalgic gluteus medius gait. Athletes with suspected synovitis should be referred to an orthopedist for complete examination. Evaluation includes x-rays and an infection workup that includes aspiration. The cause of the synovitis must be determined, but often diagnosis is one of exclusion. Frequently, the athlete requires complete bed rest or must be totally non–weight bearing on crutches until the synovitis has been properly diagnosed and treated.

Hip Joint Sprain

The symptoms of hip joint sprain are very similar to the symptoms of synovitis or stress fracture about the hip. Usually, there is a distinct history of significant twisting injury and trauma to the hip resulting in injury to the capsular ligaments about the hip, thereby causing pain.

Rotation of the leg usually causes discomfort. X-rays should be taken to rule out a fracture injury. Treatment consists of rest and protective weight bearing with crutches until walking is no longer painful. At this point, the athlete can begin progressive rehabilitation, with greater distances of walking, followed by running. When these activities can be tolerated without discomfort, the athlete can then progress to functional sports activities.

Groin Strain

The adductor muscles of the anterior groin are frequently injured during athletics. Very mild to severe strains may occur during an activity that involves running, jumping, or twisting. A sharp pain in the groin area that occurs during these activities is followed by increased pain, stiffness, and weakness on hip flexion.

The proper muscle test or stretching the affected muscle can determine which muscle group is involved. If straight-leg raising against resistance causes pain, the rectus femoris or sartorius is probably involved. Pain on resistance to hip flexion usually suggests iliopsoas injury. Adduction of the leg against resistance causes pain if the adductors are involved.

Initial treatment of groin strain includes ice packs and rest, followed by gentle range-of-motion exercises. Active stretching and progressive resistance exercises are begun when the muscle is no longer painful. Running is also allowed when range-of-motion and strength tests are performed pain free.

HIP FRACTURES AND DISLOCATIONS

Fractures or dislocations of the pelvis, hip region, and bones of the lower extremity usually result from very severe trauma. Violent trauma can cause severe, sometimes permanently disabling, injury in healthy individuals.

The general principles of splinting should always be followed—specifically, immobilization of the injured limb, including the joint above and below the suspected fracture. A general primary assessment of the athlete should be performed to determine neurological, cardiac, and pulmonary status. Serious problems such as neurovascular compromise and bleeding should be stabilized before the injured limb is evaluated and splinted. Distal neurovascular function must be evaluated immediately and monitored frequently. Bleeding is best controlled by direct compression on the wound. Application of a tourniquet is rarely necessary. A dry, sterile dressing should be applied to protect the injury from further contamination.

Dislocations

Posterior hip dislocation is caused by a direct impact to the flexed knee and hip. It immediately results in pain and the inability to walk or even move the hip. The hip remains in a flexed and internally rotated position. First-aid measures include supporting the injured limb manually or with pillows and immediately transporting the athlete to the nearest medical facility. This injury can damage the sciatic nerve, which supplies the motor and sensory function to the lower leg. The function of this nerve should be tested if hip dislocation is suspected. Dislocation may require hospitalization and general anesthesia to reduce pain so that the hip can be reduced. The athlete usually remains hospitalized following reduction.

A major concern with hip dislocation is the late onset of aseptic necrosis or death of the femoral head after this injury. This phenomenon may take up to a year to manifest, and close follow-up of the athlete by a physician is indicated after these injuries. If the athlete becomes asymptomatic during this time, rehabilitation and return to sports activities are possible under a physician's observation and care.

Fractures

Hip fractures are uncommon in young athletes. When they occur, they are often caused by a severe impact while the foot is planted and the hip twisted. A **slipped capital femoral epiphysis** can occur in an older child or a young teenager. Essentially, this injury is a disruption in the femoral head through the growth plate and can be classified as a Salter-type fracture if it occurs acutely. Ordinarily, symptoms of this serious injury develop over a period of time, starting with aching pain. Gradually, the athlete begins to limp after activity and progresses to walking with an antalgic gait with the foot externally rotated.

Examination reveals fixed external rotation and inability to internally rotate, with some loss of flexion and extension. In about 10 percent of cases, the slipped epiphysis occurs acutely, perhaps while the athlete is participating in sports. Pain is severe, and the athlete should be referred for immediate treatment.

A slipped capital femoral epiphysis is a surgical emergency. Stabilization with hip pins is required to prevent further displacement and to allow the epiphysis to fuse and become stable. Obviously, the athlete is excluded from sports during treatment. There is a significant incidence of bilateral occurrence of this phenomenon, and the other hip may be pinned prophylactically. After the hardware has been removed and the physician has determined that the epiphyses are stable, the athlete can return to a rehabilitation and sports program.

SOFT TISSUE INJURIES OF THE THIGH

Approximately 10 percent of all sports injuries are related to the thigh musculature, making these muscles among the most commonly injured muscles. Because of their large size and accessibility, the thigh muscles are subject to numerous stresses and strains.

Contusion

A contusion results from a direct impact to the soft tissue. It may vary from a mild injury to a large, deep hematoma that may take months to heal. A contusion to the anterior and lateral thigh is very common in contact sports. Rarely, loss of function, severe pain, and progressive swelling and stiffness immediately follow impact. Occasionally, an associated tear of muscle fibers may occur. A localized area of exquisite tenderness appears, and the athlete is unable to flex his or her knee.

Hemorrhage or bleeding from the injured muscle within the thigh should be controlled immediately with a compression dressing with the knee in flexion and ice applied directly to the area of trauma. Daily ice packs, very gentle active stretching of the muscle within the athlete's pain limits, and isometric exercises facilitate early rehabilitation. Heat, ultrasound, and massage after several days are sometimes advocated but may intensify the inflammatory reaction if used too soon. Passive stretching can be achieved in the prone position by pulling on the ankle to bring the knee into flexion. Passive stretching can be initiated when the athlete can actively bend the knee with minimal discomfort. As range of motion at the knee is gained, a progressive resistive quadriceps program and gradual return to jogging and running are instituted. This rehabilitation program varies from athlete to athlete, progressing according to the athlete's ability to continue without pain. Usually, 3 to 4 weeks are needed for adequate rehabilitation. Anti-inflammatory drugs may be very useful. Some physicians use oral or injectable enzymes with varying degrees of success. Enzymes are only effective in the first 24 to 48 hours after injury (if at all).

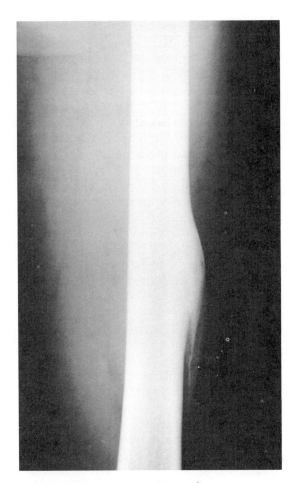

FIGURE 20.5. Late myositis ossificans on x-ray. Note formation of cortical-type bone.

Myositis Ossificans

A contusion to a muscle can result in bone deposition within the muscle. As the hematoma resolves, it is believed that periosteal tissue avulsed from bone uses the hematoma as a matrix to form ectopic ossification, a condition referred to as **myositis ossificans**. The most common sites for bone proliferation in soft tissue are the quadriceps and the brachial muscle of the arm. The process usually starts within 1 to 2 weeks after a severe contusion and can be palpated as a very hard mass within the soft tissue within 3 to 4 weeks after injury. At this time, x-rays reveal fluffy, immature bone in the soft tissue. Over a period of months, the bone matures to typical cortical-type bone (Fig. 20.5). This condition

must be recognized early because the process is self-limiting if the muscle is not irritated by active exercise or vigorous massage. If there is excessive pain, swelling, and induration (hardening) in the injury site in the first week after injury, the athlete should be referred to a physician for further evaluation and treatment.

Treatment of myositis ossificans, like that of muscle strain, consists initially of rest, ice packs to reduce swelling, and compression. This routine should be continued for 2 to 3 days. Later, modalities such as ultrasound can help decrease the proliferation of the calcification. The process is generally followed by periodic x-ray examination until the calcium deposit matures. This typically occurs in 6 to 12 months. Usually, the bony mass is no handicap once it has matured and no treatment is required other than padding. Most of the mass will resolve spontaneously in time. The mature bony mass can be excised surgically if it causes some functional disability, such as pain or limitation of motion. Excision of the bone before it has matured simply results in its reforming, sometimes larger than before.

Any severe contusion of the thigh should be treated as impending myositis ossificans. Passive stretching and massage should be avoided, and the injured limb should be rested until painless range of motion has been restored. Myositis ossificans can sometimes be prevented by a program of rest.

Muscle Strain

Muscle strains (pulls or tears) are very common injuries in all sports that involve running, jumping, or kicking. They may range from mild, first-degree strains to third-degree tears of the muscles. Hamstring strains are among the most feared injuries to athletes because they tend to recur. They are more functionally disabling than injuries to the quadriceps or the gastrocnemius musculature. The hamstrings are particularly vulnerable to strain because of the nature of their function. Athletes whose quadriceps are stronger than their hamstrings, or who have a significant imbalance between the strength of one leg and the other, are particularly vulnerable to tears.

Poor posture, inflexibility, fatigue, and poor coordination also lead to hamstring strains. As in most other injuries, it is much easier to prevent a hamstring strain through proper preventive stretching and strengthening than it is to treat it once it has occurred. Athletes with tight, inelastic hamstrings may also have low back problems. They should be instructed in a program of static stretching exercises for the hamstrings. Athletes with weaker hamstrings in one leg compared with the other should undertake a progressive resistance exercise program to balance these muscles. Rehabilitation exercises should be done two to three times daily, with progressing counts and resistance forces as the athlete's strength increases. At least 6 weeks of conditioning are required for beneficial results.

Hamstring strains are easily diagnosed by history and physical examination. The athlete feels an immediate pain locally in the posterior thigh, usually while in full stride. In milder cases, hamstring strain may simply lead to some tightness of the muscle. In third-degree tears, the athlete is unable to walk after the injury. There is local tenderness and pain to palpation of the injured muscle or with any attempt to stretch the hamstrings. Hamstring tears frequently result in profuse hemorrhage and ecchymosis that appear subcutaneously a few days after the injury. Severe muscle disruption and avulsions may require open repair if there is significant functional loss; however, this is extremely uncommon. A significant palpable defect in the muscle or x-ray evidence of a large bony avulsion may indicate a need for surgical repair.

Immediate treatment consists of ice, compression, elevation, and rest. The athlete may require crutches for mobilization. After an initial period of rest, gradual active stretching and progressive exercises may be started. Very mild injuries may heal within 10 days to 3 weeks, whereas severe injuries may take 2 to 6 months to heal.

Because these injuries tend to recur due to the inelasticity of the scar tissue in a torn muscle, affected athletes should not be allowed to resume full activity until they can demonstrate complete flexibility and return of strength and muscle balance.

THIGH FRACTURES

Stress Fractures

Stress fractures of the femoral shaft can occur, particularly in running athletes. Most often, they present clinically as a chronic, nonlocalized pain in the thigh.

Stress fractures that occur in the femoral neck present as pain in the groin that increases with activity. These stress fractures may not be seen on initial x-ray films. Examination of the athlete with a stress fracture of the femoral shaft or neck usually reveals mild tenderness about the mid- to proximal portion of the thigh on palpation or pain with rotation of the hip in the case of stress fracture of the femoral neck. In athletes who have been symptomatic for several weeks or longer, x-rays may show a periosteal reactive bone formation. Femoral neck stress fractures are intracapsular and may never show a periosteal reaction. After several weeks, increased density of the bone at the fracture site may be seen radiographically, indicating a healing of the fracture. In early cases, a bone scan may be necessary to diagnose a stress fracture.

Treatment consists of rest until symptoms subside. Continued activity may cause displacement of the fracture, which would create an unstable and more complicated injury. Two to 3 months of rest may be required before the athlete is able to return to a reconditioning and sports program. Complete rest and protection are necessary until clinical and x-ray evaluations document acceptable healing. The athlete should then progress to a gradual rehabilitation and training program to prevent recurrence of the stress fracture.

Femoral Shaft Fractures

Fractures of the femur usually result from direct, very forceful impact. They are major injuries and require immediate medical attention. They may occur in any part of the shaft, from the hip region to just above the knee joint at the level of the femoral condyles. Clinical diagnosis is usually made by observing the marked deformity of the leg. Severe angulation or rotation at the fracture site, frequently combined with shortening of the limb, indicates disruption of the integrity of the femoral shaft.

Fractures of the femur may be closed or open, with significant bleeding at the frac-

ture site. It is not unusual for an athlete with a fracture of the femur to go into hypovolemic shock; therefore, precautions must be taken to prevent or treat shock. The injured athlete must be handled extremely carefully, because any extra movement or fracture manipulation increases the blood loss. An open fracture of the femur should, like any other open fracture, be treated with appropriate sterile pressure dressings applied over the wound.

Vascular injuries can accompany femoral fractures with impaired circulation distally, causing a pale, cold, and pulseless foot. Gentle, longitudinal traction in line with the long axis of the limb, gradually restoring the overall alignment of the limb, and splinting the limb in that position usually restore circulation. If signs of circulation return are not seen after appropriate alignment and splinting, a serious vascular injury may have occurred, indicating an even greater urgency for prompt transportation to a medical facility.

A fracture of the femoral shaft is best immobilized with a traction splint. The precise sequence of steps to apply this splint properly should be known and practiced frequently to maintain the skill (see Chapter 14).

If no splinting equipment is available, the injured leg should be straightened and splinted to the adjacent leg with padding and cloth wrapping. Multiple carriers should be used to transport the athlete on a stretcher to prevent further motion of the injured extremity.

Femoral shaft injuries are a significant orthopedic problem that may require extensive treatment and rehabilitation. Often, surgical stabilization of the fracture is indicated. Healing may take longer than a year, and the athlete will have limited activity levels during this period of time. When healing is complete, the athlete can begin a reconditioning program, which will be extensive because of the prolonged period of inactivity. In time, however, a return to the previous level of sports activities should be possible.

REHABILITATION EXERCISES

Hip Flexor Stretch

Position: lying on back

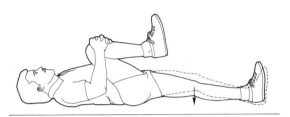

Procedure: Pull uninvolved knee to the chest and straighten the involved knee out as far as possible. Hold for 10 counts and then relax. Perform 3 sets of 10, three times a day.

Hip Extension Stretch

Position: lying over firm table or bed, with waist at the edge of the surface and uninvolved leg supported on the floor

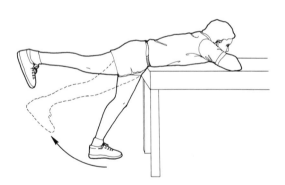

Procedure: Straighten and lift involved leg toward the ceiling. Hold for 3 to 5 counts and relax. To add resistance, secure weight around ankle. Begin with 1 pound and gradually increase to 5 pounds. Perform 5 sets of 10, three times a day.

Hip Flexion Stretch

Position: sitting on the edge of firm surface with feet resting on floor

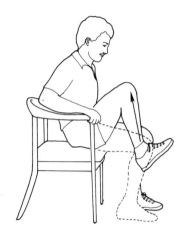

Procedure: Lift your knee toward your chest. Hold for 3 to 5 counts; lower and relax. To add resistance, secure weight on top of thigh. Begin with 1 pound and gradually increase to 5 pounds. Perform 5 sets of 10, three times a day.

Hip Abduction

Position: lying on side, with unaffected knee bent for stability

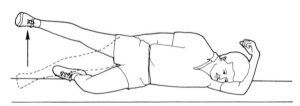

Procedure: Straighten top leg and lift upward toward ceiling. Hold for 3 to 5 counts. To add resistance, secure weight around ankle. Begin with 1 pound and gradually increase to 5 pounds. Perform 5 sets of 10, three times a day.

Hip Isometrics

Position: lying on back with a pillow between the legs and a belt secured slightly above the knees

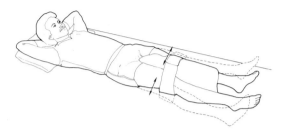

Procedure: Using your hip muscles, push both legs out against the belt. Hold for 5 counts; then pull legs together and squeeze the pillow. Hold for 5 counts and then relax. Perform 3 sets of 10, three times a day.

Iliotibial Band Stretch Standing

Position: standing beside wall, with involved leg closer to wall and crossed behind opposite leg

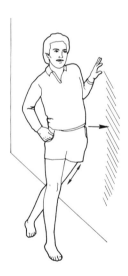

Procedure: Lean involved hip inward toward wall until you feel a stretch on the outside of leg. Hold 10 counts and then relax. Perform 3 sets of 10, three times a day.

Adductor Stretch

Position: sitting with soles of the feet together

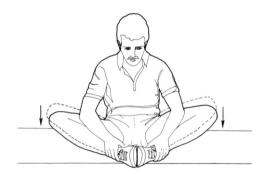

Procedure: Slide your feet toward the buttocks, and pull your knees toward the floor. Hold for 10 counts; relax and repeat. Perform 3 sets of 10, three times a day.

Supine Hamstring Stretch

Position: lying on back

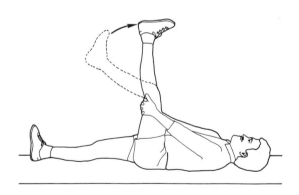

Procedure: Pull your knee to your chest with both hands clasped around the back of your thigh; slowly straighten your knee out toward the ceiling. Hold that position for 10 counts. Relax. Perform 3 sets of 10, three times a day.

Co-contraction

Position: sitting in a chair, foot supported on the floor

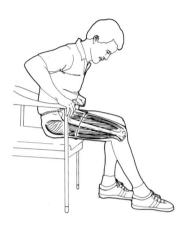

Procedure: Tighten both front and back knee muscles at the same time. Hold this isometric contraction for 5 counts. Perform 3 sets of 10, three times a day.

Straight-Leg Raise

Position: lying on back, with uninvolved knee bent

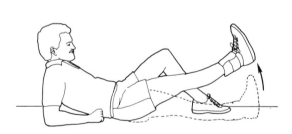

Procedure: Tighten the knee muscle performing a quad set. Lift your leg straight up, slightly lower than your bent knee, and hold 3 to 5 counts. The knee should be straight throughout the lift. Relax leg between each lift. Perform 10 sets of 10, three times a day. To add resistance, secure weight on ankle. Begin with 1 pound and gradually increase to 5 pounds. Rest 30 seconds to 1 minute between each set of 10.

Hamstring Curls

Position: standing with front part of thigh pressed against a door facing or a table

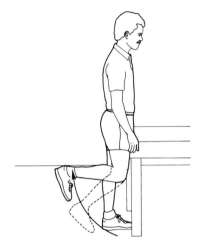

Procedure: Bring heel toward the ceiling, hold 5 counts, and relax. To add resistance, secure weight around ankle. Begin with 1 pound and slowly increase to 5 pounds. Perform 5 sets of 10, three times a day.

Quadriceps Stretch

Position: standing with hand support on wall or table

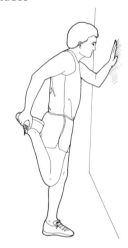

Procedure: Lift and hold foot of involved leg behind body with opposite hand. Pull foot upward to feel stretch in the front of thigh. Gradually increase upward pull and hold stretch 10 counts. Perform 3 sets of 10, three times a day.

IMPORTANT CONCEPTS

1. The articulation of the femur with the pelvis forms the hip joint.
2. The femur is the largest, longest, and strongest bone in the body.
3. The four major groups of muscles in the thigh are the flexors (hamstrings), extensors (quadriceps), abductors, and adductors.
4. Synovitis of the hip is a generalized, nonspecific inflammation of the lining of the hip joint, caused by direct injury, overuse injury, or bacterial infection.
5. A strain of the muscles of the anterior groin can occur during activities that involve running, jumping, or twisting and is first felt as a sharp pain in the groin area.
6. Posterior hip dislocation is caused by a direct impact to the flexed knee and hip and results in immediate pain and the inability to walk or even move the hip.
7. A slipped capital femoral epiphysis, which can occur in an older child or young teenager, is a disruption in the femoral head through the growth plate.
8. A contusion to a thigh muscle can result in bone deposition within the muscle, a condition known as myositis ossificans.
9. Hamstring strains are known to recur, especially among athletes whose quadriceps are stronger than their hamstrings, who have significant imbalance in leg strength, or who have poor posture, inflexibility, fatigue, and poor coordination.
10. Femoral shaft fractures result from direct, very forceful impact, and they require immediate medical attention, especially in the treatment of hypovolemic shock, which frequently follows these injuries.

SUGGESTED READINGS

Fox, James M. "Injuries to the Thigh." In *The Lower Extremity and Spine in Sports Medicine*, vol. 2, edited by James A. Nicholas and Elliott B. Hershman, pp. 1087–1117. St. Louis: C.V. Mosby, 1986.

Henry, Jack H. "The Hip." In *Principles of Sports Medicine*, edited by W. Norman Scott, Barton Nisonson, and James A. Nicholas, pp. 242–269. Baltimore: Williams & Wilkins, 1984.

Jackson, D. W., and J. A. Feagin. "Quadriceps Contusions in Young Athletes: Relation of Severity of Injury to Treatment and Prognosis." *Journal of Bone and Joint Surgery* 55A (1973): 95–105.

Lombardo, S. J., and D. W. Benson. "Stress Fractures of the Femur in Runners." *American Journal of Sports Medicine* 10 (1982): 219–227.

21

The Knee

CHAPTER OUTLINE

OBJECTIVES FOR CHAPTER 21

After reading this chapter, the student should be able to:

1. Describe the anatomy of the knee.
2. Prepare an organized method for evaluating knee injuries.
3. Describe the treatment for an acute knee injury.
4. Discuss the scheme for classifying and grading knee injuries.
5. Understand the mechanisms of ligament injury.
6. Test for knee instabilities.
7. Describe the functional capacity of the injured knee.
8. Identify patellofemoral disorders.
9. Describe meniscal disorders.
10. Recognize inflammation of the knee bursae.
11. Describe osteochondritis dissecans.
12. Describe chondral and osteochondral fractures.
13. Discuss osseous fractures about the knee.
14. Discuss the management of knee injuries.
15. Describe the process of rehabilitation following a knee injury.
16. Describe several general rehabilitation exercises and postoperative exercises for the knee.

INTRODUCTION

The knee joint is a very complex structure that is vulnerable to injury in practically all sports activities. Most knee injuries in athletic situations are first evaluated by the coach or athletic trainer, who must make a determination regarding the seriousness of the injury. Because muscle spasm and joint swelling often develop following knee injuries, the athletic trainer's initial examination may be more reliable than a subsequent exam. Therefore, it is imperative that the athletic trainer understand the basic anatomy of the knee joint and the various mechanisms of knee injury.

Chapter 21 begins with a detailed review of the functional anatomy of the knee. The chapter next describes how to evaluate an injured knee and treat an acute knee injury. A classification of knee ligament injuries, the mechanisms of ligament injury, and an explanation of how to test for knee instabilities follow. The chapter then describes the functional capacity of the injured knee. Specific knee problems, including patellofemoral disorders, meniscal disorders, inflammation of the knee bursae, osteochondritis dissecans, chondral and osteochondral fractures, and osseous fractures about the knee, are described in the next several sections. The last three sections of Chapter 21 discuss management of knee injuries, rehabilitation principles, and rehabilitation exercises. ▪

ANATOMY

The key to understanding the knee joint is in realizing that its movement is helicoid or spiral in character and not that of a simple hinge joint. The joint is formed by the articulation of the large, rounded condyles of the femur (Fig. 21.1) with the much flatter condyles of the tibia. The fibula does not take part in the joint. The patella articulates with the patellar surface of the femur, and thus the knee joint consists of three joints in one: a joint between the patella and the femur (the **patellofemoral joint**) and a joint between each tibial and femoral condyle (the **tibiofemoral joints**). The anatomical axis of the lower extremity, shown in Figure 21.2, differs from the mechanical axis, which is a line drawn from the center of the hip, knee, and ankle joints. With a wider pelvis, as in women, the inward angulation of the femur is greater, as is the outward angulation of the tibia. This condition is referred to as genu valgum, or knock-knees. The opposite condition, genu varum, refers to bowed knees.

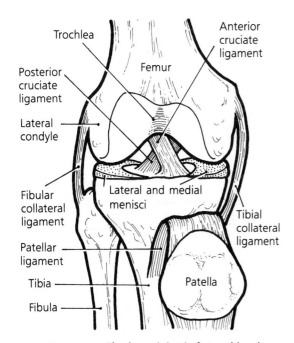

FIGURE 21.1. The knee joint is formed by the articulation of the condyles of the femur with the condyles of the tibia.

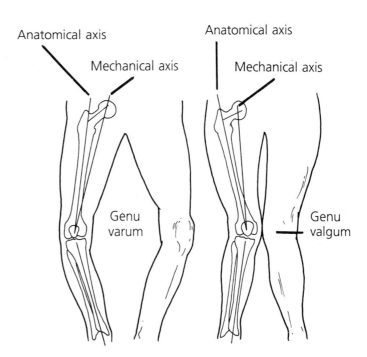

FIGURE 21.2. Anatomical and mechanical axes of the lower extremity.

The Osseous Structures

Femoral Condyles

The **femoral condyles** are two rounded prominences of the distal femur that are eccentrically curved. The anterior portion is part of an oval, and the posterior portion is a section of a sphere. The condyles project very little in front of the femoral shaft but markedly behind. The groove that runs anteriorly between the condyles (see Fig. 21.1) is the **patellofemoral groove**, or **trochlea**, which accepts the patella. Posteriorly, the condyles are separated by the **intercondylar notch**. The articular surface of the **medial condyle** is longer from front to back than that of the lateral condyle, but the **lateral condyle** is wider. The long axis of the lateral condyle is oriented essentially along the sagittal plane, but the medial condyle is usually at approximately a 22-degree angle to the sagittal plane.

Tibial Plateaus

The expanded proximal end of the tibia is formed by two rather flat surfaces, or **tibial**

plateaus, that articulate with the femoral condyles. They are separated in the midline by the **intercondylar eminence**, with its medial and lateral **intercondylar tubercles**. Anterior and posterior to the intercondylar eminence are attachment sites for the cruciate ligaments and menisci.

The lateral tibial plateau is flatter and more convex, shorter from front to back, and more oval than the medial tibial plateau. The anatomy of the tibial plateau is such that, to visualize the plateau properly on an anteroposterior radiograph, the x-ray tube must be angled about 15 degrees inferiorly, because the tibia slopes in a downward direction from front to back.

Patella

The **patella** is a rounded, triangular bone, wider at the upper (proximal) end than at the bottom (distal) end. The articular surface of the patella is divided by a vertical ridge (see Fig. 21.1) that creates two retropatellar surfaces: a smaller medial facet or surface and a larger lateral articular facet or surface. A smaller vertical ridge that lies even more medially separates the extreme medial "odd facet," which begins to contact the femur at around 135 degrees of knee flexion.

Extensor Mechanism

The **extensor mechanism** is a complex interaction of muscles, ligaments, and tendons that stabilizes the patellofemoral joint and acts to extend the knee.

Quadriceps Tendon

The **quadriceps tendon** of the **quadriceps muscle** inserts into the superior pole of the patella. There are four components of the quadriceps muscle: the **vastus medialis, vastus lateralis, vastus intermedius,** and **rectus femoris** (Fig. 21.3). Broad, fibrous expansions on both sides of the patella, made up of extensions of the vastus medialis and vastus lateralis, continue anteriorly over the knee joint to insert onto the tibia (see Fig. 21.3). These expansions are called the **medi-**

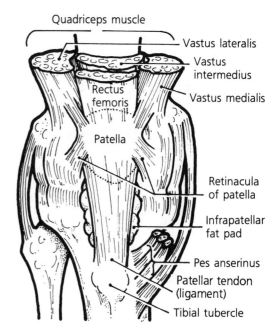

FIGURE 21.3. Anterior knee musculature.

al and **lateral patellar retinacula**. The retinacula are important because they also help extend the knee joint, even when the patellar tendon is ruptured. The fibers of the medial retinaculum, formed from the aponeurosis of the **vastus medialis obliquus,** or **VMO** (a smaller component of the vastus medialis muscle), plus the vastus medialis muscle itself, insert directly into the medial side of the patella. This fibrous insertion is the dynamic medial restraint that may prevent lateral displacement of the patella.

Patellar Tendon (Ligament)

The **patellar tendon** (also called the **patellar ligament**) is the extension of the quadriceps mechanism from the patella to the tibia (see Fig. 21.3). It is a large tendon that averages 3 inches (7.5 cm) in length. It extends from the inferior pole of the patella and courses down to attach on the **tibial tubercle** (the bony prominence of the tibia). It is readily palpable along its entire course. The **infrapatellar fat pad** extends from the lower pole of the patella to the level of the tibia, behind and on each side of the patellar tendon (see Fig. 21.3). It acts as a dynamic shock ab-

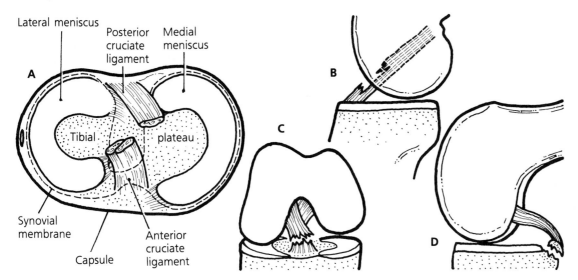

FIGURE 21.4. (a) Tibial attachments of the anterior and posterior cruciate ligaments in relationship to the synovial cavity. (b) Partial tear of the anterior cruciate ligament. (c) Mop-end tear of the anterior cruciate ligament. (d) Bony avulsion of the posterior cruciate ligament.

sorber and a source of nutrition for the tendon.

Internal Anatomy of the Knee

Menisci

The **menisci** are fibrocartilaginous structures that lie between the hyaline cartilage surfaces of the femur and tibia. Both the **medial meniscus** and **lateral meniscus** are C-shaped and conform to the shapes of the tibial surfaces on which they rest. The intricate anatomy of the menisci is discussed later when tears to these structures are considered.

Cruciate Ligaments

The **anterior** and **posterior cruciate ligaments** function in both anteroposterior and rotatory stability. They are so named because they cross each other like the arms of an X. The anterior cruciate attaches to the posterior medial aspect of the lateral femoral condyle. It has a fan-shaped attachment that corresponds to the curve of the medial margin of the lateral femoral condyle. This attachment is difficult to reach in perform-

ing ligament repairs. The tibial attachment is more compact and easily visualized.

The posterior cruciate is attached behind the intercondylar area of the posterior surface of the tibia. It is shorter, thicker, stronger, and less oblique than the anterior cruciate ligament. From its tibial attachment, it is directed in a superior, anterior, and medial direction to its femoral attachment on the lateral surface of the medial femoral condyle. The different types of cruciate tears are shown in Figure 21.4. Most commonly, the anterior cruciate is torn in its substance. The "mop-end" tear is nearly impossible to repair because the bundles of the ligament must stretch significantly before tearing, and not all the bundles tear at the same location. Because primary ligament repair is usually not possible, ligament reconstruction must be done employing autologous, homologous, or synthetic graft material. Tears at the bony attachment involve reattaching the bone, with the prognosis for function often good. The anterior cruciate blood supply through the middle geniculate artery and fat pad is usually interrupted with tears, making healing even more difficult.

Fat Pad

The infrapatellar fat pad is a relatively mobile structure that has connections with the front ends of the menisci that are fixed and which it overlaps (see Fig. 21.3). The blood supply to the patellar tendon courses through it.

Patellar Plica

In embryonic development, a septum separates the suprapatellar pouch from the knee joint. This septum usually disappears, but in approximately 20 percent of knees, it persists into adult life as a fibrous band called a **patellar plica** and may be clinically significant. The patellar plica extends from the medial wall of the knee joint obliquely downward to insert into the synovia covering the infrapatellar fat pad (Fig. 21.5). A large, thick medial patellar plica may act as a fibrous shelf and irritate the medial femoral condyle.

The athlete with a symptomatic plica may give a history of medial joint pain but usually without antecedent trauma. The symptoms often increase with activity, but the plica may also produce knee pain when

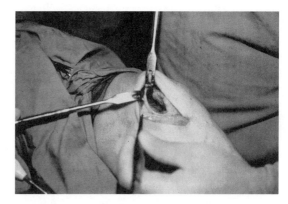

FIGURE 21.6. Open surgical procedure for the removal of a patellar plica.

the knee is kept in one position for prolonged periods, as in sitting. There may also be snapping or pseudolocking that may mimic a torn meniscus. In some cases, the medial plica can be palpated on physical examination, especially with the knee flexed to approximately 45 degrees. As the examining thumb is rolled over the medial shelf, tenderness may be produced, and the shelf may be clinically palpable. Diagnosis can sometimes be made by arthrogram but is best made arthroscopically. In symptomatic plicae, surgical excision of the shelf is recommended (Fig. 21.6).

Medial Aspect of the Knee

The major structures on the medial aspect of the knee are the medial retinaculum; the tibial collateral ligament; the medial capsular ligaments; and the pes anserinus, the combined insertion of the tendons of the sartorius, gracilis, and semitendinosus muscles (Fig. 21.7).

Ligaments and Tendons

Starting anteriorly, the patellar tendon (ligament) is evident, attaching to the anterior surface of the tibia. The **medial retinaculum** attaches along the medial border of the patella. Its primary function is to hold the patella medially. The **tibial collateral ligament** is composed of long, parallel fibers that overlie the joint capsule. Farther pos-

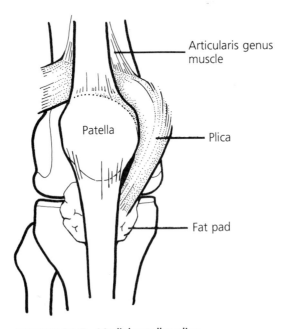

Articularis genus muscle

Patella

Plica

Fat pad

FIGURE 21.5. Medial patellar plica.

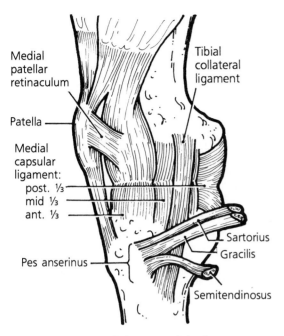

FIGURE 21.7. Medial aspect of the knee.

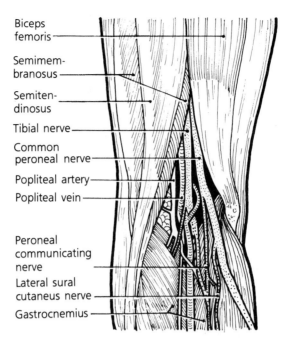

FIGURE 21.8. Posterior aspect of the knee.

terior are the three tendons of the **sartorius**, **gracilis**, and **semitendinosus** muscles, which course inferiorly to attach as the **pes anserinus** to the anteromedial aspect of the tibia. These muscles help protect the knee against rotatory and valgus stress.

The parallel fibers of the superficial tibial collateral ligament as a whole form a well-delineated, bandlike structure that inserts proximally into the medial femoral epicondyle and distally about a hand's breadth below the joint line onto the medial aspect of the tibia. This ligament glides anterior in extension and posterior with flexion. Its specific functions are discussed later in the chapter.

Capsular Ligaments

The midthird of the true capsule of the knee joint, the **medial capsular ligament**, is sometimes called the **deep medial collateral ligament**. The medial capsular ligament extends from the femur to the midportion of the meniscus and then to the tibia. The attachments of this deep structure to the medial meniscus, termed the **meniscofemoral**

and **meniscotibial** (or coronary) **ligaments**, limit excessive motion of the meniscus.

Posterior Aspect of the Knee

The hollow area that appears on the posterior surface of the knee is the **popliteal fossa**, or **popliteal space** (Fig. 21.8). Superiorly, the popliteal space is bounded by the tendon of the biceps femoris muscle laterally and the tendons of the semimembranosus and semitendinosus muscles medially. Inferiorly, the popliteal space is bounded by the two heads of the gastrocnemius muscle.

Muscles

Deep to the artery is the **popliteus muscle** (Fig. 21.9). This muscle is unusual in that it has three proximal insertions: the posterior aspect of the fibular head, the posterior horn of the lateral meniscus, and the lateral femoral condyle. It originates from the inner posterior two-thirds of the tibia. Its primary function is internal rotation of the tibia on the femur. It provides dynamic stability to the posterolateral capsular com-

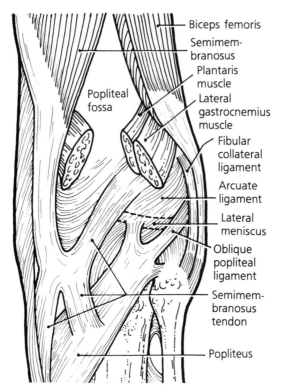

FIGURE 21.9. Popliteus and semimembranosus muscles.

plex of the knee. The popliteus muscle also pulls the posterior horn of the lateral meniscus posteriorly during knee flexion.

Medially, the **semimembranosus muscle** is an important stabilizing structure to the posterior aspect of the knee. The posterior capsule is pulled tightly around the femoral condyles in extension and helps to stabilize the knee in this position. The medial and lateral heads of the **gastrocnemius muscle** arise from the capsule of the knee and form the inferior boundary of the popliteal fossa.

Nerves

The **sciatic nerve** originates from multiple nerve roots in the lumbosacral area and provides most of the motor and sensory function in the lower extremity. It divides into the **common peroneal** and **tibial nerves** at the proximal popliteal space. The tibial nerve disappears from view as it courses

deep to the gastrocnemius muscle, whereas the common peroneal nerve, which supplies motor and sensory function to the lateral aspect of the leg, disappears by piercing the peroneus longus muscle and winding around the fibula to the anterior surface of the leg.

Vascular Structures

The femoral artery courses through the tendon of the adductor magnus muscle in the thigh and enters the popliteal fossa as the **popliteal artery**, where it is in contact with the capsule of the knee joint. With any knee surgery, such as removal of a meniscus, the artery must be protected from injury because it lies directly behind the knee joint capsule. The popliteal vein lies alongside the popliteal artery.

Lateral Aspect of the Knee

The patellar tendon (ligament) is shown anteriorly in Figure 21.3. The iliotibial tract is superficial to the capsule of the knee joint (Fig. 21.10). Posterior to the iliotibial tract are the fibular collateral ligament and the tendon of the biceps femoris muscle. The common peroneal nerve can be seen at this location as it winds around the lateral head of the gastrocnemius and the fibula to pierce the peroneus longus muscle.

Iliotibial Tract

The **fascia lata**, or **iliotibial tract**, envelops the lateral aspect of the thigh as it originates from the lateral iliac crest region, continues as a fibrous expansion over the vastus lateralis and into the lateral intermuscular septum, and continues over the lateral aspect of the knee. One major extension goes into the lateral soft tissue restraining structures of the patellofemoral joint. The **iliotibial band** is a thickening of the iliotibial tract that inserts directly into the lateral tubercle of the tibia (Gerdy's tubercle; see Fig. 21.10). The proximal attachment of this band is at the distal intermuscular septum. With knee flexion, the

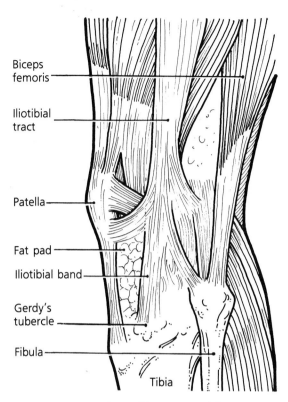

FIGURE 21.10. Lateral knee musculature.

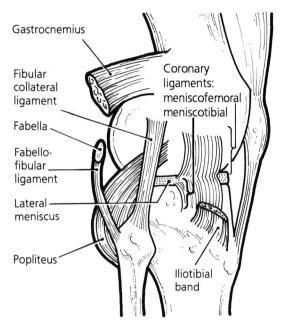

FIGURE 21.11. Lateral ligament complex.

iliotibial band moves posteriorly; with knee extension, it moves anteriorly.

Joint Capsule

Underneath the fascia lata and iliotibial band is the capsule of the joint. The capsule provides meniscal attachments as shown in Figure 21.9.

Arcuate Ligament

The posterior third of the lateral capsule, together with the popliteus attachments previously described, form the **arcuate ligament** (see Fig. 21.9). This muscular structure provides considerable stability to the posterolateral corner of the knee.

Fibular Collateral Ligament

The **fibular collateral ligament** of the knee inserts from the femoral condyle to the fibular head (see Fig. 21.9). The insertion of

the biceps muscle completely envelops the fibular insertion of the ligament.

Short Collateral Ligament

Deep to the fibular collateral ligament lies the **short collateral ligament**. If there is a **fabella** (a sesamoid bone that sometimes occurs and is located in the lateral gastrocnemius muscle tendon), this latter ligament is attached to it and is then called the **fabellofibular ligament**. It runs parallel to the fibular collateral ligament and attaches to the fibular head posterior to the tendon of the biceps. It reinforces the posterior capsule and contributes to the lateral stability of the knee (Fig. 21.11).

EVALUATION OF KNEE INJURIES

The knee, one of the most vulnerable joints of the body, has an intricate and complex anatomy. For this reason, correct diagnosis of the exact structure that has been injured is often difficult. The athletic trainer, usually the first to evaluate most knee injuries, must differentiate potentially serious injuries from minor injuries, because knee injuries with ligament damage and gross instability require immediate treatment. A common error is to assume that a knee ligament injury is less severe than it actually is. Certain features about the athlete's history and physical findings should alert the athletic trainer to the seriousness of the acutely injured knee, particularly where gross instability or fracture is not immediately obvious.

Goals of Initial Evaluation

The athletic trainer and primary care physician have the following five goals in the initial evaluation of an acute knee injury:

- Immediately exclude a limb-threatening disorder such as interruption of blood supply to the extremity or serious fracture or dislocation.
- Record the details associated with the injury that may facilitate the physician's diagnosis.
- Conduct stability tests to determine the severity of the injury.
- Provide immediate splinting and first-aid care.
- Arrange immediate transport and triage for definitive medical care.

In the less acute knee injury, such as when swelling has occurred over 3 to 4 days without a specific injury, the initial examiner can perform more diagnostic tests. In the chronically unstable knee, a variety of diagnostic tests are available to arrive at the correct diagnosis.

The secret of accurate diagnosis in the acutely injured knee is to design a standardized, systematic approach that will elicit key symptoms and physical findings and alert the examiner to the need for further tests, immediate treatment, or surgery. With the acute knee injury, pain and muscle spasm may prevent a precise examination, necessitating examination under anesthesia and, in certain instances, arthroscopy. With the chronically injured knee, the examiner can perform a variety of different tests to bring out all the subtleties of the instability. Although the examination of the acutely injured knee differs markedly from that of the chronically unstable knee, many examination techniques do not distinguish between the two.

The physical examination is designed to test methodically and specifically all of the major components of the knee joint, including the major ligaments of the knee, meniscal structures, patellofemoral joint, and muscles about the knee. Before adequate off-the-field examination can take place, the athlete must be as relaxed as possible; the extremities should be bare from the toes to the groin. During the examination, the examiner should always compare the injured knee with the opposite side. The techniques for performing the tests are described later in the chapter.

A few points of caution must be emphasized in examining the acute knee injury. First, the athletic trainer is dealing with an injury. The initial evaluation of any injury should exclude more serious or life-threatening associated injuries. The second note of caution deals specifically with the examination of the knee joint. The trainer must realize the limitations of physical examination of an acutely injured knee. The following are some points to remember:

- Be gentle.
- Do not force the knee joint through any sudden motions.
- Determine the severity of the athlete's injury and pain without producing more discomfort.
- Do not rely completely on negative findings. A joint effusion or even slight muscle spasm can block any of the laxity tests, giving a false-negative finding for knee stability.

The Evaluation Process

The initial examination includes obtaining a history, observing the limb as indicated in Figure 21.12, and palpating the joint for local tenderness. The athletic trainer

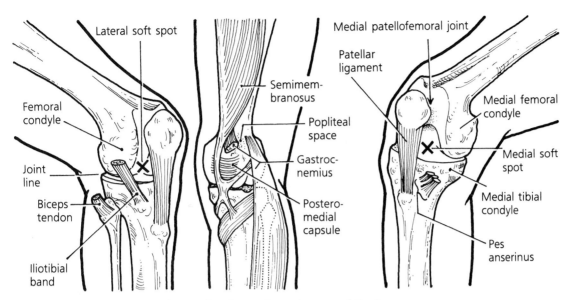

FIGURE 21.12. Anterior and posterior views of prominences of the knee.

should gently perform a simple anteroposterior drawer test and a simple abduction-adduction stress test. If the knee is grossly unstable, no other stability tests should be carried out. Instead, the limb should be immobilized and the athlete immediately transferred to a medical facility for a definitive diagnosis and treatment.

With a chronically unstable knee without the effects of an injury, a variety of stability tests can be used for evaluation. In the acutely injured knee, the treating physician eventually will have to perform similar tests, but necessarily under ideal conditions and with the athlete relaxed. Not infrequently, stability tests and knee evaluation have to be done under general anesthesia. Therefore, the athletic trainer need only initially determine gross laxity by simple anteroposterior drawer tests and abduction-adduction stress tests (Fig. 21.13). These tests are best done with the knee at 30 degrees of flexion, usually the least painful position. Negative test results, as previously discussed, do not exclude major injury. Any knee injury that disrupts an athlete's play or performance, no matter how trivial it may appear, needs comprehensive evaluation by the treating physician.

The athletic trainer should always examine the patellofemoral joint for a tendency for subluxation or dislocation. Symptoms caused by subluxation of the patellofemoral joint can be similar to those of meniscal or ligamentous origin, including giving-way episodes, generalized pain, and swelling.

History

Knee evaluation begins with a detailed history of the most recent injury and subsequent developments. The history itself very often leads to a presumptive diagnosis that the physical examination then substantiates and qualifies.

Questions to ask the athlete include the following:

1. *Did the injured knee swell acutely?* The answer to this question, along with appropriate qualifying factors of location of swelling, rate of accumulation, and amount of swelling, is extremely important. Rapid swelling is an ominous sign. It suggests hemorrhage within the knee joint and the high likelihood of a cruciate ligament tear, osteochondral fracture, or patellar dislocation.

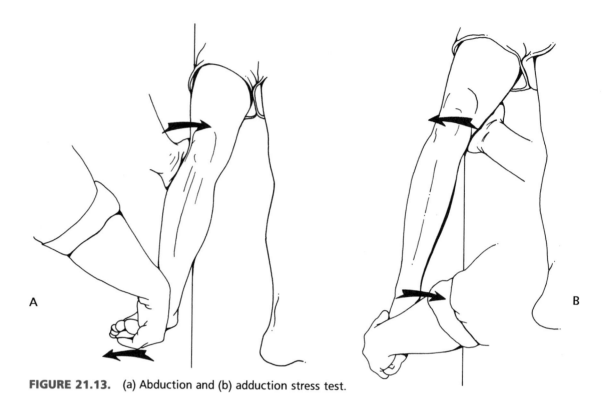

FIGURE 21.13. (a) Abduction and (b) adduction stress test.

2. *Did the athlete feel or hear a "pop"?* An audible pop or popping sensation accompanied by rapid swelling is suggestive of a torn anterior cruciate ligament. Tears of the menisci or other ligaments and intra-articular fractures are also possibilities.

3. *What was the mechanism of injury?* A medial or lateral blow causing an abnormal joint opening to the opposite side of the knee suggests injury to the collateral ligament and associated capsular ligaments, the adjacent meniscus, or a fracture at the site of impact. Anterior cruciate injuries are much more common than originally suspected, as will be discussed. Such injuries may follow a hyperextension and internal tibial rotation injury, although they more commonly result from any twisting or deceleration injury. Additional mechanisms of injury include a posterior blow to the proximal tibia, such as occurs from an illegal clip in football. Associated mechanisms of

injury that may produce particular ligament tears are described in the section on ligament function (see p. 335).

4. *Has the knee sustained a serious injury before this last accident?* On occasion, a previous injury to a meniscus or cruciate ligament has led to an internal derangement and unstable knee. The athletic trainer may be misled into thinking that the instability is secondary to an acute injury.

5. *Was the athlete able to continue playing after the knee injury?* This important question helps determine the extent of injury. More than 80 percent of athletes with serious ligament injuries are unable to continue playing after the injury. Even though approximately 20 percent are able to continue playing after the injury, the ability to walk from the playing field does not necessarily rule out a serious injury.

6. *Did the athlete's knee "give way" or "go out of place" at the time of injury?* There

are many causes for the knee's giving-way. This symptom is often found in chronic cases of instability. However, the giving-way episode may reflect an acute injury. The athlete's sensation of knee instability without its actually having given way may also indicate a ligament problem. The knee's actually going out of place or the joints separating at the time of injury may indicate a serious injury.

7. *What type of footwear was the athlete wearing?* (What type of cleats? Did the footwear have low or high tops?) Certain types of shoes such as extra long cleats or high tops can actually contribute to the severity of the injury. In sports requiring a cleated shoe the foot is fixed to the ground and the body rotates about it.

8. *On what type of surface (grass, artificial, wood floor, etc.) did the injury occur?* Surfaces that create greater traction and torque can increase the severity of the injury.

The extent of historical evaluation depends on the circumstances surrounding the injury. On the playing field, the athletic trainer can readily assess how the injury occurred and the anatomical site of the injury. Later, in a more relaxed atmosphere, closer scrutiny of all historical details is possible.

Pain

The occurrence and location of pain, particularly elicited on palpation, usually are good indicators of injury severity. In some cases pain symptoms are unreliable. In certain injuries, for example, severe capsular disruption prevents the accumulation of blood under pressure, and there may be a surprising lack of pain. Also, a few athletes may continue their sport immediately after injury, despite having sustained a major ligament tear. The athlete may only complain of a slight wobbliness to the knee, even though the knee may show gross instability on examination. Therefore, the lack of considerable pain in an acutely injured

knee does not eliminate the possibility of a serious injury. On the other hand, the finding of severe pain and inability to walk suggests a major intra-articular problem.

In the adolescent, pain and swelling may indicate a distal femoral or proximal tibial epiphyseal fracture. In the latter case, routine radiographs may not confirm the diagnosis, and stress radiographs need to be obtained. A clue to an epiphyseal fracture is the finding of localized tenderness above the joint line in the region of the medial or lateral femoral condyle. Alternatively, similar tenderness below the joint line in the region of the tibial growth plate may indicate a fracture.

Observation

If possible, it is best to begin the examination by observing the athlete's gait, limp, and functional range of motion. The examination should be tailored to the injury. In the chronic condition, the athletic trainer should observe the athlete's use of the knee joint through a variety of activities, including jumping and squatting, to note a functional deficit. An antalgic limp, guarding against an instability, or inability to perform routine functions on the knee can be noted during gait evaluation.

When swelling is observed, it is important to document the following:

1. *Location of swelling.* Restricted swelling to one side of the knee or the other does not indicate intra-articular fluid, but usually means local tissue disruption. It may indicate tearing of the tibial or fibular collateral ligaments. In an adolescent, swelling confined to the femoral condylar areas above the knee may indicate an epiphyseal fracture. Discrete swelling can also mean hemorrhagic bursitis, such as a contused prepatellar bursa. An ominous sign is a true bloody effusion, or hemarthrosis, after injury—that is, an intra-articular accumulation of blood.

2. *Rate of accumulation.* A rapid accumulation of intra-articular fluid after injury

indicates a hemarthrosis. However, after 24 hours, intra-articular swelling may not be attributable to the accumulation of blood. Aspiration by a physician may be required to evaluate the intra-articular fluid.

3. *Ecchymosis.* Occasionally, ecchymosis may be noted about the knee. This could be caused by direct trauma that results in bruising or excessive extravasation of intra-articular blood into the subcutaneous tissues. A localized deformity can be noted from hematoma formation or marked distention of the intact knee capsule. A gross deformity of the knee should alert the observer to the possibility of a fracture or significant dislocation of the knee joint.

Palpation

Palpation is performed ideally with the athlete seated or supine. Palpation for localized tenderness can detect injury to the structure. Palpation should always begin in an area distal from the suspected injury. Starting away from the injury site promotes the athlete's cooperation and prevents the ex-

aminer from overlooking a concomitant injury (see Fig. 21.12). For example, if a lesion on the medial aspect of the knee is suspected, the examiner begins by palpating all of the lateral structures: the lateral femoral condyle, the lateral aspect of the patellofemoral joint, the soft spot lateral to the patellar tendon that gives access to the lateral joint line, the entire joint line progressing to the posterolateral corner, the iliotibial band, the biceps tendon, and the lateral head of the gastrocnemius muscle. If the athlete can cooperate by crossing his or her legs, the examiner can easily palpate the fibular collateral ligament. Then the examiner proceeds to the medial aspect of the joint, palpating the medial femoral condyle, medial tibial condyle, medial portion of the patella, patellar tendon, and medial soft spot. The examiner next palpates the joint line, progressing anteriorly to posteriorly to the region of the posteromedial capsule and the semimembranosus and gastrocnemius muscles. Finally, the examiner palpates the popliteal space.

In the anterior aspect of the knee, the quadriceps attachment to the patella is palpated for a defect or localized tenderness that may indicate rupture. Tenderness directly over the patella may indicate a fracture. Pain on palpation of the patellar tendon at its attachment to the inferior pole of the patella or tibia may indicate tears. The integrity of the extensor mechanism is palpated for rupture of the quadriceps tendon, patellar fracture, patellar tendon disruption, or tibial tubercle avulsion.

The patellofemoral joint needs to be thoroughly examined at some point in the evaluation. The examiner must palpate for localized tenderness to the entire extensor mechanism as just discussed. The **apprehension test** involves lateral displacement of the patella (Fig. 21.14). The examiner attempts to subluxate the patella laterally to see if apprehension or pain is elicited. Often, localized tenderness about the medial retinacular and ligamentous supports to the patella indicates tearing of these tissues as a result of subluxation or dislocation. **Patellar**

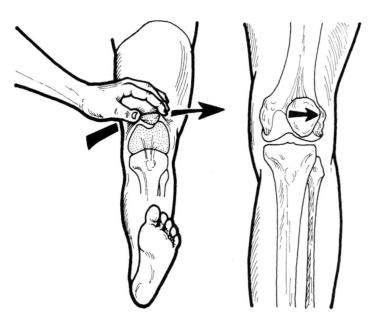

FIGURE 21.14. The apprehension test involves lateral displacement of the patella.

crepitus (a grating, grinding sensation) may also be noted during movement of the patellofemoral joint.

Joint Motion

Movement, or range of motion, is tested during examination of a chronic knee injury but not in an acute knee injury. The examiner, after asking the athlete to extend the knee, palpates the integrity of the extensor mechanism. Inability to extend the knee fully may be due to a rupture of the extensor mechanism or to pain and joint swelling. Active, as well as passive, range of motion should be documented with a goniometer; however, the knee should not be forced beyond the limits of pain. The examiner, after tracking the patella through both active and passive range of motion, should rotate the tibia internally and externally, with the knee flexed to 90 degrees, to note any blocking of rotation (a natural excursion of 5 degrees should show in each direction).

Stability Testing

The athletic trainer's initial examination of an acute knee injury need only determine gross ligamentous instability, or laxity. The treating physician will perform more specialized stability tests. The trainer first performs a gentle anteroposterior drawer test, with the knee joint at 20 to 30 degrees of flexion. This test, also termed the Lachman test, has replaced the traditional drawer test to detect anteroposterior instability. The test at 30 degrees is considered more accurate than the drawer test at 90 degrees of flexion in detecting anteroposterior laxity. Moreover, flexion to 90 degrees is usually not possible because of pain and swelling.

The athletic trainer next carries out an abduction-adduction stress test, with the knee at 30 degrees of flexion; this test may be repeated with the knee at full extension. The athletic trainer may do the abduction-adduction stress test gently at the site of injury. After the athlete has been removed, more comprehensive testing may follow,

depending on the athlete's injury and pain. These tests are described more thoroughly later in the chapter.

Meniscal Tests

The goal when evaluating the acutely injured knee is to exclude a significant fracture or ligamentous injury that requires immediate treatment. Tests of meniscal structures are inaccurate with acute injury because of pain and swelling. A meniscal tear is not an emergency. Later, if no serious ligamentous injury or fracture is found, meniscal tests such as the McMurray test and the Apley compression test (Fig. 21.15) can be done. In this latter test, the examiner places the athlete in a prone position and flexes the knee to 90 degrees. The examiner rotates the knee joint by rotating the leg while pressing the knee joint together. The result is positive if the test produces pain. The result may or may not be positive with a meniscal tear. The maneuver presses a dislodged portion of the meniscus or puts excess pressure on a damaged meniscal attachment, thereby producing pain. The pressure on the meniscal structures is re-

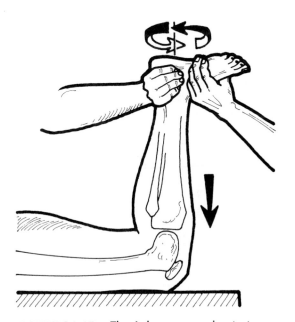

FIGURE 21.15.　The Apley compression test.

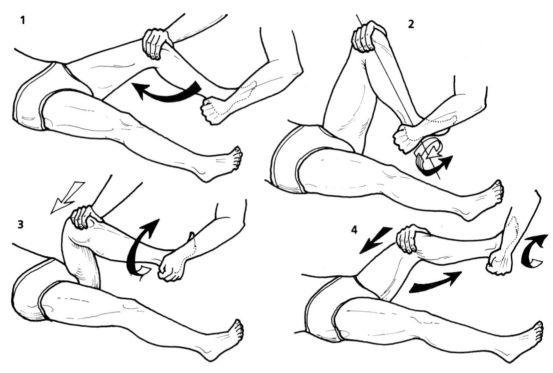

FIGURE 21.16. The McMurray test to produce click.

lieved by repeating the test with the joint distracted, and the pain is typically diminished or absent.

A modification of the Apley compression test can detect some meniscal tears. By gently flexing and extending the knee with the athlete supine, the examiner first places a valgus load on the knee joint, which produces increased compression to the lateral joint. Alternatively, the examiner places varus or adduction forces to the knee, which creates increased compression to the medial aspect of the joint. The examiner notes crepitus and pain while taking the knee through 0 to 90 degrees of motion. Crepitus detected upon palpation and heard at the joint may be a result of either a torn meniscus or surface deterioration that indicates early joint arthritis.

In the well-known McMurray test (Fig. 21.16) for a major disruption of the posterior horn of either the medial or lateral meniscus, the examiner, with the athlete's knee in full flexion, externally rotates the leg and then extends the knee. The desire is

to trap the displaced portion of the medial meniscus in the joint, producing an audible and palpable click or thud. Alternatively, with full flexion and marked internal rotation, the examiner attempts to dislodge a portion of the lateral meniscus into the joint, producing a similar sign.

Unfortunately, these tests are not highly accurate; in fact, they are frequently negative in athletes with meniscal tears. Meniscal tears in the chronically unstable knee are best diagnosed by the history and finding of localized tenderness to the joint line.

Radiographs

Radiographic studies of the knee should include routine anteroposterior, lateral, and axial patellar views. Additionally, condylar tunnel views and medial and lateral oblique views may be required in order to exclude an intra-articular fracture. Routine stress views are generally of little help unless the athlete is an adolescent with open epiphyseal growth centers and with pain

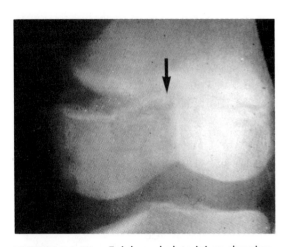

FIGURE 21.17. Epiphyseal plate injury showing opening at growth plate of femur. (From John A. Ogden. *Skeletal Injury in the Child,* 2d ed. Philadelphia: W. B. Saunders Company, 1990.)

above or below the joint line. In this instance, varus or valgus stress views may be included to rule out an injury to the epiphyseal plate. The radiographs will show opening at the growth plate of the femur or of the tibia rather than at the joint line (Fig. 21.17).

Summary of the Evaluation Process

In summary, routine evaluation of the acute knee injury establishes, in most cases, significant injury that requires immediate treatment and definitive diagnostic evaluation. If the approach outlined is performed consistently and systematically, with proper emphasis on historical and clinical findings during initial evaluation, the majority of serious injuries will be detected. While initial triage can identify those knee injuries that are emergencies, signs of severe injury may be subtle, and the severity may not be detected initially. Swelling the next day or continued pain or stiffness indicates the need for repeat evaluation. In fact, it is a good policy to reevaluate all knee injuries initially diagnosed as minor after 24 and even 48 hours. One final point requires emphasis: marked swelling in the knee joint within 24 hours of injury is an ominous sign indicating hemorrhage and possible significant intra-articular injury.

TREATMENT OF ACUTE KNEE INJURIES

First-Aid Measures

Following the initial evaluation and pending further disposition, an acutely injured knee should be protected and knee mobility decreased with a soft compression dressing combined with coaptation splinting (two slabs of plaster placed on either side of the limb and held together by an outer dressing). Commercial knee splints and knee immobilizers may also be used.

Knee dislocation, a disruption of the tibia-femoral relationship, is an infrequent but very serious orthopedic emergency. Damage to the popliteal artery occurs in at least 50 percent of cases, despite the fact that peripheral pulses may be palpable. A physician should attempt immediate reduction by extension and longitudinal traction. In addition to definitive orthopedic treatment, follow-up vascular evaluation is done. Anticipation of such emergencies is why the health care team should formulate an action plan, especially for times when the team physician is absent.

The athlete should not be allowed to bear weight on an acutely painful or swollen knee. The trainer should keep the athlete supine, with the involved leg elevated and ice packs applied to the knee intermittently before and after the compression dressing is applied. The foot and toes should always have active movement with normal color and warmth. The athlete should immediately report any increase in pain; any numbness, tingling, or weakness; or any change in skin color or warmth.

When referring an athlete to the treating physician, the athletic trainer must include a detailed report. A verbal description of the events surrounding the injury and immediate treatment is best, if at all possible. Because of developing muscle spasm and joint swelling, the initial exam is sometimes more reliable than a subsequent one.

Aspiration

Generally, aspiration of an acutely injured knee in which swelling has occurred within only 2 to 3 hours is not necessary except to relieve severe pain associated with a tense hemarthrosis. Aspiration should be avoided when possible, as it potentially introduces bacteria and may in rare cases lead to **pyarthrosis** (joint infection). A local anesthetic may be instilled on aspiration to obtain a more reliable stability examination.

CLASSIFICATION OF KNEE LIGAMENT INJURIES

Anatomical Stabilizing Systems

The stability of the knee depends on three anatomical systems. The *passive system* is composed of the ligament and capsular structures that link the femur, tibia, and patella. The *active system* is composed of the muscles that act through a functioning nervous system. The neuromuscular system coordinates muscle forces required for activity. Muscle forces provide stability to the joint and protect the ligaments from injury. Sudden turning or twisting, or a blow to the side of the knee, requires counteraction by muscle forces to keep the joint from collapsing. An athlete in superb condition in terms of muscle strength, coordination, and agility obviously responds much better to sudden, jarring movements. In contrast, an athlete with a recent injury or residual weakness from a previous injury may be at risk for repeat injury. This point cannot be overemphasized and stresses the need for proper rehabilitation of all the muscles of the extremity after injury. Neuromuscular coordination is the keystone for stability of the knee joint.

The third anatomical system providing stability relates to *joint geometry*. Some joints are exceptionally stable, such as the elbow with its interlocking bone ends. The knee joint, however, has much less inherent bony stability, because it must have more freedom for motion. Besides being able to flex and extend, the knee rotates internally and externally. Still, the geometry of the knee joint does provide considerable stability. The femoral condyles are literally pressed into the tibial surface. The tibial intercondylar notch sweeps upward, providing a bumper stop for excessive inward or outward femoral rotation about the tibia. The meniscal structures add a restraining peripheral ring and increase the concavity of the tibial surface, particularly of the lateral tibial plateau, where the convex surface slopes backward in contrast to the concave medial side.

Forces on the Knee

With activity, forces much larger than commonly realized are placed across joints. For example, walking places about three times a person's body weight across the knee joint (also hip and ankle joints); a person weighing 70 kg places up to 210 kg across the knee joint. In jumping and other strenuous activity, the forces may be as great as six to eight times body weight (a half ton in a large individual). Each muscle contraction exerts a force that moves the joint about a certain axis (e.g., flexion or extension). The muscle forces also compress the joint, which provides stability.

Loss of Joint Stability

Activity generates large external forces that act on the knee joint. These forces must be balanced and resisted by the three stabilizing systems—that is, the internal forces in ligaments, muscles, and joint geometry. If the external forces are too high and cannot be properly resisted, then ligaments or muscles may be injured or bones fractured (Fig. 21.18). With sudden external forces, such as in a clipping injury or in an unexpected fall, the muscles may not have time to contract and resist the injury forces. Full resistance is then placed on the ligaments, with ligament injury all too likely. As soon as a ligament tears, the joint can separate even farther. If the femoral condyle breaks off, then the stabilizing effect of the interlocking bone ends is lost, resulting in increased instability and probably complete

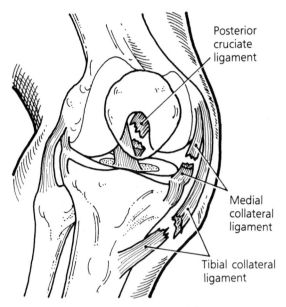

FIGURE 21.18. Sudden external forces may result in multiple disruptions to the ligamentous structures.

Posterior cruciate ligament

Medial collateral ligament

Tibial collateral ligament

collapse. Stability of the knee and any other joint is a dynamic balance between external forces and internal forces. The rationale for

many treatment programs, therefore, aims at increasing stability of the joint. All three systems for joint stability are required for proper functioning.

Classification Systems

Three different classification systems denote the type and extent of injury to the ligaments and capsular structures of the knee. Each system is somewhat separate and provides additional information.

Severity of Sprain

The American Medical Association's (AMA) standard nomenclature of athletic injuries classifies ligament injuries into *mild sprains* (few fibers torn), *moderate sprains* (a definite tear in some component of the ligament), and *severe sprains* (ligament torn completely across). The classification is based on the signs, symptoms, and severity of the injury (Table 21.1). Although the AMA classification provides an overall diagnosis of the degree of ligamentous injury, there is one criticism of this system. A

TABLE 21.1. Clinical Diagnosis of Ligament Injury

	First-Degree Sprain	Second-Degree Sprain	Third-Degree Sprain
Synonym	Mild sprain	Moderate sprain	Severe sprain
Etiology	Direct or indirect trauma to joint	Same	Severe direct or indirect trauma to joint
Symptoms	Pain; mild disability	Pain; moderate disability	Pain; severe disability
Signs	Mild point tenderness; no abnormal motion; little or no swelling	Point tenderness; moderate loss of function; slight to moderate abnormal motion; swelling; localized hemorrhage	Loss of function; marked abnormal motion; possible deformity; x-rays: stress films demonstrate abnormal motion
Complications	Tendency to recurrence, aggravation	Tendency to recurrence, aggravation; persistent instability; traumatic arthritis	Persistent instability; traumatic arthritis
Pathology	Minor tearing of ligament	Partial tear of ligament	Complete tear of ligament

Standard Nomenclature of Athletic Injuries, American Medical Association, Chicago, 1976.

sprain of a ligament is defined in medical dictionaries as only a partial tearing, without complete disruption. Also, a sprain commonly denotes no subluxation or dislocation of the joint. This is correct only for the first-degree, or mild, sprain. But in the AMA classification, a second-degree sprain indicates moderate motion or joint laxity, and a third-degree sprain, marked abnormal laxity. There is no laxity by definition with a first-degree sprain where there is only minor tearing of ligament fibers. If laxity is present, there is by definition either a second- or third-degree sprain.

Amount and Direction of Laxity

With laxity to the knee joint, a ligamentous restraint has been functionally disrupted to one degree or another, and the injury is significant. This injury can be further classified by *amount of laxity* (Table 21.2) and by *direction of laxity* (Table 21.3). The amount of laxity may not correlate in every case with the degree of ligament damage. In some ligament injuries, there may be a complete tear of a ligament (functional capacity lost) but little laxity. This is because other ligaments may block the amount of joint distraction or opening, even though a primary ligament restraint is torn. (These secondary restraints are discussed in greater detail later in the chapter.) However, an accurate grading by amount of joint opening is a useful index for defining the injury and treatment.

The classification by the direction of the laxity (see Table 21.3) is divided into the four straight laxities and the four rotatory laxities (also discussed later in the chapter).

Specific Ligaments Disrupted

The injured ligaments must be classified. A simple classification is given in the following list. The structures involved in the injury are specified based on the laxity exam, thus simply defining injury by the ligament involved. Remember, some laxities can be rather complex when one or two ligaments are torn.

A. Medial ligament injuries
   1. No associated anterior cruciate tear
   2. Associated anterior cruciate tear
   3. Associated anterior and posterior cruciate tears

B. Lateral ligament injury
   1. No associated anterior cruciate tear
   2. Associated anterior cruciate tear
   3. Associated anterior and posterior cruciate tears

C. Anterior cruciate injury: as the primary injury

D. Posterior cruciate injury: as the primary injury

In this classification, injury to the medial and lateral sides is easily identified in terms of seriousness. If the injury is confined to the tibial or fibular collateral ligaments and capsular structures, the prognosis for healing and functional stability is good. If the anterior cruciate is also injured, the prognosis is less favorable. In this context, an anterior cruciate injury, in association with any other major ligament structure disruption, has an overall poor prognosis. The presence or absence of the anterior cruciate

TABLE 21.2. Classification of Ligament Injury

	Straight Laxity	Rotatory Laxity
First-degree	Mild (less than 5 mm distraction)	Mild
Second-degree	Moderate (5–10 mm distraction)	Moderate
Third-degree	Severe (over 10 mm distraction)	Severe

TABLE 21.3. Direction of Laxity

Straight*	Rotatory
Medial	Anteromedial (anterior external rotation)
Lateral	Anterolateral (anterior internal rotation)
Anterior	Posteromedial (posterior internal rotation)
Posterior	Posterolateral (posterior external rotation)

*Denotes position of knee joint with tibia moving on fixed femur.

tear therefore immediately defines the seriousness of the injury.

With an associated posterior cruciate tear, the injury is actually a dislocation of the knee. The prognosis for return to athletic activities after tears of both cruciate ligaments is even more dismal. In severe injuries, with one or both cruciates torn, an athlete is fortunate to have a stable knee for recreational activities. Even if a stable knee is achieved through surgical reconstruction, participation in vigorous activities may not be advisable, since a repeat injury could potentially result in increased disability, making even activities of daily living difficult for the athlete.

Tears involving predominantly the anterior or posterior cruciate ligament have separate categories. These tears are not isolated in the strictest sense. Associated injuries to the capsular ligaments, meniscus, and joint are frequent. The predominant injury in these cases in terms of joint stability is to the cruciate ligament.

MECHANISMS OF LIGAMENT INJURY

The description of the mechanism of injury includes all details of the injury. Of importance is the position of the knee joint at the time of injury. The direction in which the knee displaces or rotates may suggest which ligaments have been torn. The athletic trainer may actually observe the injury—obviously, the best perspective. Did the knee bend to the inside (medial opening, abduction, or valgus position) or to the outside (lateral opening, adduction, or varus position)? Did the knee bend backward (hyperextension)? Did the femur rotate over a fixed tibia (internal or external)? Did the athlete feel as though the knee were coming apart? If so, it probably did, with tearing of the ligaments.

The athlete may remember only a few details of the injury, but even a limited description can provide important diagnostic clues. For example, most anterior cruciate tears occur in noncontact injuries, as with a sudden turning or twisting of the femur to the outside. The athlete may feel a pop. Swelling within 24 hours, often within 2 hours, means joint hemorrhage and implies a serious injury. Posterior cruciate injury may be suspected with a sudden blow to the front of the tibia, driving it backward. This injury commonly occurs in auto accidents when the knee strikes the dashboard. The same mechanism of injury can occur during a fall in any sporting activity. Remember, in cruciate injuries, the athletic trainer's findings on laxity examination may be entirely normal. All aspects of the injury mechanism, symptoms, and other data must be compiled to make a tentative diagnosis.

Table 21.4 lists common mechanisms of injury and the ligament structures that may be injured. In describing rotation of the knee, it is customary to refer to the tibia as the part that moves. Thus, a valgus external rotation injury means that the femur is fixed and the tibia is placed in a valgus position (medial joint opening) and externally rotates. Actually, in most injury situations the reverse motion occurs. The femur

TABLE 21.4.   Common Mechanisms of Knee Injury

Mechanism of Injury (Knee Position*)	Ligament Injury
Valgus (straight medial opening)	Tibial collateral plus capsular ligaments†
Valgus external rotation	Medial structures, medial meniscus, anterior cruciate, "terrible triad"
Varus (straight lateral opening)	Fibular collateral plus capsular ligaments†
Varus internal rotation	Lateral ligaments plus anterior cruciate
Varus external rotation	Lateral ligaments plus posterior cruciate
Hyperextension	Posterior capsule and posterior cruciate‡
Direct blow driving tibia backward	Posterior cruciate
Direct blow driving tibia forward	Anterior cruciate

*Tibia moving with femur fixed.
†Severe opening implies injury to either one or both cruciates.
‡Severe hyperextension may also injure the anterior cruciate ligament.

and upper body rotate about the fixed tibia and planted foot. The convention has always been to refer to the tibia as moving, and this is actually what happens in the clinical laxity exam. The tibia is moved while the femur remains stationary. Thus, there is some justification for keeping this system. Remember, the same joint position is reached and the same ligaments are stretched whether the tibia externally rotates on a fixed femur or the femur internally rotates on a fixed tibia. In describing an injury, the femur is fixed, and the position of the tibia is being described, unless otherwise stated.

TESTING FOR KNEE INSTABILITIES

Controversy exists over testing for knee laxity, specifically over which ligament structures are tested; therefore, athletic trainers may interpret identical findings differently. In view of this problem, each trainer should develop an individual approach and refine the techniques continually on the basis of experience and developing concepts. The information provided here will form the basis for such an individualized testing program.

For many years, straight anterior, straight posterior, straight medial, and straight lateral instabilities were well appreciated. In 1968, the concept of rotatory instability was first described. What appeared to be a straight anterior laxity was, in fact, the medial aspect of the tibia externally rotating out from underneath the medial femoral condyle. Since 1968, other forms of rotatory instability have been described.

Testing for knee instability must be conducted meticulously and with precision. The first observation may be more valid than subsequent ones because of the additional pain and muscle spasm which often develop after an injury. The test for medial or lateral opening of the joint is initially done with the knee in 20 to 30 degrees of flexion, because full extension is often impossible. Even when full extension can be achieved, it is often better to conduct the test first with the knee flexed to prevent initiating muscle spasm that will distort any further information obtained. One positive test result indicates a laxity. A negative test result does not necessarily exclude damage to the ligament in question, because remaining secondary restraints may block the opening of the knee. Additionally, muscle spasms may block stability testing. During testing, the athlete should be reassured, relaxed, and made as comfortable as possible while in a fully supine position with a pillow under the head.

Unidirectional Laxities

Straight Anterior Laxity

True anterior instability, or **straight anterior laxity**, is demonstrated by a straightforward motion of the tibia on the femur; it cannot occur unless the anterior cruciate ligament has been damaged (Fig. 21.19). The anterior cruciate ligament provides about 85 percent of the resisting force to anterior movement of the tibia on the femur. All of the remaining medial and lateral ligamentous structures provide a small force and are thus classified as secondary restraints. On rare occasions following medial collateral ligament and capsular ligamentous damage, a mild anteromedial rotation of the medial aspect of the tibia may give the false impression of an anterior drawer. This anteromedial rotatory instability is discussed later.

A subtle anterior laxity is often difficult to see in an acutely injured and swollen knee. The anterior drawer test conducted at 30 degrees of flexion (Fig. 21.20) is often more reliable than one at 90 degrees of flexion, because the secondary ligamentous restraints are less tight at 30 degrees of flexion and therefore allow more anterior tibial displacement when the anterior cruciate ligament is torn. The anterior drawer test at 30 degrees of knee flexion, also called the Lachman test, is very useful in acute knee injuries (see Fig. 21.20).

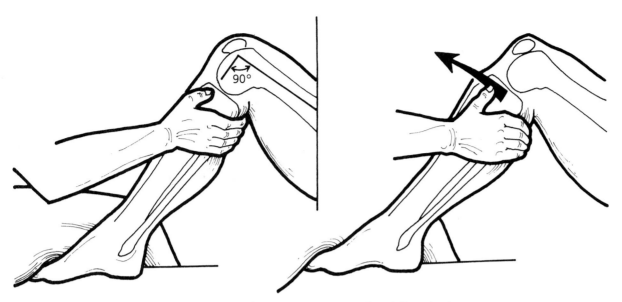

FIGURE 21.19. Anterior drawer test determines anterior cruciate instability. Flex knee to 90 degrees and stabilize foot. Note forward shift of tibia.

The Lachman test can be performed without lifting the extremity. The athlete must be relaxed. With one hand, the examiner gently grasps the lower thigh just above the patella, and with the other hand, gently grasps the proximal aspect of the tibia. The thumb may extend over the tibial tubercle to palpate the joint line. While stabilizing the thigh, the examiner carries out an anteroposterior drawer motion, with the hand

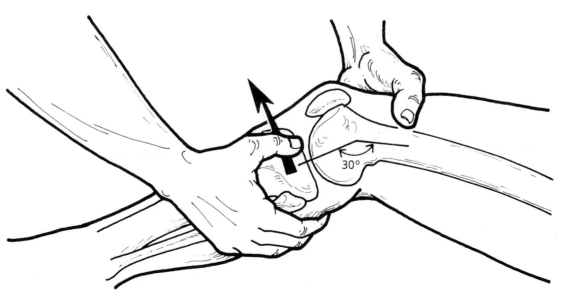

FIGURE 21.20. Lachman test for anterior cruciate instability is at 30 degrees of flexion. The extremity does not have to be lifted or the foot stabilized.

holding the proximal tibia. Subtle changes in anteroposterior displacement of the tibia can thus be detected. When this test proves positive, subsequent anterolateral rotatory instability tests are performed as described later. An increase in anteroposterior laxity means either anterior cruciate or posterior cruciate damage. On occasion, both ligaments may be damaged. Because of this possibility, any positive drawer test should be followed by a gravity drawer test.

The **gravity drawer test** is performed with the athlete supine and hips and knees flexed to 90 degrees. The athlete's foot can rest in a chair to allow relaxation of the extremity. Posterior subluxation of the tibia in this position as compared with the normal knee indicates a posterior cruciate ligament instability. When the anterior cruciate ligament is torn, anterolateral rotatory instability also occurs. This should not be confusing. The anterior cruciate ligament provides both straight anterior stability and anterolateral rotatory stability. Ligaments typically provide stability in both a straight and a rotatory plane of motion. Remember also that the amount of laxity depends on

the tightness of the remaining secondary restraints. Some knees may have only a small initial laxity. With time, the weaker secondary restraints stretch, and a grossly positive anterior drawer motion develops. Thus, the laxity of an acute knee may differ from that of the chronic knee. Occasionally, the anterior cruciate ligament may be partially torn. The anterior drawer sign may or may not be positive in such situations. When only a portion of the anterior cruciate ligament seems to be ruptured, as noted at arthroscopy, the remaining portion of the ligament usually has also sustained some microfailure.

Straight Posterior Laxity

With **straight posterior laxity**, the tibia can be displaced posteriorly in a neutral position—that is, without any rotation. The posterior cruciate ligament is the primary ligamentous restraint, providing about 95 percent of the resisting force for posterior displacement of the tibia. All of the structures provide a small remaining contribution. However, these less effective structures may still block the drawer test in acute knee injuries. Later, when stretching takes place, the amount of posterior displacement of the tibia may substantially increase.

A posterior laxity can be confused with an anterior laxity. The neutral point for the knee joint for anteroposterior laxity must be established. A posterior sag or dropping back of the tibia can often be observed with the knee flexed to 90 degrees. If the tibia has dropped back in the drawer test, the athletic trainer brings the tibia forward and may mistakenly believe the anterior drawer test is positive. In fact, the tibia started from a dropped-back position, and the real injury is to the posterior cruciate ligament.

The gravity drawer test should be performed as a routine procedure (Fig. 21.21). In this test, a ruler or straight edge is placed across the front of the knee. Any concavity compared with the normal side indicates a

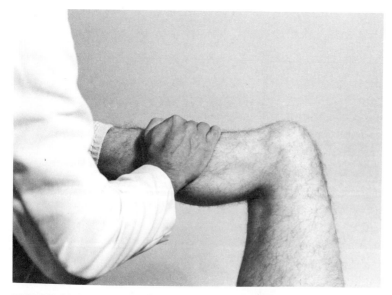

FIGURE 21.21. Gravity drawer test. Note posterior drop back of the tibia.

posterior dropping back of the tibia, and a posterior cruciate tear is suspected. The test is not accurate with long-standing Osgood-Schlatter disease, because the height of the tibial tubercle may be different on one side compared with the other.

Posterolateral rotatory instability, as will be discussed, may give a false appearance of a dropping back of the tibia when, in fact, the tibia is actually externally rotating. In posterolateral rotatory instability, the posterior cruciate may be intact or only partially damaged.

In the acutely injured knee, the posterior cruciate ligament may be completely disrupted, but the posterior drawer test is often negative. The posterior capsular structure prevents dropping back of the tibia. In the chronic posterior cruciate injury, the weak secondary restraints gradually stretch, and the test findings become grossly positive. The time for acute repair is lost if the diagnosis is not initially made. As previously indicated, the mechanism of injury may often suggest a posterior cruciate tear. Any loading on the front of the tibia which drives it backward suggests a posterior cruciate injury.

Straight Medial Laxity

In **straight medial laxity**, there is medial opening of the joint, or **valgus laxity**. This abnormal motion is different from anteromedial rotatory instability where the tibia rotates anteriorly and there is an associated medial opening. To examine for medial or valgus laxity, the athletic trainer places the knee in 30 degrees of flexion (Fig. 21.22). The physical integrity of the tibial collateral ligament is palpated while the valgus stress is applied. The knee can actually be rocked in an abduction-adduction position to test the medial and lateral sides at the same time. Placing the finger at the joint line may increase the accuracy of this test. The amount of joint opening should be estimated in millimeters to classify the amount of laxity, as discussed.

Increased medial opening at 30 degrees of knee flexion indicates damage to the primary restraint, the tibial collateral ligament. This ligament supports about 80 percent of the force applied to the knee joint at 30 degrees of flexion. Because isolated failure does not occur, opening also indicates damage to the secondary restraints, namely

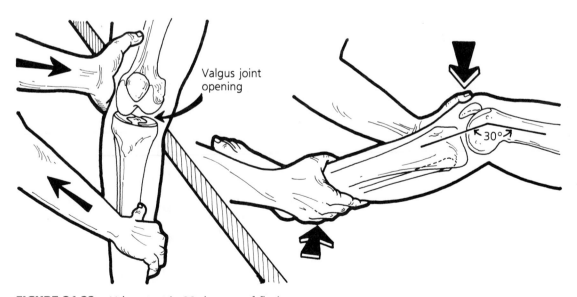

FIGURE 21.22. Valgus test in 30 degrees of flexion.

the medial capsular structures. As the knee is taken toward extension, the posterior medial capsule progressively becomes tighter and accounts for a greater force in resisting joint opening.

Joint line opening with the knee in extension also indicates damage to the posterior medial capsular structures. If the opening of the medial joint is large (over 10 mm), then damage to the anterior or posterior cruciate structures should also be suspected. After sequential rupture of the collateral ligament and capsular structures, full reliance is placed on the cruciate structures. Therefore, with significant medial opening these structures may be damaged as well. With the knee in full hyperextension, the cruciate ligaments alone lock the femur into the tibia, and no medial opening is possible. Any finding of medial opening with the knee in hyperextension might suggest a severe injury that involves all of the medial structures plus the cruciate ligaments.

An alternative way for the athletic trainer to examine medial laxity is to hold the lower leg cradled against his or her side, with the thigh supported (Fig. 21.23). To examine the right knee, the trainer gently

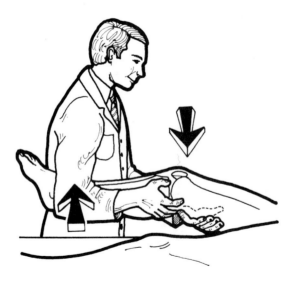

FIGURE 21.23. Alternate test for straight medial laxity.

places his or her left hand over the posterolateral aspect of the athlete's thigh, supporting the thigh. The trainer then places his or her right hand over the medial joint line of the knee. The trainer's right arm supports the foot and leg against his or her side. At 30 degrees of knee flexion, the trainer applies a gentle valgus force with the left hand. The fingertips of the trainer's right hand are placed directly over the joint line to estimate the millimeters of joint opening. In the severely swollen knee, the medial joint line is located by palpating the lower pole of the patella and proceeding directly medial and posterior to where the fingertips locate the joint line. The physical integrity of the tibial collateral ligament can also be palpated. The athlete's knee can be examined in both positions, with the leg cradled against the athletic trainer's side or with the athlete's leg over the side of the examining table.

Straight Lateral Laxity

The techniques for determining **straight lateral laxity**, or **varus laxity**, are identical to those for determining medial laxity. The athletic trainer applies a varus force to produce straight lateral opening of the joint. Varus laxity with the knee in 30 degrees of flexion indicates an injury to the fibular collateral ligament and lateral capsular structures. The fibular collateral ligament is the primary ligamentous restraint to the lateral aspect of the joint, accounting for about 70 percent of resisting force during the testing procedure. The lateral capsular structures and underlying anterior and posterior cruciate ligaments also provide varus stability. Again, when the knee is extended, the posterolateral capsular structures tighten, just as on the medial side, and any opening indicates capsular and posterior capsular damage in addition to collateral ligament damage.

With the knee fully extended, significant joint opening indicates cruciate damage as discussed for the medial side. With the knee fully extended or hyperextended, significant lateral opening indicates damage to the cruciate ligaments, as well. Additionally, any time the lateral opening is large—for example, increased 0.4 inch (1 cm) or more over the opposite side—involvement of the cruciate ligaments should be suspected, no matter what the knee flexion position tested. Cruciate laxity is verified best by a Lachman or drawer test.

Genu Recurvatum

Genu recurvatum, or the ability of the knee to bend backward, is not classified as a true instability (Fig. 21.24). However, it is not uncommon, and therefore some discussion is indicated. Three types of genu recurvatum are possible. The first type is physiologic, related to generalized laxity of the knee joint. Hyperextension to 15 degrees may be seen in the loose-jointed individual. An individual with this amount of hyperextension generally does poorly after sustaining a ligamentous injury because the knee joint lacks additional supporting ligamentous structures. Rarely, increased recurvatum may be a result of chronic stretching of the posterior capsular and ligamentous structures, and may be an infrequent reason for excluding an individual from participating in strenuous sports activities. The importance of examining both extremities is underscored in these individuals. Other joints in loose-jointed individuals may show generalized laxity as well.

The second type of genu recurvatum is actually a posterolateral rotatory instability. Instead of pure hyperextension of the joint, the tibia rotates posterolaterally. The third type of recurvatum is caused by posterior capsular and associated cruciate ligament damage. Severe hyperextension injuries to the knee joint can damage capsular and cruciate structures. The anterior cruciate, posterior cruciate, or both can be injured, depending on the type of hyperextension injury. In the true hyperextension injury, the posterior capsule and posterior cruciate ligament are injured first. If the hyperextension continues, or if any compo-

nent of the force directs the tibia forward, then the anterior cruciate ligament is also injured. Sometimes hyperextension is described, but instead the tibia is actually being displaced forward, similar to an anterior drawer. This condition causes damage predominantly to the anterior cruciate ligament. Hyperextension injuries are often associated with damage to the neurovascular system in the popliteal space.

The Multidirectional Laxities (Combined Laxities)

Anteromedial Rotatory Instability

In **anteromedial rotatory instability**, the medial plateau of the tibia rotates anteriorly. Additionally, joint opening on the medial side can be detected. The classic form of this instability involves disruption of the superficial tibial collateral ligament; adjacent capsular structures, including the posterior medial complex and medial capsule; and the anterior cruciate ligament. In a more subtle form of this injury, the predominant injury is to the superficial tibial collateral ligament and associated medial capsular structures without major involvement of the anterior cruciate ligament. In this case, there is external rotation of the tibia and medial opening. However, because the anterior cruciate ligament is intact, anterior tibial displacement is less.

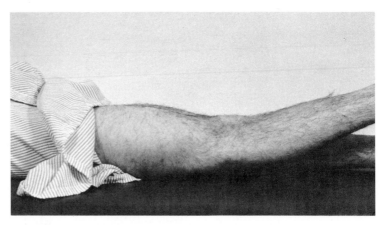

FIGURE 21.24. Genu recurvatum.

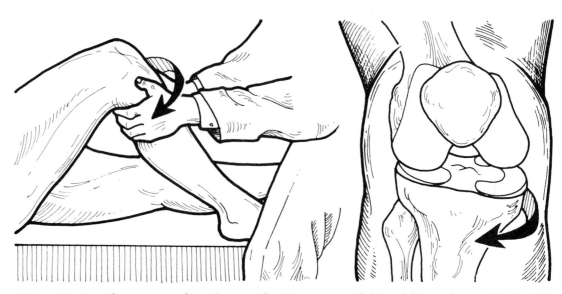

FIGURE 21.25. Slocum external rotation test showing anteromedial instability as the medial tibial plateau shifts forward and externally rotates.

There are two tests for anteromedial rotatory instability. The first is the **Slocum external rotation test** (Fig. 21.25), which is conducted with the hip flexed to approximately 45 degrees and the knee to approximately 80 degrees; the athlete's foot rests on the examining table. The normal knee is tested first for comparison with the injured knee. The athletic trainer sits on the side of the table, trapping the athlete's foot with his or her upper thigh, and gently places both hands about the lower leg below the knee. With the index finger, the trainer palpates the hamstrings to be certain they are lax and then applies a gentle forward symmetrical pull. The degree of anterior drawer in the injured knee as compared with the normal knee is recorded, with the trainer noting the amount of laxity in 5-mm increments. With a simple anterior drawer test, the neutral rotation is essential to focus on the movements of both the medial tibial condyle and the lateral tibial condyle to learn whether asymmetrical rotation is involved with the anterior tibial displacement. Moreover, if the athlete is cooperative, the basic rotational elements of the anterior drawer can also be tested. With the athlete's foot in neutral rotation, a pure rotational force is applied to the medial tibial condyle, and the anteromedial rotation is noted. A similar procedure can be performed on the lateral tibial condyle to reveal the amount of anterolateral rotatory instability.

After the neutral anterior drawer and rotational components are established, the athletic trainer repeats the test at 10 degrees of external rotation. The normal knee shows very little change in the amount of anterior drawer for the first 10 to 15 degrees of external rotation. Actually, the cruciates are unwinding, and the amount of anterior drawer may increase slightly. Thereafter, the amount of anterior drawer should progressively diminish as the amount of tibial rotation on the femur tightens the medial ligamentous sleeve. Predominantly, this maneuver tightens the tibial collateral ligament, but all of the medial capsular structures are tightened. An increasing amount of external rotation eventually blocks the amount of anteromedial excursion of the tibia, because some medial structures are tightened no matter how much damage has been produced. Thus, the amount of anter-

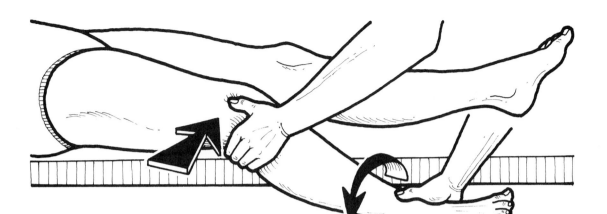

FIGURE 21.26. Alternative test for anteromedial rotatory instability. External rotation is applied to the tibia while applying valgus stress in slight flexion.

omedial excursion must be gauged in comparison with the opposite side.

The second common test for anteromedial rotatory instability, the abduction stress test, uses the same position as in the test for medial instability, where the extremity is dropped from the side of the table (Fig. 21.26). In testing for straight medial instability, only a straight valgus force is applied. In other words, only straight medial opening in one plane is elicited. In the test for anteromedial rotatory laxity, however, external rotation is applied to the tibia at the same time the valgus distraction force is applied. Therefore, increased external rotation and medial joint opening are produced together. In many knees, this test may be more sensitive for anteromedial rotation than the Slocum external rotation test, because both medial opening and increased external rotation occur simultaneously. Thus, the rotation component, as well as the medial opening component, is being tested, which increases the test's sensitivity. Because rotation is also occurring, the athletic trainer must be careful not to overestimate the amount of true medial opening. Moreover, this test is more accurate with the knee partially flexed. With full extension, other ligamentous structures

tend to tighten, which may block the findings.

Note that in Figure 21.27, the tibia rotates about an axis that is shifted to the lateral side. If the rotation axis were

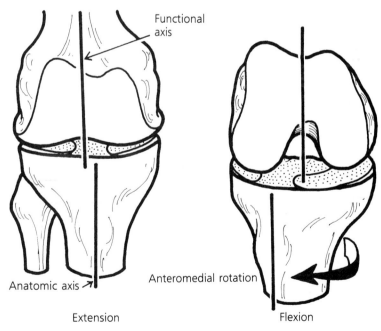

FIGURE 21.27. Tibia rotating about an axis shifted laterally in anteromedial rotatory instability.

straight through the center of the tibia, then normal external rotation would occur. With the axis shifted to the lateral aspect, both anterior displacement of the tibia and increased rotation occur—anteromedial rotatory instability.

To summarize, the primary ligamentous restraint for anteromedial rotatory instability is the tibial collateral ligament, which resists external tibial rotation and medial joint opening, assisted by secondary restraints consisting of the capsular structures. The anterior cruciate ligament provides the primary restraint for the anterior drawer component of this instability. Therefore, if marked laxity is present, there is a defect in both ligaments.

Anterolateral Rotatory Instability

Anterolateral rotatory instability is characterized by an anterior internal rotational subluxation of the lateral tibial condyle on the femur. The lateral pivot shift test is used for diagnosing this laxity. The lateral tibial condyle subluxates anteriorly from under the lateral femoral condyle. This is particularly likely to occur when an athlete makes a sudden change in direction, such as in a cutting movement or while decelerating. This subluxation is assisted by the anterior pull of the quadriceps mechanism. Also, the iliotibial band passes anterior to the flexion axis of the knee joint as the knee extends, and therefore its ability to resist the anterolateral subluxation is lessened.

The most frequent rotatory instability encountered in the knee is anterolateral. A number of clinical laxity tests can reproduce the subluxation of the lateral tibial plateau: the lateral pivot shift test, the Slocum anterolateral rotatory instability test, the Hughston jerk test, and the flexion-rotation drawer test. All of these tests produce an anterolateral subluxation of the joint followed by a reduction. The reduction is usually accompanied by a thud, jump, or jerk within the joint.

Anterior cruciate–deficient knees have mild anterolateral laxity that may be diffi-

cult to detect. These knees have no obvious jump, jerk, or thud, and the classic pivot shift test may be negative. The flexion-rotation drawer test and the Lachman anterior drawer test are often more sensitive, indicating subtle anterior cruciate laxity. These cases must be diagnosed for two reasons. First, this form of laxity is very common in the athlete. Rehabilitation and modification of strenuous activities may overcome symptoms and markedly improve knee function. Second, mild symptoms of swelling and giving way may be incorrectly attributed to a torn meniscus when the gross pivot shift sign tests are negative.

The primary restraint for anterolateral rotatory stability is the anterior cruciate ligament. The iliotibial band and, to a lesser degree, the lateral capsule provide a secondary restraint. Biomechanical studies have shown that rupture of the anterior cruciate as the primary lesion results in a mild to moderate laxity. For a severe laxity, the lateral structures must show associated laxity. This laxity may be (1) caused by a physiologic laxity without injury to the lateral structures or (2) a result of actual injury to the lateral structures. In acute injuries, hemorrhage may be noted in the lateral capsule. Damage to the iliotibial band is often difficult to detect. In the loose-jointed athlete with physiologic laxity of the supporting ligaments, including the lateral structures, rupture of the anterior cruciate alone results in severe third-degree anterolateral rotatory instability. In the more tight-jointed athlete, rupture of the anterior cruciate ligament initially results in only a mild to moderate laxity because the lateral structures provide a restraining force. If the lateral structures subsequently stretch, a severe rotatory laxity may eventually develop. The spectrum of knees that presents with this laxity underscores the need for performing more than one of the tests for anterolateral laxity.

Lateral pivot shift test. In the **lateral pivot shift test**, the athlete should be supine and relaxed (Fig. 21.28). The athletic trainer

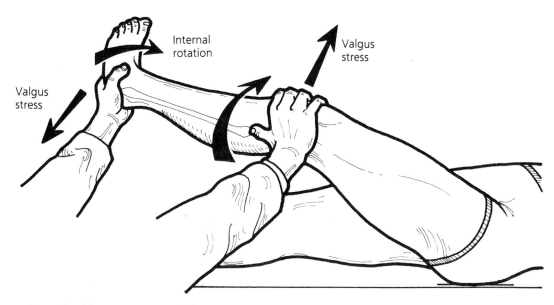

FIGURE 21.28. Lateral pivot shift test.

places the heel of the athlete's involved leg in the palm of his or her hand. To test the left knee, the trainer places the left hand under the left heel. The right hand is placed over the lateral tibia, with the thumb behind the fibular head. The trainer takes the knee to approximately 5 degrees of flexion and uses both hands to internally rotate the lower leg on the femur. At the same time, the trainer pushes the proximal tibia anteriorly with the proximal hand. Lifting the fibular head gently with the thumb will help. At this point in a markedly positive test, the lateral tibial plateau subluxates anteriorly out from under the femoral condyle. Using the right hand as a fulcrum, the athletic trainer applies a gentle valgus stress with the left hand to compress the lateral compartment. The iliotibial band acting as an extensor in this position becomes a flexor as it passes over the lateral femoral condyle at about 20 degrees of flexion. In a positive test, the tibia markedly reduces, both visibly and palpably. The key elements of a positive lateral pivot shift test are internal rotation of the lower leg on the femur, lateral compartment compression, and excursion of the knee from an extended to flexed position.

Slocum anterolateral rotatory instability test. The **Slocum anterolateral rotatory instability test** is a modification of the lateral pivot shift test (Fig. 21.29). The athlete lies on his or her side, with the uninvolved leg flexed at the hip, while the knee and the pelvis are permitted to fall back. This position automatically produces internal rotation and a gentle valgus stress to the knee. To test the right knee, the athletic trainer places his or her right hand on the proximal tibia to provide further internal rotation and to take the knee out of hyperextension. The trainer then places his or her left hand on the femoral condylar region and, with both hands, gently increases the valgus stress on the joint. As the knee goes into about 20 degrees of flexion, the subluxation reduces visibly, palpably, and audibly. In a markedly positive test, the lateral tibial condyle is easily seen going from a subluxated position in extension to a reduced position in flexion.

Hughston jerk test. In the **Hughston jerk test** for anterolateral rotatory instability, the athlete lies supine, with the knee flexed approximately to a right angle and the hip at about 45 degrees of flexion (Fig. 21.30).

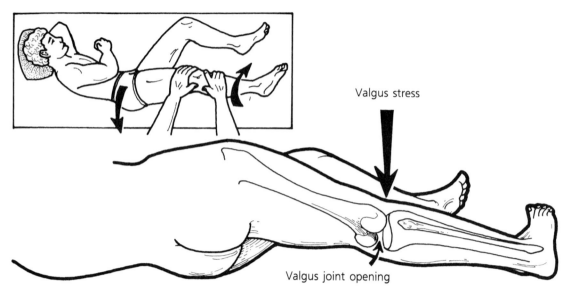

FIGURE 21.29. Slocum anterolateral rotatory instability test.

To test the left knee, the athletic trainer holds the athlete's left foot with his or her left hand and applies an internal rotational force. Simultaneously, the trainer places his or her right hand over the proximal tibia and fibula to aid the internal rotation and act as a fulcrum for the application of a valgus stress. While these forces are maintained, the trainer gradually extends the knee. Subluxation of the lateral tibiofemor-

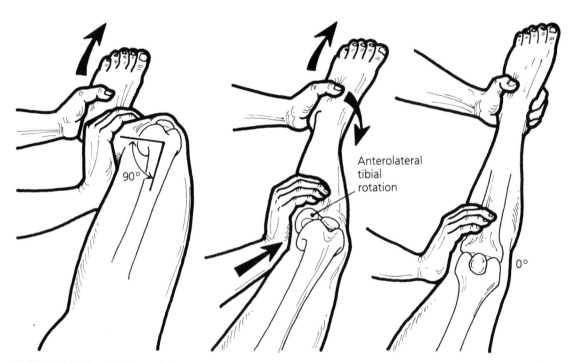

FIGURE 21.30. Hughston jerk test.

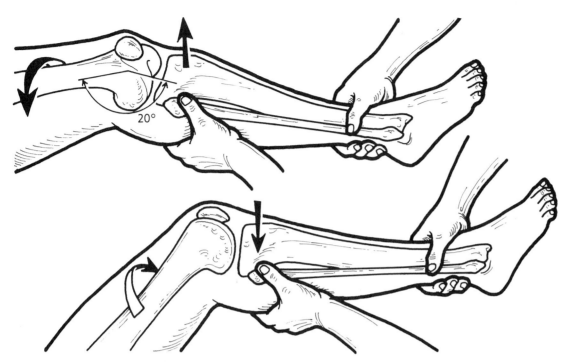

FIGURE 21.31. Flexion-rotation drawer test.

al articulation occurs at about 30 degrees. The positive test produces a snap and a pop. If the knee is carried to complete extension, reduction again occurs.

Flexion-rotation drawer test. The **flexion-rotation drawer test** is a modification of the pivot shift test and the Lachman test (Fig. 21.31). This test has proved extremely sensitive in detecting mild and moderate anterolateral rotatory instability. Again, as indicated for severe forms of instability, the pivot shift test and other tests are used.

In the flexion-rotation drawer test, the leg is held in neutral rotation at 20 degrees of knee flexion. The quadriceps must be relaxed. With anterior cruciate laxity, the weight of the thigh results in a posterior dropping back of the femur—the drawer component of the test. Very importantly, the femur also externally rotates—the rotational component of the test. This increased external rotation of the femur produces the anterolateral subluxation of the lateral tibiofemoral articulation (see Fig. 21.31). Thus, simply holding the leg produces the subluxated position of the lateral tibiofemoral joint. A gentle flexion movement of approximately 10 degrees, combined with a downward push on the tibia, produces a fully reduced position. The tibia moves posteriorly into a normal relationship with the femur. The athletic trainer gently goes between the subluxated extended position and reduced flexed position. In essence, the tibia or leg is used as the handle to flip the femur in an up-down motion.

The flexion-rotation test brings out both anteroposterior tibial translation and the rotatory motions of the femur; therefore, it can help detect the more subtle anterior cruciate laxity. It is also highly diagnostic under general anesthesia in detecting anterior cruciate tears. With the up-down rocking and gentle extension-flexion of the knee, the normal concavity of the infrapatellar tendon and tibial region is decreased in the subluxated position and increased in the flexion position, exactly as in the Lachman test. However, the femoral rotation motion can also be seen and felt during the test. A lateral valgus compressive force may

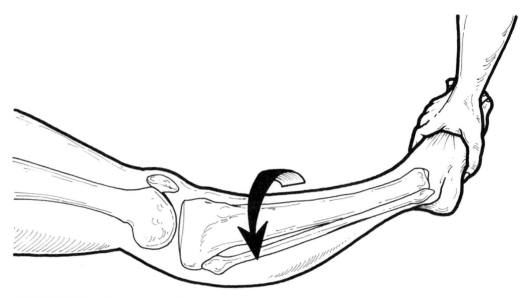

FIGURE 21.32. External rotation-recurvatum test.

or may not be applied, depending on the examiner.

In summary, tests for anterolateral rotatory instability all produce a subluxation of the lateral tibial condyle anterolaterally, with the knee in a near-extended position, followed by reduction in flexion. The Hughston jerk test is a slightly different aspect of the subluxation-reduction event in that it moves from reduction to subluxation rather than from subluxation to reduction. The rotatory tests can also detect anterolateral rotatory instability, as previously described, by noting the increase in anterolateral excursion of the lateral tibial plateau. The flexion-rotation drawer and Lachman drawer tests may be more sensitive in subtle anterior cruciate laxities.

Posterolateral Rotatory Instability

In **posterolateral rotatory instability**, the lateral tibial plateau rotates posteriorly in relationship to the femur. A force directed from the anteromedial aspect against the extended knee can cause a rupture of the posterolateral ligamentous structures that usually involves a tear in the arcuate ligament complex; the associated popliteal tendon, or its ramifications into the posterolat-

eral capsule; and the fibular collateral ligament. Some knees may also have partial or complete tears of the posterior cruciate ligament. The exact pathology in this instability is still confusing. Additionally, clinical tests for this laxity are complex. Hughston clarified the diagnosis of posterolateral rotatory instability and described the **external rotation-recurvatum test** (Fig. 21.32). For this test, the athletic trainer lifts the affected extremity by the foot and evaluates the external rotation of the lateral tibia on the femur and any associated appearance of recurvatum to the knee and tibia varus.

Another helpful test in determining posterolateral rotatory instability is the **gravity external rotation test** described by Noyes (Fig. 21.33). This test is very similar to the gravity drop-back test, where the knee, as well as the hip joint, is flexed to 90 degrees. When examining the right knee, the athletic trainer grasps the athlete's foot and ankle with his or her right hand and with his or her left hand holds the thigh with the thumb at the fibular head. The trainer rotates the tibia and foot externally and notes the excursion of the fibular head and tibial tubercle. When posterolateral rotatory instability is present, the fibular head travels farther than the normal side and proceeds

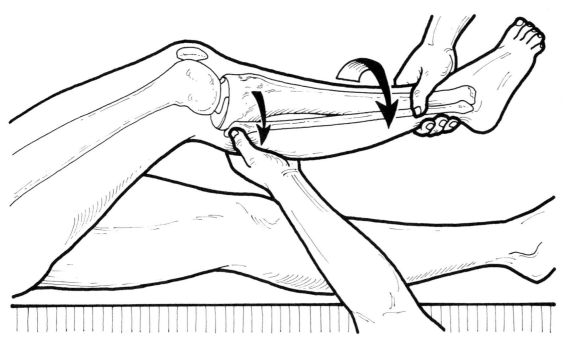

FIGURE 21.33. Gravity external rotation test.

posterior and slightly inferior to its original position. In severe cases, it may rotate into the popliteal space and not be visible. Increased external rotation of the leg can also be compared with the normal side. This test also helps detect associated injuries to the posterior cruciate ligament, since the amount of straight posterior drawer of the tibia can be distinguished from the amount of posterolateral rotation of the tibia during the test.

Posteromedial Rotatory Instability

In **posteromedial rotatory instability**, the medial tibial plateau shifts posteriorly on the femur, with associated medial opening. This injury is severe. The structures involved are the superficial tibial collateral ligament and associated medial capsular structures, plus the cruciate ligaments. There is still much confusion in reference to this laxity. A significant valgus force to the limb can disrupt all the medial structures, plus both cruciate ligaments. In such severe laxities, the posterior medial corner of the tibia sags on the femur, with valgus

opening during an abduction stress test. Actually, in such an injury the tibia can be shifted into a number of different positions, and global instability of the knee joint is common.

Combined Instabilities

All of the rotatory instabilities can occur in combination but, fortunately the frequency is low. If examination of the knee produces a confusing pattern of findings, the trainer should reevaluate the knee more carefully to determine the presence of combined instabilities. All positive findings during examination of the knee should be documented and then categorized to enumerate the types of rotatory instabilities present.

FUNCTIONAL CAPACITY OF THE INJURED KNEE

Anatomic Instability

Biomechanical information on the functional capacity of ligaments and their mechanisms of failure allows classification of injury based on the functional capacity of

TABLE 21.5. Functional Capacity of Injured Ligament

Extent of Failure	Damage*	Amount of Joint Laxity†	Residual Strength	Residual Functional Length/Capacity	Treatment
First-degree sprain: minimal	Less than ⅓ of fibers failed; includes most sprains with few to some fibers failed; microtears also exist	None	Retained or slightly decreased	*Length:* normal *Capacity:* retained	Rest until acute symptoms subside; active rehabilitation; early return to activity
Second-degree sprain: partial	⅓ to ⅔ ligament damage; significant damage but parts of the ligaments are still functional	0–5 mm increased opening, fibers in ligament resist opening	Marked decrease	*Length:* increased, still within functional range but may act as a checkrein *Capacity:* marked compromise requires healing to regain function.	When laxity is minimal, risk to complete the tear is minimal; treated by early rehabilitation and no plaster immobilization
	Microtears may exist	5–10 mm opening when damage is more considerable	At risk for complete failure		When laxity approaches higher values (5–10 mm) treated by plaster immobilization to allow healing; rehabilitation; delayed return to activity
Third-degree sprain: complete	Over ⅔ to complete failure; continuity remains in part between fibers	If 10 mm opening, remaining fibers are torn, incontinuity and complete failure exist	Little to none	*Length:* severely compromised but may provide late checkrein function *Capacity:* severely compromised or lost	Plaster immobilization, protection for healing when laxity increased 10 mm; continuity of ligament is assumed
	Continuity lost and gross separation between fibers	Depends on secondary restraints to limit amount of laxity, but they later stretch out	None	*Length:* lost *Capacity:* lost	Surgical repair required when continuity of ligament is functionally lost; usually exists when medial or lateral opening increased 10–12 mm

*Estimate of damage is often very difficult. However, the different types listed can usually be distinguished.
†Anterior and posterior cruciate tears are included with the exception that acute tears commonly exist with little to no laxity. Thus the clinical laxity exam is less accurate. In the medial and lateral exam the grading is more accurate for collateral tears.

the injured ligament (Table 21.5). Here the residual ability of the damaged ligament to provide joint stability is gauged. This information is correlated with the extent of damage, degree of sprain, and the amount of joint laxity as contained in the other classification systems. In addition, the residual strength, length, and functional capacity of the ligament are correlated. This combination of data provides the final index for treatment. In short, the estimate of functional capacity of a ligament defines the treatment.

Minimal Ligament Failure

If the extent of ligament damage is minimal, with failure of less than one-third of the fibers, the residual functional capacity is retained. The ligament can still provide stability, even though healing must take place. This point is important. There is no joint laxity in this category. The remaining intact ligament fibers resist joint opening. In fact, the seriousness of the injury can be easily underdiagnosed. The ligament has sustained a real injury that requires healing and remodeling. Return to activity is allowed only after symptoms subside and after adequate rehabilitation to overcome disuse and injury effects that produce muscular weakness. Overall, risk for completing the ligament tear or for producing further ligament damage is minimal as long as rehabilitation is complete.

Damage to the cruciate or collateral ligament structure is classified as a significant injury in which laxity of the joint can be detected. The laxity may not correspond with the degree of damage. For example, in anterior cruciate tears, the ligament observed at arthroscopy may have a rupture in one-half of its fibers—a second-degree sprain. The functional capacity is markedly compromised. Yet the increase in anterior laxity may only amount to a few millimeters because the remaining ligament fibers still provide a resisting force. Thus, in the anterior and posterior cruciate ligaments, the amount of laxity may not be a reliable indicator of the extent of damage or residual functional capacity of the ligament. In fact, either cruciate ligament can undergo complete functional disruption with little or no laxity initially on the physical examination. Weak secondary restraints block the laxity but later stretch out, and a gross laxity is then detected. In this instance, the time for acute repair has been lost.

Partial Ligament Failure

In the second-degree sprain or partial ligament injury, there are actually two different types of injuries to the tibial or fibular ligament complex (collateral plus capsular structures): those knees where the damage is partial, with 0 to 5 mm of increased laxity, and those knees in which the partial ligament injury is nearly complete, with 5 to 10 mm of increased laxity. The latter knees require protection for the remaining ligaments and to prevent a complete tear. Also, some stability (decrease in joint opening) may be regained from protection.

The clinical laxity examination is subjective, and, at times, an accurate determina-

tion of the true amount of laxity may be difficult. A second-degree sprain may not be easy to distinguish from a third-degree sprain with complete ligament disruption. In the second-degree sprain, the laxity determination is first made, based on the best estimate of straight medial or lateral opening, with the knee flexed to about 30 degrees. This maneuver relaxes the posterior capsule at the medial and lateral corners of the knee so that the amount of opening more truly reflects damage to the collateral ligaments. However, the capsular structures still provide some resistance to medial or lateral opening. A laxity of over 10 mm implies complete functional disruption. At knee extension, joint opening is always less, as the posteromedial or posterolateral capsule tightens. If joint opening is the same at knee extension, major added damage to these capsular structures has occurred. Also, remember that any time the laxity is increased over 10 mm (over the opposite, normal side), one or both cruciate ligaments may have partial or complete tears. Thus, other tests for the cruciate ligaments should be performed as discussed elsewhere. With the knee at full hyperextension, the cruciates lock or jam the femur into the tibia, and no medial or lateral joint opening is possible, even though there may be a severe collateral ligament injury. Therefore, any opening at full knee hyperextension means a serious injury that also involves the cruciate ligaments.

Complete Ligament Failure

There are two types of complete failure (see Table 21.5). In the first case, failed ligament fibers are still touching each other, even though ligament function is lost. In the second case, there is a gross separation between the ligament ends. The two conditions should be distinguished for two reasons, even though in both, the ligament's functional capacity is lost. First, ligament fibers in continuity may heal, whereas ligaments with separated ends require surgery to restore continuity for healing. Second, a ligament is out of continuity only with significant displacement of the joint. This means that other structures, including the capsule, meniscus, and cruciates, may also be damaged. The amount of laxity depends on secondary restraints, such as the capsule, after the collateral ligament has been disrupted. Thus, the greater the laxity, the greater the chance for concomitant injury and loss of ligament continuity.

Magnetic resonance imaging (MRI) is capable of documenting a ligament tear in continuity. Prior to MRI, the extent of ligamentous injuries could only be determined at the time of surgery. If the laxity is in the range of 10 to 12 mm increased over the opposite side, then immobilization is an option. Each knee injury must be evaluated individually, and many factors need to be considered in determining the need for surgery. Greater laxity implies a severe loss of continuity requiring surgery.

Functional Stability of the Injured Knee

Stabilizing Systems

All three stabilizing systems (active, passive, and joint geometry compressive forces) are required for proper function of the knee joint. A defect in one system, such as an anterior cruciate laxity or a weak quadriceps muscle, may lead to pain, swelling, and giving way and therefore loss of functional stability. If the symptoms prevent activity, then a functional disability is said to exist.

Functional Disabilities

Some ligament injuries lead to a marked functional disability and others do not. Highly coordinated athletes who retrain their neuromuscular coordination reflexes can compensate to a degree for a ligament laxity. The muscles contract at just the right time, providing knee stability. Still, a word of caution must be sounded. After serious ligament injuries, many competitive and recreational athletes have a residual laxity of the knee joint, most commonly following an anterior cruciate tear. Some athletes

compensate and take part in sports. In the past it was thought that if activity could be resumed, the athlete had "functional stability" and all was well. The ability to return to play was used to judge the success of treatment. In fact, in many knees, arthritis of the joint slowly developed, only to be discovered some 5, 10, or 15 years later.

Joint Arthritis

Great caution is needed in determining who should and should not return to competitive athletics after a major ligament injury. We now know that even minor to moderate symptoms of pain, swelling, or giving way over time may lead to **joint arthritis**, or wear and erosion of the cartilage surface. Even an occasional giving-way episode every 2 to 3 months, such as when jumping or twisting with anterior cruciate laxity, may, within a few years, lead to arthritis. Joint arthritis is often initially occult and may be totally unsuspected. Although wearing unevenly, the cartilage functions normally until it wears out, much as an out-of-alignment tire. Arthroscopy of the knee joint after serious ligament injuries often provides important information about joint arthritis and the overall condition of the knee joint. Arthroscopy is being performed earlier in symptomatic athletes to detect occult abnormalities.

The point is not to be misled about joint arthritis and an athlete's ability to perform. Any athlete who sustains a serious ligament injury or even a meniscus removal is at risk for joint arthritis. The percentage of risk varies according to the nature of the injury and many other factors and may be difficult to predict. The criteria for the athlete with a prior injury returning to competitive and recreational activities must include an analysis of the risks for future joint arthritis. The "football knee" is commonly seen today in the middle-aged athlete who is paying the price for a few added years of competitive sports. The ability of an athlete to compensate for an injury is highly individual. A "trial of function" is usually given after injury and rehabilitation to determine whether the knee joint can with-stand the rigors of competition. If symp-toms such as pain, swelling, or giving way —the "big three"—occur, a functional dis-ability exists. The athlete should not play with these symptoms which may be minor, initially ignored, or not prevent activity. These symptoms are usually persistent and may be the first evidence of joint arthritis. The following "red flags" for beginning arthritic symptoms signal the need for cau-tion and orthopedic consultation:

- Persistent, low-grade swelling in the joint, usually the first symptom.
- Persistent stiffness in a joint after ac-tivity, often 24 hours later, signaling hidden joint swelling.
- Any major joint swelling after strenu-ous activity. This requires rest and di-agnosis. An athlete should never com-pete with joint swelling.
- Persistent minor pains in the knee joint, initially only after activity but usually progressive, limiting activity more and more.
- Any giving-way episodes. Initially, this may be a complaint of weakness or feeling of instability rather than full giving way.
- Any grating in the knee joint, which means surface erosions and wear.

The "red flags" are not specific for arthri-tis and may also indicate other joint disor-ders. Persistence of any symptom indicates the need for a specific examination as to cause. Causes may include a meniscal tear, ligament laxity, patellofemoral abnormali-ties, or joint arthritis.

PATELLOFEMORAL DISORDERS

Pathology related to the patella is the single most common cause of knee pain. The discomfort may be a result of direct trauma, repetitive direct pressure (e.g., constant kneeling), constant repetitive motion with a bent knee (e.g., crew, biking), malalign-ment, or combinations of these factors. A sound understanding of patellofemoral

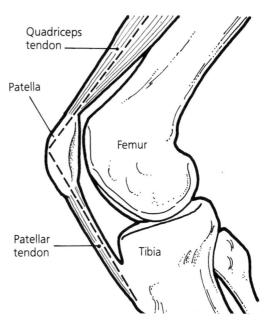

FIGURE 21.34. The patella acts as a fulcrum, increasing the extension moment of the qua-driceps muscle.

anatomy and biomechanics is required for proper diagnosis, treatment, and rehabilita-tion of patellofemoral disorders.

Anatomy and Biomechanics

Biomechanical Function

The patella is a sesamoid bone formed in the quadriceps tendon. Acting as a fulcrum, its primary function is to increase the ex-tending moment of the quadriceps muscle (Fig. 21.34). Forces transmitted from the patella to the patellofemoral groove in-crease as knee flexion increases. The patel-lofemoral compression forces are less than body weight during walking and increase to 2.5 times body weight with activities such as stair climbing.

Active and Passive Stabilizers

Normal function depends on adequate sta-bilization that is provided by both active and passive elements of the extensor mech-anism. The bone contours of the patello-femoral groove and the configuration of the patella, as well as thickening of the capsule, provide passive stabilization. The depth of the patellofemoral groove and the height of the lateral femoral condyle buttress against lateral dislocation. The patella is held in the groove superiorly by the quadriceps tendon and anteriorly by the patellar tendon as the quadriceps muscle contracts.

The passive ligamentous stabilizers consist of thickenings of the capsule, extending from the midportion of the patella to the medial and lateral femoral condyles, and are termed patellofemoral ligaments. The most important of these is the medial patellofemoral ligament. This ligament helps prevent lateral displacement. The lateral patellofemoral ligament is part of the lateral retinaculum, which is composed of two layers. The first of these is a longitudinal layer of superficial fascia. The second is a distinct, deep layer consisting of transverse fibers that form the bulk of the lateral patellofemoral ligament. These fibers are an expansion into the retinaculum of the vastus lateralis and iliotibial tract. In certain situations these ligamentous structures may be excessively tight, contributing to

lateral patellar tilt, malalignment, and excessive patellofemoral compressive forces.

The chief active stabilizer of the patella is the vastus medialis obliquus (VMO), a smaller component of the vastus medialis muscle. The importance of this muscle to knee function and patellar position was first described in the mid-19th century. More recent studies found that the primary function of the VMO is patellar alignment.

A remote stabilizer of the patellofemoral joint is the pes anserinus group of muscles: the sartorius, gracilis, and semitendinosus. Through its internal rotatory action on the proximal tibia, the pes anserinus helps to maintain alignment of the tibial tubercle with the patellofemoral groove.

As previously noted, stability provided by the patellofemoral groove through the patella depends primarily on the shape of the groove and concomitant patellar configuration. Six types of patellae have been described (Fig. 21.35). The Type I and II patellae are the most stable, with equal distribution of forces over the well-formed medial and lateral patellar facets. The other types of patellae are more prone to unequal stresses and thus lateral subluxation. Patellar type and patellofemoral groove anatomy can be determined by axial radiographic views of the patella.

The Q Angle

The **Q angle** is determined by drawing one line in the middle of the patella to the center of the tibial tubercle and a second line from the center of the patella to the center of the anterior-superior iliac spine on the pelvis (Fig. 21.36). An increase in the Q angle above 15 degrees may increase the tendency for lateral patellar malposition, but by itself it is not diagnostic. An increased Q angle, associated with another deficiency of the extensor mechanism, may allow the patella to subluxate more easily.

The Law of Valgus

The presence of the valgus Q angle and the considerably stronger and more fibrous lat-

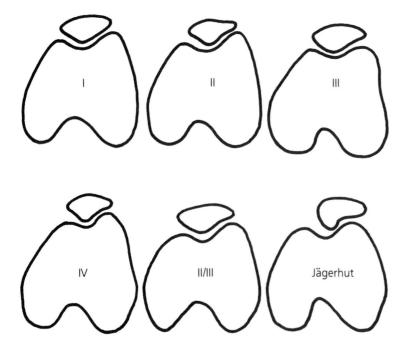

FIGURE 21.35. Six types of patellae.

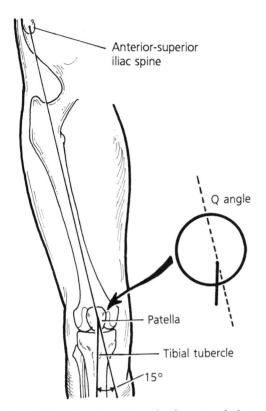

Anterior-superior
iliac spine

Q angle

Patella

Tibial tubercle

15°

FIGURE 21.36.   Q angle and valgus angulation.

eral patellar stabilizers, coupled with the physiology and biomechanics of the patellofemoral joint, is so important to understanding both normal and abnormal knee function that it has been elevated to the level of a "law." The **law of valgus** helps explain the pathophysiology involved in this joint, as well as how the delicate balance that is compatible with symptom-free function might be restored. Morphologically, this law is based on the predominant lateral trochlear surface. The more frequently found patellar form (Wiberg, Type II) has a larger lateral than medial facet. The lateral soft tissue elements reinforced by the fascia lata are balanced by similar medial soft tissue stabilizers. These medial soft tissue stabilizers, along with the congruence of the contact surfaces of the joint, offer further stability and thus tend to negate the existing valgus vector. The orientation of the lateral trochlear facet offers

further impediment to lateralization of the patella. With this understanding, then, we can discuss the pathogenesis of patellar malalignment.

Extensor Mechanism Deficiencies

Because of the law of valgus, any stabilizing deficiency in the extensor mechanism leads to patellar malposition, which is manifested by lateral patellar subluxation or dislocation. Deficiencies of the extensor mechanism can be divided into three categories: (1) abnormalities of the patellofemoral configuration; (2) deficiencies of the supporting muscles or guiding mechanisms; and (3) malalignment of the extremity relating to knee mechanics. Often deficiencies in more than one category contribute to the patellar malalignment.

Abnormalities of the Patellofemoral Configuration

Under abnormalities of the patellofemoral configuration, a combination of a low profile of the patellofemoral groove and deficiency of the medial patellar facet predisposes to patellar instability. Usually these deficiencies are developmental, caused by deficiency of the supporting muscle or malalignment that did not allow the patella and patellofemoral groove to develop normally. These deficiencies are best evaluated by radiographic studies. The lateral condyle is higher than the medial condyle and projects anteriorly an estimated 7 mm or more, therefore preventing lateral patellar displacement. The patellofemoral joint can undergo further development during the last several years of growth; thus the patellofemoral groove angle and patellar configuration can improve during treatment. This is one of several reasons why conservative treatment in the adolescent is strongly suggested. Thus, when an unstable patellar mechanism demands surgery, it should, if possible, be delayed until skeletal maturity.

Deficiencies of Supporting Structures

Deficiencies of the supporting muscles and guiding mechanisms that allow the patella to subluxate or dislocate laterally include weakness of the anterior medial retinaculum, weakness of the VMO muscle, hypermobility of the patella as a result of poor muscle tone after injury, congenital genu recurvatum, with a resultant laxity in the extensor mechanism, patella alta, and tightness of the lateral retinaculum. Lack of development of the VMO muscle, which is normally attached to the proximal one-third of the patella, allows overpull of the vastus lateralis during walking and running activities, particularly between midstance and takeoff, thus enhancing lateral subluxation or dislocation of the patella. In patella alta, only the more vertically oriented fibers that attach to the proximal portion of the medial patella are present, diminishing control of lateral patellar displacement.

The association of generalized joint laxity in recurrent patellar dislocation has been noted. Familial joint laxity is commonly the cause of recurrent dislocation.

Malalignment of the Extremity

A wide variety of structural abnormalities of the lower extremity may influence patellar tracking in the patellar groove and account for malalignment of the extremity. Certainly, genu valgum (knock-knees) increases the valgus vector to the knee, therefore setting the stage for patellar subluxation or dislocation. Likewise, lateral displacement of the tibial tubercle in relationship to the anterior-superior iliac spine enhances the tendency for the patella to displace laterally.

Femoral anteversion and internal femoral rotation cause the patellofemoral groove to be more medially placed in relation to the tibial tubercle and thus give, functionally, a more lateral insertion to the patellar tendon, enhancing the lateral pull of the quadriceps contraction or valgus vector. It is not uncommon for athletes who have patellar malalignment problems to have a history of having been treated as children for lower extremity malalignment with special orthopedic shoes and leg braces.

Foot mechanics may also alter patellar tracking. During the foot strike of a running gait, the foot pronates with subsequent external rotation of the tibia on the femur as the knee extends. Quadriceps contraction with either foot pronation or external tibial rotation enhances the lateral forces acting on the patella. For less active people who run short distances, this problem usually does not appear. However, in the long-distance runner who logs hundreds of miles per year, the abnormal lateral forces that are directed at the patella may lead to "runner's knee" or patellofemoral arthralgia.

The deficiencies discussed above are usually compensated for in the normal knee by the triangular shape of the patella, depth of the patellofemoral groove, and the restraining action of the passive ligamentous structures. However, when bone or soft tissue deficiencies occur by themselves or in combination, the potential for abnormal tracking of the patella exists, particularly when the knee suffers a secondary insult. The resultant muscle atrophy and weakness associated with even the slightest knee injury tips the delicate scales of the extensor mechanism in favor of malalignment. Pain, usually the first sign of patellofemoral difficulties, further adds to muscular atrophy and disuse. Voluntary or imposed rest to control pain and inflammation creates further muscular imbalances. Once patellofemoral arthralgia has subsided with rest, the athlete often makes the mistake of resuming full activities without proper reconditioning and restoration of muscle balance. Failure to appreciate this important principle is perhaps the most common cause of failure of conservative treatment of patellofemoral malalignment.

Patellofemoral Stress Syndrome

Patellofemoral stress syndrome, also called lateral patellar compression syndrome, is being recognized more often by physicians and athletic trainers. Essentially, either the lateral retinaculum that holds the lateral facet of the patella firmly to the femoral condyle is tight or the muscles are imbalanced so that the patella is pulled laterally. In either case, excessive pressure develops on the lateral facet and the lateral tissues about the patellofemoral joint, and pain occurs. The source of the pain is not well understood, as is sometimes the case with other patellar disorders. The lateral retinaculum, being under tension, can become tender. Also, the amount of lateral compression on the articular cartilage and underlying subchondral bone of the lateral facet may explain the pain symptoms. On evaluation, the cardinal finding is pain when the athletic trainer exerts downward pressure on the patellofemoral joint.

Additional findings in patellofemoral stress syndrome include tenderness of the lateral facet and swelling with synovial irritation. This swelling can cause crepitus on manual compression of the patellofemoral joint. The resultant pain causes the athlete to react and prevents the athletic trainer from repeating the compression test. Subluxation can coexist with this syndrome. The athlete complains of pain, usually dull and aching, in the "center of the knee." The knee is swollen, tender as described above, and can give way, presumably as a result of avoidance of pain. Treatment consists of ice, rest, and rehabilitation.

The majority of athletes with patellar pain have lateral patellar compression syndrome. Fortunately, most respond to nonsurgical treatment. Medications, exercises, support devices, and alterations of the training program usually relieve the symptoms. Mild anti-inflammatories should be used to reduce irritation of tissues in the patellofemoral joint. Support devices with padding on the lateral aspect of the patella help relieve compression and allow proper tracking of the patella. Exercises should include a quadriceps-strengthening program and, very importantly, a stretching flexibility routine for the hamstrings to decrease the imbalance between the antagonistic hamstrings and quadriceps muscula-

ture. The training programs for these athletes may need to be altered to prevent an excessive amount of bent-knee activities. Weight-training programs that load the patellofemoral joint should be avoided. Icing of the patellofemoral area after training or rehabilitation activities also helps reduce swelling and pain. After becoming asymptomatic, an athlete can return to play and get through a season by using these techniques. However, the athlete should be followed carefully to avoid irreversible damage to the articular surface.

Patellar Tendinitis

The patellar tendon (patellar ligament) can become inflamed and tender, usually because of an overuse syndrome. Recurrent forces probably produce microfailure of the collagen bundles, and pain with inflammation follows. **Patellar tendinitis** occurs in the jumping athlete, thus the term "jumper's knee." Specifically, the athlete complains of pain over the tendon, difficulty jumping or running, and pain with many of the prescribed exercises. The fat pad may even become inflamed and contribute to the symptoms. Evaluation reveals tenderness and swelling along the patellar tendon that is usually but not necessarily concentrated along the upper portion of the tendon. In the chronic case, a nodule of scar tissue, often very tender, can be palpated within the tendon or near its insertion site into the patella.

Treatment for patellar tendinitis is the same as for several other patellofemoral problems. Rest may be required initially until acute symptoms subside. Quadriceps strengthening enhances the muscles' absorption of strain. Stretching, warm-up, and icing after practice are all important. A floor that absorbs some of the stress is also important; running on concrete or asphalt increases symptoms. In the chronic case, when a nodule is present and tender, surgical resection of the nodule decreases symptoms. Also, patellar subluxation or the lateral patellar compression syndrome can coexist with this syndrome. Remember that a subtle lateral subluxation may be the cause for overloading the patellar tendon.

Tibial Apophysitis: Osgood-Schlatter Disease

Osgood-Schlatter disease was first described in 1903 by Osgood as a partial avulsion of the tibial tubercle, causing painful swelling in the knee of the adolescent (Fig. 21.37). Several months later, Schlatter described the same condition and concluded that it was an apophysitis (inflammation) of the tibial tubercle rather than a true bone avulsion fracture. Opinion since then has been divided. Traumatic separation is a distinct injury and often gives identical clinical findings. Most commonly, the condition represents an apophysitis that develops and is aggravated by activity.

This entity is commonly seen by coaches and athletic trainers. It develops during the period of most rapid growth, between the ages of 9 and 13, and is more common in boys than in girls. Bilateral involvement is noted in 20 to 30 percent of the cases.

Osgood-Schlatter disease is characterized by a painful swelling over the tibial tuberosity, exacerbated by activity, relieved by rest, and usually of several months' duration. Tenderness is most marked at the insertion of the patellar tendon. In cases of long duration, the anterior aspect of the knee appears enlarged, and a bony prominence may be palpated. The range of knee motion is not affected. Pain may be elicited toward the end of active extension or forced flexion.

Radiographic films may show an irregularity and fragmentation of the tibial apophysis. Many believe that the diagnosis is radiographic, but fragmentation can also be seen in adolescents without symptoms.

Treatment of Osgood-Schlatter disease is symptomatic. In persistently or moderately painful knees, sports activities should be restricted until the pain subsides. If the pain is particularly disabling, the knee may be immobilized in a plaster cylinder cast for 4 to 6 weeks. When the athlete returns

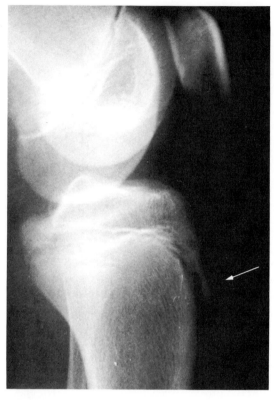

FIGURE 21.37.   Osgood-Schlatter disease is epiphyseal inflammation of the tibial tubercle, which often appears irregular, enlarged, or pulled away on x-ray.

to play, knee pads are used to avoid contusion to the prominent tibial tubercle. The symptoms usually occur from overuse or vigorous activity. Symptoms stop after growth ceases; however, the bony prominence remains.

An aggressive therapy program to increase hamstring flexibility and balance the antagonism between the quadriceps and hamstrings will markedly relieve the stress at the tibial tubercle and give significant relief of the apophysitis. Early return to sports is allowed if all symptoms have abated. The athlete should be encouraged to continue the flexibility program.

Very rarely, tumors and acute avulsion fractures may present with similar complaints and findings and must be differentiated from Osgood-Schlatter disease. Infrequently, persistent pain and failure to respond to treatment necessitate surgery, but only in severe cases after all other treatment modalities have been exhausted. In such knees often an extra bony fragment is embedded within the patellar ligament at the tibial attachment. Surgery consists of removing the accessory bone fragment and associated scar tissue. This lesion probably represents an old fracture at the patellar ligament attachment.

Patellar Dislocation

Acute **patellar dislocation** can simulate a severe collateral ligament injury of the knee. The athlete is usually cutting from the involved knee when a violent giving-way episode occurs, often with an audible pop. Usually, the patella spontaneously reduces, leaving a painful, swollen, and tender knee. Acute patellar dislocation can occur in athletes with normal or abnormal patellofemoral mechanics. Unfortunately, athletes with normal mechanics usually sustain more severe soft tissue injuries from an acute dislocation than athletes with abnormal patellofemoral mechanics. The latter have a preexisting hypermobility of the patellofemoral joint that may preclude severe injury to the tissues during a complete patellofemoral dislocation.

The athletic trainer should palpate the area to detect a defect in the medial retinaculum and vastus medialis insertion before swelling obscures it. This defect occurs as the patella dislocates laterally, tearing the medial restraints. Furthermore, pain along the lateral femoral condyle is suggestive. Obviously, if a ligament examination can be done, normal results exclude the possibility of a ligament disruption. Finally, examination of the opposite knee may reveal a tendency for patellar dislocation (hypermobile patella, loose patellofemoral ligaments)—another clue for a correct diagnosis.

Immediate care of patellar dislocation consists of ice, elevation, compression, and a splint, with physician evaluation to follow. Treatment is usually one of three modes. First, in recurrent cases of dislocation, treatment consists of rehabilitation to provide better dynamic stability, wearing a patellar support brace, and modification of activities. A second treatment regimen calls for cast immobilization or the use of a lateral restraining pad with a knee immobilizer splint if this is the first episode or if medial patellar restraints have torn. Cast or splint immobilization allows healing of the soft tissue restraints. Occasionally, a third mode, surgery, is necessary to repair the restraints or remove an osteochondral fracture. Surgery is followed by rehabilitation and a support brace. Special radiographs, such as axial or oblique views, are often required to exclude a fracture of the patella or lateral femoral condyle. Arthroscopy can determine the diagnosis and evaluate the entire knee if necessary.

Rehabilitation is aimed at decreasing the symptoms initially, followed by strengthening the quadriceps muscles, especially the VMO, to hold the patella in place. When the athlete is ready to return to activity, a patella support brace is helpful with all activities to decrease the risk of another dislocation. Each dislocation does more damage to the patellar cartilage surface. With multiple episodes, traumatic arthritis can be expected. Therefore, if multiple episodes of dislocation occur, despite taping and rehabilitation, the athlete must either give up the offending activity or undergo surgical correction.

Patellar Subluxation Syndrome

Although not as dramatic as patellar dislocation, the more common **patellar subluxation syndrome** can be just as disabling. Here, the patella repetitively subluxates laterally and places strain on the medial restraints and excessive stress on the patellofemoral joint. Symptoms are related to the amount of activity. The normal patellar posture for exerting deceleration forces in the functional position of 45 degrees of knee flexion places the patellar articular surface squarely against the femur. A higher posture, or patella alta, is often associated with patellar subluxation. The excessive superior posturing of the patella allows it to track out of the intercondylar groove of the femur, making it susceptible to lateral displacement.

Commonly, the athlete complains of pain and giving-way episodes that suggest ligamentous or meniscal problems. True locking does not occur, but stiffness of the patellofemoral joint is not unusual. Evaluation shows tenderness of the medial restraints; swelling of the knee with synovial irritation; disuse atrophy of the quadriceps muscles, particularly the VMO; and increased Q angle. Laxity of the patella—that is, its tendency to subluxate—is diagnosed when the athletic trainer notes the ease with which the patella moves laterally when pressure is applied on its medial side (Fig. 21.38). The athlete with patellofemoral stress syndrome without associated patellar subluxation will not be apprehensive with this maneuver, whereas the athlete with patellar pain on the basis of recurrent subluxation will be very concerned and voluntarily and involuntarily resist any attempt to displace the patella laterally.

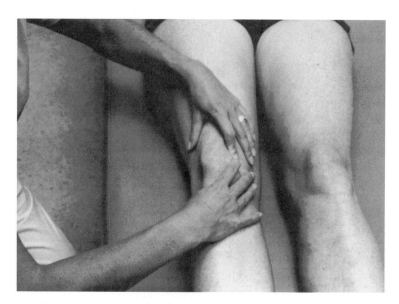

FIGURE 21.38. Lateral subluxation of the patella.

The treatment for patellar subluxation is the same as for patellar dislocation, except cast immobilization is rarely used. If symptoms still occur following an appropriate rehabilitation program, surgical realignment of the patellofemoral joint may be necessary. Here again, rehabilitation should emphasize strengthening of the VMO, because this muscle holds the patella medially to prevent subluxation. Patellar support braces or taping is extremely helpful. Most athletes with mild lateral patellar subluxation do well with proper rehabilitation. Often, decreasing activity is enough to cause symptoms to subside. In other knees, the condition can be progressive, with increasing patellofemoral crepitus and continuing symptoms despite all treatment. The athletic trainer must be aware of symptoms indicating chronicity, even though they are seen in only 1 out of 15 athletes.

Surgery for Patellofemoral Malalignment

The objective of surgical treatment is realignment of the extensor apparatus and stabilization of the patella in the trochlea during function. Athletes with recurrent patellar dislocations and subluxations often have a congenital deficiency, such as ligamentous laxity. When conservative therapy fails to correct the athlete's difficulties, and when multiple deficiencies of the extensor mechanism exist with major disability, then surgical procedures are generally necessary. The determination of which surgical procedure to use must take into account the complexities of the extensor mechanism, the biomechanics of the patellofemoral joint, and the particular deficiencies. The key to successful surgery for patellofemoral malalignment lies not in applying a single technique to all athletes, but in selecting the proper combination of techniques for a given individual.

The number of techniques for patellar realignment and stabilization reported in the literature is astonishing. This multitude of surgical procedures has been categorized for the purpose of reviewing them. For our purposes, those procedures directed at correcting persistent or recurrent patellar malalignment before the development of serious **chondromalacia** (softening of articular cartilage) of the patella or patellofemoral arthrosis can be considered "reconstructive" rather than "salvage" procedures, and can be divided into three general areas for surgical technique and postoperative rehabilitation: lateral retinacular release, proximal realignment, and distal realignment of the extensor mechanism.

Lateral Retinacular Release

Lateral retinacular release, or **capsulorrhaphy**, may be sufficient for many athletes. In this procedure, the lateral retinaculum is simply weakened by surgical release to allow the patella to move more centrally in the groove. Lateral release is particularly valuable in the adolescent because it does not involve any bony structures in which surgery may interfere with growth. The procedure may be done at arthrotomy in a "Z-plasty lengthening" technique, or subcutaneously, either by direct vision through the arthroscope or by indirect vision using digital palpation.

The lateral release is extensive and includes the entire lateral retinaculum, extending from the patellar tendon superiorly, as well as the majority of the vastus lateralis tendon (Fig. 21.39). Lateral retinacular release lessens the compressive forces on the articular surface of the patella and allows a more longitudinal force of the vastus lateralis. Lessening the resistance of the lateral patellofemoral ligament reduces the valgus vector and augments the function of the VMO muscle as a result of the improved alignment.

Lateral retinacular release, by itself, has only recently become popular. The long-term results of this procedure are yet to be compiled. The key to success with this procedure lies in preventing postoperative hemarthrosis, as well as strengthening the VMO and reeducation.

Proximal Realignment

Proximal soft tissue reconstruction, or **proximal realignment**, is designed to align the muscle pull on the patella and thus enhance the active action of the VMO. It also tightens the medial capsule, which includes the medial patellar ligament. Because of the difficulty of the procedure, meticulous surgical technique is mandatory when the VMO muscle is to be changed dynamically. Those procedures employing proximal realignment combine lateral retinacular release with reimplantation of the VMO muscle laterally and distally on the patella.

Distal Realignment of the Extensor Mechanism

When the patella is not centralized in the patellofemoral groove with a lateral retinacular release, or if the tibial tubercle is ana-

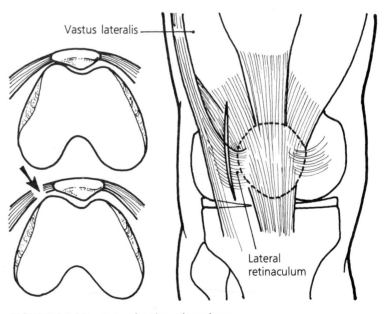

FIGURE 21.39.   Lateral retinacular release.

tomically lateral to the patellofemoral groove, producing a large valgus vector, the patellar tendon may need realignment. Several procedures are commonly being performed, and in the mature adult essentially employ moving the patellar tendon, along with its bony attachment, to a new site on the tibia. However, detachment of the tibial tubercle is not recommended in the adolescent because of the potential for growth disturbance.

Postoperative Rehabilitation Program

A postoperative rehabilitation program following patellofemoral realignment surgery must begin with straight-leg raising exercises and then progress slowly to bent-leg, progressive resistance exercises. In the bent-knee position, the patellofemoral forces are greatest, and the softened, compromised cartilage is at greatest risk. Should signs of increasing chondromalacia occur, such as anterior patellar aching, recurrent swelling, palpable synovitis, or increas-

ing patellofemoral crepitus, patellofemoral forces should be decreased immediately. This means abandonment of bent-knee progressive resistance exercises, and re-initiation of straight-leg raising and isometric exercises. Running and jumping activities should also be stopped.

Prognosis

Most surgeons report 80 to 90 percent good results with procedures to prevent recurrent subluxation and dislocation. Although short-term results may be good, length of follow-up must be considered. Chondromalacia and osteoarthritis have been frequently reported in long-term, follow-up studies. Because of the erratic and uncertain results produced by patellofemoral joint surgery, the importance of conservative treatment with proper rehabilitation cannot be overemphasized.

MENISCAL DISORDERS

Anatomy of the Menisci

The menisci are C-shaped, intra-articular structures that are wedge-shaped in cross section. Macroscopically, they are opaque, firm, and fibrous. Microscopically, the menisci are composite structures that contain fibrous collagen bundles for strength and are embedded in homogeneous ground substance typical of articular cartilage. The cells in the meniscus have the appearance of chondrocytes. The collagen fibers in the meniscus are basically arranged in a circumferential direction, although some are perpendicular and radial in orientation. Circumferential fibers aid in resisting the stresses to which a meniscus is subjected. The tibia and femur push the curved meniscus outward like a washer being pushed out of place. The greatest meniscal tensile strength is in the circumferential fibers.

The peripheral 2 to 3 mm of the menisci is nourished directly by blood supplied from the branches of the medial and lateral inferior geniculate arteries (Fig. 21.40). Menisci have the same nutritional diffusion

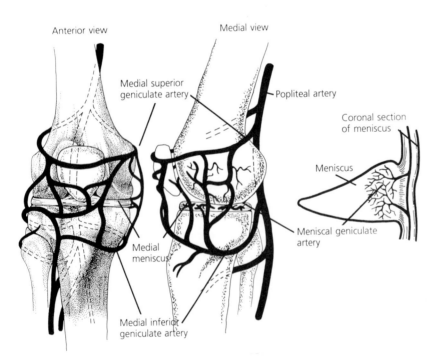

FIGURE 21.40. Meniscal geniculate arterial blood supply.

pattern as articular cartilage, because the intra-articular surfaces derive nutrition from the synovial fluid in which they are bathed. The critical depth of nutrition to articular cartilage by physiologic diffusion is 3 mm. The medial meniscus varies in width and thickness from anterior to posterior. The lateral meniscus does not vary much in width, but does increase in thickness as it progresses from anterior to posterior. This increased thickness becomes important when analyzing a cross section of this segment for nutrient supply. The central portion of this segment is at, or above, the upper limits for efficient diffusion of nutrients. This could explain the high incidence of early microscopic tears in this region.

Medial Meniscus

The anterior horn of the medial meniscus is usually attached to the nonarticulating area of the tibia, just anterior to the anterior horn of the lateral meniscus and the anterior cruciate ligament. The second attachment is known as the transverse ligament. It extends from the anterior horn of the medial meniscus to the anterior border of the lateral meniscus, or it may extend posteriorly into the attachment area of the anterior cruciate ligament.

The midportion of the meniscus is attached to the tibia and the femur at its periphery via the meniscofemoral and the meniscotibial ligaments. The posterior horn is attached firmly to the nonarticular area of the tibial plateau, between the tibial spine and the origin of the posterior cruciate ligament. The meniscal arm of the semimembranosus attaches to the posterior horn and helps retract the meniscus during knee flexion to prevent impingement. As mentioned, the width of the medial meniscus changes. The anterior half is narrow, and the posterior half is very broad.

Lateral Meniscus

The anterior horn of the lateral meniscus is attached to the tibia directly anterior to the intercondylar eminence. Additionally, it may have an attachment to the anterior cruciate ligament. The midportion of the lateral meniscus is also attached at the periphery by the meniscofemoral and meniscotibial ligaments. An opening in these peripheral attachments allows passage of the popliteal tendon.

In the posterolateral portion of the lateral meniscus the arcuate complex is attached to the meniscal border. The popliteus is strongly attached to the arcuate ligament and the meniscus through the popliteal aponeurosis. These two attachments aid in posterior displacement of the posterior segment during medial rotation.

The posterior horn is firmly attached in the medial portion of the tibial plateau, between the spines of the tibia. Occasionally, there is a second group of attachments from the posterior convex border of the lateral meniscus and the posterior horn. They insert on the tibia just anterior and posterior to the posterior cruciate ligament. These attachments are the ligaments of Humphry and Wrisberg, respectively. The width of the lateral meniscus is greater and more uniform throughout when compared with the medial meniscus, and the periphery is thicker.

Anatomic Differences Between the Menisci

Some differences between the menisci must be detailed. The lateral meniscus is more mobile than the medial meniscus, as explained by careful anatomic assessment. The attachments of the anterior and posterior horns of the lateral meniscus are close together. This proximity allows more mobility than in the medial meniscus with its widely spaced end attachments of the anterior and posterior horns. The increased mobility results in less stress on the lateral meniscus, thus leading to a decreased incidence of injury.

Contour differences are also found between the menisci. The lateral meniscus is almost the entire circumference of a small

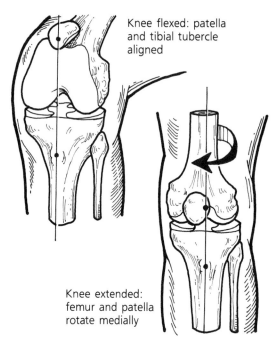

Knee flexed: patella and tibial tubercle aligned

Knee extended: femur and patella rotate medially

FIGURE 21.41. Screw-home mechanism. Femoral condyle rotates around tibial spine.

circle. By comparison, the medial meniscus is a small section of a larger circle.

In flexion, extension, and rotation of the knee joint, the menisci move with the tibia. Most motion of the knee joint occurs between the menisci and the femur. Still, some motion does occur between the tibia and the menisci, particularly with rotation. The final motion of the femur before full extension is medial rotation—which is commonly known as the **screw-home mechanism** (Fig. 21.41). The motion is caused by the larger medial femoral condyle rotating around the tibial spine after full excursion of the lateral condylar articular surface. This terminal rotation may be blocked if a portion of the meniscus is caught in the joint, as discussed later in this chapter.

Functions of the Menisci

The functions of the menisci are accepted generally as being nutritional, weight bearing, and joint movement and stabilization. The nutritional function aids in spreading a thin film of synovial fluid over the articular cartilage and in circulating that fluid throughout the joint.

Thirty to 55 percent of joint weight is carried by the menisci, which form a major portion of the weight-bearing surface of a joint. Following meniscectomy, between two and three times more compressive deformation occurs than in a normal joint. The menisci aid in joint function by deepening the tibial articular surfaces. This fills in potential dead spaces at the periphery of tibiofemoral contact, thus increasing joint stability.

The menisci, because of their figure-eight arrangement on the tibia, participate in joint movement. They guide the femur and assist its tracking during the final screw-home motion of extension.

Pathology of the Menisci

The most common meniscal pathology is a tear or disruption of the normal anatomy of the meniscus. Tears usually occur after trauma to the knee that overloads the menisci and are often associated with ligamentous injuries. Attritional tears can develop from continued use or stress overload activities as the aging meniscus becomes less pliable.

The signs and symptoms of meniscal tears are relatively uniform. Pain, often localized, is accentuated by activity. Recurrent swelling may be present. Catching and locking may occur, and the knee can buckle or give way with activity.

Classification of Meniscal Tears

Meniscal tears can be classified according to age, location, and axis of orientation (Fig. 21.42). Although the degenerative horizontal tear is more common, the acute longitudinal tear that occurs in youth is more disabling. The usual history of the longitudinal tear is a twisting injury to the knee when the foot is fixed and the knee is flexed, producing compression and rotation on a meniscus trapped in the joint. This injury

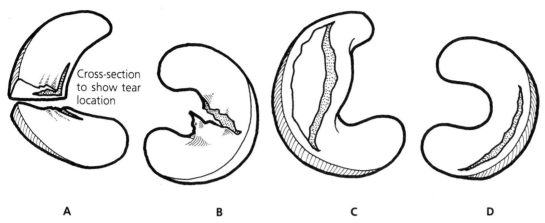

FIGURE 21.42. Types of meniscal tears: (a) horizontal; (b) parrot-beak, or radial; (c) bucket-handle; (d) longitudinal.

usually demands immediate attention and urgent surgical intervention. These lesions will therefore be considered first.

Longitudinal Tears

In order to have a **longitudinal meniscal tear**, the posterior medial segment of the meniscus must be displaced to some extent. Longitudinal tears are of two types: peripheral or extraperipheral. The meniscus can remain intact during compression and rotation, and the tear can occur through the posterior peripheral attachment or in the substance of the meniscus itself. These tears can be partial (confined to the posterior segment only) or complete. With a partial tear through the substance of the meniscus, central displacement of the medial fragment is temporary. Repeated episodes may lead to multiple partial tears of the posterior segment or progression of the tear into the anterior segment. With a **bucket-handle tear**, the entire central segment is displaced medially during the injury.

The complete longitudinal tear of the meniscus may produce locking of the knee joint, or the meniscus may return to its normal position in the knee joint following injury. Locking of the knee occurs when the meniscus or a segment of a meniscus becomes interposed between the femur and the tibia at a point anterior to the coronal plane of the knee. Locking occurs in only about one-third of complete tears of the meniscus.

Longitudinal tears limited to the anterior segment of a meniscus are rare. They occur most often in the lateral meniscus. The anterior horn of the lateral meniscus is situated more posteriorly than the corresponding portion of the medial structure. It is therefore more prone to trapping in hyperextension and rotation.

Horizontal Tears

Horizontal meniscal tears, also called **horizontal cleavage tears**, are basically due to cartilage degeneration. Presumably, nutrition of the central portion of the meniscus decreases with age. Rotation in the knee joint also causes shear forces between the superior and inferior surfaces of the meniscus. The initial tears can be entirely in the substance of the meniscus, not visible on the meniscal surface. Repeated traumatic episodes may complete the single tear or cause multiple tears in the horizontal plane. The tears may occur in the substance rather than on the meniscal surface because of less nutrition and the less tightly woven arrangement of collagen fibrils in the interior as compared with the surface.

Horizontal cleavage lesions are most frequent in the posterior medial portion of the meniscus. They can be confined to the posterior segment alone, or they can extend to the anterior segment. Once cleavage is complete, the inferior portion can detach, usually posteriorly, which can lead to episodes of momentary locking with associated pain and instability.

The **parrot-beak tear**, or **radial tear**, of the lateral meniscus is listed under horizontal cleavage lesions, but it is different for several reasons. It is usually a traumatic tear of youth and is almost always located in the middle segment of the lateral meniscus. Usually, it is associated with previous pathology and is actually a combination of tears.

The parrot-beak tear occurs in the thicker portion of the lateral meniscus. This area has usually been previously traumatized, and the meniscus has become fixed at its periphery due to cystic degeneration or some other fibrosis-producing pathology. Because of the fixation and cartilage thickness, two horizontal tears occur. The relative increased mobility of the lateral meniscus during flexion and extension causes the central medial portion between the two tears to attenuate and, finally, to connect. The meniscal superior and inferior surfaces finally attenuate, and a transverse connecting tear occurs, thus completing the complex parrot-beak tear.

Traumatic and Degenerative Meniscal Tears

Acute meniscal tears can be traumatic or degenerative in origin. A traumatic meniscal tear may occur in association with other knee injuries, and generally results in moderate to severe pain, swelling, and disability. The degenerative meniscal tear generally is an isolated injury and has less pain, disability, and reactive swelling. Degenerative tears that extend are usually related to episodes of minimal trauma and may have almost no pain or swelling. This decreased swelling is due to less synovial reaction following a smaller injury, and it also indicates minimal or complete absence of hemorrhage seen in degenerative and chronic meniscal extended tears. If the central fragment of the meniscus is displaced into the joint, the joint will lock as extended, usually 10 to 40 degrees short of full extension. Once impingement has occurred, further extension is achieved at the expense of the medial portion of the femoral condyle. If the fragment is dislocated into the notch, the normal screw-home mechanism of the knee is disrupted.

The terminal rotation is regained by stretching the anterior cruciate ligament. This stretching by fragment impingement in full extension and medial rotation can lead to chronic instability. Repeated episodes of joint impingement by fragment displacement can lead to damage of the cartilage surfaces. This accelerated wear can progress through all the stages of chondromalacia. It is not possible to predict which knees will have deterioration of the cartilage surfaces. In many chronic instances of locking, arthroscopy has surprisingly shown no surface deterioration.

The Discoid Meniscus

An anomalous (congenital) variation of the normal semilunar meniscus is the **discoid meniscus**, which probably is found more often in females than males. This condition may present in childhood but may not cause problems until the meniscus is injured or becomes degenerative. The lateral meniscus is more often the discoid (Fig. 21.43). Classically, persons with this condition have a loud snap at the lateral joint line with flexion and extension of the knee.

Because of the abnormal discoid shape, stresses and forces are absorbed by the meniscus in an abnormal, unbalanced way, cystic degeneration occurs, and tears develop without the usual mechanism of injury. Presence of a discoid meniscus and whether it is torn are confirmed by arthrography or arthroscopy. Surgical excision is performed in symptomatic cases.

Diagnosis of Meniscal Tears

Signs and Symptoms

In a knee with a torn meniscus, pain can be a variable finding. Chronic meniscal tears in the absence of degenerative joint disease may have point tenderness only over the site of the lesion. With associated degenerative joint disease, chronic pain increases with activity, and there is more local tenderness at the site of the lesion, particularly at night. The cause of night pain in meniscal tears is uncertain. It may be produced by unguarded knee rotation while turning in bed. Because little joint compression occurs in bed, the fragment can more easily displace and become entrapped, thereby producing pain. Chronic local inflammation is often more painful or is more easily perceived at night when there are fewer distractions. Of interest, some athletes report that the weight of the bed sheet increases local pain.

More commonly, the athlete with a torn meniscus complains of catching and occasional locking of the knee with activities. Locking can also be caused by momentary displacement of the torn fragment. This catching or locking can cause the knee to buckle and give way, making the athlete stumble and fall. Recurrent effusions can develop in the knee after an episode of catching or locking.

Physical Findings

Diagnosis of an internal derangement of the knee involving a meniscus can be difficult. Several physical findings are helpful.

- *Effusion.* Effusion is usually due to synovial inflammation. It can be associated with an acute injury but usually is seen with chronic meniscal lesions.
- *Locking.* True locking of the knee joint is a restriction of knee joint ex-

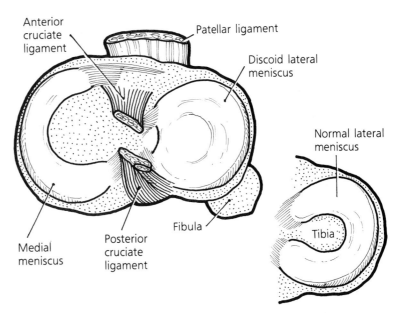

FIGURE 21.43. Lateral discoid and normal medial meniscus.

tension, generally secondary to a displaced bucket-handle tear of the meniscus. Usually about 10 degrees of extension is lacking, and joint motion is painful. An episode of locking may follow severe or apparently insignificant trauma. If it follows minor trauma, there have usually been multiple episodes of minor trauma. The effusion associated with locking in the knee may be correspondingly small.
- *Joint line tenderness.* In a person who has had repeated episodes of minor meniscal tears, joint line tenderness may be the only positive sign.
- *Quadriceps atrophy.* Quadriceps atrophy is usually present in acute and chronic injuries.
- *Incomplete flexion.*
- *Tibiofemoral clicking on stairs.*
- *A click by a McMurray test.* The click caused by a McMurray test (see Fig. 21.16) is usually secondary to a posterior horn tear.

In order to test anterior horn tears, the athletic trainer has the athlete stand and perform internal and external rotatory movements with the knee extended. This weight bearing causes anterior impingement.

Another test, the Apley compression test (see Fig. 21.15), can separate meniscal tears from other internal derangements. This test is valuable for detecting meniscal tears in the middle portions, and it also elicits crepitus to the lateral or medial joint, which is indicative of surface arthritis.

Initial Treatment

Once a meniscal tear has been diagnosed, treatment must be considered. If the athlete has a locked knee, the dislodged meniscus must often be removed if spontaneous reduction assisted by rotation or joint dislocation is not successful. If the athlete only has pain and effusion, the standard program for knee effusion is undertaken—rest, ice, compression, elevation, and early rehabilitation. Ice should be applied immediately following injury. A bulky pressure dressing from the toes to the inguinal region provides compression. Elevation controls swelling. If the joint is painfully swollen, aspiration for athlete comfort may be performed. The athlete is placed on crutches and isometrics are started. As soon as major pain subsides, weight bearing and quadriceps exercises are increased. Return to full weight bearing is not recommended until swelling has resolved and range of motion and exercise are pain free.

Surgical Treatment

Surgery is indicated for torn menisci that are causing symptoms—that is, pain, effusion, giving way, and/or locking. In contrast to past literature, recent investigations of the function, biomechanics, and blood supply of the menisci, as well as clinical observations with arthroscopic surgery, have shown that partial meniscectomy is preferable, if possible, to total meniscectomy. Additionally, certain peripheral meniscal tears seem amenable to surgical repair, as opposed to excision, in late as well as

acute cases. Preoperative arthrography is helpful in defining the tear and planning the surgical repair. Magnetic resonance imaging can provide even greater detail of the lesion and can be helpful in planning treatment.

In bucket-handle tears, excision of the bucket-handle segment only is preferred. Meniscal regeneration does not follow excision of the centrally displaced portion of a longitudinal tear. Morbidity and rehabilitation time following meniscectomy are lessened with partial meniscectomy. With the advent of arthroscopic surgery, a partial or total meniscectomy can be performed with little morbidity.

INFLAMMATION OF THE KNEE BURSAE

Athletes frequently develop inflammation of the bursae, or **bursitis**, about the knee. Bursitis is usually recognized without difficulty, but because of the close proximity to tendons and ligaments, the diagnosis may be confusing at times. Bursae are closed, fluid-filled sacs lined with synovium, similar to that lining the joint space. Their elegant but simple function is to reduce the friction between adjacent tissues, such as where skin and tendons pass over a bony prominence. Although many bursae are found about the knee, problems with only a few are consistently encountered (Fig. 21.44). The bursae are subject to a variety of conditions, including trauma, infections, metabolic abnormalities, rheumatic afflictions, and neoplasms.

Classification

Bursitis can usually be classified as either acute or chronic. In acute bursitis, the cause is usually traumatic, although an acute infectious bursitis must always be considered. Acute traumatic bursitis occurs in those bursae subject to direct injury. A typical example is prepatellar bursitis. The bursal sac becomes distended, often with a bloody effusion.

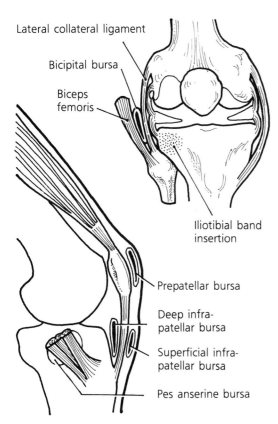

Lateral collateral ligament

Bicipital bursa

Biceps femoris

Iliotibial band insertion

Prepatellar bursa

Deep infra-patellar bursa

Superficial infra-patellar bursa

Pes anserine bursa

FIGURE 21.44. Bursae of the knee.

Chronic traumatic bursitis is encountered more frequently than the acute type. Because of repeated insults to the bursa, the bursal wall becomes thickened, and the sac volume increases so that the bursa extends far beyond its usual confines.

Acute bursitis secondary to infection is seen in the athlete who sustains a penetrating injury. Bacteria are inoculated into the bursa and rapidly produce a clinical picture of swelling, erythema, and exquisite tenderness. Infectious bursitis differs from the traumatic variety because of the added constitutional symptoms of fever and malaise. However, there can be local inflammation, redness, and pain in both the acute traumatic and the infectious bursitis. Since it may be very difficult to distinguish between the two, a high index of suspicion is necessary to diagnose the infectious type early. Usually, with infection, more redness and in-

flammation are present. A scratch or break in the skin may precede the onset of symptoms. If there is any question, a physician should be consulted immediately. Bacteria can spread by way of the lymphatics to the joint, causing pyarthrosis. This highlights the necessity for prompt first aid of lacerations to prevent a deep-seated infection, in this case an infectious bursitis. Also, extensive laceration of a bursa, such as the prepatellar bursa over the knee, requires formal cleansing, irrigation, and closure, often over a drain, as done in outpatient surgery.

Inflammation of Specific Bursae

Prepatellar Bursitis

The prepatellar bursa lies anteriorly between the skin and the outer surface of the patella. This location makes it particularly susceptible to direct trauma. Acute prepatellar bursitis presents as a tender, erythematous area of swelling over the patella. With knee flexion, increased skin tension directly over the bursa produces pain. Direct pressure over the bursa is also painful. The localization of signs and symptoms in front of the patella allows prepatellar bursitis to be distinguished from problems within the knee joint. Again, the first principle is to make the correct diagnosis and exclude an infectious cause of the swelling.

For acute traumatic bursitis, treatment consists of ice packs if bursal swelling arises within 24 hours after injury, followed by compression and rest until acute symptoms subside. On occasion, the bursa requires aspiration. When aspiration is performed, cultures should be taken. Rarely, operative drainage or excision is necessary. Recurrence of an effusion is likely in any knees subjected to direct trauma. For this reason, athletes should wear protective knee padding to prevent reinjury.

Chronic prepatellar bursitis is more frequent than the acute type. It results from repeated episodes of slight trauma, and the inflammation is usually recalcitrant to conservative therapy (Fig. 21.45). Treatment

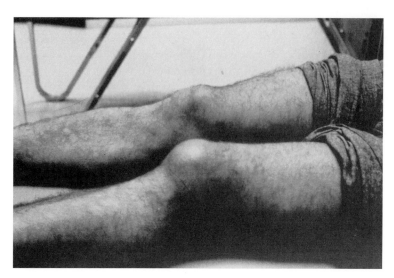

FIGURE 21.45. Chronic prepatellar bursitis that did not respond to conservative measures. Surgical excision is the treatment of choice.

consists of fluid aspiration and application of a pressure bandage. Again, padding is required to prevent recurrent trauma. Infrequently, the bursa becomes so distended that nothing short of surgical excision will suffice. As with the acute inflammation, the hallmark of effective treatment is to prevent direct trauma through protective padding. Local corticosteroid injection is reserved for those bursae that are inflamed as a result of trauma, where infection can be absolutely excluded, and where all other means of treatment have not decreased inflammation. Corticosteroid is administered into the bursa itself by a physician, with care to prevent injection into any neighboring structures. Because steroids seriously weaken tendons, they are not injected close to or about any tendons or ligamentous structures.

Deep Infrapatellar Bursitis

The deep infrapatellar bursa is positioned beneath and behind the patellar tendon and in front of the infrapatellar fat pad that lies on the anterior surface of the tibia. These neighboring structures make direct injury to the bursa difficult. Deep infrapatellar

bursitis may be an overuse syndrome due to friction between the patellar tendon and bone. Because of its deep location, the deep infrapatellar bursa is only rarely the cause of symptoms. Localized pain and tenderness in this region are more frequently due to Osgood-Schlatter disease. The diagnosis is by local palpation to find the area of maximum tenderness. Treatment is as previously described.

Superficial Infrapatellar Bursitis

The superficial infrapatellar bursa rests between the skin and the anterior surface of the infrapatellar tendon. It becomes inflamed secondary to direct trauma, and may be clinically indistinguishable from Osgood-Schlatter disease. The symptoms of superficial infrapatellar bursitis are localized pain and tenderness just over the patellar tendon and the tibial tubercle. Treatment is as described, with local protection to prevent recurrent trauma.

Pes Anserine Bursitis

The anserine bursa lies between the pes anserinus tendons (sartorius, gracilis, and semitendinosus) and the tibial collateral ligament on the medial aspect of the tibia. Bursitis develops because of friction or from direct injury. Pain and tenderness are localized to the anteromedial aspect of the tibia. Rotation motion and contraction of the pes anserinus muscles aggravate symptoms. Anserine bursitis must be distinguished from an injury to the medial collateral ligament, medial tendons, or tear of the medial meniscus. Crepitus can be elicited (a feature of bursitis), and there is tenderness beneath the pes tendons. A valgus stress usually produces much more pain in a medial collateral ligament injury than in bursitis. With meniscal tears, there is localized tenderness directly at the joint line. The anserine bursa lies about 2 cm distal to the medial joint line. Tenderness is noted on palpation of an inflamed anserine bursa and is below the level of the joint line. Stress fractures of the proximal tibia can also manifest as tenderness in this area, but they are usually more diffuse and may not have the localized swelling that is noted with anserine bursitis. Treatment is principally symptomatic, consisting of ice, anti-inflammatory agents, and steroid injections as indicated.

Bicipital Bursitis

The lateral aspect of the knee contains many small bursae that reduce friction between the interdigitations of the biceps tendon and the fibular collateral ligament and other lateral structures. Whereas most of these bursae are inconsistent in location, the bicipital bursa consistently lies between the fibular collateral ligament and the fibular attachment of the biceps tendon. The inflammation of bicipital bursitis ensues after overactivity and, infrequently, after direct trauma. The diagnosis again rests with excluding ligament or meniscal injuries. Local swelling, so typical of bursitis, is the only real differential. Treatment is symptomatic as previously described.

Iliotibial Band Friction Syndrome

An acute inflammatory condition called **iliotibial band friction syndrome** occurs where the iliotibial band repeatedly rubs against the bony prominence of the lateral femoral epicondyle. This condition is common with running, especially downhill, or any activity with repetitive flexion and extension of the knee. Symptoms are worse climbing hills or stairs. The band drops posteriorly with knee flexion and rubs against the femoral epicondyle. The person often walks with the knee in full extension, preventing knee flexion.

The exact site of inflammation is often in the soft tissue, presumably as a result of the mechanical friction. Treatment is symptomatic, with rest or a decrease in activities, ice, and use of anti-inflammatory medication. In persistent conditions, a local corticosteroid injection is occasionally prescribed. With lateral knee pain on running, a malalignment problem, such as knee varus that places stress on the lateral tissues, may be present.

Popliteal Cyst (Baker's Cyst)

The term **Baker's cyst** is a catch-all for localized fluid accumulation in the posterior fossa of the knee. The cyst may be due to actual bursitis (such as seen in the semimembranosus bursa) or a structural defect in the posterior capsule that permits synovial herniation. There may be as much as a 50 percent incidence of communication between the joint space and the popliteal (semimembranosus) bursa in asymptomatic individuals. With chronic knee effusions, torn menisci, or swelling due to any cause within the knee, synovial fluid accumulates within the communicating bursae.

Most athletes who have a Baker's cyst complain of a mass behind the knee that may or may not be painful. The mass is particularly bothersome at full flexion and extension. Furthermore, many athletes report periods during which the mass disappears. It is of utmost importance to exclude other causes of a popliteal mass. Rarely, rheumatoid arthritis, arterial aneurysm, arteriovenous fistula, thrombophlebitis, or tumor may be present.

Treatment of the symptomatic cyst rests on correcting the underlying cause of joint swelling, after which the cyst often disappears. Arthrography, MRI, or arthroscopy can often help diagnose the cause of chronic joint effusion. Occasionally, in long-standing cases, the cyst requires excision after the primary internal derangement of the knee has been corrected. In general, cyst aspiration and injection, as well as joint immobilization, are not regarded as satisfactory modes of treatment because they do not treat the primary cause of the cyst. In children, this situation is different, and the cyst can appear spontaneously, with no intra-articular abnormality, and later disappear without recurrence. However, in adults, the presence of the fluid-filled bursa often denotes intra-articular abnormalities (meniscal tear, arthritis, etc.) as described.

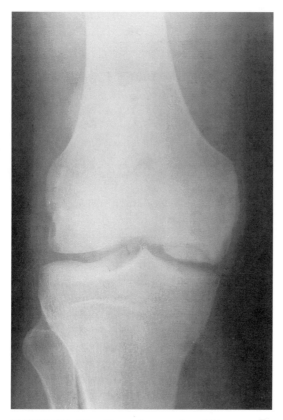

FIGURE 21.46.   X-ray of osteochondritis dissecans.

OSTEOCHONDRITIS DISSECANS

Osteochondritis dissecans is a condition of adolescents and young adults in which a part of the articular surface of a joint separates because of a cleavage plane through the subchondral bone (Fig. 21.46). The true cause of osteochondritis dissecans is not definitely known, although several theories have been proposed. A familial tendency and an association with certain skeletal or endocrine abnormalities have been noted, but in most cases a combination of factors, including trauma, nonunion of a fracture line, and ischemic necrosis, seems to be involved. Clinically and experimentally, osteochondral fractures are seen wherever osteochondritis dissecans is seen. Either direct exogenous trauma to the articular surface or indirect endogenous trauma from one bony surface forcefully striking another produces an acute osteochondral fracture. Some believe that a very prominent tibial spine may impinge against the intercondylar portion of the medial femoral condyle, producing the fracture. This site is the classic and most common site for the lesion. More recently, in the hyperflexed knee, the odd facet of the patella has been shown to impinge against this region and, with enough force, can cause a fracture. The fracture may be undiagnosed and, with repeated trauma, it fails to unite. The fracture fragment becomes walled off from the remainder of the epiphysis by fibrous tissue. As a result, the blood supply becomes interrupted and the bone dies. The cartilage of the articular surface remains alive, however, because it receives nutrition from the synovial fluid. The result is the typical lesion of osteochondritis dissecans—viable articular cartilage with underlying dead subchondral bone, separated from the remainder of the epiphysis by a layer of fibrous tissue.

Two additional observations may explain the particular association of this lesion with the adolescent age group. First, an adult joint has a junction between calcified and uncalcified cartilage called the *tide mark*, where the cartilage surface gains attachment to the underlying bone. This junction is absent in the juvenile joint. When shearing forces are applied in the adult, they are transmitted through the tide mark, causing a chondral fracture but sparing the subchondral bone, resulting in the typical osteochondral fracture. Second, irregular ossification centers frequently occur in normal children. Minor trauma may cause a cleavage plane that interrupts an already tenuous blood supply and results in the typical lesion.

The typical lesion consists of a separated fragment of dead subchondral bone covered by live cartilage. A cleavage plane of fibrous and inflammatory tissue separates the dead bone from the underlying normal, viable epiphyseal bone.

Three stages of lesions are based on the degree of separation from the underlying epiphysis: (1) nondisplaced with continuity of the articular cartilage, (2) partially displaced with disruption of the articular cartilage, and (3) completely detached (i.e., loose body in the joint). The nondisplaced or partially separated lesion may heal. Capillaries invade from the periphery, bringing in viable osteoclasts and osteoblasts that remodel and lay down new bone on top of the necrotic trabecular bone. In the totally detached lesion, the raw bony surfaces of both the loose body and the cavity are covered with a fibrous tissue that becomes fibrocartilage.

Clinical Presentation

The peak incidence of osteochondritis dissecans is in the adolescent and young adult. Males are more commonly affected than females. About half of the athletes give a history of trauma. In 10 percent of cases, additional sites may be involved, including the other knee, elbow, or ankle. The occurrence of many anatomical sites supports the theory of anomalous ossification or disturbances in growth.

The clinical presentation of osteochondritis dissecans is usually chronic knee pain and/or swelling with exertion. The pain is aching and poorly localized. If there is a loose body, the knee may momentarily lock. Physical examination reveals signs of chronic limitation and disuse, perhaps with synovial thickening and atrophy of the quadriceps muscles. With the classic lesion on the lateral portion of the medial femoral condyle, the region may be tender to palpation when the knee is acutely flexed.

In some athletes a clinical sign (Wilson's) may be specific for the classic lesion of osteochondritis. To perform this test, the athletic trainer flexes the athlete's knee to 90 degrees, internally rotates the tibia, and then extends the knee. At approximately 70 degrees of flexion, pain is elicited about the region of the medial femoral condyle. About 25 percent of athletes show align-

ment deformities of the knee, such as genu valgum (knock-knees), genu varum (bowleg), or genu recurvatum (back knee). The significance of these growth abnormalities is not known.

A definitive diagnosis can only be made by roentgenograms. A well-circumscribed area of sclerotic (dense), subchondral bone is separated from the remainder of the epiphysis by a radiolucent line. Since most lesions are noted in the intercondylar notch region of the medial femoral condyle, a tunnel view often shows this area to the best advantage.

Arthroscopy, MRI, and arthrography are additional diagnostic procedures that can be utilized if routine radiographs are inconsistent. These tests are also helpful in staging the lesion to determine the correct treatment.

Treatment

For the early, nonseparated symptomatic lesion, immobilization by cast or soft knee immobilizer and diminished weight bearing for 4 to 6 weeks may be necessary. The leg should be casted in a position that protects the lesion from tibiofemoral contact. The initial period of immobilization is followed by refraining from strenuous activities. This is the prescribed treatment until radiographs demonstrate satisfactory healing. The younger the child and the shorter the duration of symptoms, the more likely is satisfactory healing. Occasionally, an entirely asymptomatic athlete may have a small osteochondral defect on a radiograph taken for another reason. In these cases, treatment consists of close follow-up and repeat radiographs; immobilization is unnecessary.

In the older athlete or the more chronic lesion, surgery is frequently the treatment of choice. Certainly, surgical removal of a loose fragment is necessary. For the lesion still attached, treatments available include simple drilling, curettage and drilling, and pinning in situ by metallic pins or cortical bone pegs. Some procedures can be performed by arthroscopic surgery. Whatever method is used, cast immobilization for 6 to 8 weeks follows. If metallic pins are used, a second operative procedure is required to remove them. The overall prognosis is generally good to excellent, depending on the size of the lesion. Older athletes have less favorable results, especially when degenerative joint changes have already developed before surgery.

OSTEOCHONDRAL FRACTURES

An **osteochondral fracture** is an intra-articular fracture in which part of the articular surface is separated from the remainder of the epiphysis by a fracture line through the subchondral bone (Fig. 21.47). The fracture may result from exogenous trauma with a direct, tangential blow to the knee or from endogenous trauma where one bony structure hits another as a result of forceful rotation and axial compression. Each type of trauma produces predictable fracture

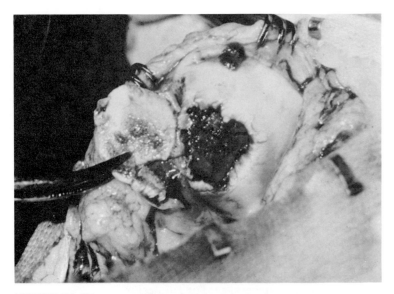

FIGURE 21.47. An osteochondral fracture demonstrated at open arthrotomy. Note the disruption of a large portion of the articular surface. (From Don H. O'Donoghue. "Treatment of Acute Dislocations of the Patella." In American Academy of Orthopaedic Surgeons: *Symposium on the Athlete's Knee.* St. Louis: The C. V. Mosby Co., 1980.)

sites in the involved bones. Exogenous trauma causes fractures in any exposed location, such as the medial or lateral aspect of the femoral condyles or the margins of the tibia. These fractures may be large, involving a considerable portion of the articulating surface. Endogenous trauma usually produces smaller lesions in the interior protected areas of the joint—for example, the intercondylar notch region of the medial femoral condyle or the patellofemoral joint.

A common area of fracture due to patellar dislocation is the anterolateral aspect of the lateral femoral condyle or medial aspect of the patella. With patellar dislocation, the patellar undersurface strikes the lateral femoral condyle, fracturing one or both surfaces. An underlying malalignment of the extensor mechanism may be the cause of the acute patellar dislocation.

Pathology

In osteochondral fractures an acute fracture line through the subchondral bone produces a fragment consisting of articular cartilage and viable subchondral bone. If the fragment becomes separated, the defect begins to fill in with fibrous tissue, usually within 10 days. If the fragment remains in place, the hematoma is invaded by capillaries that bring fibroblasts and other cells involved in bony healing. Just as likely, however, a fibrous nonunion may develop from inadequate immobilization or the repeated trauma of weight bearing. In this case, the fracture appears very much like osteochondritis dissecans. Because of this similarity, many orthopedists believe that the osteochondritis lesion is an ununited osteochondral fracture. The bony portion becomes necrotic, the articular cartilage remains viable, and the fracture line fills in with fibrous tissue. The entire piece may later separate and be caught in the joint.

Clinical Evaluation

The fracture usually occurs in the adolescent with no preexisting knee abnormalities. There may be a history of a direct blow to the knee or a violent twisting motion that produced an audible snap or pop. Intra-articular swelling due to blood in the joint occurs within hours. The athlete may be unable to bear weight on the extremity due to pain. On aspiration, the effusion is bloody. Severe muscle spasm or the fragment displaced as a loose body in the joint may cause the knee to lock in the flexed position. If the fracture is a result of patellar dislocation, an associated tear of the medial retinaculum may produce medial joint line tenderness. The presence of joint line tenderness may lead the athletic trainer to diagnose the condition erroneously as a meniscal tear. Ligamentous instability may be associated with osteochondral fractures. These defects were reported in as many as one-fifth of knees with acute anterior cruciate tears. If the athlete does not present acutely, symptoms may become chronic, with vague knee pain and recurrent swelling, the typical picture of osteochondritis dissecans.

Role of Radiographs and Arthroscopy

The definitive diagnosis depends on visualizing the fragment on radiographs or arthroscopically. Since cartilage is not visualized on routine radiographs and the bony fragment is usually small, the lesion is commonly missed. Multiple views of the knee may be necessary to rotate the fragment into view where overlap of other bony structures does not obscure it. The usual views are anteroposterior, lateral, right and left obliques, tunnel, and axial patella (sunrise). If the diagnosis remains in doubt, arthroscopy usually defines the extent of injury and resolves any questions on the cause of the hemarthrosis in acute injuries.

Treatment

The treatment of osteochondral fractures is usually surgical. If the fracture fragment is very small and on a non-weight-bearing surface, it may be simply excised. Larger fragments and those situated on a weight-bearing surface are anatomically reduced and fixed in place. Afterward, the knee is placed in a cylinder cast and protected from weight bearing. Full weight bearing on the knee is usually not allowed until healing and incorporation of the fracture fragment into the fracture bed. Healing may take 12 to 16 weeks from the time of surgery. Arthroscopic visualization of the joint surface is sometimes used to determine the extent of healing.

If surgical treatment is delayed past 10 days, achieving an anatomic reduction may be difficult because of fibrous tissue ingrowth about the fracture bed. In long-standing lesions it may be impossible to replace the separated fracture fragment. This problem underscores the urgency of diagnosis and treatment.

Prognosis

The prognosis for the acutely treated lesion is good to excellent. The prognosis for lesions not treated until the chronic phase is reasonably good but not as favorable as the prognosis for acutely treated lesions because of difficulties in restoring the articular surface anatomically. With less than ideal restoration of the joint surface, degenerative changes may occur, and the prognosis is poor. Any extensive fracture of the joint surface carries the risk of surface deterioration and future joint arthritis.

OSSEOUS FRACTURES ABOUT THE KNEE

Distal Femoral Fractures

The supracondylar area extends from the femoral condyles to the junction of the femoral metaphysis and diaphysis. The condylar area is the region from the top of the femoral condyles to the knee joint line (Fig. 21.48).

Displacement of fractures in this area can be predicted on the basis of the muscle

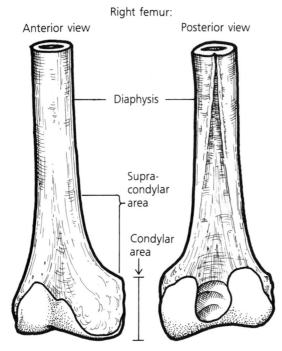

Right femur:
Anterior view   Posterior view

Diaphysis

Supra-
condylar
area

Condylar
area

FIGURE 21.48. Areas of the femur.

attachments. Generally, fractures of the distal femur angulate and displace posteriorly. The adductor muscles tend to rotate and shorten the femoral shaft, whereas the quadriceps, hamstrings, and gastrocnemius contribute to posterior displacement of the condylar fragment.

Severe valgus or varus stress, coupled with axial loading or rotational forces, produces fractures of the distal femur. Although vehicular accidents as in auto racing account for most of these fractures, they may also be produced by a fall on the flexed knee, particularly in the older, osteoporotic, recreational athlete.

Initial treatment of distal femoral fractures is splinting and immobilization. Neurovascular status should be evaluated and treated, if necessary. Closed treatment includes application of skeletal traction with maintenance of the fracture in a reduced position as documented by serial x-rays. After early healing has occurred, the athlete can progress to a spica cast treatment protocol.

Surgical treatment includes an open reduction and internal fixation with plates and screws or metallic rods, as indicated. After initial healing has occurred from nonsurgical treatment or stabilization and wound healing has been achieved from surgical treatment, the athlete should begin a progressive, active range-of-motion rehabilitation program to prevent soft tissue fibrosis and ankylosis of the hip and knee joint.

Supracondylar Fractures

Supracondylar fractures may be undisplaced, impacted, or displaced. Displaced fractures may be transverse or oblique in the orientation of the fracture line, and accompanied by comminution. History includes major trauma, followed immediately by painful swelling and deformity of the distal thigh. Usually there is gross motion and crepitus at the fracture site. Neurovascular damage associated with this injury is uncommon, but disruption of a major vessel can occur, and circulatory status of the lower leg should be carefully evaluated.

Evaluation of a supracondylar fracture requires anteroposterior and lateral radiographs of the knee, as well as anteroposterior and lateral x-ray films of the femoral shaft and hip to avoid overlooking serious associated injuries.

Treatment may be closed or surgical. Closed methods entail traction for reduction, followed by application of a long leg cast, spica cast, or cast brace. In open treatment, traction is followed by operative reduction and fixation with metallic plates and screws or with intramedullary rods. After operative treatment, external immobilization by cast or by cast brace is usually required. Early knee motion is advised to prevent fibrous ankylosis.

Intercondylar Femoral Fractures

Fractures of the femoral metaphysis with extension into the knee joint may be represented as a T or Y fracture, depending on the configuration of the fracture lines, although a variety of fracture configurations may be present. Neer's classification, the most widely accepted, is based on displacement and comminution of the supracondylar extension of the fracture line (Fig. 21.49).

In addition to deformity, intercondylar femoral fractures are associated with a marked knee effusion and crepitus on passive knee motion. In general, the same mechanism of injury accounts for these injuries as in supracondylar fractures—a blow to the flexed knee, as well as varus or valgus combined with rotational forces.

While treatment of these fractures may or may not be operative, the intra-articular relationship of the knee must be reestablished. Surgical intervention is often necessary to achieve this goal. Postoperatively, a cast or cast brace is required, again with a goal of early knee motion.

Femoral Condyle Fractures

Isolated fractures of the femoral condyle are not as common as supracondylar and intercondylar fractures. They are the result of abduction or adduction forces or axial loading.

Following injury, crepitus with knee motion and varus or valgus instability may be apparent. A large hemarthrosis develops. While anteroposterior and lateral radiographs should be obtained to evaluate this injury, oblique views are often necessary to appreciate the full extent of the fracture.

Treatment may be operative or nonoperative. The nondisplaced fracture treated nonsurgically must be carefully observed for any tendency to displace. Open reduction and internal fixation are usually required for displaced or comminuted fractures, again with the goal of early knee motion to prevent fibrous ankylosis.

Proximal Tibial Fractures

Fractures of the proximal tibia may be articular or nonarticular, but loss of knee function is the primary consideration in both. The proximal tibial metaphysis flares from

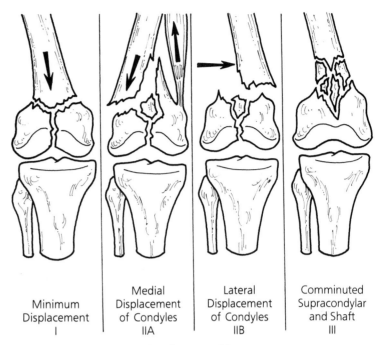

| Minimum Displacement I | Medial Displacement of Condyles IIA | Lateral Displacement of Condyles IIB | Comminuted Supracondylar and Shaft III |

FIGURE 21.49.   Neer's classification of fractures.

the diaphysis to provide a large, relatively flat surface to articulate with the distal femur. The intercondylar eminence is a nonarticular region between the two tibial condyles to which the anterior cruciate is attached.

Fractures to the tibial condyles are known as "bumper" injuries, but falls from heights and twisting falls also produce these injuries. Forces in vertical compression produce characteristic fractures of a T or Y configuration. Pure varus or valgus forces tend to cause ligament injury, whereas, when combined with axial loading forces, they cause various types of fracture configurations. The location and the amount of depression of the fracture depend to some extent on the amount of knee flexion at the time of injury. With the knee extended, the compression force is exerted anteriorly. With flexion, the middle or posterior third of the articular surface may be involved.

Undisplaced fractures are those that show less than 4 mm of depression or plateau widening. Displaced fractures are

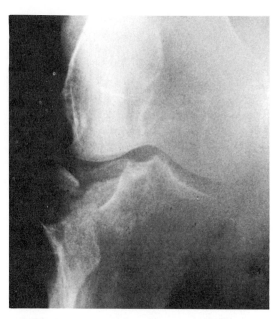

FIGURE 21.50. Compression fracture of the lateral tibial condyle with disruption of the articular surface and severely depressed bone.

compression fractures, split fractures, or total plateau fractures.

Compression fractures are divided into two distinct subtypes. In one, the compression is localized to an area roughly shaped to the corresponding femoral condyle. In the second type, compression occurs with splitting off of a fragment of the metaphysis and articular surface (Fig. 21.50).

Proximal tibial fractures produce acute pain and swelling of the knee. The athlete may be aware that the knee was deformed at the time of injury. While hemarthrosis is common, sometimes the capsule tears and hemorrhage drains spontaneously into the soft tissues of the knee. Limited motion and pain over the tibial metaphysis are present. Relative varus or valgus instability may be noted with stress testing, which is secondary to the loss in height of the tibial articular surface. Stress x-rays are often necessary to locate an associated ligamentous injury.

Treatment may be operative or nonoperative, depending on the severity of the fracture. Of paramount importance is restoring the normal articular surface with early knee motion and delayed weight bearing. When the articular surface has been severely depressed, bone grafting may be necessary in order to maintain the depressed articular surface in a reduced position. Traction is an alternative form of treatment in displaced fractures.

In nondisplaced fractures, plaster immobilization or cast brace immobilization may be employed. Again, weight bearing is delayed, but knee motion is encouraged early in the course of treatment. With severe depression of the articular surface, open reduction usually is necessary.

Tibial Spine Fractures

Violent twisting or abduction-adduction injuries may cause fractures of the tibial spine. Avulsion of portions of the intercondylar eminence adjacent to the tibial spine indicates cruciate ligament avulsion.

The athlete with a tibial spine fracture may present with effusion and often cannot fully extend the knee. Signs of anterior or posterior cruciate ligament insufficiency may be present. Cycling injuries in children commonly cause tibial spine fractures.

Closed treatment is indicated when the avulsed fragment is minimally displaced. If closed reduction cannot be performed, arthrotomy and open reduction with fixation by any number of available methods are performed. Postoperatively, cast immobilization with the knee held in nearly full extension for 5 to 6 weeks is necessary, followed by rehabilitation.

Patellar Fractures

The patella protects the anterior articular surface of the distal femur and increases the force of the quadriceps mechanism by improving the lever arm. Patellar fractures constitute 1 percent of all skeletal injuries and occur in all ages. The leading causes of injury include falls, direct blows, traffic accidents, and falls from heights. Bilateral fractures are uncommon. Ipsilateral fractures (in the same extremity) occur in 15 percent of athletes with patellar fractures.

Patellar fractures are classified into three types: (1) transverse (60 to 75 percent in frequency), (2) comminuted and stellate (28 to 34 percent in frequency), and (3) longitudinal (12 to 20 percent in frequency). Stress fractures, while rare, may occur in the lower patella and result in detachment of the extensor mechanism.

The mechanism of injury and the position of flexion at the time of trauma influence the type of fracture produced. Indirect violence produces a transverse fracture, as does a sudden, forced contraction of the quadriceps when the knee is flexed (eccentric muscle contraction). The patella is literally "pulled apart," fracturing through the plane of tensile stress, which is perpendicular to the muscle pull.

Direct violence is commonly caused by dashboards in auto accidents but may also occur in any athletic endeavor. These fractures are usually comminuted, with or without separation of the fragments. Direct blows may also produce serious ligamentous injuries besides the obvious patellar fracture. A thorough physical and roentgenographic examination is necessary to evaluate the knee and extremity properly.

The diagnosis of patellar fractures usually presents little problem. Often an indentation is palpable over the anterior aspect of the knee, and the athlete is unable to perform a straight-leg raise. Radiographic diagnosis is usually made in frontal, lateral, and axial views. Differential diagnosis includes the bipartite patella, found in 1 to 6 percent of adolescents. Bipartite patella, often bilateral, occurs in the proximal and lateral aspect of the patella and is nine times more common in men than in women.

The treatment of patellar fractures is based on the nature of the injury and the type of fracture. Nonoperative treatment is recommended for nondisplaced fractures where the extensor mechanism is preserved. A separation of 2 to 3 mm is acceptable, provided the articular surface is without a stepoff. The knee is immobilized in a cylinder plaster cast or knee immobilizer splint for 4 to 6 weeks. Then partial weight bearing is followed by rehabilitation. The prognosis is generally excellent for nondisplaced fractures.

Operative treatment is indicated when the fracture fragments are displaced more than 4 mm or with major disruption of the quadriceps extensor mechanism requiring repair. Different surgical treatments are based on the type or severity of fracture. **Osteosynthesis**, a fixation designed to internally fix and reduce the fracture fragments with wire, screws, and pins, is used to obtain bony union. Alternative treatments include partial **patellectomy**, where one large fragment of the patella is retained to save patellar function and the smaller fragments are excised. The extensor mechanism is repaired as indicated. Total patellectomy is a last resort for comminuted fractures when no large fragment can be retained.

Rehabilitation is most important after all forms of treatment, operative or nonoperative. Duration of immobilization may vary, but muscle strength and power must be regained to return the athlete to the preinjury level of function. Bone and soft tissue healing requires a number of weeks of protection before any strenuous quadriceps exercises are instituted.

Injuries to the Growth Plate

The seriousness of bony injuries about the knee in growing children cannot be overemphasized. Not only are these injuries critical in terms of locomotion, but the growth centers about the knee determine approximately 65 percent of the longitudinal growth of the lower extremity—40 percent in the distal femoral epiphysis and 25 percent in the proximal tibial epiphysis.

The growth plate is often the weakest link in the growing child. With angular displacements about the knee, a fracture occurs across the cartilage growth plate, which may injure the cellular component and lead to cessation of growth and a short limb.

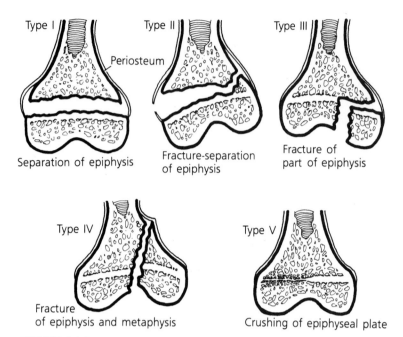

FIGURE 21.51. Salter-Harris classification of fractures.

The diagnosis of growth plate injury is made by finding local tenderness about the growth plate region and from varus and valgus stress x-ray views of the knee. With fracture, the growth plate opening can be seen on stress radiographs.

Because of the stout periosteal layer in the bones of the growing child, joint alignment can usually be obtained by closed means. An anatomical restoration of the growth plate, however, is essential, even if surgery is the only option. Traditionally, the Salter-Harris classification has been used as a guide for prognosis and treatment (Fig. 21.51). The Type I, or shear injury, has traditionally been given the best prognosis and Type V, or compression injury, the worst prognosis for continued growth.

MANAGEMENT OF KNEE INJURIES

Protocol for Injury Management

Proper and appropriate care of the knee begins immediately on injury. Although initially the degree of damage and involve-

ment may not be ascertained in every detail, early evaluation and proper care are necessary for optimal recovery. In the protocol for knee management, the following steps should take place:

- Determine how the injury occurred, either from the injured athlete or another individual (player, official, etc.) if the trainer did not see it.
- Determine the area and degree of pain.
- Determine if there is injury to other areas by checking:
  1. Sensation and circulation in the extremity.
  2. Position of the limb.
  3. Stability of the knee.
  4. Active and passive motion of the joints.

The degree of pain and involvement dictates initial care. All of the above information may not be collected immediately. Obviously, if the athlete is down on the field of play and in intense pain and a quick glance indicates an obvious deformity, the course of action is different from the case of an athlete's limping off the field and seeking assistance.

Treatment Schedule

The injured athlete presents in one of five categories:

- *Category I*: Injured athlete on the field.
- *Category II*: Injured athlete who limps off the field.
- *Category III*: Injured athlete who is still participating but summons help during the course of competition or practice.
- *Category IV*: Athlete seen after the game.
- *Category V*: Athlete with next-day evaluation.

These categories may in no way indicate severity. The injury seen the next day may be as severe as that seen on the field.

Category I

The athletic trainer pinpoints the problem by asking the injured athlete where the pain is located. In some cases, a severe injury may be apparent and appropriate first-aid steps are then important. The following injuries fall into this category:

- Severe ligamentous injury.
- Dislocations (determined by observation).
- Fractures (determined by observation).
- Multistructure involvement (determined by observation).
- These injuries should be handled as outlined in Chapter 14.

Category II or III

When the athlete comes off the field under his or her own power, the athletic trainer should direct the person to an area where a thorough examination can be conducted. The trainer begins by collecting a complete history. Questions include: Where does it hurt? How did it happen? Did you hear anything? What does it feel like? The athletic trainer should already be familiar with any history of injury.

In deciding whether immediate return to competition is possible or if a serious injury requires treatment, the trainer must consider the following factors:

- Is there adequate stability?
- Is there adequate strength?
- Is there adequate mobility?
- Is the athlete ready (mentally)?
- Is added support or taping necessary?

The extent of injury may not be evident immediately, so ice may be applied initially. Later, after the pain has subsided, the athlete should be allowed to move around. The athletic trainer observes the athlete for a limp or any inability to use the extremity fully. If the repeat examination reveals no serious injury, the athlete tries the knee along the sidelines by light jogging. The trial can progress until the athlete has proven the ability to participate fully, without limitation. Any question regarding the ath-

lete's condition should be referred to a team physician.

Injuries treated on the sidelines need to be followed very closely and definitely re-evaluated after the contest or practice. The course of ICE (ice, compression, and elevation) should be followed. Splinting and crutches may even be warranted.

Category IV or V

Serious knee injuries may present after play or the next day. For example, in one study, approximately 15 percent of those sustaining an anterior cruciate tear after a twisting injury continued to play. After the game or during the next day, knee effusion and stiffness brought the athlete to the athletic trainer or physician. Continued participation in sports places the athlete at increased risk for the knee to give way and produce further damage.

The athletic trainer should reinforce the necessity of having every "knee sprain" examined. The usual error is to assume the condition is not serious. The trainer must continually observe for any limp, stiffness, knee swelling, or knee complaints, even those thought to be minor. Additionally, even minor ligament sprains (first-degree, no laxity) require vigorous rehabilitation to restore normal muscular strength, endurance, and coordination and to prevent more serious injury. Subtle patellofemoral subluxations can produce a gradual weakness and lead to a full giving-way episode and serious injury.

Suggested Treatment Plan

- Acute treatment: first 24 hours
  1. ICE (appropriate ice treatment with compression and elevation).
  2. Crutches (non-weight-bearing).
  3. Pressure wrap (toe to upper two-thirds of the thigh).
  4. Splint or knee immobilizer.

- 24 hours after injury
  1. Appropriate cold therapy.
  2. Crutches.

3. Pressure wrap (toe to upper two-thirds of the thigh).
4. Splint or knee immobilizer.
5. Exercise protocol.
6. Factors that determine when active range of motion is allowed.

   a. Absence of laxity or minimal laxity as found by physician.
   b. No effusion.
   c. Absence of or minimal pain.
   d. Minimal patellar crepitus.

■ Early mobilization period to progressive range of motion

1. Appropriate cold therapy twice a day with active range of motion within pain limits.
2. Patellar mobilization (medial-lateral and proximal-distal).
3. Crutch walking (progression).

   a. Functional range (two crutches).
   b. Absence of effusion (one crutch or cane).
   c. Absence of pain and limp (discard cane or crutch).
   d. Adequate strength (maintain knee extension while weight bearing).
   e. Supportive devices (braces).

4. Exercise protocol.

REHABILITATION OF THE KNEE

To rehabilitate an injured knee, pain, swelling, and the effects of acute injury must first be relieved. Damaged tissue requires time to heal. This is true for both surgically and nonsurgically treated knees. Pain is an important guideline to the extent of healing. Remaining pain is a clear warning of further damage. In the early-injury or postoperative phase, immobilization (splint or cast) and crutches provide the rest necessary for healing and relief of pain.

Decreasing Inflammation and Pain

Every injured or postoperative knee has some degree of inflammation. Inflamma-

tion of the synovial tissues can be secondary to a hemarthrosis. Blood acts as an irritant, causing the synovial tissue to become edematous, and this swelling increases the pain. Decreased swelling and effusion are important signs of improvement. To relieve swelling and inflammation, follow an ICE program. Initially use ice for 20 minutes, four to eight times per day, placing a towel over the knee and under the surrounding ice bags to avoid burning the skin. Cotton cast padding and Ace wraps provide compression. Rewrap the compressive dressing two to three times per day. Elevation is best supine, with the knee elevated higher than the heart. Aspirin in adequate doses (two tablets four times per day) is commonly the first medication, but nonsteroidal, anti-inflammatory medication may be required. Steroids have too many systemic effects for use in this setting.

Neuromuscular Reeducation

After measures to combat pain and inflammation, the next goal is reeducating the knee's neuromuscular system. Contraction of muscles in an injured or postoperative knee often causes pain. A reflex response acts to diminish muscle contraction and pain but also causes loss of muscular tone, resulting in considerable, rapid atrophy. To minimize this problem, exercise has to begin early. Exercise should be pain free. If exercise evokes pain, then either the repetitions or the intensity has to be reduced. Electrical muscle stimulation or transcutaneous nerve stimulation may be required if rehabilitation is delayed or initially painful. Muscle stimulation retards atrophy, and in some studies it produced hypertrophy. Once neuromuscular reeducation and muscle tone are established, pain sometimes diminishes dramatically, especially in disorders of the extensor mechanism and patellofemoral joint.

Cautions

While specific exercise techniques for strength, power, and endurance are discussed in the next section, a word of caution is required. Too vigorous an exercise or improper exercises can damage the knee. The patellar surface is most vulnerable. Tremendous loading forces of many times the body weight develop between the patella and femur with exercise. Frequently, exercising the quadriceps from 90 to 30 degrees produces pain in the patellofemoral joint. Therefore, initial exercises are often prescribed from 0 to 30 degrees of knee flexion.

Pain and swelling during the exercise program must be carefully followed. Added time for healing is often necessary before any vigorous exercises. After knee surgery, soft tissue must be allowed to heal before exercising begins. During immobilization, certain exercises may be done in the cast or splint.

Exercise programs must be designed to maintain the athlete's interest, as the recovery period is often long and tedious. After serious ligament injury and surgery, as long as 1 year's recovery may be necessary. Continued encouragement maintains motivation required for proper rehabilitation and a well-functioning knee.

Besides specific knee exercises, the rest of the lower extremity must not be ignored. The athletic trainer must be careful not to focus all the attention on the injured knee, only to find later that the hip and ankle musculature is weak from disuse, preventing full return to activity or potentially leading to another injury. A comprehensive exercise program should include back, hip, knee, and ankle exercises of the injured and uninjured extremities. Upper body exercise programs are also prescribed.

Proper rehabilitation is the key to good results, whether in acute nonsurgical knee injuries, chronic knee conditions, or surgically repaired knees.

Rehabilitation Programs

Orderly Sequence of Rehabilitation Program

Muscular weakness develops in all injured knees. After the relief of pain and recession

TABLE 21.6.   Rehabilitation Progression

Range-of-Motion Progression		
Active pain-free ROM* with appropriate modality		
Patellar mobilization (knee)		
Active assistive ROM with PNF†		
Resistive ROM		
Passive ROM		

Strength Progression		
Straight leg raising	8 × 10 to 10 lbs	
Short arc knee extensions	8 × 10 to 10 lbs	−30 to 0°
Full ROM PRE	4–8 × 10	90° to 0°

*Range of Motion
†Peripheral nerve facilitation

of inflammation and swelling, the first goal is to regain range of motion and then strength. Range of motion and strength must be achieved before power, endurance, speed, agility, and coordination are developed, because without range of motion and strength these other functions cannot be obtained (Table 21.6).

Achieving Range of Motion

Initial range-of-motion exercises consist of a gravity-aided active range-of-motion program, with the athlete sitting or standing. The knee should be taken to the extremes of resistance and pain in flexion and extension, with a goal of 0 to 90 degrees. Some assistance, such as peripheral nerve stimulation and careful manual assistance to the tolerances of pain, may be required. Once an acceptable range of motion of 0 to 90 degrees is achieved, resistance can be initiated, with light weights used to develop extension and aid in flexion of the knee. Finally, after pain and resistance have abated, passive manipulation and flexion and extension are used to develop the extremes of range of motion.

Achieving Strength: Basic Principles

Many techniques are cited for obtaining strength (Table 21.7). Whatever method is

TABLE 21.7. Rehabilitation Exercise Programs for Common Knee Problems

Diagnosis	Rehabilitation Areas to Stress	Method	Cybex or Orthotron
Chondromalacia patella Subluxating patella S/p‡ surgery for chronic dislocations or chronic irritative processes	Strengthening the quads, particularly VMO*, without putting additional stress on patellofemoral surface Achieve or maintain full ROM† General strengthening of hamstrings, ab- and adductors and lower leg musculature	Quad sets, straight lifts, lifts, short arcs with progressive resistance ROM and strengthening of hamstrings, ab- and adductors can be done conventionally	Only for strength testing
Anterior cruciate deficient knees, chronic/acute; s/p casting; s/p reconstruction, intra-articular or extra-articular	Achieve full ROM Emphasis is placed on strengthening secondary stabilizers to the anterior cruciate	Active ROM exercises Hamstring strength aims to equal quad strength of the nonaffected leg, done with programs of isometrics, isotonic with concentric and eccentric contractions; isokinetics Quad strength to be elevated by use of isometrics at 90°, 60°, 30° and full extension; isotonic resistance done only in 90°–45° flexion	For strength For hamstring strengthening For quad strengthening 90°–45° only
Medial collateral ligament sprains, chronic/acute, s/p reconstruction; s/p immobilization	Special emphasis should be placed on strengthening quads and adductors General ROM General strengthening of hamstrings, adductors and lower leg musculature	Achieve or maintain full ROM Quad sets Straight leg lifts with progressive resistance in hip flexion and adduction Isotonics for quads and hamstrings Isokinetics for quads and hamstrings	For testing and workouts

*Vastus medialis obliquus muscle
†Range of Motion
‡Status/post

used, the basic principle remains: the more demand on the muscle, the greater the resultant strength. There are many methods for progressively increasing this demand—some by daily methods, some weekly. All may be termed **progressive resistance exercises (PREs)**. Suffice it to say that some guidelines and goals must be set for every exercise period to see improvement.

Achieving Strength: Exercise Techniques

In the initial phases of knee rehabilitation, strength building is often started with isometric exercises for several reasons. First, moving the joint through a range of motion may cause pain. Second, isometrics can be done with the leg in a splint or cast. Third, isometrics in full extension put little or no force on the patellofemoral joint, which is important if patellofemoral chondrosis exists. Isometric exercises are started immediately after injury or surgery, and often exercise alone is sufficient to prevent further problems, particularly in the case of patellofemoral disorders. The athlete is taught simultaneous contraction of the quadriceps and hamstrings. This develops strength in both muscle groups without joint motion and can be done in any position of immobilized knee flexion.

To teach quadriceps isometrics, the athletic trainer positions the athlete on a table or bed, lying or sitting, with the knee extended or partially flexed if more comfortable. The athlete places his or her hand over the quadriceps muscle and palpates the muscle contraction. Usually, the vastus medialis obliquus is the most neglected and atrophied portion of the quadriceps muscle. The athlete specifically palpates the vastus medialis, feeling for a firm, sustained contraction. The "Rule of Tens" is followed: a 10-second contraction, 10 seconds of relaxation, repeated ten times each exercise period, six to ten times daily. If there is pain and reflex inhibition of the muscles, only a poor contraction is obtained.

In isometric exercises, the "shrug" principle is used. As the athlete contracts the muscle, he or she feels for the tone that is developed. In the middle of the 10-second contraction, the athlete may feel the tone diminish, requiring added contraction to regain a firm, hard muscle; the athlete "shrugs" the muscle to increase the tension. This maintains a near maximal contraction for a full 10 seconds.

Hamstring contractions can be done sitting, standing, or lying (prone or supine). The knee is placed in some degree of flexion to obtain a firm hamstring contraction. The therapist or trainer, a fixed object (table, wall, chair, or the athlete's cast), or simply co-contraction of the quadriceps muscle offers resistance. Other isometric exercises added to the program include hip abductor and adductor and flexion isometrics. Ankle extensor and flexor isometrics may also be done.

Straight-leg raises are an important adjunct to isometrics. The athlete lies supine on the table. After first doing a maximal isometric quadriceps contraction, the athlete lifts the leg off the table to a height of 1 to 2 feet. The athlete "shrugs" the quadriceps during the leg lift to further increase muscle tension. The extremity is held with the knee extended for 5 seconds, then slowly lowered while the quadriceps shrug is maintained. Full extension (no lag) must be maintained for complete contraction of the quadriceps muscle. If 10 to 15 straight-leg raises can be completed with no extensor lag, then weights may be placed at the knee or ankle.

Terminal extensions are another method for early quadriceps rehabilitation. A rolled towel is placed under the knee to give 5 to 10 degrees of knee flexion. The athlete then extends the knee straight and holds to a count of five. This exercise may also be done with ankle weights. If terminal extension is painful or if the athlete cannot lock the knee in extension, eccentric exercises with the leg over the side of the table may be prescribed. With the knee in full extension, a maximum isometric contraction is performed. The athlete gradually allows knee flexion. The athletic trainer may assist the exercise, or ankle weights may be used. Terminal extensions, whether in a concentric or eccentric mode, provide some protection of the patellar surface as the joint is not taken into full flexion.

Side step-ups can also be used if terminal extensions are painful. The athlete stands beside a step, usually 4 to 6 inches in height (low enough to keep the knee from flexing beyond 20 degrees to 30 degrees). He or she then steps up sideways and fully extends the knee, progressing to a toe raise. In coming down, the knee is slowly flexed, with the body weight over the knee until the opposite foot reaches the ground. This exercises the hip, knee, and ankle muscles, using body weight. It is a very effective exercise, yet simple and easy to do; furthermore, it requires no fancy equipment.

As the situation permits and strength improves, the athlete can progress to heavier weights and more sophisticated exercise equipment. The previously described exercises may be done at home. However, the use of equipment requires trainer supervision. Advancement to the exercise machines begins when the athlete is able to do exercises with 10 pounds of ankle weights. The first weight setting on many machines is around 10 pounds, and the exercise program will therefore progress smoothly. The

TABLE 21.8.   Progression of Activity (Endurance)

Phase I	4 inch step-ups daily	walk 30 min M, W, F	swim 30 min T, Th, Sa		
Phase II	8 inch step-ups daily	rapid walk 30 min M, Th	swim 30 min T, Sa	bike 30 min W, F (when 90° + range of motion at- tained at the knee)	
Phase III	12 inch step-ups daily	walk/jog 30 min M, Th	swim 30 min T, Sa	bike 30 min W, F	
Phase IV	18 inch step-ups daily	jog 30 min M, W, F	swim 30 min T, Th, Sa	bike 30 min T, Th, Sa	quads PRE at 30 lbs × 10 reps
Phase V	18 inch step-ups daily	full speed sprints 30 min, M, W, F	swim 30 min T, Th, Sa	bike 30 min T, Th, Sa	
Phase VI	18 inch step-ups daily	full speed sprints, cutting			quads PRE at 45 lbs × 10 reps
Phase VII	return to competition				

Criteria for Return to Activity After Lower Extremity Injury

Full, pain-free range of motion

Strength and power equal to uninjured side
  (80%+ may be used in season)

Endurance equal to uninjured side

Cardiovascular endurance complete

Cerebromuscular rehabilitation complete

Running tests without limp
  Full speed/straight ahead at preinjury times
  Full speed cutting left and right
  Full speed crossover or carioca

Able to control any instability

No effusion or swelling

Physician, trainer, and athlete agree on return to activity

Note: In progression of activity, all exercise should be pain-free, without a limp. In patellofemoral problems, eliminate step-ups over 8 inches.

patellofemoral joint is protected, if required, by blocking the machines to work only in a 0-degree to 30-degree extension range for quadriceps exercises. For hamstring exercises, no restriction of motion is necessary since the patellofemoral joint is not loaded.

Achieving Power, Endurance, Speed, Agility, Flexibility, and Coordination

As the PRE program begins to improve strength, attention can be directed to developing power, endurance, speed, agility, flexibility, and coordination (Table 21.8). Power is developed by doing the same amount of work faster, or more work at the same speed. This is controlled by putting a limit on the time allowed for one exercise period and requiring the athlete to complete his or her total exercise program in that allotted time.

Endurance is gained by exercising the muscle to fatigue with low weights and multiple repetitions. For the knee, this can be done by cycling or by careful use of isokinetics. Too much isokinetic resistance causes thrusting and injurious forces on the patellar surface or in healing ligaments. Exercising to fatigue (thigh burn) encourages endurance. Cardiovascular endurance for general body conditioning can be maintained by swimming or a running program in the swimming pool. Exercise in the pool is an excellent way to provide low forces on the joint by using the buoyancy of water to maintain balance and also to provide mild resistance to knee motion. Cycling may also be started, as long as the seat of the cycle is raised to a high level, decreasing the amount of flexion at the knee during the pedaling motion.

Running activities or individual sports activities are resumed gradually. The running program starts with straight-ahead running only. The athlete gradually progresses to figure-eight drills and faster running drills over weeks to months. Speed, agility, and coordination are developed by specific skill drills relative to the individual's chosen sport in the latter phases of rehabilitation.

Flexibility is an important aspect of knee rehabilitation. Flexibility exercises are begun early in rehabilitation as the range of motion improves. A good flexibility program includes exercises for the back, hip, knee, and ankle. The safest method is a slow, constant stretching at extremes of motion. A bouncing technique should not be used since it may produce small tears in a tight muscle. Bouncing also stimulates firing of the muscle spindles, thereby increasing muscle tension. This effect is the opposite of what is desired—namely, to stretch out the passive element in muscles. Flexibility programs should also be done before and after exercise periods.

Included in the flexibility program are active and passive range of motion. In the early phases of knee rehabilitation, pain and joint stiffness limit the range of motion. Mobilization of the patella is important to achieve complete range of motion. Active range of motion in which the athlete flexes and extends the knee under his or her own power is the safest. In passive range of motion, great care must be taken to avoid manually forcing the knee and causing damage. To perform passive motion, the athlete sits on the edge of the table and, with support from the good leg, gradually flexes the knee. This exercise should be done without pain. The athletic trainer may assist passive range of motion, but only

with gentle pressure and pushing. As the range of motion and strength increase and as pain decreases, the PRE program advances to include exercises performed through a full range of knee motion.

Return to Activity

As strength increases and enough time has elapsed for adequate tissue healing, the athlete is evaluated for return to activity. Strength and power are measured isotonically, isokinetically, or isometrically (manual muscle test). A strength of 80 to 85 percent of the uninjured knee is necessary before the rehabilitated athlete can resume activity that involves running. Hamstring strength should be 60 percent of the quadriceps muscles, except in the case of anterior cruciate ligament injuries, when the quadriceps and hamstring strength levels should be equally balanced.

The final stage of rehabilitation is often termed the "return to activity and maintenance stage." There can be no pain, swelling, or subjective knee instability. The return to activity is gradual, and the athlete must continue to build strength and endurance. Muscles may function adequately for the first 15 minutes or so in practice; then fatigue may set in due to loss of endurance. By continuing to practice, the athlete risks a repeat injury. Muscle strength and endurance should at least be 80 to 85 percent of the opposite, normal extremity before any strenuous activity is begun. Skill and running drills and practice situations involving sudden turning or twisting are gradually resumed over weeks to months, depending on the specific knee injury or condition. Agility and proper neuromuscular condition take time to build. These qualities must be finely developed, since they ultimately provide dynamic stability to the knee joint. To function athletically or in routine daily activities, knee strength must be maintained. This can be done with exercise periods two to three times per week. Other drills that develop fine skill, endurance, coordination, and agility are tailored to the individual.

REHABILITATION EXERCISES

General Knee Rehabilitation

Stationary Bike

Adjust seat height so that affected leg is almost straight with only a slight bend in the knee when the ball of the foot is on the lowest pedal. Tension should be set to allow minimum to moderate resistance. Begin riding for 10 minutes and progress to 30 minutes, two times daily.

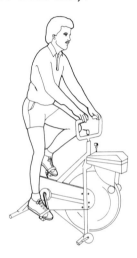

Resisted Knee Flexion

Sit in a chair facing pulley setup. Secure ankle strap around involved lower leg. Slide foot back as far as possible along floor against resistance. Hold for a count of five, relax and repeat. Perform 5 sets of 10, three times daily.

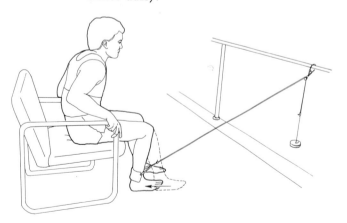

Assisted Knee Flexion

Sit in a chair with a rung. Secure rope around the ankle. Loop the free end of the rope under the rung and bring it over the top of the chair. Actively, bend the knee as far back as possible. Assist bending by pulling on the rope. Hold for a count of 10, relax, and repeat. Perform 3 sets of 10, three times daily.

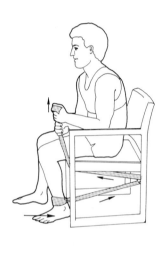

Active Knee Flexion

Sit in a chair with the involved foot flat on the floor. Slide the foot as far as possible using the hamstring muscle. Hold for a count of 5, relax, and repeat. Perform 3 sets of 10, three times daily.

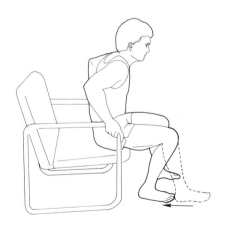

Side Step-Up

Stand sideways with the involved leg toward a step. Place the foot up on the step. Lift the body weight while pushing off with the toe of the uninvolved leg. Progress to standing on the heel of the uninvolved leg and lifting the entire body weight with no push-off. The height of the step should increase from 3 to 7 inches. Perform 5 sets of 10, three times daily.

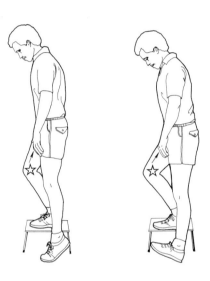

Postoperative Knee Rehabilitation

Terminal Knee Extension

Lie on back and place a towel roll under the involved knee, allowing it to bend slightly. Lift the heel and straighten the leg. Hold for a count of five and then relax. Perform 5 sets of 10, three times daily.

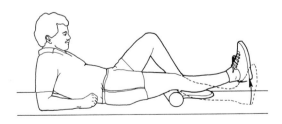

Flexion-To-Extension (70 to 40 degrees)

In a sitting position, with foot flat on floor, thigh completely supported, straighten the involved knee out until brace locks. Hold for a count of 5, then relax. Repeat 10 times; rest for 1 minute. Do 5 sets of 10, three times a day.

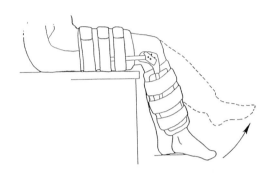

Hip Flexor Strengthening

In a sitting position, with foot flat on floor, thigh completely supported, lift the involved knee straight up while sitting straight. Hold for count of 5, then relax. Repeat 10 times; rest for 1 minute. Do 5 sets of 10, three times a day. To add resistance, begin with 1 pound of weight and gradually increase to 5 pounds of weight.

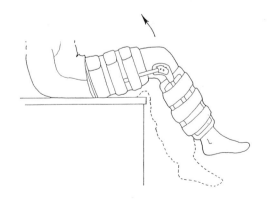

IMPORTANT CONCEPTS

1. The knee consists of three joints in one: a joint between the patella and the femur and a joint between each tibial and femoral condyle.

2. The extensor mechanism of the knee is a complex interaction of muscles and patellar ligaments that stabilize the patellofemoral joint and, through their formation of the patellar ligament (tendon), act together to extend the knee.

3. The menisci are fibrocartilaginous structures that lie between the hyaline cartilage surfaces of the femur and tibia.

4. The infrapatellar fat pad extends from the lower pole of the patella to the level of the tibia, behind and on each side of the patellar tendon.

5. The major structures on the medial aspect of the knee are the medial retinaculum, the tibial collateral ligament, the medial capsular ligaments, and the pes anserinus.

6. The hollow area that appears on the posterior surface of the knee is the popliteal space.

7. The major structures on the lateral aspect of the knee include the iliotibial tract, the iliotibial band, the joint capsule, the arcuate ligament, the fibular collateral ligament, and the short collateral ligament.

8. Knee injuries with ligament damage and gross instability require immediate treatment.

9. The physical examination is designed to test all major components of the knee joint, including the major ligaments, menisci, patellofemoral joint, and the muscles of the knee.

10. Marked swelling in the knee joint within 24 hours of injury is an ominous sign indicating hemorrhage and a potential significant intra-articular injury.

11. Ligament injuries to the knee are classified according to the severity of the sprain, the amount and direction of laxity, and the specific ligaments disrupted.

12. Knee stability depends on three systems: the passive system, which comprises the ligamentous and capsular structures that link the femur, tibia, and patella; the active system, which comprises the muscles that act through a functioning nervous system; and the system that allows joint geometry, or the ability to flex and extend and to rotate externally and internally.

13. Patellofemoral disorders include extensor mechanism deficiencies, patellofemoral stress syndrome, patellar tendinitis, Osgood-Schlatter disease, patellar dislocation, and patellar subluxation.

14. Meniscal tears of the knee can be longitudinal or horizontal and can be caused by acute injury or by cartilage degeneration.

15. Bursitis of the knee can be acute (from direct injury that causes the bursal sac to become distended) or chronic

(from repeated insults to the bursa so that the bursal wall thickens and the sac volume increases causing the bursa to extend beyond its usual confines).

16. Osteochondritis dissecans is a condition of adolescents and young adults in which part of the articular surface of a joint separates because of a cleavage plane through the subchondral bone.

17. An osteochondral fracture is an intra-articular fracture in which part of the articular surface is separated from the remainder of the epiphysis by a fracture line through the subchondral bone.

18. Osseous fractures about the knee include distal femoral fractures, supracondylar fractures, intercondylar fractures, femoral condyle fractures, proximal tibial fractures, tibial spine fractures, patellar fractures, and fractures across the cartilage of the growth plate in children.

19. Management of knee injuries includes initial evaluation of the injury, treatment according to the severity of injury, and a program of rehabilitation.

20. The goals of rehabilitation are to regain range of motion and strength first; then power, endurance, speed, agility, and coordination are developed.

SUGGESTED READINGS

Baker, B. E., A. C. Peckham, F. Pupparo, et al. "Review of Meniscal Injury and Associated Sports." *American Journal of Sports Medicine* 13 (1985): 1–4.

Baugher, W. H., and G. M. White. "Primary Evaluation and Management of Knee Injuries." *Orthopedic Clinics of North America* 16 (1985): 315–327.

Beck, J. L., and B. P. Wildermuth. "The Female Athlete's Knee." *Clinics in Sports Medicine* 4 (1985): 345–366.

Bentley, G., and G. Dowd. "Current Concepts of Etiology and Treatment of Chondromalacia Patellae." *Clinical Orthopaedics and Related Research* 189 (1984): 209–228.

Bertin, K. C., and E. M. Goble. "Ligament Injuries Associated with Physeal Fractures About the Knee." *Clinical Orthopaedics and Related Research* 177 (1983): 188–195.

Blazina, M. E., R. K. Kerlan, F. W. Jobe, et al. "Jumper's Knee." *Orthopedic Clinics of North America* 4 (1973): 665–678.

Bloom, Marvin H. "Traumatic Knee Dislocation and Popliteal Artery Occlusion." *The Physician and Sportsmedicine* 15 (October 1987): 142–155.

Boland, Arthur L., Jr. "Soft Tissue Injuries of the Knee." In *The Lower Extremity and Spine in Sports Medicine*, Vol. 1, edited by James A. Nicholas and Elliott B. Hershman, pp. 983–1012. St. Louis: C. V. Mosby, 1986.

Bradley, G. W., T. C. Shives, and K. M. Samuelson. "Ligament Injuries in the Knees of Children." *Journal of Bone and Joint Surgery* 61A (1979): 588–591.

Cahill, B. "Treatment of Juvenile Osteochondritis Dissecans and Osteochondritis Dissecans of the Knee." *Clinics in Sports Medicine* 4 (1985): 367–384.

Clanton, T. O., J. C. DeLee, B. Sanders, et al. "Knee Ligament Injuries in Children." *Journal of Bone and Joint Surgery* 61A (1979): 1195–1201.

Colville, J. M., and D. W. Jackson. "Reasonable Expectations Following Arthroscopic Surgery." *Clinics in Sports Medicine* 4 (1985): 279–293.

Dehaven, K. E. "Injuries to the Menisci of the Knee." In *The Lower Extremity and Spine in Sports Medicine*, Vol. 1, edited by James A. Nicholas and Elliott B. Hershman, pp. 905–928. St. Louis: C. V. Mosby, 1986.

Dehaven, K. E., W. A. Dolan, and P. J. Mayer. "Chondromalacia Patellae in Athletes. Clinical Presentation and Conservative Management." *American Journal of Sports Medicine* 7 (1979): 5–11.

DeLee, J. C., and R. Curtis. "Anterior Cruciate Ligament Insufficiency in Children." *Clinical Orthopaedics and Related Research* 172 (1983): 112–118.

DePalma, Bernard F., and Russell R. Zelko. "Knee Rehabilitation following Anterior Cruciate Ligament Injury or Surgery." *Athletic Training* 21 (1986): 200–204.

Drez, D., Jr. "Arthroscopic Evaluation of the Injured Athlete's Knee." *Clinics in Sports Medicine* 4 (1985): 275–278.

Feagin, J. A., Jr. "Operative Treatment of Acute and Chronic Knee Problems." *Clinics in Sports Medicine* 4 (1985): 325–331.

Fulkerson, J. P. "The Etiology of Patellofemoral Pain in Young, Active Patients: A Prospective Study." *Clinical Orthopaedics and Related Research* 179 (1983): 129–133.

Gecha, S. R., and E. Torg. "Knee Injuries in Tennis." *Clinics in Sports Medicine* 7 (1988): 435–452.

Grana, W. A., and L. A. Kriegshauser. "Scientific Basis of Extensor Mechanism Disorders." *Clinics in Sports Medicine* 4 (1985): 247–257.

Henard, D. C., and R. T. Bobo. "Avulsion Fractures of the Tibial Tubercle in Adolescents. A Report of Bilateral Fractures and a Review of the Literature." *Clinical Orthopaedics and Related Research* 177 (1983): 182–187.

Henning, Charles E., Mary A. Lynch, and Karl R. Glick, Jr. "Physical Examination of the Knee." In *The Lower Extremity and Spine in Sports Medicine*, Vol. 1, edited by James A. Nicholas and Elliott B. Hershman, pp. 765–800. St. Louis: C. V. Mosby, 1986.

Henning, C. E. "Semilunar Cartilage of the Knee: Function and Pathology." *Exercise and Sport Sciences Reviews* 16 (1988): 205–213.

Hohl, Mason, Robert L. Larson, and Donald C. Jones. "Fractures and Dislocations of the Knee." In *Fractures in Adults*, 2d ed., Vol. 2, edited by Charles A. Rockwood, Jr., and David P. Green, pp. 1429–1591. Philadelphia: J. B. Lippincott, 1984.

Holden, D. L., and D. W. Jackson. "Treatment Selection in Acute Anterior Cruciate Ligament Tears." *Orthopedic Clinics of North America* 16 (1985): 99–109.

Howe, James, and Robert J. Johnson. "Knee Injuries in Skiing." *Clinics in Sports Medicine* 1 (1982): 277–288.

Hughston, J. C., P. T. Hergenroeder, and B. G. Courtenay. "Osteochondritis Dissecans of the Femoral Condyles." *Journal of Bone and Joint Surgery* 66A (1984): 1340–1348.

Insall, J. "Current Concepts Review: Patellar Pain." *Journal of Bone and Joint Surgery* 64A (1982): 147–152.

Jensen, J. E., R. R. Conn, G. Hazelrigg, and J. E. Hewett. "Systematic Evaluation of Acute Knee Injuries." *Clinics in Sports Medicine* 4 (1985): 295–312.

Jones, R. E., M. B. Henley, and P. Francis. "Nonoperative Management of Isolated Grade III Collateral Ligament Injury in High School Football Players." *Clinical Orthopaedics and Related Research* 213 (1986): 137–140.

Kaye, Jeremy J., and E. Paul Nance, Jr. "Pain in the Athlete's Knee." *Clinics in Sports Medicine* 6 (1987): 873–883.

Kelly, D. W., V. S. Carter, F. W. Jobe, et al. "Patellar and Quadriceps Tendon Ruptures—Jumper's Knee." *American Journal of Sports Medicine* 12 (1984): 375–380.

Kennedy, J. C., ed. *The Injured Adolescent Knee*. Baltimore: Williams & Wilkins, 1979.

Klein, Karl K. "Developmental Asymmetries and Knee Injury." *The Physician and Sportsmedicine* 11 (August 1983): 67–72.

Kujala, U. M., M. Kvist, and O. Heinonen. "Osgood-Schlatter's Disease in Adolescent Athletes. Retrospective Study of Incidence and Duration." *American Journal of Sports Medicine* 13 (1985): 236–241.

Leach, R. E., S. James, and S. Wasilewski. "Achilles Tendinitis." *American Journal of Sports Medicine* 9 (1981): 93–98.

Lipscomb, A. B., and A. F. Anderson. "Tears of the Anterior Cruciate Ligament in Adolescents." *Journal of Bone and Joint Surgery* 68A (1986): 19–28.

Losee, R. E. "Diagnosis of Chronic Injury to the Anterior Cruciate Ligament." *Orthopedic Clinics of North America* 16 (1985): 83–97.

Manzione, M., P. D. Pizzutillo, A. B. Peoples, et al. "Meniscectomy in Children: A Long-Term Follow-up Study." *American Journal of Sports Medicine* 11 (1983): 111–115.

Martens, M., P. Wouters, A. Burssens, et al. "Patellar Tendinitis: Pathology and Results of Treatment." *Acta Orthopaedica Scandinavica* 53 (1982): 445–450.

McCarroll, J. R., A. C. Rettig, and K. D. Shelbourne. "Anterior Cruciate Ligament Injuries in the Young Athlete with Open Physes." *American Journal of Sports Medicine* 16 (1988): 44–47.

McCarthy, Paul. "Prophylactic Knee Braces: Where Do They Stand?" *The Physician and Sportsmedicine* 16 (December 1988): 102–115.

Micheli, L. J., J. A. Slater, E. Woods, et al. "Patella Alta and the Adolescent Growth Spurt." *Clinical Orthopaedics and Related Research* 213 (1986): 159–162.

Minkoff, J., and O. H. Sherman. "Considerations Pursuant to the Rehabilitation of the Anterior Cruciate Injured Knee." *Exercise and Sport Sciences Reviews* 15 (1987): 297–349.

Montgomery, J. B., and J. R. Steadman. "Rehabilitation of the Injured Knee." *Clinics in Sports Medicine* 4 (1985): 333–343.

Nicholas, J. A. "Injuries to the Menisci of the Knee." *Orthopedic Clinics of North America* 4 (1973): 647–664.

Nisonson, Barton, Elliott Hershman, W. Norman Scott, and John Yost. "The Knee." In *Principles of Sports Medicine*, edited by W. Norman Scott, Barton Nisonson, and James A. Nicholas, pp. 270–341. Baltimore: Williams & Wilkins, 1984.

Olson, Daniel W. "Iliotibial Band Friction Syndrome." *Athletic Training* 21 (1986): 32–35.

Pascale, Mark S., and Peter A. Indelicato. "Anterior Cruciate Ligament Insufficiency of the Knee." *Advances in Sports Medicine and Fitness* 1 (1988): 183–216.

Paulos, L., F. R. Noyes, E. Grood, et al. "Knee Rehabilitation after Anterior Cruciate Ligament Reconstruction and Repair." *American Journal of Sports Medicine* 9 (1981): 140–149.

Prentice, William E. "A Manual Resistance Technique for Strengthening Tibial Rotation." *Athletic Training* 23 (1988): 230–233.

Quillen, William S., and Joe H. Gieck. "Manual Therapy: Mobilization of the Motion-Restricted Knee." *Athletic Training* 23 (1988): 123–130.

Ray, J. M., W. G. Clancy, Jr., and R. A. Lemon. "Semimembranosus Tendinitis: An Overlooked Cause of Medial Knee Pain." *American Journal of Sports Medicine* 16 (1988): 347–351.

Silfverskiold, J. P., J. R. Steadman, R. W. Higgins, et al. "Rehabilitation of the Anterior Cruciate Ligament in the Athlete." *Sports Medicine* 6 (1988): 308–319.

Singer, K. M., and J. Henry. "Knee Problems in Children and Adolescents." *Clinics in Sports Medicine* 4 (1985): 385–397.

Solomonow, M., R. Baratta, and R. D'Ambrosia. "The Role of the Hamstrings in the Rehabilitation of the Anterior Cruciate Ligament-Deficient Knee in Athletes." *Sports Medicine* 7 (1989): 42–48.

Steiner, Mark E. "Hypermobility and Knee Injuries." *The Physician and Sportsmedicine* 15 (June 1987): 159–165.

Steiner, M. E., and W. A. Grana. "The Young Athlete's Knee: Recent Advances." *Clinics in Sports Medicine* 7 (1988): 527–546.

Walter, N. E., and M. D. Wolf. "Stress Fractures in Young Athletes." *American Journal of Sports Medicine* 5 (1977): 165–170.

Zarins, B., and M. Adams. "Knee Injuries in Sports." *New England Journal of Medicine* 318 (1988): 950–961.

Zarins, Bertram, and Victor A. Nemeth. "Acute Knee Injuries in Athletes." *Clinics in Sports Medicine* 2 (1983): 149–166.

22

The Leg

OBJECTIVES FOR CHAPTER 22

After reading this chapter, the student should be able to:

1. Comprehend the general musculoskeletal and neurovascular anatomy of the leg.
2. Understand the examination, diagnosis, and treatment for overuse syndromes in the leg.
3. Identify major traumatic injuries of the leg.

INTRODUCTION

The leg is the portion of the lower extremity between the knee and the ankle. It includes the tibia, fibula, and large muscles vital to locomotion. The athletic trainer should understand the functions of the leg and the pathological conditions that might affect it.

Chapter 22 begins with the anatomy of the lower extremity. The chapter then explains how the athletic trainer conducts an evaluation of the injured leg. Injuries from overuse syndromes are discussed next, followed by traumatic injuries to the soft tissues and fractures. ■

ANATOMY

Osseous Structures

The **tibia** is the second largest bone in the body. It is slightly cup-shaped at its proximal end and is generally cylindrical through most of its shaft (Fig. 22.1). At the distal end it widens to include the ankle mortise. Posteriorly and laterally, it is covered by musculature. Anteriorly, the tibia is protected only by skin through most of its length and is vulnerable to direct impact. It articulates proximally with the distal femur proximally in the knee joint, and the talus and fibula distally in the ankle joint.

The **fibula** is a long slender bone lying lateral to the tibia. It forms an arthrodial joint proximally and a syndesmosis distally with the tibia. A limited weight-bearing bone, it serves primarily for muscle attachments. It is also the lateral buttress of the ankle joint. The tibia and fibula are connected by a thick **interosseous membrane** whose fibers course distally and laterally. This membrane dissipates the forces of weight bearing to the tibia and divides the leg into compartments.

Soft Tissue Structures

The muscles of the leg are divided into three distinct compartments and separated by thick fascial planes (Fig. 22.2). The anterior compartment contains the **tibialis anterior muscle** and the extensor muscles to the great and small toes, the **extensor hallucis longus** and the **extensor digitorum longus**. The posterior compartment contains the **gastrocnemius, soleus, tibialis posterior, flexor digitorum longus,** and **flexor hallucis longus** muscles. The peroneal compartment contains the **peroneus longus** and **peroneus brevis** muscles, which evert the ankle, and the superficial peroneal nerve. The posterior compartment muscles are innervated by the tibial nerve, and the anterior and lateral compartments are innervated by the peroneal nerve.

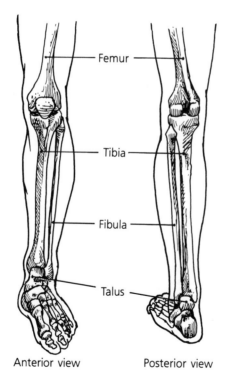

Femur

Tibia

Fibula

Talus

Anterior view   Posterior view

FIGURE 22.1. Leg portion of lower extremity.

EVALUATION

History

An appropriate history is mandatory prior to examination of the injured lower extremity. If the injury is traumatic, it should be noted whether direct contact or indirect forces were involved. The presence of open wounds and the mechanism of injury should be noted to assess the athlete's risk of infection. Any previous leg injury should be included in the medical history.

Overuse syndromes of the leg most often occur in distance runners, but they can also occur in athletes who participate in other sports. These problems result from accumulative impact loading of the lower extremity. The athletic trainer evaluating these injuries should be familiar with the language of the sport in order to take an adequate history and perform a physical examination. An adequate history frequently discloses the cause of injury, which helps in its treatment.

When obtaining a history from an athlete with an overuse syndrome, the trainer should ask questions regarding the athlete's training program. Up to two-thirds of all problems associated with overuse syndromes are caused by training program errors rather than abnormal biomechanics. Training errors contributing to overuse syndromes include excessive mileage, intense workouts, dramatic changes in training routines (e.g., switching too rapidly from cross-country to interval workouts), running hills, and running on hard surfaces.

Physical Examination

Routine physical examination includes complete evaluation of the lower extremities. Leg-length discrepancies are frequently associated with overuse syndromes. Excessive activity can cause symptoms in the longer leg (Table 22.1). Other subtle anatomic abnormalities that may lead to overuse syndromes are femoral anteversion, with excessive internal rotation of the hips and little external rotation; tight ham-

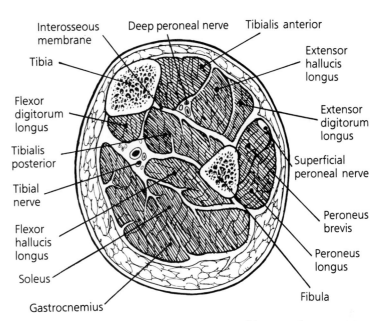

FIGURE 22.2. Three distinct compartments of leg muscles are separated by thick fascial planes.

strings; genu varum (bowlegs) or genu valgum (knock-knees); excessive Q angles of the patella; patella alta; tibia vara; functional shortening of the gastrocnemius-soleus group; and functionally pronated feet.

Alignment and Unit Analysis

When examining the runner, the athletic trainer notes the alignment of the leg to the heel and the heel to the forefoot. Functionally, the foot should be positioned so that, with weight bearing, the vertical axis of the heel is parallel to the longitudinal axis of the distal tibia. Likewise, the forefoot should be perpendicular to the vertical axis of the heel. Deviation from normal alignment usually causes compensatory motion through the subtalar joint. These compensatory motions place additional stress on the joints, ligaments, and musculotendinous units of the lower extremity, resulting in overuse problems.

The most common compensatory movement is excessive and prolonged pronation of the foot during the stance phase of run-

TABLE 22.1. Relation of Physical Anomalies to Overuse Syndromes

				Syndrome			
		Tenosynovitis					
Anomaly	Muscle Cramps	A.T.*	F.H.L. & P.T.**	Achilles Tenosynovitis or Degeneration	Periostitis Tibia	Stress Fracture	Plantaris Syndrome
Leg-length discrepancy					+	+	
Femoral anteversion			+		+	+	
Excessive internal hip rotation		+			+	+	
Tight hamstrings	+						
Genu varum or valgum						+	
Excessive Q angle						+	
Patella alta						+	
Tibia vara		+	+				+
Functional shortening of gastrocnemius-soleus muscle	+	+		+			+
Functionally pronated feet		+	+	+			

* anterior tibialis
**flexor hallucis longus and posterior tibialis

ning. This occurs most frequently with mild tibia vara, heel varus, and tight gastrocnemius and soleus muscles. Prolonged pronation creates internal tibial torsion, which puts excessive stress on the posterior tibial muscles and the structures around the knee. Treatment may include changing the individual training program, reducing mileage, and changing surfaces and/or shoes.

OVERUSE SYNDROMES

The leg is subject to a number of overuse syndromes, particularly in the jogger and distance runner. Overuse syndromes are pathognomonic to certain sports such as shinsplints in football and dancing, compartment syndrome in hiking, and Achilles tendinitis in soccer and basketball. The athlete with an overuse syndrome usually presents with leg pain with no history of a specific injury. These syndromes can occur in the novice or the well-trained athlete. Their common denominator is that they are all associated with exercise. Initially, they may present as pain only after activity, but eventually they can develop into continuous pain during and after activity.

Overuse syndromes include acute muscle cramps; tenosynovitis (inflammation of the tendon sheath) of the tibialis anterior, flexor hallucis longus, tibialis posterior, or Achilles tendon; periostitis of the tibia; stress fractures of the fibula or tibia; cystic degeneration of the Achilles tendon; "plantaris syndrome" (tear of the musculotendinous junction of the medial head of the gastrocnemius); or acute anterior or peroneal compartment syndromes.

The term "shinsplints" has long been used to describe any sort of leg pain associated with exercise. This term does not identify the specific pathology associated with the symptoms. If it is used, it should be reserved for anterior or posterior tibial tendinitis.

Muscle Cramps

The simplest and most common overuse syndrome affecting the leg is muscle cramping in the gastrocnemius-soleus group. An acute spasm in the muscle may occur during the late stages of prolonged physical exertion or during the night after a day of strenuous activity. The precise cause of the cramp is unknown. It may be due to electrolyte imbalance or dehydration, or to simple muscle fatigue. Some persons are predisposed to cramps and get them regularly with any physical exertion. Acute cramps are treated with ice, massage, and gradual stretching. Preventive measures include a regular stretching program of the gastrocnemius-soleus complex with a slant board and adequate fluid and electrolyte intake during prolonged physical activity.

Anterior Compartment Syndrome

The anterior compartment contains the tibialis anterior, extensor hallucis longus, and extensor muscles to the toes, as well as the deep peroneal nerve and the anterior tibial artery. Because the muscles are encased in a compartment bounded by the tibia and fibula, tough interosseous membrane medially and laterally, and a tough fibrous fascia sheath anteriorly, they are vulnerable to increases in tissue pressure.

Mechanism of Injury

In the **anterior compartment syndrome**, soft tissue pressure is increased to the point of jeopardizing the viability of the muscles and nerves. The syndrome results most commonly from a direct blow, such as a kick in soccer. It may develop insidiously, however, through minor trauma such as running or marching. Classically, the individual sustains a direct blow to the anterior lateral side of the leg, resulting in hematoma (Fig. 22.3). The pain progresses and eventually leads to decreased sensation over the superficial peroneal distribution of the foot, and then to total foot drop, with no active eversion or dorsiflexion of toes and foot as the muscles in the compartment become paralyzed. Less frequently, the athlete limps after exercise for a period of time, sometimes for several months, before seeking treatment.

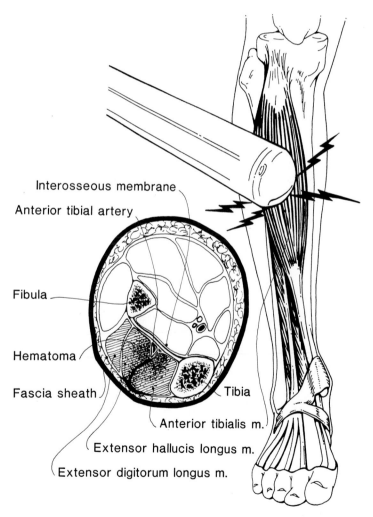

FIGURE 22.3. Hematoma causing artery impingement in anterior compartment syndrome.

The amount of pressure required to produce a compartment syndrome depends on a number of factors, including the duration of elevated pressure, the metabolic rate of the tissues, local blood pressure, and vascular tone. Functional abnormalities of the nerve are produced within 30 minutes after onset of ischemia, and irreversible loss may occur after 12 to 24 hours. Compartment syndromes lasting longer than 12 hours are likely to produce chronic functional abnormalities, such as contractures, sensory aberrations, and motor weakness.

The clinical features include a firm, sometimes stony induration over the anterior compartment of the leg and exquisite tenderness to palpation or to plantar flexion of the ankle. In the late stages of the syndrome, sensation over the dorsum of the foot decreases. In the end stage, there is total foot drop.

Treatment

An athlete who presents with severe pain and swelling in the anterior compartment area must be watched carefully by someone skilled in managing this problem. Continuity of care is critical, since close observation for changes in signs and symptoms is important. Rest and elevation of the leg are necessary during the observation period, and limited icing may be helpful. The extremity should be left unwrapped rather than wrapped to decrease the risk of further compression.

If the foot becomes numb, surgical decompression of the leg through fasciotomy of the entire length of the compartment is indicated. This is a true surgical emergency. Once signs of paralysis develop, the muscles involved seldom recover completely. This is one of the few conditions in which watchful observation or continued conservative treatment has no place. Remember that palpable pulses in the foot are lost late in the syndrome, and occasionally not at all. The athlete with palpable pulses can still suffer irreversible tissue damage. It is imperative that compartment syndromes be diagnosed as early as possible and a

fasciotomy, when indicated, be performed without undue delay.

One factor present in any compartment syndrome is increased tissue pressure. Normal tissue pressure is approximately 0 millimeters of mercury (mm Hg). Tissue pressures are usually measured with needle devices such as the wick manometer. This testing should be done by a skilled professional. Ischemia may begin at tissue pressures 10 to 30 mm Hg less than the athlete's diastolic pressure.

Acute Peroneal Compartment Syndrome

A less common but related condition is the **acute peroneal compartment syndrome**. This is essentially the same pathologic condition localized to the peroneal musculature on the lateral aspect of the leg. The pain phenomenon is localized to this compartment. Numbness may also occur in the distribution of the peroneal nerve since it is compressed with this phenomenon. Treatment for acute peroneal compartment syndrome is the same as that described for the anterior compartment syndrome.

Posterior Tibial Syndrome

In the **posterior tibial syndrome**, pain occurs along the medial border of the tibia, usually in the distal third, and is associated with running. Characteristically, the pain is severe as the individual warms up or begins running, then disappears after a short time, only to recur once activity stops. The condition occurs primarily in the novice runner. When it is seen in the well-conditioned athlete, it is usually secondary to some mechanical abnormality, such as prolonged pronation of the foot during the stance phase of running.

Physical examination reveals a tenderness of the posterior tibial musculature where it attaches along the posterior medial border of the tibia (Fig. 22.4). The tenderness may be confined to a small area in the distal third of the tibia, or extend through the length of the muscle.

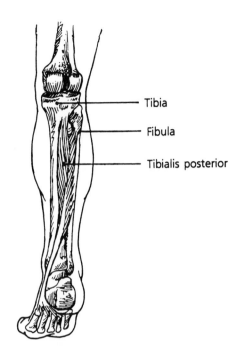

FIGURE 22.4. Posterior tibial musculature.

Tibia

Fibula

Tibialis posterior

Opinions differ regarding the pathology of this condition. Some authorities believe posterior tibial syndrome is actually a periostitis of the tibia caused from pull of the muscles. Others believe it is a pressure phenomenon much like the anterior compartment syndrome where muscles are expanding within a closed compartment.

Differential Diagnosis

Differentiating the posterior tibial syndrome from an early stress fracture involving the tibia is sometimes difficult; both may present as pain localized along the posterior medial border of the tibia associated with some bony tenderness. A stress fracture, however, upon healing, usually leads to some periosteal reaction that becomes evident on x-ray films several weeks after symptoms have begun.

Treatment

Treatment of the posterior tibial syndrome consists of decreasing the individual's mileage, ensuring proper foot alignment, changing surfaces, and possibly, changing shoes.

Anti-inflammatory drugs, such as aspirin in therapeutic doses, usually relieve symptoms. Ice packs or cold water whirlpool to the legs immediately after running, and compressive dressings occasionally help.

Rehabilitation includes stretching exercises both before and after running, particularly for the gastrocnemius-soleus group, and strengthening of the posterior and anterior tibial muscles through progressive resistance exercise. The posterior tibial syndrome usually subsides with this conservative program as the athlete becomes better conditioned. Any biomechanical abnormalities of foot strike should be corrected with functional orthoses.

Rarely, a chronic posterior tibial syndrome is unresponsive to any conservative program, even prolonged rest. Surgical intervention may then be necessary. A fasciotomy of the overlying fascia is performed through a small incision along the medial border of the tibia.

Achilles Tendinitis

Repetitive overextension or overuse of the Achilles tendon, such as jumping in basketball or distance running, may cause the overlying sheath to become inflamed and thickened. This results in chronic pain and tightness over the Achilles tendon. The condition, called **Achilles tendinitis,** may be chronic and incapacitating, particularly to the competitive athlete.

Achilles tendinitis usually comes on insidiously from a change in training, such as hill running or increasing mileage too rapidly. The predisposing problem in almost all cases is excessively tight gastrocnemius-soleus muscles, but tibia vara, cavus foot, and heel and forefoot varus deformities may also be predisposing factors.

Symptoms

Symptoms include pain both during and after running and with any stretching of the tendon. Examination reveals either diffuse or localized swelling and tenderness to palpation of the tendon. In chronic tendinitis a nodule composed of mucoid degeneration may form inside the tendon. Occasionally, motion of the ankle produces crepitus, indicating friction between the tendon and its overlying sheath.

Treatment

Treatment includes rest until acute inflammation subsides, ice to the affected area, and oral nonsteroidal anti-inflammatory drugs. A 1/2- to 3/4-inch heel lift should be inserted into shoes to decrease tension on the tendon. An orthosis may be required to correct biomechanical abnormalities of foot strike, such as with pronated feet. Active stretching and strengthening of the gastrocnemius-soleus muscles begin after acute symptoms subside.

Occasionally, the condition persists for a long time and does not respond to conservative measures. The underlying problem in this case may be a partial tear deep in the Achilles tendon itself, usually as a result of preexisting degenerative changes within the tendon. Surgery may then be necessary. The overlying tendon sheath, which is usually thickened, fibrotic, and constricting the tendon itself, is stripped. If evidence of a partial tear is present, the degenerative area is excised and the tendon repaired.

After postoperative rest, the athlete begins gradual stretching exercises and progressive resistance exercises for the calf muscle, which frequently atrophies after surgery. When running is begun, the athlete should use a heel lift and well-padded running shoes for several months. Athletes who have only the Achilles sheath stripped and who show no evidence of any tear within the tendon can usually start running within 3 to 6 weeks after surgery. Those with partial tears require longer healing times. Rehabilitation of this injury is therefore slower and more prolonged than in a simple case of tendon sheath excision.

Stress Fractures

The tibia and fibula frequently sustain stress fractures as a result of overuse. A stress fracture is a partial or complete disruption of bone produced by rhythmic, repeated, subthreshold stress. Stress fractures do not occur at any particular instant in time but are rather the end product of an adaptive process in which the bone attempts to remodel itself rapidly along the lines of increased stress. A repetitive stress leads to muscle fatigue in the leg. The resulting loss of shock-absorbing ability increases stress of the bone and periostitis. The pain produced causes involuntary disuse of the extremity, which then leads to further muscle atrophy, and the process compounds itself. The final result, if stress is not relieved, is fracture of the bone.

Stress fractures are most common in distance runners, but they are also seen in basketball and soccer players. Although they are infrequent in football players, kickers can sustain stress fractures of the fibula.

Symptoms

The symptoms of a stress fracture usually begin with mild discomfort. Stress fractures of the tibia can occur in the lower shaft, but they can also occur proximally, where they may mimic anserine bursitis. Simple rest relieves the symptoms. With continued activity, the pain becomes more persistent and lasts from day to day. Ultimately, the pain is severe enough to prohibit activity.

Diagnosis

Diagnosis is by clinical examination, which shows localized tenderness to palpation directly over the fracture site. A tuning fork applied to the bone can localize a fracture site by accentuating pain symptoms. Frequently, x-rays are negative early in the course of stress fractures, but reveal periosteal reaction or cortical thickening 2 to 4 weeks after the onset of symptoms. A bone scan may be positive before x-ray changes are present. Osteolysis after cortical disruption develops late after a stress fracture and may never show on plain x-rays. Callus, or the new bone formation of healing, may take weeks before it can be seen on routine x-rays. Therefore, a bone scan may be necessary for diagnosis when x-rays are negative.

Stress fractures may occur at any level of conditioning, but they are more common in women than in men. The most common site is the proximal third or distal third of the tibia. Stress fractures of the fibula also occur in sports activities that require chronic muscle tension, such as aerobic dance, kicking, and running.

Treatment

Treatment of the stress syndrome or fracture includes rest, changing the training program if indicated, and correcting all mechanical abnormalities that may have led to the fracture. The stressful situation, such as running, must be eliminated during healing, but total rest is not necessary. The athlete may continue cardiovascular activities by substituting swimming or cycling. Specific weight training for overall body conditioning and the lower extremity in particular should be encouraged within the athlete's pain tolerance. It is seldom necessary to keep the athlete non–weight bearing or immobilized in plaster. Tibial stress fractures take 4 to 8 weeks to heal, while fibular stress fractures take 3 to 6 weeks to heal. An athlete should be completely asymptomatic from a stress fracture before being allowed to return gradually to play.

TRAUMATIC INJURIES

The anterior aspect of the leg is a common site for direct trauma. When the blow occurs over the anterior lateral aspect of the leg, it may cause an anterior compartment syndrome. Large hematomas that may be painful and difficult to heal often result. Soft tissue wounds in this area are frequently ragged and dirty, usually as a result of cleats or spikes. Because the blood supply to the wound often is poor, the wound may be slow to heal and break down with repeated trauma. Traumatic injuries are usually straightforward on examination, with wounds and deformities being quite apparent. The athlete's neurovascular status should always be evaluated during examination of the traumatized leg.

Soft Tissue Injuries

Achilles Tendon Rupture

Acute rupture of the Achilles tendon usually occurs 1 or 2 inches above the insertion of the tendon on the calcaneus (Fig. 22.5). The athlete feels a sudden tearing sensation and severe pain. Often, he or she may describe a feeling of being kicked in the tendon area, although no apparent injury has occurred. The athlete experiences a sudden loss of function and inability to stand on tiptoes. Active plantar flexion is weakened but may still be present because

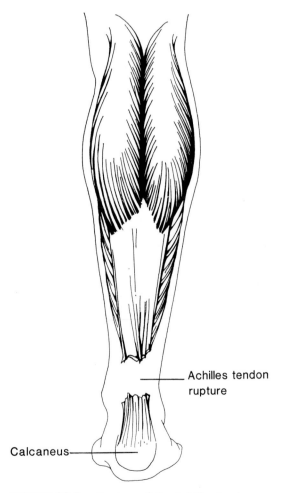

Achilles tendon rupture

Calcaneus

FIGURE 22.5. Rupture of the Achilles tendon.

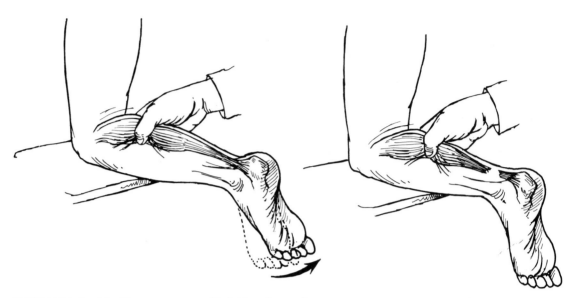

FIGURE 22.6. The Thompson test will yield a plantar flexion response if the gastrocnemius-soleus complex is intact. Lack of this response indicates a rupture.

of action in the tibialis posterior and flexor hallucis longus muscles. Achilles tendon rupture is disabling, and the injured athlete should be seen by an orthopedist as soon as possible.

Physical examination of complete tears reveals swelling and ecchymosis in the posterior aspect of the leg and heel. There is frequently a palpable gap between the tendon ends, and the athlete has no active plantar flexion.

A simple test to determine whether the gastrocnemius-soleus group is intact is the **Thompson test**. The individual kneels in a chair with the feet hanging free. The examiner squeezes the calf muscle between his or her thumb and fingertips (Fig. 22.6). If there is continuity between the gastrocnemius-soleus muscles and the Achilles tendon, plantar flexion of the foot will occur. Lack of plantar flexion indicates rupture of the tendon mechanism.

Although conservative management of complete Achilles tendon ruptures is sometimes advocated, surgical repair may be considered for the athlete. If an orthopedic surgeon is not readily available, the athletic trainer should splint the leg and foot in a posterior splint and compressive dressing, with the foot in relaxed plantar flexion.

Partial Achilles tendon ruptures are more difficult to diagnose. The symptoms may be insidious and associated only with activity. A partial rupture should be considered in anybody over the age of 30 with symptoms of chronic Achilles tendinitis. Partial ruptures may be treated conservatively with a long leg cast for 3 to 4 weeks, followed by a heel lift for several months.

Muscle Strains

The most commonly strained muscle in the leg is the medial head of the gastrocnemius. Most of these cases used to be called the ruptured plantaris syndrome. Because this strain is so frequently seen in the middle-aged tennis player, it is sometimes called "tennis leg."

The symptoms of muscle strain are classic. The athlete feels a sudden, painful snapping or tearing sensation in the calf when the plantar flexed foot is suddenly dorsiflexed, usually with the knee in extension. It almost always occurs in active athletes over 40. The individual is unable to continue playing, and subsequently marked swelling and ecchymosis of the leg extends down into the ankle and foot.

Examination immediately after injury reveals pain to palpation over the medial gastrocnemius. Occasionally, the athletic trainer can feel a palpable defect at the musculotendinous junction of the medial head of the gastrocnemius. By the time the athlete is examined by a physician, sometimes a day or two later, edema and hematoma may mask this defect.

As with other muscle tears, degrees of injury may vary. In some cases, swelling is minimal, and symptoms subside rapidly. In other cases, swelling is massive, and the individual is totally incapacitated for an extended period of time.

Most strains are classified as first- or second-degree and can be managed by elevation of the heel, with gradual active stretching and progressive exercise as tolerated. Some physicians advocate surgical repair if the muscle has a severe third-degree tear or if the individual is unable to sustain his or her body weight on tiptoes. Others prefer plaster immobilization of the foot in plantar flexion to approximately 50 to 60 degrees, and the ankle in plantar flexion to 15 degrees for 3 to 4 weeks. Third-degree injuries can be treated with crutches and wrapping without immobilization if the athlete is willing to follow the treatment protocol. The muscles should be protected with a heel lift for several months after the person resumes athletic activities.

Plantaris Muscle Rupture

The small, ribbonlike plantaris muscle originates over the posterior lateral aspect of the knee joint and then curves medially and distally between the two heads of the gastrocnemius to a very small, ribbonlike tendon that inserts along the medial aspect of the calcaneus. It has long been thought to be the culprit when older people feel pain in calf muscles during strenuous activities. Complete rupture of the plantaris muscle tendon complex has not been documented anatomically, however, and most plantaris muscle ruptures are probably tears of the medial head of the gastrocnemius muscle. Occasionally, individuals feel a sharp or tearing pain in the upper midcalf but have little swelling or tenderness. This may be a tear of the plantaris. Since it is a very small muscle with little vascularization, substantial ecchymosis or swelling is unlikely. Treatment consists of symptomatic relief, including crutches, rest, ice, and heel lift. Activities may be resumed as symptoms subside.

Fractures

The tibia and/or fibula may be fractured acutely during collision sports by direct impact, or by twisting or torque forces to the body when the foot is planted. The latter frequently results in long, oblique, spiral fractures of the distal tibia with fracture of the proximal fibula.

Deformity, immediate loss of function, pain, and motion at the fracture site make the diagnosis easy. Open fractures are an orthopedic emergency because of the risk of infection and potential loss of blood.

Tibial fractures should be splinted, preferably with an air splint to prevent excessive swelling, and the athlete promptly transported to the nearest medical facility.

Fractures of the fibular shaft can occur from direct trauma. They are occasionally overlooked since the symptoms can mimic a deep bruise from the blunt trauma. Fractures of the distal fibula usually require a short leg walking cast for 4 to 6 weeks. Fracture of the midshaft and upper portions of the fibula may be treated with a simple compressive dressing and crutches. All fractures should be evaluated by a physician.

IMPORTANT CONCEPTS

1. The two bones of the leg are the tibia and the fibula.
2. The muscles of the leg are divided into the anterior compartment, posterior compartment, and peroneal compartment.
3. With normal leg alignment, the vertical axis of the heel is parallel to the tibia, and the forefoot is perpendicular to the axis of the heel; deviation from normal alignment usually causes compensatory motion through the subtalar joint, placing additional stress on the joints, ligaments, and muscles.
4. Overuse syndromes include acute muscle cramps, anterior compartment syndrome, acute peroneal compartment syndrome, posterior tibial syndrome, Achilles tendinitis, and stress fractures.
5. Soft tissue injuries to the leg include Achilles tendon rupture, muscle strains, and plantaris muscle rupture.
6. The tibia, fibula, or both at once can be fractured from direct impact, or by twisting or torque forces to the body when the foot is planted.

SUGGESTED READINGS

Bryk, Eli, and S. Ashby Grantham. "Shin Splints: A Chronic Deep Posterior Ischemic Compartmental Syndrome of the Leg?" *Orthopaedic Review* 12 (April 1983): 29–40.

Clement, D. B., J. E. Taunton, and G. W. Smart. "Achilles Tendinitis and Peritendinitis: Etiology and Treatment." *American Journal of Sports Medicine* 12 (1984): 179–184.

Curwin, Sandra, and William D. Stanish. *Tendinitis: Its Etiology and Treatment.* Lexington, Mass.: Collamore Press, 1984.

D'Ambrosia, R. D., and D. Drez, Jr., eds. *Prevention and Treatment of Running Injuries.* Thorofare, N.J.: C. B. Slack, 1982.

Detmer, D. E. "Chronic Leg Pain." *American Journal of Sports Medicine* 8 (1980): 141–144.

————. "Chronic Shin Splints: Classification and Management of Medial Tibial Stress Syndrome." *Sports Medicine* 3 (1986): 436–446.

Hunter, S. C., and R. M. Poole. "The Chronically Inflamed Tendon." *Clinics in Sports Medicine* 6 (1987): 371–388.

Jones, D. C., and S. L. James. "Overuse Injuries of the Lower Extremity: Shin Splints, Iliotibial Band Friction Syndrome, and Exertional Compartment Syndromes." *Clinics in Sports Medicine* 6 (1987): 273–290.

Leach, Robert E. "Fractures of the Tibia and Fibula." In *Fractures in Adults*, 2d ed., vol. 2, edited by Charles A. Rockwood, Jr., and David P. Green, pp. 1593–1663. Philadelphia: J. B. Lippincott, 1984.

Leach, R. E., G. Hammond, and W. S. Stryker. "Anterior Tibial Compartment Syndrome. Acute and Chronic." *Journal of Bone and Joint Surgery* 49A (1967): 451–462.

Michael, R. H., and L. E. Holder. "The Soleus Syndrome; A Cause of Medial Tibial Stress (Shin Splints)." *American Journal of Sports Medicine* 13 (1985): 87–94.

Miller, A. P. "Strains of the Posterior Calf Musculature ("Tennis Leg")." *American Journal of Sports Medicine* 7 (1979): 172–174.

Puranen, J., and A. Alavaikko. "Intracompartmental Pressure Increase on Exertion in Patients with Chronic Compartmental Syndrome in the Leg." *Journal of Bone and Joint Surgery* 63A (1981): 1304–1309.

Rorabeck, C. H., R. B. Bourne, and P. J. Fowler. "The Surgical Treatment of Exertional Compartment Syndrome in Athletes." *Journal of Bone and Joint Surgery* 65A (1983): 1245–1251.

Smart, G. W., J. E. Taunton, and D. B. Clement. "Achilles Tendon Disorders in Runners: A Review." *Medicine and Science in Sports and Exercise* 12 (1980): 231–243.

Stanitski, C. L., J. H. McMaster, and P. E. Scranton. "On the Nature of Stress Fractures." *American Journal of Sports Medicine* 6 (1978): 391–396.

Styf, J. "Diagnosis of Exercise-Induced Pain in the Anterior Aspect of the Lower Leg." *American Journal of Sports Medicine* 16 (1988): 165–169.

Styf, J. R., and L. M. Körner. "Diagnosis of Chronic Anterior Compartment Syndrome in the Lower Leg." *Acta Orthopaedica Scandinavica* 58 (1987): 139–144.

Sullivan, D., R. F. Warren, H. Pavlov, et al. "Stress Fractures in 51 Runners." *Clinical Orthopaedics and Related Research* 187 (1984): 188–192.

23

The Ankle

OBJECTIVES FOR CHAPTER 23

After reading this chapter, the student should be able to:
1. Understand the anatomy of the ankle.
2. Understand the mechanisms of ankle injuries.
3. Discuss the initial evaluation of an ankle injury.
4. Describe the different types of ligament injuries in the ankle.
5. Identify other soft tissue injuries of the ankle.
6. Identify bony injuries to the ankle.
7. Discuss how to rehabilitate the athlete with an ankle sprain.

INTRODUCTION

The ankle, the linkage joint between the foot and the leg, is critical in the performance of all running and jumping sports. The ankle joint is at significant risk for injury during sports activities and, when injured, creates significant disability. Knowledge of the ankle's anatomy and function allows the athletic trainer to understand the mechanisms of ankle injuries, diagnostic approaches, treatment protocols, and rehabilitation techniques.

Chapter 23 begins with the anatomy of the bones, ligaments, and musculotendinous structures of the ankle. The chapter then discusses the mechanisms of ankle injuries and the initial assessment of injuries. Next, the classification and evaluation of ligament injuries are described. The chapter then discusses specific ankle injuries, dividing them into soft tissue and bony injuries. The last section of Chapter 23 focuses on rehabilitation of ankle injuries and presents several rehabilitation exercises. ■

ANATOMY

Bony Architecture

The ankle joint is formed by three bones: the **tibia**, **fibula**, and **talus**. The dome of the talus fits into the mortise (cavity) formed by the tibia and fibula. The **medial** and **lateral malleoli** project downward to articulate with the sides of the talus. The lateral malleolus projects down to the level of the subtalar joint, considerably farther than the medial malleolus, and thus provides greater bony stability for the lateral side of the ankle joint (Fig. 23.1).

The ankle joint moves, essentially, in one plane, up and down, about a central axis of rotation. The talus is wider anteriorly than posteriorly; the lateral wall slopes outward instead of being parallel to the medial wall. The tibial portion of the joint is also wider anteriorly than posteriorly.

When the foot is dorsiflexed, the wider anterior portion of the talus is brought into contact with the narrower portion between the malleoli and, therefore, is gripped more tightly. As the ankle goes into plantar flexion, the narrower posterior portion of the talus is brought into contact with the wider anterior portion of the tibia. This permits a small amount of free play in the ankle joint, as the wedge effect noted in dorsiflexion is lost. This bony arrangement also helps to promote anterior stability of the ankle

joint. As the tibia is driven forward on the plantar-flexed talus, the narrower part of the tibia impinges on the widened anterior portion of the talus, blocking forward dislocation of the tibia on the talus.

Ligaments of the Ankle Joint

The relationship of the tibia, talus, and fibula is maintained by three groups of ligaments: the **deltoid ligament** medially,

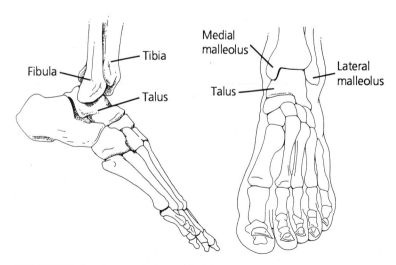

FIGURE 23.1. Bones of the ankle joint.

the **lateral collateral ligament**, and the **tibio-fibular syndesmosis**.

Deltoid Ligament

The deltoid ligament, the strongest of the three ligaments, is a broad, triangular or delta-shaped band with bony insertions on the navicular, talus, and calcaneus (Fig. 23.2). It is functionally divided into a deep and superficial portion. The deep portion attaches to the talus and is horizontal and, therefore, resists lateral displacement of the talus. In coronal sections through the ankle joint, the vertical position of the superficial portion and the horizontal position of the deep portion are clearly seen. Also, the deep portion is placed posteriorly.

Lateral Collateral Ligament

The lateral collateral ligament of the ankle is T-shaped and consists of three distinct ligaments (see Fig. 23.2). The **posterior tal-ofibular ligament** arises from the posterior portion of the tip of the fibula and runs backward and slightly downward to attach to the lateral tubercle of the posterior process of the talus. This ligament is the strongest of the three and helps to resist forward

dislocation of the leg on the foot. The **calcaneofibular ligament**, the longest of the three, passes inferiorly in a posterior direction to insert on the lateral surface of the calcaneus. When the foot is in plantar flexion, the calcaneofibular ligament is almost perpendicular to the axis of the fibula. It is extracapsular, but may be associated with the peroneal tendon sheath. On its lateral and dorsal aspects, the calcaneofibular ligament is covered for almost its entire length with the thin inner wall of the tendon sheath. This ligament is completely relaxed when the foot is in a normal standing position. It does not become taut until the calcaneus makes a strong supination movement. The **anterior talofibular ligament** arises from the anterior border of the lateral malleolus and passes forward and somewhat medially to attach to the neck of the talus. Its direction corresponds to the longitudinal axis of the foot and is taut in all positions of plantar flexion.

Tibiofibular Syndesmosis

The tibiofibular syndesmosis, an arrangement of dense fibrous tissues between the osseous structures just above the ankle joint, maintains the relationship of the distal tibia and fibula. It consists of the **anterior** and **posterior tibiofibular ligaments** and the **interosseous membrane** and **ligament** (see Fig. 23.2). The anterior and posterior tibiofibular ligaments arise respectively from the anterior and posterior caliculi on the lateral side of the tibia. These ligaments actually hold the fibula snug in a groove on the tibia, where the fibula rotates about its vertical axis as well as rises and falls with dorsiflexion and plantar flexion. There is 6 degrees of medial rotation of the fibula with dorsiflexion and 6 degrees of lateral rotation with plantar flexion. These two ligaments blend into the interosseous membrane 2 to 3 cm above the ankle joint.

Musculotendinous Structures

Important musculotendinous structures relate to the deltoid and lateral collateral

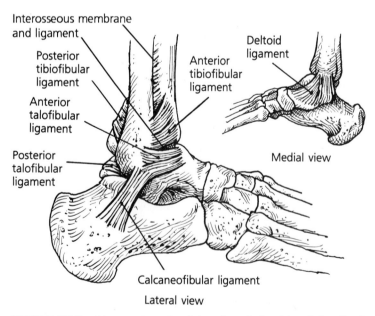

FIGURE 23.2. Ligaments maintaining the relationship of the distal tibia, fibula, and talus.

ligaments. Understanding the functions of these muscles is important in preventing ankle injuries as well as in rehabilitating the athlete after an ankle injury.

Medial Stabilizers

The medial stabilizers of the ankle are the tendons of the **tibialis anterior, tibialis posterior, flexor digitorum longus,** and the **flexor hallucis longus** muscles. The latter three tendons originate from the posterior compartment of the leg and pass posterior and inferior to the medial malleolus. They are important for plantar flexion and supination of the foot. The tendon of the tibialis posterior is adjacent to the posterior and middle parts of the deltoid ligament. This explains why this tendon is often trapped between the talus and medial malleolus with severe deltoid ruptures. The tendon of the tibialis anterior arises in the anterior crural compartment of the leg and then passes downward and medially to insert on the first cuneiform and base of the first metatarsal.

Lateral Stabilizers

The lateral stabilizers of the ankle are the peroneal muscles that make up the lateral compartment of the leg. The **peroneus brevis** and **peroneus longus** pass distal and inferior to the lateral malleolus. The brevis inserts on the base of the fifth metatarsal; the longus passes under the cuboid bone in its own groove to insert on the inferior surface of the medial cuneiform and base of the first metatarsal.

As mentioned earlier, the peroneal tendon sheath covers the posterior and lateral portion of the calcaneofibular ligament. When this ligament is ruptured, the overlying inner wall of the peroneal tendon sheath is also torn because it lies adjacent to this ligament. Thus, the peroneal tendon sheath communicates with the ankle joint in this situation. The peroneal tendons are important for pronating and everting the foot. Because of the intricate relationship of these muscles to the stabilizing ligaments of the ankle joint, they are capable of ab-

sorbing stress and protecting these ligaments from injury.

MECHANISMS OF INJURY

Inversion

Injuries to the ankle must be considered in relation to the magnitude and direction of forces applied to the ankle. In sports requiring a cleated shoe, the foot is usually fixed to the ground and the body is rotating and angulating about it. The anatomy and the activity of the running foot are predisposed toward **inversion injuries.** As mentioned earlier, bony stability is greater laterally than medially, thereby predisposing the ankle to inversion rather than eversion injuries. Once inversion has been initiated, the ankle loses the bony stability of its neutral position. As inversion increases, the medial malleolus may lose its stabilizing function and act as a fulcrum for further inversion. If the everting muscles (peroneals) are not strong enough, the tensile strength of the lateral ligaments may be exceeded, resulting in injury. Inversion stress is usually the mechanism in lateral ligament injuries, lateral avulsion fractures, and medial shear fractures.

The way athletes use their ankles may also predispose them to inversion injuries. A cutting or turning maneuver, often the initiating factor in these injuries, involves pushing off to the side from the opposite lead foot. For example, to cut to the left, the direction change is initiated off the fixed right foot, inverting the ankle and internally rotating and plantar flexing the right foot. Another common mechanism of injury is landing on an irregular surface such as another player's foot in basketball or stepping into a hole in a poorly prepared playing field (Fig. 23.3). This usually results in an inversion mechanism of injury.

Plantar Flexion

Plantar flexion makes the ankle more susceptible to injury because of increased laxity of the joint and the position of the

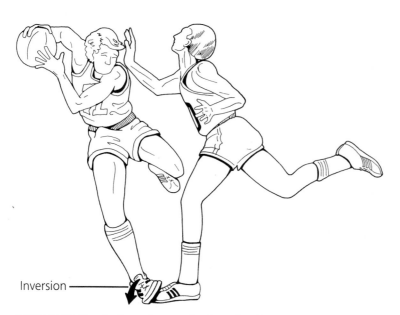

Inversion

FIGURE 23.3. An inversion mechanism of ankle sprain.

calcaneofibular ligament. Lateral ligament injuries are particularly common with plantar stress. As the ankle goes into plantar flexion, this ligament goes from a vertical to a horizontal position, resulting in less resistance to inversion. The opposite mechanism of injury may occur, although statistically it is far less likely.

Eversion

An external rotation mechanism, or **eversion**, can occur when the planted leg receives a lateral blow. Eversion stress can damage medial structures such as the deltoid ligament or rupture the syndesmosis. Medial avulsion fractures and lateral shear fractures can also occur. This same mechanism may also result in knee injuries.

INITIAL ASSESSMENT

At initial evaluation of an acute injury, the neurological and vascular function of the extremity must be assessed. The athletic trainer palpates the dorsalis pedis pulse on the dorsum of the foot and the posterior tibial pulse behind the medial malleolus. Evaluation of capillary refill of the toes, as

well as warmth and color, is helpful. Once the neurovascular function has been determined to be intact, then the athlete should be transported to the appropriate treatment facility. If the ankle appears stable, crutches will suffice. However, if there is any question of stability, a well-padded posterior short leg splint should be used.

Initially, a fracture must be differentiated from a sprain. Many fractures about the ankle are obvious, with the exception of the undisplaced spiral fracture of the fibula or the avulsion fracture of the distal tip of the fibula. Fibular pain with compression or on heel tap often indicates fracture. Following an inversion ankle injury, a fracture at the base of the fifth metatarsal must also be considered. Often, careful palpation of these structures helps locate the injury.

Routine x-ray views of the ankle, including oblique views, can identify fractures. If a fracture of the base of the fifth metatarsal is suspected, then x-ray views of the foot are indicated.

EVALUATION OF LIGAMENT INJURIES

Classification

Ligament sprains, the most common ankle injury, are classified as first-, second-, or third-degree before treatment and prognosis are determined (Table 23.1). A first-degree sprain is a minor ligamentous injury in which the ligament is partially torn and the joint is stable. A second-degree sprain is a more severe injury in which the joint remains stable. A third-degree sprain is a ligamentous injury resulting in an unstable joint.

Clinical Evaluation

Ankle instabilities can be classified as collateral ligament injuries in which the talus has excessive tilt in the ankle mortise on stress testing, or as interosseous ligament injuries in which there is widening of the ankle mortise as seen on x-ray. The importance of clinical recognition of these insta-

TABLE 23.1. Clinical Diagnosis of Ligament Injury

	First-Degree Sprain	Second-Degree Sprain	Third-Degree Sprain
Synonym	Mild sprain	Moderate sprain	Severe sprain
Etiology	Direct or indirect trauma to joint	Same	Severe direct or indirect trauma to joint
Symptoms	Pain; mild disability	Pain; moderate disability	Pain; severe disability
Signs	Mild point tenderness; no abnormal motion; little or no swelling	Point tenderness; moderate loss of function; slight to moderate abnormal motion; swelling; localized hemorrhage	Loss of function; marked abnormal motion; possible deformity; x-rays: stress films demonstrate abnormal motion
Complications	Tendency to recurrence; aggravation	Tendency to recurrence, aggravation; persistent instability; traumatic arthritis	Persistent instability; traumatic arthritis
Pathology	Minor tearing of ligament	Partial tear of ligament	Complete tear of ligament

Standard Nomenclature of Athletic Injuries, American Medical Association, Chicago, 1976.

bilities cannot be overemphasized. Physical examination, stress x-ray views, and arthrography are all useful in making the diagnosis.

All ligament structures about the ankle are first palpated. Localized tenderness laterally, medially, or anteriorly determines the site of injury to specific ligaments. Stability can be tested with manual inversion, eversion, and anterior drawer tests of the foot. The most common injury, involving the anterior talofibular ligament, results in anterior instability only, demonstrated by a positive anterior drawer test of the ankle (Fig. 23.4). If instability is suspected on clinical examination, stress testing is repeated under x-ray. Local anesthesia is needed in acute injuries because muscle spasm secondary to a painful injury can hide instability. If local anesthesia is unsuccessful, a general anesthetic may be necessary. Tilting of the talus within the mortise with supination of the foot is diagnostic of lateral instability. Usually the ankle opens between 5 and 15 degrees on the anteroposterior view with an isolated tear of the

anterior talofibular ligament. However, if the foot is forced forward, the talus will subluxate anteriorly (anterior drawer test), as documented on a lateral x-ray view. If, on a straight anteroposterior x-ray view, the talus opens 15 to 30 degrees laterally, the diagnosis is rupture of both the anterior talofibular and the calcaneofibular ligaments (Fig. 23.5). Gross lateral instability means complete rupture of all three parts of the lateral collateral ligament.

An injury to the deltoid ligament must always be suspected with any fracture of the fibula or any pronation mechanism of injury. Palpation of the deltoid ligament can detect pain and swelling, and stress x-rays may reveal widening of the medial joint space pathognomonic of a deltoid ligament injury associated with the fibular fracture.

X-ray Evaluation

Routine plain films, including anteroposterior, lateral, and inversion stress views of the ankle, are important to the evaluation. A widening between the tibia and fibula on

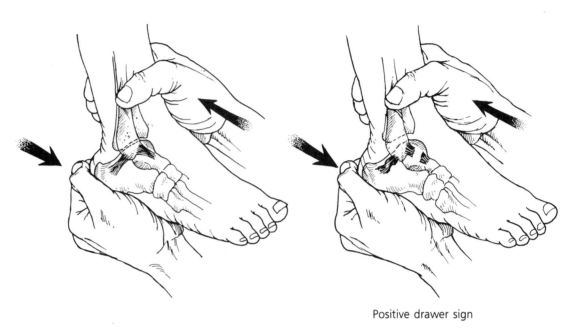

Positive drawer sign

FIGURE 23.4. Positive anterior drawer test.

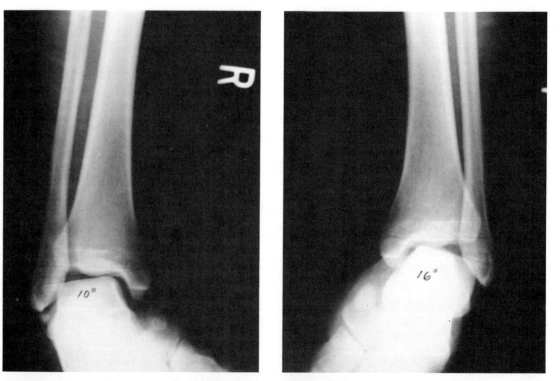

FIGURE 23.5. Inversion stress film to determine front talar tilts; normal (left) shows 10-degree talus opening versus abnormal, with 16-degree opening.

the oblique view indicates an injury to the syndesmosis. An avulsion of the very tip of the lateral malleolus is diagnostic of a major injury to the lateral collateral ligament. Osteochondral fractures of the dome of the talus may accompany any injury resulting in instability.

An arthrogram of the ankle offers little information over and above stress x-ray views. It may help localize the specific ligament injured. For instance, if dye escapes from the joint and is seen in the peroneal tendon sheath, there is a tear in the calcaneofibular ligament. Whether this test has true practical value will eventually be determined by further experience and data.

SPECIFIC INJURIES

Ankle injuries can be classified anatomically as soft tissue injuries of the ligaments and tendons, and bony injuries or fractures.

Soft Tissue Injuries

Lateral Ligament Sprain

Lateral ligament sprains are the most common ankle injuries. They vary in degree and are predictably progressive in the anatomic pathology involved. As the injurious stress forces are applied to the ankle, the anterior talofibular ligament stretches and tears. Continuing forces and deformity then cause stretching and progressive tearing of the calcaneofibular ligament. With the most severe injuries, the posterior talofibular ligament is involved.

The injured athlete experiences pain, localized swelling, and, sometimes, instability of the ankle laterally. Clinical examination can detect a palpable ligament defect and instability on stress testing. Stress x-ray views confirm the degree of instability.

A first-degree ankle sprain may be treated symptomatically with protective support, nonweight bearing, and early rehabilitation. Treatment of second-degree sprains depends on the amount of soft tissue injury and requires various amounts of time for ligament healing, but is basically the same

as for a first-degree sprain, only longer. Also, immobilization or splinting is more frequent than with first-degree sprains.

The treatment of the unstable third-degree sprain of the lateral collateral ligaments is controversial. The choices are a short leg cast for 4 to 6 weeks, a cast-brace, or surgical repair. Most experts agree that a torn anterior talofibular ligament with anterior subluxation may be treated conservatively by a cast with the foot at a right angle for 4 to 6 weeks or a cast-brace with plantar flexion stop. Complete tears of the anterior talofibular and calcaneofibular ligament result in ankle instability; they show 15 to 30 degrees of talar tilt on stress x-ray films. These gross instabilities in competitive athletes often must be repaired surgically. The athletic trainer should note this degree of instability, splint the athlete's ankle, and defer definitive care to the team physician or orthopedic surgeon.

Peroneal Tendon Injury

Peroneal tendon injuries can occur when the adjacent lateral ankle ligament structures are injured. Acute dislocation of the peroneal tendons is possible with this injury. The mechanism is forceful plantar flexion and valgus of the foot. The groove behind the fibula in which the peroneal tendons slide may be shallow, thereby predisposing the tendons to injury. Clinically, the athlete has pain and swelling over the lateral malleolus. The peroneal tendons are usually palpable on the outer aspect of the fibula. Eversion is very painful. Treatment in the athlete frequently requires repair of the torn retinaculum posterior to the fibula, along with cast immobilization for 6 weeks.

Usually, peroneal tendinitis symptoms are those of chronic overuse. The condition manifests as pain and swelling, pathognomonic of tendinitis and tenosynovitis. Where these structures pass behind the lateral malleolus, stress forces can cause irritation, resulting in swelling, pain, and dysfunction of the tendon.

Unique to the peroneal tendon is the possibility of subluxation or dislocation

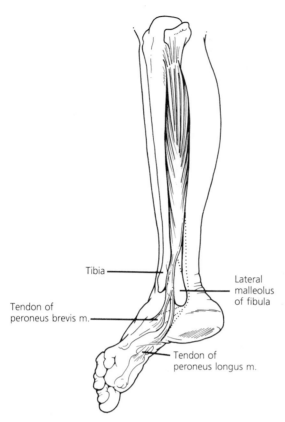

Tibia

Tendon of
peroneus brevis m.

Lateral
malleolus
of fibula

Tendon of
peroneus longus m.

FIGURE 23.6.   Peroneal tendon dislocation.
Dotted line shows normal location of tendon.

from behind the lateral malleolus (Fig. 23.6). Attrition or an acute tear of the tendon sheath allows this phenomenon. The tendon can intermittently subluxate and spontaneously relocate or remain dislocated. Either condition results in pain, deformity, and dysfunction on the lateral aspect of the ankle.

Simple strain of the peroneal tendon is treated conservatively with rest, heat and/or ice modalities, strapping support, and, eventually, progressive strengthening rehabilitation modalities. Recurrent peroneal tendon subluxation warrants more aggressive treatment. External padding and strapping may help stabilize the tendon, but often surgical reconstruction of the stabilizing tendon sheath is required. Adhesions and loss of function are complications of the surgery and make the functional results less than perfect.

Medial Ligament Sprain

Medial ligament injuries are not as common as lateral ligament injuries. Often, they are associated with fractures of the lateral malleolus. Eversion forces on the ankle create lateral malleolar fractures. If the forces continue after the fracture occurs, the talus shifts laterally. The medial ligament is then stretched and possibly torn. Localized pain and swelling characterize these injuries and, if a fracture is present, symptoms are also noted laterally. Clinically, the athletic trainer should concentrate on detecting localized tenderness, defects, and instability.

Treatment of medial ligament injuries is dictated by the degree of injury. Minor sprains are treated symptomatically, while tears that elicit minimal instability on stress testing are treated with splinting or cast immobilization. Progressive weight-bearing activities encourage early healing, and progressive therapy after remobilization of the ankle encourages rapid return to function. If fractures are associated with medial ligament injuries, surgical repair is generally indicated for the fracture and for the ligaments.

Interosseous Ligament Sprain

Twisting injuries of the talus and the ankle mortise may cause a sprain of the interosseous ligament which holds the ankle mortise in continuity. Minor sprains present as localized pain and tenderness with no evidence of instability. These injuries can be treated conservatively with rest, followed by rehabilitation when symptoms have abated. Distal tibiofibular interosseous ligament sprains can occur after considerable trauma to the ankle that has caused other ligamentous and bony injuries. If massive ankle trauma has occurred and repair is indicated, lesions of the interosseous ligaments are repaired incidentally along with the other injuries. Restoration of the anatomical alignment and stability of the distal tibiofibular configuration are important. Instability or malalignment results in functional disability in the ankle.

Injuries to the tibiofibular ligament sustained in football players often ossify, and this ectopic ossification can be detected radiographically. Usually it causes no functional disability unless impingement occurs in the interosseous space.

Achilles Tendon Injury

At the level of the ankle, the Achilles tendon can sustain an acute injury from direct trauma or stress and can be stressed chronically by repetitive overloading. These injuries are covered in Chapter 22. It should be noted that recovery from these injuries is long and difficult and requires extensive rehabilitation. Contusion and strain of the distal Achilles tendon are best treated with rest, heat modalities, and progressive therapy rehabilitation routines.

Tibialis Posterior Tendon Injury

More problems arise in the tibialis posterior tendon than are recognized and treated. This structure is often irritated as it courses behind the medial malleolus. Pain and mild swelling of tendinitis and synovitis result from this irritation. If attrition occurs, the tendon can actually rupture, resulting in functional disability. Pain, tenderness, and some weakness on push-off are noted by athletes with tibialis posterior injuries. With acute ruptures, a pop can be felt, and pain, swelling, and increasing loss of function are noted (Fig. 23.7). In the chronic case of a partial tear or a complete rupture, a painful, palpable nodular scar builds up in the tendon sheath. Collapse of the midfoot and hyperpronation are also clinical findings.

Treatment of tibialis posterior injuries also depends on the degree of severity. While tendon strains can be managed with rest, oral nonsteroidal anti-inflammatory drugs, heat modalities, and taping for support, acute ruptures warrant an attempt at surgical repair. Chronic injuries may require surgical débridement of the tendon and the inflamed tendon sheath. If secondary degenerative changes have occurred in the midfoot, arthrodesis may be indicated.

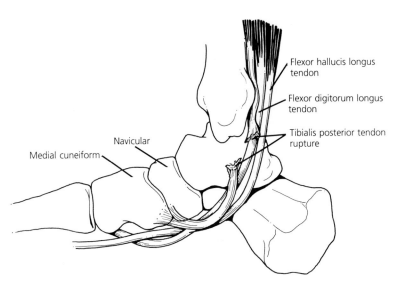

FIGURE 23.7. Posterior tibialis tendon rupture.

This surgery is usually only performed for the relief of chronic pain, and return to high-performance levels is doubtful with these problems.

Chronic Synovitis

Occasionally, an athlete who has a history of multiple minor injuries to the ankle from direct trauma and sprains presents with a swollen, stiff, and painful ankle. When no history of trauma is noted, an evaluation for a systemic arthritic condition should be performed. Traumatic or idiopathic loose body formations in the ankle joint can also cause a chronic reactive synovitis.

Initial treatment consists of rest, immobilization, and, possibly, the use of oral nonsteroidal anti-inflammatory medications. Taping or brace support should be used when the athlete begins rehabilitation and returns to functional activities. Continued support may be indicated when unrestricted athletic activities are resumed.

Bony Injuries

The same forces that cause ligament injuries about the ankle can cause fractures of the osseous structures. Nondisplaced, these

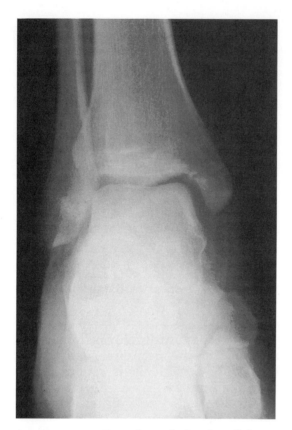

FIGURE 23.8. X-ray of nondisplaced medial malleolar fracture.

injuries can be treated conservatively with immobilization. However, any disruptions of the finely aligned architecture of the ankle joint must be reduced and stabilized to prevent the loss of normal function.

Medial and Lateral Malleolar Fractures

Many of the same forces that cause ligament injuries about the ankle can create osseous fractures. It often is a matter of which yields first to the forces—the ligaments or the bones. Inversion or shear forces often cause medial malleolar fractures (Fig. 23.8). Usually, these fractures are level with the talar dome or spiral end of the distal tibial metaphysis. Lateral ligament or bony injuries often accompany these medial injuries.

Nondisplaced medial malleolar fractures usually heal or fibrose in situ (healing with scar tissue but no bony union) with conservative treatment. Anatomic congruity of the ankle mortise is essential in conservative treatment of these ankle injuries.

Lateral malleolar fractures are usually caused by eversion and/or twisting injuries. Most lateral malleolar fractures are spiral fractures and can be comminuted. In severe eversion injuries, the tip of the medial malleolus can avulse.

Many malleolar fractures actually require open reduction and internal fixation because of incongruity, displacement, and persistent instability. Healing after surgery or conservative treatment usually takes 2 to 3 months or longer, and extensive therapy is required.

Fracture-Dislocations

To differentiate the spiral fracture and the avulsion fracture of the distal fibula from a sprain is usually possible by careful clinical palpation to locate the tenderness. An appropriate x-ray view, of course, ultimately confirms the diagnosis.

Severe fracture-dislocations and dislocations of the ankle are usually dramatic events. Fracture-dislocations often occur after a jump, such as in basketball or volleyball. How the athlete lands on the foot determines the type of injury. For instance, landing on an everted foot in plantar flexion can produce an open dislocation of the ankle. The medial malleolus may be exposed through the skin and the foot displaced relative to the lower leg. The athletic trainer should immediately remove the shoe and evaluate the athlete's circulation, sensation, and motor function. In an open wound with bone showing, closed reduction should not be attempted because of the contamination of the exposed bone. Usually, the skin is buttonholed around the bone and blocks reduction. This injury should be covered with a sterile dressing, and a well-padded, short leg splint should be applied. The athlete should be transported to the

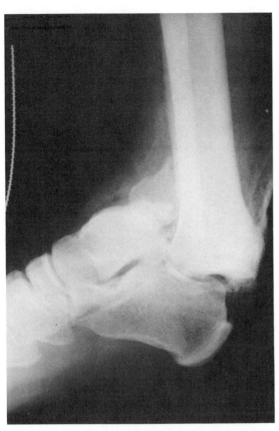

FIGURE 23.9. Fracture-dislocation of the ankle.

foot on the end of the tibia. However, if the fracture cannot be easily reduced, then the ankle should be splinted in its displaced position, and the athlete transported immediately to an emergency facility. A well-padded, short leg splint (or air splint) should be applied before transportation.

Fractures of the ankle differ from sprains in that they all require cast or cast-brace immobilization and may require surgical stabilization. Rehabilitation is more difficult and prolonged due to injury severity and the muscle atrophy resulting from cast immobilization. Rigid internal fixation of these fractures may offer a shorter period of immobilization and, hence, a faster recovery. The ultimate prognosis in ankle fractures is related to the damage to the articular surface that may not be apparent for some time after the injury.

Osteochondral Fracture of the Talus

Acute or chronic subluxation of the talus in the ankle can allow the edge of the talar dome to impinge against the malleolus on either side. The edge of bone, along with its cartilaginous cover, can be chipped away, creating osteochondral fragments that can remain in situ or float freely in the joint (Fig. 23.10).

An osteochondral fracture causes pain and swelling, and, if the fragment is free-floating, intermittent locking can occur. A nondisplaced fragment often heals following ankle immobilization and rest. Loose fragments should be removed surgically; this can be done arthroscopically.

Osteochondritis dissecans, which is a condition of fragmentation and loosening of a portion of the osteochondral surface of the talus, can create loose bodies that float free in the ankle joint. These, too, can become symptomatic, causing catching, locking, pain, and swelling in the ankle joint. Athletes having the symptoms of intra-articular loose bodies in the ankle should be referred for diagnostic evaluation and treatment. After surgical removal of loose bodies, most ankles can be rehabilitated, and the athlete

nearest emergency department, and the team orthopedist must be notified immediately. An open wound must be débrided surgically as soon as possible to minimize the chance for infection.

Closed fracture-dislocations of the ankle are usually either bimalleolar fractures or a fibular fracture with a ruptured deltoid ligament (Fig. 23.9). In some instances, these can be severely displaced. As with other ankle injuries, the circulation, sensation, and motor function of the foot must be assessed immediately. A severe fracture-dislocation will usually be displaced laterally to the lower leg. This abnormal position can compromise the posterior tibial artery and nerve. In instances of obvious circulatory compromise, the athletic trainer should flex the knee and apply gentle linear traction to reduce (or reposition) the

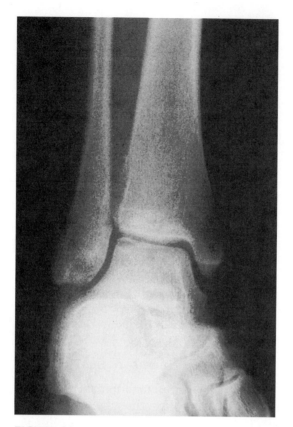

FIGURE 23.10. Osteochondral fracture.

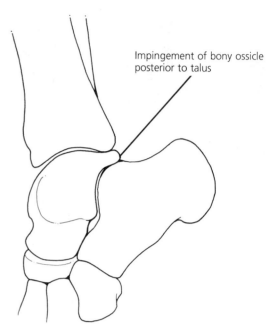

Impingement of bony ossicle posterior to talus

FIGURE 23.11. Os trigonum syndrome.

allowed to return to sports activities. An obvious defect is left in the talus after this injury and can alter ankle function. However, recovery and return to activities are expected if the lesion is not too large.

Os Trigonum Syndrome

A bony ossicle posterior to the talus is present in some athletes (Fig. 23.11). It is usually asymptomatic but can become inflamed with overuse of the foot, especially in activities involving repeated plantar flexion. Certain sports activities such as dancing, skating, and kicking can cause this phenomenon, called **os trigonum syndrome**. Persistent pain should be treated with rest, medication, and splinting. Rarely, surgery is required in cases that resist conservative care because of impingement of the fragment in the tibiotalar joint.

REHABILITATION OF ANKLE SPRAINS

Rehabilitation of ankle sprains begins almost simultaneously with the onset of treatment. The goal is to obtain a stable, painless, mobile ankle that can undergo the rigors of the athlete's sport.

Strengthening Program

Strengthening of the medial and lateral stabilizers may begin as soon as pain-free exercise is possible. Full weight bearing is not permitted until it can be done without a limp and the athlete has nearly full range of motion without pain. Swimming may begin before weight bearing. Strengthening exercises are initially isometric, progressing dynamically as the athlete is able to bear weight. Isometric, isotonic, and isokinetic exercises for dorsiflexion, plantar flexion, inversion, and eversion strengthen the four major muscle groups of the lower leg. Walking is followed by jogging, running, figure-eights, and various maneuvers of the sport before return to competition is allowed. Exercises to regain proprioception are also important and can be done on a tilt board or by the athlete's balancing on the injured leg with the eyes closed.

Return to Sport

Some form of external support, such as taping, an air splint, or a cast-brace, is necessary when the athlete with a second- or third-degree sprain returns to play. Taping or brace support may be required throughout the remainder of the season to prevent reinjury.

The athlete with recurrent ankle problems indicating chronic instability should have his or her ankle taped or braced for all practice sessions and games, and should be on an ankle-conditioning program. If this is not successful, reconstructive surgery should be considered. Rehabilitation following fractures is similar but prolonged relative to the length of immobilization.

Rehabilitation Exercises

Peroneal (Eversion) Strengthening

Position: Attach a 1-pound weight on forefoot. Lie on your uninvolved side so your involved foot is over the edge.

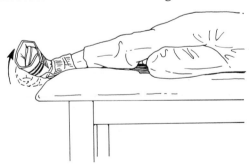

Procedure: Raise lateral side of foot up toward ceiling, with toe pointed. Hold for a 5 count. Relax and repeat 2 sets of 10, three times daily. Progress to 5 pounds, 5 sets of 10, three times daily.

Dorsiflexion Strengthening

Position: Attach a 1-pound weight on the forefoot. Sit so foot is off floor.

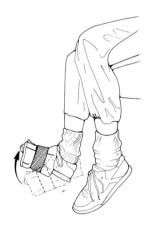

Procedure: Pull foot straight up. Hold for a 5 count. Relax and repeat 2 sets of 10, three times daily. Progress to 5 pounds, 5 sets of 10, three times daily.

Tibialis Posterior (Inversion) Strengthening

Position: Attach 1-pound weight on forefoot. Lie on your involved side so involved foot is over the edge.

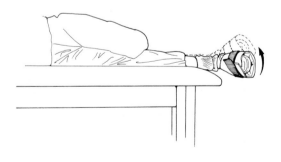

Procedure: Raise the medial side of your foot up toward the ceiling as high as possible with toes pointed. (This may be done sitting with legs crossed.) Hold for a 5 count. Relax and repeat 2 sets of 10, three times daily. Progress to 5 pounds, 5 sets of 10, three times daily.

Heelcord Stretch—Incline Board

Position I: Stand on incline board with higher edge toward wall.

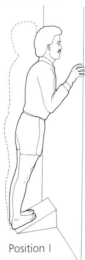

Position I

Procedure: With feet pigeon-toed and knees straight, lean toward wall. Hold for 10 counts. Perform 3 sets of 10, three times a day.

Tibialis Posterior (Plantar Flexion) Strengthening

Position: Stand with feet slightly pigeon-toed using a wall or table for balance.

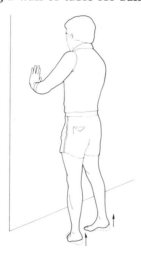

Procedure: Push up on toes and lift heels. Hold for a count of 5, lower, relax, and repeat. Perform 3 sets of 10, three times a day.

Position II: Stand on incline board with higher edge away from wall.

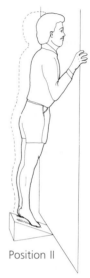

Position II

Procedure: Heels should be lifted toward wall. Hold for 10 counts. Perform 3 sets of 10, three times a day.

IMPORTANT CONCEPTS

1. The bones of the ankle joint are the tibia, fibula, and talus.
2. The relationship of the tibia, talus, and fibula is maintained by the deltoid ligament, the lateral collateral ligament, and the tibiofibular syndesmosis.
3. The medial stabilizers of the ankle are the tibialis anterior, tibialis posterior, flexor digitorum longus, and the flexor hallucis longus.
4. The lateral stabilizers of the ankle are the peroneal muscles.
5. Because the stability of the ankle is greater laterally than medially, the ankle is predisposed to inversion injuries rather than eversion injuries.
6. Anteroposterior, lateral, oblique, and stress (inversion and drawer) x-ray views are used to diagnose ligament injuries of the ankle.
7. Soft tissue injuries of the ankle include lateral and medial ligament sprains, peroneal tendon injuries, interosseous ligament sprains, Achilles tendon injuries, tibialis posterior tendon injuries, and chronic synovitis.
8. Bony injuries of the ankle include medial and lateral malleolar fractures, fracture-dislocations, osteochondral fracture of the talus, and os trigonum syndrome.
9. A protocol for rehabilitation of ankle injuries starts with isometric exercises when the athlete is pain free, and progresses to isotonic and isokinetic exercises for dorsiflexion, plantar flexion, inversion, and eversion.

SUGGESTED READINGS

Arrowsmith, S. R., L. L. Fleming, and F. L. Allman. "Traumatic Dislocations of the Peroneal Tendons." *American Journal of Sports Medicine* 11 (1983): 142–146.

Balduini, Frederick C., and John Tetzlaff. "Historical Perspectives on Injuries of the Ligaments of the Ankle." *Clinics in Sports Medicine* 1 (1982): 3–12.

Black, H. M., R. L. Brand, and M. R. Eichelberger. "An Improved Technique for the Evaluation of Ligamentous Injury in Severe Ankle Sprains." *American Journal of Sports Medicine* 6 (1978): 276–282.

Brodsky, A. E., and M. A. Khalil. "Talar Compression Syndrome." *American Journal of Sports Medicine* 14 (1986): 472–476.

Cox, J. S., and T. F. Hewes. "'Normal' Talar Tilt Angle." *Clinical Orthopaedics and Related Research* 140 (1979): 37–41.

Derscheid, G. L., and W. C. Brown. "Rehabilitation of the Ankle." *Clinics in Sports Medicine* 4 (1985): 527–544.

Harrington, K. D. "Degenerative Arthritis of the Ankle Secondary to Long-Standing Lateral Ligament Instability." *Journal of Bone and Joint Surgery* 61A (1979): 354–361.

Hontas, M. J., R. J. Haddad, and L. C. Schlesinger. "Conditions of the Talus in the Runner." *American Journal of Sports Medicine* 14 (1986): 486–490.

Ihle, C. L., and R. M. Cochran. "Fracture of the Fused Os Trigonum." *American Journal of Sports Medicine* 10 (1982): 47–50.

Inman, Verne T. *The Joints of the Ankle.* Baltimore: Williams & Wilkins, 1976.

Jackson, D. W., R. L. Ashley, and J. W. Powell. "Ankle Sprains in Young Athletes: Relation of Severity and Disability." *Clinical Orthopaedics and Related Research* 101 (1974): 201–215.

McManama, G. B., Jr. "Ankle Injuries in the Young Athlete." *Clinics in Sports Medicine* 7 (1988): 547–562.

Nemeth, Victor A., and Elliott Thrasher. "Ankle Sprains in Athletes." *Clinics in Sports Medicine* 2 (1983): 217–224.

Nicholas, J. A. "Ankle Injuries in Athletes." *Orthopedic Clinics of North America* 5 (1974): 153–175.

Peiró, A., J. Aracil, F. Martos, et al. "Triplane Distal Tibial Epiphyseal Fracture." *Clinical Orthopaedics and Related Research* 160 (1981): 196–200.

Quillen, William S., and Leon H. Rouillier. "Initial Management of Acute Ankle Sprains with Rapid Pulsed Pneumatic Compression and Cold." *The Journal of Orthopaedic and Sports Physical Therapy* 4 (1982): 39–43.

Rovere, G. D., T. J. Clarke, C. S. Yates, et al. "Retrospective Comparison of Taping and Ankle Stabilizers in Preventing Ankle Injuries." *American Journal of Sports Medicine* 16 (1988): 228–233.

St. Pierre, R. K., L. Andrews, F. Allman, Jr., et al. "The Cybex II Evaluation of Lateral Ankle Ligamentous Reconstructions." *American Journal of Sports Medicine* 12 (1984): 52–56.

Scheller, A. D., J. R. Kasser, and T. B. Quigley. "Tendon Injuries about the Ankle." *Orthopedic Clinics of North America* 11 (1980): 801–811.

Smith, R. W., and S. F. Reischl. "Treatment of Ankle Sprains in Young Athletes." *American Journal of Sports Medicine* 14 (1986): 465–471.

Stover, C. N. "Air Stirrup Management of Ankle Injuries in the Athlete." *American Journal of Sports Medicine* 8 (1980): 360–365.

Vegso, Joseph J., and Louis E. Harmon, III. "Nonoperative Management of Athletic Ankle Injuries." *Clinics in Sports Medicine* 1 (1982): 85–98.

Walsh, W. M., and T. Blackburn. "Prevention of Ankle Sprains." *American Journal of Sports Medicine* 5 (1977): 243–245.

24

The Foot

OBJECTIVES FOR CHAPTER 24

After reading this chapter, the student should be able to:

1. Understand the function of the osseous structures and the soft tissue anatomy of the foot.
2. Describe the biomechanics of foot function.
3. Identify abnormalities that can cause foot problems.
4. Discuss the diagnosis and treatment of minor and major foot problems.
5. Provide first aid to the athlete with a foot injury.
6. Plan a rehabilitation program for the athlete with a foot injury.

INTRODUCTION

The foot is the terminal appendage of the lower extremity and functions as the contact point between the body and terrain in locomotion. It is a complicated structure with a complicated function. Understanding the injuries and the disorders of the foot and their treatment is a challenge to the athletic trainer.

Chapter 24 begins with the anatomy of the foot and the biomechanics of walking and running. The chapter next describes the deformities and pathological conditions of the foot. Specific injuries to the soft tissues and bones are described next. The last two sections of Chapter 24 briefly discuss first-aid measures in the event of a foot injury and rehabilitation that should begin following an injury. ■

ANATOMY

Bones

The bony skeleton of the foot is composed of 26 bones (Fig. 24.1). The **talus** articulates with the **tibia** and **fibula** to make up the ankle joint. Movement at the ankle is basically dorsiflexion and plantar flexion, with simultaneous anterior and posterior sliding motions of the talus and the ankle mortise.

Because the talus is wider in front, the tibiofibular joint spreads with dorsiflexion and narrows with plantar flexion. The inferior surface of the talus articulates with the **calcaneus** (heel bone), making up the subtalar joint. The head of the talus articulates with the **navicular bone** on the medial side of the foot, and the calcaneus (anterior process) articulates with the **cuboid bone** on the lateral side of the foot. The combination of movements of these three articulations —talocalcaneal, talonavicular, and calcaneocuboid—results in the complex foot movements of eversion, inversion, pronation, and supination.

The remaining bones of the foot are the three **cuneiforms**, five **metatarsals**, and the **phalanges** (three for each of the lateral four toes and two phalanges for the great toe). The midtarsal joints, navicular-cuneiform and cuneiform-metatarsal, are stable joints that produce very little movement. The metatarsals and proximal phalanges form the metatarsophalangeal (MP) joints that function during push-off. The small toes have two interphalangeal (IP) joints between their three phalangeal bones, and the great toe has a single IP joint between its two bones. The two small **sesamoid bones** located beneath the first metatarsal head function as extra weight-bearing structures and leverage points for the mechanics of the great toe.

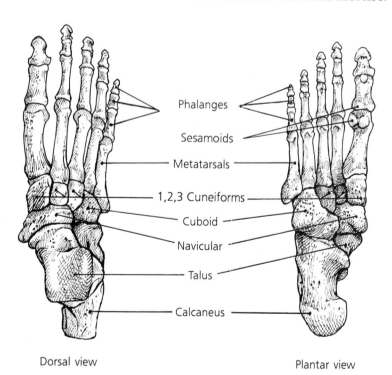

Phalanges

Sesamoids

Metatarsals

1,2,3 Cuneiforms

Cuboid

Navicular

Talus

Calcaneus

Dorsal view

Plantar view

FIGURE 24.1. Bony skeleton of the foot.

Arches

The bones of the foot are arranged structurally to form two arches: the **longitudinal arch** and the **transverse arch**. The bones are mortised together to form the architecture of these two arches (Fig. 24.2). The ligaments of the foot provide intrinsic support, and the muscles of the leg provide extrinsic support to the arches.

Longitudinal Arch

The longitudinal arch starts at the weight-bearing surface of the calcaneus and ends at the metatarsal heads. It is supported intrinsically by the **plantar calcaneonavicular ligament** (spring ligament). This ligament supports the head of the talus. The talus is also supported by the **plantar fascia**, which runs from the calcaneal tuberosity to the phalanges. The plantar fascia acts as a bowstring for the longitudinal arch and supports the muscles on the plantar surface of the foot.

The extrinsic support comes from the **anterior tibial tendon** pulling on its insertion at the first cuneiform and from the **posterior tibial tendon** and **peroneus longus tendon** that pass under the foot. These structures create a dynamic sling supporting the longitudinal arch.

Transverse Arch

The metatarsal bones form a transverse arch when the foot is non–weight bearing and at rest. There is no transverse arch at the metatarsal heads on weight bearing, as each of the lateral four metatarsal heads bears one-sixth of the body weight and the first metatarsal head (with two sesamoid bones) bears two-sixths of the body weight.

Muscles, Arteries, and Nerves

The three main muscle groups of the lower leg all insert on the foot, thus controlling the action of the foot.

Posterior Compartment

The **gastrocnemius-soleus group** is located in the superficial part of the posterior com-

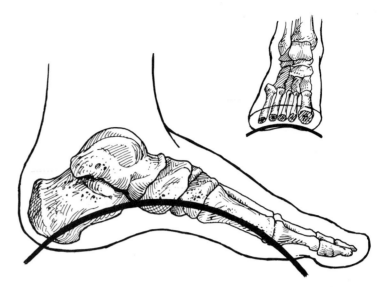

FIGURE 24.2. Longitudinal arch and transverse arch of the foot.

partment. It leads to the **calcaneal**, or **Achilles**, **tendon** and inserts on the posterior aspect of the calcaneus (Fig. 24.3a). The deep portion of the posterior compartment contains three muscles: the **tibialis posterior**, the **flexor digitorum longus**, and the **flexor hallucis longus** (Fig. 24.3b). The tibialis posterior muscle supports the longitudinal arch and inverts the foot. The flexor digitorum longus flexes the lateral four toes, and the flexor hallucis longus flexes the great toe (Fig. 24.3c).

These three muscles enter the foot through a ligamentous tunnel behind the medial malleolus, along with the posterior tibial nerve, artery, and vein. The posterior tibial nerve divides into the medial and lateral plantar nerves and supplies sensation to the plantar surface of the foot while innervating the plantar muscles.

The posterior tibial tendon attaches directly on the tuberosity of the navicular bone and indirectly on the plantar surface of the navicular and middle cuneiform bones (see Fig. 24.3c). The flexor digitorum longus attaches to the plantar surface of the lateral four toes. The flexor hallucis longus passes between the two sesamoid bones under the first metatarsal head and thus between the two heads of flexor hallucis

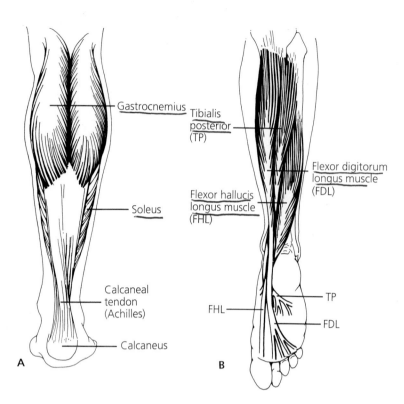

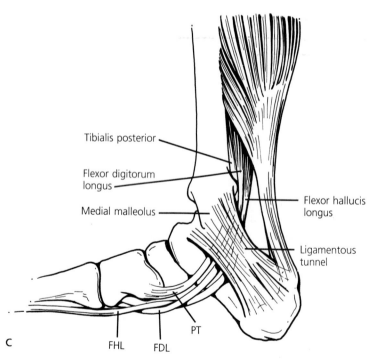

FIGURE 24.3. The muscles of the posterior compartment of the foot: (a) the superficial position; (b) the deep portion; and (c) the medial view.

brevis and inserts on the plantar surface of the distal phalanx of the great toe.

Lateral Compartment

The lateral compartment is composed of two muscles: the **peroneus longus** and the **peroneus brevis** (Fig. 24.4). The peroneus longus crosses under the longitudinal arch from lateral to medial and inserts on the plantar surface of the first cuneiform and first metatarsal. The peroneus brevis inserts on the base of the fifth metatarsal. These muscles evert and plantar flex the foot.

Anterior Compartment

The anterior compartment consists of (1) the **tibialis anterior**, which inserts on the medial cuneiform; (2) the **extensor digitorum longus**, which divides and inserts on the dorsum of the small toes; and (3) the **extensor hallucis longus**, which inserts on the dorsum of the great toe (Fig. 24.5). This

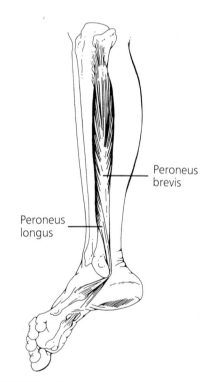

FIGURE 24.4. Muscles of the lateral compartment of the foot.

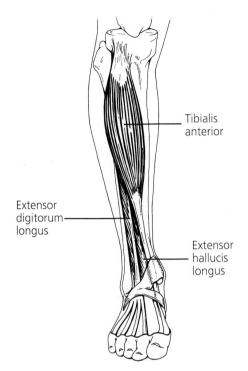

FIGURE 24.5. Muscles of the anterior compartment of the foot.

group dorsiflexes the foot and toes. The tibialis anterior and extensor hallucis longus muscles are invertors, and the extensor digitorum longus is an evertor. The **peroneus tertius** is essentially a lateral slip of the extensor digitorum longus muscle.

Intrinsic Foot Muscles

The intrinsic muscles of the foot are primarily related to toe function. There is only one muscle on the dorsum of the foot—the short toe extensor, or **extensor digitorum brevis**. There are 15 small muscles on the plantar surface of the foot arranged in layers, all related to toe function (Fig. 24.6). They fill in the space between the longitudinal arch and the plantar fascia.

Fat Pad

The **fat pad** is a specialized soft tissue structure designed specifically for weight bearing and absorbing impact. It consists of specialized fat globules located between the plantar skin and the underlying calcaneus and plantar fascia. These fat globules are contained between vertical fibrous septa. The fatty tissue is packed into multiple fibrous walled compartments that are capable of withstanding the pressure of weight bearing.

BIOMECHANICS: GAIT ANALYSIS

Understanding the normal biomechanics of the gait and the forces applied to the foot facilitates understanding the mechanism of injury. The normal gait is divided into a stance, or support, phase and a swing phase. The major difference between running and walking is that in the support phase in walking one foot is always on the ground, whereas in running there is an airborne period where neither foot is in contact with the ground.

Walking

The walking stance phase begins when the foot strikes the ground. Initial contact called *heel strike*, is usually made with the calcaneus. Thus, all the weight-bearing force is absorbed initially by heel contact. The foot then proceeds into *midsupport phase*. Weight-bearing force passes along the lateral border of the foot to the metatarsal heads. As this occurs, the normal foot is inverted at heel strike and then pronates (rolls inward) as the weight passes from the lateral side of the foot and is spread out along the entire longitudinal arch. This complex series of movements through the subtalar and midtarsal joints absorbs and dissipates the force of heel strike. The foot then progresses from midsupport to *toe-off*. The other foot then goes through the identical activity.

Running

In running, the same activity occurs during the midsupport, or midstance, phase until

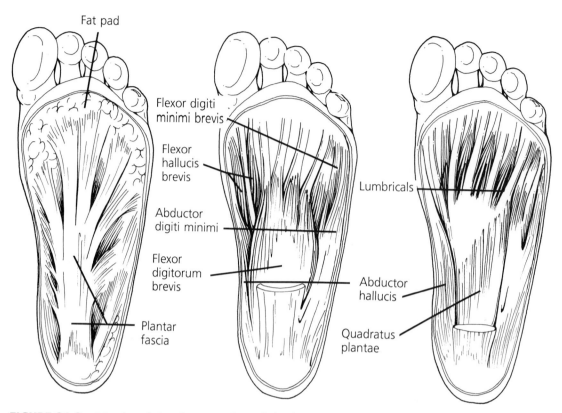

FIGURE 24.6.   Muscles of the plantar surface of the foot.

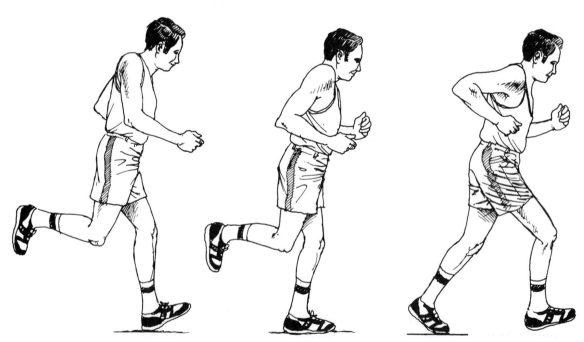

FIGURE 24.7.   Three phases of the normal running gait: heel strike, midsupport, and toe-off.

push-off occurs (Fig. 24.7). The gastrocnemius-soleus muscle group forcefully contracts to assist toe-off as the runner enters the airborne phase (Fig. 24.8).

The trailing leg is in swing phase and is just completing follow-through as the stance phase leg is in heel strike. The swing phase leg then begins an acceleration phase as the thigh and knee flex and are brought forward. The pelvis rotates around the hip joint of the stance phase leg. Initially, the pelvis rotates backward (external rotation of the stance phase hip) as the pelvis follows the swing phase leg in follow-through. As the swing phase leg comes forward, the pelvis rotates forward with it. Thus in midsupport phase, the center of gravity is directly over the weight-bearing foot, and the pelvis is in neutral rotation. The swing phase leg continues forward and begins its deceleration phase as the knee extends and the foot is preparing for heel strike. At this time, the stance phase leg has completed toe-off and the runner is momentarily airborne. These complex movements and forces in running explain why some subtle foot deformities and muscle imbalances can cause problems in the foot. The interrelationships between the foot, the knee, and the hip in walking, jogging, and running are extremely complex.

DEFORMITIES AND DISEASES

The foot is a part of the anatomy that is accessible to examination, palpation, and mechanical evaluation. Several foot deformities and diseases are sources of potential problems. Treatment options exist that attempt to correct or alter the abnormality discovered from the history and physical examination (Table 24.1).

Cavus Foot

The **cavus foot** has an excessively high longitudinal arch. This deformity may range from an elevated longitudinal arch to a full-blown deformity, consisting of a varus

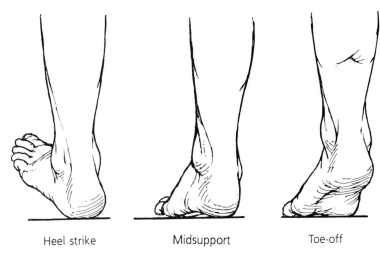

Heel strike   Midsupport   Toe-off

FIGURE 24.8. Contraction of the gastrocnemius-soleus group of muscles at toe-off.

heel and clawing of the toes (Fig. 24.9). Subtalar motion (inversion/supination and eversion/pronation) is frequently restricted, which limits the foot's ability to absorb the forces encountered during heel strike. Athletes with cavus feet frequently complain of plantar fascia pain due to the tripod effect of the deformity and the increased bow-string pull of the fascia. Cavus feet often result in painful callosities on the lateral aspect of the heel, under the metatarsal heads, and on the dorsum of the IP joints if the toes are clawed. An orthosis, a properly placed metatarsal pad, and special attention to footwear may eliminate or prevent symptoms.

Flat Foot (Pes Planus)

The **flat foot**, also called **pes planus**, is pronated with a flattened longitudinal arch. The hindfoot may be in valgus. Occasionally, there is an associated accessory navicular bone. In this congenital deformity, the ossification center of the navicular tuberosity fails to fuse to the main bone and remains a bony prominence on the medial side of the foot. These are often locally symptomatic and require protection or surgical excision.

Flat feet are classified as flexible or rigid. A flexible flat foot (or pronated foot) has

TABLE 24.1. Treatment Options for Foot Problems

Abnormality	Orthotic	Pad	Shoe Modification	Splint	Surgery
Cavus foot	X				
Flexible flat foot	X				
Rigid flat foot	X				X
Metatarsus varus	X		X	?	
Metatarsus valgus	X		X	?	
Morton's foot	X				
Hallux valgus				?	
Claw toes		X	X		X
Hammertoes		X	X		X
Tailor's bunion		X	X		X
Avascular necrosis				X	
Sesamoiditis		X			
Plantar wart		X			X

full range of motion in the midtarsal joints. The arch of the foot can be developed by dynamic input through the tibialis posterior. This can be seen when the athlete stands on his or her toes. A rigid flat foot has a fixed deformity, and the flattening of the longitudinal arch is unchanged by dynamic extrinsic input to the foot (Fig. 24.10). The flexible flat foot is the most common and is usually asymptomatic in the milder forms. Moderate to severe deformities may be symptomatic. Proper attention to footwear and longitudinal arch supports are helpful. The rigid flat foot is a much more difficult problem and may prohibit such activities as long-distance running. A rigid flat foot is often due to congenital tarsal coalition, which is a fusion of some of the bones in the hindfoot and midfoot. Some of the more common fusion sites are talonavicular and calcaneocuboid; the most common are calcaneonavicular and talocalcaneal. Other combinations are possible. Symptoms from this phenomenon may be delayed until adolescence or later.

Metatarsus Varus and Valgus

Metatarsus varus (metatarsus adductus) is a congenital deformity of the forefoot, in

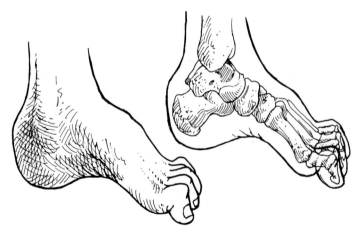

FIGURE 24.9. Cavus foot with elevated longitudinal arch and clawing of the toes.

which the forefoot is angulated and rotated medially in relation to the hindfoot. **Metatarsus valgus (metatarsus abductus)** is the opposite deformity of the forefoot, in which abnormal stress is placed on the foot, resulting in painful callosities. With these deformities, as with the others, proper footwear and orthoses may prevent problems. The hindfoot may also be in varus (angulated medially) or valgus (angulated laterally). These deformities are usually associated with a cavus (heel varus) or flat foot (heel valgus) deformity.

Morton's Foot

Deformities of the toes are also common. **Morton's foot** is characterized by a short first metatarsal. Excessive weight bearing is then shifted to the relatively elongated second toe, causing an imbalance in the transverse metatarsal arch. This deformity interferes with the normal weight-bearing stresses in the forefoot and places greater stress on the second metatarsal head, which often results in pain. An orthosis in the shoe may help correct the imbalance and relieve pain.

Hallux Valgus

Bunions, or **hallux valgus deformities**, are not common in young athletes. A widening between the first and second metatarsal bones produces a prominence of the first metatarsal head medially, which becomes the bunion. The great toe then shifts laterally, forming the hallux valgus deformity, which eventually can become rigid and nonfunctional in this position. The metatarsal splay is an inherent factor in the development of bunions and hallux valgus, but improper footwear creates additional deforming forces that cause the deformities to progress. Once the deformities have occurred, pain may be avoided by proper footwear that has an adequate toe box to relieve pressure over the bony prominences. Surgical correction may be indicated in severe cases.

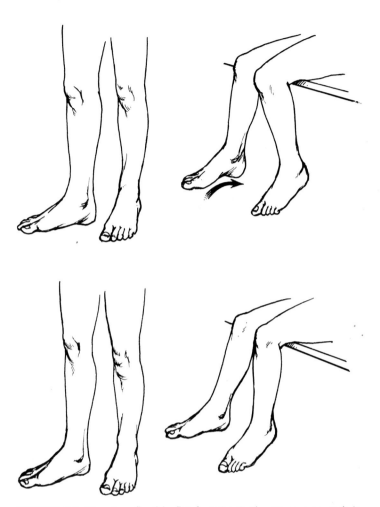

FIGURE 24.10. In a flexible flat foot (top), the transverse arch is present in a non-weight-bearing position. With a rigid flat foot (bottom), there is no change in the flattened longitudinal arch when in a non-weight-bearing position.

Claw Toes

The **claw toe** deformity is a hyperextension of the MP joint and a hyperflexion of the IP joints (Fig. 24.11). This deformity can be congenital, but it can also be the result of subtle muscle imbalances in the foot or of neurological disorders such as cerebral palsy or Charcot-Marie-Tooth disease. Painful callosities often develop on the dorsum of the IP joints from pressure against the shoe and under the metatarsal heads where they press against the sole of the shoe. Proper placement of a metatarsal pad can usually control these symptoms.

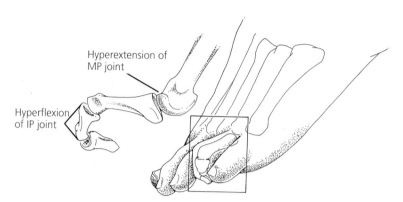

FIGURE 24.11.   Claw toe deformity.

Hammertoes

Hammertoe is a deformity of flexion of the distal IP joint, resulting in pressure on the nail and the end of the toe from contact against the sole of the shoe (Fig. 24.12). This deformity can be congenital or it can be caused by intrinsic and extrinsic muscle contractures that create a hyperflexion of the distal toe joint.

These deformities are difficult to control conservatively and may require surgical correction. Fusion of the joint is usually necessary to correct the deformity. After 2 to 3 months of healing, the athlete should be able to rehabilitate, retrain, and return to sports.

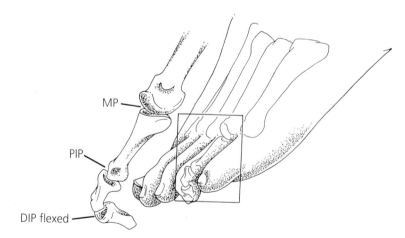

FIGURE 24.12.   Hammertoe deformity.

Bunionette (Tailor's Bunion)

A **bunionette (tailor's bunion)** is a prominence of the lateral aspect of the fifth metatarsal. It is usually the result of a splay posture of all of the metatarsals. A malunion of a fracture of the fifth metatarsal may also cause prominence of the metatarsal head. Improperly fitting footwear can then cause pressure against the bony prominence, which creates the irritation and pain. Footwear that does not create pressure over the bony prominence affords relief of these painful symptoms.

Avascular Necrosis

Certain bones in the body have the tendency to lose a portion of their blood supply, and consequently, become nonviable. This phenomenon is called **avascular necrosis.** The bone can recover its blood supply and will regenerate into a living osseous structure in time. **Freiberg's disease** is a specific avascular necrosis that occurs in the head of the second metatarsal in some adolescents (Fig. 24.13). It manifests as functional pain in the forefoot. Diagnosis is by the radiographic findings of the sclerotic bone corresponding to the area of tenderness. After the pain is controlled by conservative means (padding and restricted activity), the athlete may return to competition.

Plantar Warts

Plantar warts, like other warts, are a skin growth caused by a localized viral infection. They become symptomatic when subjected to pressure in footwear, particularly if they are located in the heel area or beneath the metatarsal heads. Pain can be relieved by trimming the excess skin tissue over the wart and, also, by padding with soft orthotic devices. Topical medications that can kill the viral infection causing the wart formation are available. Occasionally, surgical excision or cauterization by a physician is required to remove particularly resistant warts.

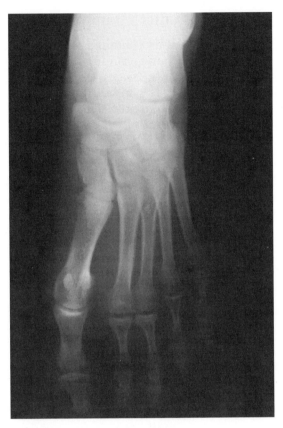

FIGURE 24.13. Freiberg's disease.

MECHANISMS AND TYPES OF INJURY

Foot injuries may result from direct trauma during competition or from minor stresses associated with repetitive training. Foot contusions, sprains, and fractures are caused frequently by external forces, such as an improper landing from a jump, striking an object on or near the playing surface, or the direct trauma of being stepped on. Overuse injuries of the foot caused by indirect trauma are more difficult to diagnose than acute traumatic injuries, but are equally disabling.

Soft Tissue Injuries

Blisters

Blisters are caused by friction resulting in the separation of skin layers. Fluid accumu-

lates between the layers. Blisters can be very painful and can become infected.

Avoiding or reducing the friction is the key to preventing blisters. Shoes should be properly fitted and broken in gradually. Multiple pairs of socks, petroleum jelly, Spenco Second Skin, and magnesium carbonate–based powders may also help prevent blisters. Applying thin adhesive felt (moleskin) over known blister sites prior to their development may also be effective.

If a blister forms, padding and protection may be needed during competition. Felt donuts can relieve pressure on small blisters. Larger blisters may require pads that cover a large area of the foot while avoiding the blister. After the pads have been taped in place, petroleum jelly may be applied to the outside of the taping, over the blister, for more protection from friction.

If a blister is large, it may be necessary to drain it. Unless it drains spontaneously, a physician should perform this task. The skin should not be removed for several days; it provides natural protection for the sensitive underskin. An antiseptic and/or antibiotic ointment may be applied to the area. A sterile dressing can be taped over the blister and checked frequently for signs of infection. Should infection occur, the athlete should be seen by a physician who can clean the area and prescribe antibiotics. Soaks in warm, soapy water may also be used for blister care.

Bursitis

A **bursa** is a flattened synovial sac that may be located over bony prominences throughout the body. It functions as a lubricating device to allow tissues to move freely over bony prominences. It is potentially a space that can fill with synovial fluid when irritated. External pressure from a poorly fitting shoe may cause inflammation, called **bursitis**, that is manifested by local pain, swelling, and erythema (abnormal redness of the skin). An example is the inflammation that can develop over an underlying bony abnormality and as a bunion due to pressure from the shoe against this abnormal bony structure. Shoe modification or corrective surgery may be necessary.

The retrocalcaneal bursa, located between the Achilles tendon insertion and the calcaneus and posterior aspect of the talus, is often irritated in athletes. Pain, the presenting symptom, is localized in the soft tissues just anterior to the Achilles tendon. This pain can be elicited on palpation and also on plantar flexion and push-off during gait, because this action compresses and irritates the retrocalcaneal bursa. Treatment consists of rest from the offending activity, use of a heel lift, anti-inflammatory medication, and occasionally, a short leg walking cast for complete rest. Stretching exercises of the gastrocnemius-soleus muscle group may increase flexibility and decrease the pressure that is exerted on the bursa during gait.

At times, bursitis may develop between the Achilles tendon and overlying skin. This swelling can be detected on palpation and can become quite thickened and erythematous. It is usually related to footwear and can be corrected by shoe modification.

Calluses

A **callosity**, or **callus**, is an area of thickened skin overlying a bony prominence. A callus on the foot usually indicates abnormal pressure between the shoe and the bony protrusion, such as is sometimes seen over the proximal IP joints and claw toes. In this condition, the MP joint is hyperextended, pushing the head of the metatarsal into the sole of the foot. Abnormal pressure can develop under the metatarsal head or at the flexed IP joint of the corresponding toe. Pain can often be relieved by placing a felt pad in the shoe just proximal to the metatarsal heads. The felt pad spreads the weight-bearing pressures across the metatarsal heads, relieving the stress point. Also, the pad lifts the metatarsal heads in relation to the proximal phalanges of the toes and partially corrects a claw toe deformity.

Neuritis

Neuritis, the inflammation or irritation of a nerve, can be a troublesome problem for athletes. **Morton's neuroma**, a common neuritis, is classically characterized by localized pain between the third and fourth metatarsal heads that often radiates into the third and fourth toes (Fig. 24.14). The medial and lateral plantar nerves converge between the third and fourth toes where the junction becomes enlarged. Tight shoes compress the metatarsal heads against the nerve, producing a painful neuroma. The plantar nerves and other interspaces of the foot may also be involved. The pain is increased by tight shoewear and is relieved by going barefoot. Once the pain starts, it is often difficult to control. Wider shoes with a low heel and a metatarsal pad may help. Surgical excision is often required.

The **tarsal tunnel syndrome** is another neuritis. The posterior tibial nerve passes through a soft tissue tunnel behind the medial malleolus to enter the foot (Fig. 24.15). The nerve may become inflamed from pronation or direct trauma, causing swelling and increased pressure in this area. The pain radiates along the course of the nerve. Some athletes may manifest numb-

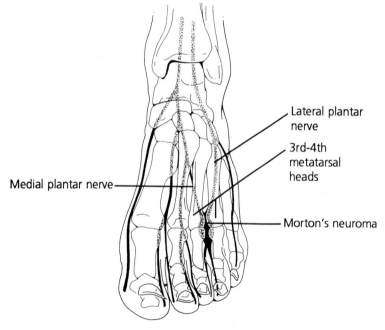

Lateral plantar nerve

3rd-4th metatarsal heads

Medial plantar nerve

Morton's neuroma

FIGURE 24.14. Morton's neuroma.

ness in the sensory distribution of the posterior tibial nerve. Treatment with rest, anti-inflammatory drugs, shoe correction, and occasional local cortisone injections is usually successful. Surgical release of the tarsal tunnel ligament may be required if symptoms persist despite conservative care.

Neuritis can develop along the course of other superficial sensory nerves of the foot, usually on the dorsum of the foot, because of pressure from footwear. Local cortisone injections and modification of shoes usually correct these problems.

Fasciitis

The plantar fascia is dense fibrous tissue that runs from the calcaneal tuberosity along the plantar surface of the foot and inserts on the plantar aspect of the metatarsal heads. This fascia can become irritated from overuse, particularly in running or jumping, and may be especially vulnerable in runners with cavus feet. The pain from **plantar fasciitis** is most severe at the calcaneal tuberosity, but may spread along the course of the fascia. Occasionally, in chronic cases, excessive ossification occurs at the insertion of the fascia on the calcaneal tuberosity. This manifests as a traction phenomenon of bone, or so-called **heel spur**. Treatment is usually conservative: rest until the athlete can walk or run without discomfort; therapy modalities, including alternating ice and heat to relieve acute symptoms; stretching exercises that relieve tension in the Achilles tendon and the plantar fascia; a heel-pad orthosis; and possibly a local injection of cortisone. Rarely, in refractory cases, surgical release of the fascia at its insertion may be indicated.

The heel pad may be injured from direct trauma, resulting in a **stone bruise**. The history of direct trauma can help differentiate the contused heel-pad injury from plantar fasciitis, a stress-related phenomenon. Rest usually resolves this problem.

Sprains

Sprains may occur in the foot without associated bony injuries. These sprains usually

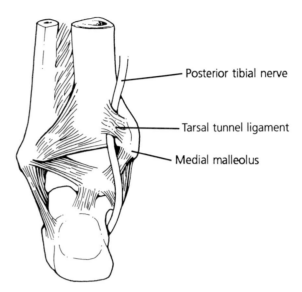

FIGURE 24.15. Posterior view of the foot showing tarsal tunnel syndrome.

involve the ligaments and/or capsule about the calcaneocuboid joint, the sinus tarsi, the midtarsal joints, and occasionally the transverse and longitudinal arches. The diagnosis is usually made by finding local tenderness and swelling in the presence of a normal x-ray film. Treatment consists of protected weight bearing and protective strapping until painful symptoms of the sprain resolve. Ice and heat modalities often help control pain. Strengthening exercises for the intrinsic musculature of the foot will help the athlete return to sports activities.

Sesamoiditis

Sesamoiditis is an inflammation of the sesamoid bones of the great toe and their encasing fibrous tissues. Symptoms include pain with weight-bearing activity that is localized beneath the great toe joint and tenderness on palpation in this area. Treatment is symptomatic with rest, anti-inflammatory medications, and a splint orthosis, which would limit the pressure and motion about the MP joint of the great toe. Once the athlete becomes asymptomatic, return to sports activities is possible.

Fractures and Dislocations

Stress Fractures

Stress fractures, also called **fatigue fractures**, can be disabling problems for athletes. Stress fractures of the lower extremity are related to overuse and are often seen in long-distance runners. Other running sports such as soccer and track can cause stress fractures in the foot. Although the neck of the second metatarsal is the most common location of stress fractures, they can occur in any other bone of the foot. A negative x-ray film does not rule out a stress fracture, because the osteolysis of the fracture or the new bone formation from healing may not be visible for a period of time after the fracture occurs. A bone scan may be needed for a definitive diagnosis. Stress fractures do not require a cast and usually respond to rest from the offending activity.

Stress fractures that occur in the tarsal navicular are disabling, difficult to treat, and require astute diagnostic skills. The athlete may present with vague foot pain that persists with any attempt at activities. Defects in the tarsal navicular are difficult to visualize on routine films, and a bone scan or possibly computed tomography (CT) may be necessary to make this diagnosis. Tarsal navicular fractures that are resistant to conservative management may require surgical treatment, including bone grafting. Recovery is slow, and the athlete's foot may have to be protected for months before the athlete is allowed to rehabilitate and return to sports.

Avulsion Fractures

A common avulsion fracture in athlete is that of the base of the fifth metatarsal. Inversion is often the mechanism of injury, creating the overpull of the peroneus brevis muscle, which fractures the bone at the tendinous insertion. Treatment may require a short leg walking cast initially to help relieve pain. The athlete then can progress to a protective brace in order to return to sports activities. Transverse fractures into the proximal shaft of the fifth metatar-sal are more troublesome and require diligent care. These **Jones fractures** occur at a stress site and manifest during an overload trauma. Healing is often delayed, causing prolonged disability. Occasionally, surgical bone grafting is required to achieve healing. These fractures are often missed when an ankle sprain occurs simultaneously and the concomitant fracture is not suspected.

Other Traumatic Fractures

Direct trauma may cause fractures of any of the bones in the foot. All the bones are vulnerable, and the site of the fracture depends on the amount of force and its direction. A fractured phalanx is usually a minor injury, although fracture of the first toe may be more serious. If the injured toe is in good alignment, it can simply be taped to the adjacent toe, taking care not to obstruct circulation. If the phalanx is displaced, the toe must be aligned under local anesthesia and then taped to the adjacent toe. Fractures of the metatarsal and midtarsal bones may require a short leg walking cast or hard-soled shoe. This rigid support effectively protects the foot. Fractures of the first and fifth metatarsals take longer to heal and may cause more disability.

Fractures of the sesamoids can occur from both direct trauma and stress activities. Pain, swelling, and localized tenderness are noted at the site of injury. X-rays are used to confirm the diagnosis. It should be noted that some sesamoid bones are congenitally bipartite and may appear as fractures on x-ray. These injuries usually respond to conservative treatment consisting of rest and splinting, and the athlete can return to sports activities when the symptoms subside.

The neck of the talus may be fractured by a forceful dorsiflexion injury. Prompt reduction is mandatory. Since the blood supply to the talus may be lost following the fracture, this injury requires prolonged protection and follow-up. Major fractures of the calcaneus are rare in athletics. However, avulsion fractures at the site of ligamentous and tendinous attachments do occur with

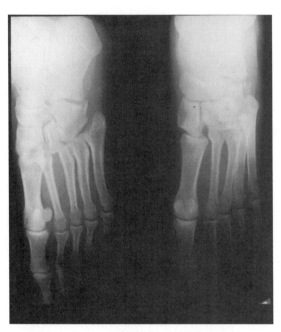

FIGURE 24.16. A Lisfranc fracture occurs at midfoot.

inversion injuries—for example, on the anterior process of the calcaneus at the calcaneocuboid joint. The Achilles tendon sometimes ruptures at its insertion in the calcaneus, avulsing a bone fragment with it, usually requiring surgical repair.

Lisfranc Fractures

A **Lisfranc fracture**, a rare but severe fracture-dislocation, can occur in the midfoot (Fig. 24.16). Originally described in equestrians as an eversion injury that occurs when a rider is dragged with his or her foot caught in the stirrup, a Lisfranc fracture can be chronically disabling if undiagnosed or mistreated. Trauma that causes midfoot eversion produces this injury. Pain and swelling in the area should be carefully evaluated by a physician using stress x-ray views if necessary to rule out this instability. Treatment may include surgery and an extended recovery period.

Other Dislocations

Dislocations in the foot are most common at the MP joints and the IP joints. Closed reduction and protection for 10 to 14 days are usually sufficient treatment. A more common injury to the MP joint of the great toe is the so-called **turf toe**. This is a hyperextension injury, with partial tearing of the joint capsule, usually corrected by rest and protective taping. A more severe dislocation is that of the subtalar joint. This dramatic injury may result from a fall from a height (as in basketball or volleyball) with the foot in inversion. This injury may be open and can seriously impair the blood supply to the foot. Prompt reduction is required to save the foot, usually under a general anesthetic. The usual precautions for open injuries must be followed. Dislocations of the IP joints of the toe also occur and may be difficult to reduce if the joint capsule is buttonholed by a phalanx.

FIRST AID

Most acute injuries to the foot require no more than crutches, ice, and a compression dressing until a physician can perform a follow-up evaluation. Although foot injuries do not usually constitute an emergency, an open dislocation or a significantly displaced fracture-dislocation of the hindfoot is a real emergency. Because the blood supply to the foot may be impaired, these injuries must be treated in a hospital as soon as possible. A sterile dressing should be placed over any open wounds. Splints should be applied prior to transport to decrease the athlete's risk of further vascular compromise.

REHABILITATION

The rehabilitation of foot injuries must be individualized. In some instances, weight bearing must be avoided, yet early range-of-motion exercises may be beneficial—for example, in the case of midfoot injuries. On the other hand, exercise to strengthen the toes may be possible while a hindfoot injury is immobilized in a walking cast. When it is not detrimental to the healing process, early motion should be initiated to avoid joint stiffness and muscle atrophy.

After cast immobilization is discontinued, protected weight bearing is desirable. Swimming is a good early exercise, followed by biking, walking, jogging, and then the activity of the athlete's sport. Protective taping may be required for a period following injury. The goal is to regain complete ankle, subtalar, midtarsal, and toe motion with normal muscle strength before returning to competition.

IMPORTANT CONCEPTS

1. The 26 bones of the foot are the talus, calcaneus, navicular, cuboid, 3 cuneiforms, 5 metatarsals, and 14 phalanges (3 for each of the four toes and 2 for the great toe).
2. The two arches of the foot are the longitudinal arch and the transverse arch.
3. The three main muscles of the lower leg all insert on the foot and thus control the action of the foot.
4. Normal gait is divided into a stance, or support phase (foot is on the ground), and a swing phase (foot is airborne).
5. Among the major deformities of the foot are cavus foot, flat foot, metatarsus varus and valgus, Morton's foot, hallux valgus, claw toes, hammertoes, bunionette, avascular necrosis, and plantar warts.
6. Soft tissue injuries to the foot include blisters, bursitis, calluses, neuritis, fasciitis, sprains, and sesamoiditis.
7. Common stress fracture sites in the foot are the second and fifth metatarsals, tarsal navicular, and calcaneus.
8. Dislocations of the foot are most common at the MP joints and the IP joints.
9. Most foot injuries are not emergencies, with the exception of open dislocations and fracture-dislocations of the hindfoot.
10. The goal of rehabilitation of foot injuries is to regain complete ankle, subtalar, midtarsal, and toe motion with normal muscle strength.

SUGGESTED READINGS

Bordelon, R. L. "Management of Disorders of the Forefoot and Toenails Associated with Running." *Clinics in Sports Medicine* 4 (1985): 717–724.

Frederick, E. C., ed. *Sport Shoes and Playing Surfaces.* Champaign, Ill.: Human Kinetics, 1984.

Hunter, S. C., W. L. Capiello, G. P. Hess, and D. Joyce. "Foot Problems." In *The Team Physician's Handbook*, edited by M. B. Mellion, W. M. Walsh, and G. L. Shelton, pp. 452–463. Philadelphia: Hanley and Belfus, Inc., 1990.

Lillich, J. S., and D. E. Baxter. "Common Forefoot Problems in Runners." *Foot and Ankle* 7 (1986): 145–151.

Marti, R. "Dislocation of the Peroneal Tendons." *American Journal of Sports Medicine* 5 (1977): 19–22.

Sammarco, G. James. "Soft Tissue Conditions in Athletes' Feet." *Clinics in Sports Medicine* 1 (1982): 149–155.

25

The Skin

OBJECTIVES FOR CHAPTER 25

After reading this chapter, the student should be able to:
1. Describe the major functions of skin.
2. Describe the anatomy of skin.
3. List and describe closed soft tissue injuries and their management.
4. List and describe open soft tissue injuries and their management.
5. Explain the etiology, presentation, and treatment of common, nontraumatic dermatological conditions.

INTRODUCTION

The skin, the largest organ in the body, is essential to normal somatic functioning. The skin is also the location of many athletic injuries. The athletic trainer should understand the anatomy of the skin, its role in maintaining bodily processes, and the evaluation and treatment of common soft tissue injuries and dermatological conditions.

Chapter 25 begins with the physiology and anatomy of the skin. The chapter then describes types of closed and open soft tissue injuries and their management. The last section of Chapter 25 discusses several dermatological conditions, including acne, infections, allergies, and infestations. ■

PHYSIOLOGY AND ANATOMY OF THE SKIN

Functions of the Skin

The skin, the largest organ in the body, serves three major functions: (1) to protect the body from the outside environment, (2) to regulate the temperature of the body, and (3) to transmit information from the outside environment to the brain.

The protective functions of the skin are numerous. The skin serves to keep the balanced internal chemical solution of the body intact. The skin also protects the body from the invasion of infectious organisms, such as bacteria, viruses, and fungi. Germs cannot pass through the skin unless it has been broken by injury. Thus, the skin provides a constant protection against outside invaders.

Chemical reactions (metabolism) in the body must occur within a very narrow temperature range. If the body temperature is too low, these reactions cease. Conversely, if the temperature is too high, the rate of metabolism is high. Either a high or low metabolic rate can result in permanent tissue damage and death.

The major organ for regulation of body temperature is the skin. Blood vessels in the skin constrict when the body is in a cold environment and dilate when the body is in a warm environment. In a cold environment, constriction of the blood vessels shunts the blood away from the skin to decrease the amount of heat radiated from the body surface. When the outside environment is hot, the vessels in the skin dilate, the skin becomes flushed or red, and heat radiates from the body surface. Also, in a hot environment, sweat is secreted to the body surface from the sweat glands. Evaporation of the sweat requires energy. This energy, in the form of body heat, exits the body during the evaporation process, which causes the body temperature to fall. Sweating alone will not reduce body temperature; evaporation of the sweat must also occur.

Information from the environment is carried to the brain through a rich supply of sensory nerves that originate in the skin. Nerve endings that lie in the skin are adapted to perceive and transmit information about heat, cold, external pressure, pain, pleasurable stimuli, and the position of the body in space. The skin thus recognizes any changes in the environment.

Layers of the Skin

Anatomically, the skin is divided into two layers: the superficial **epidermis**, which is composed of several layers of cells, and the deeper **dermis**, which contains the specialized skin structures. Below the skin lies the subcutaneous layer of fat (Fig. 25.1a, color insert). The cells of the epidermis are sealed to form a watertight protective covering for the body (Fig. 25.1b, color insert).

Epidermis

The epidermis is actually composed of several layers of cells. At the base of the epidermis is the **germinal layer**, which continuously produces new cells that gradually rise to the surface. On the way to the surface, these cells die and form a watertight covering. The epidermal cells are held together securely by an oily substance called **sebum**, which is secreted by the sebaceous glands of the dermis. The outermost cells of the epidermis are constantly rubbed away and replaced by new cells produced by the germinal layer. The deeper cells in the germinal layer also contain pigment granules that, along with the blood vessels lying in the dermis, produce skin color.

Dermis

The deeper part of the skin, or the dermis, is separated from the epidermis by the layer of germinal cells. Within the dermis lie many of the special structures of the skin: sweat glands, sebaceous (oil) glands, hair follicles, blood vessels, and specialized nerve endings.

Sweat glands produce sweat for cooling the body. The sweat is discharged onto the surface of the skin through small pores or ducts that pass through the epidermis onto the skin surface. The **sebaceous glands** produce sebum, the oily material that seals the surface epidermal cells. The sebaceous glands lie next to hair follicles and secrete sebum along the hair follicle to the skin surface. In addition to providing waterproofing for the skin, sebum keeps the skin supple so that it does not crack.

Hair follicles are the small organs that produce hair. There is one follicle for each hair, connected with a sebaceous gland and also with a tiny muscle. The muscle serves to pull the hair into an erect position when the individual is cold or frightened. All hair grows continuously and is either cut off or worn away by clothing.

Blood vessels provide nutrients and oxygen to the skin. The blood vessels lie in the dermis. Small branches extend up to the germinal layer (there are no blood vessels in the epidermis). A complex array of nerve endings also lie in the dermis. These specialized nerve endings are sensitive to environmental stimuli and send impulses along the nerves to the brain.

Beneath the skin, immediately under the dermis and attached to it, lies the **subcutaneous tissue**, which is largely composed of fat. The fat serves as an insulator for the body and as a reservoir for the storage of energy. The amount of subcutaneous tissue varies greatly from individual to individual. Beneath the subcutaneous tissue lie the muscles and the skeleton.

The skin covers all the external surface of the body. The various openings to the body (mouth, nose, anus, and vagina) are not covered by skin. Called **orifices**, these openings are lined with **mucous membranes**. Mucous membranes are quite similar to skin in that they provide a protective barrier against bacterial invasion. Mucous membranes differ from skin in that they secrete **mucus**, a watery substance that lubricates the openings. Thus mucous membranes are moist, whereas the skin is dry. A mucous membrane lines the entire gastrointestinal tract from the mouth to the anus.

SOFT TISSUE INJURIES

Because the soft tissues are the first line of defense against most injuries, they are often damaged. Soft tissue injuries or wounds are divided into two types: closed and open. A **closed wound** is one in which soft tissue damage occurs beneath the skin, but the surface remains intact. An **open wound** is one in which a break occurs in the surface of the skin.

Closed Soft Tissue Injuries

Closed soft tissue injuries are characterized by a history of injury, pain at the site of injury, swelling and bleeding beneath the skin, and discoloration of the skin. Closed soft tissue injuries may be mild or quite extensive.

Contusions

A blunt object that strikes the body will crush the tissue beneath the skin. This injury is called a **contusion**, or more commonly, a bruise. The epidermis remains intact. Damage beneath the epidermis will extend to varying depths, depending on the force of injury. In the dermis, cells are damaged, and small blood vessels are usually torn. Varying amounts of tissue fluid and blood leak into the damaged area. As blood accumulates in the damaged area, a characteristic discoloration occurs. Usually the discoloration is black or blue and is called an **ecchymosis**.

Hematomas

When large amounts of tissue are damaged beneath the outer layer of the skin, large blood vessels may tear and cause rapid bleeding. The pool of blood that results, called a **hematoma**, will collect within the damaged tissue. Hematomas are not limited to soft tissue injuries; they can also occur following fractures or when blood vessels to any organ in the body are damaged. When a large bone such as the femur or pelvis fractures, the hematoma that forms may contain more than a liter of blood.

Blisters

A **blister** usually forms when heat generated by the skin's rubbing against a hard or rough surface causes the epidermis to separate from the dermis. Fluid then accumulates in the dermal layer. Treatment consists of a sterile bandage and occasional lancing by a physician if the blister is large.

Management of Closed Soft Tissue Injuries

Small bruises require no special medical care. With more extensive closed injuries, swelling and bleeding beneath the skin can be considerable. Bleeding and swelling in the deep soft tissues can be controlled to some degree by applying ice and local com-

pression immediately following the injury. Ice or cold packs will cause the blood vessels to constrict, which will slow the bleeding. Firm manual compression over the area of injury will compress the blood vessels and also decrease bleeding. Immobilizing the soft tissue injury with a splint is another way to decrease bleeding. Elevating the injured part to a level just above the level of the athlete's heart decreases the amount of swelling in the region. Therefore, when treating an athlete with a closed soft tissue injury, the athletic trainer can think of **ICES** (ice, compression, elevation, and splinting) to remember the four steps in treatment.

Open Soft Tissue Injuries

Open soft tissue injuries differ from closed wounds in that the protective skin layer is damaged. More importantly, once the protective skin layer has been violated, the wound becomes contaminated and may become infected.

Types of Open Soft Tissue Wounds

There are four types of open soft tissue wounds: abrasions, lacerations, avulsions, and puncture wounds (Fig. 25.2).

An **abrasion** is the loss of a portion of the epidermis and part of the dermis as a result of the skin being rubbed or scraped across a rough or hard surface. Abrasions usually do not penetrate completely through the dermis. Extremely painful, abrasions are known by a variety of common names: road burn, strawberry, mat burn, etc.

A **laceration** is a cut produced by a sharp object. The cutting object may leave a smooth or jagged wound through the skin and may penetrate into the subcutaneous tissue, the underlying muscles, and associated nerves and blood vessels.

An **avulsion** is an injury in which a piece of skin is either torn completely loose from all of its attachments or is left hanging as a flap. Avulsed tissues ordinarily separate at

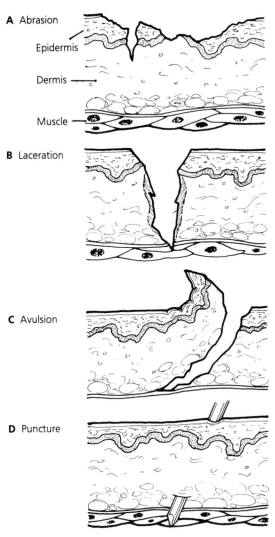

A Abrasion

Epidermis

Dermis

Muscle

B Laceration

C Avulsion

D Puncture

FIGURE 25.2. The four general types of open soft tissue injuries: (a) abrasions involve variable depths of the dermis and epidermis; (b) lacerations are cuts produced by sharp objects; (c) avulsions raise flaps of tissue, usually along normal tissue planes; (d) puncture wounds may penetrate to any depth.

normal anatomical planes, usually between the subcutaneous tissue and the muscle fascia.

A **puncture wound** results from an invasion of the skin by a pointed object. Because the entrance wound is usually relatively small, the bleeding is minimal. But the wounding object may damage deeper structures, such as in the region of the abdomen and chest, causing serious injury.

Management of Open Soft Tissue Injuries

Three general rules govern the management of open soft tissue injuries: (1) control bleeding, (2) prevent further contamination, and (3) immobilize the part. The first priority in the management of an open wound is to control the bleeding by applying a dry sterile compression dressing to the entire wound. Initially, pressure is applied by hand, followed by continual pressure from a firmly applied roller bandage. The sterile bandage will also prevent further contamination of the open wound. If the open wound is large or deep, splinting may minimize further damage and facilitate movement of the athlete.

OTHER DERMATOLOGICAL CONDITIONS

Common dermatological problems are related to the athlete's skin type as well as to environmental influences such as heat, humidity, athletic gear, and sporting activity. Therapeutic problems include acne vulgaris, fungal infections, viral infections, bacterial infections, contact allergy and irritant dermatitis, and infestations.

Acne Vulgaris

Acne vulgaris is most commonly a hereditary disorder of the oil glands and hair follicles that is influenced by the bacterial flora in these structures (Figs. 25.3 and 25.4, color insert). Clinically, the disease presents as multiple blackheads, inflammatory papules, pustules, or cysts. Acne lesions appear on the face, chest, shoulders, back, arms, and, in severe cases, the lower extremities. Seborrheic dermatitis (dandruff) is frequently associated with acne vulgaris and can be seen on the face as well as the scalp. Acne flares during athletic seasonal activities, probably due to increased heat, perspiration, and, ultimately, oil production.

The treatment of acne consists of topical drying agents and topical antimicrobial agents as well as oral antibiotics. The common topical drying and antimicrobial agent is benzoyl peroxide, which comes in 5 to 10 percent dilution. This agent reduces the number of bacteria responsible for the acneiform lesions. Reducing bacteria is helpful since the bacteria produce an enzyme that breaks down into a highly irritating free fatty acid that inflames the skin.

Benzoyl peroxide increases tissue oxygenation as well as healing. Drying or oil-removing agents such as astringent lotions and soap and water can aid healing. Mechanical and surgical removal of blackheads, while useful, must be done by a dermatologist or a trained nurse. Topical abrasive pads can be used for blackhead acne, but with the more inflammatory acnes they can worsen the condition.

Antibiotic therapy, both topical and oral, is highly effective in treating all forms of acne. The basic antibiotic used is tetracycline, in doses between 250 and 1,000 mg daily for control of bacteria, oil production, and inflammation. The worse the acne, the higher the dose of tetracycline. The newer topical tetracycline and erythromycin lotions seem effective when applied once or twice a day to areas of skin involvement and appear to equal approximately 500 mg of oral tetracycline. Topical antibiotics can be used when oral antibiotics are contraindicated, such as in a preadolescent athlete or a pregnant woman. In the growing fetus and the preadolescent, oral tetracycline may cause pigmentation of the permanent teeth. For this reason, oral tetracyclines are avoided in these age groups.

Another therapeutic modality for blackhead acne is topical vitamin A acid, which can be obtained in various concentrations and in cream, lotion, gel, or alcohol forms. Applying this treatment daily for at least 6 weeks reduces keratinization of the hair follicle, thereby reducing the formation of blackheads.

Low-dose systemic corticosteroids, estrogens, and tranquilizers, as prescribed by a physician, are adjunctive therapies used in severe resistant acne and cystic acne.

Fungal Infections

Ringworm

Ringworm infections are caused by a variety of different fungi—essentially, microscopic plants that grow on humans. On examination, this skin disease may resemble a well-defined, slightly reddened patch with some fine scaling at its periphery. Occasionally, if the athlete is allergic to the fungus, blisters may be observed. When the fungal infection involves the feet, the sole of the foot may look like dry skin or may again have some redness, swelling, and even blisters. Microscopic examination of the scale or the blister top reveals vegetating parts of the fungus. Bacterial and fungal cultures and Wood's light examination are diagnostic.

Ringworm infections are treated with antifungal agents such as tolnaftate (Tinactin cream or solution), miconazole nitrate (Micatin 2 percent), or clotrimazole (Lotrimin cream 2 percent, Lotrimin cream or solution, and Mycelex cream). Antifungal therapies are applied twice a day for at least 2 to 4 weeks. In addition, the areas must be kept dry and clean. If large areas of the skin are affected or if the fungus infection is blistered, oral antifungal agents are often used to reduce the infection. Treatment consists of griseofulvin (Fulvicin), 500 mg to 1 gm a day for at least 1 month. Inflammatory conditions of the groin may be due to fungus, bacterial infection, contact allergy, or irritant reactions. Since all of these conditions may resemble each other, if a condition fails to respond to the antifungal treatment, dermatologic consult is indicated.

Tinea Versicolor

Tinea versicolor is a ringworm infection of the skin caused by *Pityrosporon orbiculare*, a yeast fungus (Fig. 25.5, color insert). This yeast infection is found in the keratin of the horny layer of the skin as well as in the horny layers of the hair follicle. It may appear as a salmon-pink, finely scaling patch that fails to pigment when exposed to the sun; it leaves a white patch. This cutaneous fungus infection is noncontagious but highly visible because of its brown or white patches, usually on the trunk. Tinea versicolor is treated with antidandruff shampoo at least once a week for 2 weeks; treatment should be repeated as necessary.

Viral Infections

Herpes

The most common viral infection is a **herpes infection**, or cold sore. These infections can occur in the mouth or on the lips, face, trunk, or genital area. The disorder is highly contagious. It presents as a blister on a reddened base and is associated with pain locally. Frequently, groups of blisters on a reddened base ulcerate and become infected with bacterial organisms. Herpes simplex can be diagnosed on inspection, but microscopic examination of the blister base confirms the diagnosis.

The disorder is treated by destruction of the blisters by mechanical excoriation or the use of topical drying agents, including some of the acne medications such as the benzoyl peroxide agents. Anti-inflammatory agents with hydrocortisone may be used and appear to reduce the skin inflammation and increase comfort. The usual duration of the herpes infection is 2 weeks. Treatment is directed at reducing the skin pain and discomfort and decreasing the healing time. Acyclovir is an effective antiviral therapy. During active blistering and ulceration, this condition is highly contagious and should be considered a disqualifying contagious disorder in contact sports.

Molluscum Contagiosum

Molluscum contagiosum is another viral disorder characterized by flesh-colored pink papules with a central dimpling (Fig. 25.6, color insert). The skin surrounding these papules is not inflamed. Papules may occur anywhere on the body but especially on the trunk, axilla, face, perineum, and thigh, appearing singly or in multiple groups. This disorder is also contagious and is frequently passed from one athlete to another in frictional contact sports such as wrestling. Careful examination of the skin lesions by an experienced physician confirms the diagnosis. A physician should treat this disorder using destructive agents such as cryotherapy, electrodesiccation, and a variety of topically applied acids, such as trichloroacetic acid.

Warts

Warts, also a viral infection of the skin, are caused by a papillomavirus found within the skin of the body as well as the mucous membranes (Fig. 25.7, color insert). Normal incubation time for a wart virus from contact to the formation of a lesion is approximately 6 months. The lesions are discrete, raised, flesh-colored to pink papules with a rough surface. On the feet they tend to grow inward, causing pain similar to a corn on walking.

The treatment of warts, especially on pressure points during the athletic season, should be only palliative, with paring of the keratotic lesion for comfort. The use of 40 percent salicylic acid plasters applied daily reduces the raised keratotic lesion. If the lesion does not disappear, it can be treated later with 40 percent salicylic acid pads and a locally destructive procedure such as cryotherapy and electrodesiccation. Surgical excision and superficial x-ray are contraindicated as treatment. Warts on pressure points and on areas of movement should not be treated during the athletic season, since treatment produces inflammation and a wound that heals slowly.

Bacterial Infections

Impetigo

Impetigo is one of the most common contagious disorders in the athlete. It is caused by two organisms: streptococcus and staphylococcus. In the younger child or adolescent, impetigo frequently presents as a blister, but in older individuals the characteristic appearance is a superficial ulcer with a yellow crust, similar to that in older herpes lesions. Visual inspection and bacterial culture can identify this disorder.

Treatment consists of local cleansing with soap and water, or astringents or alcohol solutions. Topical antimicrobial agents can be used, but oral antibiotics are preferred. The preferred antibiotic is erythromycin, 250 mg four times a day for 2 weeks.

Staphylococcal folliculitis, a form of impetigo, is a common infection in bearded men, especially black men. The curly facial or scalp hair reenters the skin, causing a small, inflammatory lesion that becomes a pustule. This condition can be treated with astringent lotions or drying agents such as those used in acne vulgaris. Broadspectrum antibiotics given for 7 to 10 days are helpful in controlling the folliculitis. Using an abrasive facial pad may prevent reentry of the facial or scalp hair.

Other Bacterial Skin Infections

A **furuncle**, caused predominantly by a staphylococcal organism, is a tender inflammation around the hair follicle that becomes a fluctuant mass. It is treated by topical application of warm to hot packs and topical benzoyl peroxide in 10 percent dilution. Other therapy includes oral penicillin antibiotics for 7 to 14 days. Incision and drainage are usually not necessary if treatment is initiated early. An athlete with an active abscess or furuncle should be disqualified from participation until the lesion has cleared, because the condition is highly contagious.

Other superficial bacterial infections or fungal infections may develop in skin abrasions, such as seen in mat burns, Astroturf burns, and cinder burns. Treatment is routine first aid, cleansing with soap and water, topical drying agents, or topical antibiotic ointments. Systemic antibiotic medication is rarely indicated.

Contact Allergy and Irritant Dermatitis

Substances to which an athlete is allergic or those that irritate the skin can cause inflammatory skin disorders. **Contact irritant dermatitis** is a nonallergic reaction of the skin after exposure to irritating or caustic substances or to a physical agent that damages the skin, producing pain and ulceration (Fig. 25.8, color insert). **Contact allergy** is an allergic response of the skin that produces inflammation in those who have an allergy to an external agent.

In athletes, irritant skin reactions are usually secondary to physical and mechanical agents such as:

- Dry Ice burns.
- Abrasions from Astroturf.
- Poorly fitting gear, including football helmets.
- Callus formation in gymnasts and bicyclists.
- Striae (skin stretch marks) in weight lifters.
- Increased sweating in hockey players.
- Loss of skin secondary to the application of caustic agents, such as adhesive tape, and direct contact injuries.

The contact allergy skin reactions appear to be due to given contactants—for example, the following:

- Rhus (poison ivy, oak, and sumac).
- Paraphenylenediamine (blue and black dyes).
- Nickel compounds (jewelry, metal protective gear).
- Rubber compounds and chromates (tanned leather and metal parts).

The use of topical medications in the treatment of skin disorders is limited because of their increased allergy-inducing capabilities. These topical medications include benzocaine, topical antihistamine preparations, ammoniated mercury, neomycin, penicillin, and sulfonamides. In the athlete, tincture of benzoin and araminobenzoic acid are potent skin sensitizers. Allergic skin dermatitis may present as an acute, blistering rash on a red, swollen base or as chronically dry, thickened skin. Itching or pain is common to all contact skin rashes, whether due to irritant or allergic agents.

Contact dermatitis of both allergic and irritant origin is best dealt with by avoiding the contactant responsible for the skin reaction. In addition, it is helpful to recognize early potential contact irritants or allergy.

Acute skin reactions are treated with cool compresses or soaks and topical corticosteroid preparations in forms that promote drying, such as aerosol sprays, gels, lotions, solutions, or creams. Systemic antihistamines reduce itching but have an undesirable sedative effect. Aspirin is effective in reducing itching and pain and may be given in doses of 300 to 600 mg every 4 hours while the athlete is symptomatic. A short course of corticosteroids, prednisone, 30 mg a day for 7 to 14 days, with rapid reduction, is helpful but should be prescribed by a physician. Disqualification of the athlete from total participation depends on the degree of skin involvement, the site of involvement, the severity of the symptoms, and the specific sport.

The chronic form of contact dermatitis can also be managed by avoiding the contactant or establishing a barrier. For example, contact dermatitis secondary to rubber materials in footgear can be treated by applying topical corticosteroid cream to the foot and then powdering it with talcum powder and wearing a heavy white sock. The sock has to be changed frequently during the day, because a damp sock allows the rubber material to leach from the shoe onto the foot.

Topical corticosteroids are helpful in treating chronic contact dermatitis. Corticosteroids should be in cream or ointment form so that the cortisone reduces the inflammation and the cream or ointment lubricates the skin. Secondary bacterial infections should be treated with antibiotics and skin-cleansing techniques.

Infestations

The most common infestations observed in athletes are crab lice and scabies.

Pediculosis Pubis (Crab Louse)

Pediculosis pubis (crab louse), more commonly referred to as "crabs," is contracted through intimate contact with affected individuals. For athletes, direct contact in the sporting event as well as in the dressing rooms through showers, towels, and clothing may allow passage from one individual to another. Crab louse is observed in the areas of the genitals, the trunk, and occasionally, the underarms and eyelashes. The lice cause extreme itching of the involved sites and, on occasion, red spots. Diagnosis is made by visually identifying the louse or its eggs. The eggs, attached to the hair shafts, appear as clear, translucent, small masses.

Treatment consists of gamma benzene hexachloride (Kwell) lotion or shampoo applied after bathing to the affected areas for 6 to 24 hours. This treatment is repeated in 1 week if viable lice are still identified. Occasionally, the hairy areas must be shaved or combed to remove the eggs. A fine-toothed comb is used, but first it is rinsed with white vinegar in a dilution of 1:4. The clothing of an affected individual should be washed, disinfected, and set aside for 7 days. All suspected contacts should be examined and treated. On occasion, every athlete on the team may have to be examined for lice.

Scabies

Scabies is caused by a mite, *Sarcoptes scabiei*. This mite infestation is characterized by itching and elevated burrows on the skin surface. In most people, mites are observed on the hands, but in the athlete the scabies are equally common on the trunk and genital area. The female mite makes these burrows in which she lays her eggs. Long-standing infestation may present as an acute dermatitis with severe itching. Diagnosis is made by scraping the burrow, examining the scraping under a microscope, and then visualizing the mite.

The treatment of choice is the application of gamma benzene hexachloride lotion or shampoo to the whole body for 6 to 24 hours. The treatment is repeated if viable mites are seen at a later time. Clothing and bed linen have to be changed, washed, and put aside for 14 days. Team members and other contacts are treated prophylactically. Gamma benzene hexachloride is a known neurotoxin and should not be misused or overused.

Table 25.1 summarizes allergy and contact dermatitis conditions discussed in this chapter and their treatments.

TABLE 25.1. Treatment Summaries for Dermatological Conditions

Condition	Treatments
Acne vulgaris	Astringent lotion, liquid cleansing agents; benzoyl peroxide 5% or 10% once or twice a day; topical vitamin A acid daily (at night); tetracycline, 500 mg a day for 6 weeks gradually reduced to maintenance dose of 250 mg a day; topical antibiotics twice a day
Ringworm	Soap and water cleansing twice a day; topical antifungal agents twice a day for 1 month (Tinactin powder, solution, cream, Micatin cream, Lotrimin cream, solution, Mycelex cream); griseofulvin, oral fungistatic and fungicidal antibiotic, 1 gm daily for 3 to 4 weeks
Tinea versicolor	Soap and water cleansing; application of antidandruff shampoo, repeat weekly as necessary, or Tinver solution applied daily for 3 to 4 weeks, or other antifungal agents (Lotrimin, Micatin, Mycelex cream or solution) twice a day for 1 month
Herpes	Soap and water cleansing; topical drying agents three times a day (benzoyl peroxide 5% or 10%, tincture of benzoin, Camphophenique, Blistex); oral salicylates, aspirin, every 3 to 4 hours for pain; acyclocir
Warts and molluscum contagiosum	Salicyclic acid plaster 40% applied daily for 4 months; topical caustic agents (25% podophyllin in compound tincture of benzoin, applied weekly, Duofilm applied daily for 2 to 4 months); physician therapy (cryotherapy, electro-dessication or topical compounded acids)
Impetigo	Cleansing of skin; topical antibiotics; oral erythromycin 250 mg four times a day for 14 days
Contact dermatitis	Avoidance of cause; acute: wet dressings two or three times a day, topical corticosteroids, lotions, gel or cream; chronic: topical corticosteroid cream or ointment, aspirin 300–600 mg every 4 hours for itching
Infestations	Wash skin and clothing (set aside clothing for 7 to 14 days); gamma benzene hexachloride (Kwell) lotion or cream for 6- to 24-hour application, repeat as necessary; other therapies with lesser cure rates: Eurax cream twice a day for 48 hours, 6% precipitated sulfur in Vaseline, twice a day for 3 days

IMPORTANT CONCEPTS

1. The functions of the skin are to protect the body from the outside environment, to regulate the temperature of the body, and to transmit information from the outside environment to the brain.

2. The skin is divided into the epidermis, whose cells form a covering for the body, and the dermis, which contains the special structures of the skin.

3. A closed soft tissue injury is one in which soft tissue damage occurs beneath the epidermis, which remains intact; an open wound is one in which a break occurs in the skin surface.

4. The four types of open soft tissue injuries are abrasions, lacerations, avulsions, and puncture wounds.

5. Acne vulgaris is a hereditary disorder of the oil glands and hair follicles that presents as multiple blackheads, inflammatory papules, pustules, or cysts.

6. Ringworm and tinea versicolor are fungal infections.

7. Herpes, molluscum contagiosum, and warts are viral infections.

8. Impetigo, staphylococcal folliculitis, and furuncles are bacterial infections.

9. Contact irritant dermatitis is a nonallergic reaction of the skin to exposure to irritating or caustic substance, and contact allergy is an allergic response of the skin that produces inflammation in those who have an allergy to an external agent.

10. Crab lice and scabies are the most common infestations observed in athletes.

SUGGESTED READINGS

Eaglstein, W. H., and D. M. Pariser. *Office Techniques for Diagnosing Skin Disease.* Chicago: Year Book Medical Publishers, 1978.

Maddin, S. ed. *Current Dermatologic Therapy.* Philadelphia: W. B. Saunders, 1982.

Moschella, S. L., and H. J. Hurley, eds. *Dermatology,* 2d ed. Philadelphia: W. B. Saunders, 1985.

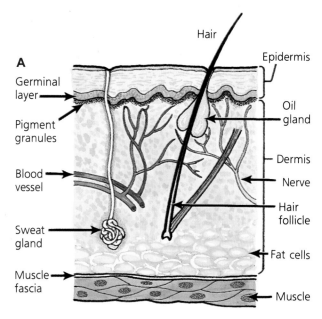

A

Germinal layer

Pigment granules

Blood vessel

Sweat gland

Muscle fascia

Hair

Epidermis

Oil gland

Dermis

Nerve

Hair follicle

Fat cells

Muscle

B

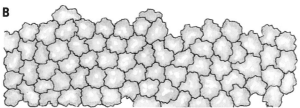

FIGURE 25.1. (a) The skin has two layers: the epidermis and the dermis. All of the major structures lie in the dermis. A layer of subcutaneous fat lies below the dermis. (b) Cells of the epidermis are fitted closely together on the skin surface to form a watertight protective layer.

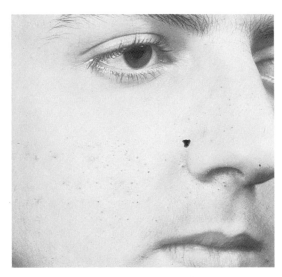

FIGURE 25.3. Acne vulgaris on the cheek and nose, presenting as multiple blackheads and papules.(Courtesy of Dr. Wilma F. Bergfeld, Department of Dermatology and Pathology, Cleveland Clinic Foundation.)

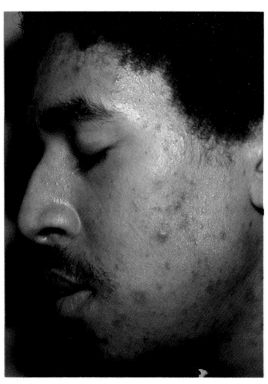

FIGURE 25.4. Severe acne vulgaris of the face and neck with multiple blackheads, inflammatory papules, pustules, and cysts. (Courtesy of Dr. Wilma F. Bergfeld, Department of Dermatology and Pathology, Cleveland Clinic Foundation.)

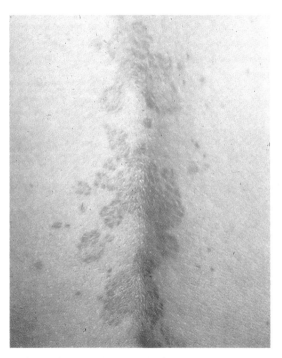

FIGURE 25.5. Tinea versicolor, appearing as salmon-pink, finely scaling patches on the athlete's back. (Courtesy of Dr. Wilma F. Bergfeld, Department of Dermatology and Pathology, Cleveland Clinic Foundation.)

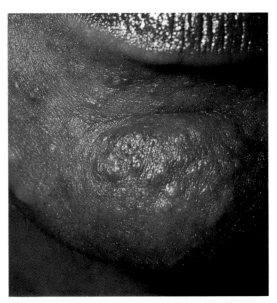

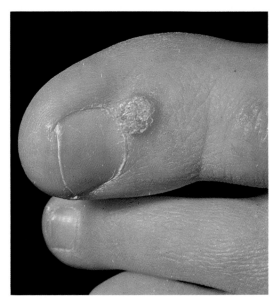

FIGURE 25.6. Molluscum contagiosum on the patient's chin shows the central dimpling of the flesh-colored papules characteristic of this disorder. (Courtesy of Dr. Wilma F. Bergfeld, Department of Dermatology and Pathology, Cleveland Clinic Foundation.)

FIGURE 25.7. Warts, such as the wart seen on the anteromedial aspect of this great toe, tend to grow inward when they occur on the foot. (Courtesy of Dr. Wilma F. Bergfeld, Department of Dermatology and Pathology, Cleveland Clinic Foundation.)

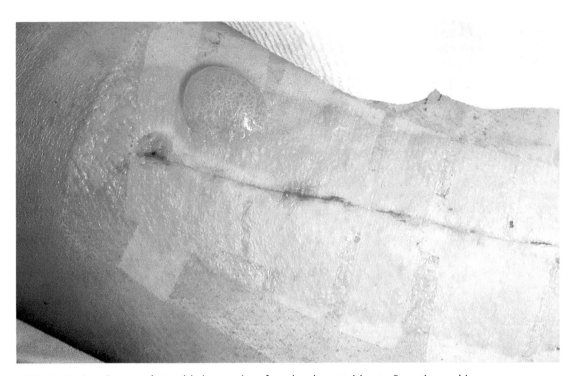

FIGURE 25.8. Contact dermatitis in a patient found to be sensitive to Benzoin used in combination with Steri-strips for skin closure. (Courtesy of Dr. Wilma F. Bergfeld, Department of Dermatology and Pathology, Cleveland Clinic Foundation.)

PART

B

THE CARDIORESPIRATORY
SYSTEM

26

The Cardiovascular System

OBJECTIVES FOR CHAPTER 26

After reading this chapter, the student should be able to:
1. Understand how blood circulates throughout the body.
2. Explain the cardiac cycle and the sequence of electrical and mechanical events.
3. Understand the determinants of cardiac output and the oxygen demands of the heart.
4. Understand how vessel size, viscosity, and the autonomic nervous system affect blood circulation.
5. Explain the effects of exercise on the heart.

INTRODUCTION

Chapter 26 explains the anatomy and function of the cardiovascular system. It begins by explaining how blood circulates in the body and how the cardiac cycle is a sequence of electrical and mechanical events. It discusses how cardiac output is the measure of the heart's performance and is calculated by multiplying the heart rate times the stroke volume. The chapter also explains how heart rate and stroke volume, along with adequate coronary blood flow, are the major determinants of the heart's oxygen needs. Discussed next are factors that influence the circulation of blood, including vessel size, viscosity, and the autonomic nervous system. Finally, Chapter 26 describes exercise and the heart—how cardiac output is increased and distributed during exercise, which exercises are best, the dual role of exercise, and how to achieve cardiovascular fitness through exercise. ■

CIRCULATION OF THE BLOOD

The cardiovascular, or circulatory, system is a complex arrangement of connected tubes that include arteries, arterioles, capillaries, venules, and veins. At the center of the system is the heart.

Blood circulates throughout the body under pressure generated by the heart, a hollow, muscular organ. The heart, or **myocardium**, is divided down the middle by a wall called the **septum**. Each side is divided again into an upper chamber called the **atrium** and a lower chamber called the **ventricle**. Thus the four sections of the heart are referred to as the left atrium, the left ventricle, the right atrium, and the right ventricle.

The **systemic circulation** carries oxygenated blood from the left ventricle of the heart throughout the body and back into the right atrium of the heart. The **pulmonary circulation** carries unoxygenated blood from the right ventricle through the lungs and returns oxygenated blood back into the left atrium.

In the systemic circulation, as blood passes through the tissues and organs, it gives up oxygen and nutrients and absorbs cellular wastes and carbon dioxide. In the pulmonary circulation, as blood passes through the lungs, it gives up carbon dioxide and absorbs oxygen.

Oxygenated blood flows from the left ventricle through the **aorta**, the major artery leaving the left ventricle (Fig. 26.1), and into the **arteries**, the tubular vessels that carry blood from the heart to the body tissues. From the arteries, the blood flows

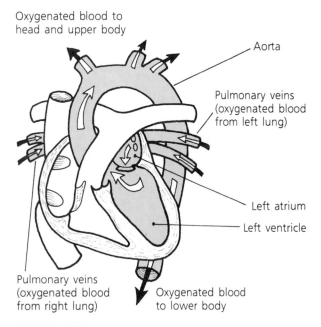

FIGURE 26.1. Oxygenated blood flows out from the left ventricle of the heart through the aorta to pass to the body in general.

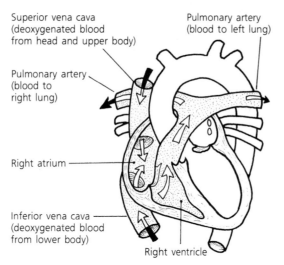

Superior vena cava
(deoxygenated blood
from head and upper body)

Pulmonary artery
(blood to left lung)

Pulmonary artery
(blood to
right lung)

Right atrium

Inferior vena cava
(deoxygenated blood
from lower body)

Right ventricle

FIGURE 26.2.   Blood is delivered to the right atrium of the heart through the superior and inferior venae cavae and passes to the right ventricle, where it is pumped through the pulmonary artery into the lungs.

into **arterioles**, which are small branches of the arteries, and into the small, thin-walled **capillaries**, in which individual red blood cells can make close contact with the individual cells of the body.

Blood passes through the capillaries into small veins, or **venules**, which unite to form larger **veins**. The veins deliver blood to the right atrium of the heart through the **superior** and **inferior venae cavae**, the two largest veins. The blood then passes into the right ventricle and is pumped to the lungs (Fig. 26.2), where it passes through the pulmonary capillaries and then into the left side of the heart, thus completing the cardiac cycle.

THE CARDIAC CYCLE

The **cardiac cycle** is the electromechanical sequence of events that occurs with one contraction (systole) and relaxation (diastole) of the heart muscle (Fig. 26.3). Knowledge of the physical events of the cardiac cycle is fundamental to understanding the heart as a pump.

Sequence of Electrical Events

A network of specialized tissue, which is capable of conducting electrical current, runs throughout the heart muscle. The flow

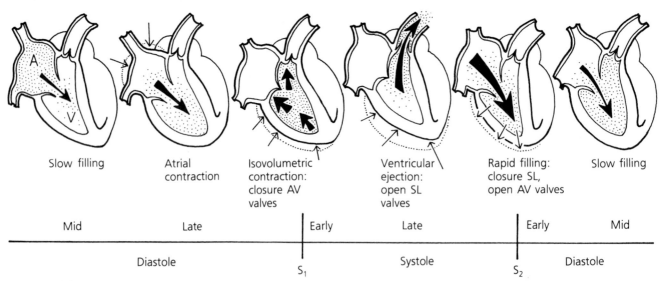

| Slow filling | Atrial contraction | Isovolumetric contraction: closure AV valves | Ventricular ejection: open SL valves | Rapid filling: closure SL, open AV valves | Slow filling |

| Mid | Late | | Early | Late | | Early | Mid |

| | Diastole | S_1 | | Systole | | S_2 | Diastole |

FIGURE 26.3.   The cardiac cycle is the electromechanical sequence of events that occurs with contraction (systole) and relaxation (diastole) of heart muscle.   (Modified from Marielle Ortiz Vinsant, Martha I. Spence, and Diane Chapell, *A Commonsense Approach to Coronary Care*, 2d ed. [St. Louis: The C. V. Mosby Co., 1975.])

of electrical current through this network causes smooth, coordinated contractions of the heart. These contractions produce the pumping action of the heart.

Each cardiac cycle is initiated by an electrical impulse that starts over the atria and the ventricles of the heart and results in depolarization (change in electricity) and contraction of the individual myocardial (heart) cells (Fig. 26.4). Under normal conditions, the impulse originates in the sinoatrial node, which is located in the upper part of the right atrium close to its junction with the superior vena cava. Upon leaving the sinoatrial node, the impulse depolarizes the surrounding atrial muscles, producing atrial contraction, and then travels rapidly via specialized conduction tissue to the left atrium and to the atrioventricular (AV) node.

An **electrocardiogram** (**ECG** or **EKG**) is a recording of the electrical current that flows through the heart. The body acts as a conductor of electrical current. Any two points on the body can be connected with electrical leads to record the electrical activity of the heart. The tracing produced by the electrical activity of the heart, as it depolarizes and repolarizes, forms a series of waves and complexes that are separated by regularly occurring intervals. The waves of the ECG are called the P wave, the QRS complex, and the T wave. The electrocardiographic correlate of atrial contraction is the **P wave**. Ventricular activation is expressed by the **QRS complex,** followed by the **T wave** that represents ventricular repolarization (Fig. 26.5).

Sequence of Mechanical Events

The mechanical events that follow electrical activation of the heart are easily explained by observing the pressure changes that occur in the atria and in the ventricles (Fig. 26.6). Following the P wave, the atrium contracts, increasing the atrial pressure and propelling blood across the mitral and tricuspid valves. At approximately the peak of the QRS complex, ventricular pressure

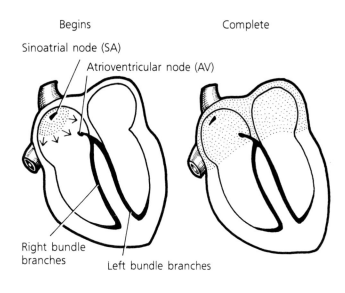

ATRIAL EXCITATION

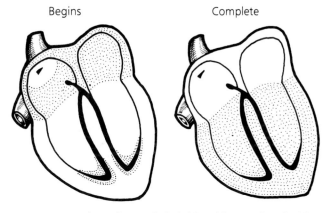

VENTRICULAR EXCITATION

FIGURE 26.4. Each cardiac cycle is initiated by an electrical impulse that starts over the atria and ventricles of the heart and results in depolarization and contraction of the individual myocardial cells.

begins to rise rapidly, initiating ventricular systole (contraction). When ventricular pressure exceeds atrial pressure, the AV valves close and may even bulge back into the atrium to some degree. After the closure of the mitral valve and before the opening of the aortic and pulmonary valves, the pressure in the ventricle rises rapidly due to ventricular contraction against its volume of blood.

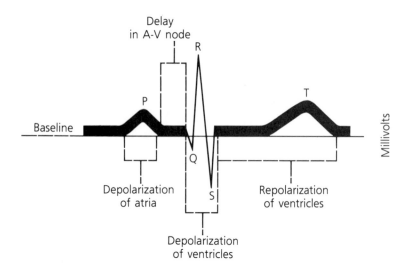

FIGURE 26.5. Sequence of electrical events in the cardiac cycle: the P wave represents atrial depolarization; the QRS complex expresses ventricular activation; and the T wave represents ventricular repolarization. (From Jules Constant, *Learning Electrocardiography*, page 3. © 1973 by Jules Constant. Reprinted by permission of Little, Brown and Co.)

When the pressure of the ventricle exceeds that of the aorta or pulmonary artery, the semilunar valves open, and blood is ejected rapidly out of the heart across these valves (rapid ejection phase). Ventricular pressure continues to rise briefly; then, as the ventricular muscle begins to relax, the pressure starts to fall rapidly. Due to the kinetic energy of the blood, there is still flow across the semilunar valves, even though a pressure gradient no longer exists. Soon, vessel pressure exceeds the energy of the outcoming blood, however, and the flow tends to reverse. This reversal causes the semilunar valves to close suddenly, ending the systolic phase, which is followed by a brief rise in aortic and pulmonic pressure (see Fig. 26.6).

When the pressure in the left ventricle drops to a point below the atrial pressure, the mitral valve opens, and blood from the atria rushes into the ventricles, initiating the rapid filling phase of the ventricle. Atrial pressure drops rapidly as blood leaves, which reflects this rapid filling phase. As the ventricle accepts this rapid filling, it becomes distended with the in-rushing blood, and the pressure begins to rise rapidly. As this occurs, the ventricular and atrial pressures begin to equilibrate, and blood flow into the ventricle becomes much slower. Following this slow filling phase, atrial systole occurs and initiates the cardiac cycle once again.

CARDIAC OUTPUT

The Determinants of Cardiac Output

Cardiac output, a measure of the heart's performance, is the product of stroke volume and heart rate, and refers to the amount of blood (in liters) ejected by the heart per minute. **Stroke volume** is the amount of blood ejected per beat, and **heart rate** is the frequency of contraction.

Stroke Volume

Stroke volume is dependent on preload, afterload, and contractile states of the heart.

Preload. **Preload** is a reflection of muscle quality. For example, an elastic, distensible ventricle in a young person propels more blood more rapidly than the stiffer, less distensible ventricle in an older individual because the stretch in the ventricular muscle fibers from the same volume of blood is greater in the young person.

Afterload. **Afterload** is the impedance of forward flow of blood from the ventricle and relates, therefore, directly to the resistance in the arterial system as manifested by aortic pressure. Left ventricular pressure must exceed aortic pressure before forward flow can occur. Thus, high blood pressure is injurious because it greatly increases the workload of the left ventricle by resisting forward flow. So, too, are obstructing lesions, such as narrowing of the aortic valves, injurious, because they impede flow out of the left ventricle.

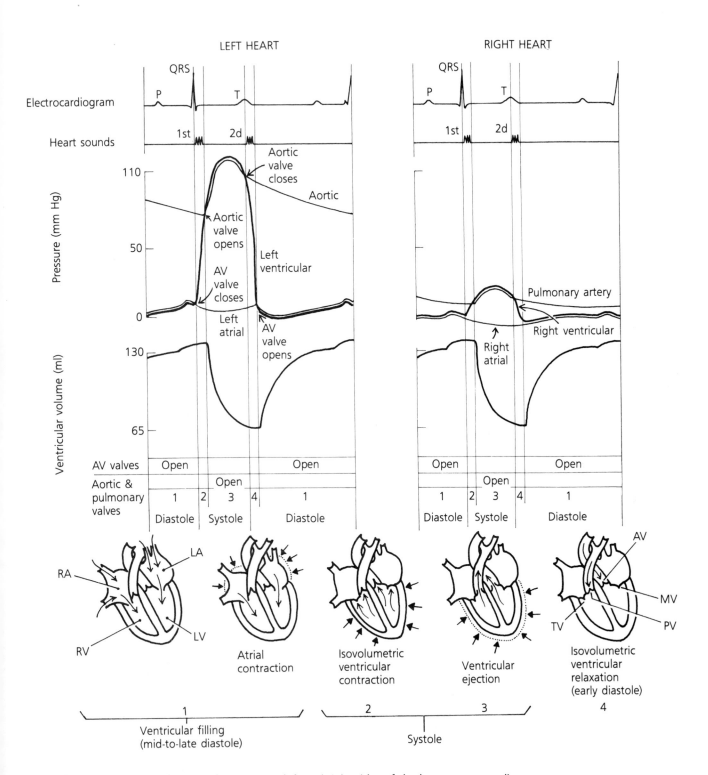

FIGURE 26.6. Atrial and ventricular events in left and right sides of the heart corresponding to systolic and diastolic contractions and relaxations. (AV = aortic valve, MV = mitral valve, PV = pulmonic valve, TV = tricuspid valve) (Reprinted with permission from W. F. Ganong. *Review of Medical Physiology*, 11th ed., by Appleton & Lange, Norwalk, Conn./San Mateo, Calif., 1983.)

Contractility. **Contractility** is the most difficult concept to portray, since it cannot be measured directly. Conceptually, it refers to the overall capacity of the muscle fibers of the ventricles to shorten and to do useful work. Contractility can be very poor in people who have severely diseased or damaged hearts. On the other hand, it can be quite vigorous in trained athletes who have exceptional output.

Heart Rate

The final major determinant of cardiac performance is heart rate. Heart rate is determined by the firing rate of the sinus node as modulated by the constant flow of neural signals (sympathetic increases rate; parasympathetic decreases rate) from the cardioregulatory centers in the brain, in the chemical (humoral) substances circulating in the blood such as adrenalin, and from the thyroid hormones. Heart rate varies with age, sex, and level of fitness. It also changes with demands of activity, temperature, flu-

id status, drug and hormone levels, and dietary state.

Oxygen Demands of the Cardiac Muscle

These four parameters of cardiac performance—preload (end-diastolic volume or pressure), afterload (aortic pressure), contractile state (inherent power to develop force), and heart rate—not only define the pumping capabilities of the heart, but also are the major determinants of the oxygen needs of the working heart muscle itself (Fig. 26.7). This oxygen demand correlates best with the product of the heart rate and blood pressure both at rest and with exercise. More important, this oxygen demand of the heart muscle is generated by the interaction of rate, pressure, and activity, and can only be met by adequate coronary blood flow.

The Need for Adequate Coronary Blood Flow

Under resting conditions, the working myocardium uses 8 to 9 mm of oxygen per 100 gm of ventricular tissue, or about 7 percent of the body's total oxygen requirement. Increases in any of the four parameters of cardiac performance sharply increase this oxygen requirement, which can only be met by increasing flow in the coronary artery. This is because all of the available oxygen presented to the working myocardium is extracted in a single pass. Thus, increased oxygen demands in coronary beds can only be met by increased coronary blood flow. Fortunately, the normal coronary arterial bed has the capability of increasing flow sixfold or providing for an increased oxygen demand of 500 percent over base conditions.

Coronary blood flow is closely regulated by myocardial oxygen demand; it also follows certain physical laws of flow inherent in a closed-pipe system such as the circulatory system. These physical principles of flow relate to all blood vessels in the body.

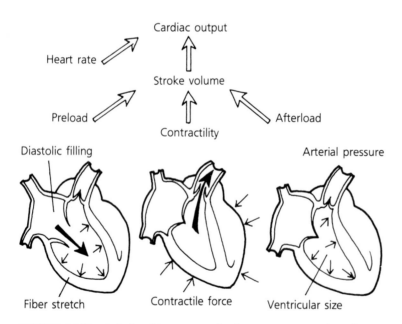

FIGURE 26.7. Relationships among the four parameters of cardiac performance. (From Sylvia Anderson and Lorraine McCarty Wilson, *Pathophysiology: Clinical Concepts of Disease Processes* [New York: McGraw-Hill, 1978]. Reprinted by permission of The C. V. Mosby Co., St. Louis.)

The Results of Impeded Coronary Blood Flow

From the prior analysis, it is clear that narrowing in one or more of the major coronary arteries can compromise coronary blood flow, even at rest, and certainly with exercise. Impeded flow may result in chest pain, or **angina**, due to lack of oxygen available to the working heart muscle. This condition is simply an imbalance between supply and demand. Complete blockage of the major coronary vessels results in total lack of oxygen to the functioning myocardial muscle cells and inevitably results in **myocardial infarction**, or heart attack, which causes permanent injury or death of the heart muscle.

FACTORS THAT INFLUENCE BLOOD CIRCULATION

Blood flows through the vessels of the body because of the pulsatile pumping action of the heart and the pressure differential across the system from the left ventricle (100 to 110 mm Hg) to the right atrium (5 to 10 mm Hg). This critical driving force permits adequate flow. Loss of pressure, such as occurs in shock, immediately compromises blood flow to critical organs such as the heart, brain, and kidneys, and if prolonged, results in death.

Influence of Vessel Size

Over a century ago, a French physician, Jean Poiseuille, studied continuous flow in small rigid tubes. He carefully delineated the elements that comply with distance and formulated the equations that govern flow in such tubes. His formula, known as **Poiseuille's law**, indicates that volume flow in a tube is directly proportional to the pressure drop along the length of the tube and to the radius of that tube to the fourth power, and is inversely proportional to the length of the tube and to the viscosity, or thickness, of the fluid flowing through the tube. Therefore, the geometry of the tube

(length and radius) is very important in determining the flow and resistance, and small changes in vessel radius can produce large changes in flow. For example, a 20 percent increase in radius will produce more than a 100 percent increase in volume flow (Fig. 26.8).

Influence of Viscosity

Poiseuille's law measures the internal friction of a fluid. Fluids of high viscosity (for example, molasses) impede flow to a much greater degree than low-viscosity fluids such as water. In humans, hematocrit is the major measure of viscosity. **Hematocrit** is the ratio of the volume of packed red blood cells to the total volume of blood. Polycythemic states, which are characterized by an increased number of red blood cells, tend to reduce flow, whereas anemia (hemoglobin less than 8 gm percent) substantially increases blood flow.

The velocity of flow through the circulation is a function of the cross-sectional area of the vessels. Thus, in the arterial system, where total cross-sectional area is small, velocities are high. In the capillary system, with its huge, total cross-sectional area, velocity is very slow. In the venous system, which also has a fairly large cross-sectional area, flows are faster than in the capillary system but slow compared with those in the arterial system.

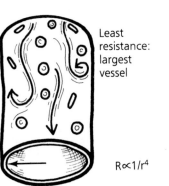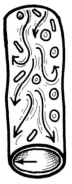

Least resistance: largest vessel

Most resistance: smallest vessel

$R \propto 1/r^4$

FIGURE 26.8. Poiseuille's law of flow through a tube.

Influence of the Autonomic Nervous System

In general, **sympathetic stimulation** (the "fight or flight" response) increases atrial and ventricular contractility, increases heart rate, and speeds the spread of excitation through the AV node and, slightly, through the ventricles. **Parasympathetic** (vagal) **stimulation** generally has the opposite effect. At any instant, the effect of the nervous system on the heart is a net balance of these two opposing controls, which usually vary reciprocally. The parasympathetic stimulation, generally inhibitory, normally predominates and maintains the usual resting heart rate of about 65 to 75 beats per minute. During exercise, however, the sympathetic nervous system becomes dominant.

Neural reflexes, particularly from stretch receptors in the carotid sinus and aorta, form a major intrinsic control mechanism that influences myocardial performance directly and indirectly. **Arterial hypotension** produces decreased carotid sinus stretch. This condition triggers the sympathetic nervous system, resulting in increased venous return and thereby increased ventricular end-diastolic fiber length. Simultaneously, **carotid sinus hypotension** produces arterial vasoconstriction, which increases peripheral vascular resistance and aortic impedance, and thus tends to increase blood pressure. Furthermore, carotid sinus hypotension elicits reflexes that increase atrial and ventricular contractility. Myocardial contractility is decreased by hypoxia (a deficiency of oxygen in the tissues of the body) and by acidosis (a condition caused by accumulation of acid or loss of base in the body).

EXERCISE AND THE HEART

The Effect of Exercise on Heart Rate and Stroke Volume

The mechanisms used to increase cardiac output during exercise vary, depending on age, health, body position, and athletic conditioning. In particular, the relative contri-bution of heart rate and stroke volume is a subject of considerable interest. When in a supine position, most normal persons without athletic conditioning appear to increase their cardiac output during mild to moderate exercise, mainly by an increase in heart rate rather than an increase in stroke volume. With more extreme exercise, these individuals increase stroke volume 10–15 percent in the supine position and 30–100 percent in the upright position, despite a considerably shortened systolic ejection. Normal persons more used to physical exercise show an earlier, more marked increase in stroke volume in both positions, and stroke volume often doubles during upright exercise. Heart rate may increase three- or even fourfold in trained athletes, whereas stroke volume increases considerably less and can even decline with extreme increases in rate.

Other Effects of Exercise

The arterial systolic blood pressure often increases 40 to 60 mm Hg during moderate or severe exercise, although the mean arterial blood pressure increases much less. The diastolic pressure may increase slightly, decrease slightly, or stay the same. Arterial resistance normally decreases considerably during exercise. The combination of vasodilation of the exercising muscles and the increased activity of the muscles and the abdominal thoracic pump increases the venous return to the heart, further contributing to the increased cardiac output.

Exercise also decreases blood volume in venous reservoirs, especially blood stored in the spleen. These shifts make more blood available to the heart, arterial vessels, and its exercising muscles. Because fluid loss is secondary to prolonged exercise, plasma volume may decrease despite these shifts, resulting in an increase in hematocrit.

Distribution of Cardiac Output During Exercise

During exercise, a major redistribution of the cardiac output takes place. During mild to moderate exercise, coronary blood flow and blood flow to the active skeletal muscle increase and cerebral flow is maintained, whereas blood flow to the kidneys and spleen diminishes. During more extreme exercise, these changes are exaggerated, and flow to the inactive muscles may actually decrease. During times of maximal exercise, brain flow may also decrease because of hyperventilation and respiratory alkalosis (a condition in which excessive breathing, as from hyperventilating, "blows off" too much carbon dioxide). Skin flow may decrease initially during exercise but then rise during continued exercise to help cool the body.

Types of Exercise

Physiologically, three types of skeletal muscular contractions put demands on the cardiovascular system. **Static exercise** occurs with isometric contraction to the point of fatigue, such as in weight lifting. Static exercise imposes a disproportionate pressure load relative to aerobic requirements on the left ventricle. **Dynamic exercise** involves rhythmical contraction of flexor and extensor muscle groups, such as in walking and jogging. Dynamic exercise causes a greater acceleration of heart rate proportional to the greater aerobic requirements. **Sustained and dynamic exercise**, such as occurs when a person walks rapidly while carrying a heavy object, creates a mixed response.

The first and third types of exercise can be hazardous if repeated in rapid sequence, particularly in persons with serious hypertension or coronary vascular disease, because of rapidly developing afterload on the left ventricle. Worse yet for such individuals is that as cumulative endogenous heart load develops and arterial pressure falls, coronary perfusion may be compromised, while demands for peripheral blood flow remain high. In addition, prolonged isometric exercise causes increased blood pressure and increased size of the cardiac muscle. Of the three types of exercise, dynamic, repetitive exercise such as walking, jogging, or swimming is best suited to developing cardiac fitness.

Dual Role of Exercise

Currently in the area of cardiovascular medicine, exercise has a dual role. By increasing the workload of the heart, exercise can uncover an imbalance between supply and demand and thus identify coronary artery disease not otherwise suspected in the resting basal state. Safe levels of exercise for athletes can be determined by the athlete's physician.

The other role of exercise, of course, is to achieve **cardiovascular fitness**. Cardiovascular fitness improves cardiac efficiency and performance by achieving workloads at less cost. Heart rate and blood pressure response at given workloads are reduced, and contractility of the heart and the blood supply to the peripheral working muscles improve.

Achieving Cardiovascular Fitness

The ability of athletes to reach a high level of performance in most sports depends in part on the supply of oxygen to the working muscle tissues, especially the heart. As the workload on the muscle tissues increases during athletic activity, the muscles' need for oxygen increases, along with a concomitant need to eliminate more carbon dioxide.

Cardiovascular fitness is the ability of the cardiovascular system to meet the oxygen–carbon dioxide transport demands of high workloads and maintain efficiency for long periods of time. When the oxygen needs are being met during activity, the athlete is working in **aerobic metabolism**. If the workload during activity becomes so great that the cardiovascular system is unable to meet the needs of the working muscles, the **anaerobic metabolism** is activated. Performance soon deteriorates, and the athlete will eventually have to stop. Both aerobic and anaerobic capacities can be increased through training.

Aerobic Training

Aerobic training involves some type of continuous muscular activity with minimal resistance for 30 to 40 minutes, three to four times a week. The intensity of the activity should be great enough to increase the heart rate by 70 to 85 percent of the athlete's maximum heart rate. The theoretical maximum heart rate can be estimated by subtracting the athlete's age from 220 and taking 70 percent of this figure. This number will provide the target heart rate during training. Thus a 20-year-old athlete would have a maximum heart rate of 200, and his or her target heart rate would be 140 beats per minute. Aerobic activities include running, cycling, cross-country skiing, swimming, and walking.

Anaerobic Training

The trained athlete, because he or she has greater cardiovascular efficiency, can exercise at a greater intensity before crossing over into anaerobic metabolism (oxygen debt). When the athlete goes into anaerobic metabolism, the muscles will continue contracting for a short period of time, but lactic acid begins to accumulate, contributing to a deterioration in athletic performance and

eventually complete muscle failure. Some experts believe that anaerobic training enables the athlete to withstand a greater buildup of lactic acid before performance deteriorates.

Anaerobic training should supplement the aerobic training for athletes likely to be involved in short bursts of speed in their sports. The relative emphasis of each type of training depends on the athlete's level of conditioning and the physical demands of the sport involved. For instance, a distance runner would concentrate primarily on aerobic training, while the sprinter would concentrate primarily on anaerobic training. One type of training, however, carries over to the other, so the sprinter should have some degree of aerobic efficiency and the distance runner, some anaerobic training for sprinting near the end of the race. When conditioning programs are established, other factors in addition to duration of activity must be considered to maximize performance safely. (See Chapter 45 for discussion of cardiovascular endurance and anaerobic and aerobic exercise.)

IMPORTANT CONCEPTS

1. Cardiac output (CO) = stroke volume (SV) × heart rate (HR).
2. At rest, the myocardium uses 7 percent of the body's total oxygen requirement.
3. Dynamic, repetitive exercise is the best way to develop cardiovascular fitness.
4. Aerobic exercise should consist of 30 to 40 minutes of activity three to four times per week, and should increase the athlete's heart rate to at least 70 percent of the athlete's maximum heart rate.
5. Maximum heart rate = 0.70 (220 − age of athlete).

SUGGESTED READINGS

Hurst, J. W., ed. *The Heart: Arteries and Veins*, 6th ed. New York: McGraw-Hill, 1986.
Little, R. C., and W. C. Little. *Physiology of the Heart and Circulation*, 4th ed. Chicago: Year Book Medical Publishers, 1989.
Smith, J. J., and J. P. Kampine. *Circulatory Physiology: The Essentials*. Baltimore: Williams & Wilkins, 1980.

27

The Hematologic System

OBJECTIVES FOR CHAPTER 27

After reading this chapter, the student should be able to:

1. Explain the primary functions of the blood cells.
2. Describe the activities of the red and white blood cells and platelets.
3. Discuss the specific functions of blood plasma.
4. Describe the functions of the spleen and bone marrow in the hematologic system.
5. Recognize normal blood parameters and describe the significance of alterations in these values.

INTRODUCTION

Proper functioning of the hematologic system—the blood, spleen, and bone marrow—is essential to physiologic well-being. Chapter 27 explores the two major components of blood: the cellular component, which consists of the red blood cells, white blood cells, and platelets; and the liquid component, or plasma. The chapter then discusses the roles of the spleen and bone marrow. The last section of Chapter 27 focuses on how alterations in normal blood parameters affect the athlete. ■

THE COMPONENTS OF BLOOD

Blood serves many vital functions in the cardiovascular system. Basically, blood consists of the liquid component (plasma) and the cellular component. All of the cellular elements are derived from bone marrow, which in the adult is primarily found within the central skeletal system—the skull, ribs, manubrium (upper portion of the sternum), vertebrae, pelvis, and proximal long bones. In the adult, the marrow cavity in the distal long bones primarily contains fat. In younger people, the long bones have active bone marrow that is replaced by fat with aging.

Functions of the Cellular Component

Blood cells have the following primary functions:

■ To distribute oxygen in adequate concentrations to body tissues that require varying levels of oxygen.
■ To maintain hemostasis (blood clotting), especially after an artery or vein has been severed.
■ To prevent, combat, and subdue infections.
■ To recognize and destroy foreign cells and cancer cells.

Red Blood Cells

Red blood cells have many functions, but the most important are delivery of oxygen and return of carbon dioxide. Under normal circumstances, carbon dioxide is released in the lungs as the blood passes through the small capillary beds found in the air sacs of the lungs. Oxygen from the ambient air crosses in the opposite direction to saturate the hemoglobin that is contained in the red blood cells. Hemoglobin then transports the oxygen to the various muscles and tissues of the body and releases it according to the oxygen demands of each tissue. Brain and myocardium (heart) tissues, for example, use much more oxygen than do eye, skin, and hair tissues, and skeletal muscles use oxygen in proportion to the amount of work they do.

Various diseases and injuries increase oxygen use, especially those conditions associated with fever, infection, or tissue injury such as burns. Persons who have anemia (decreased circulating red blood cells and hemoglobin) or alterations in their hemoglobin (such as occurs in heavy cigarette smokers when carbon monoxide displaces oxygen from the hemoglobin molecule) will not be able to deliver adequate quantities of oxygen to the tissues, and, therefore, certain tissues will suffer.

White Blood Cells

There are many different kinds of **white blood cells**. **Granulocytes** (polymorphonuclear leukocytes) search for and destroy bacteria or foreign substances which may be causing infection or inflammation. A large decrease in the number of circulating granulocytes may render an individual more susceptible to infections.

Lymphocytes, another type of circulating white blood cells, help fight infection and inflammation in a different way. B-lymphocytes (10 to 15 percent of circulating lymphocytes) make antibodies to circulate in the plasma, as well as help other cells remove foreign material, bacteria, and viruses from the body. These cells can change into plasma cells (only rarely seen in the peripheral blood) that then are capable of making antibodies in response to a particular infection. T-lymphocytes (70 to 80 percent of circulating lymphocytes) attack antigens on foreign cells and help B-lymphocytes make antibodies. The third type of lymphocyte, natural killer cells (10 to 15 percent of circulating lymphocytes), directly attack foreign cells and cancer cells.

Other white blood cells, such as basophils, eosinophils, and monocytes, have similar but lesser roles in keeping the body free from infection or inflammation, as well as roles in allergy and immune defense. The white blood cells are one of the body's many defense mechanisms against infection. Other defenses include the skin, lymphatic system, and antibodies.

Platelets

Platelets, the smallest cellular elements in the circulating blood, are critical to maintaining hemostasis (the stoppage of bleeding). The primary function of platelets is to seal tiny holes that may develop in blood vessels. Too few platelets can lead to bruising and easy bleeding, and can aggravate or prolong bleeding when a vessel is injured. Similarly, too many platelets may predispose a person to excessive blood clotting (thrombosis), or paradoxically, to bleeding.

Many diseases and drugs can affect the normal function and activity of the platelets. For instance, aspirin can interfere with the platelets' ability to stick to the vessel walls, and in some persons can accentuate bleeding abnormalities. Small doses of aspirin have been found helpful in reducing the

incidence of heart attack or stroke in certain individuals; aspirin's ability to interfere with platelet function, the first step in blood clotting, may be the underlying mechanism.

Even in normal persons, bleeding times (one of the many laboratory tests that are used to evaluate hemostasis) are usually prolonged after the ingestion of aspirin. The effect of aspirin on the platelets lasts the lifetime of the platelets involved (up to 10 days).

Functions of the Liquid Component

Plasma, the liquid component of the blood, is a sticky, yellow fluid that carries the blood cells and nutrients. It also carries wastes and potentially toxic materials from various areas of the body for excretion through the kidneys. In addition, plasma carries small quantities of oxygen to aid the red blood cells in oxygen delivery.

Plasma has several other functions in the hematologic system. For example, plasma maintains another phase of hemostasis through a system known as the plasmatic coagulation system. This system is a family of plasma proteins that, when activated, work with platelets to form blood clots. Individuals with classic hemophilia lack one of the plasmatic coagulation factors (factor VIII). Hemophiliacs tend to bleed severely, not only with trauma, but also spontaneously into joints and tissues, and occasionally into the brain. Acquired defects of coagulation may occur in severe liver disease, as the liver produces many factors necessary for clotting.

Another function of plasma is to carry vitamins, minerals, and nutrients, including fats, protein, and carbohydrates, to and from various organs (especially the liver) for processing and further use in the body's metabolic processes. These nutrients are then stored in tissues for caloric expenditure—that is, energy.

Plasma also maintains adequate circulation of electrolytes, which in turn help regulate normal water balance. Alterations in quantities of these electrolytes, especially sodium, can lead to different problems in active athletes. Contraction or reduction of the plasma volume, as seen in severe heat exhaustion with dehydration or inadequate fluid replacement, can cause delirium, a rising temperature, confusion, coma, and shock. Certain situations give rise to increased amounts of plasma and fluid within the vascular compartment. Excessive swelling in the legs, hands, or other tissues may be caused by failure of the heart, liver, or kidneys, or other alterations in proteins or electrolytes in the plasma.

ROLES OF THE SPLEEN AND BONE MARROW

The Spleen

The **spleen** is a fist-sized, solid organ situated in the left upper quadrant of the abdomen. It has no digestive function, although it lies in close association with the colon, stomach, and pancreas. When the spleen is injured, the liver and bone marrow assume its hematologic function.

The spleen is an organ of paradox. It is expendable, yet its removal increases the risk of overwhelming bloodstream infection. Simply put, the spleen is the filter of the blood. It removes foreign particles and injured or old red blood cells from the blood.

The spleen also serves as the "lymph gland" of the bloodstream. Rich in lymphocytes, the spleen helps launch the body's immune defense by trapping blood-borne bacteria and making antibodies against them.

Bone Marrow

The essence of **bone marrow** is that it contains primitive stem cells that have two functions: (1) they can renew themselves, and (2) they can differentiate (mature) into red blood cells, white blood cells, and platelets. The bone marrow, then, is the seedbed for all the cellular elements of the blood.

ALTERATIONS IN NORMAL BLOOD PARAMETERS

Alterations in Hemoglobin Content

Anemia is a condition which results from a decreased amount of circulating red blood cells and hemoglobin. Anemia, most commonly due to lack of iron, is seen in women who have heavy menstrual periods and in persons who have bleeding from peptic ulcers or other lesions in the gastrointestinal tract. **Iron deficiency anemia** is known to curtail endurance and physical performance. Iron deficiency anemia is treated by correcting any underlying medical problems and by increasing the amount of iron in the diet (see Chapter 42 for information on sources of iron). Supplemental iron tablets may also be recommended.

Although not as common as iron deficiency, **folic acid deficiency** can also cause anemia, as can the chronic administration of certain drugs. **Pernicious anemia** is caused by deficiency of vitamin B_{12} (cobalamin), a dietary vitamin. B_{12} deficiency is very rare and almost always occurs in vegans, who consume neither foods of animal origin nor dairy products.

It is important to distinguish true anemia from the hematologic effects of training, commonly called **sports anemia** or **pseudoanemia**. Extensive aerobic training tends to increase plasma volume by about 10 to 20 percent, which tends to decrease the hematocrit (the percentage of blood that is red blood cells). Even though the hematocrit is low, the athlete with this "sports anemia" (actually a false anemia) will have no adverse effects because the number of red blood cells is the same. In fact, Olympic-level training may actually increase the number of red blood cells; however, the increase in plasma volume outstrips the increase in red blood cells, so the hematocrit falls and therefore indicates the false anemia.

Another potential cause of anemia in long-distance runners is **foot strike hemolysis**, which results from multiple foot strikes on hard pavement, bursting red blood cells in the bloodstream. Treatment is better cushioning of the feet with shoes and shoe inserts and running on soft terrain.

Alterations in the White Blood Cell Count

Major alterations in the leukocyte count are much less common than anemia, unless the person has an infection, another serious disease, or a drug-induced low leukocyte count. The normal leukocyte count is usually between 4,000 and 10,000/cu mm of blood.

Persons with bacterial infections may have substantially increased leukocyte counts. Early in the course of a viral illness such as flu, measles, or chickenpox, the leukocyte count may fall and then return to normal as the disease progresses. This self-limited change is a normal response. In fact, such alterations may be clues to help identify possible causes of an otherwise unexplained fever and infection.

A **complete blood cell count** is frequently done as part of the preparticipation physical evaluation at the beginning of the school year. Table 27.1 contains normal blood cell values. Any athlete with abnormal values is screened further. It is important to know that exercise itself increases the white blood cell count for 1 to 2 hours after activity.

Alterations in the Platelet Count

The normal platelet count is 200,000 to 400,000 cells/cu mm. An athlete who has values outside this range needs further evaluation. A platelet deficiency can cause bruising and easy bleeding; a platelet surplus can predispose to either blood clotting or bleeding. A marginally low platelet count may simply be due to dilution by the increased plasma volume of an endurance athlete. If a repeat platelet count is normal and the athlete demonstrates no symptoms of bruising or easy bleeding in the absence of trauma, further evaluation may not be required.

A high platelet count may reflect the presence of dehydration rather than an actual increase in the number of platelets. The platelet count should be rechecked after the athlete is rehydrated, and if it remains elevated, further evaluation is necessary. In all cases of abnormal platelet counts, the physician should determine what type of further evaluation might be necessary.

Alterations in Plasma Volume

In the otherwise healthy person, alterations in blood plasma usually are not significant, as long as adequate hydration and electrolyte balance are maintained. As previously mentioned, normal or physiologic plasma alterations can take place in some athletes, such as long-distance runners. The plasma volume will increase, resulting in a relative decrease in hematocrit and in the concentration of hemoglobin. This phenomenon reflects a physiologic adaptation that enhances athletic performance.

TABLE 27.1. Normal Blood Cell Values

	Men	Women
Red blood cell count, cells in millions/cu mm	4.7–6.1	4.2–5.2
Hemoglobin, g%	13.4–17.6	12.0–15.4
Hematocrit, vol%	42–53	38–46
MCV, cu mm	81–96	
MCHC,[b] g%	30–36	
Total white blood cell count, cells/cu mm	4–10,000	
Granulocytes		
PMNs,[c] %	38–70	
Eosinophils, %	1–5	
Basophils, %	0–2	
Monocytes, %	1–8	
Lymphocytes, %	15–45	
Platelets, cells/cu mm	200,000–400,000	
Reticulocyte count, %	1–2	

Note: Values slightly variable to labs.
[a]Mean corpuscular volume.
[b]Mean corpuscular hemoglobin concentration.
[c]Polymorphonuclear leukocytes.
Source: Price, Sylvia Anderson and Wilson, Lorraine McCarty. *Pathophysiology: Clinical Concepts of Disease Processes* (New York: McGraw-Hill, 1978). Reprinted by permission of the C.V. Mosby Co., St. Louis.

IMPORTANT CONCEPTS

1. Blood can be divided into two parts: the liquid component (plasma) and the cellular component.
2. Red blood cells are important in the delivery of oxygen to the tissues and return of carbon dioxide to the lungs.
3. White blood cells fight infection and inflammation.
4. Platelets are critical to maintaining hemostasis (blood clotting).
5. Plasma delivers nutrients to the organs and carries toxins to the kidneys, aids in blood clotting, maintains adequate circulation of many substances, and assists in providing oxygen to the red blood cells.
6. The spleen filters foreign particles and injured or old red blood cells from the blood.
7. The bone marrow is the seedbed for all cellular elements of the blood.
8. Alterations in the quantities of red blood cells, white blood cells, platelets, and plasma volume may have serious consequences for the athlete.

SUGGESTED READINGS

Adner, M. M. "Hematology." In *Sports Medicine*, edited by R. H. Strauss, pp. 120–129. Philadelphia: W. B. Saunders, 1984.

Jandle, J. "Blood." In *Textbook of Hematology*. Boston: Little, Brown, 1987.

Williams, W. J., E. Beutler, A. Ersleb, and M. Lichtman, eds. *Hematology*, 3d ed. New York: McGraw-Hill, 1983.

28

The Respiratory System

CHAPTER OUTLINE

OBJECTIVES FOR CHAPTER 28

After reading this chapter, the student should be able to:

1. Describe the anatomy of the respiratory system.
2. Understand how oxygen enters the bloodstream and carbon dioxide is expelled from the body.
3. Be familiar with the most frequently encountered respiratory illnesses.

INTRODUCTION

The primary function of the respiratory system is gas exchange—that is, the addition of oxygen to and the removal of carbon dioxide from the venous blood. The respiratory system is complex and depends on the interaction of multiple anatomic structures. Chapter 28 discusses three areas that are important to understanding the respiratory system: anatomy, physiology, and pathophysiology. ■

ANATOMY OF THE RESPIRATORY SYSTEM

The anatomy of the respiratory system may be considered as three divisions—the airway that communicates with the environment, the lung parenchyma that acts as the primary gas exchange organ, and the skeletal structures that support these tissues, facilitating air movement into and out of the lungs. The anatomic structures that are involved in transporting air into the lungs include the nose, mouth, pharynx, larynx, trachea, bronchi, and bronchioles (Fig. 28.1).

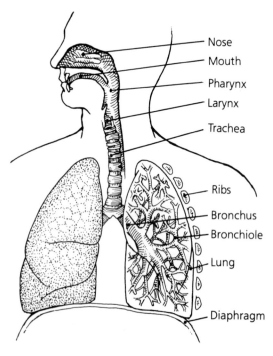

FIGURE 28.1. Anatomy of the respiratory system.

The Airways

The Nose and Upper Airways

The nose and upper airways humidify the inspired air, bring it to body temperature, and remove much of the particulate matter contained in the air. The **larynx**, which protects the trachea and lower airways from the inadvertent inhalation of liquids or swallowed particulate matter, also serves as the organ of voice. It is composed of cartilage rings and plates that give it a rigid form, muscles that act on the cartilages to vary the larynx opening, and a mucosal-covered membrane that is its lining.

The Trachea and Lower Airways

The **trachea** descends from the larynx to the **bronchi**, where it branches into the two **main stem bronchi**, which in turn branch into smaller and smaller conducting airways to the level of the **terminal bronchiole**. Beyond the terminal bronchiole are additional generations of branching in the airway system referred to as the **respiratory zone**. The air sacs, or **alveoli**, are located here, and this zone is where gas exchange occurs (Fig. 28.2).

The trachea, like the larynx, is a cartilaginous and membranous tube. The cartilaginous portion is composed of semicircular cricoid rings that are incomplete posteriorly. They are connected by the membranous portion of the trachea, which is composed of muscle and connective tissue. The semicircular cartilages surrounding the anterior portion of the trachea become disclike in

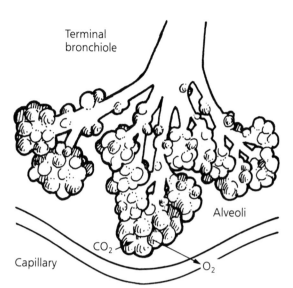

FIGURE 28.2. Terminal bronchiole and alveoli for gas exchange of oxygen and carbon dioxide.

the smaller bronchi and finally disappear at the level of the bronchioles.

The trachea and bronchi are lined by mucosal cells, including columnar ciliated cells, to the level of the terminal bronchiole. Capillaries and mucus-secreting glands are located in the submucosa. The cilia and mucus have an important protective role in forming what has been referred to as the **muco-ciliary escalator**. The approximately 1,000 ml of mucus normally formed every day is swept upward by the ciliary action, carrying particulate matter or cellular debris that has been trapped. Mucus is swallowed when it reaches the pharynx (throat). The walls of the airways also contain certain connective tissue and smooth muscle that give additional support.

The Lung Parenchyma

The **lung parenchyma** is an additional support for conduction airways smaller than 2 mm in diameter. The primary components of this portion of the respiratory system are the alveoli, or air sacs, which number about 300 million in each lung. They have an internal surface area between 40 and 80 square meters. It is in these air sacs that

blood gives up carbon dioxide and absorbs new oxygen.

The right ventricle of the heart pumps blood into the lungs via the pulmonary arteries. The pulmonary artery in each lung approximately follows the branching of the airways; the pulmonary artery branches into the pulmonary arterioles, which in turn branch into the pulmonary capillaries that lie within the walls of the alveoli. This fine network of capillary vessels allows a transfer of oxygen from the alveolar space into the blood, and transfer of carbon dioxide from the blood into the alveolar space. Blood then returns to the heart via pulmonary venules that join to form larger veins that run adjacent to the pulmonary arteries (Fig. 28.3).

The Musculoskeletal Structures

The musculoskeletal structures that surround the lungs protect and support the contents within the chest cavity and make inspiration and expiration possible.

The Ribs and Their Connections

The bony ribs of the chest wall articulate posteriorly with the spinal column and with the sternum anteriorly. On each side, seven **vertebrosternal ribs** articulate directly with the sternum via their costal cartilages; three **vertebrochondral ribs** connect indirectly by articulating with the adjacent cartilages; and two ribs are free floating (Fig. 28.4). The ribs are interconnected by intercostal muscles, and a neurovascular bundle that runs along the lower side of the ribs provides the blood supply and nerve innervation to the chest wall.

The Pleura

The **pleura** is the serous membrane lining of the lung and chest wall. Two layers of pleural tissue allow for the smooth movement of the lung against the chest wall during inspiration and expiration. The **visceral pleura** covers the outer surface of the lung, and the **parietal pleura** lines the inner surface of the

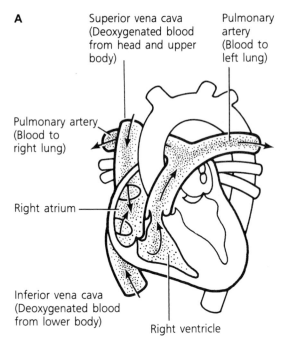

A

Superior vena cava (Deoxygenated blood from head and upper body)

Pulmonary artery (Blood to left lung)

Pulmonary artery (Blood to right lung)

Right atrium

Inferior vena cava (Deoxygenated blood from lower body)

Right ventricle

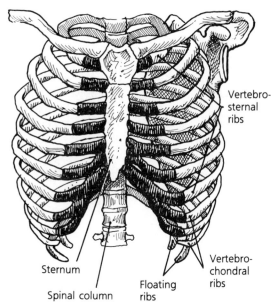

Vertebrosternal ribs

Vertebrochondral ribs

Sternum

Spinal column

Floating ribs

FIGURE 28.4. Musculoskeletal structures surrounding the lungs.

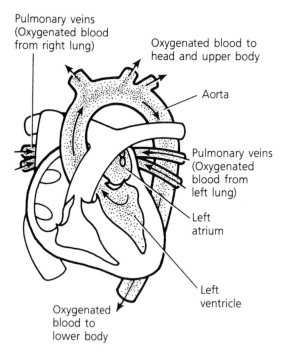

B

Pulmonary veins (Oxygenated blood from right lung)

Oxygenated blood to head and upper body

Aorta

Pulmonary veins (Oxygenated blood from left lung)

Left atrium

Left ventricle

Oxygenated blood to lower body

FIGURE 28.3. (a) The right ventricle pumps blood into the lungs via the pulmonary arteries. (b) Oxygenated blood from the lungs returns to the heart through the pulmonary veins.

chest wall. The potential space between these pleural layers is called the **pleural cavity**.

The Diaphragm and Other Muscles

The lungs are separated from the abdominal cavity by the **diaphragm**, a musculomembranous partition through which the major blood vessels (aorta and inferior vena cava) pass, as well as the esophagus.

Other anatomic structures important to respiratory system functioning include the accessory inspiratory muscles; the scalene muscles, which elevate the first two ribs; the sternocleidomastoid muscles, which raise the sternum; and the primary muscles of expiration in the abdominal wall.

PHYSIOLOGY OF THE RESPIRATORY SYSTEM

The Mechanics of Breathing

The mechanics of movement of air from the atmosphere into the lungs and back out again are complex and fascinating.

Resting Negative Pressure

A resting negative pressure in the pleural space between the visceral and parietal pleura keeps the lung inflated. The natural tendency of the lung to collapse inward and the chest wall to expand outward creates this negative pressure (Fig. 28.5). This property of the lung and chest wall becomes apparent when air leaks from the atmosphere into the pleural space—a condition called **pneumothorax** (see Chapter 29). When pneumothorax occurs, the lung collapses and the chest wall expands outward.

Inspiration

When the ribs are lifted in a "bucket-handle" type of motion by the intercostal muscles and the contracting diaphragm flattens during **inspiration**, an increasingly negative pressure is generated within the lung, resulting in airflow from the atmosphere through the conducting airways into the alveoli.

Expiration

When the intercostal muscles relax, the lung and chest wall return to their resting positions, and air is expired from the lung. During exercise and hyperventilation, **expiration** is active and is facilitated by the contraction of the intercostal and abdominal muscles.

Pulmonary Function Studies

Pulmonary physiologists interested in the mechanics of breathing have studied the characteristics of a curve representing the flow rate of the expired air at different lung volumes throughout a forced expiratory maneuver from total lung capacity to residual volume. This measurement is obtained with a spirometer, which provides a timed measurement of the volume of air expired during the maximal forced expiratory maneuver (Fig. 28.6). From the data generated, various determinations allow comparison of the pulmonary function of a given sub-

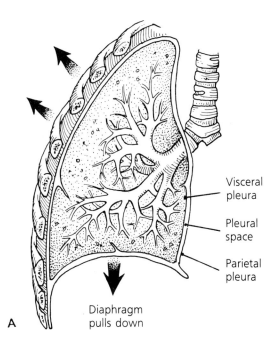

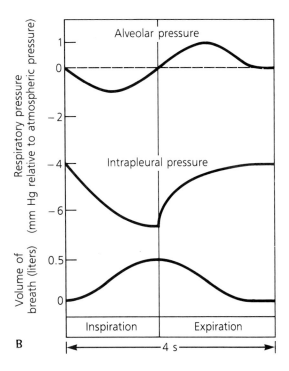

FIGURE 28.5. (a) Negative pressure in the pleural space keeps the lungs inflated. (b) Alveolar and intrapleural pressure in the respiratory cycle. (Part [b] from Vander et al., *Human Physiology: The Mechanisms of Body Function*, 3d ed. [New York: McGraw-Hill, 1980]. Reprinted by permission.)

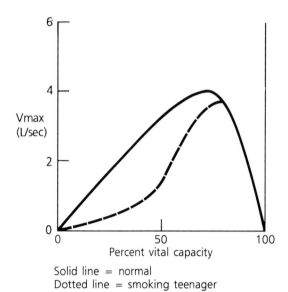

Solid line = normal
Dotted line = smoking teenager

FIGURE 28.6. Expired air volumes measured with spirometry.

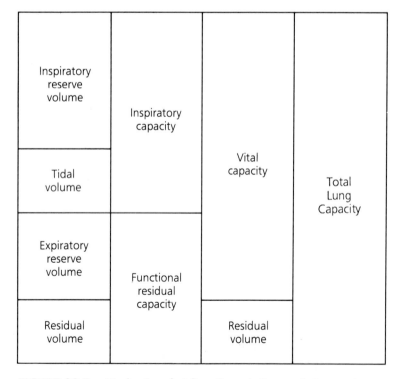

FIGURE 28.7. Mechanics of airflow through the respiratory system.

ject with predetermined normal values based on the subject's age, height, and sex.

Some important parameters measured with pulmonary function testing include inspiratory and expiratory reserve volumes, vital capacity, residual volume, functional residual capacity, tidal volume, total lung capacity, and forced expiratory volume.

Inspiratory reserve volume is the maximum volume of gas which can be inspired at the end of a normal inspiration, and **expiratory reserve volume** is the maximum volume which can be expired at the end of a normal expiration. **Vital capacity** is the maximum volume of gas that can be expired after a maximum inspiration. Air remaining in the lungs after maximal expiration is the **residual volume**. It is approximately 30 percent of the total lung capacity. During normal breathing, the volume of air remaining in the lung at the end of expiration is the **functional residual capacity**. The volume of gas inspired or expired with each breath is the **tidal volume** and is considerably less than the vital capacity. The volume of gas contained in the lungs at the end of full inspiration is the **total lung capacity** (Fig. 28.7). The volume of air expired during the first second of the forced vital capacity maneuver is the **forced expiratory volume** (**FEV**). In the athlete with suspected airway disease, these measurements allow evaluation of pulmonary function as it pertains to the ability to force air out of the lungs rapidly.

Gas Exchange

With inspiration, air (which at sea level contains approximately 21 percent oxygen) is brought into contact with the network of capillary vessels within the walls of the alveoli (air sacs), and the exchange of gases takes place. Oxygen moves into the blood, and carbon dioxide moves out of the blood into the alveolar space, where it is expired into the environment. Most of the oxygen in the blood combines with hemoglobin, though some dissolves in the blood. Carbon dioxide is carried in the blood in three forms: in solution (6 percent), as bicarbonate (70 percent), and attached to protein such as hemoglobin-forming carbamino compounds (24 percent). The effectiveness of gas exchange depends to a great extent on the critical matching of ventilation (air in the alveolus) and perfusion (blood in the capillaries surrounding the alveolus).

Diffusion

Through the process of passive **diffusion**, oxygen moves from the alveolus into the blood, and carbon dioxide moves from the blood into the alveolus. This exchange occurs because the concentration, or partial pressure, of oxygen is higher in the alveolar gas. Other factors that influence the rate of diffusion include the amount of surface area available for diffusion, the thickness of the alveolar capillary membrane through which diffusion occurs, and the diffusion constant for a given gas. The diffusion constant is proportional to the solubility of the gas in water and is inversely proportional to the square root of its molecular weight. More simply, carbon dioxide diffuses about 20 times more rapidly than oxygen in the lung, although it has a similar molecular weight because it is more soluble than oxygen (Fig. 28.8).

The Effects of Hyperventilation

In all persons, **hyperventilation** significantly reduces the level of carbon dioxide in the blood, but it does not greatly change the level of oxygen. The physiologic explanation is that oxygen and carbon dioxide have different dissociation curves. A rapid exchange of atmospheric and alveolar air allows carbon dioxide to be washed from the blood, reducing the partial pressure of carbon dioxide. The chemical characteristics of the binding of oxygen with hemoglobin do not allow the oxygen content of the blood to increase significantly. The oxygen dissociation curve becomes flat in the range of normal oxygen pressures, whereas the

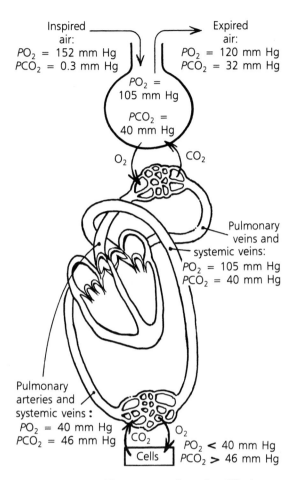

FIGURE 28.8. The process of passive diffusion. Oxygen moves from the alveolus into the blood, and carbon dioxide moves from the blood into the alveolus. (From Vander et al., *Human Physiology: The Mechanisms of Body Function*, 3d ed. [New York: McGraw-Hill, 1980], Fig. 12:18. Reprinted by permission.)

carbon dioxide dissociation curve remains steep in the physiologic range (Fig. 28.9). Hyperventilation cannot significantly increase the oxygen content of the blood.

Response to Exercise

When exercise increases oxygen demands, the frequency with which a given red blood cell travels from the lung to the heart must increase. Thus, the physiologic requirements of exercise demand the coupling of

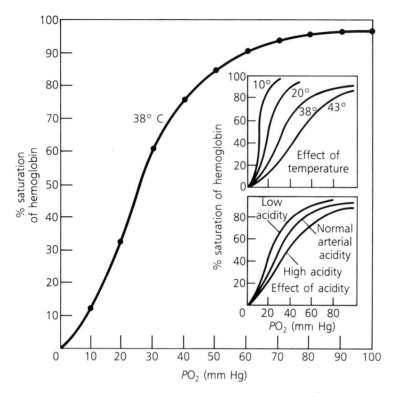

FIGURE 28.9. Hemoglobin-oxygen dissociation curve as affected by temperature and acidity. (From Vander et al., *Human Physiology: The Mechanisms of Body Function,* 3d ed. [New York: McGraw-Hill, 1980] Reprinted by permission.)

increased cardiovascular and respiratory activities to meet the gas exchange requirements. With increased oxygen demands of muscle, oxygen delivery to the cells must increase. With the increased carbon dioxide production in exercising muscle, alveolar ventilation to remove carbon dioxide from the blood must also increase. When the delivery of oxygen to the cells is inadequate to meet metabolic demands, lactic acid is released into the bloodstream. The increased acidity stimulates increased alveolar ventilation in an attempt to reduce the acidity of the blood by removing carbon dioxide, which also contributes to overall acidity. The increased production of carbon dioxide is further enhanced by the normal buffering processes of the blood, when hydrogen ions combine with bicarbonate ions to form water and more carbon dioxide.

PATHOPHYSIOLOGY OF THE RESPIRATORY SYSTEM

Chronic Obstructive Lung Disease

The umbrella term **chronic obstructive lung disease** encompasses four different conditions, each causing airway obstruction: bronchiolitis, chronic bronchitis, emphysema, and asthma.

Bronchiolitis is an inflammatory disease characterized by acute changes in peripheral airways. Infection is its most common cause, but inhalation of toxic gases and systemic diseases can sometimes be associated with this condition.

Chronic bronchitis is a nonneoplastic disorder of structure or function of the bronchi resulting from infectious or noninfectious irritation. Two elements are included in this definition: (1) obstruction to airflow during expiration; and (2) a cough, usually chronic and productive, without a known etiology. Cigarette smokers frequently develop chronic bronchitis (Fig. 28.10a).

Emphysema is defined as an anatomic alteration of the lung characterized by an abnormal enlargement of the air spaces distant to the terminal, nonrespiratory bronchioles, accompanied by destructive changes of the alveolar wall (Fig. 28.10b). Emphysema may be associated with cigarette smoking, but there is also an inherited form of emphysema (alpha-antitrypsin deficiency), which can occur in nonsmokers.

Asthma, whose hallmark is increased reactivity of the airways to various stimuli, is discussed in Chapter 53.

Chronic bronchitis and emphysema often coexist, but usually one or the other dominates the clinical picture. Pulmonary function testing results, combined with clinical manifestations of the athlete's lung disease, enable the physician to define accurately which of the obstructive conditions is present in an affected individual.

Exercise limitations found in association with these disorders are due to increased work of breathing, gas exchange impairment, or some combination of the two. Depending on the severity of these diseases, physical conditioning may improve exercise tolerance.

Respiratory Tract Infections

Before considering the anatomic site and different causes of upper and lower respiratory tract infections, the following generalizations can be made. Symptoms of mild to moderate severity and a few days' duration, such as sore throat, stuffy nose, cough, tiredness, and intermittent fever, need not keep an athlete from competing. Most often these symptoms are caused by viral infections, are self-limited, and do not respond to antibiotics. Analgesics, such as aspirin or acetaminophen, may help relieve aches and pains.

Upper Respiratory Tract Infections

Upper respiratory tract infections involve the throat, tonsils, nose, middle ear, sinuses, and/or lymph nodes in the neck.

The Common Cold. The common cold viruses cause any or all of the following symptoms: increased nasal congestion and secretions; sore throat; stuffy head; and sore, swollen lymph nodes. General symptoms may include tiredness, malaise (feeling lousy), headache, and intermittent fever. Treatment for the common cold is symptomatic with nonprescription analgesics and possibly decongestants.

Associated Sinus or Ear Infections. Bothersome aching pain localized over the cheeks or about the eyes may indicate a complicating sinus infection. Likewise, earache or a persistent blocked ear may indicate a serious ear infection. Both of these secondary infections may be caused by bacteria. Management includes physician consultation for specific diagnosis and possible antibiotic treatment.

Pharyngitis/Tonsillitis. The terms **pharyngitis** and **tonsillitis** are used interchangeably. Although most throat infections are

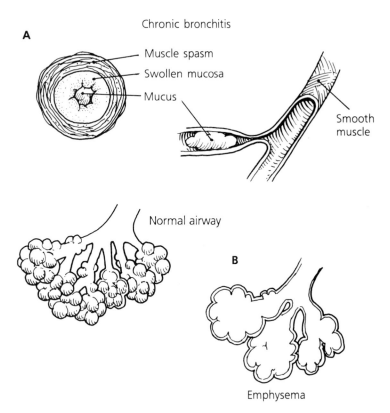

FIGURE 28.10. (a) Narrowing of airways by contraction of smooth muscle in chronic bronchitis compared to normal airway. (b) In emphysema, air spaces are overinflated.

viral, a specific diagnosis cannot be made from symptoms or physical examination. Any athlete with a sore throat that is particularly bothersome, lasts more than a few days, is associated with a persistent fever or with tender, swollen neck lymph nodes, causes pain, or restricts opening of the mouth should be more completely evaluated for one of the following four most common causes of pharyngitis: viral throat infection, streptococcal bacterial infection, infectious mononucleosis, and peritonsillar abscess.

Viral throat infection is suspected on the basis of milder symptoms and a "normal" throat on examination in association with a negative throat culture for bacteria. The treatment is symptomatic, and the athlete usually does not miss very much competition. Streptococcal bacterial infection is confirmed by throat culture. Treatment consists of antibiotics (penicillin, if possible). Athletic activity can resume when the athlete feels better, usually within 1 to 3 days.

Infectious mononucleosis is a mildly contagious viral disease primarily affecting the respiratory system. However, other lymphatic organs (spleen, liver, and lymph nodes) can be infected simultaneously, resulting in their enlargement. This disease is confirmed by serologic testing. The mainstay of treatment is rest and adequate intake of fluids. If the spleen is involved in mononucleosis, the athlete should refrain from athletics until asymptomatic and repeat examination reveals a nontender, normal-size spleen. An enlarged spleen may rupture with athletic trauma.

Peritonsillar abscess is a bacterial infection that is suspected because of pain and inability to open the mouth fully (trismus). It is diagnosed by examination of the throat. Treatment consists of close medical supervision, antibiotics, and sometimes drainage of the abscess. The athlete usually misses competition for 7 to 10 days.

Lower Respiratory Tract Infections

Lower respiratory tract infections involve the larynx, bronchial tubes, and lungs.

Laryngitis. **Laryngitis** is recognized by hoarseness and sore throat. Laryngitis caused by viruses requires only symptomatic treatment and usually does not limit athletic participation.

Viral Bronchial Infections. The vast majority of lower respiratory tract infections are viral bronchial infections, commonly referred to as **bronchitis** or chest colds. Symptoms include cough, which is aggravated by exercise or lying down. Athletes may have an intermittent fever and varying malaise. An upper respiratory tract infection or head cold generally lasts 7 to 10 days, but viral bronchitis often lasts several weeks. The treatment is symptomatic for aches and cough. Cough suppression is often possible with a codeine-containing cough medicine. Unless bronchitis symptoms are very bothersome or the athlete has a persistent fever, competition is acceptable.

Influenza is a specific viral bronchitis due to influenza viruses A or B. It occurs in epidemics and is often severe, requiring medical consultation for diagnosis or treatment of complications.

Pneumonia. **Pneumonia**, an infection of the alveoli, produces coughing, often accompanied by fever and malaise, as well as discolored sputum. Stethoscopic examination is sometimes unrevealing but may disclose localizing moist sounds called **rales**. A chest x-ray is necessary to diagnose pneumonia. An x-ray will show increased density in the lung fields. It is frequently difficult to determine whether pneumonia is caused by bacteria, viruses, or other viruslike organisms such as Chlamydia. A physician should decide whether antibiotics are advisable. The acute phase of most types of pneumonia lasts 7 to 10 days, and competition may be possible thereafter.

IMPORTANT CONCEPTS

1. The primary function of the respiratory system is gas exchange.
2. The nose and upper airway humidify the inspired air, bring it to body temperature, and remove particulate matter contained in the air.
3. The most important functional component of the alveolar wall is the network of capillary vessels within it.
4. The major musculoskeletal structures that surround and protect the lungs are the ribs, the pleura, and the diaphragm.
5. Inspiratory and expiratory reserve volumes, vital capacity, residual volume, functional residual capacity, tidal volume, total lung capacity, and forced expiratory volume are all important parameters measured during pulmonary function testing.
6. Diffusion is the process by which oxygen moves from the alveolus into the blood and carbon dioxide moves from the blood into the alveolus.
7. Hyperventilation reduces the level of carbon dioxide in the blood but does not greatly change the level of oxygen.
8. Bronchiolitis, chronic bronchitis, emphysema, and asthma fall into the category of chronic obstructive lung disease.
9. Most respiratory infections are caused by viruses, are self limited, and do not respond to antibiotics.

SUGGESTED READINGS

Åstrand, P.-O., and K. Rodahl. *Textbook of Work Physiology: Physiological Bases of Exercise*, 2d ed. New York: McGraw-Hill, 1977.

Fick, R. B., Jr., ed. *Clinics in Chest Medicine*, vol. 9, no. 4. Philadelphia: W. B. Saunders, 1988.

Fishman, A. P., ed. *Assessment of Pulmonary Function*. New York: McGraw-Hill, 1980.

———. *Pulmonary Diseases and Disorders*. New York: McGraw-Hill, 1980.

Harper, R. W. *A Guide to Respiratory Care: Physiology and Clinical Applications*. Philadelphia: J. B. Lippincott, 1981.

Snider, G. L., ed. *Clinics in Chest Medicine*, vol.4, no. 3. Philadelphia: W. B. Saunders, 1983.

Wasserman, K., J. E. Hansen, D. Y. Sue, et al. *Principles of Exercise Testing and Interpretation*. Philadelphia: Lea & Febiger, 1987.

29

Injuries to the Chest

OBJECTIVES FOR CHAPTER 29

After reading this chapter, the student should be able to:

1. Recognize the signs and symptoms of chest injuries.
2. Understand the various types of chest injuries and their resulting complications.
3. Know how to provide emergency medical treatment for chest injuries.

INTRODUCTION

Chest injuries may result from automobile accidents or gunshot or stab wounds. They may also occur with falls, blows, or compression on the athletic field. Whatever their cause, injuries to the chest are serious because of the likelihood of internal bleeding or direct injury of the heart or lungs. Unless they are properly and promptly treated, chest injuries may be fatal. Chapter 29 begins by classifying chest injuries as open or closed. The chapter lists the signs and symptoms of chest injuries and the initial steps that should be taken by trainers who must respond to a possible chest injury. The rest of the chapter discusses types of chest injuries and the conditions that can result from chest injuries. ■

CLASSIFICATION OF CHEST INJURIES

Chest injuries are divided into two categories: open and closed. In **open chest injuries**, the chest wall has been penetrated, as by a knife, bullet, or sharp piece of equipment. Open chest injuries may also be associated with severe rib fractures where the broken end of the rib has lacerated the chest wall and the skin. These injuries may be concurrent with contusions or lacerations of the heart, lungs, or major blood vessels.

In **closed chest injuries**, the skin is not broken. However, major damage from fractured ribs or a contusion may exist within the chest. The heart or lungs may be lacerated. Serious closed chest injuries include compression of the chest and severe contusions, such as might result from the blunt trauma of hitting a steering wheel, being struck by a thrown object, or being buried in a football pileup.

SIGNS AND SYMPTOMS OF CHEST INJURIES

The following are important signs of chest injuries, either open or closed:

- Pain at the site of the injury.
- Pleuritic pain aggravated by or occurring with breathing, localized around the site of a chest injury.
- Dyspnea (difficult or painful respiration).
- Failure of one or both sides of the chest to expand normally with inspiration.
- Hemoptysis (coughing up blood).
- Shock (a rapid weak pulse and low blood pressure).
- Cyanosis (blue color) of the lips, fingertips, or fingernails from poor oxygenation of the circulating blood.

Pain

Pain in the chest at the site of an obvious fracture or bruise indicates an injury of the chest wall and perhaps lung damage. Pain aggravated by breathing or on inhalation indicates irritation of the pleural surfaces of the lung or the chest wall. Pleural irritation can result from some severe disease processes, as well as from injury.

Change in Respiratory Pattern

Any change in a person's normal breathing pattern is a particularly important sign of chest injury. A normal, uninjured person breathes from 6 to 20 times a minute without difficulty and without pain, depending on his or her level of physical fitness. Very well trained athletes usually breathe very slowly with large tidal volumes of air. Respiratory rates in excess of 24 per minute are in the range of distress.

Dyspnea

The depth of respiration and difficulty in taking a breath are reliable indicators of respiratory distress. Difficulty in breathing is called **dyspnea**, and it may result from several causes. In the injured individual, it may arise because the chest cannot expand properly, the person has lost normal nervous system control of breathing, the airway is obstructed, or the lung itself is being compressed from within the chest by accumulated blood or air.

Loss of Chest Wall Muscle Function

It is extremely important to observe whether the chest wall fails to expand when the athlete inhales. This failure indicates that the muscles of the chest have lost the ability to act appropriately. Such loss of muscular function may result from a direct injury of the chest wall itself, from a severe injury of the nerves controlling the chest wall, or from a severe brain injury.

Hemoptysis

Hemoptysis (coughing up blood) usually indicates that the lung has been lacerated. In such cases, blood enters the bronchial passages within the lungs and is promptly coughed up as the person tries to clear the passages.

Shock

Shock is a state of inadequate circulatory perfusion, which means that not enough oxygen is reaching the tissues of organs because of inadequate blood flow to the organs. Shock may be caused by damage to the heart muscle, loss of circulating blood volume, or dilation of the peripheral vascular system. (See Chapter 38 for a more detailed discussion of shock.)

Cyanosis

Cyanosis (blue color around the lips, fingernails, or fingertips) indicates that blood is being insufficiently oxygenated. Finding cyanosis in an individual with severe injuries means the person is unable to bring adequate oxygen to the blood through the lungs. Therefore, a chest injury should be suspected.

INITIAL CARE OF CHEST INJURIES

Chest injuries occur because of the possibility of internal bleeding or direct injury to the heart or lungs. Since the body has no capacity to store oxygen, any injury that seriously interferes with the constant replenishment of oxygen through normal breathing must be treated without delay. Therefore, emergency medical care of all chest injuries is directed at making sure the athlete is able to breathe and is adequately ventilated. The trainer should perform the following steps in sequence when treating an athlete with a chest injury:

1. Clear and maintain the airway.
2. Use supplemental oxygen and be prepared to administer respiratory support promptly with mechanical aids or mouth-to-mouth breathing.
3. Observe and record vital signs every 5 minutes.
4. Control all obvious external bleeding.
5. Promptly cover penetrating wounds into the chest cavity.
6. Carefully monitor the effect of treatment and be ready to institute changes, transport rapidly, or offer resuscitation promptly. A person's status may deteriorate very rapidly after a chest injury, or the person may stabilize and respond to support very well.
7. Transport the athlete promptly to the emergency department, and if possible, notify the hospital in advance about the type and severity of the injury.

TYPES OF CHEST INJURIES

Rib Fractures

Rib fractures are usually caused by direct blows or compression injuries of the chest. The upper four ribs are rarely fractured, since they are protected by the shoulder girdle (scapula and clavicle). The fifth through the ninth ribs are those most commonly fractured. The lower two ribs (eleventh and twelfth) are harder to fracture because they are attached only to the thoracic vertebrae and have greater freedom of movement.

Symptoms

The common finding in all individuals with fractured ribs is pain localized at the site of the fracture. Asking the athlete to place a finger on the exact area of the pain often determines the location of the injury. There may or may not be a rib deformity, a chest wall contusion, or a laceration. Deep breathing, coughing, or movement is usually very painful. The athlete generally wants to remain still and may often lean toward the injured side, covering the fractured area with a hand to prevent the chest from moving and to ease local pain.

X-rays are usually taken to confirm rib fractures. Initially, however, nondisplaced single rib fractures may be difficult to visualize radiographically, and the athlete may need repeat films in several weeks if the symptoms persist. If shortness of breath is associated with localized rib tenderness, a standard chest x-ray is typically ordered to make certain there is not an associated pneumothorax (air inside the chest cavity) or hemothorax (blood inside the chest cavity) from a fractured rib puncturing or lacerating a lung or the lining of the chest cavity. These two conditions may result from chest injuries and are discussed later in this chapter.

Treatment

Simple rib fractures ordinarily are not bound, strapped, or taped. For an athlete who has multiple fractures and is considerably more comfortable with the chest immobilized, the best bandage is a swathe in which the arm is strapped to the chest to limit motion on the injured side (Fig. 29.1). A swathe of the arm with the forearm in a sling is most effective in immobilizing the

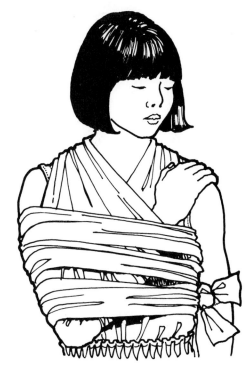

FIGURE 29.1. In multiple rib fractures, a swathe will immobilize injuries.

chest. It may be necessary to immobilize both arms if the fractures are on both sides. Traditionally, wide strips of adhesive plaster were often used to immobilize the chest wall in order to lessen the person's discomfort. However, the tight bandage of adhesive plaster applied to the skin of the thorax acts as an unyielding corset and hinders whatever expansion the injured chest can achieve. It is better to help the individual to breathe than to try to make the person more comfortable by not allowing the chest to expand.

Occasionally, the end of a fractured rib may puncture or lacerate the lung or the skin of the chest wall (Fig. 29.2). In such an instance, some degree of pneumothorax or hemothorax usually occurs (Fig. 29.3).

Flail Chest

When three or more ribs break, each in two places, the segment of the chest wall lying between the breaks will collapse rather than

A Laceration of chest wall

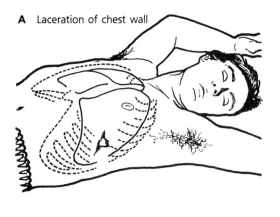

A Pneumothorax

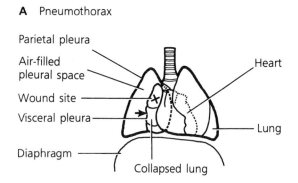

B Perforation of lung

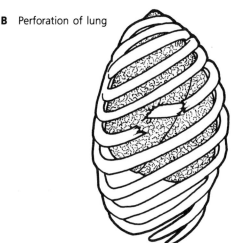

FIGURE 29.2. Fracture of the rib may cause the end of a fractured rib to (a) lacerate the skin of the chest wall or (b) perforate the lung.

B Hemothorax

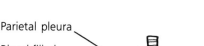
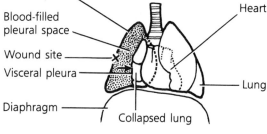

C Hemopneumothorax

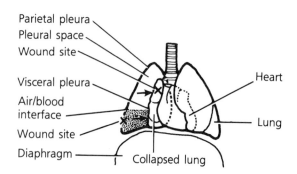

FIGURE 29.3. (a) A pneumothorax is a collection of air in the pleural space between the visceral and parietal pleural surfaces. (b) A hemothorax is a collection of blood in the pleural space between the visceral and parietal pleural surfaces. (c) When hemothorax occurs in conjunction with a pneumothorax, it is called a hemopneumothorax.

expand normally with the chest wall on each inhalation. When the individual exhales, this segment protrudes while the rest of the chest wall contracts. The motion of the segment is paradoxical because it is opposite to the normal movement of the chest wall, and is therefore called **paradoxical motion**. The portion of the chest wall lying between the fractures is called the **flail segment** (Fig. 29.4a). Several terms, such as *crushed chest* or *stove-in chest*, are used to describe this injury, but the proper term is **flail chest**. Ordinarily, the paradoxical motion of the flail segment produces considerable pain.

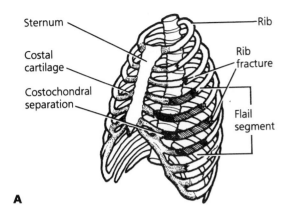

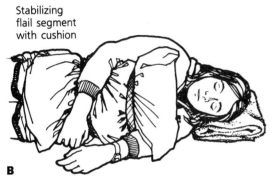

FIGURE 29.4. (a) Flail chest segment and (b) stabilization with cushion.

Flail chest is a particularly serious injury. Obviously, the lung immediately underneath the flail segment does not expand properly on inhalation, and the person loses that amount of available lung volume. Much more important, however, is that the degree of force exerted on the chest wall needed to fracture several ribs and produce a flail chest segment is almost always enough to cause severe contusion damage, or bruising, of the lung itself underneath the flail segment. The contusion injury of the lung may be far more serious than it appears.

Symptoms

Flail chest is relatively easy to diagnose through observation. The chest does not rise properly despite the person's desperate efforts to inhale deeply. In some people, signs indicating lack of oxygen follow rap-

idly. In an acute situation, immediately after injury, the major factor limiting adequate respiration is pain on breathing.

Treatment

The athlete with a flail chest may breathe more comfortably if positioned with the fractured ribs down or against a bed rail. The athlete who has a central flail segment with a fracture of the sternum and fractures in either hemithorax may hug a pillow to help stabilize the segment when motion causes pain (see Fig. 29.4b). Occasionally, sandbags are propped against the chest wall to lessen paradoxical motion and pain. If breathing is inadequate, and especially if cyanosis is present, the trainer must assist respiration and give supplemental oxygen if it is available. Oxygen should be started promptly, since individuals with flail chest may die quickly without it. The trainer must assist respiration and maintain it until arrival at the hospital. These athletes must be transported as promptly as possible.

Compression Injuries

Injuries of the chest can result from sudden **circumferential compression** of the chest and an accompanying rapid increase in intrathoracic pressure. Multiple rib fractures can occur along with a flail chest. In extreme instances of circumferential compression, the upper part of the body may be cyanotic (bluish) as well as edematous (swollen), the neck veins distended, and the eyes bulging.

Injuries to the Chest Wall

Injuries to the chest wall, other than rib fractures, are usually muscle strains, contusions, abrasions, lacerations, or penetrating wounds. Penetrating wounds present with pain and tenderness locally at the wound site. They should be examined for impaled or embedded objects. Such objects should not be removed. Impaled objects may be cut off, if necessary, a few inches from the skin for more comfortable transportation to the emergency department. Individuals with penetrating injuries should always be checked for an injury of the spine (see Chapter 32). While awaiting emergency transport, the athlete may be more comfortable in a prone position; however, the preference for this posture varies from person to person.

A bad contusion, hemorrhage, or laceration over the posterior region of the shoulder should raise the possibility of a scapula fracture (see Chapter 16). Major injuries to the back of the chest may also cause pulmonary contusion or any of the previously discussed problems within the thorax.

Costochondral and Costosternal Injuries

A direct blow to the anterior region of the chest, which can occur in sports such as rugby, skiing, football, and boxing, can cause either sternal fracture or costochondral injury, with or without separation. The costochondral region is very tender, and chest motion causes sharp pain. The athlete may feel the rib "slipping out" and/or a snapping sensation. Despite seeming to be minor, these injuries heal slowly, and usually the athlete is unable to participate for 4 to 6 weeks.

CONDITIONS RESULTING FROM CHEST INJURIES

Open or closed injuries to the chest may result in pneumothorax, hemothorax, hemopneumothorax (a combination of hemothorax and pneumothorax), subcutaneous emphysema, pulmonary contusion, myocardial contusion, pericardial tamponade, or dyspnea.

Pneumothorax

Pneumothorax refers to the presence of air within the chest cavity in the pleural space, but outside the lung (see Fig. 29.3a). In this condition, the lung separates from the chest wall and is said to be collapsed. The volume of the lung is diminished, and so the amount of air that can be inhaled to exchange oxygen and carbon dioxide with the blood is reduced. Hypoxia (oxygen deficiency) follows, and as the degree of pneumothorax increases, respiratory distress becomes evident.

Pneumothorax can occur if air enters the chest directly through a sucking wound open to the outside. In an intact chest, it can also occur if air leaks out from a lung that has been lacerated by a fractured rib. In pneumothorax, the normal mechanism by which the lung expands—that is, capillary adhesion to the inside of the chest wall—is lost, and the affected, or collapsed, lung cannot expand with inhalation. In athletes with an open wound of the chest, the trainer can minimize the amount of pneumothorax by rapidly sealing the hole prior to transportation.

Spontaneous Pneumothorax

Some people have congenitally weak areas on the surface of their lungs. Occasionally, this weak area will rupture, allowing air to leak into the pleural space. Such an event, called **spontaneous pneumothorax**, is not usually related to any major trauma and commonly occurs while the individual is sitting quietly. When the air leakage is significant, the person experiences a sudden sharp chest pain and increasing difficulty in breathing. The affected lung collapses and loses its ability to expand normally.

All degrees of spontaneous pneumothorax exist. Some people notice no particular discomfort or difficulty in breathing, while others require emergency transportation to the hospital because of respiratory distress. In the latter instance, the trainer will not be called on to make a diagnosis but must administer respiratory support while transporting the athlete promptly to the emergency department.

Tension Pneumothorax

If a spontaneous pneumothorax fails to seal when the lung collapses, a **tension pneumo-**

thorax might develop. In this condition, air continuously leaks out of the lung into the pleural space, expanding the space with every breath the athlete takes (Fig. 29.5). Hence, with each breath the affected lung collapses more, until it is completely reduced to a small ball, 2 or 3 inches in diameter.

At this time, pressure in the affected side of the chest cavity begins to rise, and the collapsed lung presses against the heart and the opposite lung. The remaining lung in turn now begins to compress. As the pressure in the chest cavity rises, the pressure may exceed the normal pressure of blood in veins returning to the heart. Blood can then no longer travel back to the heart to be pumped out. Death can follow rapidly.

Tension pneumothorax is not limited to closed chest injuries. An athlete with a fractured rib who has sustained a sucking chest wound (discussed later in this section) may also have a severe lung laceration. If the external wound is effectively bandaged and thus sealed and the lung continues to leak, a tension pneumothorax may develop. The condition cannot exist without an intact or well-sealed chest wall.

The signs of tension pneumothorax are severe, rapidly progressive respiratory distress; a weak pulse; fall in blood pressure; bulging of the tissue in the chest wall between the ribs and above the clavicle; distension of the veins in the neck; and cyanosis. The diagnosis is best made by a physician, who can immediately relieve the tension in the chest by passing a large-bore, 13- or 14-gauge hypodermic needle through the chest wall into the chest cavity to release the built-up air. The athlete will require ventilatory support, although relief of the tension within the chest often allows normal or near normal respiration to return immediately. For the athlete with a bandaged chest wound and a tension pneumothorax, simple release of the dressing is often effective.

It must be emphasized that tension pneumothorax is one of the very few true minute-by-minute emergencies. Prompt treat-

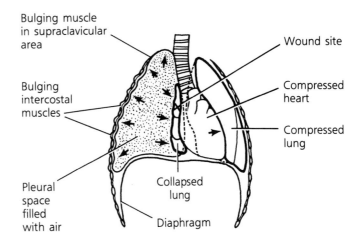

Tension pneumothorax

FIGURE 29.5. Air collects in pleural space, creating a tension pneumothorax.

ment can save the athlete's life. People with severe tension pneumothorax can die in a very few minutes.

Hemothorax

Hemothorax refers to the presence of blood in the chest cavity within the pleural space, outside the lung (see Fig. 29.3b). Hemothorax may occur in open or closed chest injuries and frequently accompanies a pneumothorax, in which case it is called a **hemopneumothorax** (see Fig. 29.3c). The bleeding may come from lacerated vessels in the chest wall, from lacerated major vessels within the chest cavity itself, or (rarely) from a lacerated lung. If bleeding in the chest is severe, the athlete may show signs of shock from blood loss. Shock (see Chapter 38) is manifested by pallor; apprehension; cold, clammy skin; chills; a rapid, weak pulse; a fall in blood pressure; and thirst.

Hemothorax, like pneumothorax, fills the chest up with something other than the lung. Normal lung expansion cannot occur, and the lung compresses and loses its volume. Less air can be inhaled, and there may be substantially less blood to carry the reduced amount of oxygen available to the organs of the body.

The athlete with hemothorax requires immediate ventilatory support, administration of oxygen, and control of obvious bleeding by means of pressure dressings. The athlete must then be transported promptly to the emergency facility.

Sucking Chest Wounds

In open chest injuries, air enters the chest cavity through the wound when the person inhales and the chest expands in the normal respiratory cycle (Fig. 29.6a). Ordinarily, the pressure inside the chest cavity is maintained at somewhat less than atmospheric pressure. Inhalation markedly reduces this pressure.

When the chest cavity has been opened, air moves through the wound just as it moves through the nose and mouth during normal respiration. This air remains outside the lung in the pleural space to create the conditions of a pneumothorax, and the lung's function is compromised. Air passes back through the wound to the outside when the person exhales, and pressure within the thorax rises. Such an open chest wound is called a **sucking chest wound** because of a sucking sound at the wound caused by the passage of air through it each time the person breathes.

As an initial emergency step, it is imperative that a sucking chest wound be sealed with an airtight dressing (see Fig. 29.6b–c). Several sterile materials may be used, such as sterile aluminum foil, Vaseline gauze, or a folded universal dressing held in place by a pressure dressing. The size of the dressing must be large enough so that the dressing itself does not get sucked into the chest cavity.

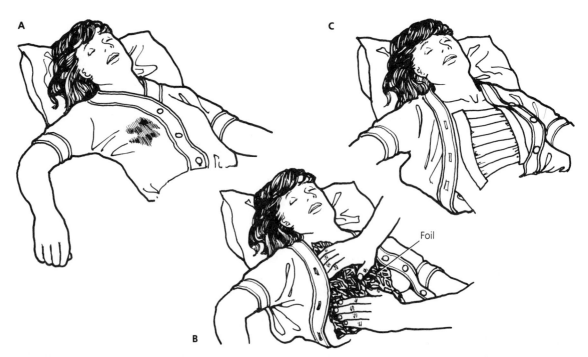

FIGURE 29.6. (a) A sucking chest wound allows free passage of air from the outside to the pleural space. (b) This wound must be sealed promptly with an airtight or impermeable sterile material such as foil. (c) Final bandaging over the seal prevents air from entering the chest through the wound.

Subcutaneous Emphysema

If a lung laceration from a fractured rib has allowed air to escape into the tissues of the chest wall, the trainer will feel a crackling sensation under his or her fingertips when the area of the fracture is examined. The name given to this finding is **subcutaneous emphysema**. In very severe instances, it can involve the entire chest, neck, and face. It indicates that air is being forced out of the lung into the tissues and confirms the presence of fractured ribs and a lacerated lung. An athlete with subcutaneous emphysema should be transported as quickly as possible to the hospital for further observation and evaluation.

Pulmonary Contusion

A **pulmonary contusion** is a bruise of the lung. It behaves in much the same way as bruises of any other tissues in the body. The blood vessels in the lung are injured, and a considerable amount of blood escapes into the lung tissue. Depending on the size of the pulmonary contusion, the person may or may not be in respiratory distress. Pulmonary contusions are almost uniformly associated with blunt injuries of the chest seen in automobile accidents, severe falls, or a direct blow that may occur in contact sports.

Pulmonary contusions may not develop until several hours following an injury. They should be suspected in an athlete who develops shortness of breath or rapid respiration following a direct blow to the chest. Some pulmonary contusions, however, are so severe initially that the athlete is in respiratory distress almost from the moment of injury. Severe chest contusions may require ventilatory support with supplemental oxygen. If the pulmonary contusion is associated with several rib fractures, artificial ventilation may be required. A physician should immediately evaluate any athlete who complains of shortness of breath or pain with breathing, or whose pulse increases or respiratory rate increases or decreases following a chest injury.

Myocardial Contusion

Blunt injuries of the chest (such as a blow to the chest from a softball, baseball, or helmet) may produce a **myocardial contusion**, which is a bruise of the heart muscle itself. This injury may not be detectable without fairly sophisticated laboratory and electrocardiographic studies. Ordinarily, a severe myocardial contusion disturbs the electrical conduction system that controls the heart rate. In such circumstances, the heart is said to be "irritable." The signs of such injuries are extra heartbeats, which irregularly interrupt the normal pulse rhythm so the athlete has an irregular pulse with occasional pauses and occasional beats coming very close together. The trainer cannot treat this condition but should note the pulse. A physician should immediately evaluate any athlete with rapid or altered pulse or chest pain.

Pericardial Tamponade

In **pericardial tamponade**, blood or other fluid is present in the pericardial sac outside the heart, exerting an unusual pressure on the heart itself. This condition almost always results from gunshot or stab wounds of the heart that have opened one of the heart chambers so that blood leaks out each time the heart beats. The pericardial sac that encloses the heart is a very tough, fibrous membrane and cannot expand suddenly. When blood leaks out of the heart, it is caught within this unyielding sac; as it accumulates within the pericardial cavity, the blood compresses the heart so that its chambers can no longer accommodate the blood normally returned to them through the veins. This pressure must be relieved or death will occur very rapidly.

The signs of pericardial tamponade are very soft, faint heart tones (hard to hear even with a stethoscope), a weak pulse, blood pressure readings in which the systolic and diastolic pressures become closer with successive readings, and congested and distended veins in the upper part of the body. The athlete with pericardial tamponade will require very vigorous emergency respiratory support with ventilatory assistance and oxygen.

The trainer who observes or suspects pericardial tamponade must transport the athlete to the emergency department as soon as possible. The trainer should, if possible, call ahead to advise the hospital of the type of injury and the athlete's status. An emergency operation may be necessary.

Dyspnea

The state of difficult or labored breathing is called dyspnea. It is a serious condition and may be terrifying to the athlete. Dyspnea can result from either trauma or disease. Some specific causes include the following:

- The flow of air in the trachea and the bronchial tubes may be obstructed, as in many instances of trauma, by aspirated vomitus or blood or foreign bodies in the throat or windpipe.
- Air may not pass easily into or out of the air sacs in the lung, as is the case with athletes who suffer from asthma or other allergic reactions, because of spasm in the airways themselves. Generally, in this instance it is far easier to inhale than to exhale.
- A lung may be collapsed and unable to expand, as in spontaneous or tension pneumothorax or hemothorax.
- The air sacs in the lungs themselves may have become inelastic and may

no longer be responsive to the normal motions of breathing (emphysema).
- The lungs may be filled with fluid because the heart muscle has failed and is no longer able to circulate the volume of blood presented to it (pulmonary edema).

The athlete who experiences sudden dyspnea may become terrified as well as exhausted from simply struggling to breathe. The trainer must handle this person firmly and calmly and make immediate arrangements for transport to the emergency department. While awaiting arrival of the transport vehicle, the trainer should follow these steps.

1. Make certain that the airways are clear of blood, vomitus, and other foreign materials.
2. If the athlete is unconscious, support the tongue so that it does not obstruct the airway.
3. If oxygen is available, administer by mask.
4. Assist the conscious athlete to find a comfortable position for breathing. This position may be semi-reclining. When dyspnea is the result of cardiac failure, a sitting position may be best.
5. Try to find out the possible causes of the attack if an injury is not immediately apparent. Causes can include asthma, heart disease, allergy, or aspiration of foreign material.

IMPORTANT CONCEPTS

1. Chest injuries may be open (the chest wall penetrated) or closed (the skin not broken but injury inside the chest).
2. The signs of chest injury are pain at the site of injury, pleuritic pain, dyspnea, loss of chest wall muscle function, hemoptysis, shock, and cyanosis.
3. Emergency medical care of all chest injuries is directed at making sure the athlete can breathe and is properly ventilated.
4. The common finding of athletes with rib fractures is pain at the fracture site.
5. Flail chest is a very serious injury because the lung immediately under the flail segment does not expand properly on inhalation, and the person loses that amount of available lung volume.
6. In pneumothorax—the presence of air within the chest cavity in the pleural space but outside the lung—the lung separates from the chest wall and is said to be collapsed.
7. Hemothorax—the presence of blood in the chest cavity within the pleural space but outside the lung—frequently accompanies pneumothorax.
8. Subcutaneous emphysema indicates that air is being forced out of the lung into the tissues and confirms the presence of fractured ribs and a lacerated lung.
9. Pulmonary contusion—a bruise of the lung—can occur following a blunt injury to the chest and may require ventilatory support if severe.
10. Myocardial contusion—a bruise of the heart muscle—can disturb the heart rate.
11. In pericardial tamponade, blood or other fluid is present in the pericardial sac outside the heart. If the pressure of this fluid against the heart muscle is not relieved, death will occur rapidly.
12. The athlete who experiences sudden dyspnea may become terrified and exhausted from struggling to breathe.

SUGGESTED READINGS

Committee on Trauma, American College of Surgeons. *Early Care of the Injured Patient*, 3d ed. Philadelphia: W. B. Saunders, 1982.

Hughes, S., ed. *The Basis and Practice of Traumatology*. London: William Heinemann Medical Books, 1983.

Kirsh, M. M., and H. Sloan. *Blunt Chest Trauma: General Principles of Management*. Boston: Little, Brown, 1977.

Zuidema, G. D., R. B. Rutherford, and W. F. Ballinger, II, eds. *The Management of Trauma*, 3d ed. Philadelphia: W. B. Saunders, 1979.

P A R T

C

THE NERVOUS SYSTEM

30

Head Injuries

OBJECTIVES FOR CHAPTER 30

After reading this chapter, the student should be able to:

1. Briefly describe the anatomy of the head.
2. Explain the different injuries to the brain.
3. Perform an initial assessment of an athlete with a head injury and recognize which injuries need follow-up evaluation and would prevent the athlete from returning to competition.

INTRODUCTION

Most injuries sustained in sports do not result in catastrophic and irreversible damage, but the potential for injury to the brain is of utmost concern for those who care for the athlete. Chapter 30 begins with the anatomy of the head—the scalp, the skull, and the brain. The chapter then focuses on the most common head injuries, including cerebral concussions, contusions, and hematomas, and concludes with a discussion on assessing head injuries. ■

ANATOMY OF THE HEAD

The head is divided into two parts: the cranium and the face. The cranium is the area above an imaginary plane that passes across the top of the ears and eyes and separates the cranium from the face. The cranium is covered by the scalp. Inside the cranium lies the brain.

The Scalp

The scalp serves as a protective coating for the bony structure of the head. Because of its mobility, the scalp allows for some dissipation of forces applied to the skull.

The scalp consists of four layers: hair, skin, subcutaneous connective tissue, and pericranium. Because the scalp has a rich blood supply, scalp and facial lacerations often bleed profusely. This bleeding can be controlled by applying a pressure bandage until a physician can evaluate the athlete. An x-ray is needed to diagnose any underlying skull fracture that may be associated with the formation of a hematoma (a lump that develops from the pool of blood that forms at the fracture site) between the scalp and the skull. Ice and pressure techniques can reduce a hematoma (see Chapter 25 for a more in-depth discussion of hematomas), but if an underlying skull fracture is suspected, pressure should be applied judiciously.

The Skull

The skull, or cranium, is a natural helmet. Its hard outer shell protects the soft brain inside a fluid-filled cushion. The bones of

the skull are united by sutures and synchondroses, which are the interdigitated

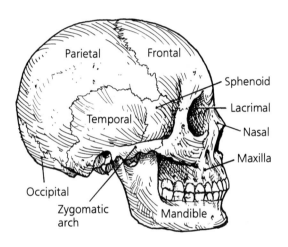

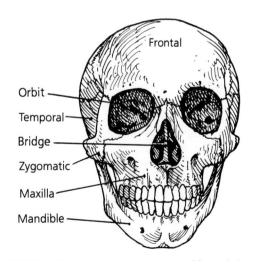

FIGURE 30.1. Anteroposterior and lateral views of the bones of the skull.

connections between the skull bones. The bones of the skull that compose the cranial cavity are the frontal, parietal, occipital, sphenoid, ethmoid, and temporal (Fig. 30.1). Of these, only the parietal and temporal are paired. The bones of the face and nasal cavities are the maxilla, zygomatic, palatine, nasal, lacrimal, inferior nasal concha, bridge, and mandible. Of these, only the bridge and mandible are unpaired.

The **foramen magnum** is the large aperture at the base of the skull through which the medulla and spinal cord pass and enter into the bony spinal canal in the neck (Fig. 30.2). The bones of the adult skull are constructed of firm outer and inner layers, or tables. Interspersed between these layers is softer bone, containing blood channels. Some of these larger vascular pathways are visible on skull x-ray films.

Whenever an athlete suffers a severe blow to the head, a skull fracture should be suspected. Although the incidence of these fractures is low, they are potentially serious injuries. Skull fractures may be described as depressed, linear, nondepressed, comminuted, and basal (Fig. 30.3). A **depressed skull fracture** occurs when the fracture causes a portion of the skull to be indented toward the brain, and **linear** and **nondepressed skull fractures** involve minimal in-

dentation of the skull toward the brain. A **comminuted skull fracture** involves multiple fracture fragments, and a **basal** or **basilar skull fracture** involves the base of the skull.

Skull fractures may be difficult to diagnose clinically. Even a depressed skull fracture may be confused clinically with a deep scalp hematoma. Therefore, x-ray evaluation is crucial for detection and management. In evaluating athletes who have sustained skull fractures, the physician must always consider associated brain injury.

The Brain

The Meninges

Layers of nonnervous tissue, collectively termed the **meninges** (Fig. 30.4), surround and protect the brain and spinal cord. These layers are the dura mater, arachnoid, and pia mater (nearest the brain). The **dura mater** is a tough, fibrous membrane that lies immediately internal to the bone. It contains venous channels, or sinuses, that carry blood from the brain to the veins in the neck. The dura mater covering the spinal cord is separated from the bone by the epidural space, which contains fat and many small veins.

The **arachnoid**, so-called because it resembles a spider web, is a thin, cellular

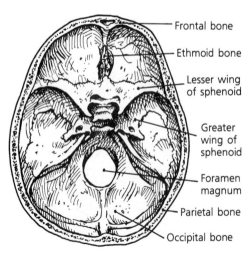

FIGURE 30.2.   Interior of the base of the skull.

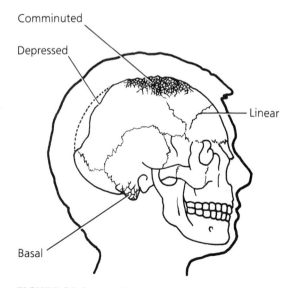

FIGURE 30.3.   Various types of skull fractures.

membrane that is separated from the dura mater by the thin subdural space. The arachnoid is very closely connected to the innermost meningeal layer, the **pia mater**, by a meshwork of connective tissue strands. The pia mater is a loose tissue that covers the brain and sheaths the blood vessels as they enter the brain. The space between the arachnoid and the pia mater is the subarachnoid space, which contains the cerebrospinal fluid. The arachnoid and pia mater are more widely separated from each other around the spinal cord than over the brain.

The Cerebrum

The largest part of the brain is the **cerebrum**, a large mass of nervous tissue distinguished by the folds or convolutions of much of its surface. The bulk of the brain is formed by two convoluted **cerebral hemispheres**. The **diencephalon** lies between the hemispheres and forms the upper part of the **brain stem**, the unpaired stalk or stem that descends from the base of the brain. The brain has four paired lobes—*frontal, parietal, occipital,* and *temporal*—plus the brain stem that connects the cerebral hemispheres with the spinal cord at the foramen magnum (Fig. 30.5).

The **cerebral cortex**, the outer part of the hemispheres, controls speech, motor, and sensory functions. The highest mental and behavioral activities of humans are functions of this portion of the brain. Only a few millimeters thick, the cerebral cortex is composed of gray matter, which largely consists of the bodies of nerve cells. In contrast, the interior of the cerebral hemispheres is composed partly of white matter, which consists largely of the processes or fibers of the nerve cells. This interior, which includes the diencephalon, also contains well-demarcated masses of gray matter, known collectively as **basal ganglia**.

The Cerebellum and Brain Stem

The **cerebellum**, sometimes called the "little brain," lies underneath the great mass of cerebral tissue. The cerebellum is important to the automatic regulation of move-

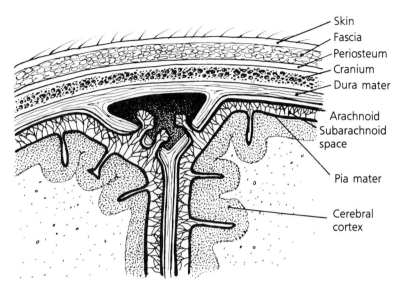

FIGURE 30.4.   The meninges protect the brain.

ment and posture, and it functions in concert with the cerebral cortex and the brain stem. It is a fissured mass of gray matter that occupies the posterior part of the cranium and is attached to the brain stem by three pairs of peduncles (stalks or bands). The cortex of the cerebellum, like that of the cerebral hemisphere, is composed mainly of white matter, although it also contains gray matter.

The brain stem contains the centers for the cranial nerves and nerves governing

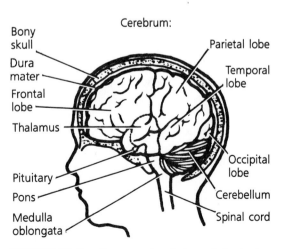

FIGURE 30.5.   Cross sectional view of the brain.

respiration, circulation, and other visceral activities. The brain stem contains nuclei in diffuse masses of gray matter.

Cerebrospinal Fluid

The **ventricles** (communicating cavities) of the brain contain a vascular portion of the pia mater, the **choroid plexus**, in which an almost protein-free **cerebrospinal fluid** forms. This fluid circulates through the ventricles, enters the subarachnoid space, and eventually filters back into the venous system (Fig. 30.6). Cerebrospinal fluid serves as a liquid cushion to minimize damage to the brain and spinal cord by protecting them from blows to the head and neck.

Pressure of the cerebrospinal fluid, when it is removed during a lumbar puncture or spinal tap, is usually between 100 and 200 millimeters of water (mm H_2O). Certain anesthetics, as well as contrast radiographic material for determining the positions of masses, tumors, ruptured discs, and displaced fracture fragments, can be administered into the space occupied by the fluid.

Cerebral Blood Supply

The cerebral branches of the vertebral and internal carotid arteries supply blood to the brain (Fig. 30.7), and the middle meningeal branch of the maxillary artery mainly supplies blood to the meninges. Vertebral arteries and segmental arteries supply the spinal cord and spinal roots, and a number of small branches along the course of the nerves supply the peripheral nerves.

Cranial Nerves

Twelve pairs of **cranial nerves** are special nerves associated with the brain (Fig. 30.8). The fibers in the cranial nerves are of two main functional types: some are composed primarily of sensory fibers, and some, primarily of motor fibers.

- Cranial Nerve I: *olfactory*—smell.
- Cranial Nerve II: *optic*—vision.
- Cranial Nerves III, IV, and VI: *oculomotor*, *trochlear*, and *abducens*—motor nerves controlling movement of the eyes.
- Cranial Nerve V: *trigeminal*—sensation of the head, face, and movement of the jaw.
- Cranial Nerve VII: *facial*—special

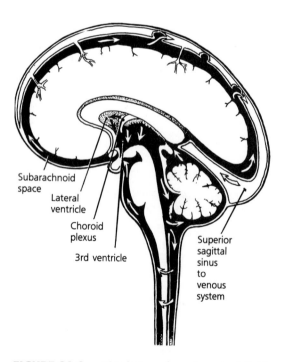

Subarachnoid space
Lateral ventricle
Choroid plexus
3rd ventricle
Superior sagittal sinus to venous system

FIGURE 30.6. Circulation of cerebrospinal fluid.

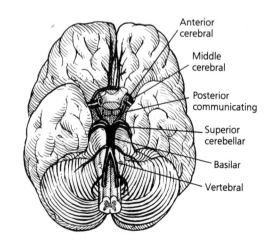

Anterior cerebral
Middle cerebral
Posterior communicating
Superior cerebellar
Basilar
Vertebral

FIGURE 30.7. Arterial circulation of the brain.

sensory, motor, and autonomic nervous components that allow taste, facial movements, and secretion of tears and saliva.

- Cranial Nerve VIII: *acoustic*—important in hearing (the cochlear part) and equilibrium (the vestibular part).
- Cranial Nerve IX: *glossopharyngeal*—sensory and motor components dealing with taste, sensation in the pharynx, and movement of the pharynx; autonomic function in secretion of saliva and sensory components in visceral reflexes.
- Cranial Nerve X: *vagus*—controls taste and sensation to the pharynx, larynx, and tracheobronchial tree; important in movements of the pharynx and larynx, secretions of the thoracic and abdominal viscera and visceral reflexes.
- Cranial Nerve XI: *spinal accessory*—motor nerve concerned with movements of the pharynx, larynx, head, and shoulders.
- Cranial Nerve XII: *hypoglossal*—primarily a motor nerve concerned with the movements of the tongue.

Medical students often learn these nerves with the mnemonic "On Old Olympus' Towering Tops, A Finn And Greek Viewed Some Hops" (olfactory, optic, oculomotor, trochlear, trigeminal, abducens, facial, acoustic, glossopharyngeal, vagus, spinal accessory, hypoglossal).

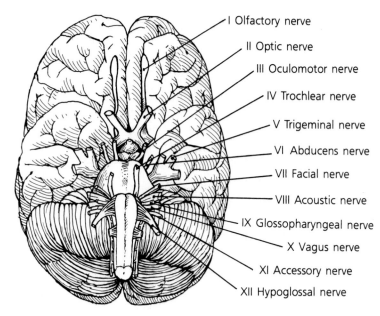

FIGURE 30.8.   The 12 cranial nerves.

INJURIES TO THE BRAIN

Cerebral Concussion

Cerebral concussion, a basic injury to the brain itself, can be classified by degree of severity: first-, second-, or third-degree concussion. These distinctions are important for treatment and prognosis. Some variations in the classification of concussions may be evident as the athlete consults different sources. Table 30.1 contains a brief comparison of the signs and symptoms of the three levels of cerebral concussions.

TABLE 30.1.   Three Levels of Cerebral Concussion

Level	Consciousness	Memory Loss	Dizziness	Tinnitus	Loss of Coordination	Recovery Time
I	No loss	May occur	May occur	May occur	No	Rapid
II	Momentary loss 10 seconds–5 minutes	Transient confusion; mild retrograde amnesia	Moderate	Moderate	May occur	Varies
III	Prolonged loss	Severe	Severe	Severe	Marked	Prolonged beyond 5 minutes

First-Degree Concussion

A **first-degree concussion**, the least severe, involves no loss of consciousness. The force of impact causes transient aberration in the electrophysiology of the brain substance, creating slight mental confusion. Memory loss, dizziness, and tinnitus (ringing in the ears) may occur, but there is no loss of coordination. Because of the rapid recovery rate, it is important to remember that an individual may suffer a minor concussion without losing consciousness.

Second-Degree Concussion

A momentary loss of consciousness results from a **second-degree concussion**. Unconsciousness may last from several seconds up to 5 minutes, and it can be associated with transient confusion, moderate dizziness, tinnitus, unsteadiness, and prolonged, mild retrograde amnesia (amnesia for the events prior to the injury). There is a wide range of findings between first- and third-degree concussions. Thus, second-degree concussions demand careful clinical observation and skillful judgment, especially regarding return to play at a later date.

Third-Degree Concussion

Third-degree concussions are more severe and result in prolonged loss of consciousness. Neuromuscular coordination is markedly compromised, with severe mental confusion, tinnitus, dizziness, and retrograde amnesia. Recovery is also prolonged beyond 5 minutes. Symptoms of concussion may be associated with more serious and progressive underlying brain injury.

Cerebral Contusion

The brain substance may suffer a **cerebral contusion** (bruising) when an object impacts with the skull or vice versa. The impact causes injured vessels to bleed internally, and there is a concomitant loss of consciousness. A cerebral contusion may be associated with partial paralysis or hemi-

plegia (paralysis of one side of the body), one-sided pupil dilation, or altered vital signs, and may last for a prolonged period of time. Progressive swelling may further endanger brain tissue not injured in the original trauma. Even with severe contusions, however, eventual recovery without intracranial surgery is usually the rule. The prognosis is often determined by the supportive care delivered from the moment of injury, including adequate ventilation and cardiopulmonary resuscitation if necessary (see Chapter 37 for basic life support techniques), proper transport techniques, and prompt expert evaluation.

Cerebral Hematoma

The skull fits the brain like a custom-made helmet, leaving little room for space-occupying lesions like blood clots. Blood clots, or **hematomas**, are of two types, epidural and subdural, depending on whether they are outside or inside the dura mater (Fig. 30.9).

Epidural Hematoma

An **epidural hematoma** in the athlete most commonly results from a severe blow to the

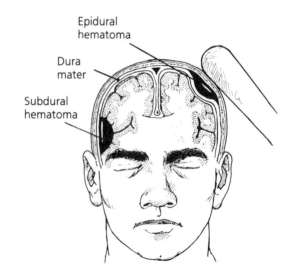

FIGURE 30.9. Epidural hematomas are blood clots outside the dura mater, and subdural hematomas are clots beneath the dura mater.

head that produces a skull fracture in the temporoparietal region. The middle meningeal artery may sever, producing an epidural hematoma. Ten to 20 minutes or longer may pass before the injured athlete's neurologic status begins to deteriorate. Immediate surgery may be required to decompress the hematoma and to control the bleeding artery.

Subdural Hematoma

The mechanism of the **subdural hematoma** is more complex. The force of a blow to the skull thrusts the brain against the point of impact. As a result, the subdural vessels on the opposite side of the brain tear, resulting in venous bleeding. As bleeding produces low pressure with slow clot formation, symptoms may not become evident until hours, days, or even weeks later, when the clot may absorb fluid and expand. Prolonged observation and monitoring are advised for any athlete who has suffered loss of consciousness or altered mental status, because additional bleeding may cause subsequent deterioration. Surgical intervention may be necessary to evacuate (drain) the hematoma and decompress the brain.

ASSESSING HEAD INJURIES

Initial Assessment

Head trauma in an athletic situation requires immediate assessment for appropriate emergency action (Table 30.2). The coach or trainer performs the initial evaluation of the athlete at the site of injury. The trainer observes respiration and cardiac status first. Next, the trainer determines the level of consciousness by asking the athlete simple questions directed toward orientation and then observing the athlete's response. After evaluating recent memory and assessing the voluntary response of muscle control in all extremities, the trainer briefly evaluates the appropriateness of response to pain and establishes whether the athlete has sensation in the extremities.

The athlete who is conscious or who was

TABLE 30.2.   Neural Watch Chart

Unit		Time
I Vital signs	Blood pressure	_____
	Pulse	_____
	Respiration	_____
	Temperature	_____
II Conscious and	Oriented	_____
	Disoriented	_____
	Restless	_____
	Combative	_____
III Speech	Clear	_____
	Rambling	_____
	Garbled	_____
	None	_____
IV Will awaken to	Name	_____
	Shaking	_____
	Light pain	_____
	Strong pain	_____
V Nonverbal reaction to pain	Appropriate	_____
	Inappropriate	_____
	"Decerebrate"	_____
	None	_____
VI Pupils	Size on right	_____
	Size on left	_____
	Reacts on right	_____
	Reacts on left	_____
VII Ability to move	Right arm	_____
	Left arm	_____
	Right leg	_____
	Left leg	_____

momentarily unconscious should be transported to the sidelines or locker room for further evaluation after the initial on-site evaluation. If the athlete is unconscious, moving and positioning should be done carefully, assuming possible associated cervical injury. A helmet does not have to be removed at this time unless in some way it compromises maintenance of adequate ventilation. Often an adequate airway can be maintained by just removing the face mask or strap. Any unconscious player must be moved with care, avoiding motion of the neck by gentle, firm support, and transported on a spine board.

Examination on the Sidelines

Once the athlete has regained consciousness and has been removed from the site of injury to an area where a more detailed examination can be conducted, a helmet can be removed (see Chapter 44 for helmet-removal instructions). The trainer can obtain a more complete history of exactly what happened, noting how the injured athlete recalls the events that caused the injury. By asking further questions, the trainer can determine the athlete's mental status. The motor functions should be examined in detail, including evaluation of strength, reflexes, and sensory and pain response. It is essential that the trainer document and record the initial findings and subsequent monitoring of any head-injured athlete.

Return to Competition After Head Injury

The question of return to competition after a head injury is handled on an individual basis, although conservatism seems the wisest course in all cases. The following are important factors to consider:

- The athlete's previous incidents of head trauma.

- Availability of experienced personnel to observe and monitor the athlete during recovery.
- Severity of the athlete's injury and potential for further neurologic deterioration.

After head trauma, the athlete should not be allowed to return to competition that day. In fact, before resuming training, a head-injured athlete must be free of headaches for 24 hours. Athletes who are unconscious for a period of time or those who have headaches require evaluation and monitoring by a physician. Although the majority of people with head trauma recover without any permanent neurologic deficit or need for surgery, major head trauma is potentially life-threatening. Following a mild concussion, an athlete who has been attended by experienced personnel, and whose status has been constantly monitored and reevaluated, may be allowed to return to competition.

The athlete who sustains repeated concussions requires special evaluation before returning to a sport with the potential for further brain injury. Most team physicians follow the "1-2-3 rule": one concussion and an athlete is out of the game; two concussions, out for the season; three concussions, he or she should no longer play.

IMPORTANT CONCEPTS

1. The scalp has a rich blood supply, and scalp lacerations often bleed profusely.
2. Skull fractures may be difficult to diagnose and may be confused clinically with a deep scalp hematoma.
3. Cerebral concussions are basic injuries to the brain itself and are classified by severity as first-, second-, or third-degree concussions.
4. Cerebral contusions occur when a head injury causes internal bleeding in the brain.
5. Cerebral hematomas are blood clots that form when the middle meningeal artery severs (epidural hematoma) or when subdural vessels tear and cause a clot to form several hours, days, or even weeks later (subdural hematoma).
6. Decisions about when and if a head-injured athlete can return to competition have to be made on an individual basis, depending on the athlete's prior incidents of head injury, the availability of experienced personnel to monitor recovery, and the severity of the injury.

SUGGESTED READINGS

Schneider, R. C. *Head and Neck Injuries in Football: Mechanisms, Treatment, and Prevention.* Baltimore: Williams & Wilkins, 1973.

Schneider, R. C., J. C. Kennedy, and M. L. Plant, eds. *Sports Injuries: Mechanisms, Prevention, and Treatment.* Baltimore: Williams & Wilkins, 1985.

Torg, J. S., ed. *Athletic Injuries to the Head, Neck, and Face.* Philadelphia: Lea & Febiger, 1982.

Youmans, J. R., ed. *Neurological Surgery: A Comprehensive Reference Guide to the Diagnosis and Management of Neurosurgical Problems,* 2d ed. Philadelphia: W. B. Saunders, 1982.

31

Soft Tissue Injuries of the Face and Neck

CHAPTER OUTLINE

Facial Fractures	Lacerations of the Mouth
Facial Bone Fractures	Injuries to the Eye
Nasal Fractures	Injuries to the Ear
Dental Injuries	Soft Tissue Injuries of the Neck

OBJECTIVES FOR CHAPTER 31

After reading this chapter, the student should be able to:

1. Describe the skeletal structures of the face and emergency care of fractures to the face.
2. Understand the initial treatment of dental injuries and subsequent evaluation.
3. Understand the treatment of mouth lacerations.
4. Describe the anatomy of the eye and recognize common eye injuries and their treatment.
5. Describe the anatomy of the ear and recognize common ear injuries and their treatment.
6. Describe common soft tissue injuries to the front of the neck.

INTRODUCTION

The face and neck are vulnerable to injury because of their relatively unprotected position, although face, mouth, and throat guards are used in several sports. Facial injuries are also commonly associated with head injuries. Chapter 31 discusses several types of facial injuries, including facial fractures, dental injuries, mouth lacerations, and injuries to the eyes and ears. The chapter also describes soft tissue injuries to the front of the neck from blunt trauma. ▪

FACIAL FRACTURES

The facial bones consist of the forehead, the orbits, the prominence of the cheek, the bony nose, and the upper and lower jaws. The **frontal bone** forms the skeleton of the forehead (Fig. 31.1). The **orbits** are the two bony cavities in which the eyes are situated. The **prominence of the cheek** is formed by the zygomatic bone. It is connected to a process from the temporal bone called the **zygomatic arch**. The upper jaw is composed of two **maxillae**, and the lower jaw consists of the **mandible**. The proximal one-third of the nose, the **bridge**, is formed by bone. The rest of the nose consists of cartilage.

Facial Bone Fractures

Facial bone fractures are often overlooked in evaluating the athlete with head trauma. Fractures may be masked by the severe swelling that often accompanies facial contusions or abrasions, as well as the inadequacy of conventional x-rays in demonstrating subtle fractures. Reduction of facial fractures is much easier in the initial hours following the injury than later. Special roentgenographic views should be obtained early on to obviate the need for technically difficult and unsatisfactory late reconstructive procedures.

Facial fractures are a common by-product of impact injuries, and they may result in severe deformities and bleeding, both of which can cause airway obstruction. Emergency care is directed at maintaining an airway and controlling hemorrhage. The application of direct pressure can often control bleeding. The trainer should check for bleeding sites inside the mouth and lacerations of the tongue. Blood that drains into the throat from cuts inside the mouth may cause vomiting and airway obstruction.

Depression of the zygomatic arch is only of cosmetic importance when it occurs as an isolated injury (Fig. 31.2). Zygomatic arch fractures can usually be easily reduced surgically and may not require internal fixation.

Fractures of the maxillae and mandible may not be obvious if undisplaced, but should be suspected with any irregularity in approximation of the teeth. Roentgenograms confirm the fracture, and reduction can often be accomplished by wiring the teeth or the bony fragments if no upper teeth are present. One crucial precaution with bilateral or comminuted mandibular

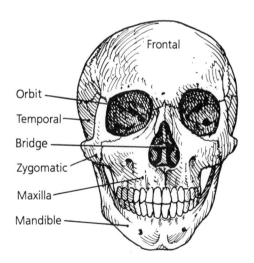

FIGURE 31.1.   The bones of the skull.

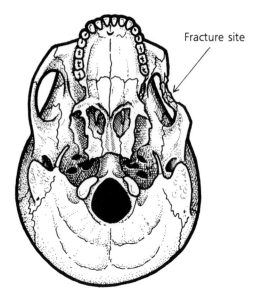

FIGURE 31.2. Compression fracture of the zygomatic arch.

fractures is to secure the airway by drawing the tongue forward (see Chapter 37). A physician may need to perform a tracheotomy if the airway cannot be secured.

Nasal Fractures

Nasal fractures are the most common facial bone fracture. They are usually recognized by palpation of the bony structures of the nose. Bleeding is profuse and may be controlled by placing an ice pack over the nose, pinching the nostrils when tolerable, or packing the nostrils with gauze. A simple nasal fracture may mean only several days' disability if a nose guard is worn, and the athlete may be allowed to return to play, depending on the discretion of the team physician.

Hemorrhage around the septal cartilage of the nose may result in necrosis (death of living tissue). Nasal fractures with septal deviation (deformity between the nasal passages) often require special treatment to prevent later problems with nasal breathing. Fractures involving the nasal cartilage as well as the bone may require packing and external and internal fixation with wires and a splint.

Fractures of the posterior aspect of the nose, which are difficult to see on x-ray films, may result in leakage of cerebrospinal fluid from the nose. The athlete with this condition has a serious problem and should be evaluated by a physician.

DENTAL INJURIES

The teeth may become loosened, chipped, or completely knocked out (avulsed) during sports activity. Capping of chipped teeth can prevent devitalization. Even loosened teeth, when still viable, can be preserved by wiring them to adjacent teeth.

If possible, the trainer should immediately replant an avulsed tooth in its socket or place it under the athlete's tongue for safekeeping if the athlete is alert and cooperative and can be trusted not to swallow the tooth. If replantation is not possible, the athletic trainer should pick the tooth up by the enamel (avoiding the root) and place it in a plastic container (with a securely fitting top) containing a preservation medium such as whole milk, saliva, or sterile saline solution. In all cases of an avulsed or damaged tooth, the athlete and the tooth should be taken to a dentist as soon as possible for treatment.

When teeth are injured by facial trauma, associated maxillary or mandibular fractures must be suspected. On the field, the trainer should palpate the gingiva and underlying bony structures directly. Barring secondary infection or retained root fragments, an athlete who has suffered trauma isolated to the teeth can generally expect rapid recovery. Athletes who have already suffered injuries to the teeth should be encouraged to wear mouth protection (see Chapter 44).

LACERATIONS OF THE MOUTH

Aside from injuries to the teeth, the most common injury to the mouth is contusion or laceration of the lip. Proper repair of lip lacerations requires exact alignment of the vermilion border, the junction of the mucous membrane and skin. Lacerations that extend completely through the lip may bleed profusely and require special suturing techniques. When loss of lip substance is excessive, the physician will refer the athlete to a plastic surgeon for immediate reconstructive flap surgery.

The only other mucous membrane lacerations of serious consequence in this region are those involving the opening of the submaxillary or parotid ducts. The parotid duct is located opposite the crown of the upper second molar tooth. The submaxillary duct opens in one to three ducts at the base of the tongue. In these cases, the physician will identify the duct, open it with a small plastic catheter, and do the repair.

Lacerations of the tongue usually result from forcible contact with the teeth. These lacerations require careful suturing to minimize scar formation and should be evaluated by a physician. A badly scarred tongue is apt to be sensitive and uncomfortable and may interfere with proper speech patterns. A physician should examine the undersurface of the tongue to determine the full extent of any lacerations.

All mouth lacerations should be monitored and require special attention to mouth hygiene. Initially, tongue lacerations should be cleaned with a water or a mouthwash gargle. Until the laceration has closed, which usually occurs within 24 hours, only liquids should be taken.

The period of disability for mouth injuries is usually brief. Most mouth injuries are preventable through the use of properly fitted mouth guards, which should be mandatory.

INJURIES TO THE EYE

The orbit of the eye is composed of the lower edge of the frontal bone of the skull, the maxilla, and the nasal bone. The bony orbit helps protect the eye from injury.

The front of the eye is covered by the **eyelid**, which contains the eyelashes and the conjunctiva (Fig. 31.3). The **eyeball** is a sphere approximately 1 inch in diameter. The **cornea** is the surface that covers the

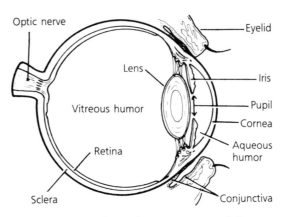

FIGURE 31.3. The major components of the eye.

front of the eye; it is clear and transparent so light can enter the eye. **Sclera** is the tough white tissue that covers the rest of the eye. The **iris**, which is visible through the cornea, regulates the amount of light that enters the eye. The space between the iris and the cornea is called the **anterior chamber**; it is filled with fluid called **aqueous humor**. In the center of the iris is a hole called the **pupil**. Behind the iris is the crystalline lens that focuses light onto the retina. The **retina** is a layer of cells on the back of the eye that changes the light image into electric impulses that can be carried by the optic nerve to the brain. The inner cavity of the eye is filled with a clear gel called the **vitreous humor**.

The eye is most commonly injured by a foreign body. The offending object should be carefully removed by thoroughly washing the eye with sterile saline solution or using copious amounts of a commercially available irrigating solution such as Dacriose. On occasion, removal of the foreign body requires inversion of the upper lid (Fig. 31.4). If the foreign body is suspected to have caused a corneal abrasion, a physician, using special lighting and a fluorescein solution instilled into the eye, will inspect the cornea carefully. If small corneal abrasions are detected, the physician will apply an antibiotic ointment and order an eye patch to be worn for a period of time. The pain of a corneal abrasion often can be

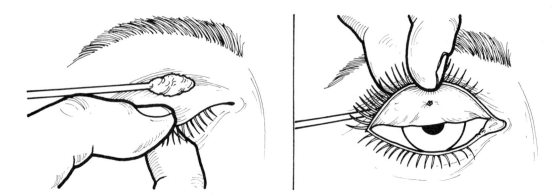

FIGURE 31.4. Removal of a foreign body by inversion of the upper lid. Holding the lid and stick in place with one hand, the examiner uses a sterile cotton swab to lift out the foreign body.

relieved by the one-time use of proparacaine ointment (0.5 percent) instilled locally into the eye by eyedropper.

The eye is subject to inflammatory conditions as well as trauma. Cortisporin ophthalmic suspension is effective in relieving inflammation, but these steroid-containing solutions should be avoided in cases of infectious conjunctivitis ("pink eye"), either bacterial or viral. Bacterial conjunctivitis can be effectively treated with Neosporin ophthalmic solution (or ointment) or sodium sulfacetamide ointment or solution instilled locally into the eye. Larger abrasions, penetrating injuries, contusions, or lacerations of the eye itself require immediate medical care, and the athlete should be transported promptly to the nearest appropriate facility. A direct blow to the eye may cause detachment of the retina.

Hyphema, or bleeding into the anterior chamber of the eye, is a serious eye injury caused by trauma. This injury can be diagnosed by examining the pupil with a small flashlight and observing a red discoloration. Comparing the suspect eye with the normal eye helps in making the diagnosis. The athlete must completely rest the affected eye and consult with an ophthalmologist.

Another frequent injury is eyelid contusion, more commonly known as "black eye." Early application of ice may limit swelling. Disability is limited to 1 to 2 days because of the body's rapid absorption of the swelling. Lid laceration, particularly in the region of the tear ducts, may require special suturing techniques, necessitating referral to an eye surgeon.

If the bones surrounding the eye are fractured, the eye may actually descend into the maxillary sinus, resulting in diplopia (double vision) and occasionally even a blowout fracture (fracture of the orbit or the bones that support the floor of the orbit). Treatment for orbital fracture includes open reduction and possibly internal fixation.

Fractures of the medial wall of the orbit may violate the ethmoid sinus. This may result in puffiness around the nose and eye, which increases markedly after blowing the nose. The athlete must be cautioned against this, and appropriate antibiotics instituted.

INJURIES TO THE EAR

The ear, whose functions include hearing and equilibration, is composed of three portions: external, middle, and internal (Fig. 31.5). The external ear consists of the **auricle** and the **external acoustic meatus.** The middle ear consists of the **tympanic membrane** and **auditory ossicles.** The internal ear comprises a series of complicated, fluid-filled spaces known as the **labyrinth.**

Foreign bodies are less common in the ear than in the eye and are usually harmless.

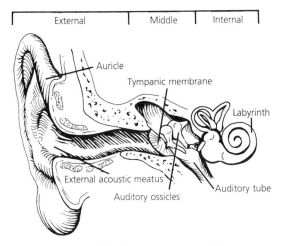

External | Middle | Internal

Auricle

Tympanic membrane

Labyrinth

External acoustic meatus

Auditory ossicles

Auditory tube

FIGURE 31.5. The basic structure of the ear.

Occasionally, water may be retained in the ear canal after swimming or bathing. Most foreign bodies in the ear are easily removed with the aid of a speculum, a device used by a physician to open the external auditory canal. The tympanic membrane itself may rupture (commonly referred to as a ruptured eardrum) as a result of a blow to the head, pressure changes, or infection. Barring complications following a tympanic membrane rupture, the disability is usually minor, but referral to an otorhinolaryngologist is suggested for further evaluation.

Basilar skull fractures may be associated with bleeding behind the tympanic membrane or from the auditory canal, and in certain extensive skull fractures, cerebrospinal fluid may even be found in the auditory canal. After head injury it is thus appropriate for the attending physician to examine the ear and the external auditory canal. If hemorrhage (blood) is seen, the athlete should be presumed to have a skull fracture until proven otherwise.

Contusions to the external ear may cause considerable bleeding around the ear cartilage, necessitating aspiration to avoid pressure and permanent cartilage damage ("cauliflower ear"). With severe lacerations, every piece of viable cartilage should be preserved. The ear has a remarkable ability to endure trauma, and resuturing is usually attempted even if circulation seems mini-

mal. Missing pieces of both the ear and nose may be restored later if they are found and preserved in chilled sterile saline solution or wrapped in a cold, moist towel and placed in a container of ice. The ice should not come in direct contact with the tissue.

SOFT TISSUE INJURIES OF THE NECK

Blunt trauma to the front of the neck can cause injury to the larynx and/or trachea and result in acute airway obstruction. Symptoms include dyspnea, coughing, pain, difficulty speaking and swallowing, and apprehension. The athletic trainer should be prepared to institute emergency medical treatment if needed. To prevent blunt trauma to the front of the neck, throat guards are recommended for athletes participating in high-risk sports such as lacrosse and field hockey (Fig. 31.6).

Other soft tissue injuries of the neck, such as cervical strains and sprains, acute cervical intervertebral disc herniation, and forced lateral deviation of the neck, are covered in Chapter 32.

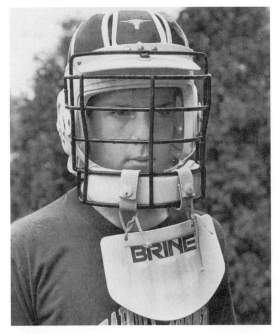

FIGURE 31.6. Throat guards help prevent blunt trauma to the front of the neck.

IMPORTANT CONCEPTS

1. A nasal fracture which results in leakage of cerebrospinal fluid is a serious injury that should be evaluated as soon as possible by a physician.
2. An avulsed tooth should be preserved by replanting the tooth in the socket; storing the tooth under the athlete's tongue if he or she is alert and cooperative; or placing the tooth in a plastic, covered container with whole milk, saliva, or sterile saline solution.
3. Treatment of mouth lacerations involves cleansing with water or a mouthwash gargle and consuming clear liquids only until the laceration has closed (about 24 hours).
4. Hyphema is a serious eye injury that must be evaluated by a physician with possible referral to an ophthalmologist.
5. Severely lacerated or avulsed ear cartilage can be successfully resutured if pieces are preserved in chilled, sterile saline solution or wrapped in a cold, moist towel and placed in a container filled with ice.
6. Blunt trauma to the front of the neck can injure the larynx and/or trachea and result in acute airway obstruction.

SUGGESTED READINGS

Freeman, H. M., ed. *Ocular Trauma.* New York: Appleton-Century-Crofts, 1979.
Torg, J. S., ed. *Athletic Injuries to the Head, Neck, and Face.* Philadelphia: Lea & Febiger, 1982.

32

The Spine

OBJECTIVES FOR CHAPTER 32

After reading this chapter, the student should be able to:

1. Describe the anatomy and function of the spine.
2. Discuss the various injuries the spine may sustain.
3. Evaluate the athlete with a possible spinal injury and provide emergency care prior to transport to the hospital.
4. Describe some basic exercises for the rehabilitation of the athlete with spinal injuries.

513

INTRODUCTION

Injury to the spine that disrupts the protection of the spinal cord can produce permanent paralysis. Therefore, athletic trainers and coaches must be able to recognize spinal injury even when the symptoms are not obvious. Chapter 32 begins with a brief anatomy of the spine. It then describes injuries to the cervical spine, the upper back and thoracic spine, and the lumbar spine. The chapter next discusses evaluation and splinting of spinal injuries on the field. The last section of Chapter 32 consists of strengthening and flexibility exercises. ■

ANATOMY OF THE SPINE

The **spine** is a segmented column of 33 vertebrae stacked one on the next and extending from the base of the skull to the tip of the coccyx. This segmented spinal column, also called the **vertebral column,** is composed of 24 movable vertebrae (7 cervical, 12 thoracic, and 5 lumbar), as well as 5 sacral vertebrae and 4 coccygeal vertebrae, which are somewhat fused (Fig. 32.1). The vertebrae become progressively larger from the skull to the sacrum, and then they become progressively smaller. The total length of the vertebral column amounts to about two-fifths of the total height of the body.

Lying between each of the cervical, thoracic, and lumbar vertebrae are the intervertebral discs. The **intervertebral disc** is a fibrocartilaginous disc whose peripheral part is composed of concentric layers of fibers called the annulus fibrosus (Fig. 32.2). The center of the disc is filled with a gelatinous pulp, the nucleus pulposus, which acts as a cushion and a shock absorber between each vertebral body.

The vertebral column completely surrounds and encases the spinal cord and partially shields the thoracic and abdominal viscera. It transmits the weight of the rest of the body to the lower limbs and to the ground when a person is standing, supports the body's weight for locomotion, and protects the spinal cord and the roots of the spinal nerves. With its muscles and joints, the vertebral column represents an axis of the body that is capable of rigidity and flexibility. The head pivots on the vertebral column, and the upper limbs are attached to it.

The vertebral column is flexible because the cervical, thoracic, and lumbar vertebrae can move slightly. Its stability depends largely on ligaments and muscles, with some stability provided by the form of the column and its constituent parts. Movement between the vertebrae is the least in

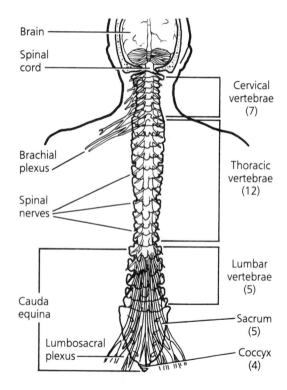

FIGURE 32.1. The vertebral column.

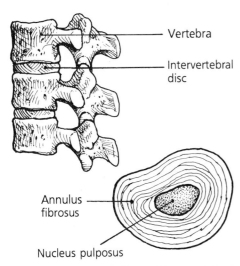

FIGURE 32.2. Normal disc and intervertebral spacing of the spinal cord.

the regions where the intervertebral discs are the thinnest—in the thoracic and pelvic cavities.

Vertebrae

The typical vertebra consists of a body, vertebral arch, and several processes for muscular and articular connections (Fig. 32.3). Each vertebra has three relatively short processes (two transverse and one spinous).

The **body** of the vertebra provides strength and supports weight. It is separated from the bodies of the vertebrae above and below by the intervertebral disc. Posterior to the body is the vertebral arch, which, with the posterior surface of the body, forms walls which enclose and protect the spinal cord.

The **vertebral arch** is composed of right and left pedicles and right and left laminae. **Superior and inferior articular processes** on each side (superior and inferior articular facets, respectively) form the small joints of the posterior elements. The lower edge of each pedicle has a deep notch, and the upper edge has a shallow notch. Two adjacent notches, together with the intervening body and the intervertebral disc, form the

intervertebral foramina that transmits the spinal nerve and its vessels.

Cervical Vertebrae

The seven cervical vertebrae are found between the skull and the thorax. They are characterized by the presence of foramina, which transmit a vertebral artery in each transverse process. The skull rests on the first cervical vertebra, the ring-shaped **atlas**. The second cervical vertebra, the **axis**, forms a pivot around which the atlas and skull can rotate. The atlas and axis are the two specialized cervical vertebrae (Fig. 32.4). The third to sixth cervical vertebrae have small, broad bodies with large triangular vertebral foramina and are similar in shape. The seventh cervical vertebra is char-

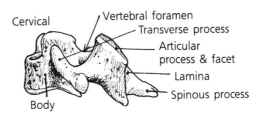

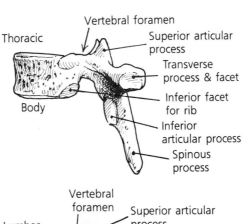

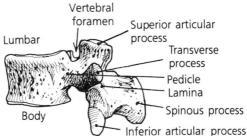

FIGURE 32.3. Anatomy of vertebrae.

acterized by a long spinous process that gives attachment to a strong cord, the **ligamentum nuchae**, that also attaches to the skull.

Thoracic Vertebrae

The 12 thoracic vertebrae are connected to the ribs at facets and form the posterior border of the chest wall. The thoracic vertebrae increase in size as they approach the lumbar region.

Lumbar Vertebrae

The five lumbar vertebrae are located between the thorax and the sacrum and are distinguished by their large size and absence of costal facets.

Sacral Vertebrae

The sacrum consists of five vertebrae that are fused in the adult into wedge-shaped bones forming the back of the pelvis.

Coccygeal Vertebrae

Below the sacrum, the coccyx lies slightly above and behind the anus. Like the sacrum, it resembles a wedge, and it usually consists of four segments.

Spinal Cord

The spinal cord is a continuation of the central nervous system and provides pathways to and from the brain. It is widest in the midcervical region, narrows in the thoracic area, and ends in the upper lumbar area in the L1–2 intervertebral space (Fig. 32.5). Nerve roots emanate from the ventral and dorsal portions of the spinal cord and combine to form the spinal nerves. There are 31 pairs of spinal nerves: 8 cervical, 12 thoracic, 5 lumbar, 5 sacral, and 1 coccygeal. Roots of the upper sacral nerves which have not exited the spinal canal extend beyond the termination of the spinal cord. This bundle of filament lying within the spinal canal is called the **cauda equina**.

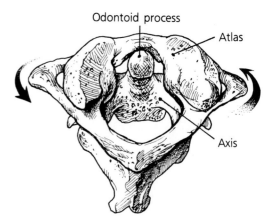

FIGURE 32.4. The axis forms a pivot for the atlas to rotate the skull.

Some nerves in the head and neck come directly from the brain.

Many of the cells of the spinal cord, as well as the brain stem, control reflexes. A **reflex** may be defined as a fairly fixed pattern of response or behavior similar for any given stimulus. The **reflex pathway** consists

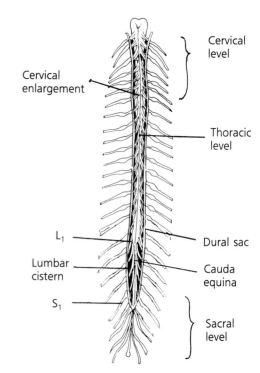

FIGURE 32.5. The spinal cord at the cervical, thoracic, lumbar, and sacral levels.

of sensory fibers bringing impulses into the spinal cord and motor fibers capable of effecting a response, as well as all the interconnections between the two (Fig. 32.6).

Autonomic Nervous System

The **autonomic**, or **involuntary**, **nervous system** is that portion of the nervous system which regulates the activity of the cardiac muscle, the smooth muscle, and the glands. The involuntary nervous system lies outside of the central nervous system and utilizes a "switch box" or **ganglion** to conduct its functions. The autonomic nervous system has two parts: the sympathetic system and the parasympathetic system. The **sympathetic**, or **thoracolumbar**, part of the autonomic system is comprised of fibers from the length of the spinal cord. The **parasympathetic**, or **craniosacral**, part of the autonomic system is comprised of fibers from the brain stem and the sacral portion of the spinal cord. The autonomic system keeps the internal environment of the body constant by maintaining temperature, fluid balance, and the ionic composition of the blood. The sympathetic system is particularly important to the athlete's "fight-or-flight" response to stress.

Curvature of the Spine

The cervical, thoracic, lumbar, and sacral portions of the vertebral column all have characteristic curves. Abnormal curves are called **curvatures**. Accentuation of the normal curve is called **lordosis** in the lumbar region and **kyphosis** in the thoracic area (Fig. 32.7). While there is normally kyphosis in the thoracic area and lordosis in the lumbar area, these terms more commonly refer to exaggeration of the normal curve resulting from a pathologic condition. These curvatures may be associated with underlying developmental problems in the young athlete. The athlete with curvatures may be subject to increased incidence of injury, dysfunction, and pain. In severe cases, curvatures may also cause dysfunction of the internal organs, such as decreased lung capacity.

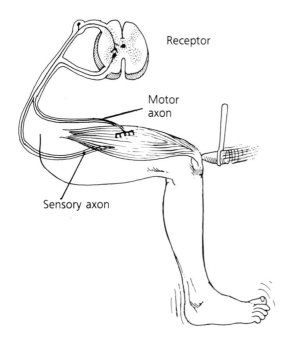

FIGURE 32.6. Reflex arc through sensory arc receptor and motor axon.

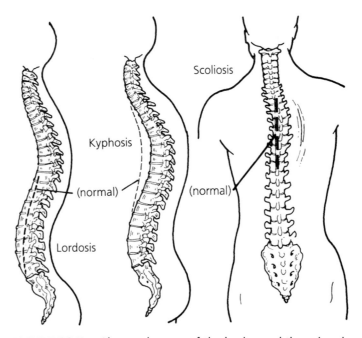

FIGURE 32.7. Abnormal curves of the lumbar and thoracic spines.

Lateral curvature of the spine to the left or right is termed **scoliosis** (see Figure 32.7). The most common type of scoliosis is idiopathic (of unknown cause), which occurs with greater frequency in girls than in boys. Scoliotic curves may first be detected during the adolescent growth spurt when rib cage deformity and postural changes become apparent. Therefore, the preparticipation physical evaluation should include screening for scoliosis.

Mild cases of scoliosis can be treated conservatively with strengthening exercises for the supporting musculature, and athletes usually do not need to restrict their sports participation. More severe or rapidly progressing cases, however, may require bracing and/or operative correction. All cases of scoliosis should be evaluated by a physician.

CERVICAL SPINE INJURIES

Soft Tissue Injuries

The esophagus lies in front of the vertebral bodies and behind the trachea and larynx. The carotid arteries carrying blood to the brain are found on each side of the trachea and are easily palpable just under the sternocleidomastoid muscles. The muscles and ligaments that control the motion of the neck can be divided into the posterior group attached to the lamina, extending from the skull to the shoulders, and the anterior group, consisting of a deep set of muscles attaching to the skull, vertebral bodies, and the upper ribs. The most superficial and largest anterior muscle is the **sternocleidomastoid**, which arises from the clavicle and sternum below and attaches to the base of the skull at the mastoid process above (Fig. 32.8).

Strains and Sprains

A **cervical strain**, an injury to the musculotendinous unit, may or may not be associated with a **cervical sprain**, which is a ligamentous injury. Cervical sprains and strains are common injuries in athletes.

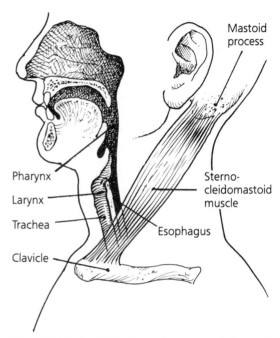

FIGURE 32.8. Soft tissue structures of the neck.

They can occur at the extremes of motion, such as hyperflexion, hyperextension, or excessive rotation, or in association with violent muscle contraction. Cervical strains can lead to easily palpable spasms in the injured muscles. Active contraction of the injured muscle with or without resistance or a passive stretch of that muscle causes pain that helps to localize the injury. Facet joint dysfunction may cause pain on movement of the head and trigger muscle spasm.

Rest, cervical collar support when necessary, and cryotherapy (use of ice) should be the initial first aid for strains and sprains. Once initial symptoms have subsided, moist heat, gentle stretching, and light isometric exercises can be started. Athletes who play contact sports must continue to strengthen their neck muscles through progressive resistance exercise, with the use of either free weights or machines. The football player may need extra bracing when blocking and tackling begin.

Injuries to the ligamentous structures about the cervical spine are numerous. Not only is there a plentitude of connective tissue stabilizing the neck; there are also capsular ligaments about each facet joint. A cervical sprain can be caused by forces ranging from those delivered in a jarring tackle or violent twist, to hyperflexion or extension of the neck, to those generated by faulty posture or an awkward sleeping position.

Differentiating between a ligamentous sprain and musculotendinous strain in the neck can be difficult. Both types of injuries can occur simultaneously. Active and passive movements may elicit symptoms. Any neurological symptoms indicate the need for further medical evaluation.

Generally, muscle strain symptoms subside within 3 to 7 days. If they persist, an underlying ligament injury may be prolonging the symptoms. As the injured connective tissue heals, resulting stiffness prohibits the normal joint motion—a condition that may elicit muscle spasm, cause nerve-ending irritation in the ligaments, and bring about referred pain in the extremities. Decreased cervical range of motion and facet joint movement are signs of this dysfunction.

Early range of motion done gently by the athlete may prevent the stiffness. Intermittent cervical traction may be beneficial in the subacute and chronic phases. Manual therapy techniques for mobilization and manual traction may also help reduce stiffness. Early institution of treatment can eliminate the pain-spasm, weakness-pain cycle. Progressive modality treatments, including cold to heat, selective stimulation, ultrasound, and a flexibility and strengthening program are useful here, as they are in the treatment of the cervical strain.

Cervical sprains and strains which are associated with muscle spasm, limited or painful motion, radiating pain, or numbness or tingling into the upper or lower extremities require further evaluation, including roentgenographic studies to ascertain the stability of the cervical spine. Flexion-extension views, cinematography, or traction studies may be required.

Acute Cervical Intervertebral Disc Herniation

Acute cervical intervertebral disc herniation (rupture) may occur in sports. An athlete who has such an injury may present with signs and symptoms as noted for strains and sprains. If the symptoms are not simply reduced range of motion, but include pain, radiating pain, spasm, numbness, tingling, weakness, or reduced or absent reflexes, a disc injury may have occurred. Violent motions of the head may have caused this injury, which may become a medical emergency.

Diagnosis in severe cases is based on objective findings, including specific areas of numbness, decreased response to the deep tendon reflex, and a reduction in muscle strength when the specific manual muscle test is done. Routine roentgenograms, although usually not helpful in making this diagnosis, should be obtained to rule out the possibility of bony injury. If conservative measures, including bed rest and traction, fail, a magnetic resonance imaging (MRI) study or computerized tomography (CT) scan may be necessary to confirm the diagnosis, to plan further treatment, and to give a more accurate prognosis.

Repeated injury to the cervical intervertebral discs may be associated with degenerative changes at the involved level. These changes can even occur in young athletes; they appear on roentgenograms as narrowing of the space occupied by the intervertebral disc, with osteophyte formation at the vertebral margins. These chronic changes are most often seen in the disc spaces of the lower cervical and lumbar spine and may become associated with symptoms related to the impingement of the neural elements as they exit the spinal canal.

Forced Lateral Deviation of the Neck

One of the most common cervical injuries seen in athletes, especially football players, is forced lateral deviation of the neck (Fig. 32.9). This injury is often associated with pain and numbness or tingling into the upper extremity and is commonly called a "stinger," "burner," or "nerve pinch."

The neck not only may be driven laterally, but also may sustain associated rotation or anterior and posterior motion. This displacement may be associated with a stretch injury to the nerve trunks of the upper portion of the brachial plexus. In rare instances, these nerves may be pulled completely away from the spinal cord. A complete nerve root avulsion results in permanent paralysis of the muscles innervated by those specific nerves. Nerve avulsions can be diagnosed by cervical myelography.

In general, most injuries to the upper brachial plexus are brief, transient episodes of paresthesia ("pins and needles" feeling) and pain extending into the upper extremities. The initial cause is usually a stretch of the neural elements of the opposite side to which the head is driven. Common symptoms are pain and weakness that extend out into the shoulder and down the extremity. The athlete usually describes a burning sensation and says that his or her arm "has gone numb."

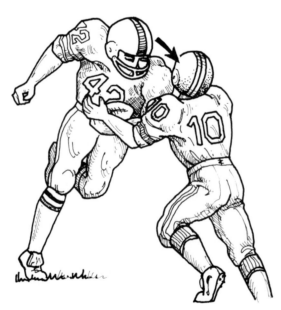

FIGURE 32.9. Forced lateral deviation of the neck, commonly called a "stinger," "burner," or "nerve pinch."

Posterior shoulder subluxation may also bring on symptoms of a numb or "dead" arm. The lower brachial plexus is affected, and symptoms are usually transient in nature. "Stingers" and "burners" most frequently involve areas innervated by the fifth and sixth cervical roots and may result in weakness of the deltoid and biceps muscles and depression of the biceps reflex. The pain is usually transient, lasting only a few minutes. When the symptoms pass, the athlete typically wishes to resume competition. If an episode is severe or there are recurrent episodes, neurologic changes may persist for variable periods of time.

In football, wearing a collar that restricts the extremes of cervical motion may offer some degree of protection. The collar must fit well on the shoulder pads and provide an effective block beneath the helmet. Off-season strengthening of cervical musculature and improved blocking and tackling techniques are recommended.

Blunt trauma to the front of the neck can be associated with injury to the larynx and trachea, resulting in acute airway obstruction. Basic life support should be provided and the athlete promptly transferred to the emergency department.

Cervical Fractures and Dislocations

Violent force in flexion or extension may cause fractures of the cervical vertebrae. Perhaps the most frequent cause of spinal cord injury is that of axial loading of the cervical spine during spearing.

A cervical fracture or dislocation is a medical emergency. Whenever an athlete has a head injury, the trainer should always consider the possibility of a cervical spine fracture or injury and protect the conscious athlete from random movements. If cardiopulmonary resuscitation must be administered, the trainer must remember that a cervical spine injury may be present. The conscious athlete can assist the athletic trainer in assessing movement, sensation, and muscle power. The player may complain of neck pain and radiating symptoms.

If x-rays are positive for cervical fracture the physician will stabilize the fracture to prevent further neurologic damage and determine if surgery will be required to treat the injury. Not all fractures result in quadriplegia; neurologic deficit can range from zero to paralysis.

A cervical spine fracture can only be diagnosed and confirmed by roentgenographic evaluation. Remember, any athlete who sustains a head or neck injury may have incurred a cervical spine fracture and should be handled appropriately until the status of the neck injury has been fully assessed. A cervical spine fracture is often accompanied by instability of the cervical spine and injury to the spinal cord and nerve roots. Thus, even if the neural elements were not injured at the time of the fracture, injudicious movement of the head and neck in an unstable spine can cause permanent spinal cord or nerve root injury.

A subluxation or dislocation of the cervical vertebrae results in loss of the normal anatomic alignment with associated ligament, tendon, muscle, disc, bone, and neural element injuries. Paralysis and even sudden death can occur.

Mechanisms of injury to the cervical spine are complex and usually represent a combination of forces rather than one single force. Mechanisms include flexion and extension in the anteroposterior plane, lateral flexion, rotation, and compressive axial loading of the vertebral column. The most common severe fracture-dislocations of the cervical spine in athletic participation occur with flexion and compression loading.

First Cervical Vertebra

The first cervical vertebra is atypical. It is composed primarily of a large ring in which there is usually more than adequate room for the spinal cord. This extra room often allows the spinal cord to escape injury in fractures, causing only minor displacement. A burst fracture of this ring of C1 (the so-called **Jefferson fracture**) occurs when the condyles of the occiput are driven down against the ring of the atlas, splitting

this fragile bone (Fig. 32.10). The danger is that this injury may be difficult to detect clinically and may be overlooked on roentgenographic examination without special views to demonstrate widening in this ring. Even without neurologic damage, the clinical presentation of paracervical muscle spasms associated with pain and resistance to rotation on examination should alert the trainer to the possibility of this injury. It is important to stabilize the neck and promptly transfer the athlete to the emergency department.

Second Cervical Vertebra

Fractures and dislocations of the atlantoaxial joint result in altered alignment between the first two cervical vertebrae. The odontoid process of the second cervical vertebra may rupture the transverse ligament of the first cervical vertebra, allowing the atlas to slide forward on the second cervical vertebra and encroach on the space occupied by the spinal cord. A fracture of the odontoid process may also occur, and like all injuries in this area, can only be

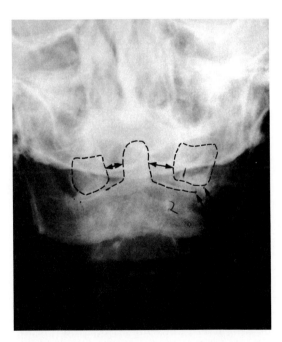

FIGURE 32.10.   A burst fracture of the ring of C1, the so-called Jefferson fracture.

confirmed with special roentgenographic views. The **hangman's fracture** is a fracture of the pedicles of C2 (Fig. 32.11). Damage to the upper cervical vertebrae of the spinal cord is a life-threatening injury because the respiratory control centers are located in this area.

Lower Cervical Spine

Fractures and dislocations of the lower cervical spine associated with spinal cord injuries in athletes are most commonly observed at the fourth, fifth, and sixth cervical levels. Like fractures and dislocations of the upper cervical spine, these injuries may be associated with varying degrees of damage to the neural elements and can cause transient or permanent paralysis. This potential for neurologic damage makes appropriate emergency care of the athlete with the injured cervical spine critical.

UPPER BACK AND THORACIC SPINE INJURIES

Soft tissue injuries to the thoracic spine are few and far between. The stability of this area is greatly enhanced by the rib cage. There is very little flexibility for that same reason. Bony problems, however, are common.

Posterior Rib Fractures

Posterior rib fractures are usually caused by a direct blow. Because they result in bleeding, swelling, and tenderness at the site of the injury, they can be easily confused with muscle contusions. Pain referred to the site of injury from pressure over an uninvolved portion of the same rib is indicative of a fractured rib. Sometimes only an x-ray can differentiate between a fracture and a muscle contusion. A correct diagnosis is important because a fractured rib can puncture the pleural lining of the chest cavity or even the lung itself, allowing air or fluid (blood) to leak into this potential space, which collapses the lung.

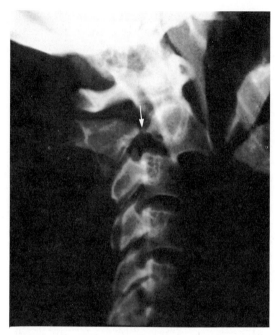

FIGURE 32.11. A fracture of the pedicles of C2, the so-called hangman's fracture.

Thoracic Spine Fractures

Thoracic, or dorsal, spine fractures can result from either direct or indirect force. The nature of thoracic spine injuries differs from that of cervical and lumbar spine injuries because of the protective effects of the rib cage. Fractures from direct blows are extremely rare and are usually the result of vertical loading of the spine or a rotational force. Fractures generally occur at the lower levels of the dorsal spine or at the thoracolumbar junction, where forces tend to concentrate at the transition from the thoracic kyphosis to the lumbar lordosis and where the ribs no longer afford added stability.

Spinal fractures are classified as stable or unstable, depending on their potential to shift and cause further injury to the spinal cord or nerve roots. The **vertebral body compression**, or **wedge fracture**, is the most common thoracic fracture. Although the bone is compressed, the ligamentous structures are intact, making this a stable fracture. In the unstable **chance**, or **slice, fracture**, there is horizontal disruption of the vertebral body and ligamentous structures.

Stress Fractures and Apophysitis

The potential for spinal injury from recurrent microtrauma sustained through repetitive flexing or extending of the spine is becoming increasingly apparent. The young athlete, particularly during the adolescent growth spurt, appears to be especially susceptible to irritation of the apophysitis, or the growth centers of the vertebral body, from repetitive loading of the anterior longitudinal ligament that inserts on them. Symptoms of **apophysitis** begin gradually, with pain occurring only during certain maneuvers and usually not hindering performance. With progression of symptoms, pain becomes localized and severe, resulting in diminished performance. X-rays and other imaging techniques may be used to confirm the diagnosis. Rest and physical therapy are indicated for up to 6 weeks. Treatment of multiple-level apophysitis is rest from activity until symptoms disappear, with strengthening of the abdominal muscles and paravertebral muscles before the athlete returns to activity.

Upper Back Contusions and Sprains

Contusions of the upper back muscles are fairly common in contact sports. Swelling, tenderness upon palpation, and ecchymosis (bruising) indicate a contusion. If the tissues that were hurt move or stabilize an extremity, there will be pain and dysfunction on movement of that extremity. Spasms may result from this injury also. Both back motion and shoulder motion can be affected.

As with any contusion of large muscle groups, immediate ICE (ice, compression, elevation) management helps to minimize disability. Active pain and swelling can also be controlled by high voltage or interferential treatment (a type of electric stimulation). After the acute symptoms have subsided, moist heat, ultrasound, and massage will help eliminate the soreness and swelling. Active and passive exercises will return strength and flexibility. If the shoulder gir-

dle muscles are involved, a sling on the involved side may increase comfort. Musculotendinous strains in this area result either from excessive extrinsic stretch of the back muscles, such as from twisting, or from a sustained overloading contraction of the muscles.

Thoracic Sprains

Upper back sprains can be difficult to distinguish from musculotendinous strains, particularly when a sprain is followed by extensive protective muscle spasm of the dorsal muscles. Usually, however, no anatomic area of muscle tenderness can be palpated with a sprain, although "trigger points" of increased sensitivity can sometimes be identified. In addition, with a sprain the athlete may strongly resist lateral or rotational motion. Upper back sprains may show dramatic improvement in 24 to 48 hours, while a true musculotendinous strain of the dorsal musculature may take 3 to 4 weeks or more to resolve.

LUMBAR SPINE INJURIES

The most common lumbar injuries seen in athletes are contusions, muscle strains, and ligament sprains. Although temporary, these injuries may be extremely painful. They generally heal without disability. If following an injury an athlete has pain that persists despite several weeks of modalities, anti-inflammatory medication, and rest, or if the athlete has pain associated with neurologic signs or symptoms, further evaluation beyond the normal history, physical examination, and routine roentgenograms is warranted.

Injuries to Discs

A young athlete whose low back pain is associated with radiating pain into the lower extremities may have a **herniated** (ruptured) **disc** (Fig. 32.12). Symptoms may begin after vigorous activity or come on slowly, though there may be intense pain in the lower back area. The distal extremity symptoms indicate the seriousness of a herniated disc. Evaluation may show weakness in the foot, ankle, or knee, depending on the level of injury. Reflexes at the Achilles tendon, patellar tendon, and semitendinosus may be diminished or absent. Specific areas of the lower extremity may have diminished or absent sensation. The athlete may present with a slightly crouched position, a lateral shift away from the lesion. Forward flexion may produce significant pain and an increase in distal symptoms. Diagnosis of disc problems is made by a careful physical exam and confirmed by special radiographic studies (CT scan or MRI).

A disc need not be completely herniated to give symptoms. The annulus may simply bulge, putting enough pressure on the neural elements to cause symptoms. If extension of the spine does not increase distal symptoms, the disc bulge or herniation is not displaced far enough to be impinged. Extension of the spine will apply pressure to move the disc forward, away from the nerve roots. The differential diagnosis of lesions mimicking a herniated lumbar disc in an athlete includes neoplasms, bony

compromise of the nerve root canal or foramina, and other rare conditions irritating the neural elements.

The key to treating the disc problem acutely is to rest the area and do everything possible to decrease distal symptoms. Sitting is to be avoided, because sitting loads the disc. The physician will undoubtedly insist on good posture while performing all activities.

Treatment of a lumbar disc injury initially consists of rest from impact load or flexion/extension activities, physical therapy modalities, strengthening exercises for the paravertebral and abdominal muscles, and medications to decrease inflammation and relax muscle spasm. Traction may also be used. A posterior or lateral disc herniation pressing against the adjacent neural elements may be temporarily incapacitating, but full recovery is the rule.

In the few cases where all conservative measures fail to relieve symptoms, operative removal of disc material may be required. However, young athletes with prolonged irritation of the neural elements may have great difficulty returning to their previous performance level or tolerance for activity. They may have to select another sport or a less demanding position in the same sport.

Recovery from an acute disc rupture may take months and cannot be rushed. Once distal symptoms resolve, total flexibility of the spine and hamstring must be obtained. Back extension strength is most important; abdominal strength is secondary. If a herniated disc is treated surgically, it is hard to predict whether the athlete will be able to return to his or her sport since conditioning programs like weight training place a load on the disc. Varying amounts of instability may also occur in the lumbar spine after disc rupture.

Spondylolysis and Spondylolisthesis

Chronic pain confined to the lumbar spine may be caused by segmental instability associated with lumbar pars interarticularis

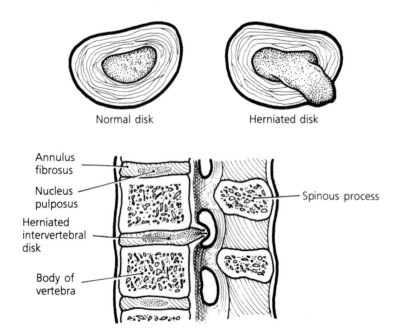

Normal disk　　　Herniated disk

Annulus fibrosus

Nucleus pulposus

Herniated intervertebral disk

Body of vertebra

Spinous process

FIGURE 32.12.　Normal and herniated intervertebral discs.

defects. **Spondylolysis** is a defect in the pars interarticularis. The cause of this defect is not known. Some argue it is congenital; others believe it results from sustained repetitive stress to the area as from an unhealed stress fracture. If both the right and left pars interarticularis of a vertebra are defective, the affected vertebra can slip anterior to the one below it—a condition called **traumatic spondylolysis**. Spondylolysis occurs in approximately 2 percent of the general population.

Spondylolisthesis is the actual displacement of one vertebra on another through the spondylitic defect of the pars, which usually occurs at L5–S1 (Fig. 32.13). Spondylolisthesis, or slippage, occurs in 5 percent of people with spondylolysis.

Most individuals with these spinal defects are unaware that they have them. The defects are frequently noted on routine films taken for some other reason. In a few individuals the degree of spondylolisthesis is progressive during the teenage years and results in a narrowed neural canal (spinal stenosis). Frequently, surgery is needed to correct this condition if pain or neurologic symptoms accompany the x-ray findings.

Because a slight slip or spondylolysis without a slip is not usually associated with low back pain, these x-ray findings should not be blamed for the athlete's symptoms unless all other causes are first eliminated. The exception is the rare occurrence of an acute spondylolysis that results from repetitive stress to the pars interarticularis (stress fracture), sometimes seen in athletes in whom the spine is repetitively loaded in a flexion or extension mode (e.g., football linemen, gymnasts, or ice skaters).

Vertebral slippage in the lower lumbar spine, commonly seen at the L5–S1 level, occurs most often between the ages of 9 and 13 in athletic women. A more vertical sacrum with hamstring tightness and loss of flexibility are signs of a possible spondylolisthesis. Symptoms of this pathology may be chronic pain in the low back, especially with increased activity and with forced hyperextension of the lumbar spine. If the pathology progresses, distal neuro-

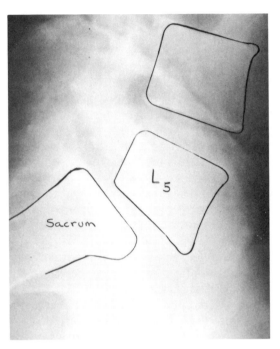

FIGURE 32.13. Spondylolisthesis, forward subluxation of the lower lumbar vertebrae (in this case L5 on S1), may cause chronic leg and back pain.

logic symptoms may appear. Treatment consists of increased trunk control, good posture, and modification of lifting technique. In extreme cases, surgery may be used to stabilize the lumbar spine.

An acute pars defect can be differentiated from a chronic one by a bone scan. This study should be ordered for those athletes with acute nonradicular low back pain who demonstrate a previously unknown defect on routine films. If the scan is positive, these athletes should rest from sports activity and may need to be protected in a splint until they are asymptomatic. They then should proceed with a back strengthening and flexibility program before returning to sports.

Sacroiliac Joint and Lumbar Joint Dysfunction

Another case of both acute and chronic pain and dysfunction is stiffness in the sacroiliac (SI) joint and the lumbar joint. This condition may result from a single maneuver, twist, awkward movement, or trauma which sprains the supporting ligaments. Sacroiliac joint and lumbar joint dysfunction may also come about as an overuse injury associated with poor posture, lifting techniques, or sportive maneuver repeated strenuously many times (i.e., swinging a golf club, pitching a ball, hitting a serve). Many times this injury can occur when the athlete reaches a fatigue level (as in a long baseball or basketball season) and the joint structures are not able to recover. Also, the athlete's conditioning levels will have decreased.

Symptoms include a consistent soreness over the SI joint area that is better in the morning but gets worse as the day goes on. There are no neurologic signs, but referred pain into the leg may be found on questioning the athlete. Heat and activity may diminish the discomfort during activity, but the pain returns as soon as cool-down occurs. Specific manual therapy techniques easily point out this dysfunction. In fact, those lower back pain situations with a negative finding on herniated nucleus pulposus exam, yet unresponsive to rest, are probably SI joint and lumbar joint dysfunctions.

Treatment is mobilization of the offending joints to free them up (not manipulation but special gentle stretch by a knowledgeable therapist). Then rest for several days is essential to allow the joint structures to heal. If the stiffness can be controlled for 3 to 7 days, a gently progressive exercise program in order to increase back extension strength and flexibility is instituted. The athlete who is in good physical condition prior to injury can be returned quickly to sport.

Lumbar Fractures and Dislocations

Transverse process or spinous process fractures, from either direct blows or violent muscle contraction, occur occasionally in the athlete and may lead to periods of disability. Pain is most acute with palpation over the area of injury. Treatment is rest from activity until symptoms disappear.

Compression fractures of the lumbar vertebrae are most frequently seen at L1 due to the mechanical vulnerability of the thoracolumbar junction. These fractures are usually caused by vertical loading and flexion.

Fracture-dislocations of the lumbar spine with or without neural injury are rare in athletic participation. The termination of the spinal cord at L2 means that fractures or dislocations of the lumbar spine below this point may injure spinal roots but not the cord and therefore, the degree of neurologic impairment is less severe.

RESPONDING TO SPINAL INJURIES ON THE FIELD

The athletic trainer who examines the spinally traumatized athlete must remember that the absence of paralysis does not negate the possibility of a severe head or spine injury. If the athlete complains of numbness or tingling, buzzing sensations, inability to move a body part, or pain in the cervical, thoracic, or lumbar region, the trainer must take appropriate precautions and immobilize the athlete to prevent further injury during transport to the emergency department. An athlete with an unstable spinal fracture may be rendered paraplegic or quadriplegic by injudicious movement.

A force strong enough to cause unconsciousness may also be strong enough to damage the cervical spine. Therefore, every traumatic episode resulting in an unconscious athlete should be assumed to have also resulted in an associated injury to the cervical spine, with neurologic damage possible until proven otherwise.

The unconscious athlete who has a concurrent respiratory or cardiac arrest may need to be promptly positioned so resuscitation can be initiated. Although immobilization and splinting of all spinal injuries should normally be accomplished without twisting or bending the spine in any direction, in the athlete whose head and neck position is obstructing the airway, one should apply gentle traction on the head followed by positioning of the head and neck into normal alignment. The chin-lift or jaw-thrust maneuver should be used to open the airway, but the neck must not be hyperextended or hyperflexed while CPR is being performed (see Chapter 37). The trainer should not try to straighten the deformity simply to make splinting easier or more convenient, but only to establish an airway.

STRENGTHENING AND FLEXIBILITY EXERCISES

At the present time, no protective athletic equipment is adequate to prevent trauma to the spinal column or the spinal cord. The helmet protects the head, but does nothing to protect the cervical, thoracic, or lumbar spine from potential injuries. Proper conditioning, good technique, and minimizing exposure to risks are the athlete's best protection against spinal injury. The strengthening and flexibility exercises that follow are recommended for both the prevention and treatment of spinal injuries.

Strengthening Exercises

Head Bobs

Purpose: for neck flexor strengthening
Position: lying on back, knees slightly bent

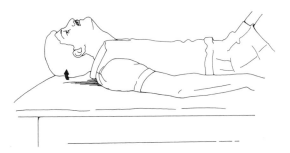

Lift head straight off the table, exhaling as you lift. Do not move head from a neutral position. Hold for ____ seconds. Lower. Relax and repeat. Perform ____ times, ____ times daily. Increase to ____ times, ____ times daily.

Chin Retractions

Purpose: for neck extensor strengthening, posture control
Position: lying on back, sitting, or standing

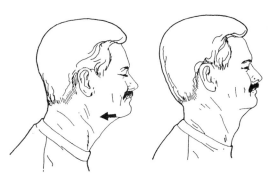

Pull chin into throat, sliding head straight backward. Do not allow head to move up or down. Hold for ____ seconds. Relax and repeat. Perform ____ times, ____ times daily. Increase to ____ times, ____ times daily.

Prone Neck Extension

Purpose: for neck extensor strengthening
Position: lying on stomach, shoulders even with edge of table, head relaxed

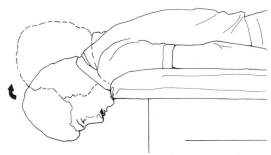

Lift head up to a neutral position, keeping chin tucked in. Hold ____ seconds. Relax and repeat. Perform ____ times, ____ times daily. Increase to ____ times, ____ times daily.

Shoulder Shrugs

Purpose: for trapezius strengthening
Position: standing, arms at side

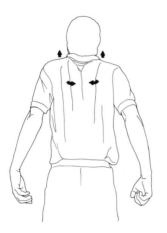

Squeeze shoulder blades back and together as tightly as possible. Hold for 2 seconds. Shrug shoulders up slightly without allowing shoulder blades to separate. Hold for 3 seconds. Relax shoulders to normal position. Repeat. Perform ____ times, ____ times daily. Increase to ____ times, ____ times daily. Gradually increase weight from ____ lbs. to ____ lbs.

Flexibility Exercises

Levator Stretch

Purpose: for stretching spasms on the levator scapular muscle and decreasing trigger points in neck
Position: sitting or standing

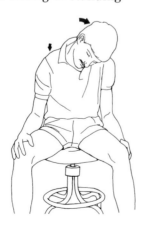

Begin by stretching right ear toward right foot, then slightly pull left shoulder down. Hold for ____ seconds. Relax. Repeat by stretching left ear toward left foot, then slightly pull right shoulder down. Hold. Alternate right and left sides. Perform ____ times, ____ times daily.

Chest Stretch in Corner

Purpose: for stretching tight pectoralis major muscles
Position: standing, facing a corner, one foot in front

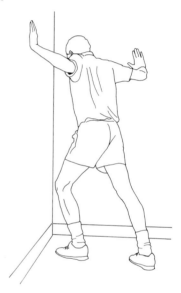

Place one hand on each wall creating the corner, elbows bent. Lean into the corner, keeping head in neutral position. Hold for ____ seconds. Relax. Repeat. Hand position may be raised or lowered to stretch the entire pectoralis muscle. Perform ____ times, ____ times daily.

Hip Flexor Stretch

Purpose: for iliopsoas stretch
Position: lying on back, one leg straight

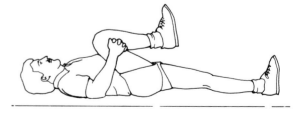

Clasp both hands under the other knee, with hip bent to 90 degrees. Pull bent knee to the chest and straighten the other knee as far as possible. Hold for ____ seconds. Relax, but do not release knee. Repeat. Perform ____ times, ____ times daily.

Standing Side Bends

Purpose: for paraspinous muscle flexibility
Position: standing with feet apart for balance

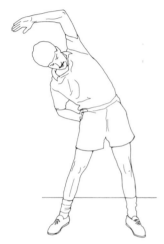

With arms overhead, bend sideways at the waist. Do not allow your hips to twist. Hold for ____ seconds. Return to upright position. Repeat to the other side. Perform ____ times, ____ times daily. Increase to ____ times, ____ times daily.

Sitting Bendovers

Purpose: for stretching lumbar extensors
Position: sitting in a chair

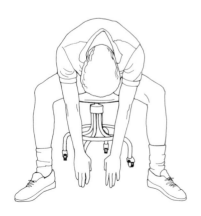

Gradually bend forward by rounding back until gentle stretch is felt in the low back. Keep head and arms relaxed. Hold for ____ seconds. Slowly arise to an upright sitting position. Repeat. Perform ____ times, ____ times daily.

Cobra Stretch

Purpose: for flexion and extension stretch of lumbar spine
Position: crouching on hands and knees

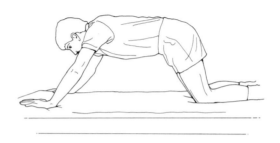

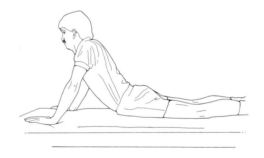

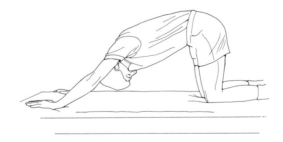

Rock forward onto extended arms allowing back to sag with head up. Hold for ____ seconds. Rock back and sit on bent knees with arms extended and head tucked in. Hold. Repeat. Perform ____ times, ____ times daily.

Pelvic Rotation

Purpose: for lumbar and sacroiliac flexibility
Position: Lying on back, both knees bent

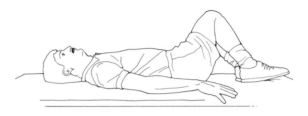

Slowly allow knees to rotate to the right. Hold for ____ seconds. Now rotate knees to the left. Hold. Repeat. Perform ____ times, ____ times daily. Increase to ____ times, ____ times daily.

Extension in Standing

Purpose: a lumbar extension exercise for discs
Position: standing, hands in small of back, feet apart for balance

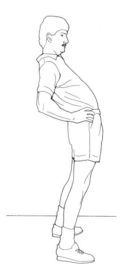

Gently lean backward keeping knees straight and head in neutral position. Hold this position briefly. Return to upright position. Repeat. Perform ____ times, ____ times daily. Increase to ____ times, ____ times daily.

Prone on Elbows

Purpose: a lumbar extension exercise for discs
Position: lying on stomach, arms bent over head

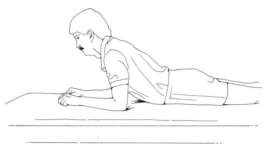

Raise head and upper back by pulling elbows in so you are propped up on your forearms. Keep low back relaxed. Hold for ____ seconds. Lower. Repeat. Perform ____ times, ____ times daily. Increase to ____ times, ____ times daily.

Double Knee to Chest

Purpose: for lumbar flexion
Position: lying on back, knees bent

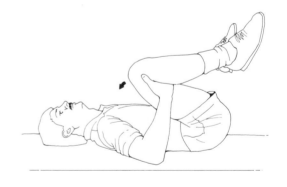

Clasp one hand underneath each knee. Gently pull both knees to chest. Hold for ____ seconds. Relax, but do not release knees. Repeat. Perform ____ times, ____ times daily. Increase to ____ times, ____ times daily.

Supine Hamstring Stretch

Purpose: for stretching hamstrings when it hurts to sit and stretch
Position: lying on back, one leg straight

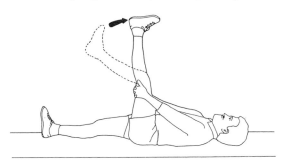

Clasp both hands under the other knee with hip bent 90 degrees. Slowly straighten knee to feel a gentle stretch in back of thigh. Keep toes pulled, back toward you. Hold for ____ seconds. Relax, but do not release leg. Repeat as indicated next with both legs. Perform ____ times, ____ times daily.

Single-Leg Lowers

Purpose: a mild abdominal exercise
Position: lying on back, one knee bent and other leg straight

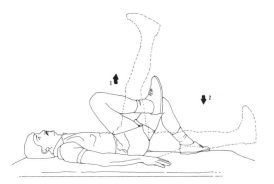

Pull the straight leg to your chest, bending the knee and using abdominal muscles. Now, straighten this knee and flatten low back against floor. Slowly lower extended leg as far as possible keeping low back flat. Hold for ____ seconds. Repeat. Complete exercise using other leg. Perform ____ times, ____ times daily. Increase to ____ times, ____ times daily.

Double-Leg Lowers

Purpose: a mild abdominal exercise
Position: lying on back, both knees bent

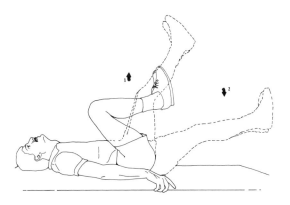

Pull both knees to chest using abdominal muscles. Extend knees. Slowly lower legs as far as possible, keeping low back flat against floor. Hold for ____ seconds. Repeat. Perform ____ times, ____ times daily. Increase to ____ times, ____ times daily.

Torso Rotations

Purpose: a lumbar flexibility exercise
Position: sitting, with proper back posture

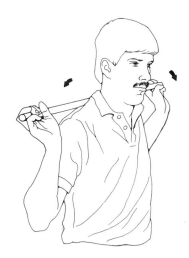

Rotate torso to the right as far as possible. Hold for 3 seconds. Rotate torso to the left as far as possible. Hold for 3 seconds. Repeat. Perform ____ times, ____ times daily. Increase to ____ times, ____ times daily.

Wall Slides

Purpose: a lumbar strengthening exercise
Position: standing, back against wall and feet about 12 inches from the wall

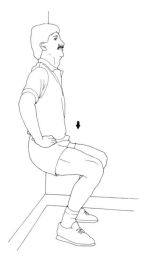

Tuck pelvis under so low back is flat against the wall. Slowly slide down the wall by bending knees. Stop when your knees are bent 90 degrees. Hold for _____ . Relax. Repeat. Perform _____ times, _____ times daily. Increase to _____ times, _____ times daily.

Squats

Purpose: a low back, hip, and hamstring strengthening exercise
Position: standing, feet shoulder-width apart and hands on hips

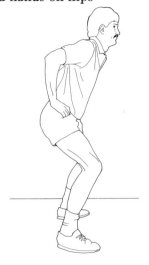

Slowly bend knees to a 90-degree angle with head up and back straight. Hold briefly, then return to starting position. Repeat. Perform _____ repetitions, _____ times daily. Increase to _____ repetitions, _____ times daily.

Bridges

Purpose: a mild lumbar strengthening exercise
Position: lying on back, both knees bent

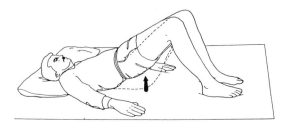

Tuck stomach in to flatten low back against the floor. Raise hips toward ceiling. Hold for _____ seconds. Lower hips slowly. Relax. Repeat. Perform _____ times, _____ times daily. Increase to _____ times, _____ times daily.

Alternate Arm and Leg Lift on Stomach

Purpose: a back extension strengthening exercise
Position: lying on stomach, arms extended overhead

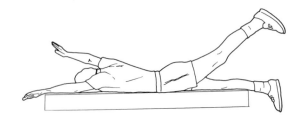

Lift right arm overhead and left leg behind you, keeping both extremities straight. Hold for _____ seconds. Lower slowly. Relax and repeat with alternate arm and leg. Perform _____ times, _____ times daily. Increase to _____ times, _____ times daily.

Prone Leg Lifts

Purpose: a hip extension, lumbar extension strengthening exercise
Position: lying on stomach, arms by sides

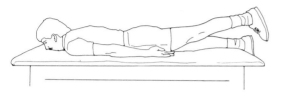

Lift one leg behind you, keeping knee straight. Do not allow hips to lift off the table. Hold for ____ seconds. Lower leg slowly. Relax. Repeat. Perform ____ times, ____ times daily. Increase to ____ times, ____ times daily.

Upper Back Exercise

Purpose: for spine extension strengthening
Position: lying on stomach, and arms at sides

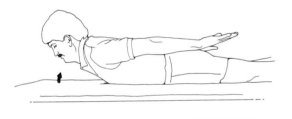

Pinch shoulder blades together and lift arms up, keeping elbows straight. Lift head and upper back with chin "tucked in." Hold for ____ seconds. Relax. Repeat. Perform ____ times, ____ times daily. Increase to ____ times, ____ times daily.

Pelvic Tilt

Purpose: for lumbar flexibility, both extension and flexion
Position: lying on back, knees bent

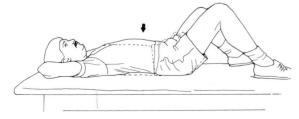

Tighten stomach muscles and tilt pelvis so lower back becomes flat against the table. Hold for ____ seconds. Relax. Repeat. Perform ____ times, ____ times daily. Increase to ____ times, ____ times daily.

Abdominal Curls

Purpose: for abdominal strengthening
Position: lying on back, knees bent

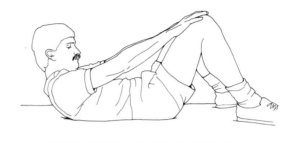

Perform a pelvic tilt, then reach with both hands toward knees. Hold for ____ seconds. Remember to exhale as you sit up. Lower slowly. Relax. Repeat. Perform ____ times, ____ times daily. Increase to ____ times, ____ times daily.

Oblique Abdominal Curls

Purpose: for abdominal strengthening
Position: lying on back, both knees bent

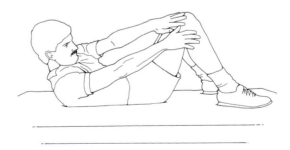

Perform a pelvic tilt; now twist slightly and reach with both hands to the outside of one knee. Hold for ____ seconds. Remember to exhale as you sit up. Lower slowly. Relax. Repeat. Perform ____ times, ____ times daily. Increase to ____ times, ____ times daily.

IMPORTANT CONCEPTS

1. Any lateral curvature of the spine is called scoliosis.
2. The intervertebral disc aids in limited motion between the vertebrae and acts to dissipate compressive forces that might injure the spinal cord.
3. The vertebral column supports body weight, encloses and protects the spinal cord, and composes the central attachment of the peripheral skeleton.
4. The central nervous system controls voluntary function of the body, and the autonomic system controls involuntary body function.
5. Cervical strains and sprains are minor injuries and must be differentiated from structural and neurologic injuries of the neck.
6. Because unsuspected neck injuries may accompany athletic head injuries, extreme caution should be taken during initial evaluation of the head-injured athlete.
7. Any athlete with spine injuries manifesting neurologic symptoms should be seen immediately by a physician.
8. The rib cage gives extra protection and stability to the thoracic spine.
9. The lumbar region is massively constructed and thus infrequently sustains serious injury.
10. A structural spondylolitic defect should be suspected in athletes with chronic low back pain aggravated by their sportive activities.
11. With even the slightest indication of an acute spine injury, the athlete must be immobilized until a definitive evaluation can be made.

SUGGESTED READINGS

Albrand, O. W., and G. Corkill. "Broken Necks from Diving Accidents: A Summer Epidemic in Young Men." *American Journal of Sports Medicine* 4 (1976): 107–110.

Albright, J. P., J. M. Moses, H. G. Feldick, et al. "Nonfatal Cervical Spine Injuries in Interscholastic Football." *Journal of the American Medical Association* 236 (1976): 1243–1245.

Andrish, J. T., J. A. Bergfeld, and L. R. Romo. "A Method for the Management of Cervical Injuries in Football. A preliminary report." *American Journal of Sports Medicine* 5 (1977): 89–92.

Bailey, R. W. "Fractures and Dislocations of the Cervical Spine: Diagnosis and Treatment." *Current Practice in Orthopaedic Surgery* 4 (1969): 132–166.

Cailliet, R. *Low Back Pain Syndrome.* Philadelphia: F. A. Davis, 1988.

Carter, D. R., and V. H. Frankel. "Biomechanics of Hyperextension Injuries to the Cervical Spine in Football." *American Journal of Sports Medicine* 8 (1980): 302–309.

Chrisman, O. D., G. A. Snook, J. M. Stanitis, et al. "Lateral-Flexion Neck Injuries in Athletic Competition." *Journal of the American Medical Association* 192 (1965): 613–615.

Clancy, W. G., Jr, R. L. Brand, and J. A. Bergfeld. "Upper Trunk Brachial Plexus Injuries in Contact Sports." *American Journal of Sports Medicine* 5 (1977): 209–216.

Cyriax, J. *Textbook of Orthopaedic Medicine*, 11th ed. Vol 2: *Treatment by Manipulation, Massage and Injection*. London: Bailliére Tindall, 1984.

Emergency Care and Transportation of the Sick and Injured, 4th ed. Park Ridge, Ill.: American Academy of Orthopaedic Surgeons, 1987.

Finneson, B. E. *Low Back Pain*, 2d ed. Philadelphia: J. B. Lippincott, 1980.

Funk, F. F., and R. E. Wells. "Injuries of the Cervical Spine in Football." *Clinical Orthopaedics and Related Research* 109 (1975): 50–58.

Leidholt, J. D. "Spinal Injuries in Athletes: Be Prepared." *Orthopedic Clinics of North America* 4 (1973): 691–707.

McKenzie, R. *Treat Your Own Back*. Auckland, New Zealand: Spinal Publications, 1985.

Macnab, I. *Backache*. Baltimore: Williams & Wilkins, 1977.

Paris, S. V. *Course Notes: The Spine: Etiology and Treatment of Dysfunction, Including Joint Manipulation*, 1979.

Schneider, R. C. *Head and Neck Injuries in Football: Mechanisms, Treatment, and Prevention*. Baltimore: Williams & Wilkins, 1973.

Yessis, M. "Absolutely Ripped." *Sports Fitness* 2 (July 1986): 14–20.

———. "Back in Shape." *Sports Fitness* 2 (June 1986): 642–647.

P A R T

D

THE GASTROINTESTINAL AND GENITOURINARY SYSTEMS

33

The Gastrointestinal and Genitourinary Systems

OBJECTIVES FOR CHAPTER 33

After reading this chapter, the student should be able to:

1. Describe the boundaries, landmarks, and contents of the abdominal cavity.
2. Describe the organs of the gastrointestinal and genitourinary systems and understand the functions of each.
3. Conduct a physical examination of the abdomen.

INTRODUCTION

The organs of the gastrointestinal and genitourinary systems lie in the abdomen, with the exception of the male genitalia. Chapter 33 begins with the anatomy of the abdomen—its boundaries, contents, and bony landmarks. The chapter then focuses on the organs of the gastrointestinal (digestive) system and the genitourinary (reproductive and urinary) system. Chapter 33 concludes with a section on how to conduct a physical examination of the abdomen. ■

ANATOMY OF THE ABDOMEN

Boundaries of the Abdomen

The body can be envisioned as having two major cavities: the **thorax** (chest) and the **abdomen**. The abdomen is further divided into the upper cavity, or **abdominal cavity**, and the lower cavity, or **pelvic cavity**.

The **diaphragm**, the large muscle of respiration, divides the chest from the abdomen. An imaginary line drawn from the superior aspect of the pubic symphysis to the top of the sacrum divides the abdominal and pelvic cavities. The pelvic cavity, therefore, lies solely in the bony pelvis, but the iliac wings of the bony pelvis extend above the pelvic cavity to protect the contents of the lower abdominal cavity (Fig. 33.1).

Both cavities are lined by a smooth, glistening, thin, transparent layer of tissue called the **peritoneum**. The peritoneum can be thought of as dividing the upper abdominal cavity further into the **retroperitoneal space** (that space lying in front of the spine but between the posterior peritoneal reflection) and the true abdominal cavity (the space between the posterior peritoneum and the anterior peritoneum which lines the anterior abdominal wall). Similarly, the peritoneum divides the area of the lower abdomen into the true pelvic cavity and the extraperitoneal space in the pelvis. However, this division is rather complex, and therefore, for the purposes of this discussion, the upper abdomen will be divided

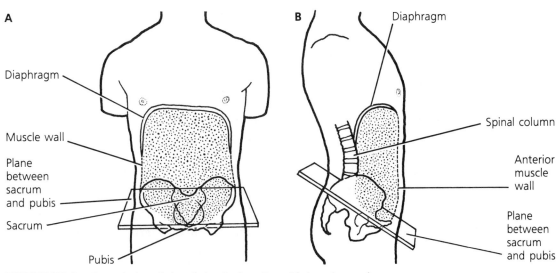

FIGURE 33.1. Boundaries of the abdominal cavity with imaginary plane.

into the abdominal cavity and the retroperitoneal space, but the true pelvic cavity and the extraperitoneal space of the lower abdomen will be grouped together under the term *pelvis*.

Contents of the Abdomen

Abdominal Cavity

The organs of the abdominal cavity include the liver, gallbladder, bile ducts, stomach, and intestines (Fig. 33.2). The spleen, although it is an abdominal organ, is not part of either the gastrointestinal or the genitourinary system. It functions in the normal production and destruction of blood and lymphatic tissue and, as such, is part of the hematologic system and is discussed in Chapter 27.

Retroperitoneal Space

The kidneys and ureter lie behind the peritoneum in the upper abdomen and, therefore, are extraperitoneal structures and are not truly considered part of the abdominal cavity (Fig. 33.3).

Pelvis

The pelvis includes the rectum, and in the female, the internal reproductive organs. The urinary bladder, urethra, and, in males, the prostate and seminal vesicles are within the pelvis but are extraperitoneal.

The Mesentery

The peritoneum not only lines the abdominal and pelvic cavities but also is reflected from the body walls to cover the organs within the cavities. These reflections of peritoneum form the **mesentery**, or suspensory ligaments for the abdominal organs. Mesenteric attachments allow the organs to be suspended fairly freely within their cavities, and hence, they can shift position with regard to one another. Blood vessels and nerves to the organs of the abdominal and pelvic cavities travel through the mesentery to reach these organs. When the peritoneum covers abdominal and pelvic organs, it is called **serosa** (see Fig. 33.3).

Nerve Supply to the Peritoneum

Peritoneum, like all other tissues, has a nerve supply. The peritoneum lining the abdominal wall (the parietal peritoneum) has the same ability to perceive sensation as the skin of the wall itself because it is directly supplied by the same somatic nerves that innervate the skin. The peritoneum that forms mesentery and serosa (the **visceral peritoneum**) perceives only one sensation—stretch—and is innervated by the autonomic rather than the somatic nervous system. The autonomic system cannot localize pain and can only perceive tension. The visceral innervation gives rise to the phenomenon of **referred pain**, which is pain felt on a distant body surface associated with the same area of the spinal cord as the organ causing pain.

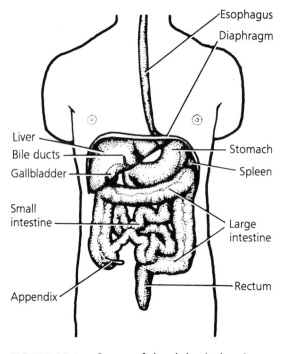

Esophagus
Diaphragm
Liver
Bile ducts
Gallbladder
Stomach
Spleen
Small intestine
Large intestine
Appendix
Rectum

FIGURE 33.2. Organs of the abdominal cavity.

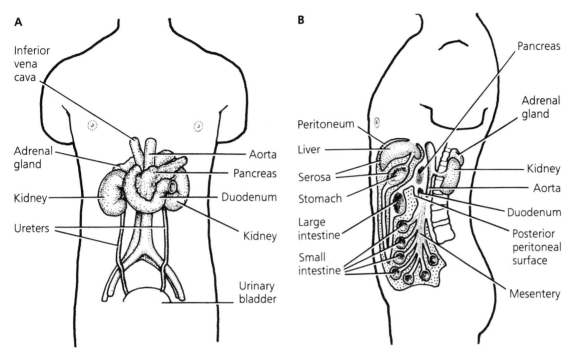

FIGURE 33.3. (a) Major retroperitoneal organs seen in frontal view. (b) Relationship of retroperitoneal organs in side view.

Bony Landmarks in the Abdomen

Bony landmarks in the abdomen include the pubic symphysis, the costal arch, the iliac crests, and the anterior superior iliac spines. The major soft tissue landmark is the umbilicus, which overlies the fourth lumbar vertebra, or the junction of the fourth and fifth vertebrae in some persons. For ease of description, the abdomen is arbitrarily divided into quadrants by two perpendicular lines intersecting at the umbilicus. (See Fig. 9.8 on page 132 for a visual representation of the quadrants.)

In the right upper quadrant, the liver lies very well protected by the eighth through twelfth ribs. Normally it is entirely under the costal arch and not palpable. Similarly, in the left upper quadrant, the stomach and the spleen are protected by the lowermost ribs, and only a very small portion of the stomach is not covered by bone and cartilage.

The aorta and vena cava divide to form the common iliac arteries and veins at the level of the fourth lumbar vertebra or underneath the umbilicus. The pubic symphysis lies immediately anterior to the bladder and forms the anterior-most portion of the bony ring that surrounds and protects the organs within the pelvic cavity.

Hollow and Solid Organs

In general, the organs of the abdominal cavity, the retroperitoneal space, and the pelvis are regarded as either hollow or solid. **Hollow organs** are tubes through which materials pass. For example, the stomach and intestines conduct food through the body, and the ureters and bladder conduct and store urine until it is expelled. The stomach, duodenum, small intestine, large intestine (colon), rectum, appendix, gallbladder, bile ducts, urinary bladder, and ureters are the hollow organs (Fig. 33.4).

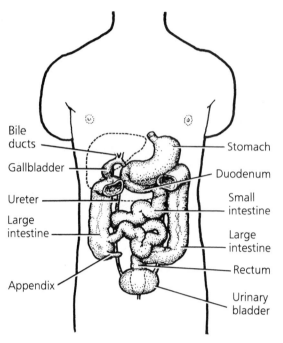

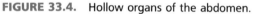

FIGURE 33.4. Hollow organs of the abdomen.

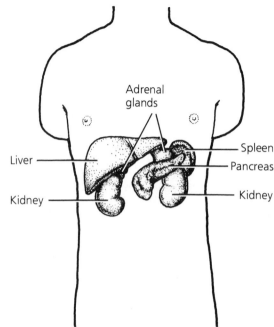

FIGURE 33.5. Solid organs of the abdomen.

Solid organs are solid masses of tissue where much of the chemical work of the body takes place. The liver, spleen, pancreas, kidneys, and adrenal glands are the solid organs (Fig. 33.5).

Injuries within the abdomen can involve either hollow or solid organs. In general, hollow organs discharge their contents into the abdominal cavity or adjacent tissue when they are lacerated, while solid organs tend to bleed copiously. Spilled contents usually cause an intense, painful inflammatory reaction called **peritonitis**. Bleeding from solid organs frequently causes shock and may be rapidly fatal. Mesentery that support hollow organs can be lacerated. Bleeding from torn mesentery can be severe, and the organ that is torn away loses its blood supply.

THE GASTROINTESTINAL SYSTEM

The digestive system is composed of the gastrointestinal tract (stomach and intestines), mouth, salivary glands, pharynx,

esophagus, liver, gallbladder, pancreas, rectum, and anus (Fig. 33.6). The function of this system is to process food to nourish the individual cells of the body.

The Process of Digestion

Digestion of liquid and solid food, from the time it is taken into the mouth until essential compounds are extracted and delivered by the circulatory system to nourish all the cells of the body, is a complicated chemical process. In succession, different secretions are added by the salivary glands, stomach, liver, pancreas, and small intestine to convert food into basic sugars, fatty acids, and amino acids. These products are then carried in the venous blood from the intestine to the liver, where they are further changed to simpler materials that nourish individual tissues and cells. The products are then pumped in the blood through the heart and arteries to the capillaries, where they pass through the capillary walls and the cell walls to feed the body's cells.

Digestion that occurs within the small

bowel produces many poisonous chemical compounds that cannot be passed safely into the general circulation until the liver has transformed them. The fact that all the blood leaving the intestine must first pass through the liver protects the body as a whole against such compounds.

Peristalsis

Two layers of involuntary or smooth muscle form the wall of the entire intestinal tract from the esophagus to the rectum. The outer layer is oriented longitudinally, and the inner layer is circular. Involuntary muscle is so called because it continues to contract rhythmically, regardless of conscious will. Involuntary muscle handles the work of all the internal organs except the heart. Blood vessels constrict or dilate in response to heat or cold, workload or rest, fright, and a number of other stimuli. Smooth muscle fibers in the vessel walls perform this action. The bronchi and bronchioles (air passages in the lung) dilate or constrict in response to cold or inhaled irritants because of involuntary muscle action in their walls.

The involuntary muscles of the gastrointestinal tract are stimulated to contract when they are stretched by food that is swallowed. **Peristalsis,** the coordinated wavelike contraction of the involuntary muscles, starts at the stomach and proceeds to the anus, propelling food through the digestive tract (Fig. 33.7). Swallowing initiates peristalsis in the esophagus. In the gastrointestinal tract, peristalsis is initiated by gastric distention. Once started, a wave passes through the entire system.

When peristaltic waves are especially strong or when they are interrupted by an obstruction so that the contents in the gastrointestinal tract cannot be propelled along, the contraction causes a painful cramp, called **colic.** Normal peristalsis is responsible for the bowel sounds that are heard when one listens to the abdomen with a stethoscope. These sounds represent the passage of gas and fluid through a narrow hollow organ.

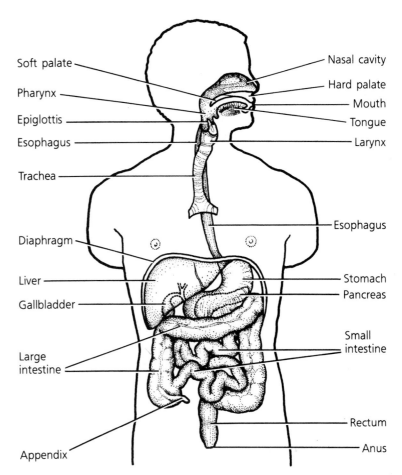

FIGURE 33.6. The digestive system extends from the head to the anus.

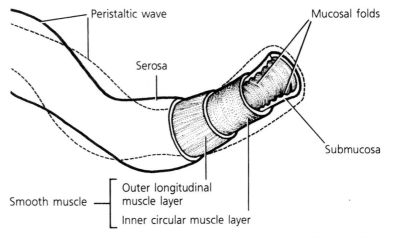

FIGURE 33.7. Smooth muscle layers or individual fibers allow tubular organs (intestine, blood vessels, or bronchi) to contract or dilate, producing a peristaltic wave of intestinal contraction.

Involuntary muscles are constantly responding to changes in their immediate surroundings, although the person does not consciously perceive many of the specific stimuli. These stimuli and their muscular surroundings keep us automatically in balance and maintain much of the body's routine work.

Organs of the Gastrointestinal System

Mouth

The mouth consists of the lips, cheeks, gums, teeth, and tongue. A mucous membrane lines the mouth, and hard and soft palates form the roof of the mouth (see Fig. 33.6). The hard palate is a bony plate that lies anteriorly, and the soft palate is a fold of mucous membrane and muscle that extends posteriorly into the throat. The soft palate is designed to hold food that is being chewed within the mouth and to initiate swallowing.

Salivary Glands

Three paired **salivary glands** are located under the tongue, on each side of the lower jaw (just below the angle of the mandible), and on each cheek (in the tissue just in front of the ears). They produce nearly 1.5 liters of saliva daily to keep the mouth and pharynx moist. **Saliva**, which enters the mouth through the salivary ducts, is approximately 98 percent water. The remaining 2 percent is composed of mucus, salts, and organic compounds. Mucus serves as a binder for chewed food and as a lubricant within the mouth.

Digestive enzymes actually accomplish the chemical conversion of food within the gastrointestinal tract, breaking it down from starch, fat, and protein into simple sugars, fatty acids, and amino acids. Saliva contains only one digestive enzyme—ptyalin. Ptyalin initiates the digestion of starch, converting it to a simple sugar. Otherwise, in the mouth, food is converted into a soft mush that mixes with mucus and saliva for easy swallowing.

Pharynx

The **pharynx**, or throat, is a tubular structure about 5 inches long that extends vertically from the back of the mouth to the esophagus and trachea. The **trachea**, or windpipe, lies just in front of the esophagus. It is connected with the pharynx by the **larynx**, or voice box. The larynx is covered by a leaf-shaped valve called the **epiglottis**. An automatic movement of the pharynx permits the epiglottis to close over the larynx when swallowing is initiated so that liquids and solids move into the esophagus and away from the trachea.

Esophagus

The **esophagus** is a collapsible tube about 10 inches long. It extends from the end of the pharynx to the stomach, and lies just anterior to the spinal column in the chest. Contractions of the muscle in the esophagus propel food through it toward the stomach. Liquids pass with very little assistance. Semisolid foods seldom take more than 10 seconds to pass through the esophagus to the stomach.

Stomach

The **stomach**, a hollow abdominal organ that is located in the upper left quadrant of the abdominal cavity, is largely protected by the lower left ribs. The major function of the stomach is to receive food in large, intermittent quantities, store it, and provide for its movement into the small bowel in regular small amounts. Muscular movement in the walls of the stomach and gastric juice, which contains much mucus, convert ingested food to a thoroughly mixed, semisolid mass. Only one digestive enzyme, pepsin, is produced in the stomach. Pepsin initiates the digestion of protein.

In 1 to 3 hours, muscular contractions propel the entire semisolid food mass, along with approximately 1.5 liters of gastric juice, into the first division of the small intestine, the duodenum. Poisoning or any reaction to trauma may paralyze gastric muscular action and cause the retention of food in the stomach. In these instances, only vomiting or insertion of a stomach tube can empty this organ.

Pancreas

The **pancreas**, a flat, solid organ, lies below and behind the liver and stomach, and behind the peritoneum on the spine and muscles of the back. It is oriented transversely in the upper abdomen. Because the pancreas is firmly fixed in position, deep within the abdomen, it is not easily damaged.

The pancreas contains two kinds of cells. **Acinar cells** secrete nearly 2 liters of pancreatic juice daily. This secretion, which is very important in the digestion of food, contains many enzymes that digest fat, starch, and protein. Pancreatic juice flows directly into the duodenum through the pancreatic ducts. The other cells that the pancreas contains are called the **islets of Langerhans**. They do not connect to any duct but instead secrete their products into the bloodstream across the capillaries. These islets produce a hormone, **insulin**, that regulates the amount of sugar in the blood. The islets also secrete several other regulatory hormones.

Liver

The **liver** is a large, solid organ that takes up most of the area immediately beneath the diaphragm on the right upper quadrant of the abdomen. It is largely protected by the lower right ribs and the costal arch. It is the largest solid organ in the abdomen and consequently the one most often injured.

The liver is a vital organ with several functions. Poisonous substances produced by digestion are brought to it by the blood and rendered harmless. Factors necessary for blood clotting are produced by the liver. In another function, the liver makes between 0.5 and 1.0 liters of bile daily to aid in the normal digestion of fat. The liver is also the principal organ for storing sugar for immediate use by the body. Finally, the liver also produces many of the factors that aid in regulating immune responses.

Essentially, the liver is a large mass of blood vessels and cells packed tightly together. For this reason, it is very fragile and easily injured. Blood flow in the liver is very high, since all of the blood that is pumped from the gastrointestinal tract passes through the liver before it returns to the heart. In addition, the liver receives a generous arterial blood supply of its own.

Gallbladder

The liver is connected to the intestine by a duct system consisting of the **gallbladder** and the **bile ducts**, properly considered hollow organs. The gallbladder acts as a reservoir for bile that is received from the liver. The gallbladder discharges the bile into the duodenum through the common bile duct. The presence of fat, food, or acid peptic juice in the duodenum triggers a contraction of the gallbladder so that it can empty. It usually contains 2 to 3 ounces of bile. The liver is connected directly to the duodenum by the bile ducts, while the gallbladder is a pouch that is connected to the side of the common bile duct. Stones can form in the gallbladder and then pass into the common bile duct to obstruct it. Injuries of the gallbladder and bile ducts are not common, since these organs are fairly small and well protected.

Small Intestine

The **small intestine**, the major abdominal hollow organ, is so named because of its diameter in comparison with the large intestine and stomach. The duodenum, jejunum, and ileum are all part of the small intestine.

The **duodenum** is the first part of the small intestine into which food passes from the stomach and mixes with secretions from the pancreas and liver that enter the duodenum through the pancreatic ducts and the bile ducts. About 12 inches long, most of the duodenum lies behind the peritoneum and closely curls around the head of the pancreas (see Fig. 33.3). The duodenum is thus well protected and is rarely injured. However, injuries of the duodenum do occur, particularly from a severe impact against the abdomen.

The second and third parts of the small intestine are the jejunum and ileum. Together, they measure more than 20 feet on the average.

The small intestine empties into the large intestine through the ileocecal valve. This valve allows passage of bowel contents in only one direction—into the colon of the large intestine. The junction of the small and large intestines is normally in the right lower quadrant of the abdominal cavity.

The small intestine lies entirely free within the abdomen, supported by its mesentery, which is attached to the back wall of the body. Arteries that lead from the aorta to the intestine and veins that carry blood to the liver lie within this supporting tissue. These vessels may be damaged in abdominal injury.

Within the small intestine are the bile, pancreatic juice, and small bowel secretions. Some 3 liters of small bowel juice containing mucus and potent enzymes are secreted daily.

Bile, which is produced by the liver and stored in the gallbladder, empties as needed into the duodenum. Bile is greenish-black, but it changes color during digestion to give feces its typical brown color. The major digestive function of bile is to emulsify and digest fat. Pancreatic juice and small bowel juice each contain the powerful chemical enzymes that carry out the final processes of digesting protein, fat, and carbohydrate.

Within the small bowel, food is digested —that is, it is broken down into its basic chemical constituents. The products of digestion, including water, ingested vitamins, and minerals, are then absorbed across the walls of the lower end of the ileum for transport through the veins to the liver.

Large Intestine

The large intestine, another major hollow organ, consists of the cecum, the colon, and the rectum. About 5 feet long, the large intestine encircles the outer border of the abdomen around the small bowel. It lies partly behind the peritoneum and partly on a mesentery, hanging free like the small bowel. It is most susceptible to injury at those areas where it changes from a fixed to a freely movable organ.

The contents of the small intestine empty into the first portion of the large intestine, the cecum, through the ileocecal valve. Then the matter enters the colon, which extends from the cecum to the rectum. The major function of the colon is to absorb the final 5 to 10 percent of water remaining in the fluid fecal matter to form solid stool, which is stored in the rectum and passes out of the body through the anus. The rectum, the lowermost end of the large intestine, lies in the hollow of the sacrum within the pelvic cavity.

Anus

At the terminal end of the rectum is the anus, a canal that is lined by normal skin and is approximately 2 inches long. The rectum and anus are supplied with a complex series of circular muscles, called sphincters, that control the escape of liquids, gases, and solids from the digestive tract. In general, the most distal anal sphincter, voluntarily controlled, can prevent or permit the escape of gas and some liquid. True rectal control is given by a broad shelf of muscle called the levator ani, which forms the entire pelvic floor.

Sensation within the rectum and anus is very specialized. The rectum is adapted to expand and, at a critical point, to expel its contents. Some rectal tumors fill up the organ and trigger this expelling reflex but cannot, in turn, be expelled. The resulting urge to defecate, which cannot be satisfied, is called tenesmus. Within the short terminal anal canal, sensation is exactly like that of the skin. Ulceration, irritations, and lacerations are as painful as on a finger or toe. Because the anus is so richly supplied with nerves, an irritation here may result in profound systemic reactions.

Appendix

The **appendix** is a small tube that opens into the cecum (the first part of the large intestine) in the lower right quadrant of the abdomen. This tubular organ, about 3 to 4 inches long, is closed at the other end. It may easily become obstructed, and as a result, inflamed and infected. **Appendicitis**, the term for this inflammation, is one of the major causes of severe abdominal distress.

The appendix has no major function in the human, although some researchers believe it may play a role in early life in developing a normal immune response. It has no role in the usual processes of digestion.

THE GENITOURINARY SYSTEM

The genital and urinary systems are commonly discussed together—hence the term **genitourinary system**—because their various organs and passages develop from the same embryologic beginnings, and they thus share many structures. The **genital system** controls the reproductive processes, and the **urinary system** controls the discharge of certain waste materials filtered from the blood.

Organs of the Urinary System

The urinary system lies in the retroperitoneal space behind the organs of the digestive system. In the urinary system, the kidneys are solid organs, and the bladder and ureters are hollow organs (Fig. 33.8).

Kidneys

The body has two **kidneys** that lie on the posterior muscular wall of the abdomen behind the peritoneum. These vital organs rid the blood of toxic waste products and control the balance of water and salt. If the kidneys are destroyed or, for any reason, no longer function adequately, **uremia** occurs. Waste accumulates within the bloodstream, the balance of salt and water is disturbed, and death may result.

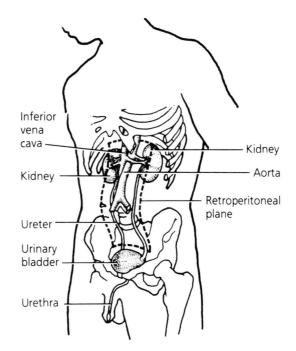

FIGURE 33.8.   The organs of the urinary system.

Nearly 20 percent of the output of blood from the heart each minute passes through the kidneys. Large vessels attach the kidneys directly to the aorta and the inferior vena cava. Blood flow in the kidneys is high. The kidneys constantly filter waste products and water from the blood to form urine. The kidneys continuously concentrate this filtered urine by reabsorbing the water as it passes through a system of specialized tubes within them. These tubes finally unite to form the **renal pelvis**, a cone-shaped collecting area that connects the ureter and the kidney. Under normal conditions, each kidney drains its urine into one ureter, through which the urine passes to the bladder.

Ureters

A **ureter** passes from the renal pelvis of each kidney along the surface of the posterior wall to drain into the urinary bladder. The ureters are small (diameter 0.5 cm), hollow, muscular tubes. Peristalsis in these tubes moves the urine to the bladder. Injuries of the ureters are rare because they are small and well protected.

Urinary Bladder and Urethra

The **urinary bladder** is situated immediately behind the pubic symphysis in the pelvic cavity. It is covered by peritoneum and hence lies outside the abdominal cavity and in front of it. The ureters enter the bladder posteriorly at its base. The bladder empties to the outside of the body through the **urethra**. In men, the urethra passes from the anterior base of the bladder into the penis (Fig. 33.9). In women, the urethra opens at the front of the vagina (Fig. 33.10).

The bladder is formed of smooth muscle with a specialized lining membrane. Smooth muscle reacts to automatic stimuli transmitted by the autonomic nervous system. Urination is largely an autonomic function that can, however, be controlled voluntarily. Ordinarily, bladder contraction and the stimulus to void are the automatic results of stimulation of the bladder at a certain critical point of fullness. This is another regulatory function of smooth muscle. Sensory cells then send messages to the brain, notifying it that the bladder is ready to empty, and the bladder contracts, forcing urine through the urethra to the outside of the body. The normal adult forms 1.5 to 2 liters of concentrated urine every day. This waste is extracted and concentrated from the 1,500 liters of blood that circulate through the kidneys daily.

Organs of the Genital System

The genital system controls the reproductive process from which life is created.

The genitalia include the male and female reproductive organs and the male urethra. The **male genitalia**, except for the prostate gland and seminal vesicles, are outside the abdomen (see Fig. 33.9). The **female genitalia**—the uterus, ovaries, fallopian tubes, and vagina—are contained entirely within the pelvis (see Fig. 33.10). The male and female reproductive organs produce sex hormones, as well as being the

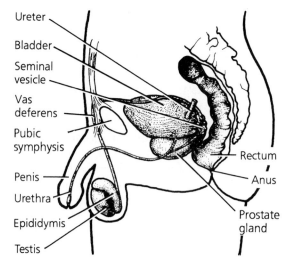

FIGURE 33.9. The male genital system is outside the abdomen, except for the prostate gland and seminal vesicles.

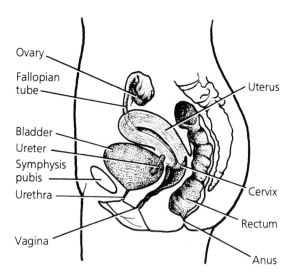

FIGURE 33.10. The female genital system is entirely contained within the pelvis.

source of sperm and eggs. They make possible sexual intercourse and, ultimately, reproduction.

Male Reproductive System

The male reproductive system includes the testicles, vasa deferentia, seminal vesicles, prostate gland, urethra, and penis (see Fig. 33.9). Each **testicle**, or **testis**, contains specialized cells and ducts. Certain cells produce male hormones and others develop sperm. The hormones are absorbed directly into the bloodstream from the testicles. The **epididymis** is a cordlike structure along the posterior border of the testis where sperm is stored. The sperm cells from each of the two testicles enter a duct called the **vas deferens**. The two ducts (vasa deferentia) travel from the testicles up beneath the skin of the abdominal wall for a short distance. They then pass through an opening into the abdominal cavity and down into the prostate gland where they meet the urethra. The **seminal vesicles** are small storage sacs for sperm and seminal fluid. These vesicles also empty into the urethra at the prostate. **Semen** (seminal fluid) contains sperm cells that were carried up through each vas deferens from a testis where they mix with fluid from the seminal vesicles and prostate gland.

The **prostate gland** is a small gland that surrounds the urethra where it emerges from the urinary bladder. Fluids from the prostate gland and from the seminal vesicles come together during intercourse. During the act of intercourse, special mechanisms in the nervous system prevent the passage of urine into the urethra. Only seminal fluid, prostatic fluid, and sperm pass from the penis into the vagina during ejaculation.

The **penis** is a special type of tissue called **erectile tissue**. This tissue is largely vascular and, when filled with blood, distends the penis into a state of erection. As the vessels fill under pressure from the circulatory system, the penis becomes a rigid organ that can enter the vagina. Certain spinal injuries, some diseases, and certain drugs cause a permanent and painful erection called **priapism**.

Female Reproductive System

The female reproductive organs include the ovaries, fallopian tubes, uterus, and vagina (see Fig. 33.10). The **ovaries**, like the testi-

cles, produce sex hormones and specialized cells for reproduction. The female sex hormones are absorbed directly into the bloodstream. A specialized cell, called an **ovum**, is produced with regularity during the adult female's reproductive years. The ovaries release a mature egg, or ovum, approximately once every 28 days. This egg travels through the fallopian tubes to the uterus.

The **fallopian tubes** connect with the uterus and carry the ovum to the cavity of the uterus. The **uterus** is a pear-shaped, hollow organ with muscular walls. A narrow opening from the uterus to the vagina is called the **cervix**.

The **vagina** is a muscular, distensible tube that connects the uterus with the **vulva**, the external female genitalia. The vagina receives the male penis during intercourse, and semen and sperm are deposited into the vagina during ejaculation of the penis. The sperm may pass into the uterus and fertilize an egg, causing pregnancy. Should the pregnancy come to completion at the end of 9 months, the baby will pass through the vagina and be born. The vagina also channels the menstrual flow from the uterus out of the body.

The **menstrual period** is the end of the monthly female reproductive cycle. A woman has monthly periods of menstruation from the start of the first menstrual period at about age 12 until menopause at about age 50. Each month the **endometrium** (lining of the uterus) is stimulated by the female sex hormones to form a special bed. This bed is prepared so that, if a sperm and ovum unite to make a fertilized egg, the uterus is ready to receive it and provide a place for it to grow. Approximately 14 days after a menstrual period ceases, one ovary produces an egg. This egg travels into the uterus through the fallopian tubes.

If a sperm is able to travel from the vagina through the cervix to fertilize the egg, either in the uterus or in the fallopian tubes, the fertilized egg settles in the uterus and begins to grow in the lining there. If the egg is not fertilized, the uterus sheds its recently formed special lining, a very thin layer of cells and blood, and the menstrual period takes place. The lining, in the form of the menstrual flow, passes out of the uterus into the vagina and out of the body. The flow lasts about 5 days. After it ceases, the uterus begins to prepare a new lining as a bed to receive a new egg, and the cycle repeats itself.

PHYSICAL EXAMINATION OF THE ABDOMEN

The trainer is not expected to be able to give a thorough examination of athletes who have abdominal complaints or injuries. However, having at least some knowledge of an abdominal examination is helpful in understanding the management of abdominal injuries and on-the-field evaluation of athletes with abdominal injuries.

Examining the Abdomen

A thorough examination of the abdomen entails six major steps, which are carried out in the following order: (1) general appearance of the athlete, (2) vital signs, (3) inspection of the abdomen, (4) auscultation, (5) percussion, and finally, (6) palpation. An expert examiner is reassuring, organized, knowledgeable, and complete.

General Appearance and Vital Signs

The examiner should always begin by noting the general appearance of the athlete. Once the initial brief assessment has been performed (see Chapter 11), the examiner should obtain and record vital signs. To avoid any confusion later, the date and time should always be written next to each vital sign. Temperature, pulse, respirations, and blood pressure are "musts" for all thorough examinations.

Inspection of the Abdomen

To inspect the abdomen, the examiner must look not only at the abdomen, but also at the neck, back, and groin. The examiner should explain to the athlete what is about to happen and then try to make the person as comfortable as possible. Placing pillows beneath the head and knees frequently helps to induce relaxation. Modesty should be respected by covering areas not being examined with a towel or blanket. When a female athlete is being examined, the examiner should ask her if there is any chance she is pregnant.

As the examination begins, the examiner should start by asking the athlete to point out any specific areas of discomfort. Then the examiner looks at the skin, taking care to notice its color, presence of stretch marks (striae), bruising, redness, or rashes. Scars and dilated veins should be searched for as well. The overall size and symmetry of the abdomen should also be noted. For example, are all quadrants of equal size? Are any masses or pulsations apparent?

Auscultation of the Abdomen

Inspection should be followed by **auscultation**—that is, listening very carefully with a stethoscope for the presence or absence of bowel sounds and their character and frequency. Normally, the bowel makes an occasional "gurgling" sound. It is not necessary to listen to all four quadrants, since sounds are easily transmitted throughout the abdomen.

Percussion of the Abdomen

The fifth part of the abdominal inspection is **percussion**, which is performed by placing one's nondominant hand lightly on the athlete's abdomen to determine the presence and location of hollow versus solid organs or masses. The examiner's middle finger is pressed more firmly against the belly than the other fingers. The distal interphalangeal joint is struck sharply with a quick motion, using one or two fingers from the examiner's dominant hand (Fig. 33.11). Sounds described as tympanic (hollow) or dull (full) result. A hollow organ such as the stomach will sound tympanic, and a solid organ such as the liver will sound dull.

All four quadrants must be percussed, and facial expressions should be observed for signs of discomfort. Percussion may be a difficult technique for beginners to master and it requires practice.

Palpation of the Abdomen

For the last portion of the abdominal examination, **palpation**, the examiner first places the palmar aspect of his or her fingers on the athlete's abdomen. By pressing lightly and using a circular motion to feel, the examiner covers all four quadrants, feeling for muscle resistance and superficial masses. Next, the examiner places the free hand on top of the examining hand and presses downward with slightly more force. This technique is used for palpation of deeper structures. Keep in mind the anatomy of structures beneath the skin. It will be difficult to palpate organs and masses in an athlete who is obese or has very developed abdominal muscles. Reassuring the athlete during deep palpation is helpful.

During palpation, the examiner should note any resistance or rigidity, as well as any masses and their exact location, size, and shape. Kidneys are usually only palpable in thin women. Structures that may be mistaken for pathologic masses are bowel, a full bladder, pregnant uterus, and sacral promontory. An enlarged liver can be detected by palpating firmly in the upper right quadrant and asking the athlete to breathe deeply in and out. Gradually, the examiner edges his or her hands toward the ribs, repeating the above maneuver. If an enlarged liver is present, the examiner may feel a mass "flip" across the fingertip of the examining hand.

If the abdomen seems more tender than usual, the examiner should check for **rebound tenderness**. The examiner puts slow, deep pressure on the abdomen and then quickly withdraws both hands. Pain elicited upon withdrawal of both hands is rebound

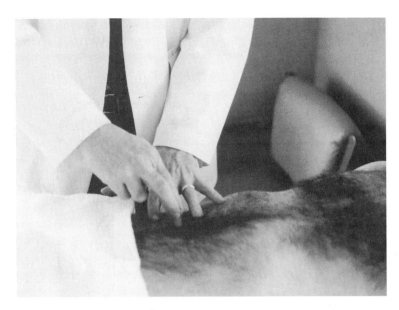

FIGURE 33.11.   Percussion.

tenderness and may be a sign of inflammation of the lining of the abdominal cavity.

Evaluating the Genitourinary System

The kidneys may be checked for discomfort by placing an open hand over the area of the back where the lower ribs exit from the spine. The examiner firmly strikes the hand with his or her fist. If pain is elicited, contusion of the kidneys may have occurred; if there is pain but no history of trauma, kidney infection may be present.

In evaluating the remainder of the genitourinary system, the examiner's responsibility is generally limited to inspection and palpation of the external genitalia. Contusions and hematomas of the scrotum in the male and the labia in the female do occur during sports participation and should be recognized so that first-aid care (cold compresses generally) can be given, and referral to a physician recommended if the swelling is severe.

IMPORTANT CONCEPTS

1. The abdomen is divided into the upper cavity, or abdominal cavity, and the lower cavity, or pelvic cavity, and both cavities are lined with a smooth, glistening, transparent layer of thin tissue called peritoneum.

2. In addition to lining the abdominal and pelvic cavities, the peritoneum is reflected from the body walls to form mesentery, or suspensory ligaments for the abdominal organs.

3. The phenomena of referred pain is pain felt on a distant body surface associated with the same area of the spinal cord as the organ causing pain.

4. When lacerated, hollow organs generally discharge their contents into the abdominal cavity or adjacent tissue, while solid organs tend to bleed copiously.

5. The products of digestion are carried in the venous blood from the small intestine to the liver where they are changed to simpler nutrients that nourish individual tissues and cells.

6. The coordinated wavelike contraction of peristalsis propels food through the digestive tract.

7. The organs of the gastrointestinal system are the mouth, salivary glands, pharynx, esophagus, stomach, pancreas, liver, gallbladder, small intestine, large intestine, and anus.

8. The organs of the urinary system are the kidneys, ureters, urinary bladder, and urethra.

9. The organs of the genital system are the testicles, vasa deferentia, seminal vesicles, prostate gland, urethra, and the penis (in the male), and the ovaries, fallopian tubes, uterus, and vagina (in the female).

10. A general examination of the abdomen should include general appearance, vital signs, inspection of the abdomen, auscultation, percussion, and palpation.

SUGGESTED READINGS

Bates, Barbara. *A Guide to Physical Examination*, 3d ed. Philadelphia: J. B. Lippincott, 1983.

Cope, Sir Zachary. *Cope's Early Diagnosis of the Acute Abdomen*, 17th ed. Revised by William Silen. New York: Oxford University Press, 1987.

Sleisenger, M. H., and J. S. Fordtran, eds. *Gastrointestinal Disease: Pathophysiology, Diagnosis, Management*, 4th ed. Philadelphia: W. B. Saunders, 1989.

Smith, D. R., ed. *General Urology*, 10th ed. Los Altos, Calif.: Lange Medical Publications, 1981.

Walsh, P. C., R. F. Gittes, A. D. Perlmutter, et al., eds. *Campbell's Urology*, 5th ed. Philadelphia: W. B. Saunders, 1986.

Wyngaarden, J. B., and L. H. Smith, Jr. *Cecil Textbook of Medicine*, 18th ed. Philadelphia: W. B. Saunders, 1988.

34

Common Gastrointestinal and Genitourinary Complaints

OBJECTIVES FOR CHAPTER 34

After reading this chapter, the student should be able to:

1. Identify and describe common gastrointestinal and genitourinary complaints.
2. Recognize gastrointestinal and genitourinary conditions that require emergency treatment.

INTRODUCTION

The athletic trainer often has to deal with complaints indicating gastrointestinal (GI) and genitourinary (GU) disease. Frequently these complaints interfere with the person's normal daily habits. In some cases, emergency help and transportation to the emergency department may be advisable. GI complaints such as vomiting, diarrhea, and blood in the stools are discussed in the first half of Chapter 34. The remainder of the chapter concentrates on GU complaints such as blood in the urine, incontinence, and urethral discharge. ■

GASTROINTESTINAL SYSTEM COMPLAINTS

Within the GI system, emergency complaints not associated with injuries or an acute abdomen include dysphagia (difficulty in swallowing), vomiting, hematemesis (vomiting of blood), diarrhea, melena (dark, black stools indicative of blood), hematochezia (bright red blood in the stool), jaundice, and colic.

Dysphagia

Dysphagia is the sensation of difficulty in swallowing. Obstructing lesions in the esophagus range from swallowed foreign bodies to carcinomas (cancerous growths). In general, the athlete complains of a sensation of food sticking under the breastbone or at the back of the throat. In many instances, the dysphagia slowly progresses, starting with difficulty in swallowing chunks of meat and becoming more severe, so that only liquids or very soft gruel can be swallowed. Many people ignore dysphagia until it becomes very severe. Drinking water at meals eases difficult swallowing, and the person tends to forget about the problem until the next meal, since this condition does not cause pain.

Dysphagia usually represents long-standing disease, and professional help should be obtained promptly. Generally, dysphagia is not an emergency condition, but it can be associated with a number of very serious ailments.

Vomiting

Vomiting, the response of the stomach to a stimulus such as irritation, infection, or obstruction, should be distinguished from **regurgitation**, the result of overfilling or overdistending the stomach with air and fluid. The "burp" is an example of regurgitation. Any situation that reduces peristalsis (wavelike contractions that propel food through the digestive tract) may result in vomiting. Any disease or situation that causes a specific inflammation of the lining of the GI tract, especially the stomach, can also result in vomiting.

Causes of Vomiting

Vomiting is one of the most common GI complaints, and it results from a multitude of causes. **Gastroenteritis**, of viral or bacterial origin, is a very common cause of vomiting, as is the ingestion of irritating agents, most commonly seen in the athlete who has indulged very heavily in alcohol. Alcohol stimulates gastric juice as well as irritates gastric mucosa. Food poisoning often causes vomiting when the stomach attempts to rid itself of the noxious agent, as does the excessive use of an irritant drug such as aspirin. Any mechanical obstruction to the passage of material through the GI tract will also cause vomiting.

Vomiting is always serious, and the trainer may not know its cause. Rarely, however, is vomiting an emergency in itself, unless it goes on for several days and the affected person has not eaten or drunk enough fluid to replace that lost in the vomitus. In such situations, the person may actually go into shock because of the amount of fluid and salt lost from the body. This particular state is termed **metabolic shock** (see Chapter 38).

Care of the Vomiting Athlete

Care of the vomiting athlete is usually straightforward unless the athlete is semiconscious. The alert athlete who is vomiting because of an illness is rarely, if ever, in danger of **aspiration** (inhaling vomitus into the lungs), since all the reflexes guarding the airway are active. The somnolent or semiconscious athlete may vomit in bed or when supine (lying on the back with the face upward) and frequently does aspirate vomitus. Clearing and protecting the airway of this person are of paramount importance. The vomiting athlete who is in shock constitutes a genuine emergency. The airway must be cleared and protected, and the person must be transported as promptly as possible to the emergency department.

Vomiting as a consequence of injury is discussed in chapters dealing with specific trauma. The athletic trainer should anticipate vomiting in these situations and be prepared to take appropriate measures to protect the airway.

Hematemesis

Hematemesis, or the vomiting of blood, is a particular concern. In general, it is associated with problems arising in the esophagus or the stomach. Hematemesis can consist of small quantities of **coffee grounds vomitus** (dark-colored, digested blood that looks like coffee grounds) or large quantities of bright red blood. Among the causes of hematemesis are peptic ulcer, esophageal varices, gastritis, and rupture of the stomach or esophagus.

Peptic Ulcer

Probably the most common disease in the United States associated with hematemesis is **peptic ulcer** in the stomach. Peptic ulcers in the duodenum that bleed usually do not produce hematemesis because the pylorus, the muscle that separates the stomach from the duodenum, prevents the blood from returning into the stomach. In these instances, the blood passes down the GI tract and out with the feces rather than up and out as vomitus. Ulcers in the stomach, however, do produce hematemesis.

Coffee grounds vomitus indicates a very slow rate of gastric bleeding. Small quantities of blood are ingested in the stomach and turned dark brown by hydrochloric acid. A very briskly bleeding ulcer may produce large quantities of bright red blood. Whatever the cause, an athlete with hematemesis requires prompt transport to the emergency department. If possible, the amount of blood vomited should be estimated and recorded and a sample collected to take to the hospital with the athlete.

Esophageal Varices

Another very common cause of upper GI tract bleeding is **esophageal varices**. In this situation, a result of long-standing alcohol abuse, cirrhosis of the liver causes blood flow from the GI tract to be shunted around the liver instead of through it. Because of the shunting, huge collateral veins (varices) develop in the esophagus. These veins are distended, and very thin, and contain blood at three or four times the normal pressure for this type of vessel. Bleeding from esophageal varices is copious, bright red, and represents a very severe, frequently fatal, medical emergency.

Ordinarily, a person with esophageal variceal bleeding has a long history of alcohol abuse, may be on a drinking binge, and generally has blood in the vomitus from the first moment of vomiting. There is little or no pain associated with variceal bleeding, but the extent of the hemorrhage makes the emergency nature of the situation obvious. Prompt transport to the emergency department is mandatory, and treatment en route may be required for hypovolemic shock (shock from loss of blood) as well as protection of the airway.

Gastritis

Another fairly common cause of GI bleeding is **gastritis**, or inflammation of the lining of the stomach. This complex disease has a number of causes. Specific agents in everyday use, such as aspirin, alcohol, and a number of related compounds, can irritate the gastric mucosa to the extent that diffuse gastritis and hemorrhage develop. Stress can also cause gastric bleeding. Some medications, such as cortisone, are also associated with this type of bleeding. Hemorrhage is often copious, and vital signs may be unstable. The person with gastritis usually has vague, indefinite epigastric and left upper quadrant pain. Again, prompt transport with treatment for shock and airway protection is needed.

Rupture of the Stomach or Esophagus

Very rarely, forceful or prolonged vomiting will completely rupture the stomach or esophagus. The athlete suddenly has excruciating severe pain in the left side of the chest and left upper quadrant abdominal pain in association with the vomiting. By the time the trainer arrives to evaluate the situation, the athlete will usually be in shock and desperately ill. Using all measures to combat hypovolemic shock and provide respiratory support, the trainer should transport the athlete immediately.

Diarrhea

Diarrhea is a condition of abnormally frequent and liquid bowel movements. Just as vomiting has many causes, so does diarrhea. Anxiety, gastroenteritis (the common flu), severe bacterial infections such as ty-

phoid fever, or parasitic infestations such as an amoeba can all cause diarrhea. Inflammatory processes in the bowel of unknown causes, including ulcerative colitis, granulomatous colitis, or enteritis, can also result in diarrhea. In the elderly, one of the most common causes of diarrhea is a partial obstruction of the bowel by fecal impaction. Only liquid material can pass beyond the impacted feces, and this liquid material produces the diarrhea.

Very rarely does diarrhea cause an acute problem for an athlete. If it has been present for several days and if the athlete has been unable to take sufficient food or fluid to balance the amount of fluid lost, then obvious evidence of dehydration and electrolyte imbalance or starvation may be present. The athlete may have unstable vital signs and be in metabolic shock. The trainer will not see this condition in an athlete very frequently. Remember, however, that uncontrolled diarrhea or vomiting over several days or weeks can result in a desperately ill individual. Ordinarily, the athlete with diarrhea necessitating an emergency call should be transported to the hospital to assess the cause of the problem. It is not generally, however, a first-priority emergency.

Melena

The term *melena* is derived from a Greek term meaning black. **Melena** is the passage of a dark black stool that is very tarry or sticky in consistency. It has a characteristic, particularly foul odor. The black color is due to blood in the stool that has been digested within the GI tract. In general, melena is associated with slow, continuous bleeding in the upper GI tract, such as with peptic ulcer in the duodenum or ulceration within the small bowel or proximal large bowel.

Melena does not constitute an emergency unless it has been ignored for many weeks and the athlete exhibits signs of hypovolemic shock. It is, however, a cause for grave concern, and the bleeding source must be identified as quickly as possible. Some medications, such as bismuth and iron-containing compounds, impart the same dark black color to the stool. In general, however, the trainer will not be required to make this differential diagnosis.

Hematochezia

The passage of bright red blood in the stool is called **hematochezia**. This condition also has several causes, ranging from colon and rectal cancer to hemorrhoids and anal fissures. Bright red blood in the stool does not ordinarily constitute an emergency, and usually bleeding is not severe. Hematochezia is, however, distinctly abnormal and requires immediate identification of the cause. An athlete who complains of hematochezia should be taken to the emergency department for examination and diagnosis as expeditiously as possible. A recorded estimate of the volume of bloody stool passed will aid the evaluating physician.

Jaundice

Jaundice, derived from a French word meaning yellow, implies a yellow color of the skin. Many diseases cause jaundice, almost all from some malfunction of the liver or the biliary tract. To form bile within its cells, the liver uses the products of the destruction of worn-out red blood cells. The bile is secreted through the common bile duct into the duodenum, where it plays an essential role in digesting fat in the GI tract. A considerable portion of the excreted bile is reabsorbed in the GI tract and returned to the liver.

Any disease that overloads the liver with red cell destruction products causes jaundice, as does any disease that interferes with the function of the normal liver cell so that bile cannot be made or excreted properly. In the latter case, jaundice will result if the outflow of bile from the liver to the GI tract is blocked.

Ordinarily, jaundice does not constitute an emergency, but the athlete should be transported to the hospital for immediate medical attention. Jaundice is most readily detected by looking at portions of the body that are normally white, such as the sclera (white portion) of the eye. In Caucasians jaundice is easily detected, but in pigmented individuals, jaundice may be evident only by examining normally pale areas, such as the undersurface of the tongue, the conjunctiva of the eyes, the scleral surfaces of the eyes, or the palms of the hands.

Colic

Colic implies a characteristic intra-abdominal pain associated with obstruction of largely muscular hollow tubes. The pain is intermittent, rises sharply to an excruciating peak, and relents suddenly as the muscle relaxes. Colic can accompany obstruction of the GI tract by tumors, polyps, foreign bodies, or adhesions. When a urinary stone is obstructing a ureter, there is a characteristic radiation of pain from the flank and into the genitalia. Colic is a very common complaint in children. It is caused by active peristalsis in the GI tract when a wave of contraction catches up with the immediately preceding wave, subjecting the segment of bowel between the two waves to extreme tension. In the adult, colic often accompanies the viral flu syndrome and diarrhea, and again is associated with extreme hyperperistaltic activity of the GI tract. Frequently, the athlete describes colic as a cramp or a gas pain.

The trainer should be familiar with the term *colic* and be able to recognize this type of pain when described. It is a very distressing complaint for the athlete, and its cause must be assessed by a physician. Thus the athlete should be seen by a physician, but the situation is usually not urgent.

GENITOURINARY SYSTEM COMPLAINTS

Within the GU system, complaints include dysuria (painful or burning urination), hematuria (blood in the urine), urinary frequency, incontinence, urethral discharge, or renal colic.

Dysuria

Dysuria is the sensation of pain, burning, or itching that occurs during urination. It generally indicates an inflammatory process or infection within the lower urinary tract (external urethral opening, urethra, and bladder). Urinary tract infections are found much more frequently in women than in men. While dysuria is a symptomatic indication of a problem that should be treated, it does not constitute an emergency. An athlete whose major complaint is dysuria should be referred to a physician for diagnosis and treatment.

Hematuria

The passage of blood in the urine is called **hematuria**. While occasionally it is visible to the naked eye, much more frequently, blood in the urine can be identified only upon microscopic examination of urinary sediment. The causes of hematuria include tumors within the urinary tract, stones that cause abrasions, bleeding from the kidney or the ureters, infection, and trauma. An athlete with hematuria should be seen as soon as possible by a physician for the appropriate diagnostic workup. Hematuria that is easily visible to the unaided eye points to a very serious problem within the urinary tract that needs prompt diagnosis by a physician. Any urine voided by an athlete with urinary complaints should be brought to the physician as well. Hemastix testing of voided urine specimens may also be helpful in diagnosing the presence of blood.

Urinary Frequency

Urinary frequency refers to an abnormally high number of voiding episodes during a 24-hour period. Frequency may be associated with dysuria and bladder infections. Commonly, very small quantities of urine are passed at very frequent intervals. Generally, this urine has a foul odor. In the aging male, the prostate gland, which surrounds the upper portion of the urethra and is adjacent to the bladder, can enlarge and encroach on the urethral passage, partially obstructing it. A sign of this obstruction is urinary frequency that persists not only during the day but also throughout the night. The person with urinary frequency has to get up to void frequently during the night, a condition called **nocturia**.

While urinary frequency may be distressing to the athlete, it is not an emergency and is associated with a number of problems of the lower urinary tract. The trainer should recognize this condition and realize it indicates an underlying disorder which requires evaluation.

Incontinence

The uncontrolled passage of urine or feces and soiling of clothing is called **incontinence**. While not an emergency, it occurs in association with many emergency conditions. Athletes are frequently incontinent during epileptic seizures, but this does not indicate major urinary or bowel disease. The athlete who has suffered a severe spinal injury resulting in paraplegia may lose control of both urinary and fecal discharge. Ordinarily, incontinence in this athlete takes the form of an obligatory overflow from a distended bladder that can no longer contract in a coordinated fashion or respond to the stimulus of being full. Episodic incontinence is frequently associated with unconsciousness or semiconsciousness, as in an alcoholic binge. An older person may be incontinent as a result of generalized senile degeneration.

Incontinence is not ordinarily considered an emergency. However, if it is sudden, unexpected, and not associated with any obvious cause, the athlete may have a serious underlying disorder in the lower urinary tract and should be seen by a physician.

Urethral Discharge

The most common indication of venereal infection in the man is a **penile urethral discharge**. In women, these infections result in an intrapelvic inflammation about the fallopian tubes and the ovaries called **pelvic inflammatory disease**. The discharge in the male may be thin and serous, or it may be grossly purulent (containing pus). Any material passed out of the male urethra other than urine or semen is abnormal and requires medical attention.

Sexually transmitted diseases are extremely common in the United States today, and the athlete with urethral discharge may wish to consult the trainer. The cause of the urethral discharge should be treated immediately. Venereal diseases can become chronic and may have devastating, long-term effects for the individual.

Renal Colic

A fairly common problem is a **renal stone**, or **kidney stone**, usually formed from a combination of calcium and oxalate crystals. Once formed, virtually no agent is able to dissolve these stones. Much less common, but next in frequency, are renal stones that are formed of uric acid in athletes with **gout** (a hereditary form of arthritis that causes extreme pain in one joint). As long as the stones stay in the kidney, they are asymptomatic or may produce hematuria, only apparent on microscopic examination of the urine. If a stone passes from the kidney into the ureter, however, it can quickly obstruct the very small caliber tube.

Urine is formed continuously in the kidney, and each kidney passes approximately 1 liter of urine into the bladder every day. Since there is no reservoir capacity for urine above the bladder and since the volume within the ureters and the collecting system of the kidney is very small, it is absolutely necessary for this liter of urine to pass constantly into the bladder without impediment. When a stone obstructs a ureter, a characteristic colicky sharp pain in the flank on either side of the back ensues, as the muscular ureter tries to overcome the obstruction by vigorous peristalsis proximal to the stone. As the stone progresses down the ureter, the pain may radiate down to either side of the external genitalia in both men and women. Renal colic is one of the most severe forms of pain and requires vigorous measures for immediate relief.

The athlete suffering from renal colic may give a typical history of the type of pain and its location and radiation. This athlete is generally restless, forever seeking a position of some comfort, getting up or lying down. While not life-threatening, this situation is urgent because the athlete demands and requires relief from pain. This athlete must be promptly transported to the emergency department. Ordinarily, no major measures for support of other body systems are necessary. If possible, any urine that is discharged should be collected for analysis at the hospital.

(Important Concepts appear on next page.)

IMPORTANT CONCEPTS

1. Dysphagia is usually a sign of long-standing disease.
2. The vomiting athlete who is in shock constitutes a genuine emergency.
3. Athletes with hematemesis should be promptly transported to the emergency department.
4. Uncontrolled diarrhea may result in dehydration, electrolyte imbalance, or starvation.
5. Melena is generally associated with slow, continuous bleeding in the upper GI tract.
6. Hematochezia is not an emergency, but it does require immediate identification of the cause.
7. Jaundice represents some malfunction of the liver or biliary tract.
8. Colic in an adult often accompanies the viral flu syndrome and diarrhea and is often described as a cramp or gas pain.
9. Dysuria generally indicates inflammation or infection of the lower urinary tract.
10. Hematuria may be grossly visible or apparent only on microscopic examination of urinary sediment.
11. Urinary frequency is associated with dysuria and bladder infections.
12. Incontinence is usually not an emergency, unless it is sudden, unexpected, and not associated with an obvious cause.
13. Urethral discharge is a sign of venereal infection, and it should be treated as quickly as possible.
14. Renal colic is the cause of one of the most severe forms of pain, and it requires immediate treatment for relief of the pain.

SUGGESTED READINGS

Sleisenger, M. H., and J. S. Fordtran, eds. *Gastrointestinal Disease: Pathophysiology, Diagnosis, Management,* 4th ed. Philadelphia: W. B. Saunders, 1989.

Smith, D. R., ed. *General Urology,* 10th ed. Los Altos, Calif.: Lange Medical Publications, 1981.

Walsh, P. C., R. F. Gittes, A. D. Perlmutter, et al., eds. *Campbell's Urology,* 5th ed. Philadelphia: W. B. Saunders, 1986.

Wyngaarden, J. B., and L. H. Smith, Jr. *Cecil Textbook of Medicine,* 18th ed. Philadelphia: W. B. Saunders, 1988.

35

Injuries to the Abdomen and Genitalia

OBJECTIVES FOR CHAPTER 35

After reading this chapter, the student should be able to:
1. Distinguish between blunt and penetrating injuries of the hollow and solid organs of the abdomen.
2. Describe injuries to the male and female genitalia.
3. Provide initial evaluation and care to the athlete with injuries to the abdomen or genitalia.

INTRODUCTION

Abdominal injuries can be fatal as a result of peritonitis or hemorrhage, and therefore prompt medical attention is essential. Injuries to the male and female genitalia are rarely life-threatening, but they can be painful and often require treatment in the emergency department. The first section of Chapter 35 focuses on blunt and penetrating injuries to the hollow and solid organs of the abdomen. The second section of Chapter 35 discusses injuries to the male and female genitalia. It also provides the athletic trainer with guidelines regarding initial evaluation and management prior to the athlete's transfer to the emergency department. ▪

INJURIES TO THE ABDOMEN

Any of the hollow and solid organs of the abdomen can be injured. The hollow organs usually contain a stream of food that is being digested, and when they are ruptured or lacerated, their contents spill into the peritoneal cavity. Digested or undigested food, the bowel contents, gastric juice, or other digestive enzymes cause an intense inflammatory reaction called **peritonitis**. This reaction produces prompt and severe abdominal tenderness, muscular rigidity, and intense pain. Bowel movement is paralyzed, and the abdomen distended. (See Chapter 36 for a discussion of peritonitis.)

Injuries of the solid organs, such as the spleen, usually cause severe hemorrhage due to their rich blood supply. The first signs of these injuries may be changes in pulse and blood pressure, together with other signs indicating shock, such as an ashen, pale color and cold, clammy skin. (See Chapter 38 for further description of the signs and symptoms of shock.)

Closed and open abdominal injuries may involve injury to the aorta, inferior vena cava, or other large blood vessels. The resulting hemorrhage may be severe and fatal.

Types of Abdominal Injuries

Abdominal injuries may be closed (blunt) or open (penetrating), and they may involve hollow or solid organs.

Blunt Abdominal Injuries

In **closed**, or **blunt**, **injuries**, the abdomen is damaged by a severe blow, but the skin remains intact—the kind of injury that can result from being tackled in football. In addition to causing severe bruises of the abdominal wall, blunt trauma can do much damage within the abdomen. The liver and spleen may be lacerated, the intestines may be ruptured, supporting mesenteries may be torn and their vessels injured, or the kidneys may be ruptured or torn from their arteries and veins. The bladder may be ruptured, especially in an athlete who has been consuming lots of fluids and whose bladder may have been full and distended. This individual may have severe intra-abdominal hemorrhage as well as peritoneal irritation and inflammation from the ruptured hollow organs.

Penetrating Abdominal Injuries

In **open**, or **penetrating**, **injuries**, a foreign body has entered the abdomen, opening the peritoneum-lined cavity to the external environment. Stab wounds or gunshot wounds are two examples of open injuries. Some penetrating injuries may only lacerate the abdominal wall itself. Whether the abdominal cavity has been penetrated may not be evident. In the case of a gunshot or stab wound, it can always be assumed that the bullet or knife has entered the abdominal cavity, and emergency care should be rendered accordingly. The only certain way to determine if the abdominal organs have been injured is through exploratory surgery. Emergency medical care for penetrating abdominal wounds is based on the assumption that penetration has occurred and that one or several internal organs have been injured.

Signs and Symptoms of Abdominal Injuries

Abdominal injuries may be very easy to perceive or quite subtle. In general, the overriding complaint of an athlete with abdominal injury is pain. Blunt injury may leave bruises as clues to the nature of the wounding agent. An athlete with penetrating injuries generally has obvious abdominal wounds, through which bowel or fat may be protruding—a condition called **evisceration**. In addition to pain, the athlete frequently will feel nauseated and may want to vomit. In general, when peritonitis is developing because of irritation of the peritoneal surface, the individual will prefer to lie still because it hurts too much to move.

The signs of an abdominal injury are generally obvious. A clinical **sign**, as opposed to a **symptom**, is a finding that can be elicited by the examiner. Tenderness when the abdomen is palpated is a sign, while pain within the abdomen, of which the athlete complains, is a symptom. Abdominal tenderness—and specifically, localized abdominal tenderness—is a very important clinical sign. Difficulty in moving because of abdominal pain is another sign. Obvious wounds of both entry and exit are excellent clues for determining the nature of an injury, as are bruises. Altered vital signs such as low blood pressure, a rapid pulse, and rapid, shallow respirations are also important indicators. Table 35.1 lists the signs and symptoms of blunt and penetrating abdominal injury.

Initial Evaluation and Care of Abdominal Injuries

The method of evaluating an abdominal injury is basically the same for both blunt and penetrating injuries. The athlete should lie supine (on the back with the face up), as comfortably as possible, with the knees slightly flexed and supported. The trainer should remove or loosen the athlete's clothes, and rapidly assess the athlete's condition by simple inspection. Next, the trainer should record the vital signs, especially the pulse, blood pressure, and rate of respiration. Many abdominal emergencies, aside from those that cause severe bleeding, can cause a rapid pulse and low blood pressure. It is absolutely necessary that a record of vital signs be made as early as possible and that they be recorded at regular intervals thereafter to help the physician evaluate the progress and severity of the problem.

At first inspection, the trainer should take note of how the athlete is lying. The athlete with severe abdominal disease or injury who prefers to lie still usually lies with the legs drawn up. Rapid, shallow breaths limit movement of the abdominal contents. An individual with acute pancreatitis or a ruptured appendix may be lying on the right side with the legs drawn up. Motion of the body or the abdominal organs

TABLE 35.1. Abdominal Injuries: Blunt or Penetrating

Signs	Symptoms
1. Bruises	1. Pain (abdominal)
2. Lacerations or stab wounds	2. Pain (referred)
3. Lowered blood pressure	3. Nausea
4. Elevated pulse	4. Anxiety
5. Rapid, shallow respirations	5. Desire not to be moved
6. Ashen color	
7. Local or diffuse abdominal tenderness	
8. Distention	
9. Shock	
10. Vomiting	

irritates the inflamed peritoneum and causes additional pain, which the athlete instinctively tries to avoid.

The athlete with an abdominal injury may feel nauseated or may vomit. The person's stomach may have been full of food or drink. If vomiting occurs, especially in an athlete who is comatose or nearly so, the throat must be kept clear of vomitus so that it is not aspirated into the lungs. The trainer should turn the athlete's head to one side, and try to keep it lower than the chest. The trainer should also note the material vomited: was it undigested food, blood, mucus, or bile?

Never should the athlete with an abdominal injury be given anything to eat or drink. Food or water not only may worsen symptoms, but also may increase the risks of surgery if an operative procedure becomes necessary.

The purpose of the initial evaluation is to determine the type of injury (whether it is blunt or penetrating), its possible extent, and the presence of shock. The athlete should be transported as promptly as possible to the hospital.

Blunt Abdominal Wounds

Bruises help determine the cause and severity of any blunt injury. The location of bruises or wounds is a clue to the organs that may be injured underneath. The trainer should place the athlete supine in a comfortable position with the head turned to one side. Any signs of shock—pallor, a cold sweat, a rapid, thready pulse, or low blood pressure—should be noted and appropriate measures taken to combat shock. The trainer may have to assist respiration by clearing the airway of vomitus and using oxygen if available. The athlete should be transported promptly and gently to the emergency department.

Penetrating Abdominal Wounds

In the care of a penetrating abdominal wound, it may be very difficult to deter-mine without surgery if the object has penetrated all the way through the abdominal wall and, if it has, what organs are injured. The trainer should always assume major damage has occurred, even if no obvious signs are present immediately, because such signs often develop slowly. With penetrating injuries, the hollow organs are usually lacerated, causing their contents to discharge into the abdominal cavity with resulting inflammation. If major blood vessels are cut or if major solid organs are lacerated, hemorrhage may be rapid and severe.

The first step in the care of the athlete with a penetrating abdominal injury is to note which area of the abdomen was penetrated, including any exit wounds. The penetrating instrument should be left in place and bandaged so that external bleeding is controlled and the instrument is stable. With severe lacerations of the abdominal wall, inner organs may protrude through the wound. The athletic trainer should not try to replace the abdominal contents, but rather cover them with a moist, sterile dressing. The dressing can be protected even further with a layer of aluminum foil (if foil is readily available) securely taped to the abdomen.

In all cases of penetrating abdominal injuries, the trainer can control other obvious external bleeding with direct pressure. The athlete's airway must be maintained and kept free of vomitus that might be aspirated. Respiratory support might be needed, along with oxygen if it is available. In any case, the trainer should make the athlete as comfortable as possible and arrange for prompt transportation to the emergency department.

INJURIES TO THE MALE AND FEMALE GENITALIA

The male and female genitalia are susceptible to injury. Because the male genitalia are entirely external, they are injured more frequently. Although not life-threatening, injuries to the male genitalia are extremely painful and frightening to the male athlete.

Injuries to the Male Genitalia

Soft Tissue Wounds

Injuries of the external male genitalia include all types of soft tissue wounds: avulsions, lacerations, abrasions, penetrations, and contusions. Although rarely life-threatening, these wounds are extremely painful and generally a source of great concern to the injured athlete.

Direct Blows

Direct blows to the scrotum and its contents can rupture a testis or cause a substantial accumulation of blood about the testes. An ice pack can be applied to the scrotal-perineal area while the athlete is being transported.

Other Potentially Disabling Conditions

Other conditions that have the potential of disabling the athlete are hydroceles and varicoceles, hernias, and the absence of a testicle.

Hydroceles and varicoceles. A **hydrocele** is a condition of fluid accumulation in the scrotal sac. A **varicocele** is a varicose enlargement of the veins of the spermatic cord in the scrotum. A urologist should see athletes who have either of these problems to institute appropriate treatment. Frequently, an appropriate athletic supporter is all that is necessary to prevent the possibility of contusion in a swollen organ.

Hernias. A **hernia**, the protrusion of the abdominal viscera through the abdominal wall, is usually ruled out during a preseason examination or cared for at that time. However, an athlete may suffer acute herniation during the training program. A hernia produces pain, frequently felt in the testicles and groin. Palpation of the inguinal canal

and the protrusion of the hernial sac when the athlete coughs yield the diagnosis. Treatment is generally surgical. The team physician can advise whether surgery is necessary immediately or whether it can be safely postponed until the season is finished.

Absence of a testicle. The absence of a testicle indicates an undescended testicle or a testicle with a short spermatic cord that tends to protract up into the abdomen. This condition should be mentioned to the team physician. Frequently, the physician can move the testicle down into the scrotal sac. If this is impossible, then surgery may be advised to try to preserve an organ that might otherwise deteriorate. The issue of whether an athlete with an undescended testicle should be allowed to participate in sports is still open to debate. The athlete and his parents should have a discussion with the team physician about the possible consequences of further injury to the remaining testicle.

Treatment

The trainer should be able to differentiate between a contusion (bruising) of the testicle, **epididymitis** (inflammation of the epididymis), and torsion (twisting) of the testicle. Certainly, testicular torsion must be considered in any acute problem involving the testis because early recognition and treatment are important.

Protective Devices

Protective devices for the male genitalia are extremely beneficial and are mandatory in certain sports. For example, a baseball catcher certainly should wear an aluminum cup; the same is true for a hockey goaltender, as a hard hockey puck can cause severe damage to unprotected external genitalia. Athletic supporters are frequently worn for comfort in other sports, particularly in running sports, although many athletes prefer not to wear them.

Injuries to the Female Genitalia

Intrapelvic Injuries

The uterus, ovaries, and fallopian tubes are subject to the same kinds of injuries as any other internal organ. However, they are rarely damaged because they are small and well protected by the pelvis. Unlike the bladder, they do not lie adjacent to the bony pelvis and most often are not injured when the pelvis is fractured.

Injuries to the External Genitalia

The external female genitalia include the vulva, the clitoris, and the major and minor labia (lips) at the entrance of the vagina. The female urethra opens at the front of the vagina. Injuries to these genital parts include all types of soft tissue damage. Because the external female genitalia have a rich nerve supply, injuries are very painful. Lacerations, abrasions, and avulsions should be treated with moist compresses, local pressure to control bleeding, and a diaper-type bandage to hold dressings in place. Major bleeding will require control in the operating room. Under no circumstances should dressings or packs be placed into the vagina.

Although injuries to the external female genitalia are painful, they are rarely life-threatening. Bleeding may be copious, but it can usually be controlled by local ice and compression. Priority for transportation to the emergency department is dictated by associated injuries, the amount of hemorrhage, and the presence of shock.

IMPORTANT CONCEPTS

1. Abdominal injuries may be open (penetrating) or closed (blunt).
2. Hollow organs that rupture or are lacerated spill their contents into the peritoneal cavity, while injured solid organs cause severe and possibly fatal hemorrhage.
3. Bruises are signs of blunt injury, while obvious abdominal wounds, through which bowel or fat may be protruding, are signs of penetrating injuries.
4. The method of evaluating an abdominal injury is the same for both blunt and penetrating injuries.
5. Injuries to the male genitalia include soft tissue wounds and rupture of the testes from a direct blow.
6. The uterus, ovaries, and fallopian tubes of the female genitalia are rarely injured because they are small and well protected.

SUGGESTED READINGS

Cope, Sir Zachary. *Cope's Early Diagnosis of the Acute Abdomen*, 17th ed. Revised by William Silen. New York: Oxford University Press, 1987.

McAninch, J. W. "Injuries to the Urinary System." In *Abdominal Trauma*, edited by F. W. Blaisdell and D. D. Trunkey, pp. 199–227. New York: Thieme-Stratton, 1982.

Trunkey, D. "Massive Abdominal Injury." In *Critical Surgical Illness*, 2d ed., edited by J. D. Hardy. Philadelphia: W. B. Saunders, 1980.

36

The Acute Abdomen

OBJECTIVES FOR CHAPTER 36

After reading this chapter, the student should be able to:

1. Recognize the common signs and symptoms of acute abdomen.
2. Describe the types of illnesses that may produce the signs and symptoms of acute abdomen.
3. Perform a quick examination of the abdomen.
4. Provide emergency treatment to the athlete with an acute abdomen prior to transport to the hospital.

INTRODUCTION

In medicine, the term *acute abdomen* indicates an abdominal condition (pathology) of acute irritation or inflammation of the peritoneum (the lining of the stomach) and, consequently, severe pain (peritonitis). All penetrating abdominal wounds and all blunt injuries severe enough to damage abdominal organs result in the signs of the acute abdomen: abdominal tenderness, distention, and pain. Chapter 36 begins by examining the development of these signs without preceding injury. The chapter then discusses some of the possible causes of the acute abdomen: intra-abdominal causes, retroperitoneal causes, pelvic causes, and aortic aneurysm. Next is a brief discussion on how the trainer should quickly examine the abdomen. The final section of Chapter 36 covers emergency care of the acute abdomen. ■

SIGNS AND SYMPTOMS OF THE ACUTE ABDOMEN

The term *abdominal catastrophe* occasionally is used to denote the most severe form of acute abdomen. Neither term—**acute abdomen** or **abdominal catastrophe**—is exact, and neither refers to a disease of any specific organ. Both terms indicate that severe abdominal pathology is causing peritonitis, usually sudden in onset. Because several diseases in many different organs result in the same signs and complaints of pain and tenderness in the abdomen, they can all be considered under these terms. Even a skilled practitioner often has difficulty determining the exact cause of an acute abdomen. The athletic trainer, while expected to recognize such an abdominal condition, need not know its exact cause. The following are some common signs and symptoms of an acute abdomen that arise from irritation or inflammation of the peritoneum:

■ No evident abdominal injury.
■ Abdominal pain, local or diffuse.
■ Abdominal tenderness, local or diffuse.
■ An athlete who does not want to move because it hurts.
■ An athlete who is breathing rapidly and shallowly because a deep breath hurts.
■ Rapid pulse (tachycardia).
■ Low blood pressure.
■ A tense, often distended, abdomen.
■ Referred (distant) pain.
■ Fever.

The problem for the trainer is that certain conditions (for example, pelvic inflammatory disease) may present in more subtle fashion, with the signs and symptoms of the acute abdomen becoming apparent only as the peritoneal inflammation progresses. The trainer must always remain aware of the potential for serious illness, even in the absence of dramatic signs and symptoms.

Pain and Tenderness

The signs of an acute abdomen arise from irritation or inflammation of the peritoneum—**peritonitis**. The athlete complains of abdominal pain and tenderness when the abdomen is palpated or moved. The degree of pain and tenderness usually reflects the severity of the inflammation.

Nerve Supply of the Peritoneum

The supply of sensory nerves to the peritoneum is rich and twofold. The parietal peritoneum (lining of the wall of the abdomen) receives its innervation from the sensory nerves of the lower intercostal and lumbar segments that supply the trunk. The parietal peritoneum perceives sensations similar to those felt by the skin: irritation, heavy touch, stretch, pressure, and temperature change. The nerves of the parietal peritoneum can localize an irritating point with little difficulty.

The visceral peritoneum (the serosa or mesentery) is supplied by the sympathetic chain and vagus nerves—the autonomic nervous system. Visceral sensory nerves are less able to localize pain. The type of pain perceived is limited to that which arises from activation of stretch receptors, caused by distention or forceful contraction within organs. This type of activation is usually interpreted as **colic**—a severe, intermittent, and cramping pain.

Referred Pain

The autonomic peritoneal innervation gives rise to the phenomenon of **referred pain**. An irritated peritoneal surface over an organ may cause pain on a distant surface of the body that is linked to the same area of the spinal cord as the irritated organ. For example, acute cholecystitis (inflammation of the gallbladder) may cause pain in the right shoulder, since the sympathetic nerves serving the gallbladder arise in the same area as the somatic nerves that innervate the skin of the shoulder (Fig. 36.1).

Guarding

Degrees of pain and tenderness vary. Pain may be sharply localized or diffuse. When localized, pain gives a clue to its cause. Tenderness may be minimal, or it may be so great that the athlete will not allow the abdomen to be touched but instead "guards" it with the muscles so that the abdominal wall is absolutely rigid.

Position of the Athlete

The position of the athlete with acute abdomen is an important clue. In some diseases, a person can obtain comfort only by lying in one position. For example, a person with appendicitis may draw up the right knee. A person with pancreatitis may lie curled up on the right side. Each position tends to

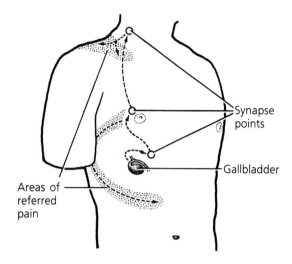

FIGURE 36.1.   Nerve pathways causing referred pain in acute cholecystitis.

relax muscles adjacent to the inflamed organ and therefore lessens pain.

Ileus

Peritonitis always causes **ileus**, which is the paralysis of normal intestinal **peristalsis** (the wavelike contractions that propel matter through the intestines). In the presence of such paralysis, nothing that is eaten can pass out of the stomach or through the bowel. Vomiting is the only way the stomach can empty itself.

Abdominal **distention** from retained gas and feces in these individuals is common. As soon as irritation causes a disturbance in the bowel action, distention develops proximal to the area of disturbance. The examiner can easily gauge distention by looking at the athlete's abdomen. Distention is apparent within a few hours after intestinal muscular activity has ceased.

Hypovolemia

In peritonitis body fluid is always lost into the abdomen. This loss decreases the volume of the circulating blood and may eventually cause hypovolemic shock. Depending on the stage of development of peritonitis, the athlete may have normal vital signs or a very rapid pulse and low blood pressure. If peritonitis is associated with hemorrhage, the signs of shock are much more acute (see Chapter 38).

Fever

Depending on the cause of the acute abdomen, fever may be evident. The person with acute appendicitis usually does not have fever until the appendix has perforated and an abscess is forming. On the other hand, persons with other acute diseases, such as diverticulitis, cholecystitis, or pelvic inflammatory disease, may have substantial temperature elevations.

Change in Vital Signs

Severe peritonitis may make breathing painful. Pulse and blood pressure, which may change drastically or not at all, usually reflect the severity of the process and its duration.

CAUSES OF THE ACUTE ABDOMEN

The solid and hollow organs in the abdominal cavity that make up the gastrointestinal and genitourinary systems are wholly covered with peritoneum, which lines the inside of the cavity and the outside of the organs. The entire cavity normally contains a very small amount of peritoneal fluid that bathes the organs. Any condition that allows pus, blood, feces, urine, gastric juice, intestinal contents, amniotic fluid, or dead or severely inflamed tissue to lie within or adjacent to this cavity can give rise to the signs of an acute abdomen.

Intra-abdominal Causes

Among the common diseases that produce the signs of an acute abdomen are acute appendicitis, perforated peptic ulcer, cholecystitis, and diverticulitis (an inflammation of pockets along the distal part of the colon). The list of diseases that can produce an acute abdomen is long, however, and includes nearly every abdominal problem. Rarely, and most often in children, a primary infection of the peritoneum occurs. This infection can also give rise to the signs of acute abdominal inflammation. Table 36.1 lists some of the common emergency problems and the location of the direct and referred pain that is produced by an acute abdomen.

Retroperitoneal Causes

Since the peritoneum is richly supplied with nerves that are sensitive to the presence of inflammation, disease or inflammation of the organs that lie behind or beneath it in the pelvic cavity can produce all the

TABLE 36.1. Acute Abdomen: Direct and Referred Pain

Disease	Localization of Pain
Appendicitis	Around navel (referred); right lower quadrant (direct)
Cholecystitis	Right shoulder (referred); right upper quadrant (direct)
Duodenal ulcer	Upper midabdomen (direct) or upper back (direct)
Diverticulitis	Left lower quadrant
Perforated peptic ulcer	Generalized
Aortic aneurysm (ruptured)	Back and right lower quadrant
Cystitis (bladder inflammation)	Lower midabdomen (retropubic)
Pancreatitis	Upper back or upper abdomen
Pyelonephritis (right or left)	Right or left angles between last rib and lumbar vertebrae (back)
Kidney stones	Either right or left sides, radiating to genitalia
Pelvic inflammation	Both lower quadrants

signs of peritonitis that accompany actual inflammation within the cavity itself. Pancreatitis can produce a severe inflammation that is difficult to distinguish from a perforated ulcer. Kidney stones that cause ureteral colic are frequently associated with paralysis of bowel action.

Pelvic Causes

One very common cause of an acute abdomen in women is pelvic inflammatory disease, a venereal infection usually involving the fallopian tubes and surrounding tissue. It is one of the major diseases that must be distinguished from appendicitis in women. Infections of the upper and lower urinary tracts, kidney and ureter, or bladder and urethra, respectively, may also cause peritoneal irritation.

Aortic Aneurysm

The aorta lies immediately behind the peritoneum on the spinal column. **Aneurysms** (weak swollen areas of the artery) are rarely associated with symptoms because they develop slowly. If the weak area ruptures, however, massive hemorrhage may occur, and some of the signs of an acute peritoneal irritation arise, along with severe back pain because the peritoneum is rapidly stripped away from the body wall. In such instances, peritoneal signs are accompanied by profound shock.

EXAMINATION OF THE ACUTE ABDOMEN

The athletic trainer should examine the abdomen quickly, using these steps:

1. Determine whether the athlete is restless or quiet, whether motion causes pain, or whether any characteristic position, distention, or abnormality is present.
2. Feel the abdomen gently to see whether it is tense (guarded) or soft.
3. Determine whether the athlete can relax the abdominal wall on command.

4. Determine whether the abdomen is tender when touched.

The trainer should not prolong this examination, as the physician will do it in much more detail at the hospital. Abdominal palpation should be carried out very gently. Occasionally an organ within the abdomen will be greatly enlarged and very fragile. Rough palpation can rupture an aneurysm of the aorta or lacerate an enlarged spleen.

EMERGENCY CARE OF THE ACUTE ABDOMEN

Conditions that give rise to acute abdominal signs and symptoms are frequently sudden in onset and rapidly progressive. If unchecked, they may quickly result in death. The overriding principle of emergency care in these conditions is to correct life-threatening problems and transport the athlete to a hospital immediately because emergency surgery may be required. The following steps should be carried out as quickly as possible prior to transport.

1. *Keep the airway clear.* The athlete often may vomit because the emergency frequently develops just after the athlete has eaten a large meal or has consumed too much alcohol. The athlete's throat and airway must be cleared of vomited material and be kept clear.

2. *Administer oxygen if it is available.* Usually the exchange of air in the lungs or in the airway is not blocked, but pain makes breathing physically difficult, and supplemental oxygen can compensate for a small respiratory volume.

3. *Do not let the athlete eat or drink anything.* Under no circumstances should an athlete with acute abdominal signs be given anything to eat or drink. Ingestion of food or fluid can only aggravate many of the symptoms. Also, if emergency surgery is required, food in the stomach makes the procedure much more dangerous. In the presence of peritoneal irritation and intestinal paralysis, food does not pass out of the stomach and only increases distention and consequent vomiting.

4. *Do not give medication for pain.* No matter how distressed the athlete is, do not give any medication for the pain or any sedatives. The examining physician must know exactly where the pain is and how much it hurts. Medication frequently masks these findings and may delay an ultimate diagnosis until it is too late to effect proper treatment.

5. *Record information.* Do not try to diagnose the athlete's disease, but listen to the description of the location of pain and tenderness and the severity of symptoms.

Record the athlete's description of how the process started and the individual's vital signs as soon as possible so the physician will have this information. Shock is common with an acute abdomen. It must be recognized early, for its presence makes prompt transport to the hospital even more imperative.

6. *Prepare to transport.* Make the athlete as comfortable as possible, conserve body heat with blankets, and arrange to transport the athlete gently and promptly to the emergency department.

IMPORTANT CONCEPTS

1. Pain and tenderness result from acute irritation of the peritoneum, a condition called peritonitis.
2. Abdominal distention and vomiting indicate ileus, or paralysis of normal intestinal peristalsis caused by peritonitis.
3. Hypovolemic shock may be present when peritonitis is associated with hemorrhage.
4. Among the intra-abdominal causes of acute abdomen are acute appendicitis, perforated peptic ulcer, cholecystitis, and diverticulitis.
5. Among the retroperitoneal causes of acute abdomen are pancreatitis and kidney stones.
6. Among the pelvic causes of acute abdomen are pelvic inflammatory disease in women and infections of the urinary tract.
7. A ruptured aortic aneurysm can cause massive hemorrhage, acute peritonitis, and profound shock.
8. Examination of an acute abdomen must be quick but with gentle palpation.
9. Because an acute abdomen can be life-threatening, the overriding principle of emergency care is rapid transport to the hospital for possible emergency surgery.

SUGGESTED READINGS

Cope, Sir Zachary. *Cope's Early Diagnosis of the Acute Abdomen*, 16th ed. Revised by William Silen. New York: Oxford University Press, 1983.
Jung, P. J., and R. C. Merrell. "Acute Abdomen." *Gastroenterology Clinics of North America* 17 (1988): 227–244.
Munn, N. E. "Diagnosis: Acute Abdomen." *Nursing* 18 (1988): 34–42.
Schöffel, U., T. Zeller, M. Lausen, et al. "Monitoring of the Inflammatory Response in Early Peritonitis." *American Journal of Surgery* 157 (1989): 567–572.

FOUR

MEDICAL EMERGENCIES

37

Basic Life Support

CHAPTER OUTLINE

OBJECTIVES FOR CHAPTER 37

After reading this chapter, the student should be able to:

1. Explain the difference between basic life support and advanced life support.
2. List and define the basic life support steps.
3. Explain when basic life support should be started and terminated.
4. Understand the principles of and know how to administer artificial ventilation.
5. Recognize airway obstruction and demonstrate the ability to alleviate this condition in a conscious or unconscious individual.
6. Understand and demonstrate the ability to perform one-person and two-person cardiopulmonary resuscitation.

INTRODUCTION

Basic life support is the emergency lifesaving procedure used to resuscitate an athlete who sustains respiratory or cardiac arrest. It requires no mechanical equipment, yet it is an effective technique for providing artificial ventilation and circulation. The effectiveness of basic life support depends on the trainer's prompt recognition of respiratory or cardiac arrest and the immediate start of treatment.

Chapter 37 begins with an explanation of why basic life support is lifesaving, when to start it, and when to terminate it. Then the chapter describes the methods of opening the airway and providing artificial ventilation. The second half of Chapter 37 focuses on artificial circulation, which is performed along with artificial ventilation in cases of cardiac arrest. ■

THE PRINCIPLES OF BASIC LIFE SUPPORT

Oxygen is essential for the life of all tissues and cells. The heart develops dangerous arrhythmias (irregular beats) within seconds after being deprived of oxygen. The brain undergoes potentially irreversible damage after the absence of oxygen for as little as 4 to 6 minutes (Fig. 37.1). The delivery of oxygen from the atmosphere to individual body cells of all types calls for two necessary processes: breathing and circulation.

The principles of **basic life support** were introduced in 1960. The specific techniques for basic life support have been reviewed and revised as necessary at national conferences on **cardiopulmonary resuscitation (CPR)** and **emergency cardiac care (ECC)** held every 6 years since then. The conference recommendations are published periodically in the *Journal of the American Medical Association*. The most recent gathering was the 1986 National Conference on

Standards and Guidelines for Cardiopulmonary Resuscitation and Emergency Cardiac Care. Recommendations in this text follow those adopted at this conference. In many instances, significant changes have been introduced since 1980.

One of the most important findings in the evaluation of the effectiveness of the basic life support training technique is that competence in administering basic life support declines rapidly after completion of a training course unless periodic retraining is provided or the individual is required to use the skills frequently. Recertification courses should therefore be taken every year.

As can be seen in Figure 37.2, prompt basic life support is indicated for

- Airway obstruction.
- Breathing (respiratory) arrest.
- Circulatory (cardiac) arrest.

Basic life support is not the same as **advanced life support**, which requires the use of complex equipment and treatment: cardiac monitoring devices, defibrillation, maintenance of an intravenous line, and infusion of appropriate drugs. Basic life support can be provided by one person alone or two together. It is the first line of treatment for respiratory or cardiac arrest. The correct application of basic life support can maintain life until transportation to a hospital is possible or until advanced life support can be delivered.

Primary Assessment

Because of the urgent need to start CPR, a prompt primary assessment must be performed on all injured or ill persons (see Chapter 11). The primary assessment is specifically designed to evaluate the need for CPR: to assess the adequacy of the airway, the quality of breathing, the quality of circulation, and the level of consciousness.

When confronted with an unconscious athlete in need of CPR, the athletic trainer must determine if the unconscious state

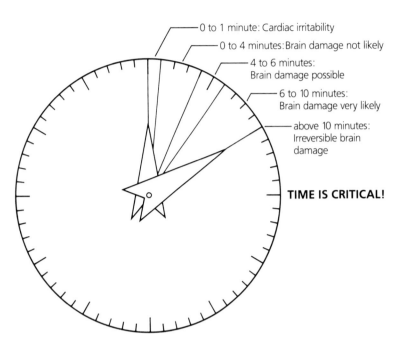

- 0 to 1 minute: Cardiac irritability
- 0 to 4 minutes: Brain damage not likely
- 4 to 6 minutes: Brain damage possible
- 6 to 10 minutes: Brain damage very likely
- above 10 minutes: Irreversible brain damage

TIME IS CRITICAL!

FIGURE 37.1.   Time is critical. If the brain is deprived of oxygen for 4 to 6 minutes, brain damage is likely to occur. After 6 minutes without oxygen, brain damage is extremely likely.

has been caused by a head or cervical spine injury. If so, special care must be taken during CPR to protect the spinal cord from further injury. The presence of a head or spinal injury is not a contraindication to CPR. It simply indicates that basic life support must be carried out within certain specific physical limits.

When to Institute Basic Life Support

The trainer should institute basic life support in all athletes who have sustained a cardiopulmonary arrest. Only two exceptions exist to this general rule. First, CPR should not be administered if obvious signs of irreversible death are present. These signs include putrefaction of the body and rigor mortis. Second, CPR is not indicated for certain persons in cardiopulmonary arrest who are known to have been in the terminal stage of an incurable disease.

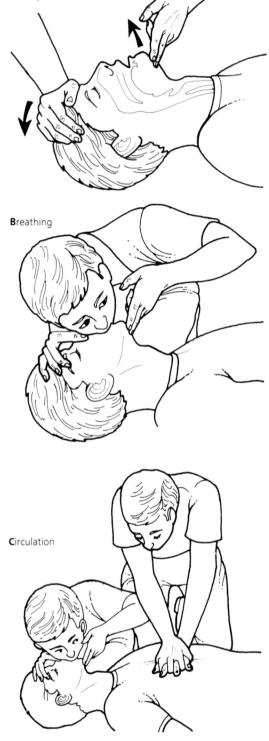

Airway

Breathing

Circulation

FIGURE 37.2. The ABCs of CPR. Basic life support is indicated for airway obstruction, breathing (respiratory) arrest, and circulatory (cardiac) arrest.

In all other circumstances, CPR is given to any individual who has sustained a partial or complete cardiopulmonary arrest. Even if a substantial amount of time has passed since the person's collapse, it is impossible to know when the last instant of effective perfusion with oxygenated blood occurred. Extrinsic factors, such as the temperature of the environment, or intrinsic factors, such as the condition of the individual's tissues and organs, may affect the person's ability to survive. Therefore, CPR should be instituted promptly in athletes who have sustained a partial or complete cardiopulmonary arrest.

When to Terminate Basic Life Support

When resuscitation is started in the absence of a physician, it must be continued until one of the following events occurs:

- Effective spontaneous circulation and respiration are restored.
- Resuscitation efforts are transferred to another person who takes charge and continues basic life support.
- A physician assumes responsibility.
- The trainer is too exhausted to continue the resuscitation efforts.

ARTIFICIAL VENTILATION

In the event the athlete is unable to breathe or unable to breathe adequately, **artificial ventilation**—that is, opening the airway and restoring breathing by mouth-to-mouth or mouth-to-nose rescue breathing—delivers oxygen to the body. Oxygenated blood is delivered to the cells, and carbon dioxide is exhaled, thus permitting bodily functions to continue, even when the athlete is unable to breathe on his or her own.

Several methods exist for opening the airway and providing artificial ventilation. All need to be instituted promptly if they are to be effective. Each method has specific applications in conscious or unconscious athletes, with or without head or spinal injury.

Positioning the Athlete

For cardiopulmonary resuscitation to be effective, the athlete must be lying face up on a firm surface. If the athlete is crumpled up or face down, repositioning will be necessary. Considerable caution is necessary when a neck or back injury is suspected. The athlete must be rolled as a single unit, including head, neck, and back. Elevating the lower extremities about 12 inches while keeping the rest of the body horizontal will promote venous blood return and assist artificial circulation if external chest compression is required.

To position an unconscious athlete, the athletic trainer kneels beside the athlete, but not in bodily contact. The trainer must be sufficiently far away so that when it is time to roll the athlete, the individual does not come to rest in the trainer's lap (Fig. 37.3a). First, the athletic trainer rapidly straightens the athlete's legs and moves the nearer arm above the head (Fig. 37.3b). Then the trainer places one of his or her hands behind the back of the head and neck of the athlete and the other on the distant shoulder (Fig. 37.3c). The trainer can then turn the athlete toward himself or herself by pulling on the distant shoulder with the head and neck controlled so that they turn with the rest of the torso as a unit (Fig. 37.3d). In this way, the head and neck remain in the same vertical plane as the back, and aggravation of any spinal injury is minimized. Once the athlete is flat on his or her back, the athletic trainer brings the athlete's farther arm back to the side (Fig. 37.3e). When possible, the athlete should be rolled onto a long spine board, which will provide support during transport and emergency room care.

Opening the Airway

Immediate clearing of the airway is the most important factor in successful CPR. Without an unobstructed airway, artificial ventilation will not succeed. The most common cause of airway obstruction in the semiconscious or unconscious person is re-laxation of the muscles of the throat and tongue, which allows the tongue to fall back into the throat to create a block (Fig. 37.4). Dentures, blood clots, vomitus, mucus, food, or other foreign bodies may also cause obstruction. Obstruction of the airway from an aspirated foreign body is discussed later in this chapter.

Head-Tilt/Chin-Lift Maneuver

Clearing the airway of obstruction from the tongue often can be accomplished easily and quickly by tilting the athlete's head backward as far as possible (Fig. 37.5). This procedure is known as the **head-tilt maneuver**. It is accomplished by placing a hand on the athlete's forehead and applying firm backward pressure with the palm. This results in extension of the neck, which moves the tongue forward, away from the posterior wall of the pharynx, clearing the airway.

An effective head tilt may be difficult to obtain with only one hand on the forehead. In this instance, the other hand can be used to apply a **chin-lift maneuver**. The head tilt is the initial and often the most important step in opening the airway.

Having achieved the head tilt, the trainer can open the airway further with the **head-tilt/chin-lift maneuver**. Trainers must be familiar with the chin-lift technique and be able to perform it well. The fingertips of the hand not on the forehead are placed under the bony part of the athlete's chin. The chin is lifted forward, bringing the entire lower jaw with it and helping to tilt the head back (Fig. 37.6). The fingers must not compress the soft tissue under the chin, as such compression could obstruct the airway. The forehead hand continues to maintain the backward tilt of the head. The chin should be lifted so that the teeth are nearly brought together; but the mouth should not be closed completely.

If the athlete has loose dentures, the trainer can hold them in position with the chin lift, making obstruction by the lips less likely. If artificial ventilation is needed, the trainer can achieve a mouth-to-mouth seal much more easily with the dentures in

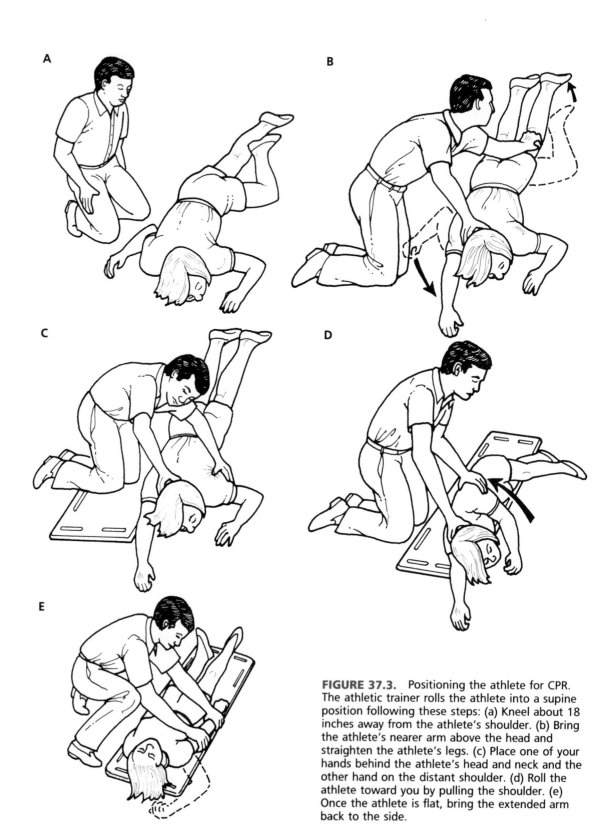

FIGURE 37.3. Positioning the athlete for CPR. The athletic trainer rolls the athlete into a supine position following these steps: (a) Kneel about 18 inches away from the athlete's shoulder. (b) Bring the athlete's nearer arm above the head and straighten the athlete's legs. (c) Place one of your hands behind the athlete's head and neck and the other hand on the distant shoulder. (d) Roll the athlete toward you by pulling the shoulder. (e) Once the athlete is flat, bring the extended arm back to the side.

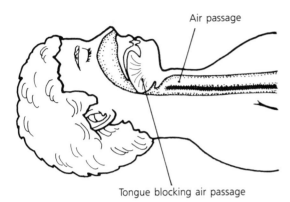

FIGURE 37.4. Muscular relaxation in the unconscious athlete may allow the tongue to fall back into the airway and obstruct it.

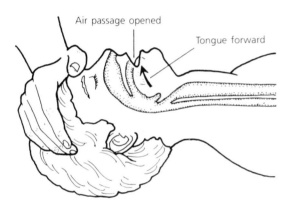

FIGURE 37.5. The head-tilt maneuver. The athletic trainer opens the airway by extending the neck with firm pressure applied to the forehead. The maneuver causes an anterior motion of the tongue to raise it from the posterior pharyngeal wall.

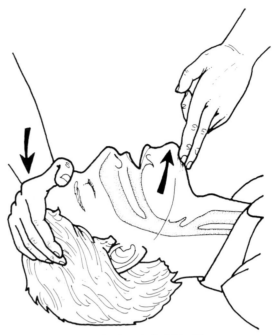

FIGURE 37.6. The head-tilt/chin-lift maneuver. The athletic trainer lifts the chin forward, bringing the entire lower jaw with it and helping to tilt the head back.

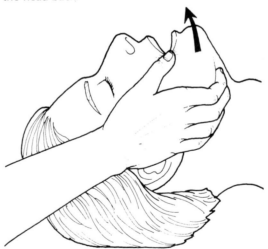

FIGURE 37.7. The jaw-thrust maneuver. The athletic trainer places his or her fingers behind the angles of the athlete's lower jaw to move the jaw forward as well as tilt the head backward without significantly extending the cervical spine.

place. If the dentures cannot be held in place, the trainer should remove them.

Jaw-Thrust Maneuver

The two methods just described are effective for opening the airway in most athletes. If they are not, an additional forward movement of the lower jaw—the **jaw-thrust maneuver**—should be done. The jaw thrust is a triple maneuver in which fingers are placed behind the angles of the athlete's lower jaw to move the jaw forward as well as tilt the head backward without significantly extending the cervical spine; the thumbs pull the lower lip down to allow breathing through the mouth as well as the nose.

The jaw thrust is performed best with the trainer kneeling by the athlete's head (Fig. 37.7). When a cervical spine injury is suspected, this simple maneuver can be modified to keep the head in a neutral position, while thrusting the jaw forward and opening the mouth as described.

Assessing Whether Breathing Has Returned

Once the airway has been opened by one of the techniques just described, the athlete may start to breathe spontaneously. To assess whether breathing has returned, the athletic trainer places an ear about 1 inch above the nose and mouth of the athlete and listens carefully (Fig. 37.8). The trainer's head should be turned to observe the athlete's chest and abdomen. If the trainer can feel and hear movement of air and can see the athlete's chest and abdomen move with each breath, breathing has returned. Feeling and hearing the actual movement of air are far more important than seeing body movements. With airway obstruction, it is possible that there will be no air movement, even though the chest and abdomen rise and fall with the athlete's frantic attempts to breathe. In addition, observing chest and abdominal movement often is difficult with a fully clothed athlete. Finally, there may

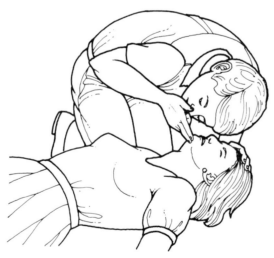

FIGURE 37.8. Respiration check. Respiration is determined by feeling and hearing movement of air and by seeing the chest and abdomen move with each breath.

be very little or no perceptible chest movement, even with normal breathing, particularly in some athletes with chronic lung disease. If there still is no movement of air after the airway has been opened by the preceding maneuvers, the athletic trainer must start artificial ventilation promptly.

Providing Artificial Ventilation

Adequate artificial ventilation requires a cycle of inspiration/expiration lasting 1 to 1.5 seconds. Inspiration lasts at least half of each cycle, occurring once every 5 cardiac compressions (12 per minute) or twice after every 15 compressions (8 per minute).

The emergency institution of artificial ventilation requires no equipment and should never be delayed while one waits to obtain devices for ventilatory assistance. Rescue breathing, done either by mouth-to-mouth or mouth-to-nose techniques, delivers exhaled gas from the athletic trainer to the athlete. This gas contains 16 percent oxygen, which is sufficient to maintain life.

Mouth-to-Mouth Ventilation

To perform **mouth-to-mouth ventilation**, the trainer opens the airway with the head-tilt/chin-lift maneuver. While continuing to exert pressure on the forehead to maintain the backward tilt of the head, the trainer pinches the athlete's nostrils together using the thumb and index finger of the same hand (Fig. 37.9a). With this technique, the thumb of the other hand, which is lifting the chin, can be used to depress the lower lip to help keep the mouth open during mouth-to-mouth ventilation. The trainer then opens the athlete's mouth widely, takes a deep breath, makes a tight seal with his or her mouth around the athlete's mouth, and exhales into it (Fig. 37.9b). The trainer then removes his or her mouth and allows the athlete to exhale passively, turning slightly to watch for chest movement and to listen and feel the air escaping from the athlete's mouth.

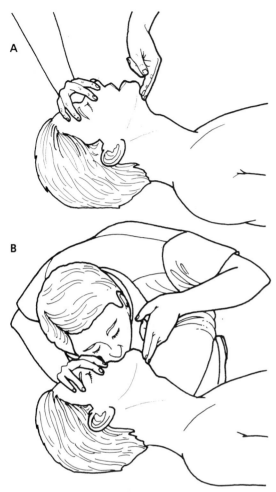

FIGURE 37.9. Mouth-to-mouth ventilation. (a) The athletic trainer seals off the athlete's nose, and (b) makes a tight seal with his or her own mouth around the athlete's mouth and exhales deeply into it.

Breaths are given slowly, in a cycle lasting 1.5 seconds for each breath. Maximum ventilation of the lung is thereby ensured.

When giving mouth-to-mouth ventilation and using the jaw thrust to maintain an open airway, the trainer must move to the athlete's side, keep the athlete's mouth open with both thumbs, and seal the nose by placing his or her cheek against the athlete's nostrils.

Mouth-to-Nose Ventilation

In some cases, **mouth-to-nose ventilation** is more effective than mouth-to-mouth venti-

lation. Mouth-to-nose ventilation is a good alternative in the following situations:

- When it is impossible to open the athlete's mouth.
- When it is impossible to ventilate an athlete through the mouth because of severe facial injuries.
- When it is difficult to achieve a tight seal around the mouth because the athlete has no teeth.

For mouth-to-nose ventilation, the trainer keeps the athlete's head tilted back, with one hand on the forehead, and uses the other hand to lift the athlete's lower jaw (Fig. 37.10). This maneuver seals the lips. The trainer then takes a deep breath, seals his or her lips around the athlete's nose, and blows in slowly until the lungs are felt to expand. Then the trainer removes his or her mouth and allows the athlete to exhale passively. The trainer can see the chest fall when the athlete exhales. It may be necessary to open the athlete's mouth or separate the athlete's lips to allow air to escape

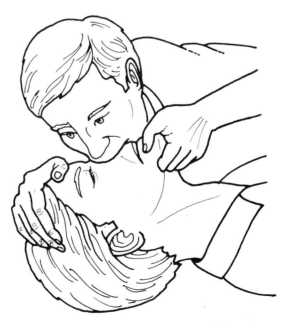

FIGURE 37.10. Mouth-to-nose ventilation. The athletic trainer seals off the athlete's mouth and, after sealing the athlete's nose with his or her lips, exhales slowly into the nose.

during exhalation. If using the jaw thrust to maintain the airway during mouth-to-nose ventilation, the trainer uses his or her cheek to seal the athlete's mouth and does not use thumbs to retract the lower lip.

The Problem of Gastric Distention

Artificial ventilation frequently causes **gastric distention** (distention of the stomach). It is most likely to appear when excessive pressures are used for ventilation or when the airway is obstructed. Slight gastric distention may be disregarded. Marked inflation of the stomach is dangerous because it causes regurgitation of gastric contents during CPR; the distended stomach can also reduce the lung volume by elevating the diaphragm.

Gastric distention has been found by investigators to occur when high ventilatory pressures are used or when several rapid breaths are administered quickly in succession. Slower, periodic ventilations at lower pressures are more likely to produce air that finds its way to the lungs.

Acute, massive gastric distention that interferes with adequate ventilation must be relieved promptly. Frequently, this can be done by exerting moderate pressure on the individual's abdomen between the umbilicus and the rib cage with the palm of the hand. The trainer must be alert to the fact that regurgitation will include air, gastric juice, and food. Pulmonary aspiration of the gastric contents must be prevented during this maneuver. The athlete's entire body should be turned to one side to minimize the risk of aspiration.

Recognizing and Relieving Airway Obstruction

Airway obstruction has several causes, including muscular relaxation in an unconscious person; vomited or regurgitated stomach contents; blood clot, bone fragments, or damaged tissue after an injury; dentures; or foreign bodies. The maneuvers to open the obstructed airway that has been caused by muscle relaxation were discussed earlier. Loose dentures and large pieces of vomited food, mucus, or blood clots should be swept forward and out of the mouth with the trainer's index finger. Once suctioning equipment becomes available, it should be used to maintain an open airway.

Recognition of Foreign Body Obstruction

On occasion, a large foreign body will be aspirated and block the upper airway. Sudden airway obstruction by a foreign body in an adult usually occurs during a meal. In a child, it occurs during mealtime or at play (sucking small objects).

Early recognition of airway obstruction is the key to successful management. The trainer must learn to differentiate primary airway obstruction from other conditions that result in respiratory failure or arrest, such as fainting, stroke, or acute myocardial infarction.

The athlete with an obstructed airway may be conscious when discovered and become unconscious, or the person may already be unconscious when discovered.

Conscious athlete. Sudden upper airway obstruction is usually recognized when the athlete who is eating or has just finished eating is suddenly unable to speak or cough, grasps the throat, appears cyanotic (bluish), and demonstrates exaggerated efforts to breathe. Air movement is either absent or not detectable. Initially, the athlete will remain conscious and be able to indicate quite clearly the nature of the problem. Frequently, the athlete will answer a simple question such as "Are you choking?" by nodding yes. Doubt about the diagnosis is then removed. If the obstruction is not removed in a short period of time, unconsciousness and death will result from the lack of oxygen.

Unconscious athlete. When an athlete is discovered unconscious, the cause is initially unknown. The unconsciousness may have been caused by airway obstruction, cardiac or cardiopulmonary arrest, or a number of other problems. Any athlete found unconscious must be managed as a person with cardiopulmonary arrest. An obstruction should be suspected in the unconscious person when standard airway maneuvers and ventilation efforts do not result in effective ventilation of the lungs.

Maneuvers to Relieve Upper Airway Obstruction

Two maneuvers are recommended for relieving foreign body airway obstruction: (1) the Heimlich maneuver, or subdiaphragmatic thrust, and (2) the finger sweep and manual removal of the object.

The Heimlich maneuver. The **Heimlich** maneuver, or **subdiaphragmatic thrust** (also called the **abdominal thrust**), is the preferred initial treatment to dislodge an aspirated foreign body in adults and children. Dislodging the object requires that energy be imparted to it to make it move. The subdiaphragmatic thrust maneuver imparts the greatest energy for the longest period of time in the proper direction to force the object out of the airway.

A series of 6 to 10 abdominal thrusts is applied until the obstructing body is dislodged. With the athlete sitting or standing, the trainer follows these steps:

1. Stand behind the athlete, with your arms wrapped around the person's waist.
2. Make a fist with one hand, grasp it with your other hand, and place the thumb side of your fist against the athlete's abdomen, just above the umbilicus and well below the xiphoid process (the lower tip of the sternum).
3. Press your fist into the athlete's abdomen with a quick upward thrust (Fig. 37.11).
4. Repeat the maneuver 6 to 10 times.

With the athlete supine (lying face up), the trainer must modify the technique as follows:

1. Kneel close to the athlete's hips or straddle either the hips or the legs of the athlete.
2. Place the heel of one hand against the athlete's abdomen, well below the xiphoid process and above the umbilicus; place your second hand on top of the first.
3. Press your hand into the athlete's abdomen with a quick upward thrust and repeat 6 to 10 times (Fig. 37.12).

This maneuver can be accomplished safely and with good results in all adults and children. Pregnancy and obesity do not con-

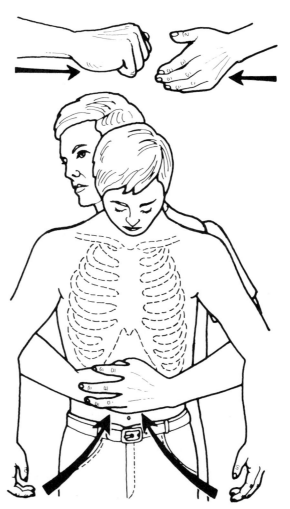

FIGURE 37.11. The Heimlich maneuver (upright).

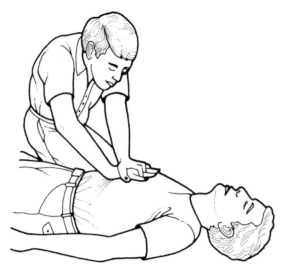

FIGURE 37.12. The Heimlich maneuver (supine).

traindicate its use; however, the chest thrust (as in cardiac compression) is recommended for women in advanced stages of pregnancy or for the very obese person.

Manual removal of a foreign body. If at any time the foreign body causing an airway obstruction appears in the mouth or is believed to be in the mouth, it should be removed cautiously with the athletic trainer's fingers. Abdominal thrust may dislodge the foreign body but not expel it. The trainer can use either a cross-finger technique or a tongue-jaw-lift maneuver combined with a finger sweep to remove the foreign material.

The **cross-finger technique** for opening the mouth includes these steps:

1. Cross your thumb under your index finger.
2. Brace your thumb and index finger against the athlete's lower and upper teeth, respectively (Fig. 37.13a).
3. Use your fingers to force the athlete's jaws open (Fig. 37.13b).

The **tongue-jaw-lift maneuver** for opening the mouth includes these steps:

1. Keep the athlete's head in the neutral position.

2. Open the athlete's mouth by grasping both the tongue and the lower jaw between your thumb and fingers and lifting them forward (Fig. 37.13c). This action will help pull the tongue back away from the throat and away from the foreign body that may be lodged there.

A **finger sweep** to remove foreign bodies includes these steps:

1. Hold the athlete's mouth open, using either the cross-finger technique or the tongue-jaw-lift maneuver.
2. Use the index finger of your opposite hand as a hook to sweep down inside the athlete's cheek to the base of the tongue.
3. Dislodge any impacted foreign body up into the mouth.
4. When the foreign body comes within reach, grasp it and carefully remove it (Fig. 37.13d).

When the finger sweep is used, the athletic trainer should be careful not to push the dislodged foreign body farther back into the airway.

Maneuvers to Relieve Partial Airway Obstruction

On occasion, a partial airway obstruction will be present. Although able to exchange some air, the athlete will still have some degree of respiratory distress. Great care must be taken to prevent a partial airway obstruction from becoming a complete airway obstruction. Abdominal thrusts generally will be ineffective in dislodging the partially obstructing object, and manual manipulation is dangerous because the object could be forced farther down the airway and completely obstruct it. In the case of a partial airway obstruction, the airway maneuvers (head-tilt/chin-lift or jaw-thrust) should be used to support the airway in its most efficient position, and supplemental 100 percent oxygen, if available, should be administered. The athlete should be transported promptly to the hospital for removal of the foreign body.

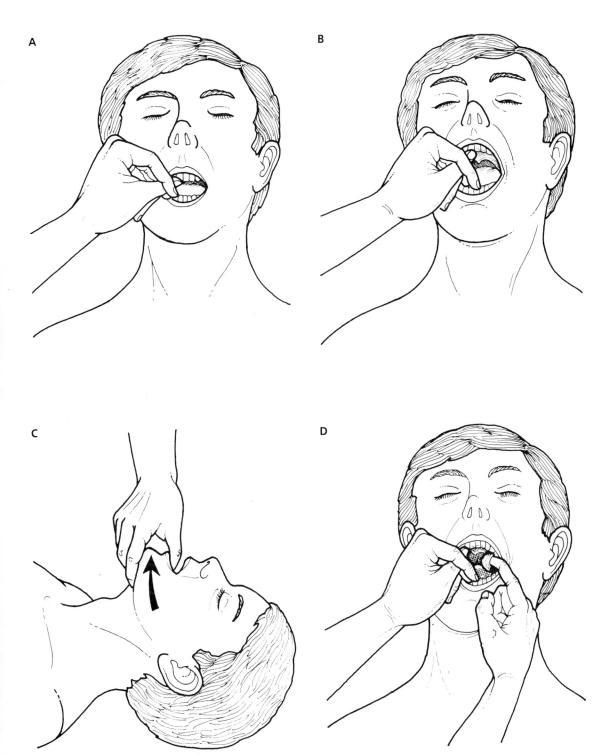

FIGURE 37.13.   The athletic trainer can follow these steps for manual removal of a foreign body. (a) Using the cross-finger technique, brace your thumb and index finger on the athlete's teeth and (b) force the jaws apart. (c) Using the tongue-jaw lift manuever, pull the tongue and jaw to open the mouth and help visualize the foreign body. (d) Use a finger sweep to sweep the foreign body out of the athlete's mouth.

Providing Basic Ventilatory Support in Infants and Children

The basic principles of CPR are the same whether the person is an infant, child, or adult. The differences in CPR for the infant and child relate to the different underlying causes of emergencies in infants and children and the smaller size of infants and children. In the great majority of instances, full cardiopulmonary arrest in infants and children results from respiratory arrest. The causes of respiratory arrest in infants and children are numerous. If uncorrected, respiratory arrest will lead to cardiac arrest and death. Some of the major crises that necessitate resuscitation in infants and children include:

- Aspiration of foreign bodies into the airway: peanuts, candy, small toys.
- Poisonings and drug overdose.
- Airway infections such as croup and epiglottitis.
- Near drowning.
- Sudden infant death syndrome (SIDS).

For the purposes of CPR, anyone under 1 year of age is considered an infant, and a child is considered as being between the ages of 1 and 8 years. Techniques used for adults can generally be applied to anyone over 8 years of age. These definitions are guidelines only, because variations in size relative to age do occur among infants and children. Small children are sometimes best treated as infants, and large children as adults. Specific information regarding life support techniques for infants and children can be found in CPR texts.

ARTIFICIAL CIRCULATION

Assessing Circulation

A disturbance of the regular electrical rhythm and activity of the heart may prevent adequate cardiac muscular contraction and result in the failure of the heart to generate sufficient blood flow to produce a pulse. The absence of a palpable central pulse, such as the carotid or femoral pulse,

indicates insufficient blood flow and hence the presence of cardiac arrest.

The carotid artery is close to the heart; it is large and readily palpable in the neck. It is found most easily by locating the larynx at the front of the neck and then sliding the index and long fingers posteriorly to the groove between the larynx and the sternocleidomastoid muscle (Fig. 37.14). Here, with light pressure the carotid pulse should be palpable. The trainer should not use excessive pressure to palpate the carotid pulse because too much pressure can obstruct the carotid circulation, dislodge blood clots, or produce marked reflexive slowing of heart activity.

The pulse may also be checked at the femoral artery in the groin. If no pulse is palpable, the absence of heart activity may be confirmed by listening over the left side of the chest for cardiac sounds.

If the athlete with respiratory arrest has been positioned for artificial ventilation, the trainer can keep one hand on the athlete's forehead to maintain the backward

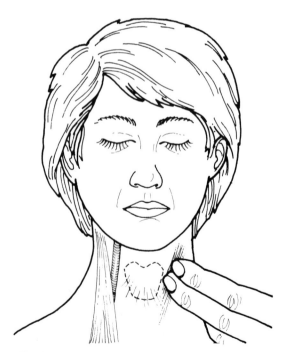

FIGURE 37.14. The carotid pulse is felt in the groove between the larynx and the sternocleidomastoid.

head tilt and use the other hand to locate the carotid or femoral pulse. If the pulse is present but breathing is absent, the trainer should ventilate the athlete twice, 1 to 1.5 seconds for each breath, and then once every 5 seconds. If the pulse is absent, the trainer should ventilate the athlete twice and begin external chest compression.

Providing External Chest Compression

The heart lies slightly to the left of the midline of the sternum (Fig. 37.15). Rhythmic pressure and relaxation applied to the lower half of the sternum, called **external chest compression** or **cardiac compression**, will compress the heart between the sternum and the spine and produce an **artificial circulation**.

Even in ideal situations, the carotid artery flow resulting from external chest compression is only about one-quarter to one-third of the normal volume. For effective cardiac compression, the athlete must be on a firm, flat surface (see "Positioning the Athlete" earlier in this chapter). Since cardiac failure precipitated the respiratory failure, external chest compression is accompanied by artificial ventilation.

Technique of One-Person CPR

The trainer should properly position the athlete and then kneel close to the athlete's side, with one knee at the level of the head and the other at the upper part of the chest. The heel of one hand should be placed on the lower half of the body of the sternum (Fig. 37.16). Great care must be taken not to place the hand on either the xiphoid process, the ribs, or the costal cartilages.

Correct positioning of the hands is achieved by sliding the index and long fingers of the hand nearer the athlete's feet along the edge of the rib cage until they reach the xiphoid notch in the center of the chest (Fig. 37.17a). The long finger is pushed as high as possible into the notch, and the index finger is then placed on the lower portion of the sternum with the two fingers touching (Fig. 37.17b). The heel of the other hand is then placed on the lower half of the sternum so that it touches the index finger of the first hand (Fig. 37.17c). The first hand is then removed from the notch in the center of the rib cage and applied over

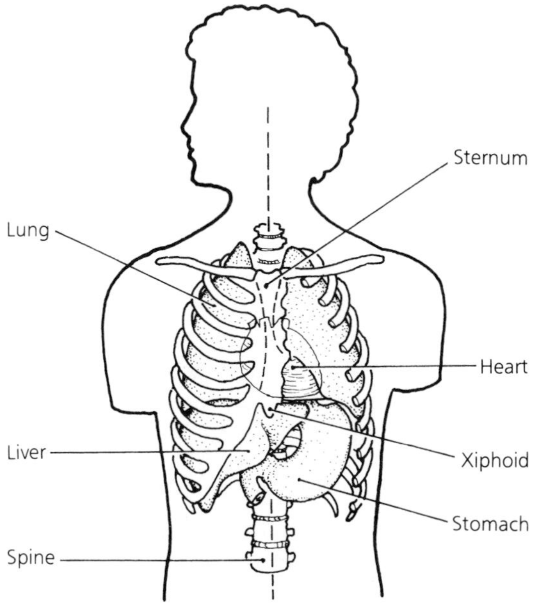

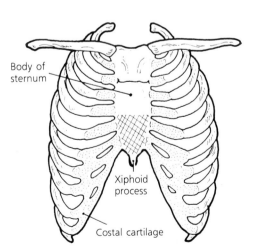

FIGURE 37.15. The heart lies slightly to the left and middle of the chest, between the sternum and the spine.

FIGURE 37.16. The xiphoid process is at the lower tip of the sternum and extends downward over the upper abdomen.

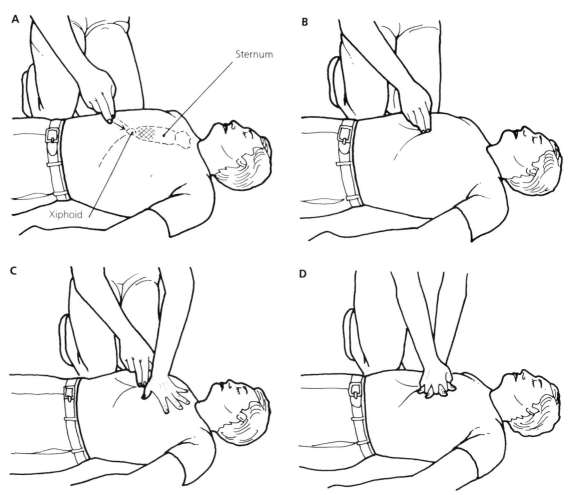

FIGURE 37.17. The athletic trainer can achieve the correct hand position for chest compression following these steps: (a) Slide your index and long fingers of the hand nearest the athlete's feet along the center of the athlete's rib cage to the notch in the center of the chest. (b) Push the long finger high into the notch, and lay the index finger on the lower portion of the sternum. (c) Then place the heel of the second hand on the lower half of the sternum, touching the index finger of your first hand. (d) Remove your first hand from the notch and place it over and parallel to the hand on the sternum.

and parallel to the hand now resting on the athlete's lower sternum (Fig. 37.17d). *Only the heel of one hand is in contact with the lower half of the sternum.* The technique may be improved or made more comfortable for the trainer if the fingers of the lower hand are interlocked with the fingers of the upper hand and pulled slightly away from the chest wall.

Pressure is exerted vertically downward through both arms to depress the adult sternum 1.5 to 2 inches for compression,

followed immediately by relaxation (Fig. 37.18). The time spent in compression is a crucial factor in determining blood flow and should be at least 50 percent of the cycle.

Motions should be smooth, rhythmic, and uninterrupted. Short, jabbing compression strokes are ineffective in producing blood flow. The heel of the hand should not be removed from the chest during relaxation, but pressure on the sternum must be completely released so it can return to its

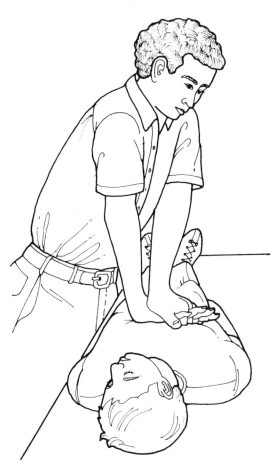

FIGURE 37.18. Pressure for external chest compression is exerted vertically downward.

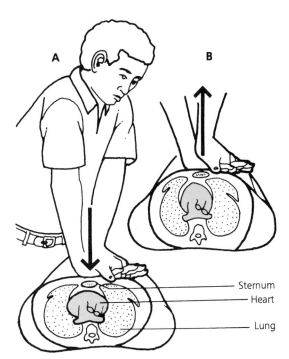

FIGURE 37.19. Chest compression should be rhythmic and uninterrupted. (a) The heel of the hand should not be removed from the chest during relaxation, but (b) pressure on the sternum must be released so it can return to its normal resting position between compressions.

normal resting position between compressions. The hand must not bounce or come away from the chest during compression (Fig. 37.19).

Even when done correctly, cardiac compression carries risks, including fractured ribs, liver laceration, splenic rupture, and sternal fracture. Proper technique will help to minimize these risks.

With one person administering CPR, the compression-to-ventilation ratio should be 15:2—that is, 15 compressions followed by 2 ventilations.

Technique of Two-Person CPR

Two people can provide more effective CPR than one because ventilation can be delivered without any pause in compression, and blood pressure never falls to zero.

If a second person becomes available after CPR is begun, the following procedure should be followed. Without stopping CPR, the first person announces that everything is ready for a switch to two-person CPR. The logical point of entrance is after a sequence of 15 compressions and 2 breaths.

The second person kneels down on the side of the athlete opposite the first person, in position to perform artificial ventilation. The second person checks the athlete's pulse to make sure the condition has been correctly diagnosed and that a pulse is felt after each compression. If a pulse is felt, the second person first says, "Stop compression," and then checks for a spontaneous pulse. If the pulse cannot be felt, two-person CPR begins.

The second person opens the airway and delivers two breaths. The entire process, from the moment the second person arrives to the point when the breaths are delivered, should be done within 10 seconds to ensure that effective CPR continues. As soon as these two breaths are delivered, CPR continues, with one breath being delivered after every five compressions. For artificial ventilation to be delivered effectively, a pause of 1 to 1.5 seconds after every five cardiac compressions is required. Therefore, the compression rate must be at least 80 to 100 per minute.

Two-person CPR should be performed with the resuscitators on opposite sides of the athlete (Fig. 37.20). They can then switch positions when necessary without significant interruption in the ventilation-compression sequence. To switch, the person who is providing ventilation, after giving a breath, moves into position to begin cardiac compression. The person performing compression, after the fifth compres-

sion, moves to the athlete's head and checks the pulse for 5 seconds but no longer. If no pulse is felt, the person at the head ventilates the athlete twice and says, "Continue CPR."

When performing CPR on a litter in an ambulance, both resuscitators must perform from the same side of the athlete. They can then switch positions using the following technique. The person ventilating the athlete rapidly moves behind the person doing compressions and assumes that role, freeing the person to move to the head of the athlete to continue ventilation (Fig. 37.21).

Effectiveness of CPR

Checking the Carotid Pulse

The carotid pulse must be palpated periodically for no more than 5 seconds during CPR to check the effectiveness of chest compression or the return of a spontaneous,

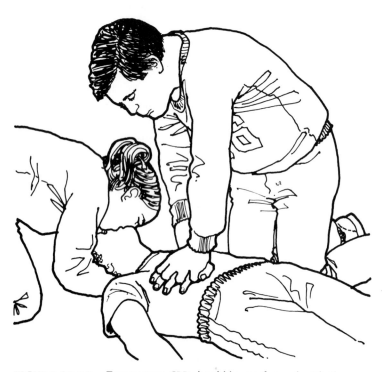

FIGURE 37.20. Two-person CPR should be performed with the resuscitators on opposite sides of the athlete.

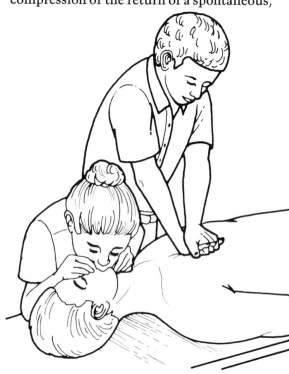

FIGURE 37.21. In an ambulance, both resuscitators must perform CPR from the same side of the athlete.

effective heartbeat. Palpation should be done after the first minute of CPR and every 5 minutes thereafter. Pupils and pulse are checked by the trainer performing the ventilation, particularly just before switching positions during CPR.

Checking the Pupils

The reaction of the pupils to light should be checked periodically, since pupil constriction provides a good indication of the delivery of oxygenated blood to the athlete's brain. Pupils that constrict when exposed to light indicate adequate oxygenation and blood flow to the brain. If the pupils remain widely dilated and do not react to light, serious brain damage may be imminent or has already occurred. Dilated but reactive pupils are a less ominous sign. However, it must be emphasized that normal pupillary reactions may be altered in the elderly and frequently are drastically changed by the use of drugs.

CPR Interruption

CPR should not be interrupted for more than 5 seconds for any reason, except when it is necessary to move an athlete up or down a stairway. When the athlete has to be moved, it is best to perform CPR at the head or foot of the stairs, then interrupt at a given signal and move quickly to the next level, where effective activity can resume. Interruptions should not exceed 15 seconds, nor should the athlete be moved until all transportation arrangements have been made.

Without advanced life support (monitoring, an intravenous line, drugs, and defibrillation), basic life support will rarely be sufficient for a person's survival, regardless of how well it is performed. If advanced life support modalities cannot be brought to the scene, the athlete must be moved promptly to the emergency department. CPR should be continued during transport to the hospital.

Providing Artificial Circulation in Infants and Children

The basic principles of CPR are the same whether the individual is an infant, child, or adult. The differences in performing CPR relate to the varied underlying causes of emergencies in infants and children and the recognition that their smaller size necessitates changes in technique.

As previously stated, in most instances, cardiopulmonary arrest in infants and children begins with respiratory arrest. Cardiac arrest results from the hypoxia produced by respiratory arrest. Therefore, initial attention must be directed to the airway and ventilation.

(Important Concepts appear on next page.)

IMPORTANT CONCEPTS

1. The brain undergoes potentially irreversible damage within 4 to 6 minutes after the absence of oxygen.
2. The purpose of the primary assessment is to evaluate the adequacy of the airway, the quality of breathing, the quality of circulation, and the level of consciousness.
3. Basic life support should be instituted in all athletes who have sustained cardiopulmonary arrest unless irreversible signs of death are present or the person is known to be in the terminal stage of a terminal disease.
4. Basic life support must continue until circulation and respiration are restored, the resuscitation efforts are transferred to another person, a physician takes over, or the resuscitator is too exhausted to continue.
5. For effective CPR, the athlete must be lying face up on a firm surface, preferably a spine board.
6. The trainer should be familiar with the head-tilt/chin-lift maneuver and the jaw-thrust maneuver of opening the airway.
7. Adequate ventilation may be provided through mouth-to-mouth or mouth-to-nose rescue breathing.
8. Airway obstruction should be suspected in an unconscious person who does not respond to standard airway maneuvers and ventilation efforts.
9. The two maneuvers recommended for relieving foreign body obstruction are the Heimlich maneuver (also called the subdiaphragmatic thrust or the abdominal thrust) and the finger sweep (manual removal).
10. The absence of a palpable pulse in a carotid or femoral artery indicates insufficient blood flow and the presence of cardiac arrest.
11. External chest compression, since it indicates the presence of respiratory failure, is always accompanied by artificial ventilation.
12. The effectiveness of CPR is determined by checking the carotid pulse and the reaction of the pupils of the eyes to light.
13. CPR should not be interrupted for more than 5 seconds.

SUGGESTED READINGS

Budassi, S. A., J. J. Bander, L. Kimmerle, et al., eds. *Cardiac Arrest and CPR: Assessment, Planning, and Intervention.* Rockville, Md.: Aspen Systems, 1980.

Heimlich, H. *Dr. Heimlich's Home Guide to Emergency Medical Situations.* New York: Simon & Schuster, 1980.

Redding, J. S. *Life Support: The Essentials: In Introduction to Sound Principles of Intensive Care in Cardiorespiratory Crises.* Philadelphia: J. B. Lippincott, 1977.

38

Shock

OBJECTIVES FOR CHAPTER 38

After reading this chapter, the student should be able to:
1. Define shock.
2. Identify the three common pathways for the development of shock.
3. List and describe seven medical conditions that can precipitate shock.
4. Describe signs and symptoms common to all types of shock.
5. Explain the initial emergency treatment of shock while arranging transport to an emergency facility.

INTRODUCTION

Shock is defined as cardiovascular collapse or the inability of the cardiovascular system to provide sufficient circulation of blood to the entire body. If the athlete is not treated quickly, blood flow to vital organs may cease and death will ensue. Chapter 38 begins with a discussion of the physiology and development of shock and the role of the cardiovascular system in maintaining adequate perfusion. The signs and symptoms of shock are listed next, followed by a discussion of the initial emergency management of shock. ▪

THE PHYSIOLOGY OF SHOCK

The cardiovascular system can be described as consisting of two parts: a container and its contents. The container is the heart and its system of blood vessels: arteries, veins, innumerable small arterioles and venules, and capillaries. The contents of the container is the blood. Normally, there is just enough blood to fill the entire system—in an average adult, 6 liters.

The heart is a muscular pump that circulates the blood through the system. The heart pumps 6 liters of blood per minute through a system that can hold just 6 liters. Thus, every part of the system receives a regular supply of blood every minute. Cardiovascular collapse, or any condition under which the system fails to provide sufficient circulation, is called **shock**.

Perfusion

The term **perfusion** refers to the circulation of blood within an organ or tissue. An organ or an area of the body is perfused if blood is entering it through the arteries and leaving it through the veins. To reach the veins, the blood must pass from the arteries through the arterioles to the connecting capillaries and into the venules. The blood gives up nutrients and oxygen and picks up waste from the organ or tissue that is being perfused. In states of shock, perfusion of organs and tissues fails.

Certain tissues or organs are more sensitive than others to a transient loss of blood flow. Lack of perfusion to the brain and the spinal cord (the central nervous system) for more than 4 to 6 minutes will result in permanent damage to nerve cells. Permanent damage to the kidney results after inadequate perfusion for a period of 45 minutes. The heart requires constant perfusion or it will not function properly. Skeletal muscle, if subjected to the loss of perfusion for 2 hours, will be permanently damaged. The gastrointestinal tract can exist with limited (but not absent) perfusion for a number of hours. No part of the body can exist without adequate perfusion for an indefinite period of time. An organ or tissue that is considerably below normal body temperature (98.6 degrees Fahrenheit or 37.0 degrees Centigrade) is much more resistant to damage from lack of perfusion since cooler temperatures slow the metabolic rate. At lower metabolic rates the cells need less oxygen and fewer waste products are accumulated.

Causes of Shock

While a number of medical conditions can precipitate shock, there are really only three pathways (Fig. 38.1) by which each of these medical conditions can induce shock:

- The heart can be damaged so that it fails to act properly as a pump.
- Blood can be lost so that the volume contained within the vascular system is insufficient for perfusion.

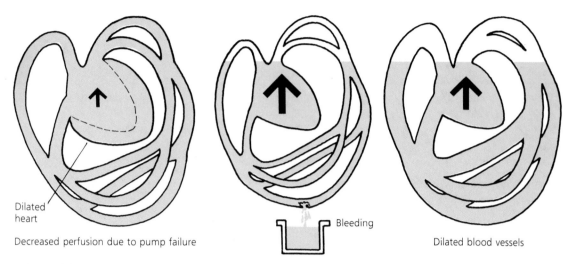

Dilated heart

Decreased perfusion due to pump failure

Bleeding

Dilated blood vessels

FIGURE 38.1.   There are three basic causes of shock and impaired tissue perfusion: (a) pump failure due to heart disease; (b) decreased blood volume, usually a result of bleeding; and (c) dilation of blood vessels, making the container too large and decreasing the blood pressure.

▪ The blood vessels of the container can dilate so that the blood within them, even though it is of normal volume, is insufficient to fill the system and provide efficient perfusion.

In all instances, the results of shock are exactly the same. There is insufficient perfusion of blood through the tissues of the body to provide adequate food and oxygen and to carry away waste. All local body processes are affected. If the conditions causing shock are not promptly arrested and perfusion to vital tissues restored, death soon follows. Table 38.1 lists the seven most common medical conditions that can precipitate shock.

THE SIGNS AND SYMPTOMS OF SHOCK

Loss of perfusion to organs and tissues results in characteristic manifestations. The following signs and symptoms are common to all types of shock.

▪ Nausea or vomiting.
▪ Restlessness and anxiety.
▪ A weak, rapid pulse ("thready" or difficult to feel).

▪ Cold, wet skin (commonly described as "clammy").
▪ Profuse sweating.
▪ Paleness, which may change to cyanosis as oxygen delivery to tissues continues to fall.
▪ Shallow, labored, rapid, or irregular gasping respirations.
▪ Dull, lusterless eyes with dilated pupils.
▪ Gradual and steadily falling blood pressure. (Although some people normally have a systolic blood pressure of only 90 to 100 mm Hg, it is best to assume that shock is developing in any adult whose systolic blood pressure is 100 mm Hg or lower.)
▪ Loss of consciousness in cases of rapidly developing or severe shock.

The trainer must remember that although shock means failure of the cardiovascular system to perfuse blood through organs and tissues at proper pressures, the blood pressure may be the last measurable parameter to change. Many mechanisms react automatically to help maintain the blood pressure. When a falling blood pressure is observed, shock is usually far along in development.

TABLE 38.1. Medical Conditions That Can Precipitate Shock

Condition	Mechanism of Shock Production	Description	Specific Treatment in Addition to Life Support Measures
Hypovolemic shock	Decreased blood volume	Acute blood loss can result from external or internal bleeding (e.g., fracture, laceration, organ rupture).	Replace blood.
Metabolic shock	Decreased blood volume through profound loss of body fluids	Can have profound fluid losses from vomiting, diarrhea, or excessive urination in some metabolic diseases such as diabetes.	Replace fluids, treat the metabolic disease.
Cardiogenic shock	Pump failure	Many diseases can cause destruction or inflammation of the cardiac muscle, resulting in the inability of this organ to serve as an efficient pump. These include coronary artery disease, viral myocarditis, and inadequate functioning of heart valves (valvular heart disease).	Provide support to the injured or diseased cardiac muscle through medication and mechanical support (repair faulty valve, bypass or open obstructed vessels).
Neurogenic shock	Increased dilation of peripheral blood vessels	With injury to the spinal cord, particularly at cervical levels, the nerve supply which controls contraction of smooth muscle in blood vessel walls is damaged. This results in all the vessels below the level of the spinal injury dilating widely, and although there is no blood or fluid loss, the available blood can no longer fill the enlarged vascular system and circulatory failure (shock) ensues.	Reverse peripheral pooling by giving medications to increase smooth muscle tone in vessel walls.

INITIAL EMERGENCY MANAGEMENT OF SHOCK

Any person who exhibits any of the signs or symptoms of shock should be immediately transported to an emergency facility. While in the process of arranging transport, the trainer should take the following measures:

1. Secure and maintain a clear airway and give oxygen if available.

2. Control all obvious bleeding by direct compression.
3. Elevate the lower extremities about 12 inches.
4. Splint fractures to lessen bleeding.
5. Avoid rough and excessive handling.
6. Prevent the loss of body heat by putting blankets under and over the person. Do not overheat the athlete. It is better that the person be cool than too warm.

TABLE 38.1.   (continued)

Condition	Mechanism of Shock Production	Description	Specific Treatment in Addition to Life Support Measures
Psychogenic shock	Increased dilation of peripheral blood vessels	In the common faint, sudden reaction of the involuntary nervous system causes a dilation of blood vessels, resulting in decreased perfusion to the brain in the upright individual. This reaction is very transient, however, and normal vessel tone is soon achieved. The vascular dilation is so transient that no other organ systems display any manifestations of this temporary loss of blood volume.	Place athlete supine to increase perfusion to the brain during this transient reversible phenomenon.
Anaphylactic shock	Increased dilation of peripheral blood vessels, decreased blood volume secondary to the fluid component of blood leaking through injured (sick) vessel walls into tissues	A dramatic example is an immediate hypersensitivity reaction to an allergen which has been injected, ingested, inhaled, or inflicted through an animal or insect bite or sting. This complex reaction affects the skin (flushing, itching, burning) and the respiratory system (wheezing, dyspnea), as well as the circulatory system. This reaction is described in more detail in Chapter 57.	The allergic reaction is treated by injecting epinephrine 0.5 to 1.0 ml of 1:1,000 dilution intramuscularly, intravenously, or subcutaneously.
Septic shock	Increased dilation of peripheral blood vessels, decreased blood volume secondary to the fluid components of blood leaking through injured (sick) vessel walls into tissue	In severe bacterial infections, the bacteria liberate toxins (poisons) into the bloodstream which dilate and injure peripheral blood vessels, causing not only the available blood volume to be pooled in the periphery, but also plasma fluid to be lost through vessel walls into tissues.	Give antibiotics to treat the infection.

7. Keep the injured athlete supine, remembering, however, that some persons in shock after a severe heart attack or with lung disease cannot breathe as well when supine as when sitting up or in a semi-sitting position. With such a person use the most comfortable position.

8. Accurately record the athlete's pulse, blood pressure, and other vital signs. Maintain a record of them at 5-minute intervals until the athlete is delivered to emergency medical personnel.

9. Do not give anything to eat or drink.

Air pressure splints, also called pneumatic trousers, are now available to treat hypovolemic shock. They force blood from the extremities centrally to preserve vital organ function. They should only be applied by those knowledgeable in their use.

Once an athlete in shock has arrived at the medical facility, hospital personnel will maintain basic life support while specifically treating the medical condition that precipitated shock. For example, transfusions are given to the person in hypovolemic shock (from acute blood loss), while the person in cardiac shock (from heart pump failure) receives medications to help the diseased or injured cardiac muscle perform more efficiently.

IMPORTANT CONCEPTS

1. Shock is defined as cardiovascular collapse. It is inadequate circulatory perfusion to meet the needs of the body's tissues.
2. The three basic causes of shock are pump failure of the heart, loss of blood from severe bleeding, and dilation of blood vessels that makes the vessels too large to fill and thus causes a decrease in blood pressure.
3. Any athlete who exhibits the signs or symptoms of shock should be transported to an emergency facility as quickly as possible.

SUGGESTED READINGS

Barrett, J., and L. M. Nyhus, eds. *Treatment of Shock: Principles and Practice*, 2d ed. Philadelphia: Lea & Febiger, 1986.

Carolan, J. M. *Shock: A Nursing Guide*. Oradell, N.J.: Medical Economics Books, 1984.

Cowley, R. A., and C. M. Dunham, eds. *Shock Trauma/Critical Care Manual: Initial Assessment and Management*. Baltimore: University Park Press, 1982.

Perry, A. G., P. A. Potter, eds.; L. Niedringhaus, A Smith-Collins, J. L. Myers, co-authors. *Shock: Comprehensive Nursing Management*. St. Louis: C. V. Mosby, 1983.

39

Control of Bleeding

OBJECTIVES FOR CHAPTER 39

After reading this chapter, the student should be able to:
1. Explain the difference between bleeding from a vein and that from an artery.
2. Briefly describe the body's normal blood-clotting mechanism.
3. Explain and demonstrate the methods used to control external bleeding.
4. Recognize the potential dangers of internal bleeding.

INTRODUCTION

Unquestionably, bleeding is a major emergency problem. The athletic trainer must recognize its existence (obvious when it is external and clearly visible but not so obvious when it is internal), assess its seriousness, and recognize when urgent medical attention will be required. In the case of internal bleeding, recognition of its existence and prompt transportation to an emergency department are paramount because the athletic trainer has very limited means to control this type of bleeding.

Chapter 39 begins with an explanation of how bleeding can be external or internal and what happens to the body when it sustains severe blood loss. The chapter then discusses blood-clotting mechanisms, five methods of applying pressure to control external bleeding, and how to control a nosebleed. The last section of Chapter 39 discusses the sources of internal bleeding, its signs and symptoms, and the urgency of getting an athlete with suspected internal bleeding to an emergency facility. ■

THE SIGNIFICANCE OF BLOOD LOSS

Bleeding, or **hemorrhage**, refers to the loss of blood from arteries, capillary vessels, or veins. Bleeding may be external or internal. Loss of blood may initially cause weakness and progress to shock and death if the bleeding is not controlled.

Sources of Bleeding

Blood is transported within the circulatory system through blood vessels. If the vessels are disrupted by injury or disease, bleeding occurs. Characteristically, blood from an artery is bright red and spurts under pressure, in time with the beat of the heart. Blood from a vein is much darker and flows steadily without spurting. Bleeding from damaged capillaries results in a continuous, slow, steady ooze (Fig. 39.1).

Blood Loss Over Time

The rapidity of bleeding is very important to note. For example, the average adult may comfortably lose a unit (500 ml) of blood donated in a blood center over 15 to 20 minutes. While the blood is being withdrawn, the body adapts to the decrease in blood volume quite well. However, if larger amounts of blood are lost, especially more suddenly, the adult may show signs and symptoms of shock.

The average adult has 6 liters of blood. The acute loss of 10 percent of the circulatory blood volume (in an adult, 600 ml; in a child, 200 to 300 ml) may be critical. In an infant, the loss of as little as 25 to 30 ml of blood can cause the signs of shock.

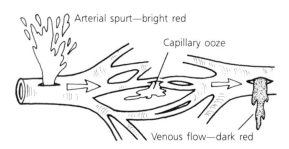

FIGURE 39.1. A capillary loop connecting an arteriole and a venule is shown in this schematic drawing. Bleeding on the arterial side is bright red and spurting; from the venous side it is dark red, or reddish-blue, with a steady flow. Bleeding from the capillaries themselves is a slow, steady ooze.

EXTERNAL BLEEDING

External hemorrhage is bleeding that can be seen coming from a wound. Some examples of external hemorrhage are bleeding from open fractures, bleeding from wounds, and nosebleeds. Several methods exist for controlling obvious external bleeding, each with varying degrees of risk.

Clotting Mechanisms

In most instances, bleeding stops naturally after 6 to 10 minutes because of the body's clotting mechanism. If a finger is cut, for instance, blood will at first gush from the cut vessels, but then the cut vessel ends will constrict to diminish the hemorrhage. A clot forms at the ends of the vessels, and bleeding stops as the clot increases in size and plugs the hole.

Clotting mechanisms are activated by body tissues and tissue fluids. Normally, blood within an artery or vein is protected from contact with body tissues or tissue fluids by the vessel wall and therefore will not clot unless the vessel is injured.

In some athletes who have undergone a severe injury, the damaged blood vessels may be so large that clots cannot occlude (block) them. Sometimes only a portion of the vessel wall may be cut; thus, the wall cannot retract or constrict. In these cases, bleeding will continue unless it is stopped by external means. Blood loss may occasionally be so rapid that there is not enough time for the body's normal protective processes to stop the bleeding. Therefore, it is imperative that the trainer know how to control bleeding. After securing an airway and being certain that the athlete can breathe, the trainer must address the second matter for immediate concern—the control of hemorrhage.

Control of External Bleeding

Frequently, external bleeding is adequately controlled by applying direct local pressure to the injury. Pressure stops the physical flow of blood and permits normal blood coagulation to occur. Methods of applying pressure to an external bleeding wound include local pressure, pressure point control, a tourniquet, splints, and air pressure splints.

Local Pressure

When pressure is applied directly over the wound, bleeding typically stops (Fig. 39.2a). Initially, pressure may be applied with the finger or hand, but a sterile gauze pressure dressing is preferred: 4-by-4-inch or 4-by-8-inch sterile gauze pads should be used for small wounds and a sterile universal dressing for larger wounds. Once bleeding is controlled using local pressure, the compression can be maintained by wrapping the wound circumferentially and firmly with a sterile, roller, self-adhering bandage. The roller bandage, stretched sufficiently tight to control the hemorrhage, should cover the entire sterile dressing above and below the wound. If sterile pads are not immediately available, a handkerchief, sanitary napkin, clean cloth, or bare hand can be used to apply pressure.

Once in place, the dressing should not be removed until the athlete has been evaluated by a physician at the emergency department. Persistent bleeding after the dressing is in place usually means that not enough pressure has been applied to the wound. In such instances, additional manual pressure should be applied through the dressing. Additional gauze pads should be applied over the first dressing and secured with a second roller bandage.

Pressure Point Control

When pressure dressings are not available or when direct pressure with reinforced dressings does not control wound bleeding, proximal arterial pressure control can sometimes be used to slow bleeding (Fig. 39.2b). Pulse points for the major arteries are described in Chapter 11. To use proximal arterial pressure correctly to control

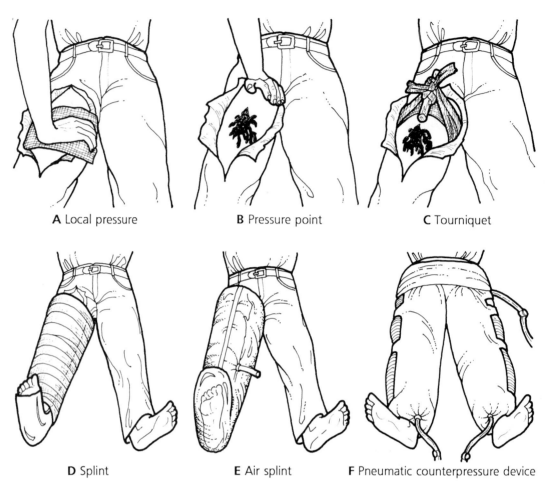

A Local pressure   **B** Pressure point   **C** Tourniquet

D Splint   **E** Air splint   **F** Pneumatic counterpressure device

FIGURE 39.2. The major means of controlling external bleeding: (a) local pressure; (b) pressure point; (c) tourniquet; (d) splint; (e) air splint; and (f) pneumatic counterpressure device.

bleeding, the trainer must know the location of these pulse points.

Because most wounds are supplied by more than one major artery, compression of a major artery rarely arrests hemorrhage completely from a wound distal to that artery. Thus, pressure point control can aid temporarily in the control of severe hemorrhage, but it should not be the primary or sole method of bleeding control.

Tourniquet

The use of a tourniquet to stop bleeding is rarely necessary. Tourniquets, if they are used improperly, can crush the soft tissue of an injured extremity and cause permanent damage to nerves and blood vessels. If a tourniquet is left on for an extended length of time, all tissues distal to the tourniquet will die from a lack of perfusion. The use of a tourniquet is not indicated in wounds of the trunk or for wounds distal to the elbow or knee. Thus, the range of injuries for which a tourniquet may be effective is quite limited.

Nevertheless, a properly applied tourniquet may be lifesaving for a person whose bleeding from a major vessel cannot be controlled in any other way. For example,

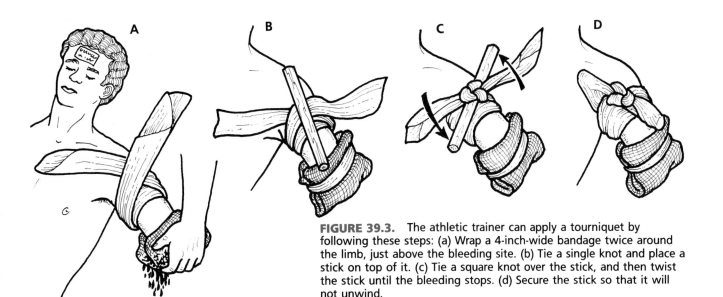

FIGURE 39.3. The athletic trainer can apply a tourniquet by following these steps: (a) Wrap a 4-inch-wide bandage twice around the limb, just above the bleeding site. (b) Tie a single knot and place a stick on top of it. (c) Tie a square knot over the stick, and then twist the stick until the bleeding stops. (d) Secure the stick so that it will not unwind.

the tourniquet is useful for the individual who has severe bleeding from a traumatic amputation, either partial or complete, or for whom local pressure supplemented by proximal pressure point control has failed to arrest the hemorrhage.

If a tourniquet must be used, it should be applied in the following manner (Fig. 39.3):

1. Fold a triangular bandage until it is 3 to 4 inches wide and six to eight layers thick.
2. Wrap this long, 4-inch-wide bandage twice around the extremity, at a point proximal to the bleeding but as far distally on the extremity as possible (Fig. 39.3a).
3. Tie one knot in the bandage. Place a stick or rod on top of the knot and tie the ends of the bandage over the stick in a square knot (Figs. 39.3b, c).
4. Use the stick as a handle and twist it to tighten the tourniquet until the bleeding has stopped. Once the bleeding has ceased, stop turning the stick. Secure the stick in place and make the wrapping neat and smooth (Fig. 39.3d). The technique of using a rod passed through a bandage to achieve pressure is called the **Spanish windlass.** Occasionally, the Spanish windlass is also used to apply traction.

A blood pressure cuff, if available, can also serve as an effective tourniquet (Fig. 39.4). The cuff should be applied proximally (closer to the trunk) to the bleeding point and inflated to a pressure just in excess of that required to arrest the bleeding.

Anyone who uses a tourniquet must observe the following precautions:

1. Use as wide a bandage as possible.
2. After the tourniquet has been applied, make certain it is secure and will not become loosened when the athlete is moved during transport to an emergency facility. Never use wire or any other material that will cut into the skin.
3. Do not loosen the tourniquet. A physician in the emergency department will loosen it after measures have been taken to control the expected bleeding.
4. Never cover a tourniquet with a bandage. Leave it open and in full view. Always signify that the athlete has had a tourniquet applied by writing "TK" and the time the tourniquet was applied on a piece of adhesive tape securely fastened to the athlete's forehead (see Fig. 39.4).

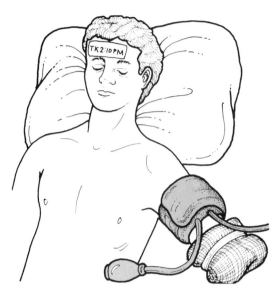

FIGURE 39.4. A blood pressure cuff can be used effectively as a tourniquet. With all tourniquets, a note must be made, usually taped to the athlete's forehead, of the time of application.

The emergency department personnel must be notified that a tourniquet is in place.

5. Never place a tourniquet below the knee or elbow. In these more distal areas in the extremity, nerves lie close to the skin and may be injured by compression. Furthermore, rarely, if ever, does one encounter bleeding distally to the knee or elbow that will require tourniquet control.

6. If a blood pressure cuff is used, continuously monitor the gauge to be certain that the pressure is not being gradually lost.

Splints

Bleeding from injured extremities can occur because muscles are damaged by the sharp ends of broken bones or because vessels lying near the fractured bone continue to bleed. Stabilization of the fracture by the proper application of a splint helps to diminish bleeding from these sources (see Fig. 39.2d). The principles of applying splints are given in Chapter 14.

Air Pressure Splints

Many ambulances throughout the United States carry **air pressure splints** (see Figs. 39.2e, f). Air pressure splints are used to control severe soft tissue hemorrhage when fractures or severe soft tissue lacerations have occurred. Air splinting allows a pressure bandage to be applied to an entire extremity rather than to a single laceration or a given area on the extremity. At the same time, effective splinting of the coexisting fracture, if such exists, can be accomplished (see Fig. 39.2e).

Control of Nosebleed (Epistaxis)

Nosebleed, or **epistaxis**, is a common emergency. A person may lose enough blood in a nosebleed to cause shock. The blood seen coming from the nose may represent only a small amount of the total loss, since much blood passes down the throat into the stomach as the athlete swallows. A person who swallows a large amount of blood may become nauseated and may vomit.

Bleeding from the nose may be caused by the following conditions:

A fractured skull.
Facial injuries, including those caused by a direct blow with the fist, helmet, or racket.
Sinusitis, infections, or other abnormalities of the inside of the nose.
High blood pressure.
Bleeding diseases.

Bleeding from the nose or ears following a head injury may mean that a skull fracture is present. Sterile gauze pads should be placed gently over the nose or ears and the athlete promptly transported to an emergency facility for further evaluation and treatment.

Nosebleeds resulting from all other causes should be initially treated at the scene. The following techniques are successful in stopping most nosebleeds:

1. Apply pressure by pinching the nostrils together or by placing a rolled 4-by-4-

inch gauze bandage between the upper lip and the gum and pressing against it with the fingers. The athlete can sometimes apply enough pressure to stop the bleeding by stretching the upper lip tightly against the rolled bandage.

2. Keep the athlete in a sitting position with the head tilted forward whenever possible so that the blood trickling down the back of the throat will not be aspirated into the lungs.

3. Keep the athlete quiet. This rule is particularly important if the athlete suffers from high blood pressure or is anxious. Anxiety will tend to increase the blood pressure, and the nosebleed will worsen.

4. Apply ice over the nose. Local cooling treatment is helpful in controlling hemorrhage.

If these measures fail to control the nosebleed, the athlete should be transported promptly to the emergency department. Although most nosebleeds arise from injury of the mucous membrane covering the nasal septum, anterior in the nose, and therefore can usually be controlled by the local measures listed above, a few nosebleeds arise posteriorly, in the nasopharynx, and cannot be stopped by these usual emergency methods. This kind of nosebleed may require application of a nasopharyngeal pack, which should be done by a physician.

An athlete who suffers from frequent nosebleeds should be evaluated by a physician to determine the cause of the nosebleeds so that appropriate treatment may be instituted.

INTERNAL BLEEDING

Although not usually visible, **internal hemorrhage** can be very serious. The athlete with severe internal hemorrhage may develop hypovolemic shock before the trainer realizes the extent of the blood loss.

Sources of Internal Bleeding

Bleeding from any body orifice is of concern to the trainer because it may indicate internal hemorrhage. A bruise or contusion indicates hemorrhage into the soft tissues and may be seen after a slight or severe injury. Internal hemorrhage can also result from a stomach ulcer, a closed fracture, a lacerated spleen or liver, a ruptured bowel, a contused or ruptured kidney or bladder, or an acute muscle or tendon rupture.

Signs and Symptoms of Internal Bleeding

Signs and symptoms that may point to internal bleeding are the same as those indicating the development of hypovolemic shock:

- The pulse becomes weak and rapid ("thready").
- The skin becomes cold and moist ("clammy").
- The eyes are dull; the pupils may be dilated and slow to respond to light.
- The blood pressure falls (a late sign).
- The athlete is usually thirsty and anxious, with a feeling of impending doom.
- The athlete may be nauseated and may vomit.

Control of Internal Bleeding

There is little the athletic trainer can do in the field to control internal hemorrhage within the body cavities or organs. If the trainer suspects internal bleeding based on the mechanism of injury or the athlete's signs and symptoms, basic life support should be provided and the athlete transported immediately to the emergency department. Internal bleeding into the extremities can be initially managed by the trainer by the same methods used to control external bleeding of the extremities.

IMPORTANT CONCEPTS

1. The acute loss of 10 percent of the circulating blood volume may precipitate shock.
2. Bleeding from an open artery is bright red and spurts with the beat of the heart; bleeding from an open vein is dark red and flows steadily; bleeding from damaged capillaries is a slow, steady ooze.
3. External bleeding can usually be controlled by applying di-

rect local pressure; rarely, if ever, is a tourniquet necessary.
4. Bleeding from the nose or ears may indicate a skull fracture.
5. There is little a trainer can do to control internal bleeding other than administer basic life support and arrange for prompt transportation to an emergency facility.

SUGGESTED READINGS

Franks, M. R. *The American Medical Association's Handbook of First Aid and Emergency Care.* New York: Random House, 1980.

Bergmann, et al. *Musculoskeletal Trauma.* English Language edition edited by M. A. Rinehart and T. Sutton. Rockville, Md.: Aspen Publishers, 1987.

Gilbert, G. G. *Teaching First Aid and Emergency Care.* Dubuque, Iowa: Kendall/Hunt, 1981.

Grant, H. D., R. H. Murray, Jr., and J. Bergeron. *Emergency Care,* 3rd ed. Bowie, Md.: R. J. Brady Co., 1982.

Hughes, S., ed. *The Basis and Practice of Traumatology.* London: William Heinemann Medical Books, 1983.

40

Acute Chest Pain

OBJECTIVES FOR CHAPTER 40

After reading this chapter, the student should be able to:

1. Understand how arteriosclerotic heart disease develops.
2. Recognize the cardiac causes of acute chest pain, including angina pectoris and acute myocardial infarction.
3. Describe the emergency treatment of acute chest pain.

INTRODUCTION

Heart disease reportedly affects 25 percent of the United States population and currently causes more than one million deaths annually. Heart disease may present as angina pectoris or acute myocardial infarction, and both of these conditions present as acute chest pain. Although rare in high school, collegiate, and professional athletes, acute chest pain does occur in recreational athletes.

Chapter 40 begins with a brief explanation of arteriosclerotic heart disease. The chapter then focuses on two causes of acute chest pain, angina pectoris and acute myocardial infarction, in order that the trainer can become familiar with these entities and their emergency treatment. ■

ARTERIOSCLEROTIC HEART DISEASE

To carry out its pumping function, the **myocardium** (heart muscle) needs a continuous supply of oxygen and nutrients, both of which are provided by the blood circulating through the coronary arteries (Fig. 40.1). When the heart muscle must increase its work, as during periods of physical exertion and stress, the myocardium requires more oxygen and therefore greater blood flow. In the normal heart, this increased flow is supplied by dilation of the coronary arteries.

In individuals with **arteriosclerotic heart disease**, lipid deposits (cholesterol) in the coronary artery wall prevent normal dilation of the coronary arteries. The heart muscle, unable to receive sufficient oxygen, becomes ischemic (lacking in oxygen), and a condition called **cardiac ischemia** develops (Fig. 40.2). Cholesterol deposits can begin to accumulate in vessel walls as early as age 18, and therefore arteriosclerotic heart disease, although reaching its peak incidence in individuals aged 40 to 70, can also occur in younger people.

Risk factors have been identified to determine those individuals more prone to arteriosclerotic heart disease. These factors can be divided into controllable and uncontrollable factors. The major *controllable factors* are high blood pressure, an elevated level of blood cholesterol, obesity, and smoking. The *uncontrollable* factors are age, sex, heredity, personality traits, and the presence of other diseases such as diabetes.

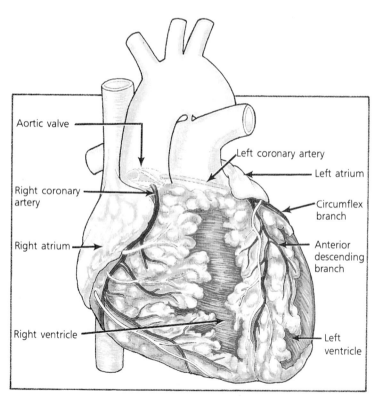

FIGURE 40.1. The coronary arteries carry the blood supply to the heart. The right coronary artery supplies the right ventricle, and the left coronary artery supplies the left ventricle.

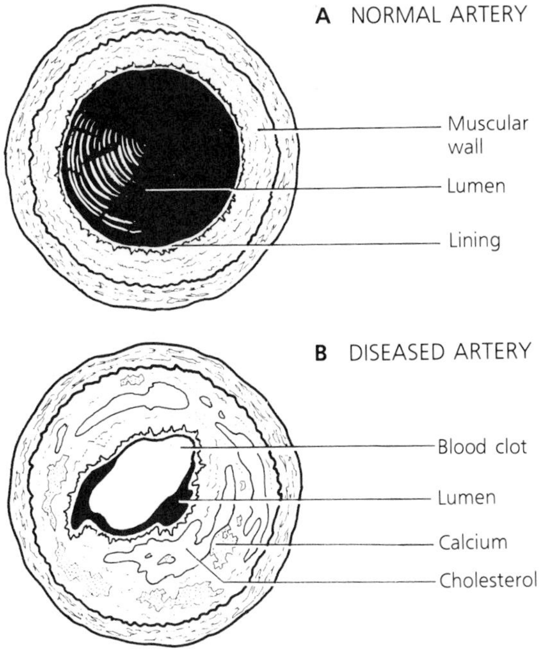

A NORMAL ARTERY

—— Muscular wall

—— Lumen

—— Lining

B DISEASED ARTERY

—— Blood clot

—— Lumen

—— Calcium

—— Cholesterol

FIGURE 40.2. Cross section of a coronary artery: (a) a normal artery is unobstructed; (b) a diseased artery is narrowed by cholesterol and calcium deposits and eventually obstructed by a blood clot.

CAUSES OF ACUTE CHEST PAIN

Angina pectoris, chest pain caused by an inadequate flow of blood to the heart muscle, and **acute myocardial infarction** (AMI), the death of the heart muscle, are conditions that occur from too little oxygen. Each represents a form of arteriosclerotic heart disease, and each presents as acute chest pain.

Angina Pectoris

The presentation of angina pectoris pain, usually called simply *angina*, is varied. In its extreme form it is described as crushing —"it takes one's breath away"—or as a squeezing feeling—"like someone standing on your chest." Angina may also present as chest tightness, a vague sense of chest discomfort, or apparent indigestion.

Angina generally occurs when the heart increases its workload—that is, increases its need for more oxygen—such as occurs during periods of physical or emotional stress. The principal characteristic of angina pectoris is pain that comes on with exertion and is relieved by rest. The pain is usually felt under the sternum, but it can radiate to the jaw, to the arms (typically the left arm), or to the epigastrium (the upper-middle region of the abdomen). The pain usually lasts from 3 to 8 minutes and rarely longer than 10 minutes. It may be associated with shortness of breath, nausea, and sweating. Pain disappears promptly when the increased workload of the heart diminishes (the individual rests) or when more oxygen is supplied to the heart (medication is taken to dilate the coronary arteries).

Treatment of Angina

Angina is treated with **nitroglycerin**, a medication dispensed as a small white pill about one-half the size of an aspirin tablet. The pill is placed under the tongue and works in seconds. Nitroglycerin relaxes vascular smooth muscle, dilates coronary arteries, and increases blood flow and the supply of oxygen to the heart muscle, relieving the pain. Because nitroglycerin dilates blood vessels in the brain, one common side effect is a severe headache.

Significance of Angina

It is important to recognize the symptoms of angina and institute treatment for coronary artery disease before cardiac ischemia progresses to the point of cardiac muscle death or AMI.

Anyone experiencing anginal pain should be evaluated by a physician. If the pain is only experienced with exercise, a stress electrocardiogram should be done to look for cardiac ischemia.

Coronary arteriography confirms coronary artery disease. Treatment depends on the extent and location of cholesterol deposits in the vessel walls and varies from limited arterial dilation (balloon angioplasty) to replacement of a section of damaged coronary artery with a vein graft (coronary artery bypass graft).

Acute Myocardial Infarction

Although the development of AMI may be preceded by several episodes of angina, it can also occur in an individual who has not previously been symptomatic—that is, the person's first episode of cardiac ischemia may be severe enough to cause muscle death.

The pain of AMI differs from the pain of angina pectoris in that AMI pain lasts longer and is not relieved by rest or by taking nitroglycerin. Anginal pain typically lasts from 3 to 10 minutes, whereas the pain of AMI may last from 30 minutes to several hours.

Physical Findings of AMI

The physical findings of AMI are variable and will depend on the extent and severity of heart muscle damage. The following are the most frequent physical findings seen in AMI:

Pulse. Generally, the pulse rate increases as a normal response to stress, fear, or the injury of the myocardium. Since **arrhythmias** (irregular heartbeats) are the rule rather than the exception, an irregularity of the pulse may be noted. In some cases of acute infarction, **bradycardia** (an abnormal slowing of the pulse) develops rather than **tachycardia** (an abnormally rapid pulse).

Blood pressure. Blood pressure falls as a result of diminished cardiac output and diminished capability of the left ventricle to pump.

Respiration. Respirations are normal unless pulmonary edema (abnormal accumulation of fluid in the lungs) occurs. In this case, rapid shallow respirations are seen.

General appearance. The person with AMI appears frightened. A cold sweat is frequently present. The individual may feel nauseated and may vomit. The skin is often ashen as a result of poor cardiac output and the loss of skin perfusion. Occasionally, cyanosis (bluish color of the skin) may be observed as a result of poor oxygenation of the circulating blood.

Mental state. One of the unexplained aspects of AMI is that most victims report having an almost overwhelming feeling of impending doom. These individuals are convinced—almost resigned—that they are about to die.

Consequences of AMI

AMI has three major and serious consequences: sudden death from arrhythmia, congestive heart failure, or cardiogenic shock.

Sudden death. Approximately 40 percent of all people with AMI die before they reach the hospital. These deaths occur because of arrhythmias, which prevent any effective pumping action of the heart. The chance of an arrhythmia occurring after AMI is greatest within the first hour after the event; it diminishes to a very small risk after 3 to 5 days. Arrhythmias may produce completely disorganized quivering, called **fibrillation**, or no heartbeat at all, called **asystole** (Fig. 40.3). In either case, the heart is described as being in **cardiac arrest**. These situations require immediate cardiopulmonary resuscitation (CPR). (See Chapter 37 for a complete discussion of basic life support techniques.)

Congestive heart failure. **Congestive heart failure (CHF)** refers to the condition that occurs when the heart muscle is so damaged by infarction that it is no longer able to pump enough blood for all the needs of the body. Venous pressure increases, resulting in tissue edema commonly presenting as swelling in the feet and ankles or as fluid in

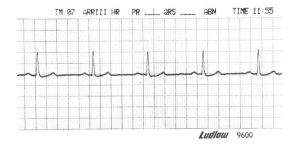

TM 07 ARRIII HR PR _I_ QRS ____ ABN   TIME 11:55

Ludlow 9600

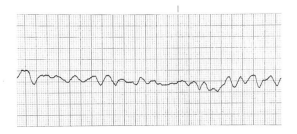

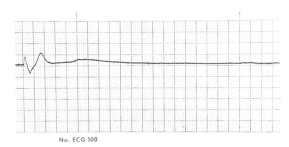

No. ECG 100

FIGURE 40.3. ECG (electrocardiogram) tracings show (a) normal heart rhythm, (b) arrhythmia from fibrillation, and (c) asystole (cardiac arrest).

the lungs (pulmonary edema). Difficulty in breathing accompanies pulmonary edema.

Cardiogenic shock. **Cardiogenic shock**, an early complication of AMI seen in the first 24 hours, results when the heart has been so damaged that it is unable to sustain a blood pressure adequate to perfuse the tissues of the body. Death results unless recovery of the heart can be achieved through medical management.

Treatment of Suspected AMI

When treating a conscious athlete in whom heart disease or AMI is suspected, the trainer should take the following steps while awaiting emergency transportation to the hospital.

1. *Reassure the athlete.* Act professionally and stay calm. Speak in a voice that is not too loud or too soft. Inform the athlete that trained individuals are present to provide care and that he or she will soon be taken to the hospital. Remember, all persons with acute chest pain are frightened. Some may act carefree, and some may be demanding, but all are frightened. The professional attitude of the medical personnel may be the single most important factor in securing the person's cooperation.

2. *Take a brief history.* If time permits, take a brief history from the athlete. Friends or family members who are with the athlete might provide helpful information.

3. *Position the athlete.* If AMI is suspected, place the athlete in a comfortable and well-supported position, usually sitting. Make sure the athlete has no difficulty breathing and has no airway obstruction.

4. *Institute CPR if needed.* The athletic trainer should record the athlete's vital signs at regular intervals and be prepared to institute CPR if needed.

(Important Concepts appear on next page.)

IMPORTANT CONCEPTS

1. Cholesterol deposits can prevent normal dilation of the coronary walls and prevent adequate blood flow to the heart, resulting in the pain of angina pectoris or AMI.
2. The pain of angina pectoris usually lasts 3 to 8 minutes and is relieved by rest or nitroglycerin. The pain of AMI usually lasts 30 minutes or longer and is not relieved by rest or nitroglycerin.
3. Consequences of AMI are sudden death from arrhythmia, congestive heart failure, or cardiogenic shock.

SUGGESTED READINGS

Corbett, S. J., and J. E. Watson. *Cardiac Rehabilitation: An Interdisciplinary Team Approach.* New York: Wiley, 1984.

Little, R. C. W. C. Little. *Physiology of the Heart and Circulation*, 4th ed. Chicago: Year Book Medical Publishers, 1989.

Smith, J. J., and J. P. Kampine. *Circulatory Physiology: The Essentials.* Baltimore: Williams & Wilkins, 1980.

41

Sudden Loss of Consciousness

OBJECTIVES FOR CHAPTER 41

After reading this chapter, the student should be able to:

1. Explain initial emergency treatment for the unconscious athlete.
2. Describe briefly some of the causes of unconsciousness in the athlete.

INTRODUCTION

No matter what the cause, all unconscious athletes require initial emergency evaluation and basic life support. While administering emergency treatment, the trainer should be alert to any information that may disclose the cause of unconsciousness. Chapter 41 explains the six steps in the emergency medical care of the unconscious athlete and briefly describes some of the causes of unconsciousness. ■

INITIAL EMERGENCY CARE OF THE UNCONSCIOUS ATHLETE

All unconscious athletes require similar emergency medical treatment, regardless of the specific cause of the unconsciousness. In general, the trainer should follow these six steps:

1. Secure and maintain an airway.
2. Institute cardiopulmonary resuscitation (CPR) if necessary.
3. Record the history from bystanders, if possible; note any items that might serve as evidence regarding the cause of the unconscious state.
4. If possible, attempt to define the specific cause of unconsciousness in the athlete.
5. Observe and record vital signs and the level of consciousness.
6. Transport the athlete promptly to the emergency department.

Respiratory Support

For every unconscious athlete, the first and foremost treatment is to ensure an open airway and to provide respiratory support when necessary. A supine (lying flat, face up) unconscious person is in danger of aspirating (taking into the lungs) vomitus or other oral contents, or of suffocating from an obstructed airway. The airway should be opened and the unconscious athlete placed on one side with the head lower than the feet. The trainer must take steps to keep the airway open and then arrange to transport the athlete in this position with continued monitoring of respiration and vital signs.

When a neck injury is suspected following an accident, the first step in emergency care is to stabilize the spine (see Chapter 14). Then the trainer must direct attention to the airway.

Cardiopulmonary Resuscitation

If the unconscious athlete has sustained a cardiopulmonary arrest, CPR must be started. (See guidelines in Chapter 39 for instituting CPR.)

Gathering and Recording Information

Once cardiopulmonary function has been restored and stabilized, the trainer should try to retrieve and accumulate information concerning the cause of an athlete's problem. If the trainer did not witness the event preceding the athlete's development of unconsciousness, he or she should question teammates and bystanders about the events immediately before the athlete became unconscious. Did the athlete fall? Was the individual struck by another person or object? Is there any history of previous episodes of unconsciousness, epilepsy, or any recent medical illness? Details of drug use, the possibility of a drug overdose, or any type of poisoning also must be considered. The trainer who is not familiar with the athlete's history should look for medical identification symbols that may suggest the cause of the unconscious state.

The trainer should record vital signs and note and describe any obvious injuries. The time of the onset of unconsciousness and the rapidity of its development should also be recorded, if known, along with any subsequent changes in mental status. A determination should be made as to whether the pupils of the eyes are constricted or widely dilated. The pupillary response to light should be evaluated and recorded (see Chapter 11). The trainer should also arrange for prompt transportation of the athlete to the emergency department.

CAUSES OF UNCONSCIOUSNESS

Unconsciousness can be caused by diseases, injuries, emotional reactions, environmental causes, or injected or ingested agents. Table 41.1 lists the pathophysiology and emergency medical treatment of the most common causes of unconsciousness. Some of these problems are discussed in more detail in the following sections.

Diseases

The common diseases that may precipitate a loss of consciousness are diabetes and arteriosclerosis.

Diabetes Mellitus

In the diabetic, a headache, followed by unconsciousness, may develop if too much insulin is taken without enough food so that the amount of glucose in the blood (blood sugar level) drops below a level needed for adequate brain functioning (**insulin shock**). If permanent brain injury is to be avoided, insulin shock must be treated immediately by administering glucose orally or by injection to offset the excessive insulin.

Unconsciousness can also occur from the opposite state—insufficient insulin. This condition, called **diabetic coma** or **diabetic ketoacidosis**, develops more slowly. With insufficient insulin, the amount of glucose in the blood rises and causes excess fluid and sugar loss from the kidneys. This results in dehydration and a gradual accumulation in the blood of metabolic waste products. Insulin shock and diabetic coma are discussed more fully in Chapter 54.

Arteriosclerosis

Arteriosclerosis can develop in any blood vessel. When the disease damages and subsequently blocks the arteries that supply the heart muscle, a heart attack may follow. The lack of oxygen precipitates pain and arrhythmias (abnormal heart rhythms). A loss of consciousness can occur if the arrhythmia results in a lack of oxygen to the brain. In this case, CPR may be lifesaving. Heart attack and its many presentations are discussed more fully in Chapter 40.

Similarly, when arteriosclerotic vascular disease damages the arteries that supply blood to the brain, a **thrombus** (blood clot) may develop, obstructing blood flow to the brain and thus precipitating unconsciousness (a **stroke** or **cerebrovascular accident**). A ruptured aneurysm of a vessel supplying the brain may also alter the brain's blood flow and result in a partial or complete loss of consciousness.

Injuries

Many injuries result in loss of consciousness. All injuries that cause excessive blood loss, and thus, a loss of blood flow to the brain and heart, may result in a loss of consciousness from **hypovolemic shock**. The athlete in hypovolemic shock is critically ill and requires the most rapid possible transport to an emergency room.

Injuries of the Respiratory System

Unconsciousness can also result from insufficient oxygen intake following injuries to the chest wall or lungs. Injuries of the chest wall cause severe pain, which restricts breathing. **Hemothorax** (the presence of blood in the chest cavity) or **pneumothorax** (the presence of air in the chest cavity) from a perforated chest wall or lung reduces the

TABLE 41.1. Causes of Unconsciousness and Emergency Medical Management

Problem	Cause	Pathophysiology	Management
General loss of consciousness	Injury or disease	Shock, head injury, other injuries/diabetes, arteriosclerosis	Need for CPR; triage, priority one
Diseases: Diabetic coma	Hyperglycemia and acidosis	Inadequate use of sugar, acidosis	Transport; complex treatment for acidosis
Insulin shock	Hypoglycemia	Excess insulin	Sugar, transport
Acute myocardial infarction	Damaged myocardium	Insufficient cardiac output	O_2, CPR, transport
Stroke	Damaged brain	Loss of arterial supply to brain or hemorrhage within brain	Support, gentle transport
Injury: Hemorrhagic shock	Bleeding	Hypovolemia	Control external bleeding, recognize internal bleeding, CPR, transport
Respiratory insufficiency	Insufficient inspired O_2	Paralysis, chest wall damage, airway obstruction	Clear airway, supplemental O_2, CPR, transport
Cerebral contusion, concussion, or hematoma	Blunt head injury	Bleeding into or around brain, concussive effect of blow	Airway, supplemental O_2, CPR, careful monitoring, transport
Emotions: Psychogenic shock	Emotional reaction	Sudden drop in cerebral blood flow caused by vasodilation	Place supine, make comfortable, observe for injuries
Neurological problems: Epilepsy	Brain injury, scar, genetic predisposition, disease	Excitable focus of motor activity in brain	Support, protect athlete, transport in status epilepticus

actual volume and capacity of the lung to accept and transport oxygen (see Chapter 29). Cervical spinal cord injuries may result in paralysis of some or all of the muscles of respiration, leading to respiratory arrest and unconsciousness.

Injuries of the Head

Injuries of the head which produce cerebral concussion, contusion, or hematoma are probably the most common causes of loss of consciousness. In treating the athlete who has sustained a head injury, the trainer must observe the level of consciousness at the time the athlete is first seen and at intervals thereafter. Changes in the level of consciousness may occur very rapidly following injury. For this reason an athlete with a head injury should be transported to the emergency department as rapidly as possible. During transport the airway should be maintained, the cervical spine should be protected, and oxygen should be given if available.

Emotional Reactions

The common faint is an emotional reaction that results in a temporary but sudden general dilation of blood vessels without an

TABLE 41.1. (continued)

Problem	Cause	Pathophysiology	Management
Injected or ingested agents:			
Alcohol	Excess intake	Cerebral depression	Support, CPR, transport
Drugs	Excess intake	Cerebral depression	Support, CPR, transport (bring drug)
Plant poisons	Contact, ingestion	Direct cerebral or other toxic effect, local irritant effect	Support, recognition, CPR, identify agent, local wound care, transport
Animal poisons	Contact, ingestion, injection	Direct cerebral or other toxic effect, local irritant effect	Recognition, support, CPR, identify agent, local wound care, transport
Environment:			
Heatstroke	Excessive heat, inability to sweat	Brain damage from heat	Immediate cooling, support, CPR, transport
Anaphylaxis	Acute contact with agent to which athlete is sensitive	Allergic reaction, bronchospasm, excess bronchial secretions	Intramuscular epinephrine, support, CPR, transport
Electric shock	Contact with electrical current	Cardiac abnormalities (fibrillation, standstill)	CPR, transport, do not treat until current controlled
Systemic hypothermia	Prolonged exposure to cold	Diminished cerebral function, cardiac arrhythmias	CPR, rapid transport, warming on the way
Drowning	$O_2 \downarrow$, $CO_2 \uparrow$, breath holding, H_2O inhalation	Cerebral damage	CPR, rapid transport
Air embolism	Intravascular air	Obstruction to arterial blood flow by air bubbles	CPR, transport, recompression
Decompression sickness	Intravascular nitrogen	Obstruction to arterial blood flow by nitrogen bubbles	CPR, recompression

increase in cardiac output. Momentarily, inadequate blood flow is supplied to the brain, causing impairment of function. In general, full alertness is restored promptly once the athlete increases the flow of blood to the brain by lying supine. The athletic trainer must be alert for injuries that may have been incurred if the athlete fell during a fainting episode.

Environmental Causes

Environmental causes for loss of consciousness include excessive heat or cold, electricity, and water.

Extreme Heat or Cold

Generally, unconsciousness due to extremes of heat (**heatstroke**) or cold (**systemic hypothermia**) is easily diagnosed by virtue of the circumstances and the athlete's body temperature. Basic life support is mandatory, in addition to appropriate cooling or warming of the individual. Specific details of these environmental problems are discussed in Chapter 52.

Electrical Shock

With athletes who have sustained electrical shock, the trainer must think first of self-protection. If still charged, the athlete is a good electrical conductor and may transmit the full volume of current to the trainer. The power source must be turned off and the electrical circuit disconnected before any treatment can be given. The athlete may have sustained a cardiopulmonary arrest as a result of the shock and may require CPR.

Water Emergencies

Drowning victims require basic life support measures and immediate transport to an emergency department. Athletes who are suspected of having either air embolism or decompression sickness usually require treatment in a hyperbaric chamber. They may need basic life support. Prompt transportation to the emergency department, where the recompression treatment can be arranged, is mandatory. Further details concerning these problems are presented in Chapter 52.

Injected or Ingested Agents

Injected or ingested substances, such as alcohol, drugs, and plant and animal poisons, have a direct toxic effect on the brain. Some are very toxic in minute amounts. Emergency medical care for injection or ingestion of toxic agents includes basic life support and prompt transport to the emergency department.

IMPORTANT CONCEPTS

1. The first and most important step in administering emergency medical care to an unconscious athlete is to clear the airway and provide respiratory support.

2. Unconsciousness may result from a variety of conditions, including diseases, injuries, emotional reactions, environmental causes, and injected or ingested agents.

SUGGESTED READINGS

Aloia, J. F., P. Donohue-Porter, and L. Schlussel. *Diabetes: The Comprehensive Self-Management Handbook.* Garden City, N.Y.: Doubleday, 1984.
Cantu, R. C. *Diabetes and Exercise.* New York: E. P. Dutton, 1982.
Kapp, J. P., and H. H. Schmidek, eds. *The Cerebral Venous System and Its Disorders.* Orlando, Fla.: Grune & Stratton, 1984.
Wade, D. T., et al. *Stroke: A Critical Approach to Diagnosis, Treatment, and Management.* Chicago: Year Book Medical Publishers, 1985.

FIVE

PREVENTING INJURY

42

Sports Nutrition

CHAPTER OUTLINE

OBJECTIVES FOR CHAPTER 42

After reading this chapter, the student should be able to:

1. Describe the caloric requirements of the athlete and how to meet these requirements by combining fats, carbohydrates, proteins, vitamins, and minerals.
2. Recognize that replacement of fluid is essential to the athlete and must be done in a timely manner, and that the most essential fluid to be replaced is water.
3. Know how to advise the athlete regarding special dietary requirements such as weight gain and weight loss programs, pre-game meals, and carbohydrate loading for endurance activities.
4. Describe the impact food can have on athletes who take medications.
5. Recognize the effects of caffeine.
6. Understand the seriousness of eating disorders such as anorexia and bulimia.

INTRODUCTION

Proper nutrition is an important consideration for athletes who seek to maximize their performance. While an adequate diet will not directly increase strength, power, or endurance, it will provide the necessary raw material to allow a good training program to build and run the human machine. Chapter 42 focuses on the scientific rationale for good nutritional practices, as well as on practical information concerning the nutritional needs of athletes. ■

THE ROLE OF DIET IN ATHLETICS

Many factors, including the athlete's physical condition, nutritional status, age, and genetic background, affect nutrient needs and nutrient availability. In addition, the presence and concentration of other substances, as well as the chemical form of the nutrient itself and the environment, play a role.

Diets must be individualized. Athletes come from many different backgrounds, with widely varying beliefs regarding diet. The age, sex, physical condition, and metabolic rate of each player must be considered. For example, adolescent athletes have increased needs to support growth, and female athletes have a lower basal metabolic rates than do male athletes.

The many influences on nutritional needs and physical performance make it difficult to measure how a change in dietary intake affects performance. Lack of knowledge, coupled with the desire for a magic formula that guarantees success, leads to many nutritional myths and fads among athletes.

Diets do not create strong bodies or increase speed. Strength, power, and endurance come only through training. The diet merely provides the necessary raw material that allows a good training program to improve athletic performance.

Caloric Balance and Weight Control

Weight and Body Composition

The focus of weight control in the athlete should be on body composition rather than on weight. An assessment of body fat percentage is far more useful than a simple scale weight measurement. The percentage of body fat and its complement of lean body weight should be assessed at regular intervals throughout the season so that if corrective measures such as changes in training and diet are needed, they may be initiated in a timely fashion.

The body fat percentage recommended for the average man is 15 percent and for the woman, 26 percent. Body fat stores of most athletes are below these averages because extra pounds of fat create more work for the body without increasing its efficiency. Male gymnasts and runners have reported body fats as low as 5 to 8 percent, while women involved in the same sports have reported body fats of 10 to 12 percent. Table 42.1 lists levels of body fat observed in athletes in various sports.

In general, the percentage of body fat for male athletes should be 8 to 10 percent, and 12 to 14 percent for females. The optimal body fat percentage may vary according to the sport and the athlete. It should be strongly emphasized that many athletes perform very well at higher body fat percentages. The goal is improved athletic performance—not a specific percentage of body fat. Women should not drop below 10 percent body fat because of the risk of cessation of menses (see Chapter 59).

Measuring Body Fat

The amount of body fat can be calculated by the skinfold method, underwater weighing, or more recently, measuring electrical impedance flow through tissues. Underwater weighing, which requires calculating

TABLE 42.1. Body Composition Values for Male and Female Athletes

Sport or Position	Sex	Relative Fat %
Baseball	m	11.8–14.2
Basketball	f	20.8–26.9
	m	7.1–10.6
Football		
Defensive backs	m	9.6–11.5
Offensive backs	m	9.4–12.4
Linebackers	m	13.4–14.0
Offensive linemen	m	15.6–19.1
Defensive linemen	m	18.2–18.5
Quarterbacks, kickers	m	14.4
Gymnastics	m	4.6
	f	9.6–17.0
Ice hockey	m	13.0–15.1
Jockeys	m	14.1
Rowing	m	8.5–11
	f	14.0
Skiing		
Alpine	m	7.4–10.2
	f	20.6
Cross-country	m	7.9–12.5
	f	15.7–21.8
Soccer	m	9.6
Speed skating	m	11.4
Swimming	m	5.0–8.5
	f	17.1–26.3
Tennis	m	15.2–16.3
	f	20.3
Track and field	m	8.8
Distance running	m	6.3–13.6
	f	15.2–19.2
Discus	m	16.3
	f	25.0
Weight lifting	m	9.8–12.2
Power	m	15.6
Body building	m	8.3
Wrestling	m	4.0–10.7

Source: Jack H. Wilmore, "Body Composition and Athletic Performance," in *Nutrition and Athletic Performance*, edited by William Haskell, James Skala, and James Whittam (Palo Alto, Calif.: Bull Publishing Co., 1981). Reprinted by permission.

lung volume, is probably the most accurate, but it is not generally available. Skinfold calipers are less expensive and more easily obtained. Calipers are used to "pinch" the fat layer at various designated areas (triceps, subscapula, and abdominal areas). Standard values are supplied with the caliper and are used to translate caliper measurements into body fat percentage measurements. Changes in skinfold thickness are a fairly sensitive indication of changes in total body fat. This method is reasonably accurate and is described in greater detail in Chapter 5.

Equipment to measure body fat percentage calculated by impedance flow of an electrical impulse through tissue is marketed by several companies. Charts can be used to translate impedance to percentage of body fat; many of the instruments make this calculation within the equipment, providing the trainer with a readout of total body fat—not the rate of impedance.

Caloric Requirements

A calorie is a measurement of energy. The energy sources in food and the body's energy expenditure can both be measured in calories. One calorie is defined as the amount of heat needed to raise the temperature of 1 gm of water 1 degree Centigrade. One calorie is a very small amount of energy; therefore, when discussing the energy expended during exercise or the energy available in food, it is more convenient to use kilocalories, abbreviated as Calories with a capital "C," or 1,000 calories.

Weight maintenance is accomplished by balancing caloric intake with caloric output. Calories are provided by carbohydrates, fats, proteins, and alcohol. The number of calories in a given food reflects its energy potential. Protein and carbohydrate are equal in calories; 1 gm of each contains 4 calories. One gm of fat equals 9 calories. Alcohol falls in the middle, with 1 gm yielding 7 calories.

The number of calories the athlete uses (caloric output) depends on age, sex, body weight, body composition, basal metabolic rate, and physical activity levels. Caloric needs per kilogram of body weight are highest in children because of the growth and development of tissues. As individuals age, their caloric needs decrease.

Body weight affects total caloric requirements because it takes more calories to maintain a higher weight. Percentage of body fat is also important because it takes more calories to maintain muscle tissue than to maintain fat. Therefore, even if two athletes weigh the same, the one with the lower percentage of body fat has higher caloric needs. Since men have less fat than women, men's caloric needs are greater.

Individual variations in basal metabolic rate, which range from 10 to 20 percent, can either increase or decrease caloric needs. Physical activity can require an additional 1,000 to 1,500 calories. Caloric output through exercise is determined by the duration and intensity of the activity and the weight of the athlete.

All of these factors make it difficult to assess actual caloric needs from formulas and tables. The best way to determine caloric needs during a time of weight maintenance is to have the athlete keep track of food intake for 3 days and then calculate total calories consumed. Many calorie books are available to help determine this amount. Computer programs now make this calculation fairly easy. Table 42.2 lists average caloric intakes of university athletes.

TABLE 42.2. Caloric Intakes of University Athletes

Sport	Average	Minimum	Maximum
Men			
Basketball	4,762	1,600	9,270
Crew (no coxswain)	5,267	2,711	7,162
Football	5,557	2,516	13,517
Gymnastics	2,080	568	4,249
Lacrosse	3,926	2,467	8,147
Mountain climbing	3,829	2,441	5,959
Soccer	2,965	2,177	3,705
Wrestling	2,665	412	6,702
Women			
Basketball	2,835	500	3,879
Crew	2,339	1,262	3,577
Dancing	1,909	898	2,909
Lacrosse	2,219	1,438	3,059
Swimming	2,874	1,516	5,874
Volleyball	2,094	1,144	3,199

Source: Adapted from S. H. Short and W. R. Short, "Four-Year Study of University Athletes' Dietary Intake." Copyright The American Dietetic Association. Reprinted by permission from Journal of the American Dietetic Association, vol. 82:632, 1983.

Weight Loss

Calories consumed in excess of caloric need cause weight gain, regardless of whether the calories are in the form of carbohydrate, fat, protein, or alcohol. Some evidence indicates that excess fats are used more efficiently than excess proteins or carbohydrates and consequently promote greater weight gain. Alcohol intake is often underreported and can contribute as much as 25 percent of the total daily calories. Obviously, a reduction in alcohol and fat intake can contribute substantially to weight loss and improve the nutritional quality of the diet.

Estimating Calories Needed for Weight Loss. Each pound of body fat contains approximately 3,500 calories. Being 15 pounds overweight represents nearly 53,000 excess calories. If the average need for calories is about 2,000 per day, then a week of total starvation would theoretically result in only a 4-pound weight loss. The body cannot exist on calories provided by fat alone; therefore, in times of starvation or very low calorie intake, the body begins to break down body protein—namely, muscle tissue.

Fat loss and maintenance of weight loss are best achieved by reducing daily intake by 500 to 1,000 calories, thus promoting a loss of 1 to 2 pounds per week. Rapid weight losses to make weight minimums are rarely achieved through dieting but usually through water losses. These water losses can be harmful, since they make the athlete dehydrated and susceptible to muscle cramping, fatigue, weakness, and loss of concentration. The use of diuretics and laxatives for weight loss should be strongly discouraged since repeated use can be harmful.

Rate of Weight Loss. Very low calorie diets or semi-starvation techniques to cause rapid weight loss are also not recommended because a large proportion of body weight lost through such techniques is from muscle protein. Repeated use of very low calorie regimens results in adaptation to lower caloric intake, thus causing slower weight loss and faster regain.

In the first weeks of dieting, weight loss will appear rapid because of accompanying water loss. As the diet continues, weight loss slows. Weight change is not immediately related to caloric intake. An excess intake of 1,000 calories on one day does not cause a gain of half a pound on the next day. Water retention, digestive processes, and other factors cause fluctuations in weight. Athletes should weigh in only once a week, at the same time of day, preferably first thing in the morning.

Weight Gain

In order to gain weight in the form of muscle mass, a combination program of diet and exercise is essential. No hormone, vitamin, drug, or protein supplement will increase muscle mass. Muscle tissue is approximately 70 percent water and 22 percent protein; the rest consists of fat and carbohydrate. A pound of muscle tissue represents about 700 to 800 calories. To provide sufficient calories for muscle synthesis, 500 to 1,000 calories per day from a balanced diet are needed for a gain of 1 to 2 pounds a week. A high intake of protein foods is not necessary, since excess protein is broken down for energy or stored as fat. A weight-training program is essential to stimulate the growth of muscle tissue.

Diet Composition During Training

Six classes of nutrients are necessary to build and drive the human body: carbohydrates, proteins, fats, vitamins, minerals, and water. Alcohol can also be considered a nutrient since it can be used by the body for energy, but it is not essential for body functioning and can be toxic to the system.

Carbohydrates, proteins, and fats are the energy-yielding nutrients, whereas vitamins, minerals, and water regulate body processes. Through digestion in the stomach and intestines and metabolism in the liver, the energy nutrients are broken down or converted to their smaller, more usable compounds. They are then transported to the site in the body where they are needed for building, repair, energy, or energy storage (as fat or glycogen).

Carbohydrates

Carbohydrates are found in foods such as sugars, starches, and fiber. The body converts sugars and starches to glucose for energy or to glycogen for energy storage in the liver and muscle tissues. When glycogen stores are filled, excess carbohydrate is converted to fat. Glycogen stores may be increased in specific muscle tissue through a process called carbohydrate loading, which will be discussed in a later section of this chapter.

Fiber is not absorbed but is essential for gastrointestinal functioning. Low-fiber diets have been associated with several diseases, including diverticulosis, constipation, heart disease, cancer of the colon, and diabetes. Consequently, a high-fiber diet is recommended. Fiber is found in fruits, vegetables, whole-grain breads, and cereals.

While a high-carbohydrate diet is essential to good health in all individuals, it is especially important to the athlete in training who works out for 3 to 6 hours a day. Fifty to 60 percent of this athlete's caloric intake should be from carbohydrates to keep the glycogen stores filled. Carbohydrate loading, used to generate extra glycogen, requires a carbohydrate intake of 70 to 80 percent.

Proteins

Proteins are long chains of nitrogen-containing compounds called amino acids. The 22 amino acids are synthesized into structural components, enzymes, and hormones as needed, or are converted to fatty acids or glucose for energy or energy storage. The body cannot store protein; therefore, extra protein is used for energy or converted to fat.

Protein intake should be approximately 10 to 12 percent of caloric intake, or .8 gm/kg of body weight in the adult and 1.0 to 1.5 gm/kg in the adolescent. Even during intense training and buildup, protein intakes above these levels are unnecessary. Protein sources are meats, fish, poultry, eggs, dried beans, nuts, and dairy products. Animal protein sources are usually high in fat, so a high-protein diet often is a high-fat diet. Low-carbohydrate intake may be associated with this diet.

Fats

Fats in the diet that are synthesized by the body are triglycerides, fatty acids, phospholipids, and sterols. The predominate sterol is cholesterol. Cholesterol and phospholipids function as integral parts of cell membranes.

There are two types of cholesterol. **Low-density lipoprotein (LDL) cholesterol** is found in foods and is produced by the body. LDLs contribute to high circulating levels of blood cholesterol. **High-density lipoprotein (HDL) cholesterol** is produced only by the body. High blood levels of HDL cholesterol are thought to play a preventive role in heart disease.

There is still controversy about how much cholesterol and saturated fat intake should be reduced in order to reduce cholesterol levels in the general population. Since exercise increases HDL cholesterol, a protective lipid, severe reduction of cholesterol-containing foods may not be necessary unless the athlete has a family history of heart disease.

Triglycerides, the major storage form of fats, consist of a glycerol and three fatty acids (Fig. 42.1). Fatty acids are the body's alternative energy source to glucose. Fatty acids may be saturated or unsaturated, and both types contribute the same amount of calories.

High-fat intakes are associated with heart disease, cancer of the colon, breast cancer, and endometrial cancer in women. In addition, calories consumed as fat means fewer calories from carbohydrates. Therefore, 30 to 35 percent of caloric intake should come

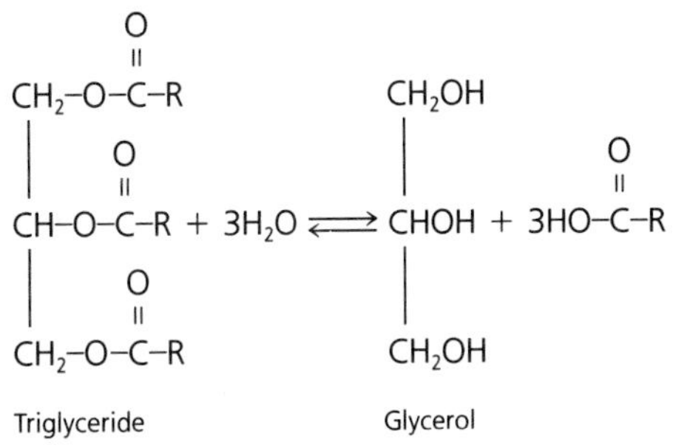

$$CH_2-O-C-R \quad\quad CH_2OH$$

Triglyceride consists of a glycerol and three fatty acids (hydrolysis reaction yielding glycerol and three fatty acids with water).

R = Aliphatic chain of various lengths and degrees of saturation.

FIGURE 42.1. Triglycerides consist of a glycerol and three fatty acids.

from fat. Meats, eggs, milk, and cheese all contain fat. Other sources are fried foods, butter, margarine, salad dressings, oils, and mayonnaise. Because of the large number of calories needed by athletes, fried foods and high-fat foods may be consumed, but only in moderation.

Recommended Servings From the Four Food Groups

Table 42.3 provides a recommended number of daily servings from the four food groups and the additional categories of vitamins, minerals, and water. The four basic food groups are (1) milk and cheese; (2) meat, poultry, fish, and eggs; (3) breads and cereals; and (4) fruits and vegetables.

Role of the Dietitian or Nutritionist

Observing athletes during training meals is one way to identify those with unusual or inadequate nutritional habits. A calorie counter and nutrient composition manual are helpful references. Seeking guidance from a dietitian or nutritionist can be especially beneficial. Those versed in sports nutrition are obviously most helpful. However, if a sports nutritionist is not available, the trainer can work with a nonsports dietitian or nutritionist to develop individual programs for athletes based on each player's sports energy requirements and eating habits.

REPLACEMENT OF FLUID DURING EXERCISE

Water

Water is the most critical element in the diet. Most of the other nutrients essential for life can function only in the presence of water. Under optimal conditions, the body can survive 60 days without food but only 10 to 18 days without water.

Under moderate environmental conditions and activity levels, the body needs approximately 2,000 ml (slightly more than 2 quarts) of water per day. Continuous sweating during prolonged exercise can

TABLE 42.3. Daily Servings from Food Groups

	Calorie Intake		
Food Group	2,800	4,300	5,500
Meats, fish, poultry, and eggs	8–10 oz	10–12 oz	16–18 oz
Low-fat milk	2 or more cups	2 or more cups	2 or more cups
Vegetables	2–4 servings*	2–4 servings	2–4 servings
Fruits and juices	4 or more servings	6 or more servings	8 or more servings
Breads, cereals, starches	10–12 servings	14–16 servings	16–18 servings
Desserts and sweets†	1–2 servings	2–3 servings	3–4 servings
Sweetened beverages	1 12 oz	4–5 12 oz	5–6 12 oz
Fats and oils	3–4 tbsp	6–8 tbsp	8–10 tbsp

*One serving is approximately ½ cup unless specified.
†Sample dessert servings: 1/8 of pie, a piece of cake 3″ × 3″, 1 cup of ice cream, 5–10 cookies.

reach a rate of 800 to 1,000 ml/hour. Under hot environmental conditions, sweating may be as great as 2,000 ml/hour. Since 1 pint of water equals 1 pound of body weight, only an athlete over 200 pounds can tolerate a continuous workout in a moderate to cold environment for 2 hours without fluid replacement. Under heated conditions, a loss of 4,000 ml is a 5 percent loss in a 160-pound athlete and a 4 percent loss in a 200-pound athlete. Both are performance and life-threatening percentages. Football players and runners can lose 8 to 10 pounds during a 2-hour workout.

Water is provided by fluids, foods (up to 90 percent of the composition of fruits and vegetables is water), and metabolic water. Metabolic water is produced when proteins, carbohydrates, and fats are broken down for energy. For every gram of glycogen stored, 3 gm of water are stored. This water is released into the body when the glycogen is broken down.

A loss of body water equaling 2 to 3 percent of body weight will begin to affect performance adversely. Loss of 4 to 5 percent of body weight results in reduced carrying capacity of the blood for nutrients, as well as reduced ability to remove heat from the body. Unless lost water is replaced, body temperature will rise, leading to heat exhaustion, heatstroke, and even death.

Sweating to make a "weigh-in" and then attempting to replace all water lost immediately prior to competition results in loss of strength and endurance and should be discouraged (see Chapter 52).

Electrolytes

The major electrolytes lost in sweat are sodium, chloride, potassium, calcium, and magnesium. Small amounts of iron and copper, as well as nitrogen and some water-soluble vitamins, are also lost. Sodium and chloride account for the greatest percentage of nutrients lost through sweat.

The body's own feedback mechanisms of decreasing electrolyte loss in the urine during periods of strenuous exercise partially compensate for losses. Research shows that an adequate diet prior to and during training, with salt allowed as desired, provides adequate electrolytes. Intake of citrus juices, fruits, and vegetables as potassium sources should be encouraged.

Athletes with hypertension or a strong potential for hypertension should have their blood pressures monitored. A mild sodium restriction (4 gm) may be indicated. Treatment should be individualized, based on blood pressures, eating habits, and sweat losses.

Electrolyte replacement during exercise is of little value. Electrolyte concentrations in the body actually increase due to the loss of body water. Even during prolonged, strenuous exercise such as marathon running, water, in combination with a balanced diet, maintains electrolyte balance. Electrolyte imbalances can occur after 4 to 7 days of hard training with inadequate food intake.

Sugar

Small amounts of glucose taken during prolonged exercise help spare glycogen and thus can increase the amount of energy available. However, high concentrations of glucose adversely affect water absorption by slowing the gastric emptying rate. High-glucose concentration formulas (10 percent or higher) are only recommended for exercising in a cold environment where sweat losses are not great. For exercising in a hot environment, fluid replacement takes precedence over glucose replacement. Glucose content of formulas should not exceed 2 to 3 percent. Glucose polymers (combinations of two or more glucose molecules) may be used at percentages of up to 5 percent without delaying gastric emptying.

Guidelines for Fluid Replacement

The following guidelines ensure adequate fluid replacement and thus lead to optimal performance.

- Drink small volumes of water frequently rather than large volumes infrequently—for example, 6 to 8 ounces every 15 minutes.
- Drink cold beverages (refrigerator temperature) to reduce core temperature.
- Have fluids accessible, since the thirst mechanism does not function adequately when large volumes of water are lost. Athletes will not seek out water if it is far away. In many cases, they need to be reminded to drink.
- After workout, replenish fluids at the rate of 1 pint for every pound lost. Weight should be back to normal prior to the next workout. Minimal body fat is lost during a workout, so weight after an event compared to weight immediately prior to an event is a good indication of total body water lost.
- Water is the ideal fluid replacement, although commercially prepared glucose, electrolyte solutions, juices, and other beverages may be used. Consider taste preferences of athletes, since whether they like a substance will govern how much they drink. The following guidelines are recommended:

  1. Glucose content of less than 2.5 gm/100 ml of water, or 25 gm/quart. This is equal to 1½ rounded tablespoons of sugar per quart.
  2. Few or no electrolytes. If included, they should be limited to a maximum of .2 gm of sodium chloride and .2 gm of potassium per quart.
  3. Juices diluted with five parts water, and sweetened sodas diluted with three parts water to reduce the glucose concentration to 2.5 percent. These could be adjusted to taste.
  4. Glucose and electrolyte solutions diluted as needed; most will need some dilution. Read product labels carefully.

- Encourage athletes to hydrate properly prior to prolonged exercise in a hot environment. Intake should be approximately 16 ounces of cold beverage, 15 to 30 minutes prior to workout. With experience, larger amounts (up to 2 pints) may be tolerated.

VITAMINS AND MINERALS

The Need for Supplementation

The Food and Nutrition Board of the National Research Council states that, even though athletic activity increases energy expenditure, the larger quantities of food consumed, if chosen wisely, meet increased needs for any essential nutrients. Some athletes always have and always will believe supplements are the key to improved performance. Currently, there is little scientific basis for any vitamin or mineral supplement above and beyond normal needs. Simply the belief that a supplement will improve performance can give the athlete increased confidence, and thereby a "mental edge." Therefore, although trainers should not encourage vitamin and mineral supplements, they may not wish to mandate their restriction unless the dosages are potentially harmful. Trainers should explain the facts to their athletes, however, as well as detail the costs and potential dangers of megadose supplementation. What should be stressed is that correct selection of food can more directly affect performance than taking supplements.

Vitamins

The standard charts used for the recommended dietary allowances of vitamins are difficult to use with an athlete whose weight and intake may be 50 percent higher than that of the reference person. Table 42.4 gives the nutrient allowances per 1,000 calories derived from the recommendations of the Food and Nutrition Council of the National Research Council. Table 42.5 lists the vitamins and their functions, sources, and toxicity.

TABLE 42.4. Nutrient Allowances per 1,000 kcal Derived from the 1989 Recommended Dietary Allowances

Age and Sex Group	Energy	Protein	Fat-Soluble Vitamins			Water-Soluble Vitamins			
			Vitamin A	Vitamin D	Vitamin E	Ascorbic Acid	Thiamin	Ribo-flavin	Niacin
	kcal	gm	μgRE	μg	mgαTE	mg			mgNE
Children									
1–3 yr	1,300	16	400	10	6	40	0.7	0.8	9
4–6 yr	1,800	24	500	10	7	45	0.9	1.1	12
7–10 yr	2,000	28	700	10	7	45	1.0	1.2	13
Males									
11–14 yr	2,500	45	1,000	10	10	50	1.3	1.5	17
15–18 yr	3,100	59	1,000	10	10	60	1.5	1.8	20
19–24 yr	2,900	58	1,000	10	10	60	1.5	1.7	19
25–50 yr	2,900	63	1,000	5	10	60	1.5	1.7	19
51 + yr	2,300	63	1,000	5	10	60	1.2	1.4	15
Females									
11–14 yr	2,200	46	800	10	8	50	1.1	1.3	15
15–18 yr	2,200	44	800	10	8	60	1.1	1.3	15
19–24 yr	2,200	46	800	10	8	60	1.1	1.3	15
25–50 yr	2,200	50	800	5	8	60	1.1	1.3	15
51 + yr	1,900	50	800	5	8	60	1.0	1.2	13

Water-Soluble Vitamins

Vitamins are either water soluble or fat soluble. The water-soluble vitamins include all of the B complex vitamins as well as vitamin C. Because these vitamins are not stored in large amounts in the body, megadoses do not increase body stores. Many of the B vitamins are used in energy metabolism, so that needs increase as more calories are burned. As long as appropriate foods are chosen, B vitamin intake increases in proportion to need. In a recent study of food intakes of university athletes participating on various sports teams, researchers found B vitamin intake to be adequate without supplementation.

Megadoses of B complex vitamins, except for niacin, do not appear to be toxic. High doses of niacin cause decreased use of free fatty acids and therefore increase fatigue. In addition, niacin supplements in the form of nicotinic acid cause tingling sensations, flushed skin, and liver damage. Megadoses of B vitamins have not been shown to improve performance. Vitamin B_{12} shots have no effect on performance.

Controversy still surrounds the need for vitamin C supplementation. The increased stress caused by exercise indicates an increased need for vitamin C. Some respected investigators in the field of physical performance have recommended intakes of 200 to 300 mg, levels easily achieved through appropriate food selection.

While megadoses of vitamin C are not harmful, the body does adapt to high levels. As the level of vitamin C supplement increases, the percentage absorbed decreases. If the athlete stops the supplement suddenly, a deficiency can occur. Trainers should discourage megadoses of 500 mg and wean athletes off high doses slowly.

Fat-Soluble Vitamins

The fat-soluble vitamins, A, D, E, and K, are stored in the body, especially in the

TABLE 42.4.   (continued)

| Water-Soluble Vitamins | | | Minerals | | | | | |
Vitamin B$_6$	Folacin	Vitamin B$_{12}$	Calcium	Phosphorus	Magnesium	Iron	Zinc	Iodine
mg	μg		mg					μg
1.0	50	0.7	800	800	80	10	10	70
1.1	75	1.0	800	800	120	10	10	90
1.4	100	1.4	800	800	170	10	10	120
1.7	150	2.0	1,200	1,200	270	12	15	150
2.0	200	2.0	1,200	1,200	400	12	15	150
2.0	200	2.0	1,200	1,200	350	10	15	150
2.0	200	2.0	800	800	350	10	15	150
2.0	200	2.0	800	800	350	10	15	150
1.4	150	2.0	1,200	1,200	280	15	12	150
1.5	180	2.0	1,200	1,200	300	15	12	150
1.6	180	2.0	1,200	1,200	280	15	12	150
1.6	180	2.0	800	800	280	15	12	150
1.6	180	2.0	800	800	280	10	12	150

Source: Adapted from *Recommended Dietary Allowances,* © 1989 by the National Academy of Sciences, National Academy Press, Washington, D.C.

liver. Excessive intakes through megadoses over long periods of time lead to toxic symptoms and, in the case of vitamin A, death. Megadoses of vitamin E appear to be nontoxic but are not recommended.

Athletes often take vitamin E supplements. Through its role as an antioxidant, vitamin E could increase oxygen and fatty acid supply and thus endurance. However, studies have not shown improved performance with vitamin E supplements.

Nonvitamins

Periodically, new "vitamins" are promoted to athletes. These substances are not truly vitamins. A vitamin is an organic compound essential to life and is involved in many specific interactions in the body. To be essential to life, a compound must be in the normal food supply of the population. Otherwise, the population would have ceased to exist or would have adapted to life without the "vitamin," in which case it would no longer be essential.

Pangamic acid is erroneously labeled vitamin B$_{15}$. This substrate is derived from apricot pits and is supposedly a mixture of dichloroacetate and dimethylglycine. It is not an essential nutrient and therefore should not be considered a vitamin.

Minerals

Minerals are grouped into two classes: major and trace. The major minerals are those needed in amounts greater than 100 mg/day. Trace minerals are those needed in very small amounts. Table 42.6 lists minerals, their sources, functions, and toxicity.

Excessive intakes of major minerals are generally nontoxic but are not recommended. Increased intake of most minerals cannot be justified as long as the diet is balanced. One possible exception is iron, as iron needs in menstruating females may

TABLE 42.5. Vitamin Sources and Functions

Fat-Soluble Vitamins

Nomenclature	Important Sources	Physiology and Functions

Vitamin A
  Retinol
  Retinal
  Retinyl ester
  Retinoic acid
  Provitamin A
    Alpha-, beta-, gamma-
    carotene, cryptoxanthin
	Animal
	  Fish-liver oils
	  Liver
	  Butter, cream
	  Whole milk
	  Whole-milk cheeses
	  Egg yolk
	Plant
	  Dark-green leafy vegetables
	  Yellow vegetables
	  Yellow fruits
	  Fortified margarines
		Bile necessary for absorption
		Stored in liver
		Maintains integrity of mucosal epithelium, maintains visual acuity in dim light
		Large amounts are toxic

Vitamin D
  Vitamin D_2
    Ergocalciferol
  Vitamin D_3
    Cholecalciferol
  Antirachitic factor
	Fish-liver oils
	Fortified milk
	Activated sterols
	Exposure to sunlight
	Very small amounts in butter, liver, egg yolk, salmon, sardines
		Synthesized in skin by activity of ultraviolet light
		Liver synthesizes $25(OH)D_3$
		Kidney synthesizes $1,25(OH)_2D_3$
		Functions as steroid hormone to regulate calcium and phosphorus absorption, mobilization and mineralization of bone
		Large amounts are toxic

Vitamin E
  Alpha-, beta-, gamma-
  tocopherol
  Antisterility vitamin
	Plant tissues—vegetable oils; wheat germ, rice germ; green leafy vegetables; nuts; legumes
	Animal foods are poor sources
		Not stored in body to any extent
		Related to action of selenium
		Humans: reduces oxidation of vitamin A, carotenes, and polyunsaturated fatty acids
		Animals: normal reproduction; utilization of sex hormones, cholesterol

Vitamin K
  Phylloquinone (K_1)
  Menaquinone
  Menadione
	Green leaves such as alfalfa, spinach, cabbage
	Liver
	Synthesis in intestine
		Bile necessary for absorption
		Formation of prothrombin and other clotting proteins
		Sulfa drugs and antibiotics interfere with absorption
		Large amounts are toxic

Water-Soluble Vitamins

Ascorbic acid Vitamin C	Citrus fruits; tomatoes; melons; cabbage; broccoli; strawberries; fresh potatoes; green leafy vegetables	Very little storage in body Formation of intercellular cement substance; synthesis of collagen Absorption and use of iron Prevents oxidation of folacin
Thiamin Vitamin B_1	Whole-grain and enriched breads, cereals, flours; organ meats, pork; other meats, poultry, fish; legumes, nuts; milk; green vegetables	Limited body storage Chiefly involved in carbohydrate metabolism

TABLE 42.5.   (continued)

	Water-Soluble Vitamins (continued)	
Nomenclature	Important Sources	Physiology and Functions
Riboflavin 　Vitamin B₂	Milk; organ meats; eggs; green leafy vegetables	Limited body stores, but reserves retained carefully; involved in energy metabolism
Niacin 　Nicotinic acid 　Nicotinamide	Meat, poultry, fish; whole-grain and enriched breads, flours, cereals; nuts, legumes Tryptophan as a precursor	Coenzyme for glycolysis, fat synthesis, tissue respiration
Vitamin B₆ 　Three active forms 　pyridoxine, pyridoxal, 　pyridoxamine	Meat, poultry, fish; potatoes, sweet potatoes, vegetables	Involved in protein metabolism; conversion of tryptophan to niacin; conversion of glycogen to glucose; requirement related to protein intake
Pantothenic acid	Meat, poultry, fish; whole-grain cereals; legumes Smaller amounts in fruits, vegetables, milk	Involved in energy metabolism
Biotin	Organ meats, egg yolk, nuts, legumes	Avidin, a protein in raw egg white, blocks absorption; large amounts must be eaten; involved in energy metabolism
Vitamin B₁₂ 　Cyanocobalamin 　Hydroxycobalamin	In animal foods only: organ meats, muscle meats, fish, poultry; eggs; milk	Requires intrinsic factor for absorption; involved in energy and cell synthesis; synthesis of DNA and RNA; formation of mature red blood cells
Folacin 　Folic acid 　Tetrahydrofolic acid	Organ meats, deep green leafy vegetables; muscle meats, poultry, fish, eggs; whole-grain cereals	Active form is folinic acid; requires ascorbic acid for conversion; synthesis of nucleoproteins, maturation of red blood cells; interrelated with vitamin B₁₂
Choline	Egg yolk, meat, poultry, fish, milk, whole grains	Probably not a true vitamin; involved in cell synthesis
Lipoic acid 　Thioetic acid 　Protogen		Probably not a true vitamin; involved in energy metabolism

Source: Reprinted with permission of Macmillan Publishing Company from *Normal and Therapeutic Nutrition,* 17th ed. by Corinne H. Robinson, Marilyn R. Lawler, Wanda L. Chenoweth, and Ann E. Garwick. Copyright © 1986 by Macmillan Publishing Company.

TABLE 42.6. Minerals: Sources and Functions

Nomenclature	Physiology and Functions	Important Sources
Calcium	Hardness of bones, teeth Transmission of nerve impulse Muscle contraction Normal heart rhythm Activate enzymes Increase cell permeability Catalyze thrombin formation	Milk, hard cheese Ice cream, cottage cheese Greens: turnip, collards, kale, mustard, broccoli Oysters, shrimp, salmon, clams
Chlorine	Chief anion of extracellular fluid Constituent of gastric juice Acid-base balance; chloride-bicarbonate shift in red cells	Table salt
Chromium	Efficient use of insulin in glucose uptake; glucose oxidation, protein synthesis, stimulation of fat, and cholesterol synthesis Activation of enzymes	Liver, meat Cheese Whole-grain cereals
Copper	Aid absorption and use of iron in synthesis of hemoglobin Electron transport Melanin formation Myelin sheath of nerves Purine metabolism	Liver, shellfish Meats Nuts, legumes Whole-grain cereals Typical diet provides 1 to 5 mg
Fluorine	Increases resistance of teeth to decay; most effective in young children Moderate levels in bone may reduce osteoporosis	Fluoridated water: 1 ppm
Iodine	Constituent of diiodotyrosine, triidothyronine, thyroxine; regulate rate of energy metabolism	Iodized salt is most reliable source Seafood Foods grown in nongoitrous coastal areas
Iron	Constituent of hemoglobin, myoglobin, and oxidative enzymes: catalase, cytochrome, xanthine oxidase	Liver, organ meats Meat, poultry Egg yolk Enriched and whole-grain breads, cereals Dark-green vegetables Legumes Molasses, dark Peaches, apricots, prunes, raisins Diets supply about 6 mg per 1,000 kcal
Magnesium	Constituents of bones, teeth Activates enzymes in carbohydrate metabolism Muscle and nerve irritability	Whole-grain cereals Nuts; legumes Meat Milk Green leafy vegetables

TABLE 42.6.   (continued)

Nomenclature	Physiology and Functions	Important Sources
Manganese	Activation of many enzymes; oxidation of carbohydrates, urea formation, protein hydrolysis Bone formation	Legumes, nuts Whole-grain cereals
Molybdenum	Cofactor for flavorprotein enzymes; present in xanthine oxidase	Organ meats Legumes Whole-grain cereals
Phosphorus	Structure of bones, teeth Cell permeability Metabolism of fats and carbohydrates; storage and release of ATP Sugar-phosphate linkage in DNA and RNA Phospholipids in transport of fats Butter salts in acid-base balance	Milk; cheese Eggs, meat, fish, poultry Legumes, nuts Whole-grain cereals
Potassium	Principal cation of intracellular fluid Osmotic pressure; water balance; acid-base balance Nerve irritability and muscle contraction, regular heart rhythm Synthesis of protein	Widely distributed in foods Meat, fish, fowl Cereals Fruits, vegetables
Selenium	Antioxidant Constitute of glutathione oxidase	Meat and seafoods Cereal foods
Sodium	Principal cation of extracellular fluid Osmotic pressure; water balance Acid-base balance Regulate nerve irritability and muscle contraction "Pump" for active transport such as for glucose	Table salt Processed foods Milk Meat, fish, poultry
Sulfur	Constituent of proteins, especially cartilage, hair, nails Constituent of melanin, glutathione, thiamin, biotin, coenzyme A, insulin High-energy sulfur bonds Detoxication reactions	Protein foods rich in sulfur-amino acids Eggs Meat, fish, poultry Milk, cheese Nuts
Zinc	Constituent of enzymes: carbonic anhydrase, carboxypeptidase, lactic dehydrogenase	Seafoods Liver and other organ meats Meat, fish Wheat germ Yeast Plant foods are generally low Usual diet supplies 10 to 15 mg

Source: Reprinted with permission of Macmillan Publishing Company from *Normal and Therapeutic Nutrition,* 17th ed. by Corinne H. Robinson, Marilyn R. Lawler, Wanda L. Chenoweth, and Ann E. Garwick. Copyright © 1986 by Macmillan Publishing Company.

exceed dietary supplies, necessitating supplementation.

Calcium and Phosphorus

Diets high in phosphorus (meat and soft drinks) and low in calcium (milk and dairy products) may cause a calcium-phosphorus imbalance (normal ratio 1:1), resulting in calcium being lost from the bones. For this condition to occur, however, very large amounts of food high in phosphorus or large amounts of artificial phosphorus sources must be consumed.

Sodium and Potassium

The need for sodium and potassium was discussed earlier. Salt tablets are not recommended because processed foods and table salt provide more than an adequate amount of sodium. Potassium depletion can occur in athletes with large sweat losses, and therefore, those athletes should be advised to include ample potassium-rich foods in their diet (bananas, orange juice, cereals).

Iron

Iron deficiency is one of the few mineral deficiencies found, mostly in women. Iron deficiency may seriously limit athletic performance, as iron is needed for hemoglobin and oxygen transport. It is also the mineral needed to form several other oxidating enzymes necessary for energy production. An intake of over 2,500 calories is needed to ensure adequate iron intake. The consumption of meat enhances the absorption of the iron found in grains and vegetables. Vitamin C enhances the absorption of iron in all foods. Athletes, especially menstruating women, with low calorie intakes may require iron supplements. Ferrous gluconate is usually best tolerated, but its prescription and dosage should be done by a physician. Excess iron can be highly toxic.

Other Minerals

The physiologic roles and daily required amounts of the other trace minerals are presently under study. However, megadoses are not recommended due to the potential for toxicity.

Absolute Dietary Requirements

The compounds the body actually requires are few. These include 8 to 10 of the 22 amino acids; glucose; 1 fatty acid, linoleic acid; approximately 20 minerals; 16 vitamins; and water. Theoretically, a body could thrive on only this handful of essential ingredients. However, the balance of chemical reactions is such that, if the correct amount and proportions are not available when needed, a deficiency or inefficiency can occur. For this reason, it is far more practical and logical to maintain health through a balanced diet than to try to outwit nature by depending on essential elements alone. In addition, since the nutrients are interdependent and the sources varied, there is obviously no advantage to any fad diet that is unbalanced.

EATING BEFORE AND DURING EVENTS

Carbohydrate Loading

In endurance competitions requiring high levels of energy over a prolonged time, maximizing the storage of glycogen in the muscle can improve performance. **Carbohydrate loading**, in combination with depletion exercise, can increase these stores. Most likely to benefit from a carbohydrate-loading program are long-distance runners, swimmers, bicyclists, and cross-country skiers. Carbohydrate loading may also benefit athletes involved in sports that require prolonged movement of varying intensities such as soccer, lacrosse, and ice hockey, as well as tournament sports such as tennis and handball.

On the day prior to going on a carbohydrate-loading diet, the athlete exercises to exhaustion to deplete glycogen stores. The workout must be identical to the competitive event in order for the appropriate muscles and muscle fibers to become depleted.

TABLE 42.7. Carbohydrate-Loading Methods

Method A		Method B	
1st day	Depletion exercise	1st day	Depletion exercise
2nd day	High-carbohydrate diet; little or no exercise	2nd day	High-carbohydrate diet; regular exercise
3rd day	High-carbohydrate diet; little or no exercise	3rd day	High-carbohydrate diet; regular exercise
4th day	High-carbohydrate diet; little or no exercise	4th day	High-carbohydrate diet; regular exercise
5th day	Competition	5th day	High-carbohydrate diet; little or no exercise
		6th day	High-carbohydrate diet; little or no exercise
		7th day	High-carbohydrate diet; little or no exercise
		8th day	Competition

Source: Adapted by special permission from Melvin Williams, *Nutrition for Fitness and Sport.* Dubuque, Iowa: Wm. C. Brown, p. 35.

For example, the athlete who is bicycling should bicycle to exhaustion. The athlete who is involved in soccer or lacrosse should do interval training, alternating between high- and low-intensity running.

Two methods of carbohydrate loading are shown in Table 42.7; both have been used successfully. The athlete's schedule and tolerances should determine which one to use.

During carbohydrate loading, the athlete's weight should increase 1 to 3 pounds, since water is stored with glycogen. During the 3 days prior to the event, 70 to 80 percent of the calories should come from carbohydrate, 10 to 15 percent from fat, and 10 to 15 percent from protein. Table 42.8 lists the number of servings which should be eaten of each nutrient.

TABLE 42.8. Carbohydrate Loading: Intake Three Days Prior to Competition

Food Groups	2,800 kcal	4,300 kcal	5,500 kcal
*Low-fat meats, fish, poultry; occasional eggs	6 oz 330 kcal	8 oz 440 kcal	12 oz 660 kcal
Milk, skim or low-fat	2 cups 220 kcal	2 cups 220 kcal	2 cups 220 kcal
Breads and cereals	10–14 servings 980 kcal	14–18 servings 1,260 kcal	18–22 servings 1,540 kcal
Vegetables	2–4 servings 100 kcal	2–4 servings 100 kcal	4–6 servings 100 kcal
Fruits and fruit juices	3–4 servings 240 kcal	5–6 servings 360 kcal	7–8 servings 480 kcal
Fats and oils	1–2 tbsp 135 kcal	1–2 tbsp 135 kcal	2–4 tbsp 270 kcal
Desserts and sweets	1–2 servings 470 kcal[†]	3–5 servings 1,200 kcal	4–6 servings 1,500 kcal
Beverages, sweetened	2–12 oz 320 kcal	4–12 oz 640 kcal	6–12 oz 960 kcal

*Chuck roasts, round steak, ground round, any cut of veal. If higher fat meats are desired (sirloin, rib eye, etc.), omit added gravies, fats, and oils.

[†] For 3,000 calories and less, avoid high-fat desserts such as pies, pastries, and doughnuts.

TABLE 42.9. Carbohydrate-Loading Menus

2,800 kcal	5,500 kcal
1 cup orange juice	2 cups orange juice
2 cups cereal	8 large pancakes with syrup
2 slices toast	1 cup milk, low-fat
2 tsp jelly	
1 cup milk, low-fat	
Turkey hoagie	2 turkey sandwiches with
Large peach	lettuce and tomato
2 cupcakes	2 large apples
Iced tea	Large slice of cake
	12 oz soda
2 cups spaghetti with 1 cup	6 oz roast beef
meat sauce	Large baked potato
1½ cups green beans	4 slices bread
1 tsp margarine	1½ cups broccoli
½ cup applesauce	1 cup fruit cocktail
	2 tsp margarine
	3 tsp jelly
	Large slice of pie
20 cookies	1 tuna sandwich
1 cup milk	20 cookies
	1 cup milk
2 12 oz sodas during day	6 12 oz sodas during day

TABLE 42.10. Sample Pre-Event Menus

Orange juice	Orange juice
Cereal with low-fat milk	Pancakes with syrup
Toast with butter and jelly	Toast with margarine and jelly
Beverage of choice	Beverage of choice
Grapefruit juice	Fruit cup
Spaghetti with meat sauce	Beef chow mein
Tossed salad with dressing	Shrimp fried rice
Italian bread with margarine	Stir-fried vegetables
Fruit cup	Sherbet
Beverage of choice	Beverage of choice

Since the carbohydrate-loading diet is necessarily low in fat, most high-fat meats, breads, desserts, and visible fats are to be avoided. The athlete may be permitted limited amounts of butter, margarine, and gravy; high-fat meats like steak; and eggs as demonstrated in the sample menus that are presented in Table 42.9.

The original carbohydrate-loading program had a carbohydrate-deficient diet inserted between the exercise and the carbohydrate loading. Research showed that very low carbohydrate intake followed by high-carbohydrate intake was not necessary. A high-carbohydrate diet alone was found to offer similar benefits.

Pre-Event Meal

The food eaten immediately before an athletic event does not generally benefit performance. As explained in the preceding nutritional section, preparation for endurance activities must begin several days in advance. High intakes of protein foods such as steak and eggs do not give the athlete extra energy; nor do they prevent muscle injury. In fact, high-protein, high-fat foods cause increased stress on the kidneys and take a long time to digest. A pre-event meal rich in carbohydrates is best. The following are general guidelines for eating prior to a competitive event:

- Plan a meal consisting of high-carbohydrate, low-fat, and protein foods (Table 42.10), either in solid form or in a liquid formula.
- Take solid food 3 to 4 hours prior to an event.
- Take liquid meals 2 to 3 hours prior to an event. They should be low in fat and high in carbohydrate, with some vitamins and minerals added. Some examples of liquid meals are Nutrament, Sustacal, and Instant Breakfast.
- Select easily digestible foods. Avoid fried foods and foods known to cause flatulence, which varies with the individual.
- Do not ingest foods and beverages high in sugar within 1 hour of the start of competition. Sugars taken at the start of a game stimulate insulin production and therefore actually

cause an accelerated use of glycogen supplies.

■ Take adequate fluids to ensure hydration. Unsweetened beverages may be taken within 15 to 30 minutes of competition.

Eating During an Event

The primary dietary concern during an event is to replenish lost fluids. Glucose feedings during athletic events of long duration of moderate to high intensity may help prevent hypoglycemia and spare glycogen stores. Marathon running, cross-country skiing, and soccer are examples of activities in which performance might benefit from replacement of fluids and glucose.

In general, a glucose solution of 2 to 3 percent is recommended to supplement normal fluid replacement. (For more specific recommendations, review the discussion on fluid replacement.)

IMPACT OF FOOD ON MEDICATIONS

Drug absorption is affected by gastrointestinal function, the relative lipophilic/hydrophilic character of the drug, gastrointestinal pH, and the drug product dissolution rate. In general, drugs are absorbed more slowly when taken with a meal because food delays gastric emptying.

In most cases, food intake does not reduce the quantity of the drug absorbed. It does affect the length of time it takes for the drug to reach peak levels. This factor is not clinically significant if the drug is used on a continual basis. However, the delay is undesirable in the following situations:

■ When rapid effect is needed to relieve acute symptoms.
■ When the delay precludes the achievement of effective plasma and tissue concentrations of drugs rapidly metabolized and excreted.
■ When drugs are inactivated in the stomach.

TABLE 42.11.   Drugs Taken with Meals

Acetylsalicylic (Aspirin)	Ketoprofen (Orudis)
Diclofenac (Voltaren)	Meclofenamate sodium (Meclomen)
Diflunisal (Dolobid)	Naproxen (Naprosyn, Anaprox)
Fenoprofen (Nalfon)	Phenylbutazone (Butazolidin)
Flurbiprofen (Ansaid)	Piroxicam (Feldene)
Ibuprofen (Motrin)	Sulindac (Clinoril)
Indomethacin (Indocin)	Tolmetin (Tolectin)

TABLE 42.12.   Drugs Taken 1 Hour before or 2 Hours after Meals

Ampicillin	Lincomycin
Erythromycin	Cephalosporins
Penicillin	Tetracycline
Enteric-coated medications	

Some drugs are recommended to be taken with food because they irritate the gastrointestinal tract. Most nonsteroidal anti-inflammatory drugs fall into this category (Table 42.11).

When food is ingested, the pH of the stomach decreases. This increased acidity may increase the destruction of antibiotics and therefore decrease the amount of active drug. Therefore, drugs like ampicillin, erythromycin, and penicillin should be taken 1 hour before meals or 2 hours after meals (Table 42.12). Because of the effect of acidity on these drugs, they should not be taken with citric juices.

The drug tetracycline is affected by iron and calcium, which bind with the drug to form a nonabsorbable complex. Therefore, tetracycline should be taken before meals and not at the same time as an iron or calcium supplement or milk and milk products.

TABLE 42.13. Caffeine Content of Beverages

Beverage	Caffeine (mg/100 ml)	mg/8 oz
Carbonated		
Coca-Cola*	18	45
Dr. Pepper*	17	43
Mountain Dew*	15	38
Diet Dr. Pepper*	15	38
Tab	13	33
Pepsi-Cola*	12	30
RC Cola*	9	23
Diet RC*	9	23
Diet Rite*	9	23
Fanta Root Beer†	0	0
Coffee		
Instant*	44	110
Percolated*	73	183
Dripolated*	97	243
Coffee: decaffeinated		
Infused‡	1–3	8–24
Instant‡	0.50–1.50	4–12
Decaf†	0.90	7.2
Nescafe†	3–6	36–47
Sanka	2	15
Tea, bagged		
Black, 5 min brew*	33	83
Black, 1 min brew*	20	50
Tea, loose		
Black, 5 min brew*	29	73
Green, 5 min brew*	25	63
Green, Japan, 5 min brew*	15	38
Cocoa; chocolate*	6	15
Ovaltine‡	0	

*Bunker, M. L., McWilliams, M. "Caffeine Content of Common Beverages." *Journal of the American Dietetic Association* 74(1979):28.
†Nutritional analysis data supplied by the manufacturer.
‡Nagy, M. "Caffeine Content of Beverages and Chocolate." *Journal of the American Medical Association* 229(1974):337.
Source: Adapted from "Caffeine Content of Beverages." *Handbook of Clinical Dietetics,* by the American Dietetic Association (New Haven: Yale University Press), p. 149. Reprinted by permission.

Products that irritate the stomach are sometimes coated with an acid-resistant, base-susceptible "enteric coating" developed to pass through the stomach and dissolve in the intestine. Foods that increase the pH of the stomach, such as milk, may dissolve the coating while the drugs are still in the stomach. Aspirin and erythromycin are sometimes coated and should never be taken with milk.

In general, medication should always be taken with a glass of water and not immediately before bed to avoid possible irritation or ulceration of the esophagus. This advice is particularly important with those known ulcerogenic drugs such as analgesics, tetracycline, and nonsteroidal anti-inflammatory drugs. The pharmacist or physician should be consulted about how to take a medication. In addition, when any medication is prescribed, it is always a good practice to inquire about its interaction with foods (see Chapter 58).

CAFFEINE

Caffeine stimulates the central nervous system as well as the heart. Intakes of 50 to 200 mg of caffeine will cause alertness, while excessive intakes of 300 to 500 mg can cause nervousness, muscular tremors, and heart palpitations. To put these amounts into perspective, an 8-ounce cup of instant coffee has 110 mg of caffeine and an 8-ounce drink of Coca-Cola has 45 mg of caffeine. With habitual intake, the body adapts to higher levels of caffeine.

Caffeine also stimulates the release of adrenaline and causes a rise in the amount of free fatty acids in the blood. Because of this increased availability of free fatty acids, caffeine may affect performance. Most research shows that caffeine has no effect on performance in events lasting under 1 hour. However, for events lasting over 2 hours, caffeine may increase energy available from fats and thus spare glycogen. Some studies show conflicting findings. Caffeine may be beneficial only in some people. More research is needed in this area.

The amount of caffeine needed to produce the rise in free fatty acids is low—200 to 300 mg, or the equivalent of two cups of brewed coffee (Table 42.13). If the athlete believes that caffeine improves his or her performance, it can be allowed and should be taken 1 hour prior to exercise. However, note that caffeine has been classified as a drug by the International Olympic Committee, and urinary levels of caffeine must not exceed 12 mg/ml.

Aside from acting as a stimulant, caffeine acts as a diuretic. It may decrease body water prior to an event and thus adversely affect performance capacity. This adverse effect should be weighed against potential benefits.

ANOREXIA AND BULIMIA

Anorexia nervosa and bulimia are two nutritional disorders of which the athletic trainer should be aware. An estimated 10 percent of all teenagers and young adult females have either bulimia or anorexia nervosa.

Anorexia Nervosa

Anorexia nervosa is a disorder of severe weight loss. A person with this disorder begins dieting sensibly, often in reaction to a stressful life event, but then loses sight of a realistic weight goal. To be as thin as possible becomes an obsession, and the person loses all concept of a normal body image despite significant weight loss. Caloric input and output become a preoccupation. The fear of losing control and gaining weight is such a concern that these people often exercise constantly in an effort to "burn up" any calories consumed that day.

Anorexia is primarily found in young women. It is frequently associated with menstrual disorders (amenorrhea or oligomenorrhea). Young men may also be affected, but less so than women (approximately a 9:1 ratio). Anorexia is a serious disorder. Psychological counseling may be necessary because anorexics can die from self-starvation. Athletes most susceptible to this disorder are those involved in activities in which low body weight and small size are advantageous—gymnasts, dancers, wrestlers, jockeys, long-distance runners, divers, lightweight boxers, and coxswains in crew.

The following signs are indicators that an athlete might be anorexic:

- The athlete feels obese, even as weight decreases.
- The athlete has an altered body image.
- The athlete experiences more than a 25 percent weight loss.
- The athlete has no desire to keep body weight over the minimum for her age and height.
- There is no physical disorder to cause such weight loss.
- The athlete is depressed.

Bulimia

Bulimia is a disorder involving a more normal weight, but the person uses vomiting, diuretics, or laxatives to prevent weight gain. The person may eat an inordinate amount of food in a binge once or twice a week or as frequently as 20 times a day. Vomiting often becomes addictive and uncontrollable.

Most bulimics are perfectionists and overachievers. The bulimic athlete often displays this behavior in practice or competition. Whereas the anorexic may become withdrawn, the bulimic has an intense desire to please everyone. Therefore, the coach and athletic trainer may be extremely influential in working with the bulimic athlete.

Hypokalemia (potassium deficiency) resulting from chronic vomiting or laxative/diuretic abuse is a major concern for bulimic individuals. Potassium is necessary for adequate muscle functioning, and a deficiency is often marked by muscle fatigue, weakness, erratic heartbeat, and kidney damage. Potassium loss aggravates dehydration and electrolyte imbalances.

The stomach normally secretes acid in response to food as it initiates digestion. Chronic vomiting causes this acid to irritate the esophagus, teeth, and mouth, resulting in ulcers, esophageal varices (dilated veins in the esophagus that can rupture and cause death), destruction of tooth enamel, and sores in the mucous membranes of the mouth. Other concerns include hiatal hernias and rupture of the esophagus.

The following signs are indicators that an athlete might be bulimic:

- The athlete engages in binge eating repeatedly.
- During a binge, the athlete eats inconspicuously.
- The athlete ends a binge with the onset of abdominal pain, sleep, self-induced vomiting, or use of laxatives.
- The athlete attempts severely restrictive diets to lose weight.
- The athlete's weight varies more than 10 pounds due to binges and fasts.
- The athlete realizes that her eating pattern is abnormal and that she is not able to stop it voluntarily.
- The athlete experiences depression after eating binges.

- There is no physical disorder to account for the weight loss.
- The behavior is not anorexic.

The Trainer's Role

Medical treatment is imperative for both the bulimic and the anorexic. The trainer can help by ensuring that the coach is not setting unrealistic weight goals for the athletes and by helping the athlete determine an ideal body weight and fat content. The trainer may also help diagnose nutritional problems and encourage the athlete to seek help from psychologists, psychiatrists, or nutritionists experienced in working with eating disorders. See page 646 for a list of support organizations for eating disorders.

IMPORTANT CONCEPTS

1. Diets must be individualized, taking into consideration the age, sex, physical condition, and metabolic rate of each player.
2. The focus of weight control should be on body composition rather than weight.
3. Weight loss is best accomplished by reducing daily intake by 500 to 1,000 calories, producing a loss of 1 to 2 pounds per week.
4. The six classes of nutrients are carbohydrates, proteins, fats, vitamins, minerals, and water.
5. Water is the ideal fluid replacement for sweat lost during prolonged exercise.
6. The athlete's vitamin and mineral needs can usually be met by a carefully chosen diet; supplementation is rarely needed.
7. Carbohydrate loading, in combination with depletion exercise, increases the storage of glycogen in the muscles and improves performance.
8. The impact of food intake on medications is such that the quantity of the drug absorbed is not reduced, but the length of time for the drug to reach peak levels often is affected.
9. Caffeine stimulates the central nervous system and the heart and increases the amount of free fatty acids in the blood.
10. Anorexia nervosa and bulimia are serious eating disorders that can be fatal if they are untreated.

SUGGESTED READINGS

Clark, N. *The Athlete's Kitchen: A Nutrition Guide and Cookbook.* Boston: CBI Publishing, 1981.

Craig, T. T., ed. *Comments in Sports Medicine.* Chicago: Department of Health Education, American Medical Association, 1973.

"Eating Disorders in Young Athletes" (A Round Table). *The Physician and Sportsmedicine* 13 (November 1985): 88–106.

Eisenman, P., and D. A. Johnson. *Coaches' Guide to Nutrition and Weight Control.* Champaign, Ill.: Human Kinetics, 1982.

Huse, D., and R. Nelson. "Basic, Balanced Diet Meets Requirements of Athletes." *The Physician and Sportsmedicine* 5 (1977): 52–56.

Moore, M. "Carbohydrate Loading: Eating Through the Wall." *The Physician and Sportsmedicine* 9 (October 1981): 97–103.

Nelson, R. A. "Nutrition and Physical Performance." *The Physician and Sportsmedicine* 10 (April 1982): 55–63.

Smith, N. J. *Food for Sport.* Palo Alto, Calif.: Bull Publishing, 1976.

Smith, N. J. "Nutrition and the Athlete." *American Journal of Sports Medicine* 10 (1982): 253–255.

Smith, N. "Nutrition and Athletic Performance." In *Principles of Sports Medicine,* edited by W. N. Scott, B. Nisonson, and J. A. Nicholas, pp. 27–31. Baltimore: Williams & Wilkins, 1984.

Vitale, J. J. "Nutrition in Sports Medicine." *Clinical Orthopaedics and Related Research* 198 (1985):158–168.

EATING DISORDER SUPPORT ORGANIZATIONS

West

Anorexia Nervosa & Related Eating
  Disorders, Inc. (ANRED)
P.O. Box 5102
Eugene, OR 97405
(503) 344-1144

Midwest

Anorexia Nervosa & Associated
  Disorders, Inc. (ANAD)
P.O. Box 271
Highland Park, IL 60035
(708) 831-3438

Bulimia Anorexia Self Help (BASH)
P.O. Box 39903
St. Louis, MO 63139
(314) 567-4080

National Anorexic Aid Society (NAAS)
1925 East Dublin-Granville Road
Columbus, OH 43229
(614) 436-1112

East and New England

American Anorexia Bulimia
  Association, Inc.
418 East 76th Street
New York, NY 10021
(212) 734-1114

Anorexia Bulimia Care (ABC), Inc.
P.O. Box 213
Lincoln Center, MA 01773
(617) 259-9767

Pennsylvania Educational Network for
  Eating Disorders (PENED)
P.O. Box 16282
Pittsburgh, PA 15242
(412) 922-5922

South

Maryland Association for Anorexia
  Nervosa and Bulimia, Inc. (MAANA)
6501 North Charles Street
Baltimore, MD 21285
(301) 938-3000

43

Taping, Bandaging, Orthotics

CHAPTER OUTLINE

INTRODUCTION

Taping and bandaging are important skills of the athletic trainer. Chapter 43 presents some general guidelines for using tape, cotton wraps, or elastic bandages, including not only some examples of various taping and bandaging techniques for the upper and lower extremities, but also a general discussion of the types of tape and bandaging materials available, how to prepare the athlete's skin prior to taping and bandaging, and how to tear tape and remove it. ■

CONSIDERATIONS IN TAPING AND BANDAGING

The Role of Taping and Bandaging

Manufacturers now supply a variety of protective braces and supports, but the athletic trainer frequently uses tape, cloth, felt, moleskin, and other basic materials to fashion protective or supportive wraps. The athletic trainer may find it helpful not only to be aware of available prefabricated support devices, but also to know how to apply the basic principles of strapping and taping for support.

Adhesive and elastic bandaging techniques, fabrication and fitting of special pads, splints, braces, and other protective devices are an important part of the trainer's responsibilities. These devices are used not only for compression and protection of acute injuries, but also for protection against initial or recurrent injury.

Adhesive Taping

Tape is available in a variety of widths. Most tape used for protection or support is a two-component material consisting of a backcloth and an adhesive mass made of a latex or acrylic base. Tapes vary in strength. Most nonelastic tape and some elastic tape can be hand torn. Tape should be stored in a cool place, as high temperatures (greater than 75 degrees Fahrenheit) may alter the latex adhesive mass.

General Guidelines

The application of adhesive taping varies from trainer to trainer, but most procedures follow these general guidelines:

■ Be sure the area is dry, clean, and free of body hair, although not always shaved when prewrap is used.

■ Use some form of tape adherent to ensure bonding of the tape to the skin (Fig. 43.1). If foam underwrap is used, one layer should be applied over the tape adherent. Underwrap helps protect the skin but decreases the efficiency of the tape.

■ In areas with potential for friction blisters or burns, apply a lubricated pad (grease pad). A pad is made by spreading a non–water-soluble lubricant over a cotton sponge or Telfa pad that is placed between the skin and the tape. Cuts, blisters, and rashes should be covered with a clean non-stick pad prior to the use of adherent or tape.

■ If anchor strips (the first strips of adhesive tape that will serve to "anchor" the rest of the tape) are used, apply them first.

■ Apply continuous circular strapping cautiously, especially with acute or recent injuries, because of the possibility of circulatory embarrassment.

■ Overlap each strip of tape to the previous strip of tape by half. Avoid spaces between tape segments, as such spaces may result in blistering.

■ Smooth and mold the tape on the natural contour of the area being taped.

■ Maintain equal pressure (tension) on the tape throughout the procedure.

■ Try to make the athlete comfortable but maintain the extremity in the correct position while it is being taped.

■ Do not permit the athlete to "test the tape" before the procedure is completed.

Tearing Tape

To tear tape, hold firmly on each side of the proposed tear line. Pull the free end away at an angle so that the force crosses the lines of the fabric at a sharp angle. For speed and efficiency, the trainer should learn to tear tape from the various positions used during taping procedures. When tape is properly torn, the edges should be straight, with no loose threads.

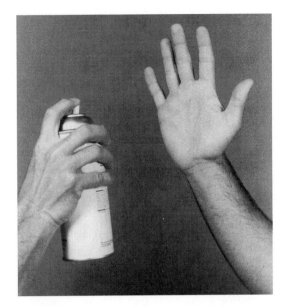

FIGURE 43.1. Tape adherent assures bonding of tape to skin.

Tape Removal

Special cutters are made for tape removal (Fig. 43.2). Alternatively, bandage scissors may be used. Applying a little petrolatum on the scissors or cutters may allow them to slide under the tape more easily. Avoid cutting over bony prominences. After cutting the tape, peel the edges back at 180 degrees, gently pulling the skin from the

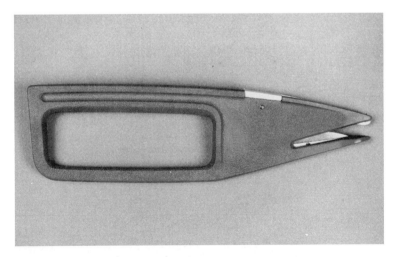

FIGURE 43.2. Tape removal cutter.

tape and not pulling the tape from the skin. Be careful to look for blisters or other skin irritation. Rubbing alcohol will remove the residue of tape adherent.

Effectiveness of Adhesive Taping

The effectiveness of adhesive taping for prevention and treatment of injury has been a matter of controversy for many years. Arguments against taping include the following:

- Tape usually becomes loose with wear.
- Because the skin is mobile, taping cannot be effective.
- Taping the ankle weakens the leg muscles.
- Moisture develops between the skin and tape, thus affecting the adherence of the tape.
- Tape tears under stress.

However, a review of recent literature concerned with effectiveness of adhesive strapping techniques on reducing the incidence of injury concluded that adhesive techniques do contribute to a lower incidence of injury and reinjury.

Complications of Adhesive Taping

Possible complications with tape use include:

- Skin allergies.
- Skin irritations.
- Blisters.
- Lacerations.
- Reactions to tape adherent (benzoin).

Some people have allergies to adhesive tape. Skin irritations commonly develop with prolonged use of taping over a sport season. Usually these irritations are minor. Proper daily cleansing of the area that has been taped can sometimes prevent irritation. Improper application techniques can result in blisters or small skin lacerations. Finally, certain athletes have skin reactions (allergies) — not to the tape itself but to the tape adherents which contain benzoin.

Elastic Bandaging

While each athletic trainer has a particular technique for applying adhesive tape, elastic bandaging techniques are less variable. Elastic bandages provide compression and support to injured tissue.

Guidelines for Applying Compression Wraps

1. When possible, wet and cool the wrap so that it can enhance the conductivity of various cold application agents.
2. Use ½-inch household sponges dipped in ice water and place them over the injured area to enhance the wrap's ability to provide compression.
3. Start the wrap distal to the injury site. For example, with a sprained ankle, start the wrap at the base of the toes.
4. The wrap should be tighter distal rather than proximal to the injury site to minimize venous congestion.
5. After the wet elastic wrap is in place, apply ice packs to assist in controlling the bleeding and swelling (Fig. 43.3).
6. Place a dry elastic wrap over the ice packs to secure them and assist in compression (Fig. 43.4).

Guidelines for Applying Soft Tissue Support

1. Spray the area to be bandaged with a tape adherent to reduce the chance of slipping.
2. Use a pad made of felt or foam rubber, approximately 1 inch larger than the injured area, to provide additional support.
3. If the wrap is applied where friction with the skin or clothing may be excessive, use a skin lubricant pad.
4. Make sure the wrapping allows for contraction and relaxation of major muscle groups.
5. Begin distal to the injury and wrap toward and beyond the injury site, applying constant, even support.
6. Check for vascular compromise after the athlete has had time to warm up.

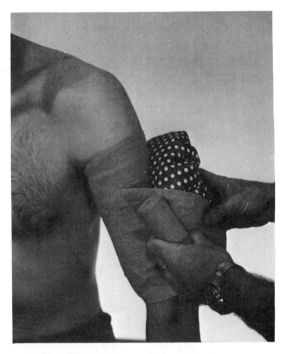

FIGURE 43.3.   An ice pack is applied to control bleeding and swelling.

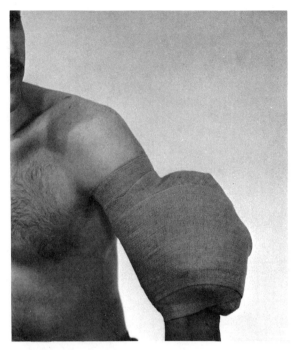

FIGURE 43.4.   A dry elastic wrap secures the ice pack and assists in compression.

Cotton Wraps

Cotton wrap may be used for ankle support. The most common cotton ankle wrap is a piece of muslin, 2 inches wide and 92 to 102 inches long (Fig. 43.5). Such a wrap combines protection with ease of application and durability. It is cost-effective when compared with tape.

Most ankle wrap procedures involve a series of figure-eight turns in combination with heel locks. The purpose of the heel locks is to limit rotational movement in the ankle. Although this technique limits rotational movement, it should not limit ankle extension or flexion. The Louisiana ankle wrap, one of the more popular techniques, is illustrated in Figure 43.6. The following are guidelines for applying cotton wraps:

1. Make sure the sock over which the wrap is applied is snugly fitted.
2. In areas where friction blisters may develop, apply grease pads between the sock and the wrap.
3. Avoid wrinkling the wrap when applying.
4. Secure the completed wrap with strips of adhesive tape which follow the contour of the wrap.

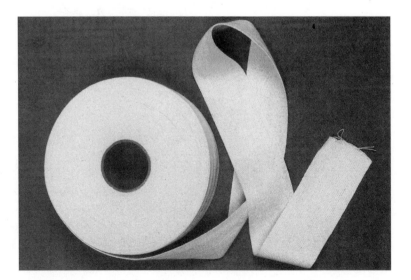

FIGURE 43.5.   Muslin is the most common cotton ankle wrap.

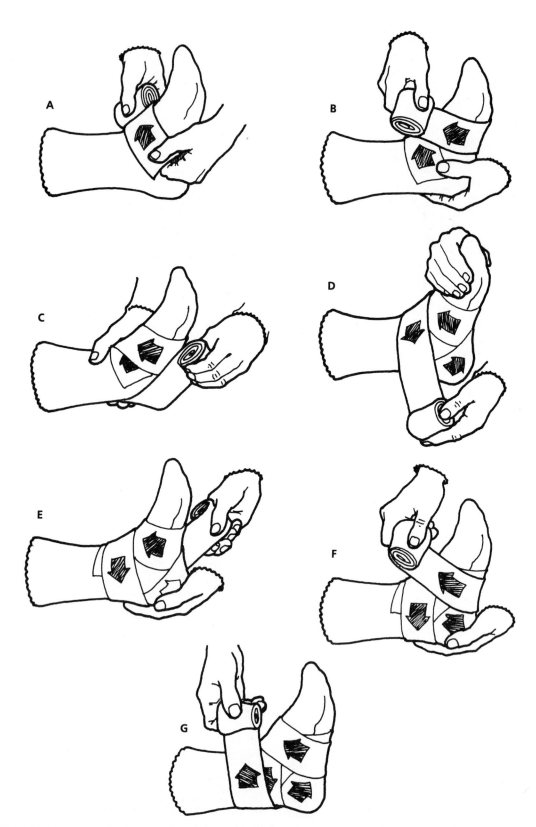

FIGURE 43.6. The Louisiana ankle wrap. The completed wrap is secured with strips of adhesive tape which follow the contour of the wrap.

UPPER EXTREMITY TAPING

Shoulder Strapping

Protective Acromioclavicular Joint Taping

Taping should stabilize the acromioclavicular articulation but allow movement of the shoulder.

MATERIAL

one ¼- to ½-inch-thick felt pad
(doughnut-shaped)
2-inch adhesive tape
tape adherent
2-by-2-inch gauze pad
3-inch elastic bandage

POSITION

The athlete sits or stands; the affected arm is resting, slightly abducted, and externally rotated (Fig. 43.7a). The trainer stands facing the athlete's abducted arm.

PROCEDURE

1. Apply three anchor strips: the first in a three-quarter circle just below the deltoid insertion; the second just below the nipple encircling half the chest; and the third over the trapezius near the neck and then attaching to the second anchor in front and back. Cover the nipple with the 2-by-2-inch gauze pad and the acromioclavicular joint with the ¼- to ½-inch felt pad to achieve greater compression at this area (Fig. 43.7b).
2. Apply the next two strips of tape from the front and back of the first anchor, crossing each other at the acromioclavicular articulation and attaching to the third anchor strip (Figs. 43.7c, d).
3. Place the third support strip over the ends of the first and second pieces, following the line of the third anchor strip.
4. Lay the fourth support strip over the second anchor strip.
5. Continue applying the tape in this basketweave pattern until the entire shoulder complex is covered (Fig. 43.7e).

Then apply a shoulder spica (figure-eight) with an elastic bandage.

Taping for Shoulder Support and Restraint

Taping should support the soft tissues of the shoulder complex and restrain the arm from abducting more than 90 degrees.

MATERIAL

one ½-inch-thick felt pad
2-inch adhesive tape
tape adherent
2-by-2-inch gauze pad
3-inch elastic bandage

POSITION

The athlete sits in a chair with the affected arm resting, slightly abducted. The trainer stands facing the abducted arm.

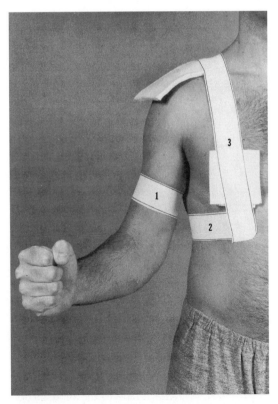

FIGURE 43.7a. Protective acromioclavicular joint taping.

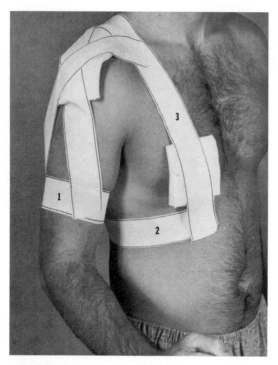

FIGURE 43.7b. Apply three anchor strips; for compression, cover acromioclavicular joint.

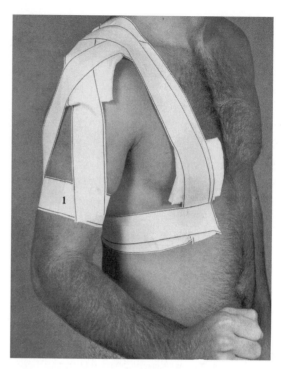

FIGURE 43.7c. Apply the next two strips of tape.

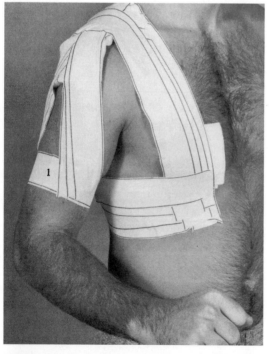

FIGURE 43.7d. Attach tape to the third anchor strip.

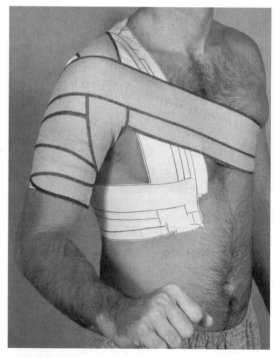

FIGURE 43.7e. Continue taping until the entire shoulder is covered.

PROCEDURE

1. The first phase of taping is designed to support the capsule of the shoulder joint. After placing a cotton pad in the axilla, apply a series of three loops around the shoulder joint. Start the first loop at the top of the scapula, pulling it anteriorly across the acromion process and around the anterior aspect of the glenohumeral joint, posteriorly under the axilla, over the posterior glenohumeral joint, crossing the acromioclavicular joint again, and terminating at the clavicle (Fig. 43.8a).
2. Next, run strips of tape upward from a point just below the insertion of the deltoid muscle and crossing over the acromion process, completely covering the outer surface of the shoulder joint (Fig. 43.8b).
3. Before applying the final basketweave shoulder taping, place a gauze pad over the nipple area. Lay a strip of tape over the shoulder near the neck and carry it to the nipple line in front and to the scapular line in back. Take a second strip from the end of the first strip, around the middle of the humerus, ending at the back end of the first strip (Fig. 43.8c).
4. Continue the above alternating pattern, overlapping each preceding strip by at least one-half of its width, until the shoulder is completely capped (Fig. 43.8d).
5. Apply a shoulder spica with an elastic wrap to keep the taping in place (Fig. 43.8e). (See the next section on elastic bandaging.)

Shoulder Dislocation Taping

Designed to support the structures around the glenohumeral joint after dislocation, this taping can also be used to support the glenohumeral joint for activity.

MATERIAL

gauze pad
skin lubricant
3-inch elastic tape

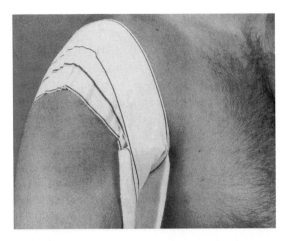

FIGURE 43.8a. Shoulder support taping begins with three loops at the shoulder joint.

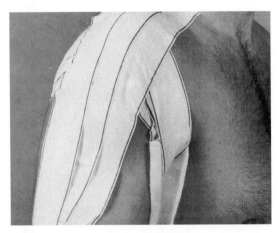

FIGURE 43.8b. Apply tape upward, to cover the surface of the shoulder joint.

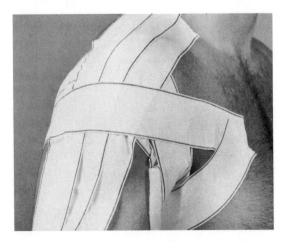

FIGURE 43.8c. Cover nipple area with gauze pad before basketweave shoulder taping.

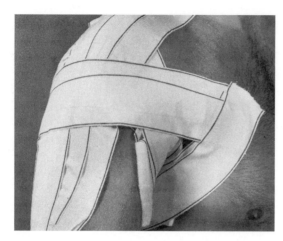

FIGURE 43.8d. Continue basketweave pattern until the shoulder is covered.

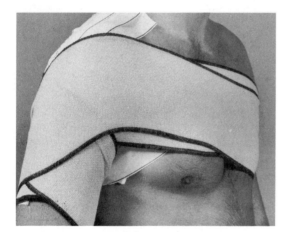

FIGURE 43.8e. Apply a shoulder spica.

POSITION

The athlete stands facing the trainer with the hand of the affected side behind the body on the buttocks area. This position internally rotates the arm and yet allows for some degree of abduction.

PROCEDURE

1. Shave the chest area if body hair is dense.
2. Place a gauze pad with skin lubricant over the nipple on the breast nearest the affected arm (Fig. 43.9a).
3. Apply two figure-eights (shoulder spicas) around the affected upper arm, using 3-inch elastic tape. Begin on the vertebral border of the scapula, cross over the affected deltoid, and encircle the upper arm from posterior to anterior. Cross the chest below the nipple line, go around the upper body, and continue on around the upper arm.
4. Overlap the tape just one-half the width of the first strip of tape, and encircle the body a second time (Figs. 43.9b, c, d).
5. Continue applying elastic tape until the entire roll is used. Ensure that the tape encircling the upper arm is not too constricting. In addition, the tape must come down far enough onto the upper arm to obtain an appropriate angle of pull to prevent external rotation and abduction (Fig. 43.9e).

In addition to taping, numerous types of shoulder harnesses have been used with varied degrees of success in preventing a recurrence of glenohumeral dislocation (see Chapter 44).

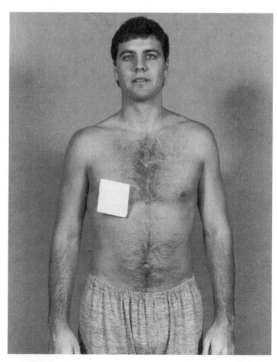

FIGURE 43.9a. Shoulder dislocation taping first protects the nipple area.

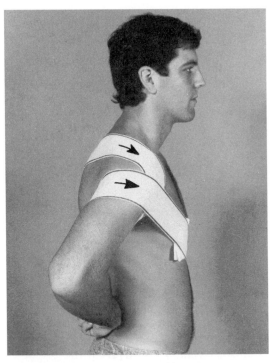

FIGURE 43.9b. Apply two figure-eights to the affected upper arm.

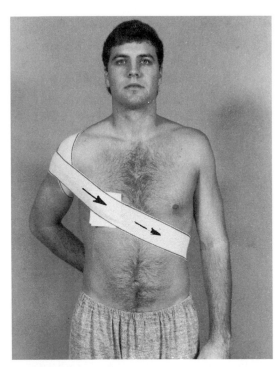

FIGURE 43.9c. Apply the tape across the chest below the nipple line.

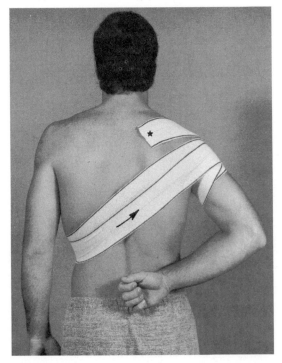

FIGURE 43.9d. Encircle the body a second time with tape.

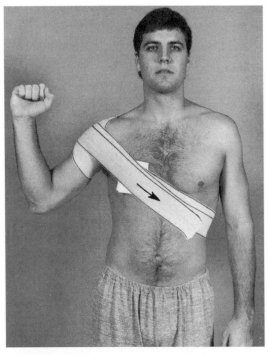

FIGURE 43.9e. Taping must not constrict yet must prevent external rotation and abduction.

Elbow Hyperextension Taping

Elbow hyperextension can be prevented by using tape as a checkrein. Two ways of taping are presented here.

Method 1

MATERIAL

1½-inch adhesive tape
tape adherent
2-inch elastic bandage

POSITION

The athlete stands with the affected elbow flexed 90 degrees and the forearm in a neutral position. The trainer stands facing the side of the affected arm.

PROCEDURE

1. Apply two anchor strips loosely around the arm, approximately 2 to 3 inches above and below the elbow joint (antecubital fossa) (Fig. 43.10a).
2. Construct a checkrein by cutting a 10-inch and a 4-inch strip of tape and laying the 4-inch strip against the center of the 10-inch strip, adhesive side to adhesive side. Next, place the checkrein so that it spans the two anchor strips, with the blanked-out side facing downward (Fig. 43.10b).
3. Place five additional 10-inch strips of tape over the basic checkrein (Fig. 43.10c). (A leather strap or a rubber bandage [AT6843, minimum length 14 feet, Fulflex, Inc., Bristol, RI 02809] can serve as the checkrein.)
4. Finish the procedure by securing the checkrein with three lock strips on each end (Fig. 43.10d).
5. Apply a figure-eight elastic wrap over the taping to close the strapping.

Method 2

MATERIAL

tape adherent
1½-inch adhesive tape
2- to 3-inch elastic tape
underwrap (optional)

POSITION

The athlete sits or stands with the elbow flexed at 90 degrees and the forearm in a neutral position. The trainer stands facing the side of the athlete's affected arm.

PROCEDURE

1. Apply two anchor strips loosely around the arm, approximately 3 inches above and below the elbow joint (antecubital fossa) (Fig. 43.11a).
2. Begin on the medial side of the forearm on the anchor strip with 1½-inch tape, bringing it obliquely upward and crossing the antecubital fossa to the superior anchor strip (Fig. 43.11b).
3. Repeat this lateral to medial, creating a crisscross fan effect over the antecubital area (Fig. 43.11c).
4. Each set of oblique strappings should move laterally and overlap the previous pair by one-half the width (Fig. 43.11d).
5. Place lock strips to secure oblique taping in place (Fig. 43.11e).
6. Close loosely with 2- to 3-inch elastic tape (Fig. 43.11f).

Wrist Taping

Wrist Band

Wrist bands are designed for mild wrist injuries where slight limitation of motion in all directions is necessary. Wrist taping can also be used for compression or to support the retinaculum of the wrist.

MATERIAL

tape adherent
1-inch or 1½-inch adhesive tape (depending on athlete's size)
underwrap (optional)

POSITION

The athlete stands with the affected wrist in a neutral position, fingers moderately abducted, elbow flexed to 90 degrees, and forearm in neutral position. The trainer stands facing the athlete's affected wrist.

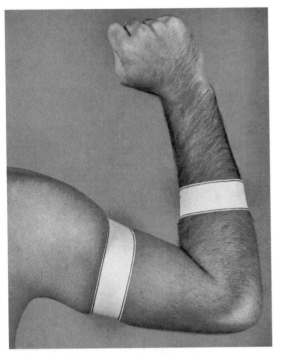

FIGURE 43.10a. Elbow hyperextension taping (method 1) begins with two anchor strips.

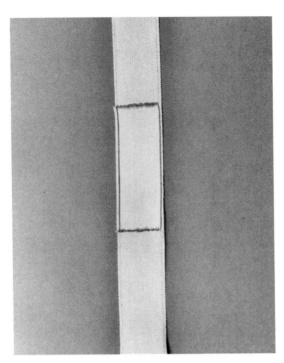

FIGURE 43.10b. Construct a checkrein, using a 10-inch and a 4-inch strip of tape.

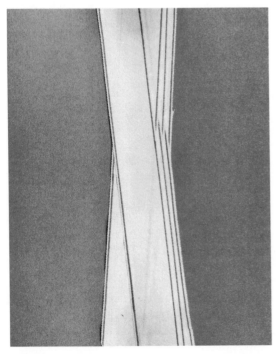

FIGURE 43.10c. Cover the checkrein with five l0-inch strips.

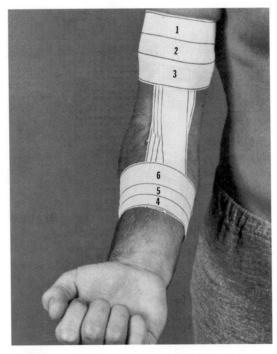

FIGURE 43.10d. Secure the checkrein with three lock strips.

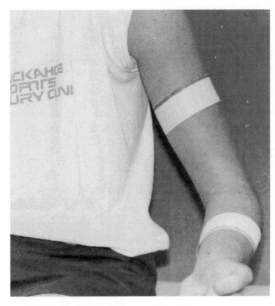

FIGURE 43.11a. Elbow hyperextension taping (method 2) begins with two anchor strips.

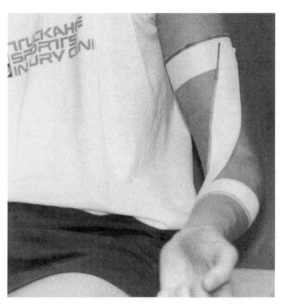

FIGURE 43.11b. Start taping on the medial side of the forearm and cross to the antecubital fossa.

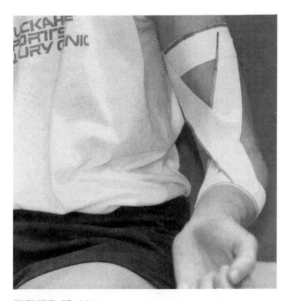

FIGURE 43.11c. Repeat pattern, creating a crisscross fan effect.

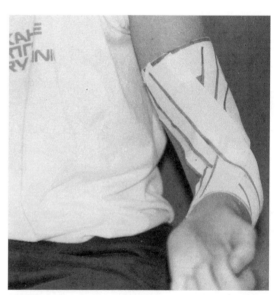

FIGURE 43.11d. Each set of strappings should move laterally and overlap the previous pair by one half width.

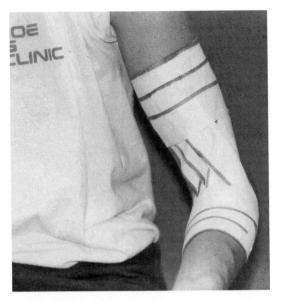

FIGURE 43.11e. Apply lock strips to secure oblique taping in place.

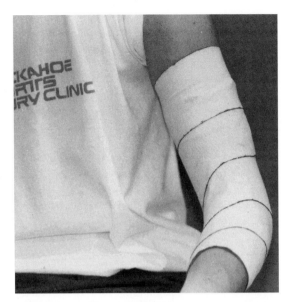

FIGURE 43.11f. Finish taping by loosely applying a 2- to 3-inch elastic tape.

PROCEDURE

1. Starting at the base of the wrist, bring a strip of tape from the palmar side upward and encircle the wrist (Fig. 43.12a).
2. In the same pattern, lay in place three additional strips with each strip overlapping the preceding one by at least one-half its width (Fig. 43.12b).

Wrist Hyperextension/Hyperflexion Taping

This taping is designed to protect and stabilize the injured wrist by limiting wrist flexion and extension. Two methods frequently used are the checkrein method and the figure-eight method.

Method 1: Checkrein Method

MATERIAL

tape adherent
1-inch or 1½-inch adhesive tape (depending on the athlete's size)
underwrap (optional)

POSITION

The athlete stands with elbow flexed at 90 degrees, forearm in neutral position, fingers abducted, and wrist placed toward injured side (either flexion or extension). The athletic trainer stands facing toward the athlete's affected wrist.

PROCEDURE

1. Place anchor strips 3 inches proximal to the styloid process, with another strip around the spread hand proximal to the base of the metacarpal heads (Fig. 43.13a).
2. With the wrist flexed, or extended, toward the injured side, take a strip of tape from the anchor strip near the little finger and carry it obliquely across the wrist joint to the wrist anchor strip. Take another strip from the anchor strip on the index finger side and carry it obliquely across the wrist joint to the wrist anchor. This forms a crisscross

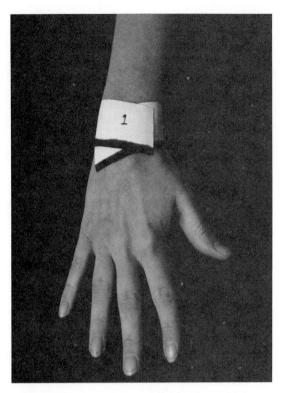

FIGURE 43.12a. Wrist taping begins at the base of the wrist, by encircling the wrist from the palmar side.

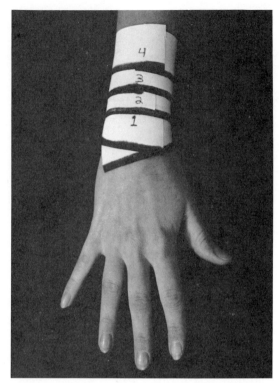

FIGURE 43.12b. Continue the pattern, with three strips overlapping the preceding one by at least one half width.

over the wrist joint (Fig. 43.13b). A series of four or five crisscrosses may be applied. A checkrein may be used instead of the crisscross, formed in a manner similar to the elbow hyperextension strapping.
3. Apply two or three series of figure-eight tapings over the crisscross taping (Fig. 43.13c).

Method 2: Figure-Eight Method
(for protection against hyperflexion)

MATERIAL

 tape adherent
 1-inch adhesive tape
 1½-inch adhesive tape
 underwrap (optional)

POSITION

The athlete stands with the elbow at the side, flexed to 90 degrees, wrist extended, and fingers abducted. The

forearm is in neutral position. The trainer stands facing the athlete's affected wrist.

PROCEDURE

1. Start a strip of 1-inch tape on the palmar aspect of the hand and bring it radially through the web space (Fig. 43.14a).
2. Continuing with the tape, move obliquely toward the ulnar styloid process (Fig. 43.14b).
3. Wrap the tape around the wrist once and continue for one-half turn, until the tape obliquely crosses the dorsal surface of the hand to the original anchor (Fig. 43.14c).
4. Cut the tape and repeat.
5. Close with 1½-inch tape around anchors to lock tape in place (Fig. 43.14d).

Method 2: Figure-Eight Method
(for protection against hyperextension)

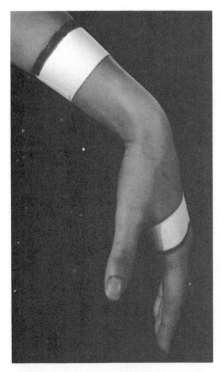

FIGURE 43.13a. Wrist hyper-extension/hyperflexion taping (check-rein method) begins with two anchor strips.

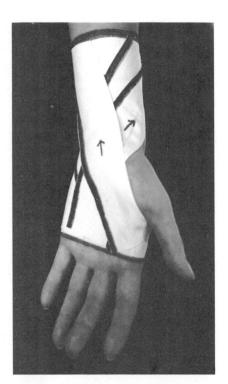

FIGURE 43.13b. With the wrist extended toward the injured side, taping forms a crisscross pattern over the wrist.

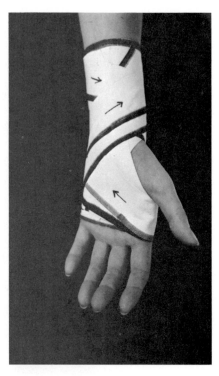

FIGURE 43.13c. The checkrein method finishes with two or three series of figure-eight tapings.

Figure-eight wrist hyperextension taping is a mirror image of the figure-eight wrist hyperflexion taping, since its purpose is to prevent wrist extension. The oblique strapping will be on the palmar surface of the hand. The wrist is held in flexion while tape is applied (Figs. 43.15a, b).

Ulnar Deviation Assist Taping

Ulnar deviation assist taping is designed to support the wrist in ulnar deviation while allowing radial deviation.

MATERIAL

> tape adherent
> 1½-inch adhesive tape
> 2-inch elastic tape
> one pair of scissors
> underwrap (optional)

POSITION

> The athlete sits with the arm supported by a table and the elbow flexed to 90

degrees. Forearm is in neutral position with wrist in ulnar deviation and fingers abducted. The trainer stands facing the athlete's affected wrist.

PROCEDURE

1. Place two anchor strips loosely—one, two-thirds of the way down the forearm, and the other around the metacarpals (Fig. 43.16a).
2. Measure and split elastic tape at both ends and wrap it around the anchor strip. The tape should pull the wrist into ulnar deviation (Fig. 43.16b).
3. Secure the elastic tape with 1½-inch adhesive tape all the way up the ulnar surface (Fig. 43.16c).
4. Lock in place with 1½-inch tape (Fig. 43.16d).
5. Close in the taping with elastic tape using figure-eights around the wrist and loose spiral strapping on the forearm (Fig. 43.16e).

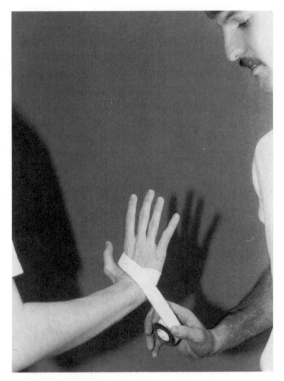

FIGURE 43.14a. Wrist hyperextension/hyperflexion taping (figure-eight method) begins taping at the palmar aspect of the hand.

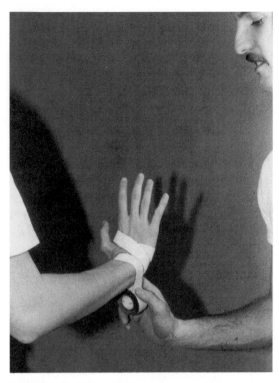

FIGURE 43.14b. Taping moves toward the ulnar styloid process.

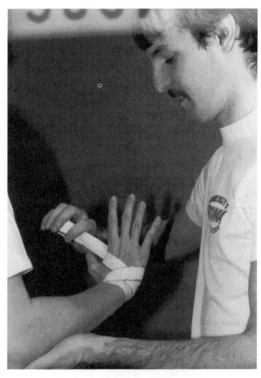

FIGURE 43.14c. Taping encircles the wrist and crosses the dorsal surface to the original anchor.

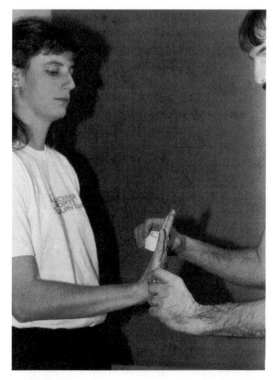

FIGURE 43.14d. Taping around anchors locks tape in place.

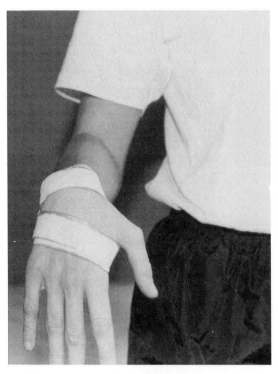

FIGURE 43.15a. Wrist hyperextension/ hyperflexion taping (figure-eight method for protection against hyperextension).

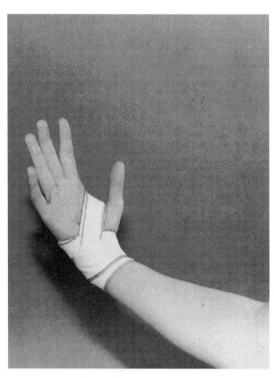

FIGURE 43.15b. The taping pattern is the mirror image of that for hyperflexion taping.

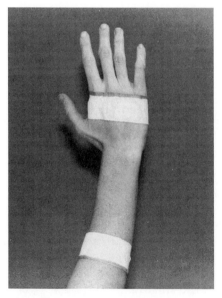

FIGURE 43.16a. Ulnar deviation assist taping begins with two anchors.

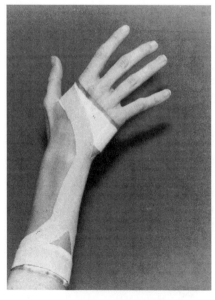

FIGURE 43.16b. Split tape at both ends and wrap it around the anchor strip, pulling wrist into ulnar deviation.

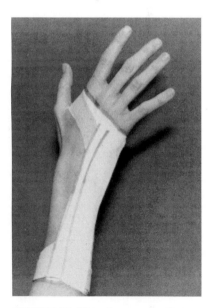

FIGURE 43.16c. Secure elastic tape with adhesive to the ulnar surface.

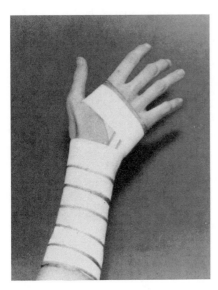

FIGURE 43.16d. Lock in place with 1½-inch tape.

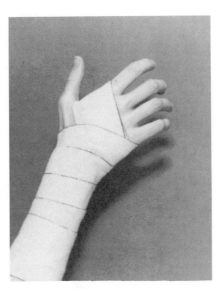

FIGURE 43.16e. Close in taping with figure-eights around the wrist and spiral strapping on the forearm.

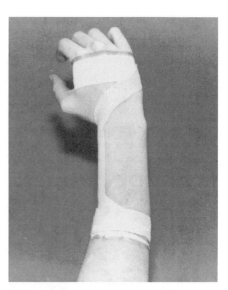

FIGURE 43.17. Radial deviation assist taping.

Radial Deviation Assist Taping

This method is similar to the ulnar deviation assist taping, but it uses radial deviation rather than ulnar deviation.

Place elastic tape on the radial side of the forearm (Fig. 43.17) and close in the tape as in the preceding steps 3, 4, and 5. Notice that these assistive taping techniques can be used for flexion or extension and/or combinations of these movements.

Thumb Taping

Thumb Spica Taping

This taping technique is designed to protect the joints of the first ray (the carpometacarpal joint, the metacarpophalangeal (MCP) joint, and the interphalangeal joints), as well as the surrounding muscles.

MATERIAL

    tape adherent
    1-inch adhesive tape
    underwrap (optional)

POSITION

The athlete should hold the thumb in a relaxed, neutral position —usually the functional position (as if holding a can). The trainer stands in front of the athlete's injured thumb.

PROCEDURE

1. Place an anchor loosely around the wrist with another around the distal phalanx of the thumb (Fig. 43.18a).
2. From the anchor at the tip of the thumb to the anchor around the wrist, apply four splint strips in a series on the side, either dorsal or palmar, and hold these strips in place by one lock strip around the wrist and the distal phalanx (Fig. 43.18b).
3. Now add a series of three thumb strips in a "spica" fashion. Start the first strip, which goes around the MCP joint, on the radial side at the base of the thumb and carry this strip under the thumb, completely encircling the thumb, and then cross to the starting point (Fig. 43.18c). Each of the following spica strips should overlap the preceding strip by at least ⅔ inch and move proximally on the thumb.
4. Figure 43.18c shows the final anchors around the tip of the thumb and wrist.

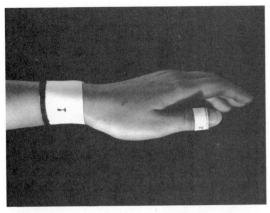

FIGURE 43.18a. Thumb spica taping loosely anchors the wrist and the distal phalanx of the thumb.

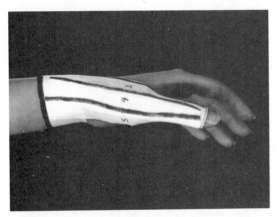

FIGURE 43.18b. Apply four splint strips in a series on the side, either dorsal or palmar, and lock in place with lock strip.

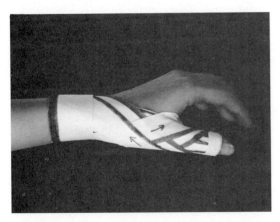

FIGURE 43.18c. Add a series of three thumb strips in a "spica" fashion and anchor taping at thumb and wrist.

Thumb Checkreins

This taping technique is a reinforcing strapping for the previous thumb taping method and can be used by itself to provide additional protection to the injured MCP joint of the thumb by limiting motion.

MATERIAL

> 1-inch adhesive tape
> tape adherent

POSITION

> The athlete spreads the fingers widely but within a pain-free range of motion. The trainer faces the athlete's injured thumb.

PROCEDURE

1. Place 1-inch anchor strips around the distal phalanx of the injured thumb and proximal phalanx of the index finger. Place a checkrein between these two connections of 1-inch tape. Leave enough slack between the thumb and second phalanx to protect the joint but still allow some function (Fig. 43.19a).
2. Encircle the center of the checkrein for additional strength (Fig. 43.19b).

ALTERNATE PROCEDURE

1. Place 1-inch anchor strips around the distal phalanx of the injured thumb and proximal phalanx of the index finger. Place a checkrein between these two anchors. Leave enough slack between the thumb and second phalanx to protect the joint but still allow some function.
2. Encircle the center of the checkrein for additional strength.

Pancake Thumb Strapping

This taping method is designed to protect the thumb from reinjury but does not allow the thumb to be used functionally for grasping.

MATERIAL

> tape adherent
> 2- or 3-inch elastic tape

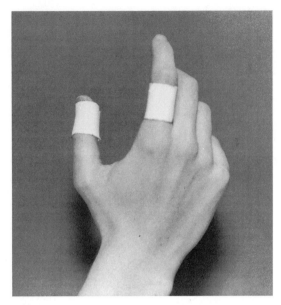

FIGURE 43.19a. Thumb checkrein: wrap anchor strips around distal phalanx of injured thumb and proximal phalanx of index finger.

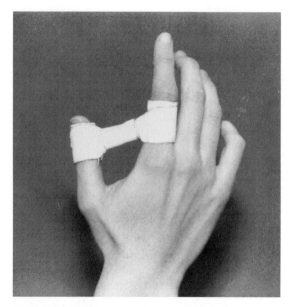

FIGURE 43.19b. Encircle the center of the checkrein for additional strength.

1½-inch adhesive tape
underwrap (optional)

POSITION

The athlete should stand with elbow flexed 90 degrees, wrist and forearm in neutral position, and thumb and fingers abducted. The trainer faces the athlete's injured thumb.

PROCEDURE

1. Begin a spiral wrap of elastic tape at the MCP joints of the fingers, holding the thumb adducted to the second metacarpal (Fig. 43.20a).
2. Continue to wrap the hand loosely, overlapping the strips by one-half until the ulnar and radial styloid processes are covered (Fig. 43.20b).
3. Close the strapping with 1½-inch adhesive tape around the wrist, covering the end of the elastic tape (Fig. 43.20c).

Hand Strapping

Skin Strapping

Hand taping is designed to protect the distal palmar skin.

MATERIAL

tape adherent
1½-inch adhesive tape
1-inch gauze roll (optional)

POSITION

The athlete should be seated with arm resting on a table, elbow flexed at 90 degrees, forearm and wrist in neutral position, and fingers and thumb abducted. The trainer faces the injured hand.

PROCEDURE

1. Apply tape adherent to palm and wrist, making sure that none is on the fingers (Fig. 43.21a).
2. Apply one layer of 1½-inch adhesive tape around the palm and wrist for anchors (Fig. 43.21b).
3. Tear thin strips of tape and place them between the fingers without rolling the edges (Fig. 43.21c), anchoring them on the wrist. (Optional: place 1-inch gauze between fingers so it covers the palm and dorsum of the hand.)
4. Place lock strips around the wrist, and

possibly the palm, to hold the thin strips in place (Fig. 43.21d).

5. For the gymnast, apply chalk over the tape as normally done.

Metacarpal Strapping

This taping supports the metacarpals and protects the heads of the metacarpals and phalanges from bruising when punching with a fist.

MATERIAL

tape adherent
1-inch adhesive tape
1½-inch adhesive tape
2-inch rolled gauze
½-inch-thick soft sponge rubber pad

POSITION

The athlete should stand, with elbow flexed 90 degrees, forearm in neutral position, and fingers abducted. The trainer faces the athlete's hand.

PROCEDURE

1. Lay the pad over the dorsum of the hand (Fig. 43.22a).
2. Wrap 2-inch rolled gauze around the styloid process of the wrist twice. Then continue the gauze distally to the web space between the fourth and fifth digits. Loop it around the fifth digit and back around the wrist for a complete turn. Repeat for the second, third, and fourth digits (Fig. 43.22b).
3. Using 1-inch tape, apply thumb horseshoes, followed by a spica (Fig. 43.22c).
4. Apply a figure-eight using 1-inch tape to hold the wrist in slight extension (Fig. 43.22d).
5. With 1½-inch tape, lock the strapping into place around the wrist and the palm, covering the metacarpal phalanges (Fig. 43.22e).

Finger Taping

Buddy Taping

With buddy taping, the injured finger is protected by taping it to the neighboring

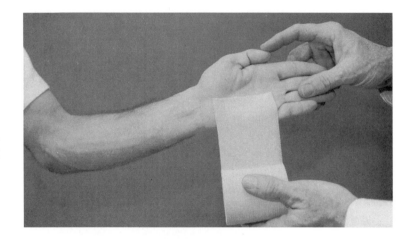

FIGURE 43.20a. Pancake thumb strapping begins with a spiral wrap.

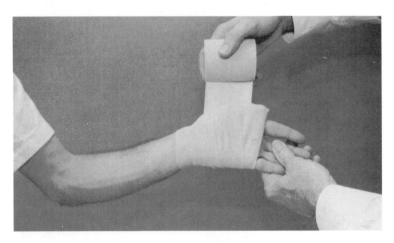

FIGURE 43.20b. Wrap loosely until the ulnar and radial styloid processes are covered.

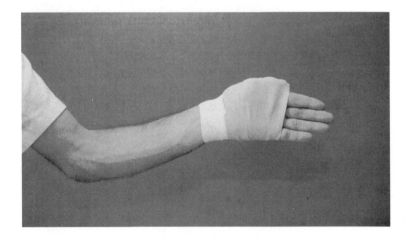

FIGURE 43.20c. Close the strapping, covering the end of the elastic tape.

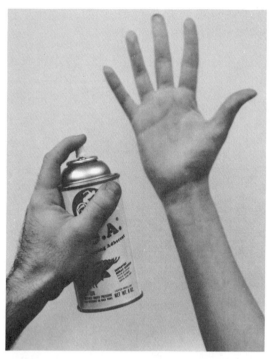

FIGURE 43.21a. Skin strapping: apply tape adherent to palm and wrist, making sure none is on the fingers.

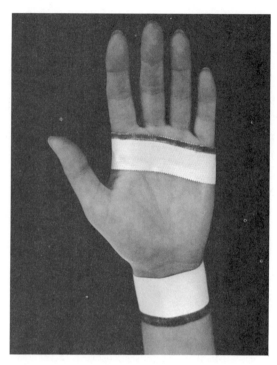

FIGURE 43.21b. Apply anchors around the palm and wrist.

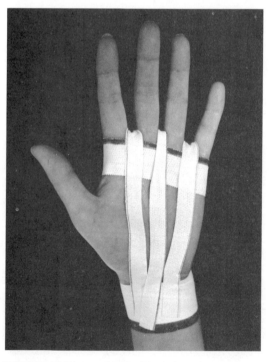

FIGURE 43.21c. Apply thin strips of tape between the fingers and anchor them on the wrist.

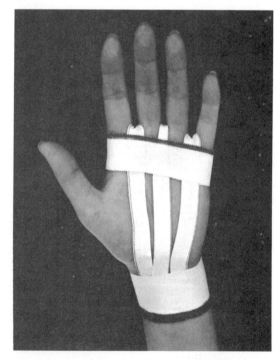

FIGURE 43.21d. Place lock strips around the wrist, and possibly the palm, to hold strips in place.

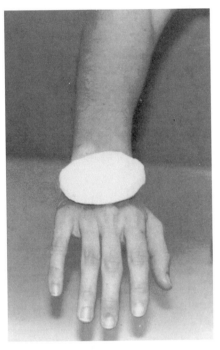

FIGURE 43.22a. Metacarpal strapping begins with application of a pad to protect the dorsum of the hand.

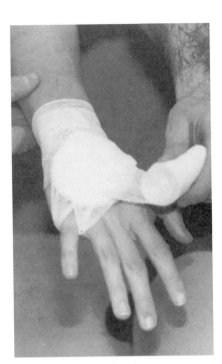

FIGURE 43.22b. Wrap the styloid process of the wrist twice and continue to the web space between the fourth and fifth digits.

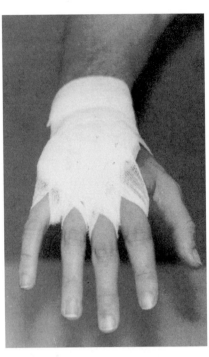

FIGURE 43.22c. Continue for second, third, and fourth digits; apply thumb horseshoes and then a spica.

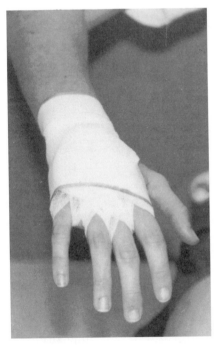

FIGURE 43.22d. Apply a figure-eight to hold wrist in slight extension.

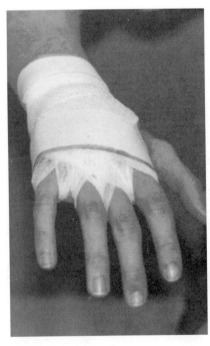

FIGURE 43.22e. Lock the strapping into place around the wrist and palm.

noninjured finger, without impeding functional range of motion.

MATERIAL

½- or 1-inch adhesive tape (depending on athlete's size)
tape adherent

POSITION

The athlete should stand with elbow at 90 degrees flexion, and wrist and forearm in neutral position, holding together the fingers that are to be taped. The trainer stands in front of the athlete's injured finger.

PROCEDURE

1. Place a ½-inch or 1-inch tape strip around the injured finger and the adjoining proximal phalanx and distal phalanx to hold them together.
2. Place tape above and below the proximal interphalangeal (PIP) joint to allow fullest mobility possible (Fig. 43.23).

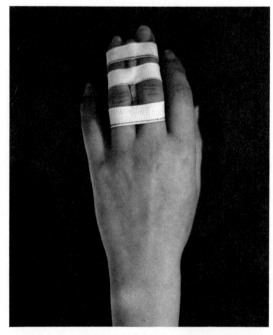

FIGURE 43.23. Buddy taping protects the injured finger without impeding functional range of motion.

Finger Joint Hyperextension/Hyperflexion Stop Strapping

This taping method is designed to restrict PIP joint motion markedly.

MATERIAL

½-inch or 1-inch adhesive tape (depending on athlete's size)
tape adherent

POSITION

The athlete stands with elbow flexed to 90 degrees, wrist and forearm in neutral position, and the injured finger in the position to be fixed. The trainer stands in front of the athlete's injured finger.

PROCEDURE

1. Wrap a ½-inch or 1-inch strip of tape around the proximal phalanx (Fig. 43.24a).
2. As the turn is completed, pull the tape obliquely across the dorsal surface (to prevent flexion) or the palmar surface (to prevent extension). Then wrap the middle phalanx twice.
3. As the second turn is completed, pull the tape down obliquely across the PIP joint, forming a crisscross over the joint.
4. Turn the wrap once around the proximal phalanx to lock it in place (Fig. 43.24b).

Single-Digit Immobilization

Immobilization of one digit is designed to use tape only to splint and limit motion of a finger in the functional position.

MATERIAL

tape adherent
1-inch adhesive tape
gauze
2-inch elastic tape

POSITION

The athlete is seated with arm resting on table, elbow flexed to 90 degrees, forearm in neutral position, wrist slightly extended, and fingers abducted and slightly flexed. The trainer stands in front of the athlete's injured finger.

PROCEDURE

1. Place anchor strips around the wrist, the palm of the hand, and the phalanx to be immobilized (Fig. 43.25a).
2. Starting at the wrist, place a strip of adhesive tape the length of the metacarpal and phalanx to be immobilized from the distal phalanx to the anchor strip at the wrist on the palmar surface (Fig. 43.25b).
3. Place a piece of gauze on the tip of the finger and continue the adhesive tape down the dorsal side until it reaches the wrist.
4. Place lock strips between the distal interphalangeal (DIP) and PIP joints, between the PIP and MCP joints, and around the palm and the wrist.
5. Close with a figure-eight elastic taping to hold in place (Fig. 43.25c).

Multiple-Digit Immobilization

Immobilization of multiple digits is designed to allow functional use of some fingers while allowing support and stabilization of others.

MATERIAL

    underwrap
    1½-inch adhesive tape
    elastic tape
    1-inch gauze

POSITION

    The athlete sits or stands with elbow flexed, wrist extended, forearm in neutral position, and the fourth and fifth digits flexed. The trainer is in front of the athlete's injured hand.

PROCEDURE

1. The athlete holds onto the 1-inch gauze with the fourth and fifth digits while the underwrap is applied around the digits, palm, and wrist (Fig. 43.26a).
2. Apply an anchor strip to the wrist with 1½-inch adhesive tape (Fig. 43.26b).
3. Place a longitudinal strip of the 1½-inch tape over the top of the fourth and fifth

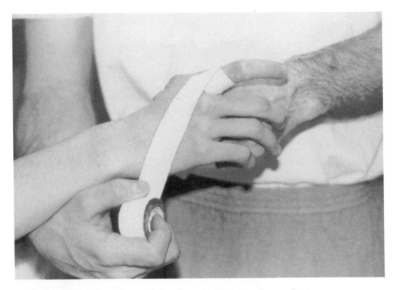

FIGURE 43.24a.   Finger joint hyperextension/hyperflexion stop strapping begins with a wrap of the proximal phalanx.

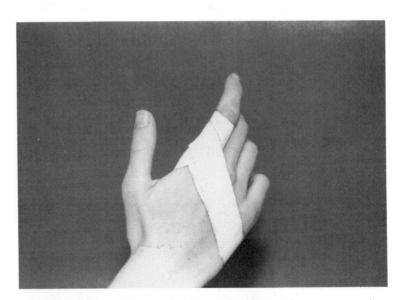

FIGURE 43.24b.   When taping is completed, turn the wrap around the proximal phalanx to lock it in place.

digits and anchor it at the wrist (Fig. 43.26c).
4. Place lock strips at the wrist and, loosely, around the palm (Fig. 43.26d).
5. Close strapping with elastic tape in a figure-eight fashion to hold in place (Fig. 43.26e).

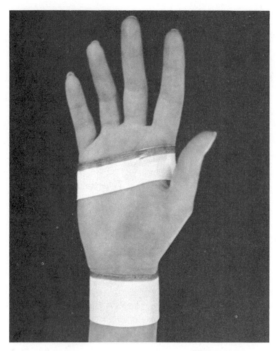

FIGURE 43.25a. Single-digit immobilization begins with anchor strips around the wrist, palm, and injured phalanx.

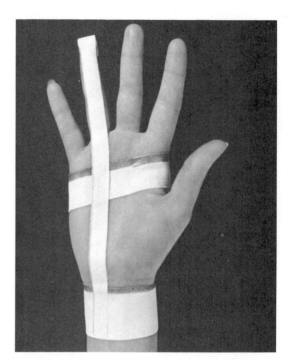

FIGURE 43.25b. Tape from the wrist, to the length of the metacarpal and injured phalanx, to the anchor strip at wrist on palmar surface.

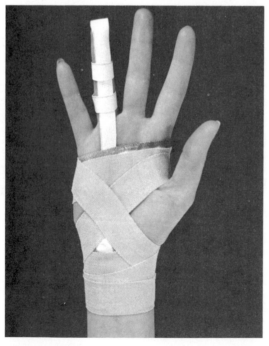

FIGURE 43.25c. Close with a figure-eight elastic taping to hold in place.

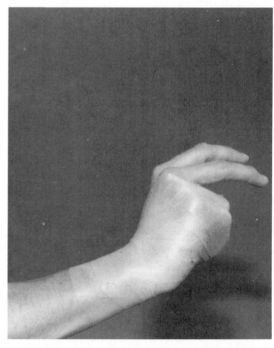

FIGURE 43.26a. Multiple-digit immobilization: underwrap around the digits, palm, and wrist.

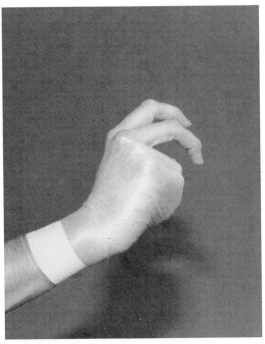

FIGURE 43.26b. Apply an anchor strip to the wrist with adhesive tape.

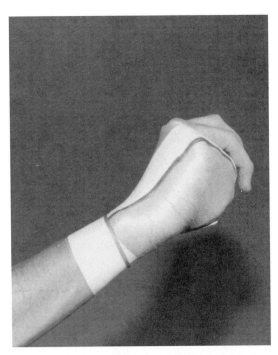

FIGURE 43.26c. Place a longitudinal strip over the top of the fourth and fifth digits and anchor to wrist.

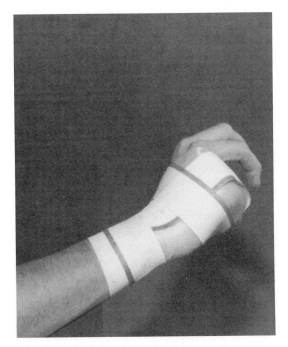

FIGURE 43.26d. Place lock strips at the wrist and around the palm.

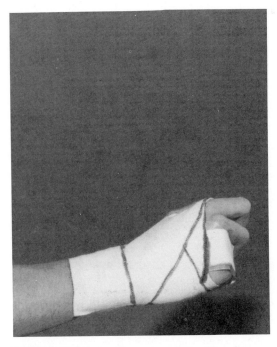

FIGURE 43.26e. Close strapping with a figure-eight pattern to hold in place.

LOWER EXTREMITY TAPING

The following general considerations apply to all lower extremity tapings:

- Select tape of proper width.
- Tape directly to the skin for maximum protection.
- Properly prepare the area to be taped. This includes covering all areas of skin irritation, protecting areas of potential irritation, and applying adherent or benzoin as needed.
- Stretch elastic tape 85 to 90 percent.
- Contour all tape strips to tapered body parts to prevent wrinkles.
- Always tape from distal to proximal— that is, toward the heart.

Knee Taping

Use tape to support the knee following injury to the medial collateral ligament (MCL) or the lateral collateral ligament (LCL), or following a hyperextension injury (Table 43.1).

When taping following MCL or LCL injury, do not apply tape simply over the side of the injured knee. Tape both sides of the knee to afford as much support as possible. Keep all tape off the patella to prevent patellofemoral complications.

Taping Following MCL Injury

MATERIAL

    tape adherent
    underwrap (optional)
    1½-inch adhesive tape
    3-inch elastic tape

POSITION

The athlete stands with heel of foot elevated on a 2-inch object. The affected knee should be in 15 to 20 degrees of flexion. The trainer stands facing the athlete.

PROCEDURE

1. Apply anchor strips at midthigh and midcalf (Fig. 43.27a).
2. Using elastic tape, apply six strips to the medial aspect of the knee (Fig. 43.27b). Begin at the lower midlateral aspect of the calf and cross the medial joint line to the midmedial aspect of the thigh. Start a second strip at the midmedial aspect of the calf, crossing the previous strip at the joint line and progressing to the midlateral aspect of the thigh. Be careful to keep the patella free of tape. Apply a second set of crossing strips in the previously described manner, overlapping the previous strips by one-half to three-fourths (Fig. 43.27c). Apply two vertical strips from midmedial calf to midmedial thigh (Fig. 43.27d).
3. Apply three strips of elastic tape to the lateral aspect of the knee. Begin at the midlateral calf, cross the lateral joint line, and progress to the midmedial thigh (Fig. 43.27e). A second strip starts at the midlateral calf, crosses the previous strip at the joint line, and progresses to the midmedial thigh. Apply a vertical strip from midlateral calf to the midlateral thigh (Fig. 43.27f).
4. Apply anchor strips to the calf and thigh to hold previous strips in place (Fig. 43.27g). The number may vary with the size of the athlete.

Taping Following Hyperextension Injury

MATERIAL

    tape adherent
    4-by-4-inch gauze or felt pad
    1½-inch adhesive tape
    6-inch elastic tape (optional)

TABLE 43.1. Basic Knee Taping Formulas

MCL Injury	LCL Injury	Hyperextension Injury
1. 6 strips inside	1. 6 strips outside	1. 3 strips posterior
2. 3 strips outside	2. 3 strips inside	2. anchors
3. anchors	3. anchors	

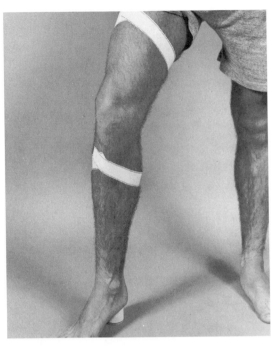

FIGURE 43.27a. Knee taping following medial collateral ligament injury: apply anchor strips at midthigh and midcalf.

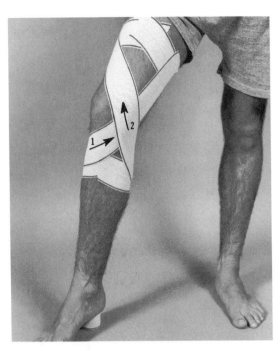

FIGURE 43.27b. Beginning at the lower midlateral aspect of the calf, apply six strips to the knee.

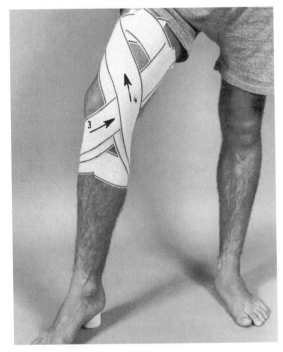

FIGURE 43.27c. Apply another set of crossing strips, overlapping the previous strips by one-half to three-fourths.

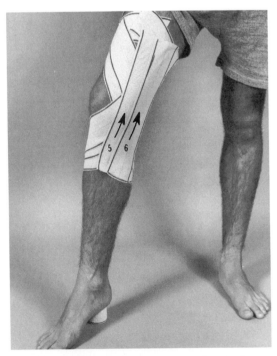

FIGURE 43.27d. Apply two vertical strips from midmedial calf to midmedial thigh.

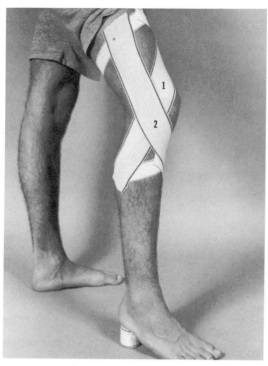

FIGURE 43.27e. Apply three strips of tape to the lateral aspect of the knee.

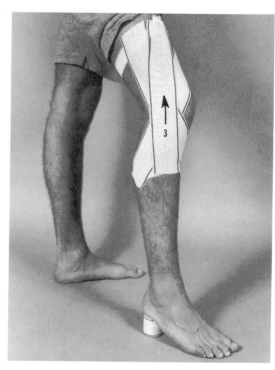

FIGURE 43.27f. Apply a vertical strip from midlateral calf to midlateral thigh.

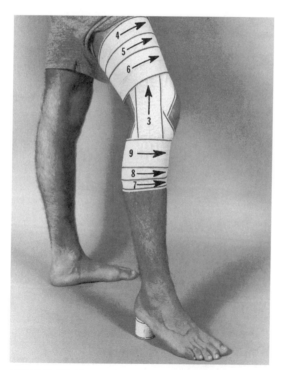

FIGURE 43.27g. Apply anchor strips to the thigh and calf.

POSITION

The athlete stands with heel of foot elevated on a 2-inch object, with knee in slight flexion.

PROCEDURE

1. Apply anchor strips at midthigh and midcalf, being careful not to apply them too tightly (Fig. 43.28a).
2. Place a 4-by-4-inch gauze or felt pad in the popliteal space.
3. Cross two strips in the popliteal area to form an X (Fig. 43.28b) and run the third strip up and down the posterior aspect of the leg. Begin the first strip in the midmedial calf and pass it through the popliteal area, ending on the midlateral upper thigh. Begin the second strip on the midlateral calf and pass it through the popliteal area to the midmedial upper thigh. These two strips form an X behind the knee. The third strip begins on the posterior calf and ends on the midposterior thigh (Fig. 43.28c).

4. Repeat this procedure as necessary, depending on the amount of restriction desired.
5. Apply anchors around the calf and thigh areas to secure longitudinal strips (Fig. 43.28d).

When placing anchor strips encircling the thigh and calf, have the athlete contract the thigh and calf musculature in turn as you encircle each area with elastic tape. If anchor strips are applied too tightly, the athlete may experience discomfort or muscle cramping.

Ankle Taping

Taping Following Lateral Inversion Sprains

The following method is used to tape the athlete's ankle following a lateral inversion sprain.

MATERIAL

heel and lace pads with lubrication (petrolatum)
tape adherent
1½-inch adhesive tape
underwrap (optional)

POSITION

The athlete sits on a table with knee extended and lower third of calf extended past the edge of the table. Athlete's foot is in dorsiflexion. The trainer faces the plantar aspect of the athlete's foot.

PROCEDURE

1. Apply heel and lace pads appropriately.
2. Apply two anchor strips. Place one at the base of the gastrocnemius heads and the second at the distal third of the longitudinal arch (Fig. 43.29a). Make sure that the base of the fifth metatarsal is not constricted.
3. Apply stirrup strips, beginning on the medial part of the calf. Pass under the foot (heel) and pull up on the lateral aspect of the leg with moderate tension (Figs. 43.29b, c). This direction of application results in slight eversion of the foot, thus counteracting the inversion sprain. Apply between three and six stirrups, depending on the amount of support desired.
4. Apply heel locks using one of several methods. One simple method is to begin the tape on the lateral lower part of the leg; cross the tibia at a 45-degree angle just above the medial malleolus; pass directly behind the ankle and down onto the lateral aspect of the calcaneus, under the foot; and pass up onto the top of the forefoot. Reverse this process for the medial lock: begin the heel lock strip on the top of the forefoot; cross in front of the lateral malleolus at a 45-degree angle, going downward, under the calcaneus and up behind the medial malleolus; cross the Achilles tendon and continue to the top of the forefoot (Fig. 43.29d). Usually, two or three heel locks in each direction are adequate.
5. Apply figure-eight strips with force to cause slight foot eversion. Start the tape strip just in front of the medial malleolus, passing the tape under the foot and up the outside of the foot. As the tape passes under the foot, use your free hand to evert the foot while applying the tape firmly. The foot should be flattened as well as everted to prevent the tape from encircling the foot too tightly. The "8s" continue on up and around the foot and around the lower leg (Fig. 43.29e). (The "8s" acquire their name from encircling both the foot and the lower leg in the figure-eight fashion.) Usually, two, three, or four "8s" produce adequate foot eversion. Encircling the foot too tightly distal to the base of the fifth metatarsal can result in foot discomfort. Applying the tape properly in conjunction with pressure to the foot, causing the foot to spread to a greater width, decreases the chances of this problem.
6. Apply fill-in strips to hold other tape components (stirrups, heel locks, figure-eights) in place. The fill-in strips encircle the lower part of the leg, the ankle area, and the foot with overlapping strips that

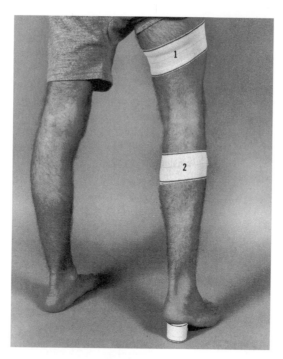

FIGURE 43.28a. Knee taping following hyperextension injury: begin taping with anchor strips at midthigh and midcalf.

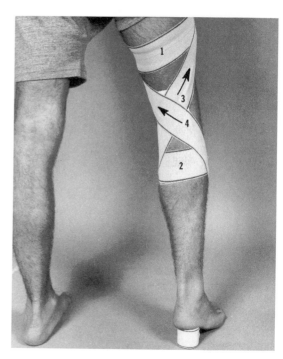

FIGURE 43.28b. Apply protective pad in popliteal space and then cover with two strips to form an X.

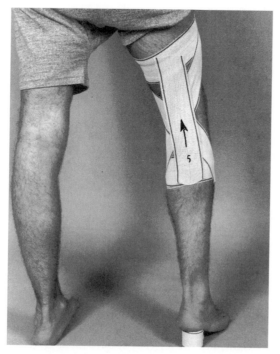

FIGURE 43.28c. Apply a third strip up and down the posterior aspect of the leg.

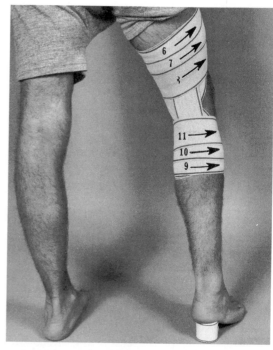

FIGURE 43.28d. Repeat the procedure as necessary; then secure with anchors around the calf and thigh areas.

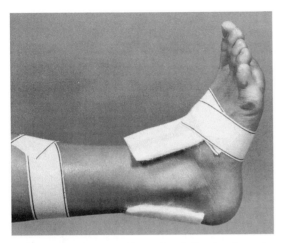

FIGURE 43.29a. Ankle taping following lateral inversion sprains: apply heel and lace pads, then apply two anchor strips.

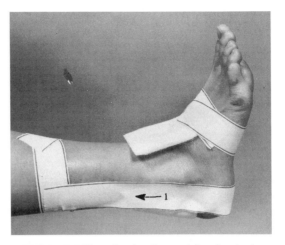

FIGURE 43.29b. Apply stirrup strips, beginning on the medial part of the calf and passing under the heel.

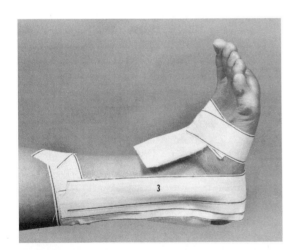

FIGURE 43.29c. Continue applying strips up on the lateral aspect of the leg; apply between three and six strips.

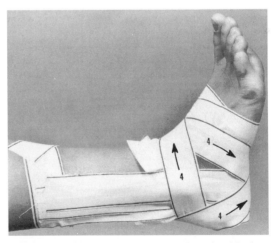

FIGURE 43.29d. Apply two to three heel locks in each direction.

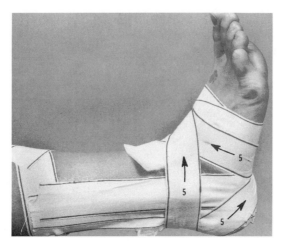

FIGURE 43.29e. Apply figure-eight strips with force to cause slight foot eversion.

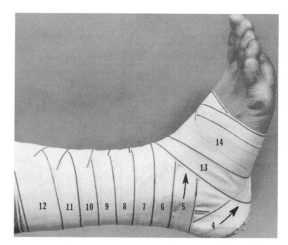

FIGURE 43.29f. Anchor tape components with fill-in strips, beginning at base stirrups and working up to proximal anchor.

encase the entire area with tape (Fig. 43.29f). They should begin at the bottom of the stirrups and encase the entire area upward to the proximal anchor.

Open Basketweave Taping

For taping that is done immediately after an injury, an open basketweave tape application is the preferred choice because it allows for swelling.

MATERIAL

heel pad with lubrication (petrolatum)
tape adherent
1½-inch adhesive tape
elastic bandage or compressive sleeve (optional)

POSITION

The athlete sits on a table with knee extended and lower third of calf extended past the table's edge; the foot is in dorsiflexion. The trainer faces the plantar aspect of the athlete's foot.

PROCEDURE

1. Apply heel pad appropriately. Apply two anchor strips. The first is placed at the base of the gastrocnemius head, three-fourths circumference with the opening in the front. The second anchor strip is applied at the level of the metatarsal heads. Apply the first stirrup, as posterior as possible, beginning on the medial aspect of the calf. Pass under the heel and pull up on the lateral aspect of the leg with moderate tension. A horizontal stirrup is added distally, beginning on the first metatarsal head portion of the anchor strip, going around the heel to the fifth metatarsal portion of the anchor strip (Fig. 43.30a).

2. Repeat the vertical stirrup, moving forward on the foot/ankle, overlapping one-half the previous strip. A second horizontal stirrup is added, moving proximal and overlapping one-half the previous strip (Fig. 43.30b).

3. Alternate vertical and horizontal stirrups are repeated, creating a weave effect. A ½- to 1-inch opening strip is left on the dorsum of the foot and lower leg, as the strips should only go three-fourths of the way around the foot and ankle. As the vertical strips are added, they will no longer create a weave effect. They should be added with one-half

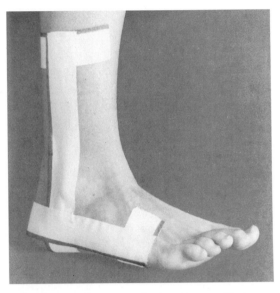

FIGURE 43.30a.   Open basketweave ankle taping: apply heel pad and two anchor strips; then apply a horizontal and a vertical stirrup.

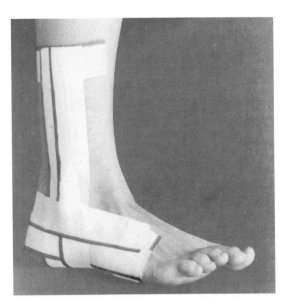

FIGURE 43.30b.   Repeat the vertical stirrup; then apply a second horizontal stirrup.

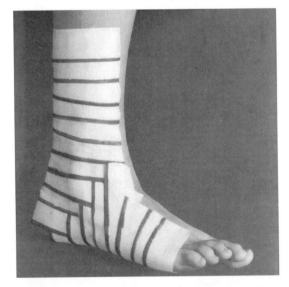

FIGURE 43.30c.   Continue alternating the vertical and horizontal stirrups, overlapping by one-half; lock ends with long strips.

overlapping the previous strip overlap and opening on the dorsum of the foot. The same general principle applies to the horizontal strips. Ends may be locked

with long strips, going from proximal to distal anchors or supplemented with an elastic bandage or compressive sleeve. Taping in this manner provides compression and allows for swelling. It is not a taping procedure for support (Fig. 43.30c).

Taping Following Eversion Sprains

Eversion sprains comprise only 5 to 10 percent of all ankle sprains. When taping for the medial (deltoid/eversion) sprain, follow the previously described routine except apply the stirrups and figure-eights in a neutral fashion, pulling equally on the medial and lateral strips. Do not pull strips in a lateral to medial direction, as this puts the ankle in an inverted position and could increase the likelihood of an inversion sprain.

Achilles Tendon Taping

Achilles tendon taping is designed to prevent extreme dorsiflexion of the ankle when Achilles tendinitis or a mild Achilles tendon strain is present.

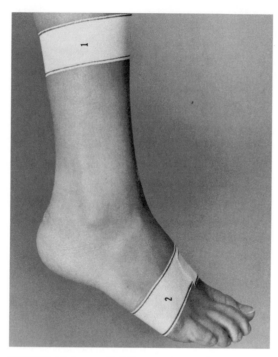

FIGURE 43.31a. Achilles tendon taping: begin procedure with two anchor strips, below the metatarsal head and at midcalf.

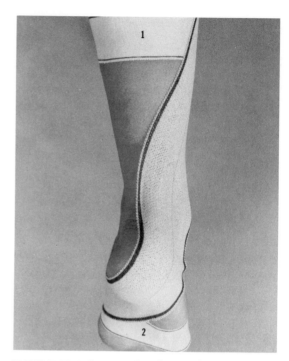

FIGURE 43.31b. Apply a longitudinal strip from the first metatarsal head to the gastrocnemius muscle.

MATERIAL

> tape adherent
> heel pad with lubricant (petrolatum)
> 2- or 3-inch elastic tape
> 1½-inch adhesive tape

POSITION

> The athlete lies prone on the table, with lower leg extending over the edge and the foot in relaxed plantar flexion. The trainer stands at the foot of the table.

PROCEDURE

1. Apply anchors below the metatarsal heads and at midcalf with 1½-inch tape (Fig. 43.31a).
2. Using 2- or 3-inch elastic tape, apply a longitudinal strip starting at the plantar surface of the first metatarsal head and ending at the lateral aspect of the gastrocnemius muscle (Fig. 43.31b).
3. Continuing to use the same material, apply a second longitudinal strip starting at the plantar surface of the fifth metatarsal head and ending at the medial aspect of the gastrocnemius muscle (Fig. 43.31c).
4. Center a third longitudinal strip between the two prior strips, beginning at the center of the metatarsal arch and ending at the posterior aspect of the calf (Fig. 43.31d).
5. Use circular strips of 2- or 3-inch elastic tape to close off the forefoot and lower part of the calf (Fig. 43.31e). Be sure these closing strips do not cause binding of the midfoot or calf.

Foot Taping

Taping of the Medial Longitudinal Arch

The purpose of longitudinal arch taping is to give support to the structures of the longitudinal arch. It is quite useful in treating (protecting) posterior tibial tendinitis, plantar fascitis, and other midfoot dysfunctions.

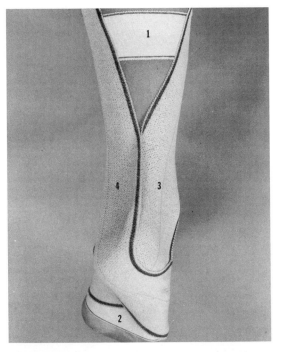

FIGURE 43.31c. Apply a second longitudinal strip, from the fifth metatarsal head to the gastrocnemius muscle.

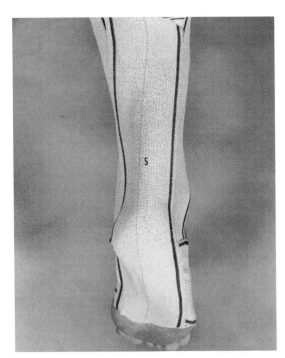

FIGURE 43.31d. Center a third longitudinal strip between the first two, from the metatarsal arch to the posterior aspect of the calf.

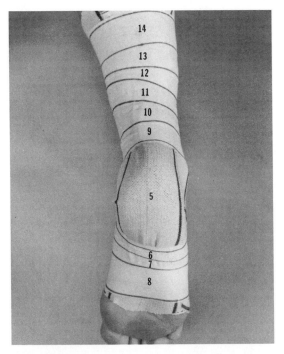

FIGURE 43.31e. Using circular strips, close off the forefoot and the lower part of the calf.

MATERIAL

tape adherent
1-inch elastic tape
1½-inch adhesive tape
underwrap (optional)

POSITION

The athlete sits on a table, with the ankle in a slightly dorsiflexed and neutral position during the procedure.

PROCEDURE

1. Prepare the area to be taped. The sole of the foot must be clean and dry before applying tape adherent. Sometimes underwrap is applied to protect the hair on the dorsum of the foot, but it should not extend beyond the anchor strip.
2. Apply anchor strips to the skin at the heads of the metatarsals, encircling the forefoot (Fig. 43.32a). The tape must be wrinkle free to avoid skin irritation and must not be too tight.

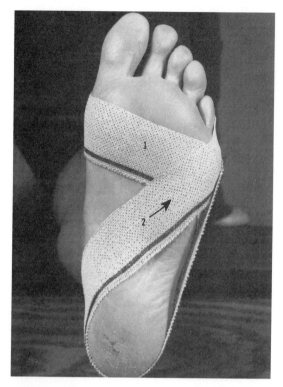

FIGURE 43.32a. Taping of the medial longitudinal arch: apply anchor strips.

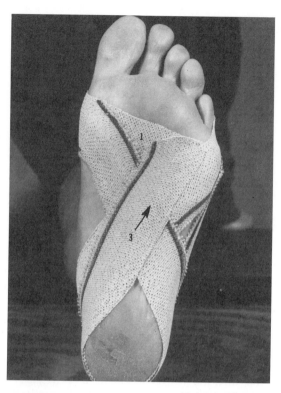

FIGURE 43.32b. Apply supportive strips to the longitudinal arch.

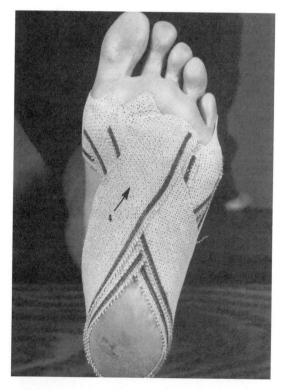

FIGURE 43.32c. Repeat the procedure until the entire foot is covered.

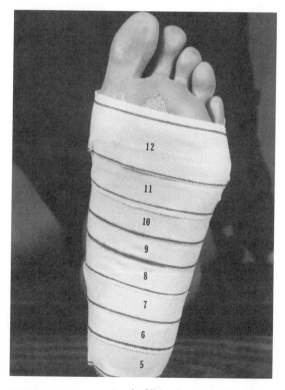

FIGURE 43.32d. Apply fill-ins by encircling the forefoot with strips of tape.

3. Apply supportive strips to the longitudinal arch (Figs. 43.32b, c), usually beginning at the fifth metatarsal head, wrapping around the heel not too tightly, and returning to the head of either the fifth or the first metatarsal. Repeat this procedure until the entire sole of the foot is covered.

4. Apply fill-ins with strips of tape that encircle the forefoot, overlapping one-third to one-half to prevent spacing between layers of tape (Fig. 43.32d). These strips are usually placed from a lateral to medial direction to give added support to the medial plantar surface of the foot. Be sure strips that encircle the midfoot do not cause binding.

Great Toe Taping

Taping of the great toe is designed to decrease range of motion at the first metatarsophalangeal (MTP) joint and to support injured structures. Depending on the application, the taping can restrict abduction, flexion, or extension.

MATERIAL

tape adherent
1-inch adhesive tape

POSITION

Athlete sits on a table, with knee in full extension and foot off the edge of table.

PROCEDURE

1. Begin the taping by applying tape adherent to the dorsum and plantar aspects of the forefoot and great toe. Tape directly to the skin for maximum protection.

2. Place an anchor around the forefoot, encircling the metatarsals (Fig. 43.33a). Allow the tape to conform to the contours of the body part to prevent wrinkles and binding.

3. Apply half figure-eight taping by starting at the superior medial aspect of the first MTP joint and encircle the great toe, ending on the superior aspect of the second MTP joint (Figs. 43.33b, c). Repeat two to three times. This technique

prevents flexion/abduction. To prevent extension, begin on the inferior medial aspect of the first MTP joint and encircle the great toe (Fig. 43.33d).

4. Close in the toe and forefoot with overlapping strips applied distal to proximal (Fig. 43.33e).

Supportive Pads for the Foot

Frequently, pads rather than tape can be used for support, especially for the lower extremity. Pads can be made from felt, foam rubber, or similar material. Felt has an advantage over foam in that it is less compressible. Sorbothane is another popular padding material. While Sorbothane is fairly noncompressible, it is more expensive than felt.

A longitudinal arch pad can be used to support the arch in cases of foot pronation (Fig. 43.34a). It is therefore useful in treat-

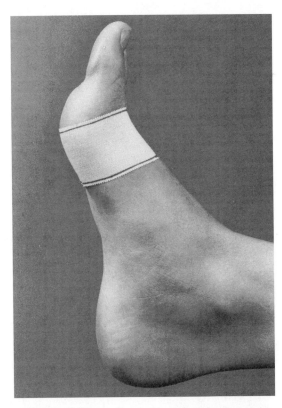

FIGURE 43.33a. Great toe taping: begin procedure by placing an anchor around the forefoot, encircling the metatarsals.

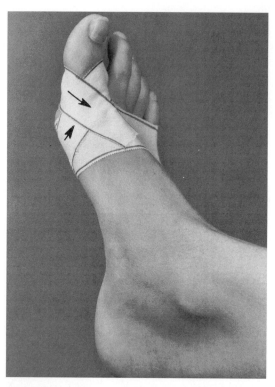

FIGURE 43.33b. Apply half figure-eight taping at the first MTP joint and encircle the great toe.

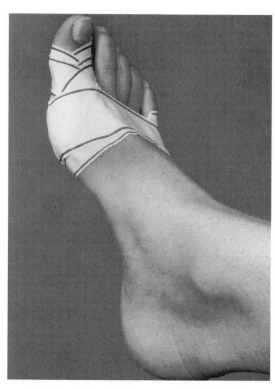

FIGURE 43.33c. To prevent extension, repeat the figure-eight procedure two to three times.

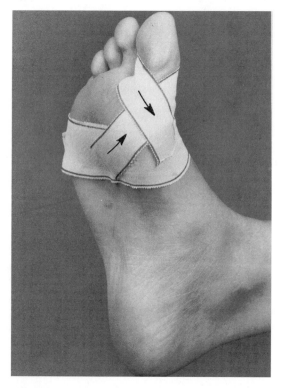

FIGURE 43.33d. Begin figure-eight taping of the first MTP joint and encircle the great toe.

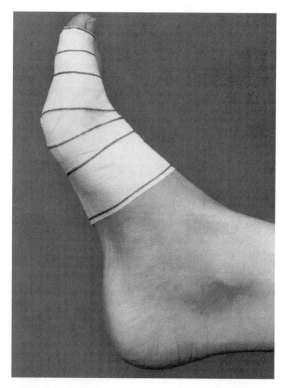

FIGURE 43.33e. Close in the toe and forefoot with overlapping strips applied distal to proximal.

ing shin splints, plantar fasciitis, and so forth.

Metatarsal cookies can take the pressure off metatarsal heads, and therefore are useful in treating metatarsalgia (Fig. 43.34b).

Heel pads may be used to elevate the heel, decreasing the tension placed on the Achilles tendon and plantar fascia in athletes with Achilles tendinitis or plantar fascitis (Fig. 43.34c).

Pads may also be used to take the pressure off a particularly painful area such as bone spurs or bone bruises (Fig. 43.34d).

To make supportive pads, follow these steps.

1. Using a magic marker or liquid adherent, draw an outline of the area to be supported—for example, the longitudinal arch—on the bottom of the athlete's foot (Fig. 43.35a).
2. Immediately place the foam, felt, or Sorbothane on the outlined area. The imprint of the drawing will remain.
3. Cut along the imprinted line and bevel the edges. This gives the padding a gradual, rather than sharp, drop-off in line with the foot's normal contour (Fig. 43.35b).
4. Covering the felt or foam pad with moleskin helps give it longevity.
5. Hold the pad in place with circular strips of tape (Fig. 43.35c).

ELASTIC BANDAGING PROCEDURES

Properly applied elastic bandages have several uses in sports medicine, including the following:

- They provide compression to retard and/or reduce swelling and hemorrhage following injury.
- They secure ice packs, dressings, splints, and protective pads.
- They provide mild support of joints.
- They provide support of large muscle groups.
- They restrict movement.

The wraps are available in widths of 2, 3, 4, and 6 inches and regular (generally 5 yards) and double lengths (10 yards). It is important to select the proper size wrap for the area. For example, a 2-inch regular wrap is best for the hand and wrist, while the 6-inch bandage is used to wrap the knee, thigh, shoulder, and groin. Extra long wraps are useful in supporting the hip, thigh, and knee.

Elastic bandages are manufactured with several grades of tension. Tension depends on the amount of rubber in the fabric and the type of weave. Mild tension is usually used for first-aid applications. Stronger tension is used to support large muscle groups.

Application/Removal Guidelines

Some basic guidelines should be followed when using elastic bandages.

1. Tape adherent may be sprayed onto the skin to prevent slippage.
2. Wraps should be anchored distally in the part being wrapped. The end of the wrap is covered with the first turn.
3. In most cases, the bandage is applied in a distal to proximal direction.
4. The wrap should be overlapped by one-half its width on each turn.
5. Do not leave skin exposed between strips.
6. Make the bandage contour to the part with equal tension on both the upper and lower edges.
7. For the greatest support and compression, take out most of the stretch in the wrap as it is applied. If less support is needed, apply with less stretch.
8. Fasten the wrap with clips only if the athlete is not going to participate (Fig. 43.36). Use tape if the athlete intends to participate (Figs. 43.37a, b).
9. The wrap should be comfortable to wear. A wrap that is too tight may cause the extremity to swell.
10. In removing tape or clips, be careful not to damage the bandage.

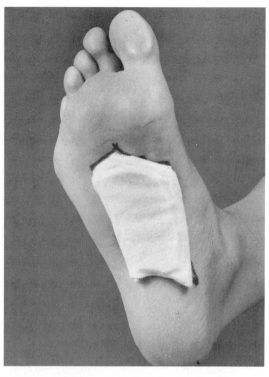

FIGURE 43.34a. A longitudinal arch pad.

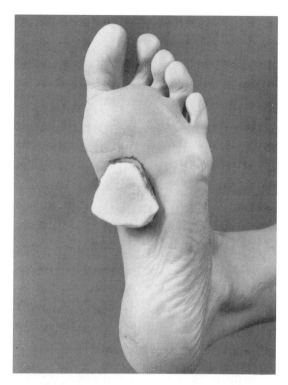

FIGURE 43.34b. Metatarsal cookies relieve pressure.

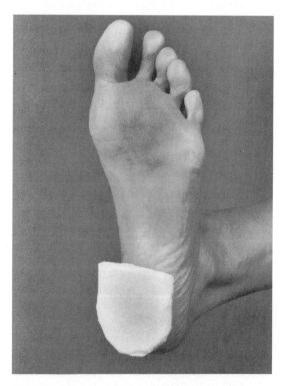

FIGURE 43.34c. Heel pads decrease tension.

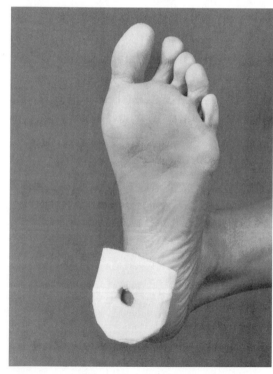

FIGURE 43.34d. Pads relieve pain from bone spurs.

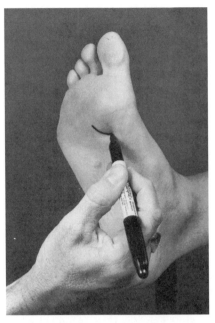

FIGURE 43.35a. To make supportive pads, begin by outlining the area to be supported.

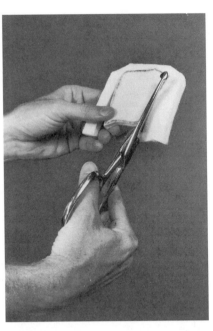

FIGURE 43.35b. Cut along the imprinted line and bevel the edges; this gives the padding a gradual slope, in line with the athlete's foot.

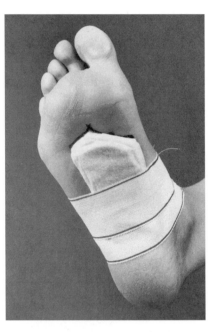

FIGURE 43.35c. Secure the pad in place with circular strips of tape.

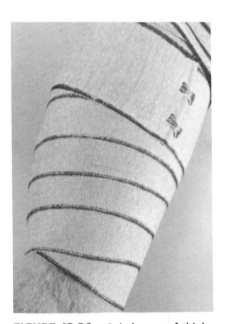

FIGURE 43.36. Spiral wrap of thigh with end secured by clips.

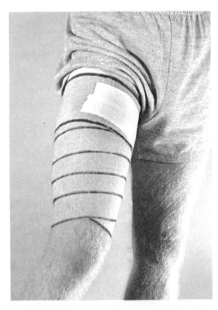

FIGURE 43.37a. Secure end of spiral wrap with adhesive tape applied halfway around the thigh.

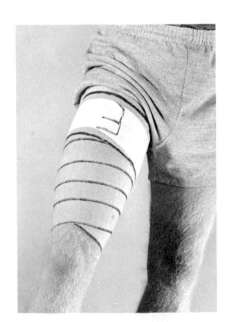

FIGURE 43.37b. Apply more adhesive tape in opposite direction to completely secure spiral wrap for activity.

11. The soiled bandage may be laundered in mild soap and warm water. It can be dried in mild heat in the dryer or in the open air. Both hot water and hot air drying tend to reduce the effectiveness of the rubber and shorten the life of the bandage.

Common Application Methods

The most common types of bandages are the spiral, figure-eight, spica, and combinations of these. Each bandage type has advantages for certain situations.

Spiral Wrap

The spiral wrap is simply anchored and spiraled around the area, overlapping each turn by one-half the width of the wrap (Fig. 43.38). It is quick and easy to apply and can cover a large area.

The wrap can be used with an ice pack as a first-aid measure. The anchor and first layer may be moistened with water and applied under the ice pack (Figs. 43.39a, b).

This manner of application provides compression directly to the skin and makes the cold pack more comfortable. The major disadvantage is that the spiral wrap tends to slip if the athlete is active.

The spiral wrap is effective over felt strip splints as a first-aid measure on the field for care of injuries such as knee sprains (Figs. 43.40a, b), or it may be used over a taping procedure to give additional support.

Figure-Eight Wrap

The figure-eight wrap is a very good bandage for many areas of the body, especially over large muscle groups such as the thigh, knee, and calf. With some practice, it is easy to apply and does not slip as easily as the spiral wrap.

The wrap is anchored, and the first turn is taken at a sharp angle (Fig. 43.41a). The returning turn is taken at a downward angle (Fig. 43.41b). The additional loops in the pattern overlap the previous loops by half the width of the wrap (Fig. 43.41c). This pattern is continued from the distal to the

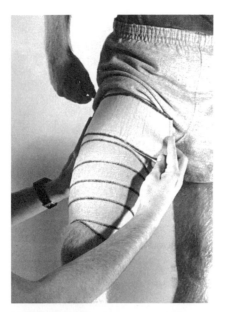

FIGURE 43.38. The spiral 4-inch elastic wrap on the thigh begins at the distal thigh and is covered by the completed wrap.

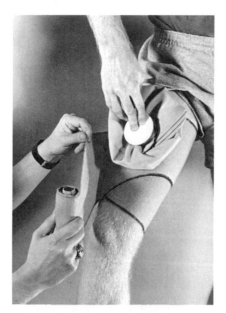

FIGURE 43.39a. Spiral wrap applied to secure an ice bag to the thigh.

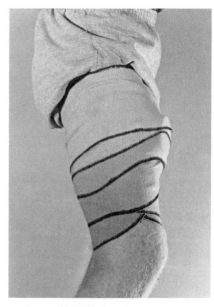

FIGURE 43.39b. Completed spiral wrap securing ice bag over thigh.

proximal portion of the body segment (Fig. 43.41d). The wrap should be secured with nonelastic tape at the top and bottom. The top tape may be carried partially onto the skin to prevent slippage (Fig. 43.41e). The securing tapes are applied in two pieces, each going only half the way around the extremity—front to back and back to front—thus preventing compromise of the circulation when the muscles expand during contraction.

The figure-eight wrap can also be used for the knee, thigh and calf, forearm, elbow, and upper arm. When applying the wrap to the knee or elbow, it is better to anchor low, carry the first turn over the joint (Figs. 43.42a–h), anchor at the top, and work the pattern down to the original anchor. Starting at the bottom and ending at the bottom may help prevent slippage.

The figure-eight wrap provides excellent compression. If adherent is not available, or if the athlete has a sensitivity to the adherent, a piece of white tape, folded lengthwise with the adhesive side out, can be used under the wrap (Figs. 43.43a, b).

Spica Wrap

The spica wrap is basically a figure-eight in which one loop is substantially larger than the other loop. This wrap is used in support of the foot/ankle, shoulder, and groin areas (Figs. 43.44a–d).

The wrap is anchored on the extremity and carried over the joint and around the body. Normally, at least two sets of loops are used. More loops can be used if additional support is desired.

Care must be taken not to apply the wrap too tightly. Also, the direction in which the spica is applied is important in obtaining maximal support. For example, with an adductor strain (groin), the first loop, after the anchor, should be pulled around the outside of the leg, across, up, and over the front of the abdomen to the opposite hip (Figs. 43.45a–f), pulling the leg into the groin, not away from it.

The opposite is true in supporting the muscles of the buttocks. The initial large loop is pulled from the leg, across, up, and over the back of the buttocks (Figs.

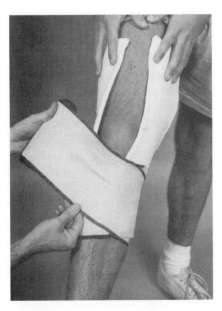

FIGURE 43.40a. Spiral wrap applied over felt strips as a splint for the knee.

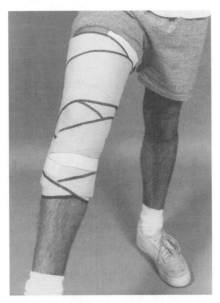

FIGURE 43.40b. Completed spiral wrap securing felt strips over the knee.

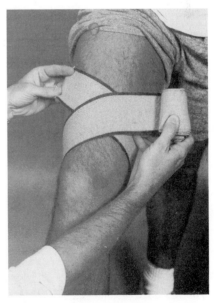

FIGURE 43.41a. To anchor the figure-eight wrap of the thigh, position the beginning of the wrap so the completed wrap will cover it.

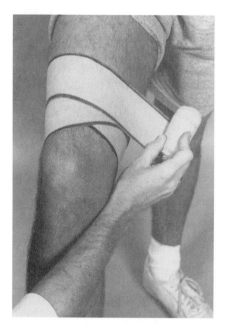

FIGURE 43.41b. The end of the first turn in the figure-eight wrap for the thigh.

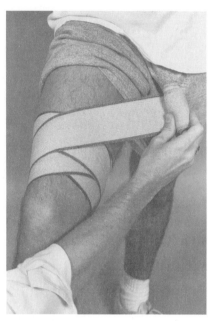

FIGURE 43.41c. The beginning of the second turn of the thigh figure-eight wrap.

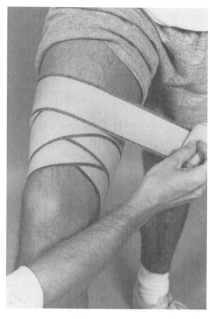

FIGURE 43.41d. Completion of the second turn of the thigh figure-eight wrap.

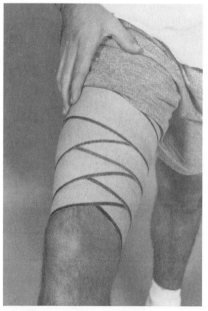

FIGURE 43.41e. Continue the figure-eight pattern up the thigh and end it at the top. Secure it by tape or clips.

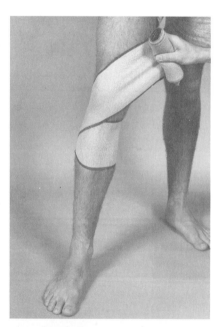

FIGURE 43.42a. To start the figure-eight wrap for the knee, anchor it below the knee and carry it up over the kneecap at a sharp angle.

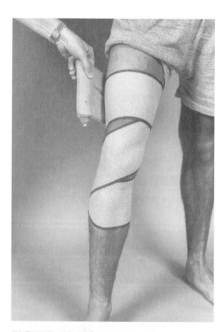

FIGURE 43.42b. Anchor the knee figure-eight around the thigh, thus providing anchors above and below the knee.

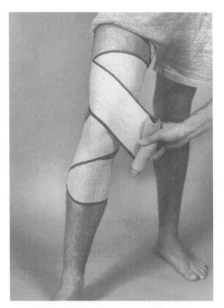

FIGURE 43.42c. Start the figure-eight pattern back down the leg by pulling the beginning of the first turn down at a sharp angle.

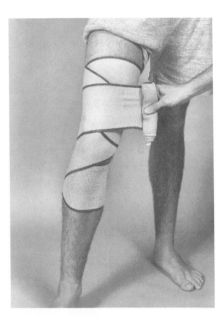

FIGURE 43.42d. Pull up at a sharp angle the end of the first turn of the knee figure-eight.

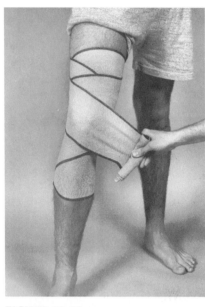

FIGURE 43.42e. The beginning of the second turn follows the first turn, overlapping by at least one half width at the same angle.

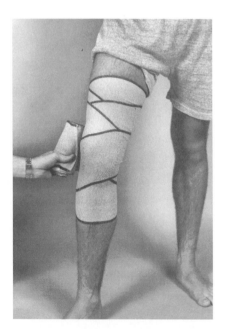

FIGURE 43.42f. Complete the end of the second turn by following the upward angle of the first turn and overlapping by at least one half turn.

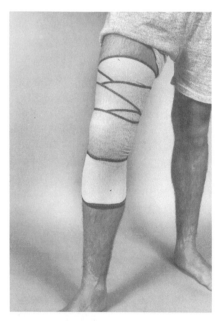

FIGURE 43.42g. Continue the knee figure-eight pattern down to the bottom anchor and complete it below the knee.

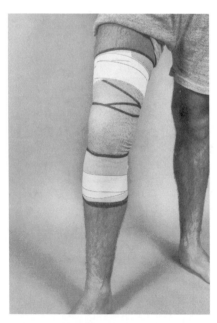

FIGURE 43.42h. Secure the knee figure-eight with adhesive tape over the top and bottom. The top tape can override onto the skin.

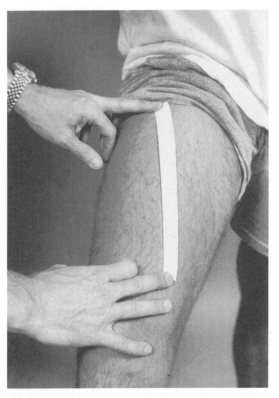

FIGURE 43.43a. Folded adhesive tape can be used in place of spray adhesive.

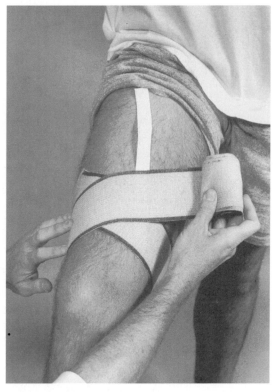

FIGURE 43.43b. Apply the wrap over the adhesive tape. The folded tape helps to prevent slippage of the wrap.

43.46a–d). This maneuver pulls the buttocks into the midline of the body. In a shoulder spica, a soft pad may be applied under the armpit to avoid chafing. In a hip spica, additional support for a groin strain may be given by incorporating a felt pad fitted into the groin.

Combinations of the preceding wraps are sometimes used for special situations. The 4 S wrap is such a combination, used as a first-aid measure for many shoulder injuries. This wrap requires a double-length, 4- or 6-inch wrap, or two or three regular length wraps. This bandage incorporates the spica bandage, the sling, the swathe, and stabilizing acromioclavicular joint straps (Figs. 43.47a–i). An ice bag may be added where necessary. The wrap supports the entire shoulder area and is especially useful when a sling is not available.

The foot/ankle pressure wrap is a combination of wrapping techniques used to retard and/or prevent swelling and hemorrhage following injury. A pressure gradient is created by applying more pressure at the toe of the bandage and gradually decreasing the pressure as the wrap continues proximally (Figs. 43.48a–h). This gradient of pressure diminishes the accumulation of swelling in the foot and toes.

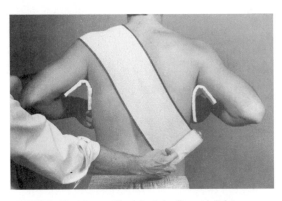

FIGURE 43.44a. The clavicle figure-eight wrap is used for emergency care of clavicle fractures. The athlete places his hands on his hips and throws his shoulders back. Start the wrap on one shoulder and carry it down and across the back.

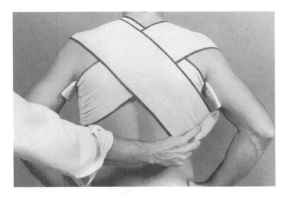

FIGURE 43.44b. Pull the wrap under the opposite shoulder, around and across the back, following this pattern at least twice.

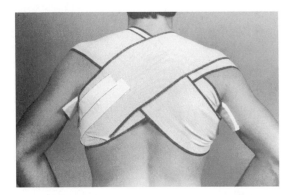

FIGURE 43.44c. Secure the completed clavicle figure-eight with tape.

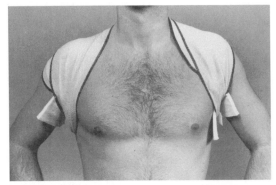

FIGURE 43.44d. In the completed clavicle figure-eight wrap, note the padding under the arms to prevent discomfort.

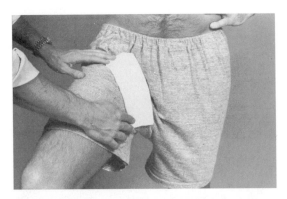

FIGURE 43.45a. A felt pad fitted for the area can provide additional support for a groin (adductor) strain. This is held in place by a hip spica wrap.

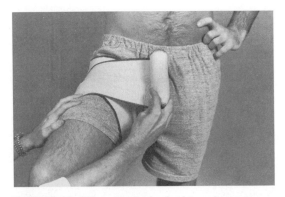

FIGURE 43.45b. To apply the hip spica wrap, pull it from the lateral aspect to the medial, pulling the leg into the groin.

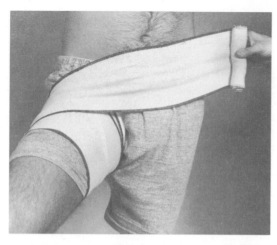

FIGURE 43.45c. After anchoring, carry the first large loop of the hip spica up and over the groin, onto the opposite hip.

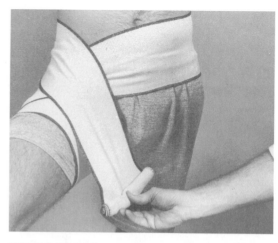

FIGURE 43.45d. Complete the first large loop of the hip spica by pulling the wrap around, behind the waist and down firmly into the groin.

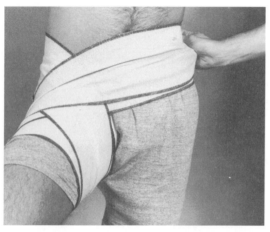

FIGURE 43.45e. The second loop of the hip spica wrap follows the pattern of the first, overlapping by at least one half width.

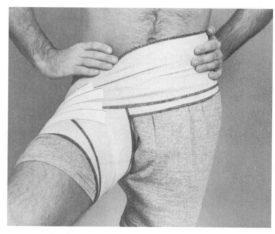

FIGURE 43.45f. The completed hip spica wrap for an adductor strain.

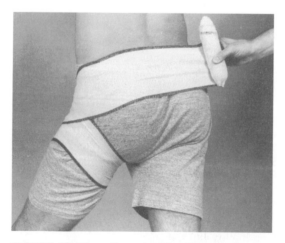

FIGURE 43.46a. To anchor the hip spica for a buttocks strain, pull the wrap from lateral to medial, into the midline of the body.

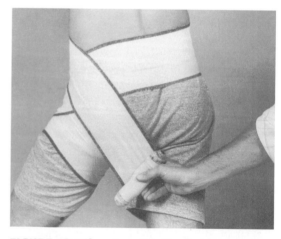

FIGURE 43.46b. Complete the first large loop of the hip spica around the waist, over and into the buttocks.

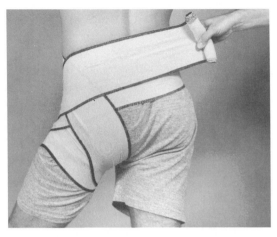

FIGURE 43.46c. The second large loop of the hip spica overlaps the first by at least one half width.

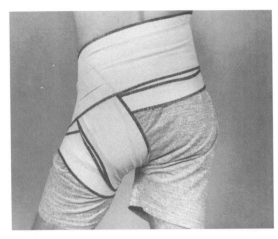

FIGURE 43.46d. The completed hip spica, supporting the buttocks. This wrap can be used to hold dressings over abrasions.

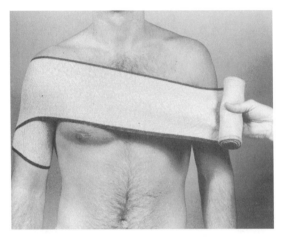

FIGURE 43.47a. The 4 S wrap starts with a shoulder spica, normally pulled from the lateral to the medial aspects.

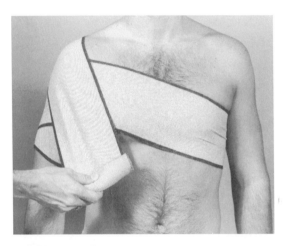

FIGURE 43.47b. Completion of the first shoulder spica in the 4 S wrap.

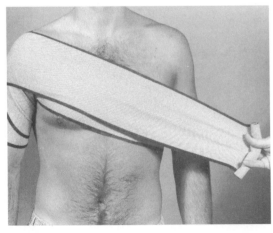

FIGURE 43.47c. Beginning of second shoulder spica in the 4 S wrap.

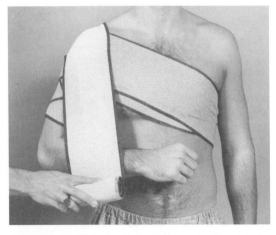

FIGURE 43.47d. Pull the wrap over the acromioclavicular joint and down under the bent forearm. This supports the joint and a sling.

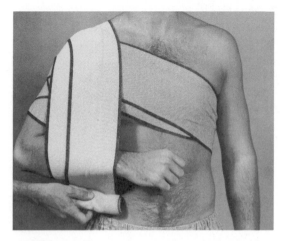

FIGURE 43.47e.   Apply a second sling loop.

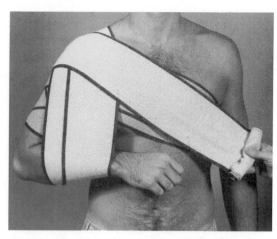

FIGURE 43.47f.   After completing the second sling loop, pull the wrap down across the chest to start the swathe portion of the wrap.

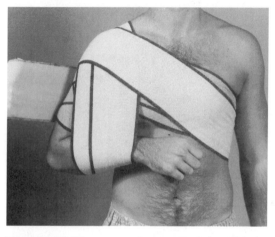

FIGURE 43.47g.   Start the swathe portion by pulling the wrap around the back.

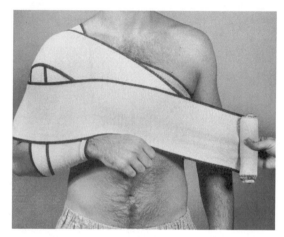

FIGURE 43.47h.   Complete the swathe portion of the wrap by going around the injured arm and around the chest (usually twice).

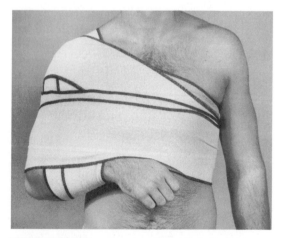

FIGURE 43.47i.   The completed 4 S shoulder wrap. It can include an ice bag and be secured with tape.

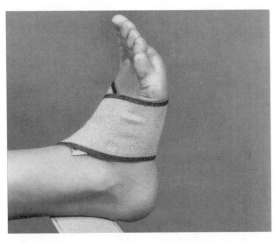

FIGURE 43.48a. Anchor the foot/ankle pressure wrap just behind the toes. Start the spica by pulling the wrap low across the medial aspect of the foot and behind the heel.

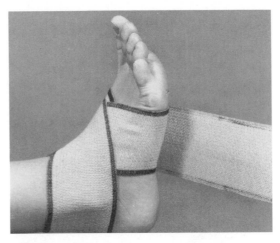

FIGURE 43.48b. Complete the first spica by covering the low, lateral aspect of the foot, then repeat.

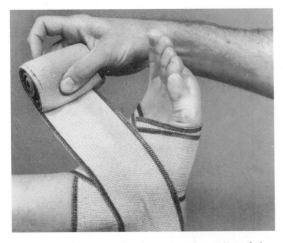

FIGURE 43.48c. After covering the point of the heel, bring the wrap up over the front of the ankle.

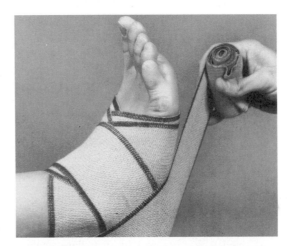

FIGURE 43.48d. Then pull the wrap behind the ankle diagonally down over the lateral aspect of the heel. This is similar to a heel lock in ankle taping.

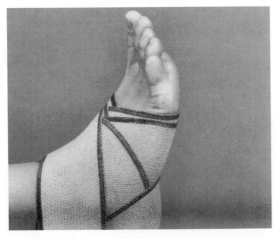

FIGURE 43.48e. Pull the wrap under the heel, over the high front of the ankle to start the inside heel lock.

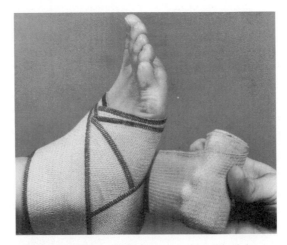

FIGURE 43.48f. Pull the second heel lock behind the heel diagonally down across the medial aspect of the ankle.

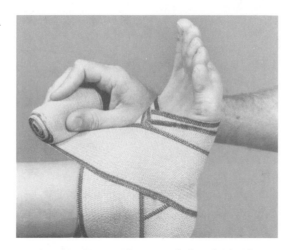 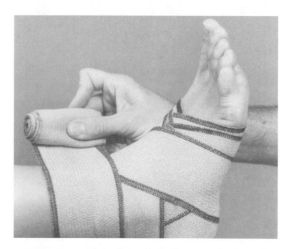

FIGURE 43.48g. After completing the heel locks, bring the wrap up over the lateral aspect of the foot and over the high front of the ankle.

FIGURE 43.48h. Complete the wrap by loosely spiraling the end of the wrap just above the ankle.

SUGGESTED READINGS

Arnheim, D. D. *Modern Principles of Athletic Training: The Science of Sports Medicine: Injury Prevention, Causation, and Management*, 6th ed. St. Louis: Times Mirror/ Mosby College Publishing, 1985, pp. 318–338.

Beiersdorf's Medical Program. *Manual of Taping and Strapping Techniques*. Agoura, Calif.: Macmillan.

Johnson & Johnson. *Athletic Uses of Adhesive Tape*, 1981.

Kulund, D. N., ed. *The Injured Athlete*, 2d ed. Philadelphia: J. B. Lippincott, 1988, pp. 180–183.

Laughman, R. K., T. A. Carr, E. Y. Chao, et al. "Three-Dimensional Kinematics of the Taped Ankle before and after Exercise." *American Journal of Sports Medicine* 8 (1980): 425–431.

Roy, S., and R. Irvin. *Sports Medicine: Prevention, Evaluation, Management, and Rehabilitation*. Englewood Cliffs, N.J.: Prentice-Hall, 1983, pp. 55–77.

Vaes, P., H. De Boeck, F. Handelberg, et al. "Comparative Radiologic Study of the Influence of Ankle Joint Bandages on Ankle Stability." *American Journal of Sports Medicine* 13 (1985): 46–50.

Viljakka, T. "Mechanics of Knee and Ankle Bandages." *Acta Orthopaedica Scandinavica* 57 (1986): 54–58.

APPENDIX: CRUTCHES

How to Adjust Crutches

- Adjust the overall length so that the shoulder portion of the crutch is approximately 1 to 1½ inches—about 2 to 3 fingers width—below the armpit (axilla) of the athlete while he or she is standing erect.
- Adjust the handgrip portion so that the elbow is bent approximately 30 degrees.
- Place the handgrip so that it is about even with the top of the athlete's hip line (the greater trochanter).

How to Use Crutches

The Non-Weight-Bearing Case

The rule is: "Crutches and the involved (injured) leg always go together."

1. The athlete begins by standing erect on the noninvolved leg and crutches.
2. The athlete leans forward slightly, placing both crutches and the involved leg forward approximately 12 inches (see Fig. 43A.1).
   Note: The shoulder pieces are held tightly to the athlete's side, and the weight is absorbed by the hands. The athlete never leans on the crutches with the arm piece pressing up into the armpit.
3. The athlete steps through with the non-involved leg as if taking a normal step.
4. The athlete repeats steps 1 and 2 above.

Going Up and Down Stairs

1. The athlete begins in the same manner as described above in steps 1 and 2.
2. To go *up* the stairs, the athlete *leads with*

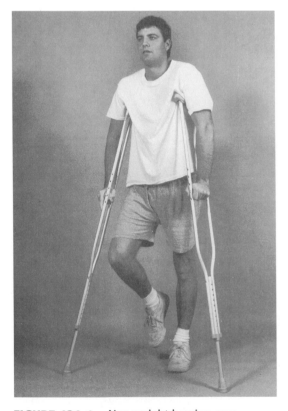

FIGURE 43A.1. Non-weight-bearing case.

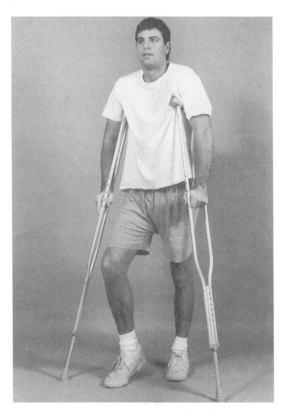

FIGURE 43A.2. Partial-weight bearing case.

the noninvolved leg first—remember by, "Go to heaven—good leg goes first."

3. To go *down* the stairs, the athlete *leads with the crutches and involved leg first*—remember by, "Go to hell—bad leg goes first."

4. If a handrail is available, the athlete may hold the rail with one hand, place both crutches in the other hand, and then go up and down the stairs as described in steps 2 and 3.

The Partial Weight-Bearing Case—Progressing to Full Weight Bearing

1. The athlete begins in the same manner as described in steps 1 and 2, "The Non-Weight-Bearing Case."

2. When the crutches and the involved leg go forward together, the athlete should place as much weight as tolerable on the injured foot and absorb the rest of the weight on his or her hands (Fig. 43A.2).

3. The athlete should be reminded to use a proper heel-toe walking pattern where the heel strikes first and then weight is shifted to the ball of the foot.

The rule is: "Do not walk on your toes."

One Crutch or a Cane

- The crutch or cane is placed on the opposite side of the involved extremity.
- The crutch or cane always goes forward with the involved extremity.
- The athlete should *not lean or list* too heavily on the crutch or cane. If there is a tendency to do so, then, the athlete should use two crutches.

44

Protective Equipment

CHAPTER OUTLINE

OBJECTIVES FOR CHAPTER 44

After reading this chapter, the student should be able to:
1. Explain the basic principles of protective equipment, including its intent, risks, construction materials, design, and proper maintenance.
2. Know the rules that govern the use of protective equipment and which agencies to consult if further information is needed.
3. Select or create protective equipment for the head and upper and lower extremities.

INTRODUCTION

The functions of protective equipment in sports are to prevent injury and to prevent reinjury. Chapter 44 discusses the general principles of protective equipment, including selection and fitting, maintenance, design and fabrication, construction materials, cost, regulations, and education of the athlete. The chapter also provides descriptions of protective equipment for the head, face, torso, and upper and lower extremities. ■

PRINCIPLES OF PROTECTIVE EQUIPMENT

Objectives of Protective Equipment

Protective equipment in sports should be designed to prevent injury and to protect injured parts against further injury. The ideal protective equipment causes minimal functional interference and is not harmful to other participants. Practicality dictates that such equipment be simple to fit and maintain, be durable and reliable, and not be prohibitively expensive.

Protection for Injury Prevention

The hazards demonstrated in each individual sport dictate the need for specific types of protection. In contact sports such as football and hockey, exposed and vulnerable areas must be protected from impact with the surface or other players. Appropriate pads must protect the primary contact points such as the shoulder, arms, and the anterior aspect of the leg. Vital areas such as the head, eyes, neck, kidneys, and genitalia must have priority for protection. In sports using sticks such as lacrosse and field hockey, players must wear protective pads to cushion inadvertent blows.

High-velocity, low-mass hazards are seen in sports that use balls or pucks, such as baseball, lacrosse, hockey, and racquet sports. Protection from these missiles is gained with helmets, face masks, and various types of eye protection for athletes with and without glasses. Dental protection by mouth guards is mandatory in football and is recommended in other sports.

The injurious effects of rigid protective equipment such as the football helmet are still a problem, because protective equipment can be abused either by players who use the equipment as a "weapon" against their opponent, or by players who take dangerous risks and rely on the equipment to protect them.

The prophylactic value of bracing or taping at susceptible joints such as the knee and ankle is well established, but the type of brace or manner of taping remains variable. The relationship of footwear to turf fixation has been recognized, and the type of shoe surface has to be tailored according to the playing surface. The condition of the playing surface also affects the choice of footwear. For example, the wear factors of the decreased impact absorption and interface friction of artificial surfaces must be considered when selecting footwear.

Protection for Injured Parts

When medical supervision indicates the athlete can return to sports activity with appropriate protection, the protective equipment is often individually chosen by training personnel. In football, improved impact absorption helmet linings provide protection after a concussion. Commercial or individualized cervical collars or straps can help prevent recurrent neck strain, but they must be properly fitted to be safe and of value. Contused areas on the body can be protected with customized resilient padding of semirigid or firm materials which can disperse the impact.

Taping procedures can restrict joint mobility. Common examples are protection against hyperextension of the knee, attempted control of rotational stresses on the knee, prevention of full abduction and external rotation of the shoulder, and limitation of either flexion or extension of the elbow. Shoulder pad extensions, as well as various types of hip padding, are available for injured areas on the rib cage and pelvic bones. All materials must be sufficiently padded on the exterior to prevent injury to other participants.

Selection and Fitting of Protective Equipment

Selection and fitting of protective equipment should be a combined effort by the equipment manager, trainer, physician, coach, and parents. Because correctly fitting equipment is of the utmost importance for injury prevention and protection, standards of correct fit should be set and adhered to. Incorrectly fitting equipment can be hazardous. Athletes will often want to wear smaller, less restrictive equipment because it makes them look better or feel faster. This practice should be discouraged. To fit athletic equipment correctly, the following factors should be considered: size, sport and position, strength, age and physical development, and skill levels.

Size

Athletic equipment that is too small or large for an athlete does not offer adequate protection (Fig. 44.1). In fitting equipment in relation to size, the person doing the measuring must first measure the area to be protected and then visualize the athlete with the pads in place. Once the appropriate size has been selected, the trainer should have the athlete try on the pads and then inspect them to ensure that they actually protect the area specified.

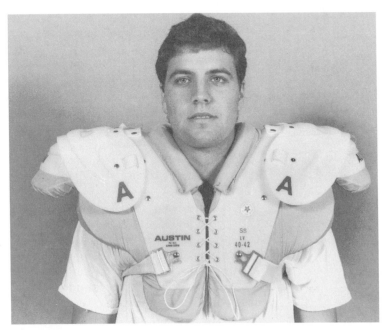

FIGURE 44.1.   Ill-fitting equipment does not offer adequate protection against injury.

Sport and Position

Equipment for sports such as ice hockey, lacrosse, football, and baseball is designed for the demands of a specific position—for example, goalie, midfielder, quarterback, and catcher. Individual needs should be evaluated closely in selecting equipment for a specific sport position.

Strength

Evaluating an athlete's strength further determines what size of equipment should be used. If the equipment is too small and restrictive, the strong athlete could be compromised; the inverse could be true of large and bulky equipment used by the weaker athlete.

Age and Physical Development

A tremendous array of equipment is manufactured for athletes of different ages and developmental stages. This equipment can be adapted for use by athletes at all levels of competition.

Skill Levels

Some equipment is manufactured to adapt to different skill levels. Equipment for the professional athlete may not be suitable for the amateur athlete.

Maintenance of Protective Equipment

Daily monitoring of all protective equipment most effectively prevents injuries due to faulty equipment. Schedules for equipment inspection, repair, and disposal are advisable.

Responsibilities for maintaining equipment should be defined and adhered to for each sport. Daily inspections, cleaning, drying, storage, and repair are maintenance procedures for which athletes can be made responsible, especially when trained maintenance people are not always available.

Although athletes and their parents are expected to assist in equipment mainte-nance, trained personnel should be designated to monitor this area. The maintenance person, along with the rest of the sports staff, should constantly watch for ill-fitting or damaged equipment and establish a weekly schedule for inspection and repair of all equipment. A weekly maintenance schedule for football helmets, for example, consists of the following program:

■ Visually inspect and stress shells to locate defects.
■ Check padding for wear and deterioration.
■ Check air cells for leaks and proper inflation levels.
■ Check face masks for bends or cracks. Also inspect screws and grommets that secure the mask to the helmet for deterioration and looseness.
■ Check chin straps and buckles for wear and looseness.
■ Send helmets to a reconditioner for inspection, certification (if required), and overall repair annually.

Football shoulder pads are another example of equipment that should be inspected and repaired in accordance with the following maintenance program:

■ Inspect the shell for cracks and loose rivets.
■ Inspect straps, laces, and buckles for wear and deterioration.
■ Inspect pads for defects in the padding and its covering; test the shock absorption capacity of the padding.
■ Inspect cantilevers to make sure they are functioning.
■ Send shoulder pads to a reconditioner for inspection, certification (if required), and overall repair annually.

These basic principles of maintenance can be applied for all other protective equipment.

Design of Protective Equipment

The following four basic principles are used in pad design:

- *Channeling.* Forces are channeled away from anatomical structures.
- *Dispersion.* Forces are dispersed over a large area.
- *Mechanical structuring.* Forces are reduced through the use of a mechanical structure.
- *Restriction.* Anatomical ranges of motion are reduced to prevent forces that cause injury.

By knowing these design principles, the athletic trainer can better fabricate protective equipment and evaluate the worth of prefabricated equipment.

Fabrication of Protective Equipment

Knowledge and mastery of fabrication techniques are essential for those constructing protective equipment. While experience, imagination, and practice are the best teachers, a good construction plan for each pad helps. Factors to consider when constructing protective padding include injury protection during fabrication; material selection; and cutting, bending, and stabilization of pads.

When using the athlete as a model to fabricate a pad, the trainer must take great care not to aggravate the injury. The injury should be protected from undue pressure, temperature, constriction, or movement. Stockinette, prewrap, or positive cast molds may be used to protect the athlete during fabrication.

When selecting materials, the trainer must make certain the materials are compatible in terms of physical properties: flexible versus inflexible, soft versus hard, and so forth. Some pads are composed of a combination of materials. Often it is better to bond the materials together before forming the pad. Bonding adhesives must be resistant to water and perspiration to maintain the pad's integrity.

The trainer should mark areas to be trimmed on an unfinished pad while it is still in place on the athlete (Figs. 44.2a, b).

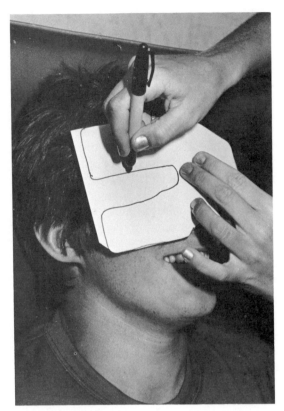

FIGURE 44.2a. A model for a nasal splint can be created with paper.

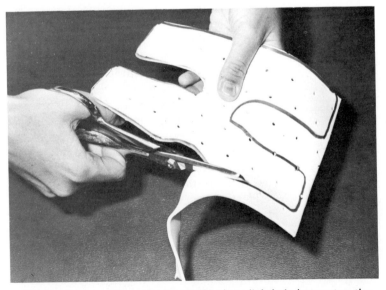

FIGURE 44.2b. After softening Orthoplast slightly in hot water, the athletic trainer cuts out the nasal splint form.

Proper tools, such as cast saws and scissors, should be sharp and in good working order.

Stabilization of padding should be determined prior to pad construction. Materials such as Velcro, elastic webbing, canvas straps, elastic wraps, elastic sleeves, rubber sleeves, and adhesive elastic or nonelastic tape can be used for this purpose. Incorporation of the pad into the uniform (pants, jersey, girdle, etc.) may be an effective technique to stabilize pads located in awkward positions.

Ridges, channels, bubbles, or donuts may be formed above an injured area to dissipate forces.

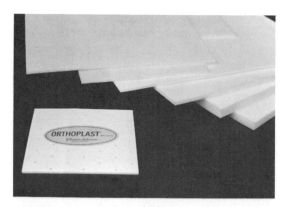

FIGURE 44.3.   Various thicknesses and densities of Plastazote (top), plus a perforated piece of Orthoplast, also available in solid sheets.

Construction Materials

One needs an understanding of the physical properties of materials used in constructing protective equipment. Shock absorption capacity, deflective properties, weight, and durability are considerations when selecting materials for purchase or use. Decisions should be based on injury location, severity, other equipment or materials involved in treatment, and the type of restriction needed. When designing protective pads, the trainer should make sure that pad design and the materials used are allowable by that sport. Most sports rulebooks list equipment restrictions.

Foam rubber products provide a variety of shock absorption and recovery properties. Commercial thermoplastics, or cast-type materials, provide flexibility as well as deflective, restrictive, or hard dispersive qualities. Pneumatic (air-filled) devices are currently being used more extensively, but problems with rupture, maintaining inflation, and stabilization have limited the use of these products.

Plastics are available to create splints and pads. Two common types are Orthoplast, a rather rigid plastic, and Plastazote, a softer, foamlike material. These are designed to pad or softly splint an injured area (Fig. 44.3).

Staying abreast of improvements made in protective equipment maintains the quality

of care. Contacting sales representatives and obtaining product literature are good ways to acquire knowledge of the latest materials, manufactured equipment, and fabrication techniques. Sports journals are good references for learning about new techniques and materials for constructing protective appliances.

Cost of Protective Equipment

Protective equipment is important for preventing athletic injuries and its quality should not be compromised because of cost. Athletic program administrators should comparison shop for materials and buy in bulk whenever feasible. No real savings are attained by purchasing cheaper but inferior equipment and materials.

Protective Equipment Regulations

Mandatory use of protective equipment, such as mouth guards, and head, eye, and throat protection, has reduced the number and severity of injuries to these areas. Standardization and improved testing of materials have resulted in increased quality of available protective equipment. Equipment that is standardized and regulated should not be altered by the player, coach, or trainer. Any modification of these devices must be done by certified reconditioners.

Regulating Organizations

Sports regulatory bodies have established certification standards through the National Operating Committee on Standards for Athletic Equipment (NOCSAE) for protective equipment such as football helmets. The Sports Equipment and Facilities Committee of the American Society for Testing and Materials (ASTM) has established testing standards for skiing equipment and is involved in establishing standards in other areas. Publications and meetings of the American Equipment Manager's Association help keep those responsible for daily maintenance of protective equipment aware of new developments and regulations.

Need for Continued Evaluation and Revision

Protective devices must be continually updated and matched to the needs of changing athletic activities. Biomechanical principles are increasingly employed in developing protective equipment to identify material with maximal impact resistance, shock attenuation, and durability under various conditions. Protective equipment will continue to improve because the materials available continue to improve, as does the understanding of the mechanical forces that affect the body in sports. The characteristics of all kinds of playing surfaces, for both indoor and outdoor sports, and their relationship to traction and footwear continue to be evaluated.

Athlete Education

Athletic trainers should instruct athletes in the use, maintenance, application, and limits of all protective equipment worn. Athletes should be encouraged to ask questions regarding equipment use. Trainers should also avoid making guarantees to athletes as to the protective powers of the equipment they use.

PROTECTIVE EQUIPMENT FOR THE FACE, SKULL, AND BRAIN

Headmasks and Helmets

Effective protection for the head and skull has improved and expanded significantly in recent years, especially in such sports as football, ice hockey, lacrosse, boxing, baseball, cycling, and automobile and motorcycle racing.

Face and Throat Protection

In several sports, the combination of face masks and helmets is used. The face mask in ice hockey, lacrosse, and baseball must limit the entry of the puck, stick, and ball. In addition, a movable pad for throat protection is desirable. The football face mask is designed to protect the facial bones, nose, and eyes. The fencing mask should be of strong, fine metal mesh with an extra shell over the top of the head and ears for exclusion of the saber. The fencing mask must be adjustable to head size and have a thick bib to protect the throat from thrusting weapons.

Fitting a Football Helmet

The football helmet must fit correctly to function properly. A football helmet should be able to absorb force levels high enough to fracture the skull. With an improperly fitted helmet, a skull fracture or concussion could result.

Helmet fit must be monitored often because the fit can be altered by factors such as environmental temperature, hair length, deterioration of internal padding, loss of air from cells, and spread of face mask. The front of the helmet should be approximately two finger-widths above the eyebrow (Fig. 44.4). This distance may vary slightly with air-inflated headgear. The back of the helmet should cover the skull base but not dig into the neck with neck extension (Fig. 44.5). Space at the neck band allows the helmet to rotate forward. The side earholes should coincide with the ear canals. The

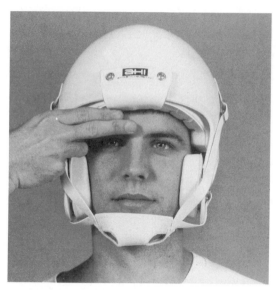

FIGURE 44.4. The front of the helmet should be about two finger-widths above the eyebrow.

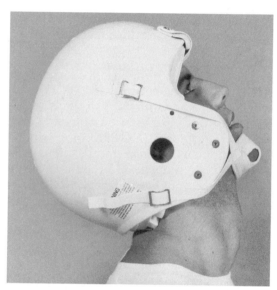

FIGURE 44.5. The back of the helmet should cover the skull base but not dig into the neck.

jaw pads should fit snugly to prevent lateral rocking (see Fig. 44.4).

The trainer checks helmet fit by having the athlete buckle the chin strap and hold his or her head straight ahead. The trainer grasps the sides of the helmet and tries to turn the helmet on the head and side to side, and then tries to rock it front to back.

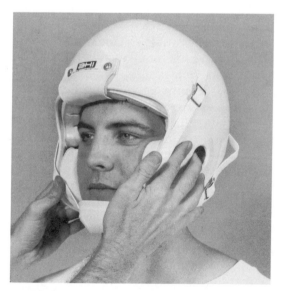

FIGURE 44.6. A properly fitting helmet moves only slightly.

A properly fitting helmet moves only slightly (Fig. 44.6).

The number of sports and variety in equipment designed for each sport make it difficult to describe the correct fit for each situation. However, adhering to the preceding principles will increase the likelihood of having equipment fit correctly.

Mouth Guards

Mouth guards are mandatory in football and are increasingly used in other contact sports. Mouth guards are manufactured to provide intraoral, extraoral, or combination protection. They can be obtained in three styles: (1) the preformed, or stock, mouth guard; (2) the form-fitted or moldable mouth guard, which is placed in boiling water and then molded to the athlete's mouth; and (3) the custom-fitted variety, which is made from a mold taken of the athlete's teeth.

Ear and Eye Protection

Eye and ear protection is needed for participants in sports using paddles or racquets with high-velocity small balls. The Nation-

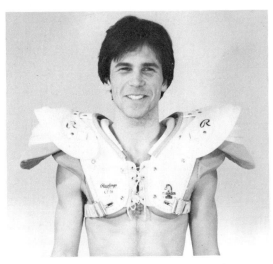

FIGURE 44.7. Commercial shoulder pads.

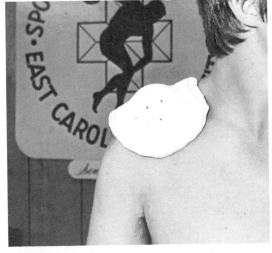

FIGURE 44.8. Customized pad provides additional protection to the athlete's acromioclavicular joint.

al Collegiate Athletic Association recommends eye protection which conforms to the standards developed by the ASTM.

PROTECTIVE EQUIPMENT FOR THE UPPER BODY

The Shoulder Girdle

Protective Pads

The shoulder girdle should be protected against forceful contact with opponents and hard surfaces and objects. Commercial shoulder pads used in football, ice hockey, and lacrosse are adequate to protect this region (Fig. 44.7).

Additional customized padding can be readily fashioned to further protect local areas of susceptibility, such as the acromioclavicular joint (Fig. 44.8). Standard shoulder protective equipment does not protect the glenohumeral joint. Tape restraints or commercial equipment that limits abduction movements can be used when an athlete requires protective restriction of motion at this joint (Fig. 44.9).

Football Shoulder Pad Fitting

Although different styles and types of shoulder pads are used in football today,

the principles used in fitting have remained the same over the years. The shoulder is measured to determine what size pad is needed. When fitted correctly, the shoulder pad should meet the following criteria:

■ The inner padding should cover the tips of the shoulders.

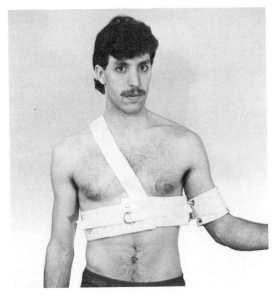

FIGURE 44.9. Commercial tape restraints to limit abduction of the athlete's glenohumeral joint.

- The neck opening should not be constrictive, yet should minimize the areas exposed to injury.
- The epaulets and cups should cover the deltoid and allow those movements required by the athlete's specific position.
- Straps and lacings should be as snug as possible without constricting breathing.
- If a split clavicle shoulder pad is used, the channel for the acromioclavicular joint should be in proper position. Collars and drop down pads can be added as adjuncts to shoulder pad protection.

Ribs and Thorax Protection

The ribs and thorax may be protected by commercially available "flak jackets." Football running backs who are exposed to repeated thoracic contusion or quarterbacks with prior rib cage injury may derive significant benefit from this padding.

Protection for the Arm, Elbow, and Forearm

Protective Pads

The humeral or arm region can be protected in any sport by commercial padding similar to types available for the elbow. Additional protective padding can be fashioned to cover broader or more specific areas. This additional padding is typically strapped on by elastic bandaging tape. The motion of the elbow can be limited by appropriate taping methods (see chapter 43). Similarly, forearm musculature and bone structures can be adequately protected with commercial cushion pads.

Elbow Anti-Friction Braces

Many players with lateral epicondylitis ("tennis elbow") report relief of symptoms from braces designed to decrease the pull of the origin of the wrist extensor muscles on

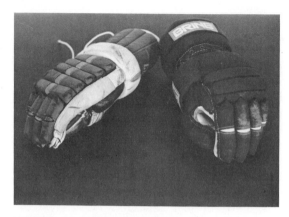

FIGURE 44.10. Padding in the form of gloves protects the athlete's hands.

the lateral epicondyle of the humerus. Many different styles of braces are commercially available.

Some players, when symptomatic, wear the brace not only for competition, but also for activities of daily living. When asymptomatic, they then may continue to wear

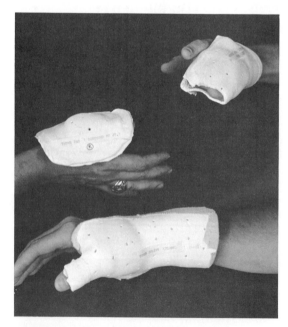

FIGURE 44.11. Orthoplast uses: (top to bottom) sandwich splint for fingers; bubble pad for thumb; thumb/wrist splint.

the brace during play as a protective device to prevent reinjury.

Hand Protection

Padded gloves to protect the hands are now part of the standard equipment for ice hockey and lacrosse players, and goalkeepers in field hockey. In boxing, the gloves protect not only the boxer's hands but also the impact site on the opponent (Fig. 44.10).

Silicone rubber is extensively used to construct protective pads for the hand, wrist, and forearm. When immobilization is needed for fractures or severe sprains, silicone casts offer an advantage over more rigid plaster and fiberglass casting materials because players wearing silicone casts are not excluded from play in most sports (Figs. 44.11 and 44.12).

PROTECTIVE EQUIPMENT FOR THE LOWER BODY

Protection for the Hip and Pelvis

Standard protective padding for the hip and pelvic area must be varied in structure, weight, and application according to the contact sport for which it is used. Commercial and custom pads can be used to protect vulnerable areas such as the iliac crest from contusions (Fig. 44.13). Commercial soft and rigid protectors are available for the genital area.

In the thigh region, the standard padding provided in the uniforms is effective, but typically coverage is limited to the most susceptible anterior region. Larger, more protective pads for this region, or pads that cover the thigh circumferentially, can be easily made.

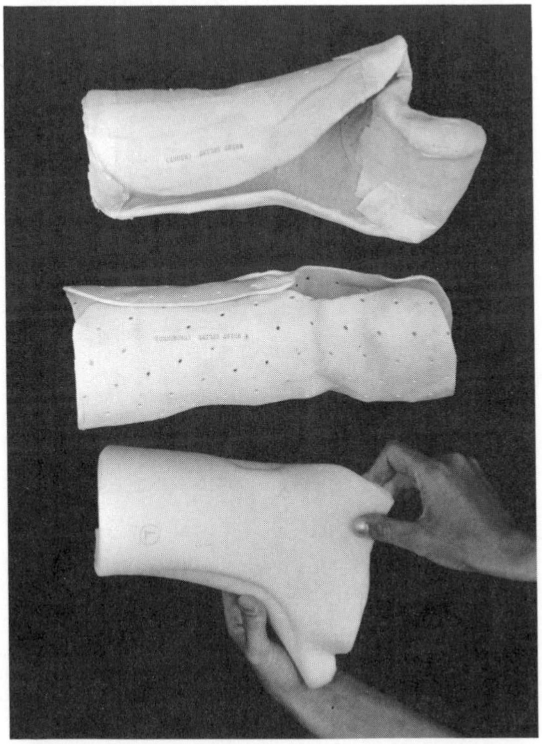

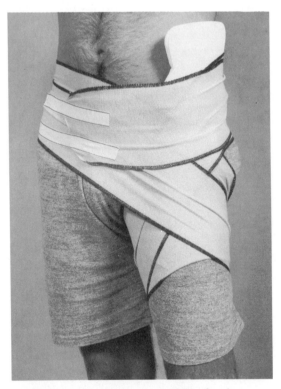

FIGURE 44.12.   Splints for the hand and wrist: (top and middle) Orthoplast; (bottom) softer Plastazote.

FIGURE 44.13.   Protective padding for the athlete's hip to protect injured areas.

Knee Protection

Protective Pads

The knee can be protected against direct blows by padding in the uniforms such as in the hockey uniform, or by leg guards, such as those worn in baseball and field hockey. Commercially available supplementary padding or custom pads can be obtained when additional protection is needed. Knee pads used in wrestling protect the prepatellar and infrapatellar bursae from friction. Pads are also available for volleyball and soccer, where players intentionally fall forward onto their knees.

Braces

The effectiveness of prophylactic knee braces for collateral ligament injury to the knee is controversial. Both unilateral and bilateral strut braces are available. Bracing is more economical than standard taping proce-dures, but at present the use of prophylactic braces remains a controversial issue.

Prophylactic braces that prevent recur-rent patellar dislocation or subluxation are acceptable alternatives to taping. Many commercial types of either Neoprene or elastic material are available. These braces may also be helpful for the athlete who is experiencing patellar pain. An alternative style brace for treating patellar pain is a strap worn under the patella (Fig. 44.14).

Functional knee braces that are designed to prevent reinjury in athletes with prior injury to the cruciate ligaments can be ordered only with a prescription from a physician. The effectiveness of these braces has been better documented than that for prophylactic knee braces.

Players with prior injury frequently wear knee sleeves of Ace or Neoprene material. The braces shown in Figure 44.15 have

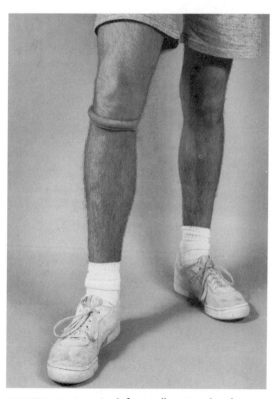

FIGURE 44.14. An infrapatellar strap is a brace that is worn under the patella for treating patellar pain.

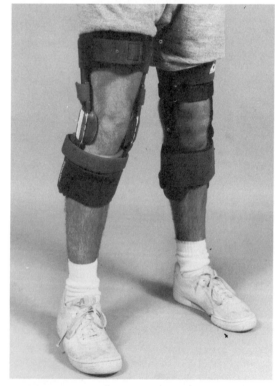

FIGURE 44.15. Two types of knee braces, or knee sleeves, that protect the collateral knee structures.

small metal side supports. The players subjectively feel more secure in these devices. The scientific rationale for this "security" is not clear, but perhaps it is related to the fact that the devices do provide warmth and increased knee awareness.

Protection for the Leg and Ankle

Protective Pads

External padding for the tibial region is available for baseball, ice hockey, field hockey, soccer, and several other sports. Such shields are designed to protect against blows from high-velocity missiles such as the balls, pucks, and sticks used in these sports. Again, supplementary customized padding is easily devised with semirigid resilient materials. Additional external padding can be used to protect contused areas about the ankle.

Ankle Support

Many commercial supports exist as an alternative to ankle taping, both for treatment of acute injury as well as for protection against initial injury or reinjury. Figure 44.16 shows examples of some of these supports. Shoes for some sports (particularly basketball) are available with

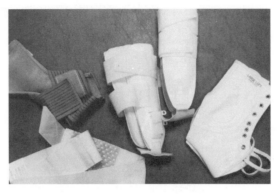

FIGURE 44.16.   Commercially available ankle supports.

built-in straps for additional ankle protection.

Foot Protection

Pads and custom-made foot orthotics may be helpful in treating a variety of foot problems, as well as other lower extremity problems involving the hip and knee. For example, athletes with patellofemoral stress syndrome or painful bunions, blisters, or corns may benefit from such devices. The effective use of available materials to meet the needs of the athlete is a skill the student in athletic training learns during apprenticeship.

IMPORTANT CONCEPTS

1. Protective equipment must be durable, easy to maintain, and simple to fit.
2. Protective equipment is used to prevent injury or protect the athlete from reinjury.
3. Trainers should not deviate from manufacturers' guidelines for fitting, maintaining, or using their protective equipment.
4. Athletes should be educated regarding the benefits, proper fit, and maintenance of protective equipment.
5. Mouth guards can be preformed, moldable, or custom fitted.

IMPORTANT CONCEPTS

1. Protective equipment must be durable, easy to maintain, and simple to fit.
2. Protective equipment is used to prevent injury or protect the athlete from reinjury.
3. Trainers should not deviate from manufacturers' guidelines for fitting, maintaining, or using their protective equipment.
4. Athletes should be educated regarding the benefits, proper fit, and maintenance of protective equipment.
5. Mouth guards can be preformed, moldable, or custom fitted.

SUGGESTED READINGS

American Academy of Orthopaedic Surgeons. *Knee Braces.* Seminar Report. Chicago: American Academy of Orthopaedic Surgeons, 1985.

Arnheim, D. D. *Modern Principles of Athletic Training: The Science of Sports Medicine: Injury Prevention, Causation, and Management,* 6th ed. St. Louis: Times Mirror/ Mosby College Publishing, 1985, pp. 179–195.

Beck, C., D. Drez, Jr., J. Young, et al. "Instrumented Testing of Functional Knee Braces." *American Journal of Sports Medicine* 14 (1986): 253–256.

Craig, Timothy T., ed. *Comments in Sports Medicine.* Chicago: Department of Health Education, American Medical Association, 1973.

France, E. P., L. E. Paulos, G. Jayaraman, et al. "The Biomechanics of Lateral Knee Bracing. Part II: Impact Response of the Braced Knee." *American Journal of Sports Medicine* 15 (1987): 430–438.

Gieck, J., and F. C. McCue, III. "Fitting of Protective Football Equipment." *American Journal of Sports Medicine* 8 (1980): 192–196.

Kulund, D. N., ed. *The Injured Athlete,* 2d ed. Philadelphia: J. B. Lippincott, 1988, pp. 178–180, 277–278, 285–286.

Meyer, R. D., W. W. Daniel. "The Biomechanics of Helmets and Helmet Removal." *Journal of Trauma* 25 (1985): 329–332.

National Collegiate Athletic Association. *NCAA Sports Medicine Handbook,* 3d ed. Mission, Kans.: National Collegiate Athletic Association, 1987.

National Operating Committee on Standards for Athletic Equipment. *NOCSAE Manual.* Kansas City, Mo.: National Operating Committee on Standards for Athletic Equiment, 1987.

Paulos, L. E., E. P. France, T. D. Rosenberg, et al. "The Biomechanics of Lateral Knee Bracing. Part I: Response of the Valgus Restraints to Loading." *American Journal of Sports Medicine* 15 (1987): 419–429.

Roy, S., and R. Irvin. *Sports Medicine: Prevention, Evaluation, Management, and Rehabilitation.* Englewood Cliffs, N.J.: Prentice-Hall, 1983, pp. 45–51.

Steele, B. E. "Protective Pads for Athletes." *The Physician and Sportsmedicine* 13 (March 1985): 179–180.

45

Basic Principles of Conditioning Programs

INTRODUCTION

Athletes with superior training and conditioning are stronger, better coordinated, and less subject to injury. Improvement in the athlete's conditioning is the factor most responsible for enhanced performance. Maximum physical and mental fitness requires training of the whole body, including every tissue and cell. This kind of conditioning helps the athlete compete effectively, prevents injuries, and speeds recovery following injuries.

Chapter 45 begins with the physiology of muscle contraction. The chapter then discusses the three basic components of conditioning: the development of muscle strength, power, and endurance; flexibility; and cardiorespiratory endurance. Maximum development of all three components is essential for safe athletic performance. ■

PHYSIOLOGY OF MUSCLE CONTRACTION

The basic unit of structure and function in skeletal muscle is the **sarcomere**, which is composed of the contractile proteins actin and myosin. According to the sliding filament theory, when a muscle contracts (either shortening or lengthening), a series of events causes the actin and myosin filaments to interact. This interaction results in the actin filaments sliding over the myosin filaments—a process that produces the force or tension of the muscle contraction. The force of contraction is transmitted to the bones to which the muscles are attached by the muscle tendons (Fig. 45.1).

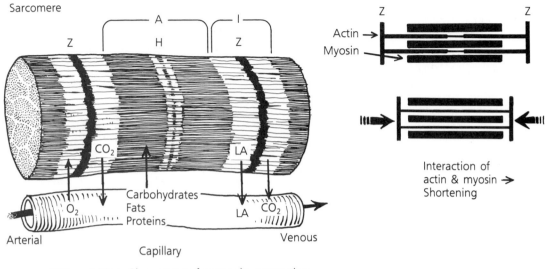

ATP   ADP + Pi + energy for muscle contraction.
Anaerobic processes
       PC   Pi + C + energy to resynthesize ATP
       Glycogen   Lactic Acid + energy to resynthesize ATP
Aerobic process
       Carbohydrates, Fats, Proteins + O_2 CO_2 + H_2O + energy to resynthesize ATP

FIGURE 45.1. A skeletal muscle cell, tissue capillary, and the energy systems that supply adenosine triphosphate (ATP) for muscle contraction.

Skeletal muscle is voluntary muscle under the control of the nervous system, and is, therefore, properly termed the **neuromuscular system**. The basic unit of structure and function is the motor unit. A **motor unit** is the nerve and all the muscle fibers it innervates. During different tensities of muscle contraction, the nervous system selectively recruits muscle fibers to fire, therefore performing the desired movement.

Types of Muscle Contraction

A muscle contracts concentrically, eccentrically, or isometrically. The **concentric muscle contraction** is most frequently used. In this contraction, tension is developed where the actin filaments slide over the myosin filaments, causing the muscle to shorten in length. In an **eccentric muscle contraction**, tension is developed with actin and myosin interaction, but the muscle lengthens. In an **isometric muscle contraction**, muscle tension is developed, but the relative length of

the muscle remains constant, neither shortening nor lengthening.

Types of Muscular Energy Systems

The immediate source of energy for muscle contraction, **adenosine triphosphate (ATP)**, is synthesized from the consumption of food nutrients and is utilized in both anaerobic and aerobic energy systems to produce energy (see Fig 45.1).

Anaerobic Systems

Anaerobic energy systems do not require oxygen to synthesize ATP; instead, they produce energy for use by the muscles in the absence of oxygen. These systems are the ATP-PC system (adenosine triphosphate-phosphocreatine) and the lactic acid system.

Phosphocreatine (PC) is stored in muscle and broken down into creatine and inorganic phosphate. This breakdown creates a release of energy readily available to the muscle. The ATP-PC system produces enough energy for short quick bursts of activity like 100-yard dashes and is exhausted in about 10 seconds.

In the lactic acid system, carbohydrates are broken down into glucose. Glucose is used immediately or stored in the liver as glycogen. The breakdown of glucose and glycogen results in a release of energy and the production of lactic acid. Lactic acid accumulates in muscle tissue and eventually causes fatigue. The lactic acid system produces enough energy to allow work from 10 seconds to 3 minutes.

Aerobic Systems

Aerobic energy systems depend on the availability of oxygen. Carbohydrates, fats, and proteins can be completely broken down with oxygen, producing carbon dioxide, water, and energy to synthesize ATP. This process occurs in the mitochondria of muscle cells and allows a release of energy for several hours.

Muscle Fiber Types

Through examination of muscle biopsy specimens, two distinct muscle types have been identified. Although both types act aerobically as well as anaerobically, Type I muscle fibers (**slow twitch muscle fibers**) are better adapted for aerobic or endurance activity, while Type II muscle fibers (**fast twitch muscle fibers**) are adapted for anaerobic activity. All muscles are made of a mixture of both fast twitch and slow twitch muscle fibers. The proportion of this mixture is genetically determined; therefore, some individuals are predisposed to be more adept at power activities, while others are predisposed to be better at endurance activities. "Power" athletes have a greater proportion of fast twitch fibers, while "endurance" athletes have a higher proportion of slow twitch fibers. Training programs are designed to develop the slow or fast twitch fibers needed for a specific sport.

STRENGTH TRAINING

The first component of a conditioning program is strength training for the development of muscle strength, power, and endurance.

Principles of Strength Training

The basic principles of strength training are overload, progressive resistance, specificity, intensity, duration, frequency, reversibility, and periodization.

Overload

Thousands of years ago, Milo of Croton began his daily routine of lifting a baby bull until it was fully grown. In the present day, a similar principle—the **overload principle** —is employed in strength and endurance development. The overload principle states that strength, power, endurance, and hypertrophy of muscle can only increase when a muscle performs workloads greater than those previously encountered. The overload principle has been incorporated into what is now known as progressive resistance exercise.

Progressive Resistance

Progressive resistance exercise (PRE), first formulated by DeLorme following World War II, is successful because it not only overloads the muscle, but it does so in a progressive, gradual manner and therefore avoids the pitfalls of overtraining and fatigue.

DeLorme's original recommended program of progressive resistance exercise was based on the 10 RM (resistance maximum). The 10 RM is the maximum amount of weight a person can successfully lift 10 times. DeLorme recommended lifting three sets of 10, starting with one-half the 10 RM weight. Each time the individual could successfully complete three sets of 10 lifts, he or she would progress to the next higher weight at the next training session.

Specificity

Specificity, another important training concept, states that training must be relevant to the demands of the sport. That is, training should (1) work the muscles involved in the sport in a manner resembling the movements to be performed during the activity, and (2) develop the predominant energy system. This concept is also known as SAID (specific adaptation to imposed demands). Analysis of both the energy system and the muscles involved is necessary prior to the design of a program.

Intensity, Duration, Frequency, and Reversibility

Intensity, duration, and **frequency** are also terms commonly heard in relation to training. **Intensity** refers to the degree of work or effort exerted by the athlete. **Duration** is the time necessary to complete the desired exercise. **Frequency** is the number of workouts completed per unit of time (that is, how many workouts per week).

Reversibility is another important training concern. **Reversibility** basically states that if you don't use it, you lose it. Muscles atrophy from disuse and will detrain if they are not consistently trained toward a set goal.

Periodization

Periodization refers to the concept of dividing the annual training plan into smaller segments, phases, or cycles. This cycle-type of training philosophy appears to have originated in the Soviet Union in the 1950s. As with any training program, the goal of periodization is to improve athletic performance. However, periodization has another feature in its design: to allow the athlete to "peak" during the competitive season rather than during a training phase.

Periodization helps to decrease the possibility of overtraining by varying exercise selection, intensity, volume, and load. Normally, a yearly training cycle can be divided into three or possibly four phases, depending on the sport. A three-phase training cycle would consist of (1) a preseason or preparatory phase, (2) an in-season or competitive phase, and (3) a postseason or transition phase. Matveyev's four-phase training cycle, consisting of (1) a preparation phase, (2) a first transition, (3) a competition phase, and (4) a second transition (active rest) is illustrated in Figure 45.2.

The preseason or preparatory phase is marked by high-volume, low-intensity workouts which focus on proper exercise technique and provide a foundation for later training. Sometimes the preparatory phase is divided into generalized and specialized phases. Strength-building exercises are introduced in the generalized preseason conditioning phase, while exercises more closely duplicating actual playing skills are employed in the specialized preseason phase. The specialized preseason phase shifts into higher-intensity workouts with lower volumes of work. Power and strength workouts are introduced in the second half of the preseason phase (first transition in four-phase model) if the sport is primarily anaerobic.

As the in-season or competitive phase approaches, more emphasis should be placed on power workouts. If the sport is generally anaerobic in nature, anaerobic endurance should be emphasized. The overload principle would be appropriate for this type of anaerobic workout.

The in-season, or competitive, phase focuses on technique during an event, bringing performance to its peak. Peak performance is maintained by high-intensity technique exercises during brief workouts. The goal during this phase is to maintain a level of intensity sufficient enough to prevent retrogression but not so intense that it leads to overtraining.

The postseason or transition phase (second transition in the four-phase model) begins the termination of the competitive season. This period is one of active rest, where the athlete should engage in recreational physical activity so that a psychologi-

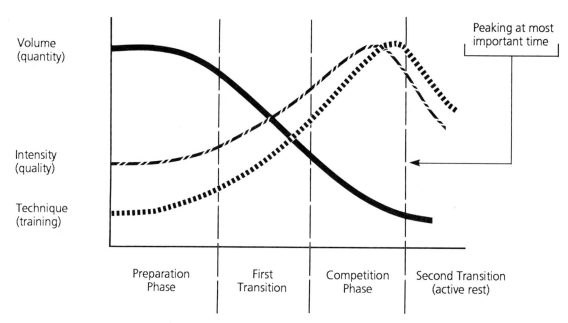

FIGURE 45.2 Matveyev's model of periodization. (From L. Matveyev. 1972. Periodisierang des sportlichen training. Berlin: Berles & Wernitz. Reprinted in Roundtable: "Periodization, Part 3," *National Strength and Conditioning Association Journal* 9, no 3 (1987). Reprinted by permission of the National Strength Conditioning Association, Lincoln, Nebraska.)

cal, as well as a physiological, break from competition occurs. Active rest consists of low-volume work and low- to moderate-intensity work, which allows the athlete enough time to heal physically and to recover emotionally.

Sample periodization models for conditioning programs for swimming, track throwing, soccer, wrestling, pole vaulting, and the various positions in football are contained in the appendix at the end of this chapter.

Specific Terminology

The following are definitions of specific terms that are used in weight-training programs.

- *Repetition (reps)*: performing the particular exercise—for example, raising and lowering the weight in the bicep curl—one time.
- *Set*: the grouping of a specific exercise into a number of repetitions—for ex-

ample, ten repetitions of the bicep curl is one set of this exercise, which is most commonly written as 1 set × 10 reps.
- *Resistance*: the opposing force to muscle contraction. Resistance can take many forms, including free weights, machines, sand bags, elastic tubing, or manual resistance provided by a partner.
- *One repetition maximum (1 RM)*: the maximum resistance that can be moved in one time through a full range of motion.
- *Movement time*: the time it takes to complete one repetition of the particular exercise.
- *Relief time (rest)*: the time interval occurring between performance of sets and repetitions.
- *Exercise order*: larger muscles should be exercised first (back, legs, chest) and smaller muscles last (bicep, tricep, abdominal).

TABLE 45.1.   Three Types of Resistive Exercise

Exercise	Resistance	Muscle Contraction Possible	Examples	Advantages	Disadvantages
Isotonic	Constant	Concentric Eccentric	N.K. table; pulleys; free weights; calisthenics	Inexpensive; easy to exercise most muscle groups	Slow speed only; is likely to cause irritation at inflamed points of range of motion
Isometric	Accommodating to the force applied	None; tension development only	The application of muscular force to any fixed point	Easily performed; least irritation to inflamed points of range of motion	Little muscular endurance developed
Isokinetic	Accommodating to the force applied	Concentric	Cybex II; Orthotron; Mini Gym; Hydra Gym; underwater exercise	Inexpensive when swimming pool is available; wide range of exercise speeds available; 100% musculoskeletal loading; extensive biomechanical information available from read out	Can be expensive; concentric contractions only

Types of Strength Training

Table 45.1 lists the similarities and differences between three basic types of resistance exercises: isometric, isotonic, and isokinetic.

Isometric Exercise

As discussed earlier, a muscle that contracts isometrically neither shortens nor lengthens. Tension develops in the muscle, but there is no range of motion utilized concurrent with the development of this tension. Substantial strength gains can be made ±7 degrees from the exercised point (Fig. 45.3). **Isometric exercises** are excellent in the early stages of rehabilitation, and their application in this area will be discussed in Chapter 49. The greatest disadvantages to training with isometrics alone are the lack of development of muscular endurance and

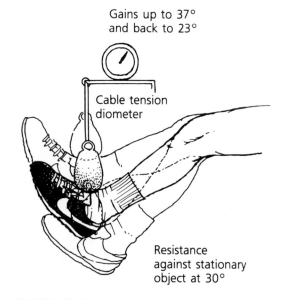

Gains up to 37° and back to 23°

Cable tension diometer

Resistance against stationary object at 30°

FIGURE 45.3.   Isometric exercise can produce strength gains up to ±7° from the exercised point.

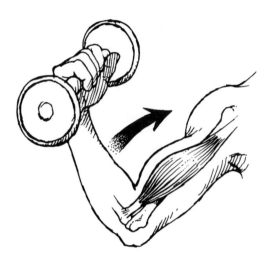

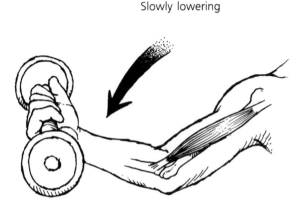

Slowly lowering

FIGURE 45.4. In concentric contraction, muscle shortens against resistance.

FIGURE 45.5. In eccentric contraction, muscle lengthens against resistance.

the limited carryover in strength to all points within the range of motion from a single contraction.

Isotonic Exercise

Isotonic exercise is performed by contracting either concentrically—that is, shortening as tension is developed (Fig. 45.4)—or eccentrically—that is, lengthening while tension is developed—against a resistance (Fig. 45.5). Isotonic exercise is probably the most common type of strength training due to its ease in performance and low cost. One disadvantage is that this type of weight training is generally performed on conventional weight devices and occurs at a very slow speed of contraction. When the speed of exercise is increased, the effective load on the muscle is reduced proportionally by the acceleration at the end of the range of motion (Fig. 45.6).

Isokinetic Exercise

Isokinetic exercise is performed on specialized machines, such as Cybex II, Orthotron, Biodex, or Kinkom, or underwater. During an isokinetic contraction, the muscle develops tension as it shortens. The machine controls the speed of contraction, which is held constant at all joint angles. The athlete

must provide force in both directions of movement, thereby working the muscle groups on both sides of the joint. Concentric contractions, of both the agonist and the antagonist muscle groups during exercise, allow for reflex relaxation of the muscles involved. This is especially important in the early phases of active exercise pro-

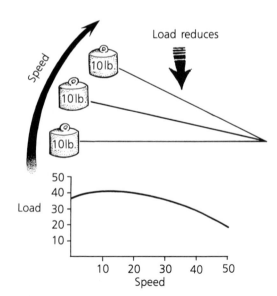

FIGURE 45.6. Effect of increased speed on muscle load with accelerations at end of range of motion.

grams since maximum blood flow through the muscles is maintained during exercise.

Many isokinetic machines are also equipped to perform eccentric exercise as well as concentric contractions. With speed control, isokinetic exercise machines accommodate 100 percent to the tension developed by the muscles. Therefore, 100 percent loading of the muscles occurs during the entire range of motion. This feature is helpful when there is pain or weakness at one or more points on the range of motion, such as occurs with an injury.

The isokinetic machine, when coupled with a computer, can record an abundance of biomechanical information. The computer frequently calculates automatically torque-motion curves, total work, average power, and torque-to-body weight measurements. This information (1) allows the athletic trainer to set standards and goals for power, strength, and endurance for various athletes on specific athletic teams; (2) establishes a comprehensive measure and standard for return to play; (3) serves as feedback to the athlete; and (4) provides objective and concrete measures for the athletic trainer and athlete to determine the status of a joint or muscle injury.

Underwater exercise is another type of isokinetic strength training, but it does not allow accurate speed control. The water lessens acceleration of body parts during the movement pattern while underwater, with the water absorbing energy. The amount of lessening is related to the surface area of the body part moved. Standing in waist-deep water, kicking one foot forward and back, produces a crude isokinetic movement of 100 degrees per second. When swim fins are attached to the foot, the speed of movement falls accordingly to the surface area of the fin. Underwater exercise can support injured limbs, and the athlete can easily perform partial ranges of motion without stress on weak or painful positions. Because water supports the weight of the body part, jogging, jumping, and balancing exercises can be performed early in the rehabilitation process.

Plyometric Exercises

Plyometric exercises are a variety of exercises that utilize explosive movements to increase athletic power. It is believed that prestretching muscles eccentrically creates tension. This tension causes increased muscular tension during the concentric phase of the movement. This effect increases the power exerted by the muscle. As the athlete progresses in the exercises, the rate at which this reflex movement occurs (eccentric prestretch to concentric power movement) increases. As the speed of the movement increases, neuromuscular efficiency increases, and the muscles are trained to switch from eccentric to concentric contractions rapidly.

Commonly performed plyometric exercises include power jumps, leaps or bounds, and throwing a weighted object such as a medicine ball or weighted baseball. Plyometrics can be easily adapted to special conditioning programs for any sport and can be worked into the athlete's normal practice routine. These exercises should not be performed on a daily basis but rather 2 to 3 days per week in order to allow proper muscular recovery from fatigue. Plyometrics should always be performed on surfaces that are conducive to jumping and landing so the surface does not cause potential injury. Soft surfaces, grass, and padding are excellent foundations for this type of activity, especially when landing. Athletes who have a current injury should avoid plyometric exercises. Only after the athlete has attained strength adequate to perform such exercise with stability should plyometrics be added into the conditioning program.

Muscle-Training Prescription

Muscle strength, power, and endurance development should begin at least 6 to 8 weeks prior to the competitive season. A maintenance program, 1 day per week throughout the season, maintains the gains made in the preseason period.

Strength, power, and endurance should follow the SAID technique previously described in this chapter. The same exercise regimen of exercising every other day, with one exhaustive workout per week, can be adhered to; however, special considerations should be given to periodization.

Muscle-training programs can be designed to develop muscle strength, muscle power, and/or muscle endurance. **Muscle strength** is the force or tension that a muscle or muscle group can exert against a resistance, and is usually measured by 1 RM. **Muscle power** is the speed of movement or the rate at which a resistance can be moved per unit of time—that is, the rate of doing work. **Muscle endurance** refers to repetitive muscle contractions carried out over time without undue fatigue.

In general, strength training and power training use high resistance and low number of repetitions. Muscle endurance training programs use low resistance and high number of repetitions. The following example is a strength program designed for muscle strength for the bench press.

Exercise: bench press
Sets: 3
Resistance: 80 to 85 percent of 1 RM
Reps: 6
Rest interval: 50 to 90 seconds

The number of repetitions is based on the percent of 1 RM employed:

Percent 1 RM	Number reps/set
90–95	1–2
85–90	3–4
80–85	4–6
75–80	6–8
70–75	8–10
65–70	10–12

The next example is a program designed for muscular endurance for the bench press.

Exercise: bench press
Set: 3
Resistance: 65 to 70 percent of 1 RM
Reps: 10 to 15
Rest interval: 40 to 70 seconds

Athletes in training often ask, "When should I add more weight?" In a strength or endurance program, once the athlete is able to perform the prescribed number of repetitions with ease, the athletic trainer adds an increment of weight, forcing the muscle(s) to fail on the last few reps. When the muscles adapt to new weight, the trainer again adds more weight (the progressive overload principle).

The trainer must include rest and recovery time in the muscle-training program. Recovery time allows the muscles to build strength. Staleness and retrogression occur when proper recovery time is not allowed. It is imperative that all trainers realize that they must not overtrain athletes.

Tables 45.2, 45.3, and 45.4 are muscle-conditioning programs designed for free weights, Universal gym, and Nautilus. Note that many of the strength experts advocate the use of a free weight program or a combination free weight and machine program.

The free weight program can be combined with the following exercises.

Nautilus	*Universal*
Leg extension	Knee extension
Leg curl	Knee curl
Hip abduction	
Hip adduction	

Muscular Response to Training

The actual muscular response to exercise is a controversial subject. Some researchers believe resistance training causes an increase in the cross-sectional area of individual muscle fibers. This increase is called **hypertrophy of muscle**. Others believe **hyperplasia** occurs—that is, the muscle fibers split and increase in number.

It is certainly possible that hypertrophy and hyperplasia both occur proportionately as a result of training, adding to the overall size and strength of the muscle. Tendons and ligaments also respond to resistance training stresses by becoming thicker and stronger.

TABLE 45.2. A Free Weight Program for Muscle Strength and Endurance

Exercise	Body Part	Weight, % 1 RM	Sets	Reps
Half squat	Thighs, hips	70	3	10–15
Heel raise	Calf	70	3	10–15
Lunge	Thighs, hips	(10–30 lbs)	3	15–20
Bench press	Chest, upper arm	70	3	10–15
Overhead press	Shoulder, upper arm	70	3	10–15
Good morning	Back	(30–75 lbs)	3	10–15
Bent over row	Upper back	70	3	10–15
Bicep curl	Arm, forearm	70	3	10–15
Tricep extension	Arm, forearm	70	3	10–15
Bent knee sit-ups	Abdominals	(5–25 lbs)	3	10–15
Trunk twists	Trunk	(10–25 lbs)	3	10–15

Note: The exercises should be performed in the order given above. The time interval between sets should be 60 to 70 seconds. Perform all three sets of each exercise before proceeding to the next. The total workout time is approximately 70 minutes. The rest between exercises should be no more than 70 to 80 seconds.

TABLE 45.3. A Universal Gym Program for Muscle Strength and Endurance

Exercise	Body Part	Weight, % 1 RM	Sets	Reps
Leg press	Thighs, hips	70	3	10–15
Knee extension	Thighs	70	3	10–15
Knee curl	Hamstrings	(10–30 lbs)	3	10–15
Bench press	Chest, arms	70	3	10–15
Overhead press	Shoulder, arms	70	3	10–15
Back hyperextension	Back	(0–15 lbs)	3	10–15
Bicep curl	Arm, forearm	70	3	10–15
Tricep extension	Arm, forearm	70	3	10–15
Lat pull-down	Back, lats	70	3	10–15
Bent knee sit-ups	Abdominals	(5–25 lbs)	3	10–15
Trunk twists	Trunk	(10–25 lbs)	3	10–15

Note: Follow the same instructions as for the free weight program.

TABLE 45.4. A Nautilus Program for Muscle Strength and Endurance

Exercise	Body Part	Weight	Sets	Reps
Hip and back	Hips, lower back	Plates*	3	10–15
Leg extension	Thigh	″	3	10–15
Leg press	Hips, thighs	″	3	10–15
Leg curl	Hamstrings	″	3	10–15
Hip abduction	Gluteus medius	″	3	10–15
Hip adduction	Adductor magnus	″	3	10–15
Lateral raise	Shoulder	″	3	10–15
Seated press	Shoulder, upper arm	″	3	10–15
Decline press	Chest, shoulder	″	3	10–15
Bicep curl	Arm, forearm	″	3	10–15
Tricep curl	Arm, forearm	″	3	10–15
Abdominal curls	Abdominals	″	3	10–15

*The proper plate allows completion of three sets of 10 to 15 repetitions for the first 3 weeks. The second 3 weeks, select a plate that allows completion of three sets of 6 repetitions.

TABLE 45.5. Guidelines for Strength Training in the Adolescent and Preadolescent

Frequency	Duration	Intensity
2–3 times per week	20–30 minutes per session plus warm-up and cool-down	6–15 repetitions per set 1–3 sets should be performed Start with no weight and work on form—progressively add 1 to 3 lbs. working from high repetitions and low weight to low repetitions and higher weights

Special Issues in Strength Training

Strength Training for Adolescents and Preadolescents

Weight training for the preadolescent is becoming a pertinent and controversial issue as fitness and weight-training programs are being targeted at younger age groups. Unfortunately, there are few scientific data concerning this topic. Much of the current thinking has been extrapolated from other populations.

Health care organizations such as the National Athletic Trainers Association, the American Orthopaedic Society for Sports Medicine, and the National Strength and Conditioning Association have addressed this issue at great length. These organizations were among those attending a conference held in Indianapolis in 1985 to outline some of the general guidelines, risks, and benefits of weight training in the adolescent and preadolescent age group (Tables 45.5, 45.6).

Those who are designing specific programs for this age group must consider certain points. First, the child should have a comprehensive medical examination prior to participation. Second, the child must be emotionally mature to receive and understand instructions from a weight-training counselor or coach. Proper supervision is imperative because improper form and unsupervised workouts can lead to serious injury in the young athlete. The program should emphasize dynamic concentric contractions as opposed to eccentric contrac-

TABLE 45.6. Comparison of Risk and Benefits of Strength-Training Programs for the Adolescent and Preadolescent

Potential Benefits	Potential Risks	No Effect
Increase in muscle strength	Acute and chronic injury to *bone* (especially due to accidents or improper form)	On flexibility, no increase or decrease has been elicited in range of motion when full range of motion was used during exercise
Increase motor performance		
Protection against acute injury	Acute and chronic *musculoskeletal* injury	
Increases in muscle endurance		
Increase in lean body mass	Acute and chronic *joint* injury	
Psychologically beneficial—"self-image improved"	Hypertension and blackout (Valsalva maneuver)	
Cardiorespiratory function improves if used as part of circuit training		
Speeds up rehabilitation after injury		
Could teach proper lifting techniques early in life		

tions. These contractions or exercises should be taken through a full range of motion. Strength training should be a part of an overall conditioning program, including warm-up and cool-down periods as well as flexibility sessions. Olympic or competitive weight lifting should be prohibited in this age group.

Strength Training for Women

Women are encouraged to participate in resistance training. Research has shown that women have great potential for gaining strength. Hypertrophy differences between men and women are significant. The lesser amount of hypertrophy that women experience has been attributed to women's lower testosterone levels. More research is needed in this area since many women have high levels of testosterone yet do not show signs of hypertrophy like their male counterparts.

FLEXIBILITY

The second component of a conditioning program is the flexibility of the muscles that cross the joint. Flexibility is increased by muscle-stretching exercises.

Physiology of Muscle Stretch

Flexibility is defined as the capacity of a muscle to lengthen or stretch. Most often a particular sport involves short, intensive movements within a small part of the full range of motion of the joint. If not fully stretched, the muscles involved progressively tighten, limiting the flexibility. Abnormally tight muscles as a result of injury can alter form, thus reducing biomechanical efficiency and creating a climate for athletic injuries, particularly muscle strains and tendinitis.

A few simple tests will determine where an athlete falls on the spectrum of muscle tightness. The sit-and-reach test indicates low back and hamstring tightness (Fig. 45.7). The athlete places his or her feet on

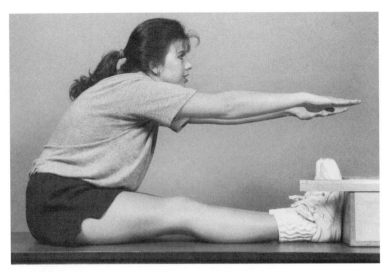

FIGURE 45.7. The sit-and-reach test indicates low back and hamstring tightness.

the box at right angles and reaches with fingertips over a ruler at the end of the box. The measurement is read in either plus or minus, depending on the tightness found. Most athletes should strive to achieve either zero or plus scores. A minus score indicates muscle tightness, and that the athlete might have to work harder than average on flexibility. Standard measures have been established as norms for elementary children. High school or older athletes should be rated according to the average formed within each athletic event and each sport.

A test of upper-extremity flexibility of the shoulders is conducted with the athlete standing, arms flexed at 90 degrees, and elbows fully extended (Fig. 45.8). The athlete externally rotates his or her arms as far as possible. Those who can rotate their palms beyond horizontal, making the hypothenar eminence higher than the thenar eminence, are considered loose.

Although time-consuming, measuring flexibility for all joints is best done using a goniometer. (See Chapter 10 for standard goniometric measurements of the shoulder, elbow, hip, knee, and ankle.)

All tests should be used to determine tightness or looseness for the individual

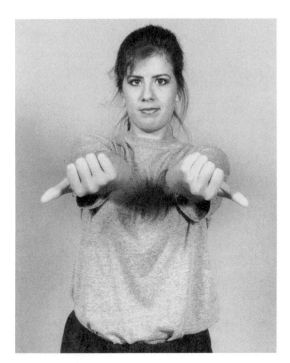

FIGURE 45.8. Test of upper extremity flexibility at the shoulder, indicating looseness.

athlete. Retesting should progress after a flexibility program is initiated. Stretching exercises should be conducted after the athlete is warmed to a mild perspiration level. Environmental temperatures determine the amount and intensity of effort required.

Types of Muscle Stretching

Appropriate stretching techniques increase the flexibility of tissues. Stretching techniques can be performed (1) ballistically; (2) statically, either actively or passively; or (3) through the use of proprioceptive neuromuscular facilitation (PNF).

Ballistic Stretch

Ballistic stretch involves the use of body momentum to bob or bounce at the end range of a stretch, which causes activation of the muscle fibers. Activation of these fibers causes the muscles to contract while the muscles are being stretched in the opposite direction. Ballistic stretching has been shown to increase flexibility; however, this stretch has the potential to cause musculoskeletal injuries such as muscle tears. For this reason, ballistic stretching is not recommended.

Static Stretch

Static stretch consists of stretching muscle tissue to a comfortable position and holding this position for a period of time. The effectiveness of static stretch depends on the intention and time of the actual stretch. Each exercise should be taken to the point of tightness and slightly beyond. For safety purposes, emphasis should be on proper form, and no motion should be forced. All exercises should be held for 5 seconds (counting "one thousand one, one thousand two, one thousand three, one thousand four, one thousand five"). When in doubt, less tension and more time are best—1 to 2 minutes for each muscle group at 15-second intervals.

Active static stretch is performed without assistance from an outside force. Passive static stretch utilizes an outside force to assist in regaining full range of motion. Passive static stretch is performed in specific situations in the physical therapy or athletic training environment, where caution and care are taken when doing the actual stretch. Athletes should not passively stretch their fellow athletes because of the potential for injury.

Proprioceptive Neuromuscular Facilitation

Proprioceptive neuromuscular facilitation (PNF) was developed by Herman Kabat, MD, Margaret Knott, RPT, and Dorothy Voss, RPT, as a way to enhance the neuromuscular response. Certain PNF techniques are designed for stretching selected muscle groups, and others are directed at relaxing the muscle so a better stretch can be attained. Two basic PNF stretching techniques are used in sports medicine: the contract-relax method and the hold-relax method.

In the *contract-relax method*, the athlete's body part to be stretched is moved passively until resistance is felt. At this point the athlete contracts the muscle group against the resistance of a partner. Resistance is applied as the body part is allowed to travel through a selected range of motion. The body part is moved to a new stretch position beyond the original stretch, and the process is repeated.

In the *hold-relax technique*, movement does not occur. The athlete actively stretches to a comfortable level. Once an original stretch position is chosen, the athlete applies force against the resistance of a partner. An isometric contraction is applied, and the partner allows no movement after holding for 10 to 15 seconds. When this phase is completed, the body part is moved to a new stretch position beyond the original stretch starting point, and the process is repeated.

Specific Stretching Exercises

The stretching exercises illustrated in Figure 45.9 are basic to most running sports. Many other stretching exercises not included in this text are acceptable substitutes for those presented. Athletes, coaches, and athletic trainers should choose exercises that are not only comfortable and effective but also comprehensive in stretching each of the muscle groups.

Stretching should be performed after the athlete has warmed up. In colder climates the warm-up period may need to be extended. Stretching exercises should also be repeated as the athlete cools down. All exercises should be held at least 5 seconds and repeated three to six times. Once the stretching routine is learned, the entire program should take no longer than 10 minutes.

CARDIORESPIRATORY ENDURANCE

Cardiorespiratory endurance, the third and most essential component of a physical fitness conditioning program, refers to the ability of the heart, blood vessels, and lungs to deliver oxygen to the tissues while re-

Seat Straddle Lotus Seated position; place soles of feet together and drop knees toward floor. Place forearms on inside of knees and push knees to ground. Lean forward, bringing chin to feet.

Seat Side Straddle Sit with legs spread; place *both* hands on same ankle. Bring chin to knee, keeping leg straight. *Hold.* Perform exercise on opposite leg.

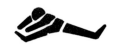

Seat Forward Straddle Sit with legs spread; place *one* hand on *each* ankle. Lean forward, bringing chest to ground. *Hold.*

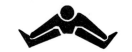

Seat Stretch Sit with legs together, feet flexed, hands on ankles. Bring chin to knees. *Hold.*

Leg Stretch Seated position; keep legs straight with hands on backs of calves. Lift and pull each leg individually to ear. *Hold.*

Leg Cross-Over Lie on back, legs spread and arms *out* to the side. Bring R toe to L hand, keeping leg straight. *Hold.* Repeat, with L toe to R hand.

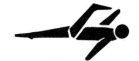

Lying Quad Stretch Lie on back with one leg straight, the other with hip in internal rotation, knee in flexion. Press knee to floor. *Hold.*

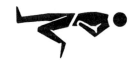

Back Bridge Lie on back; place hands behind head with palms on the ground. Push up, so the back arches and arms and legs are extended. *Hold.* Repeat.

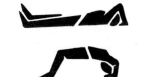

Knees to Chest Lie on back with knees bent. Grasp tops of both knees and bring them out toward the armpits, rocking gently. Repeat.

Forward Lunges Kneel on L leg; R leg forward at a right angle. Lunge forward, keeping the back straight. Stretch should be felt on the L groin. *Hold.* Repeat on opposite leg.

FIGURE 45.9. Stretching exercises for running sports. (FIGURE 45.9 continues next page)

Side Lunges Stand with legs apart; bend the L knee and lean toward the L, keeping the back straight and the R leg straight. Repeat on opposite leg.

 Cross-Over Stand with legs crossed; keep feet close together and legs straight. Touch toes. *Hold.* Repeat with opposite leg.

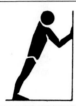 **Heel Cord Stretch** Stand 3 feet from wall, with feet pointed straight ahead. Lower hips to wall. Heels should not come off floor. *Hold.*

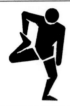 **Standing Quad Stretch** Stand supported. Pull foot to buttocks as shown. *Hold.*

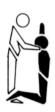 **Shoulder Stretch** Kneel/sit with arms extended overhead. Partner stands behind and grasps the athlete's arm, between the shoulder and elbow and stretches it backward. The athlete pulls forward, while the partner resists, for three to five seconds. Relax, while partner stretches the arm backward again. Repeat with opposite arm.

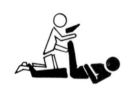 **Hamstring Stretch** Lie on back. Partner brings leg up *only* to the point of tightness and resists while the athlete pushes downward. Relax while partner pushes leg farther until tightness is felt again. Repeat with opposite leg.

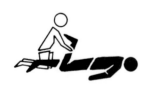 **Quad Stretch** Lie on stomach. Partner grasps lower leg and bends it until stretch is felt on the front of the thigh. The partner holds the leg while the athlete pushes against the partner for three to five seconds. Relax while the partner bends the leg again until another stretch is felt. Repeat with opposite leg.

FIGURE 45.9 (continued)

moving unnecessary materials and wastes. It has also been defined as the difference between the minimum aerobic requirement and the maximum aerobic capacity. Everyone has the same minimum aerobic requirements—that is, about 3 ml per kilogram per minute. However, maximum aerobic capacity, or the index of the ability to work, varies from person to person. Maximum oxygen consumption reflects the capacity of the heart and lungs to take up and deliver oxygen to the tissues, and it also reflects the tissues' ability to process oxygen. Therefore, consumption of oxygen reflects the effectiveness of all components of the oxygen transport system. When it is performed properly, exercise has the potential to increase cardiorespiratory endurance, thereby potentially increasing performance and the overall quality of the athlete's life.

Effects of Training

With the development of physical fitness, the cardiac output increases from 5.8 to 6.6 liters per minute, and the resting stroke volume increases the amount of blood being pumped out of the heart with each beat (about 70 ml in an untrained person and about 103 ml in an aerobically conditioned athlete). The heart empties more efficiently and requires fewer beats per minute, with the resting heart rate decreasing as a result. Stroke volume and cardiac output also increase during exercise as training continues.

Long-term aerobic exercise has several other effects. First, the actual size of the heart increases. Blood volume (plasma volume and hemoglobin) levels increase. This increases the body's ability to transport oxygen to the tissues. Exercise increases the ability of the tissues to extract oxygen from the blood. Exercise lowers both systolic and diastolic blood pressures at rest and during exercise. Exercise, therefore, increases the body's ability to take in oxygen. Finally, exercise, along with dietary considerations, can help bring about body composition changes.

Factors That Affect Cardiorespiratory Fitness Gains

Five basic factors affect the results of exercise on the body: initial fitness level, exercise intensity, duration of exercise, frequency of exercise, and type of exercise.

Initial Fitness Level

The more highly trained athletes are when they begin a specific conditioning program, the greater their chances of making significant gains in cardiorespiratory efficiency. Those individuals who start in poor condition generally show greater improvement in their cardiorespiratory status, but their eventual peak level of fitness will not be as efficient as those who start with a higher fitness base.

Intensity of Exercise

Aerobic capacity improves if exercise is intense enough to increase the heart's rate to 60 to 85 percent of its maximum rate. The formula for calculating an individual's training heart rate is to subtract the individual's age from 220 and then multiply that number by 60 to 80 percent (depending on the percentage desired of the target heart rate). As the fitness level improves, the percentage of maximum can be increased to as much as 85 percent. An accurate predicted maximum heart rate for athletes whose activities require more upper than lower body activity, such as swimming, should be determined by substituting 220 minus the athlete's age minus 13.

Duration of Exercise

Research by various exercise physiologists has shown that 20 to 30 minutes of exercise above, or at, the target heart rate is sufficient for making gains in cardiorespiratory fitness.

Frequency of Exercise

Cardiorespiratory workouts have been shown to produce optimum effects when performed at least 3 days per week. Some gains have been shown with a 2-day-per-week cardiorespiratory training program, but very minor gains are shown with once-a-week training programs. Five-day-a-week training programs have not shown to be significantly different from the recommended 3-day-per-week regimen. Consideration of overuse and fatigue injuries is strongly advised when designing a program.

Aerobic vs. Anaerobic Exercise

To improve cardiorespiratory fitness, holding all factors consistent (intensity, duration, frequency), the exercise performed must be aerobic in nature and involve large muscle groups. **Aerobic exercise** refers to those exercises performed long enough to utilize oxygen that helps burn carbohydrates and fats for fuels. **Anaerobic exercises** are those of short duration, not requiring the body's utilization of oxygen to make fuel available. Optimally, an aerobic program should be performed on days the athlete is not strength training. Bicycling, walking, running, swimming, and rope skipping are good examples of aerobic exercise.

DIET AND TRAINING

Ultimately, the fuel for energy systems comes from the food one eats. A balanced diet from the four basic food groups, plus water, provides the nutrition and calories for athletes in strength training. The four basic food groups are milk and cheese; meat (veal, pork, beef, lamb), poultry, fish, and eggs; breads and cereals; and vegetables and fruits. A balanced diet will provide an athlete with adequate vitamins and minerals.

An athlete requires 1 gm of protein per kilogram of body weight. The requirement for an athlete in strength training is 3,000–6,000 calories daily. The recommended percentages of these calories for the three types of food are protein, 10–15 percent; fats, 25–30 percent; and carbohydrates, 55–60 percent.

A more in-depth discussion of the nutritional needs of the athlete and specific nutritional programs such as carbohydrate loading are discussed in Chapter 42.

IMPORTANT CONCEPTS

1. With a concentric muscle contraction, the muscle shortens with tension; with an eccentric contraction, the muscle lengthens with tension; and with an isometric contraction, the muscle remains constant with tension.

2. The ATP-PC system and the lactic acid system are anaerobic energy systems that do not require oxygen to produce energy.

3. Aerobic systems depend on the availability of oxygen to burn carbohydrates and fats to yield energy.

4. "Power" athletes have a greater proportion of Type I muscle fibers (fast twitch muscle fibers); "endurance" athletes have a higher proportion of Type II muscle fibers (slow twitch muscle fibers).

5. According to the overload principle, strength, power, endurance, and hypertrophy of muscle only increase when a muscle performs workloads greater than previously encountered.

6. In progressive resistance exercises, the overload of muscle is done gradually and pro-gressively to avoid fatigue and overtraining.

7. According to the principle of specificity, training should work the muscles in a manner resembling the movements performed in the sport.

8. Periodization helps to decrease the possibility of overtraining by dividing the year-ly training cycle into three or four phases, depending on the sport.

9. Muscle training involves the manipulation of specificity, intensity, duration, and frequency to enhance the strength, power, and endurance of muscle.

10. Range of motion, a degree of motion permitted at a specific joint, is often influenced by flexibility of muscles which cross the joint.

11. Cardiorespiratory endurance is one's capacity to exercise at high levels for a prolonged period of time.

12. Factors that affect exercise gains include initial fitness levels, intensity of exercise, duration of exercise, frequency of exercise, and types of exercise.

SUGGESTED READINGS

Arnheim, D. D. *Modern Principles of Athletic Training: The Science of Sports Medicine: Injury Prevention, Causation, and Management*, 6th ed. St. Louis: Times Mirror/ Mosby College Publishing, 1985.

DeLorme, T. L. "Restoration of Muscle Power by Heavy-Resistance Exercises." *Journal of Bone and Joint Surgery* 27 (1945): 645–667.

Fox, E. L., and D. K. Mathews. *The Physiological Basis of Physical Education and Athletics*, 3d ed. Philadelphia: Saunders College Pub., 1981.

Kulund, D. N., ed. *The Injured Athlete*. Philadelphia: J. B. Lippincott, 1982.

McArdle, W. D., F. I. Katch, and V. L. Katch. *Exercise Physiology: Energy, Nutrition, and Human Performance*, 2d ed. Philadelphia: Lea & Febiger, 1986.

Pedemont, H. "Periodization of Strength Training." *National Strength and Conditioning Association Journal* (April–May 1982): 10–11, 60.

Stone, M., H. O'Bryant, J. Garhammer, J. McMillan, and R. Rozenek. "A Theoretical Model for Strength Training." *National Strength and Conditioning Association Journal* (August–September 1982).

Yessis, M. "The Competitive Period in the Multiyear and Yearly Training Programs." *National Strength and Conditioning Association Journal* (February–March 1983).

———. "The Transitional Period." *National Strength and Conditioning Association Journal* (April–May 1983).

APPENDIX: SPORT-SPECIFIC CONDITIONING MODELS

Strength, conditioning, and flexibility programs should all be designed following the basic principles of strength training. Programs for specific sports should follow the basic form of the classic periodization model (see Figure 45.2 on page 726) to ensure year-round training. It is important to remember that each position in each sport places unique demands on the athlete. To train an athlete adequately, the program has to be specific to the skills required for the particular sport and position. The below training programs basically follow the periodization model. It is important to remember that other programs have been designed to accomplish the same goals as those presented here. No matter which training program a coach, athletic trainer, or athlete utilizes, the program should adequately condition and train the athlete without causing overtraining.

Periodization Model for Swimmers

August 25	September 1 8 15	22	October 29 6 13 20	27	November 3 10 17	24	December 1 8 15	22 29	January 5 12 19 26	Feb/Mar
General Conditioning			Preseason Conditioning			Transition Phase	Competitive Phase			Taper and Retaper
	Hypertrophy 3	Strength 2	Power 2	Combined (Hypertrophy) 2	Strength 2	Power 2	Combined (Coordination) 2	Strength 2	Power 4	Maintenance 6

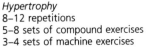

Hypertrophy
8–12 repetitions
5–8 sets of compound exercises
3–4 sets of machine exercises

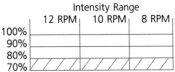

Strength
3–6 repetitions
4–6 sets of compound exercises
3–4 sets of machine exercises

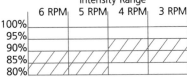

Power
1–3 repetitions
2–5 sets of compound exercises
2–4 sets of machine exercises

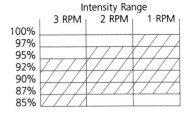

Source: R. Uebel, "Weight Training for Swimmers: A Practical Approach, *National Strength and Conditioning Association Journal* 9, no. 3 (1987). Reprinted by permission of the National Strength and Conditioning Association, Lincoln, Nebraska.

Periodization Model for Track Throwers

Variable Weight Throwing Program

| SEP | OCT | NOV | DEC | JAN | FEB | MAR | APR | MAY | JUN | JUL | AUG |

60% Heavy & 40% Light

60% Light & 40% Heavy

40% Heavy & 60% Normal

100% Normal

Sample Workout for Basic-Strength Cycle	Sample Workout for Strength-Power Cycle

Monday
 Warm-up with flexibility exercises: 10–15 min.
 Light throwing: 30–45 min.
   use light and heavy implements
 Weight lifting: 60–90 min.
   emphasis in absolute strength
 Warm-down: 10–15 min.
	Monday
	 Warm-up with flexibility exercises: 10–15 min.
	 Light throwing: 30–45 min.
	   heavy and normal implements
	 Weight lifting: 60–90 min.
	   emphasis on absolute power
	 Warm-down: 10–15 min.

Tuesday
 Warm-up with flexibility exercises: 10–15 min.
 Medium to heavy throwing: 60–70 min.
 Plyometrics: 20–30 min.
   low hurdle hopping: 3–8 hurdles
   double leg bounding: 20–30 meters
 Warm-down 10–15 min.
	Tuesday
	 Warm-up with flexibility exercises: 10–15 min.
	 Medium throwing: 45–60 min.
	 Plyometrics: 15–30 min.
	   double and single leg bounding: 30–40 meters
	 Warm-down: 10–15 min.

Wednesday Warm-up with flexibility exercises: 10–15 min. Weight lifting: 45–60 min. Warm-down: 10–15 min.	*Wednesday* Warm-up with flexibility exercises: 10–15 min. Technique drills: 45 min. Wind sprints, 80–90% intensity, full recovery: 25–35 min. 50 to 60 meters Warm-down and restorative methods: 10–15 min.
Thursday Warm-up with flexibility exercises: 10–15 min. Easy technique drills: 15–30 min. Wind sprints, 75–85% intensity, full recovery: 30–40 min. 60 to 80 meters Warm-down and restorative methods: 10–15 min.	*Thursday* Warm-up with flexibility exercises: 10–15 min. Weight lifting: 70–100 min. Warm-down: 10–15 min.

Friday
 Warm-up with flexibility exercises: 10–15 min.
 Weight lifting: 60–90 min.
 Warm-down: 10–15 min.
	Friday
	 Warm-up with flexibility exercises: 10–15 min.
	 Medium throwing: 30–45 min.
	   normal implement
	 Plyometrics: 20–30 min.
	   alternate leg bounding: 30–40 meters
	 Warm-down: 10–15 min.

Saturday
 Warm-up with flexibility exercises: 10–15 min.
 Medium to heavy throwing: 45–60 min.
   light and normal implements
 Plyometrics: 20–30 min.
   alternate leg bounding: 20 to 30 meters
 Warm-down: 10–15 min.
	Saturday
	 Warm-up with flexibility exercises: 10–15 min.
	 Weight lifting: 45–60 min.
	 Warm-down: 10–15 min.

Sunday Active Rest	*Sunday* Active Rest
Totals for week Warm-up and warm-down = 60–115 min. Throwing = 135–175 min. Technique drills = 15–30 min. Weight lifting = 165–240 min. Plyometrics = 40–60 min. Wind sprints = 30–40 min.	*Totals for week* Warm-up and warm-down = 60–115 min. Throwing = 105–150 min. Technique drills = 45 min. Weight lifting = 175–250 min. Plyometrics = 35–60 min. Wind sprints = 25–35 min.

Periodization Model for Track Throwers (continued)

Sample Workout for Competition Cycle

Early Competitive	Late Competitive

Monday
Warm-up with flexibility exercises: 10–15 min.
Weight lifting: 60–90 min.
   emphasis on explosive power
Technique drills: 30 min.
Warm-down: 10–15 min.
	Monday
	Warm-up with flexibility exercises: 10–15 min.
	Medium to hard throwing: 30–45 min.
	Wind sprints: 20–30 min.
	   10 to 30 meters
	Warm-down: 10–15 min.

Tuesday
Warm-up with flexibility exercises: 10–15 min.
Hard throwing: 45–60 min.
   95% normal, 5% light implements
Hill sprinting: 20–30 min.
   30 to 40 meters
Warm-down 10–15 min.
	Tuesday
	Warm-up with flexibility exercises: 10–15 min.
	Technique drills: 20–30 min.
	Warm-down: 10–15 min.

Wednesday Warm-up with flexibility exercises: 10–15 min. Technique drills: 30–45 min. Warm-down: 10–15 min.	*Wednesday* Warm-up with flexibility exercises: 10–15 min. Weight lifting: 45–60 min. very explosive lifting Warm-down: 10–15 min.

Thursday
Warm-up with flexibility exercises: 10–15 min.
Throwing: 15–30 min.
   4 hard stands
   6 all out throws
Light explosive lifting: 30–45 min.
Warm-down: 10–15 min.
	Thursday
	Warm-up with flexibility exercises: 10–15 min.
	Easy throwing: 15–20 min.
	   emphasis on technique only
	Wind sprints: 10–15 min.
	   10 to 15 meters
	Warm-down: 10–15 min.

Friday
Warm-up with flexibility exercises: 10–15 min.
Technique drills: 10–15 min.
Wind sprints: 10–15 min.
   10 to 15 meters
Warm-down: 10–15 min.
	Friday
	Warm-up with flexibility exercises: 10–15 min.
	Throwing: competitive situation
	   3 to 4 stands
	   3 all out competitive throws: the athlete must be
	   able to achieve a good mark in the first three in
	   order to make the finals.
	Warm-down: 10–15 min.

Saturday Competition	*Saturday* Competition

Sunday
Warm-up with flexibility exercises: 10–15 min.
Throwing: 30–45 min.
   normal implement
Wind sprints: 15–20 min.
   20 to 30 meters
Warm-down: 10–15 min.
	Sunday
	Warm-up with flexibility exercises: 10–15 min.
	Light lifting, throwing, or both or active rest: 30–45 min.
	Warm-down: 10–15 min.

Totals for week Warm-up and warm-down = 60–115 min. Throwing = 95–135 min. Technique drills = 70–90 min. Weight lifting = 90–135 min. Plyometrics = 0 Wind sprints = 45–65 min.	*Totals for week* Warm-up and warm-down = 60–115 min. Throwing = 65–90 min. Technique drills = 20–30 min. Weight lifting = will vary Plyometrics = 0 Wind sprints = 30–45 min.

Periodization Model for Track Throwers (continued)

Power Training Schedule/General Guidelines

September (60–70%)

Exercise	sets × reps
Back squat	3 × 10
Dead lift	3 × 10
Bench press	3 × 10
Military press	3 × 10
Tricep extension	3 × 10
Power clean	3 × 10
Arm curls	3 × 10
Russian twists*	3 × 10

October (75–90%)

Exercise	sets × reps
Back squat	6·5·4·3·2
Dead lift	6·5·4·3·2
Incline bench	6·5·4·3·2
Power clean	6·5·4·3·2
Russian twists	4 × 10

November (70–75%)

Exercise	sets × reps
Back squat	4 × 8
Leg press	4 × 8
Bench press	4 × 8
Push press	4 × 8
Tricep extension	4 × 8
Power clean	4 × 8
Incline situps	4 × 20
Good mornings*	3 × 15

(Fourth week) 1st workout

Power clean	2 × 2 (95%)
Incline bench	2 × 2 (95%)

2nd workout

Power clean	1 × 2 (95%)
Incline bench	1 × 2 (95%)

December (80–85%)

Exercise	sets × reps
Back squat	4 × 5
Front squat	4 × 5
Incline bench	4 × 5
Power clean	4 × 5
Bench press	4 × 5
Russian twists	5 × 15
Good mornings	3 × 20

January (70–75%)

Exercise	sets × reps
Front squat	4 × 7
Leg press	4 × 7
Incline bench	4 × 7
Power clean & jerk	4 × 7
Tricep extension	4 × 7
Twisting situps	4 × 20
Good mornings	3 × 10

February (90–95%)

Exercise	sets × reps
Power clean	5 × 3
Back squat	5 × 3
Bench press	5 × 3
Jerk from rack	5 × 3
Russian twists	4 × 20
Good mornings	3 × 20

(Second week)
Reduce second workout
by 45 pounds.

Power clean	5·3·2·1
Bench press	5·3·2·1
Back squat	5·3·2·1
Russian twists	3 × 20

March (60–85%)

Exercise	sets × reps
Power clean	10·7·5·5·7
Push press	10·7·5·5·7
Incline bench	10·7·5·5·7
Back squat	10·7·5·5·7
Incline situps	5 × 20

April (85–100%)
Reduce second workout
by 25 pounds.

Exercise	sets × reps
(Twice weekly)	
Power clean	5·4·3·2·1
Jerk from rack	5·4·3·2·1
Bench press	5·4·3·2·1
Back squat	5·4·3·2·1
Russian twists	4 × 20 fast

May (85–100%)
Reduce second workout
by 35 pounds.

Exercise	sets × reps
(First week)	
Power clean	5·3·2·1
Incline bench	5·3·2·1
Back squat	5·3·2·1
Incline situps	3 × 20

(Third week)
Reduce second workout
by 60 pounds.

Power clean	4·2·1
Incline bench	4·2·1
Back squat	4·2·1
Russian twists	2 × 20

*Russian twists: see *Sports Fitness*, May, 1985: 111–112.
*Good mornings: see *NSCA Journal*, 7(5):79.
Source: S. Auferoth, "Power Training for the Developing Thrower," *National Strength and Conditioning Association Journal* 8, no. 5 (1986). Reprinted by permission of the National Strength and Conditioning Association, Lincoln, Nebraska.

Periodization Model for Football Players

Line, Linebackers, and Fullbacks	Running Backs, Receivers, and Quarterbacks

Intensity:

LR-Light Range	MR-Moderate Range	HR-Heavy Range
8–12 Reps	5–8 Reps	1–5 Reps
65–75% Maximum	75–85% Maximum	85–100% Maximum
failure 8–12	failure 5–8	failure 1–5

Intensity:

LR-Light Range	MR-Moderate Range	HR-Heavy Range
8–12 Reps	5–8 Reps	1–5 Reps
65–75% Maximum	75–85% Maximum	85–100% Maximum
failure 8–12	failure 5–8	failure 1–5

Line, Linebackers, and Fullbacks

Abdominals
Abdominal crunches 1 × 50
Side bends w/dumbbells 1 × 50

Lower Body
Hip sled
Leg press
Sumo deadlift — Choose 1 (3 sets LR)
Squats
Quadriceps extensions
  1 set of manuals (10 reps)
Ham curls
  1 set of manuals (10 reps)
Manual groin
  1 set of manuals (10 reps)

Upper Body
Perform 2 sets (MR) 85% Maximum
  Perform 1 set (HR) 90% maximum
Bench or incline
Dumbbell bench
Chest flies — Choose 1
Manuals 1 × 10
Military press
Upright rows
Shrugs — Perform all lifts 1 set of MR
Manuals 1 × 10
Lat pulldowns
Bent-over rows
Manual towel pulls w/partner — Choose 1
Seated cable rows
Close-grip bench press
Tricep extensions — Perform all lifts 2 sets HR
Manual tricep extensions
Tricep lockouts
Hammer curls 2 sets (HR)
Manual neck resistance 2 × 10

Running Backs, Receivers, and Quarterbacks

Abdominals
Abdominal crunches 1 × 100

Lower Body
Perform 1 set (LR) and 2 sets (MR)
Sled
Leg press — Choose 1
Lunges
Quadriceps extensions
  1 set of manuals (10 reps)
Hamstring curls
Stiff-legged dead lifts — Choose 1
Manual ham curls
Manual groin 1 × 10
Hip flexors 2 × 10 each leg

Upper Body
Perform 3 sets (MR)
Bench press
Dumbbell bench
Incline bench — Choose 1
Chest flies
Manual resistance
Military press
Shoulder press — Perform both lifts 2 sets (MR)
Bent-over rows
Seated cable rows — Choose 1
Lat pulldowns
Tricep extension
Narrow-width pushups
Manual resistance — Perform 2 3 sets (MR)
Manual neck resistance 2 × 10

Periodization Model for Football Players   (continued)

DAY 1 Monday	DAY II Tuesday	DAY III Wednesday
Lower body and back	*Chest, shoulders, triceps, upper back*	*Conditioning*
Stomach crunches 100 reps	Stomach 100 reps	Stretch 5 minutes
Squats 3 × HR	High pulls 3 × LR	Skip rope Circuit Train
Front squats (Line & Linebackers) 3 × MR	Bench press 2 × LR	Medicine ball drills Alternate every 5 minutes
Lunges (Backs & WR's) 3 × MR	3 × HR	Position drills (Agilities)
Hamstring curls 1 × 8 Manual Resistance	Incline dumbbell press	Sprints: 10 minutes
Leg adductors 1 × 8 Manual Resistance	(Line & Linebackers) 3 × MR	440 yards 2 sets
Hip flexors (Backs & WR's) 2 × LR	Chest flies (Backs & WR's) 3 × MR	330 yards 2 sets
Lat pulls 4 × HR	Military press 3 × MR	220 yards 3 sets
Hyperextensions 2 × MR	Tricep lockouts on bench 2 × HR (100% max)	110 yards 5 sets
Four-way neck resistance	Tricep extensions 3 × HR	Harness runs w/partners 5 minutes •
1 × 8 each direction	Stretch 5 minutes	Rest 2 minutes
Manual Resistance		40 yard gasers 5 minutes • Rest 2 minutes
Stretch 5 minutes	Running	Stadium steps or hills 3 minutes •
	Distance 4 minutes	Rest 2 minutes
Running	Form running 15 minutes	Starts 6 minutes
Distance 8–10 minutes	Plyometrics 10 minutes	20 yards 4 sets
Medicine ball drills 5 minutes	Stretch 5 minutes	10 yards 4 sets
Stomach crunches 100 reps		5 yards 6 sets
Stretch 5 minutes		Stretch 5 minutes

DAY IV Thursday	DAY V Friday
Lower body and back	*Chest, shoulders, triceps, upper back*
Stomach crunches	Stomach crunches 100 reps
Deadlifts 3 × MR	High pulls 3 × MR
Lunges (Line & Linebackers) 3 × LR	Upright rows 3 × HR
Leg press (Backs & WR's) 3 × LR	Shrugs 3 × HR
Hamstrings: Stiff-legged deadlifts 2 × LR	Military press w/dumbbells 3 × HR
Hamstring curls (manual resistance) 1 × 8	Bench press 2 × LR
Hip flexors 2 × LR	3 × MR
Leg adductors (manual resistance) 1 × 8	Standing lateral raises 3 × MR or 1 × 8 Manual Resistance
Lat pulls 4 × MR	Tricep extensions 4 × MR
Hyperextensions 2 × MR	Stretch 5 minutes
Neck resistance (manual resistance) 1 × 8 each direction	
Stretch 5 minutes	Running
	Same as Day II
Running	Stretch 5 minutes
Same as Day I	
Stretch 5 minutes	

Source: R. Parker, ''Year-Round Conditioning for Football at Fresno State,'' *National Strength and Conditioning Association Journal* 8, no. 3 (1987). Reprinted by permission of the National Strength and Conditioning Association, Lincoln, Nebraska.

Periodization Model for an In-Season Conditioning Program for Football Players

	Movements	Objectives	Drills	
			Related	Unrelated
Agility	Back peddling Corioca Cross-over 4-point Running Shuffling	Changing directions 　Predetermined (marked) 　On reaction (sound or movement) Maneuverability 　Body control; balance 　Negotiating obstacles	Bag drills Wave drills	Side-to-side; 　point-to-point Acrobatics
Coordination	Hopping Jumping Shuffling Skipping	Improve footspeed Total body functionability Neuromuscular efficiency 　Dexterity/perception 　Quickness	Ball drills Weight training	Jump rope drills Speed shuffle (lateral) Rope runs Acrobatics Weight training
Flexibility	Extension Flexion Rotation	Enhance joint range of motion Preparation for physical exertion Means to alleviate muscle tightness 　or soreness	Position-specific	Dynamic flexibility Static flexibility Weight training
Power	Bounding Jumping Rotating Running Striking Throwing	Develop ballistic movement 　Increase efficient use of stored 　elastic energy Explosive leg drive Contact initiation 　Improve thrust action of legs, 　hip and torso	Bag drills Sled drills Weight training	Double leg and 　single leg bound/jumps Medicine ball Weight training
Reaction	Catching Hopping Running Shuffling Starting Striking	Contact initiation 　Response to audio stimulus 　Response to visual stimulus Body control Hand-eye coordination/quickness	Bag drills Ball drills Medicine ball drills Sled drills	Total body movement Weight training
Speed	Sprinting Starting	Explosive takeoff Enhance acceleration 　Contact initiation 　Attain peak velocity in 　minimal time	Off-the-ball Contact initiation 　drills	Sprints (intervals) Starts Weight training
Strength	Pulling Pressing Thrusting	Neuromuscular facilitation Creating dynamic force capacity 　Elastic energy utilization 　Contact initiation Joint range of motion and stability	Weight training*	Weight training*

*Drills listed under "Power" can be used for strength enhancement also.
Source: R. Elam, "Prime Time Football Fitness: In-Season Conditioning," *National Strength and Conditioning Association Journal* 8, no. 6 (1986).
Reprinted by permission of the National Strength and Conditioning Association, Lincoln, Nebraska.

Periodization Model for Football Linebackers

Sequence of Training Phases

Transitional (1–2 months)
Active rest
Recuperation
Recreational sports activities
Provides a "break" for the player
  psychologically as well as physiologically

General Preparatory (4 months)
Development of technique
Strength
Muscle hypertrophy
Endurance
Flexibility
High volume and low to moderate intensity

Specific Preparatory (3 months)
Specific strength
Power
Agility
Anaerobic endurance
Flexibility
Lower volume and high intensity

Competitive (3–4 months)
Focus on maintenance
Prevent retrogression
No overload
Execution of proper technique on the field
  is of primary importance
Maintain flexibility
Injury prevention

Notes: After the general preparatory phase, one week is taken off (active rest), and the following week is used for testing purposes.

Competitive Phase (Sept., Oct., Nov., and sometimes Dec.)

Monday	Wednesday
Squat 3 × 8	Bench press 3 × 8
Leg ext. 2 × 10	Shoulder press 2 × 8
Leg curl 2 × 10	Lateral raises 2 × 8
Calf raise 2 × 15	Front raise 2 × 8
Add./Ab. 2 × 20	Tricep press 3 × 8
Lat pull-down 2 × 8	Hammer curls 2 × 8
Seated low row 2 × 8	Ab. crunches 2 × 30
Ab. crunches 2 × 30	Nautilus neck 2 × 10
Nautilus neck 2 × 10	

Source: Anthony G. Smith.

General Preparatory Phase

	1st Month (M-W-F)	2nd Month (M-W-F)
Deadlift	4 × 10	4 × 8
Squat	4 × 10	4 × 8
Power clean	4 × 10	4 × 8
Shrugs	2 × 10	3 × 8
Bench press	4 × 10	4 × 8
Standing military press	3 × 10	3 × 8
Tricep press	3 × 10	3 × 8
Lat pull-down	2 × 10	2 × 8
Lat pull-down (reverse grip)	2 × 10	2 × 8
Abdominal crunches	3 × 15	3 × 20
Calf raises	—	3 × 10

ROM	3rd Month (M-W-F) full	power	4th Month (M-W-F) full	power
Deadlift	3 × 6	2 × 6	10,6	3,3,3,
Squat	3 × 6	2 × 6	10,6	3,3,3
Power clean	2 × 6	3 × 6	10,6	3,3,3
Shrugs	4 × 6		4 × 6	
Nautilus neck	1 × 10 (4-way)		2 × 10	
Bench press	4 × 6		10,6,3,3,3	
Incline press	2 × 6		2 × 6	
Standing military press	4 × 6		4 × 6	
Tricep press	3 × 6		3 × 6	
Lat pull-down	2 × 6		2 × 6	
Lat pull-down (reverse grip)	2 × 6		2 × 6	
Hammer curls	3 × 6		3 × 6	
Abdominal crunches	3 × 20		3 × 20	
Calf raises	3 × 15		3 × 15	

Bench press to be performed using a shoulder width grip to simulate actual playing situations
ROM-(range of motion) "power" indicates a biomechanically superior position to duplicate the hitting position. (For the power clean, the start is with the bar elevated slightly, to a position which places the bar just below the knees.)

Periodization Model for Football Linebackers (continued)

Specific Preparatory Phase (Monday/Thursday)

ROM	1st Month full	1st Month specific	2nd Month full	2nd Month spec/power	3rd Month full	3rd Month spec/power
Deadlift	1 × 10	3 × 8	1 × 10	3 × 8	1 × 10	3 × 6
Squat	2 × 10	3 × 8	2 × 10	2 × 10	1 × 10	3 × 8
Power clean		3 × 8		3 × 8		3 × 6
Shrugs	3 × 10		3 × 8		3 × 8	
Nautilus neck	2 × 10		2 × 10		2 × 10	
Leg extension	2 × 8		2 × 8		2 × 8	
Leg curl	2 × 8		2 × 8		2 × 8	
Abductor/Adductor	2 × 20		2 × 20		2 × 20	
Lat pull-down	3 × 8		3 × 6		3 × 6	
Seated low row	3 × 8		3 × 6		3 × 6	
Abdominal crunches	3 × 20		3 × 20		3 × 20	
Calf raises	3 × 15		3 × 15		3 × 15	

Specific Preparatory Phase (Tuesday/Friday)

ROM	1st Month full	1st Month specific	2nd Month full	2nd Month specific	3rd Month full	3rd Month specific
Bench press	10,8	6,6,6*	10,8,5	8,8*	10,8,5	8,8*
Incline bench	2 × 10		2 × 10		2 × 10	
Stand, shoulder press or	3 × 10		3 × 8		3 × 8	
(Behind neck press)						
Front delt raise	2 × 10		2 × 8		2 × 8	
Lateral delt raise	2 × 10		2 × 8		2 × 8	
Weighted forearm del.	2 × 10		2 × 8		2 × 8	
Tricep press	1 × 10	2 × 10*	1 × 10	3 × 8*	1 × 10	3 × 8*
Lying tricep ext.	2 × 10		2 × 8		2 × 8	
Hammer curls	3 × 10		3 × 8		3 × 8	
Reverse curls	2 × 10		2 × 8		2 × 8	
Abdominal crunches	3 × 20		3 × 20		3 × 20	
Calf raises	3 × 15		3 × 15		3 × 15	
Neck	2 × 10		2 × 10		2 × 10	

*Denotes a "power-set" whereby explosive power is emphasized.

Periodization Model for Pole Vaulters

Preseason

Monday	Tuesday	Wednesday	Thursday	Friday	Saturday

Warm-up
2–3 mile fartlek
Strength training
  Power cleans or jerks
  Bench press
  Squats/Hip sled
  Leg curls
  Hip flexors
  Back hyperextensions
Warm-down
	Warm-up
	3–5 mile fartlek
	8 × 200 strides
	Warm-down
		Warm-up
		2–3 mile fartlek
		Strength training
		  Power cleans
		  Bench press
		  Squats/Hip sled
		  Leg curls
		  Hip flexors
		  Back hyperextensions
		Warm-down
			Warm-up
			3–5 mile fartlek
			Pole sprints
			  (approach)
			Plant tech.
			12–15 × 75 yard
			  sprints
			Warm-down
				Warm-up
				2–3 mile fartlek
				Strength training
				  Power cleans
				  Bench press
				  Squats/Hip sled
				  Leg curls
				  Hip flexors
				  Back hyperextensions
				Warm-down
					Warm-up
					5–7 mile fartlek
					Warm-down
					
					Sunday
					Rest

Indoor-Early Competitive Season

Monday	Tuesday	Wednesday	Thursday	Friday	Saturday

Warm-up
Vault tech.
10–15 × 60-yard
  sprints
Warm-down
	Warm-up
	Approach tech.
	Strength training
	  Power cleans
	  Bench press
	  Squats/Hip sled
	  Leg curls
	  Hip flexors
	  Back hyperextensions
	Warm-down
		Warm-up
		Plant drills
		Gymnastics
		Warm-down
			Warm-up
			Vault tech.
			Strength training
			  Power cleans
			  Bench press
			  Squats/Hip sled
			  Leg curls
			  Hip flexors
			Warm-down
				Warm-up
				Approach tech.
				  (light)
				Warm-down
					Warm-up
					Competition
					Strength training
					  Power cleans
					  Bench press
					  Leg curls
					  Hip flexors
					Warm-down
					
					Sunday
					Rest

Outdoor Competitive Season

Monday	Tuesday	Wednesday	Thursday	Friday	Saturday

Warm-up
Vault tech.
  (short run)
10–15 × 75 yard
  flying starts
Warm-down
	Warm-up
	6 × 150 m
	  acceleration runs
	Strength training
	  Power cleans
	  Bench press
	  Squats/Hip sled
	  Leg curls
	  Hip flexors
	  Back hyperextensions
	Warm-down
		Warm-up
		Approach technique
		Gymnastics
		Warm-down
			Warm-up
			Vault tech.
			  (long run quality)
			Strength training
			  High pulls
			  Bench press
			  Leg curls
			  Hip flexors
			Warm-down
				Warm-up
				Approach
				  technique (light)
				Warm-down
					Warm-up
					Competition
					Strength training
					Saturday or
					Sunday
					  Power cleans
					  Bench press
					  Leg curls
					  Hip flexors
					Warm-down

Source: D. Railsback, Sports Performance Series: "The Pole Vault," *National Strength and Conditioning Association Journal* 9, no. 2 (1987). Reprinted by permission of the National Strength and Conditioning Association, Lincoln, Nebraska.

Periodization Model for Wrestlers

Off season I

Dates   June–August

Goal   Develop strength and power with emphasis on the legs, hips, and pulling muscles in the upper body.

Training Days   4 days per week

Type of Training   Power training is conducted involving full body explosive lifts, such as power cleans, squats, push press and weighted pull-ups. Rest between sets is 2–3 minutes.

Transition I

Dates   1 week

Goal   Allow the body and mind to recover from the previous mesocycle.

Type of Training   Rest.

Off season II

Dates   September–October

Goal   Same as I

Training Days   3 days per week

Type of Training   Similar to I. Possibly substitute exercise with ones that are different but develop the same muscle groups.

Transition II

Dates   1 week

Goal   Allow the body and mind to recover from the previous mesocycle.

Type of Training   Wrestling drills with no weight training.

Preseason

Dates   November–December

Goal   Maintain strength and power developed during the off-season.

Training Days   2 days per week.

Type of Training   Similar to that used during the off-season with greater emphasis placed on technique work and exercise specificity.

Transition III

Dates   1 week during Christmas break.

Goal   Allow the body and mind to recover from training.

Type of Training   Wrestling drills and practice with no weight training.

In-season (Lactic Acid)

Dates   January–Mid-February

Goal   Acclimate the body to the excessive amounts of lactic acid encountered during wrestling competitions.

Training Days   2 days per week.

Type of Training   The exercises are pre-exhaustive in nature, that is, a single joint exercise is immediately followed by a multiple joint exercise. Time between the single and multiple joint exercises is no more than 3 seconds, while the rest between sets is approximately 2 minutes. All sets are burnouts.

In-season (Circuit)

Dates   Mid-February–March

Goal   To physically peak the wrestlers in muscular strength, endurance, and conditioning.

Training Days   2–3 days per week.

Type of Training   A circuit of 12 exercises is completed with the work rest ration of 45 sec/15 sec. After completing one set of the circuit, anaerobic running is performed followed by another set of the circuit.

Active rest

Dates   April–May

Goal   Restore the athlete's body and mind to rested conditions following the long competitive season.

Training Days   2–3 days per week.

Type of Training   Very light technique work on wrestling skills, along with participation in several recreational games.

Source: G. Palmieri, Roundtable: "Periodization, Part 3," *National Strength and Conditioning Association Journal* 9, no. 1 (1987). Reprinted by permission of the National Strength and Conditioning Association, Lincoln, Nebraska.

Periodization Model for Soccer Players

Month	Weight Training	Conditioning	Flexibility
August	*In-season*	*In-season*	*Before* and
September	Maintenance program	Soccer practice	*after* practice
October			
November			
December	2 days/week		
January	Active	Rest	Period
February	Off-season		Before
March	Strength program	Over distance training Low-volume plyometric	and after
April	4 days/week	Interval training High-volume plyometric	Conditioning
May		Spring soccer	
June	Preseason	Soccer/Active rest	Individualized summer
July	Power program	Preseason Conditioning program	program
August	3 days/week		

Source: P. Ciccantelli, "Year-Round Strength and Conditioning Program for Soccer," *National Strength and Conditioning Association Journal* 9, no. 4 (1987). Reprinted by permission of the National Strength and Conditioning Association, Lincoln, Nebraska.

46

Corporate Wellness Programs

OBJECTIVES FOR CHAPTER 46

After reading this chapter, the student should be able to:

1. Understand the importance of preventive medicine and the role of corporate wellness programs in promoting healthful lifestyles.
2. Discuss how the benefits of corporate wellness programs are enjoyed not only by the individual members, but also by the corporation.

INTRODUCTION

With health care costs rising rapidly in today's world, corporate wellness programs are becoming increasingly popular. They offer benefits not only to the individual employee, but also to the corporation and to society as a whole. Chapter 46 describes the importance of preventive medicine and considerations in the organization of a corporate wellness program. ■

THE IMPORTANCE OF PREVENTIVE MEDICINE

Rising Health Care Costs

Health care costs are increasing at twice the rate of inflation and account for nearly 12 percent of the gross national product. One company, General Motors, spent $2.9 billion on employee health care in 1987, a sum that added $600 to the cost of every car manufactured by the company.

One approach to counter the financial burden of corporate health care is to promote the practice of preventive medicine. Nationally, the latter has been long neglected. For example, the overall cost of health care in the United States is over $550 billion; only 0.3 percent of that amount is spent on preventive medicine.

A national conference on health policy was held at the Carter Center in Atlanta in the mid-1980s. The conference focused on 14 health problems that account for 70 percent of hospital days, 80 percent of deaths, and 90 percent of potential years lost before age 65. About two-thirds of deaths before age 65 were believed to have resulted from potentially preventable causes. In an accompanying editorial, Dr. E. N. Brandt stated: "Prevention of disease and the promotion of health are the highest achievement of medicine. Application of the science and principles underlying these concepts will lead to decreased pain, suffering, disability, and premature death."

The Role of the Corporate Community

The corporate community has taken an active role in the practice of preventive medicine. An estimated two-thirds of U.S. companies provide some type of wellness program. For smaller companies, the American Heart Association (AHA) has made available a set of materials and action plans targeted at four risk factors for cardiovascular disease: high blood pressure, cigarette smoking, obesity, and a sedentary lifestyle.

ORGANIZATION OF A CORPORATE WELLNESS PROGRAM

Many larger companies have well-organized wellness programs, with a physical fitness component at their core. These programs are usually available to all employees, with enrollment being voluntary. In some cases, corporate wellness programs are also available to spouses and recent retirees.

Before becoming a member of a corporate wellness program, the interested employee usually must complete a medical screening process, which includes a review of the individual's past medical history and family medical history. During the fitness portion of the screening, blood pressure, height, weight, flexibility, abdominal strength, and percentage body fat are measured. A health risk appraisal questionnaire, as well as blood chemistry analysis for glucose, total cholesterol, high-density lipoprotein (HDL) cholesterol, low-density lipoprotein (LDL) cholesterol, and serum triglyceride levels, may also be included in this initial screening process.

Male employees 40 years and older and female employees 50 years and older constitute two groups at higher risk for medical problems; therefore, in addition to completing the company's medical screening process, these employees might also require referral from their personal physician for participation in the wellness program. In some instances, the company physician provides this high-risk assessment examination, which may include an exercise stress test.

Similarly, physician assessment prior to program entrance may be required for employees with at least one primary risk factor for cardiovascular disease (for example, a personal history of heart problems, smoking, hypertension, or hyperlipidemia) or several secondary risk factors (for example, a family history of coronary disease or abnormal reaction to exercise, stressful lifestyle, high percentage of body fat, or sedentary activity level).

After completion of the medical screening process, employees attend a planning and orientation session. At this time, a staff member helps eligible employees to analyze their health risks and organize their individualized wellness and exercise program. If the latter is to be done at the company exercise facility, the facility's exercise equipment is usually demonstrated during this orientation session.

Lifestyle changes are also recommended to alter risk factors such as high blood pressure, high total cholesterol level or a low HDL-cholesterol level, obesity, tobacco and alcohol use, and high levels of stress.

The Fitness Center

Most corporate programs provide an exercise facility for members. The size of these fitness centers differs markedly from corporation to corporation. Most have a locker room with showers and a sauna or steam room. Some programs provide exercise clothing and towels. One room of the facility contains the exercise equipment, such as weight machines, rowing machines, step exercisers, exercise bicycles, and free weights. Other rooms, often with specially designed shock-absorbing surfaces, are available for classes in high- and low-impact aerobics, strengthening and stretching exer-

cises, yoga, and relaxation techniques. Many corporate exercise facilities are also equipped with indoor or outdoor track facilities and courts for racquetball, handball, and squash. The hours of operation of these facilities vary. Most facilities open between 6:00 to 6:30 A.M. and offer extended evening hours to accommodate individuals who wish to use the facility after work.

Member participation in the exercise facility may be tracked by an internal computer system which permits entry and retrieval of information concerning a member's activity, interests, and fitness measurements. After entering the facility, members check in at the computer terminal, and after completing their workout, log their activities into the terminal, recording the type of activity, duration, intensity, and distance or resistance. At the end of each month, members receive a computer printout of their activities for the past month, as well as year-to-date totals. Often the fitness facility staff review these activities and make suggestions for improving or altering a member's program for the following month.

Cost of Membership

The cost to members of a corporate wellness program is typically minimal to encourage employee participation. In some corporations, a one-time registration fee covers initial blood analysis, paperwork, and fitness assessment, with monthly payroll deductions covering the cost of continued membership. In other programs, the cost depends on the total number of hours the member uses the facility. In most programs, however, the cost is fixed. An incentive rebate may be given to employees who decrease their risk factors and participate regularly in their exercise programs.

Staff of the Corporate Wellness Program

A few corporations have a physician as the medical director of the wellness program. Most programs, however, are staffed by individuals with a master's or doctoral degree in nursing, public health, exercise physiology, athletic training, or a related field. A registered dietitian and psychologist may also be full-time staff members or available on a consultant basis.

Other Features of the Wellness Program

Health education at the awareness, information, and behavorial change levels is provided to members through lectures, video and audio tapes, slides, brochures, and group meetings. Some companies provide an employee library to lend books and video and audio tapes on wellness topics.

Companies that have an athletic trainer or a physical therapist as a staff member or consultant may hold clinics on injury prevention and treatment. Providing nutritional food choices is another way that companies promote healthful lifestyles among their employees. Cafeterias in nutrition-conscious companies offer foods that are high in fiber and low in calories, fat, and cholesterol.

Encouraging Continued Motivation

The challenge of how to motivate company employees to eat properly and exercise regularly, as well as to decrease their health risk factors, is a difficult one for the wellness staff. The staff may use team and individual events scheduled throughout the year to increase employees' awareness of health issues and encourage participation in the wellness program. Special-interest groups such as a running, walking, or cycling club, or a nutritional or stress management group, with regular weekly or monthly meetings, may also help promote employee interest. Studies show that employees enjoy planned events that encourage teamwork and increase morale.

Benefit of Wellness Programs to the Company

Corporate wellness programs are committed to making a difference, not only for the individual members, but also for the company as a whole. Numerous articles in the literature of the last decade document decreases in health care costs in various companies around the country that have wellness programs. Savings have also been shown in decreased absenteeism. Such programs frequently serve as a positive influence in employee recruitment, help to decrease employee turnover, and improve job performance. In surveys of employees who participate in corporate wellness programs, 75 to 85 percent generally report that they feel better and have more endurance and more energy.

IMPORTANT CONCEPTS

1. Only 0.3 percent of the total cost of health care ($550 billion) in the United States is applied to preventive medicine.
2. Approximately two-thirds of deaths before age 65 may have potentially preventable causes.
3. The levels of health education are awareness, information, and behavioral change.
4. The benefits of a corporate wellness program to employees include improved psychological well-being, enhanced weight control, elevation in HDL-cholesterol levels, reduction in serum triglyceride levels, reduced cardiovascular risk, and prolongation of life.
5. Corporate benefits of a wellness program may include decreased health care costs, reduced absenteeism, recruitment incentive, less employee turnover, and enhanced job performance.

SUGGESTED READINGS

Bly, J. L., R. C. Jones, and J. E. Richardson. "Impact of Worksite Health Promotion on Health Care Costs and Utilization. Evaluation of Johnson & Johnson's Live for Life Program." *Journal of the American Medical Association* 256 (1986): 3235–3240.

Brandt, E. N., Jr. "Why the Carter Center?" (editorial). *Journal of the American Medical Association* 254 (1985): 1360.

Califano, J. A., Jr. "The Health-Care Chaos." *The New York Times Magazine*, March 20, 1988, p. 57.

Ferguson, E. W., L. L. Bernier, G. R. Banta, et al. "Effects of Exercise and Conditioning on Clotting and Fibrinolytic Activity in Men." *Journal of Applied Physiology* 62 (1987): 1416–1421.

Foege, W. H., R. W. Amler, and C. C. White. "Closing the Gap: Report of the Carter Center Health Policy Consultation." *Journal of the American Medical Association* 254 (1985): 1355–1358.

Fries, J. F., L. W. Green, and S. Levine. "Health Promotion and the Compression of Morbidity." *Lancet* 1 (1989): 481–483.

Goldsmith, M. F. "Risk Assessment, Management Addressed at 'Prevention 85.'" *Journal of the American Medical Association* 254 (1985): 1421–1423, 1425.

Goldsmith, M. F. "Worksite Wellness Programs: Latest Wrinkle to Smooth Health Care Costs." *Journal of the American Medical Association* 256 (1986): 1089–1091, 1095.

Hairston, J. B. "Corporate Care's Ominous Future." *Business Atlanta* 18 (1989): 56–68.

Paffenbarger, R. S., Jr., A. L. Wing, and R. T. Hyde. "Physical Activity as an Index of Heart Attack Risk in College Alumni." *American Journal of Epidemiology* 108 (1978): 161–175.

Paffenbarger, R. S., Jr., R. T. Hyde, A. L. Wing, et al. "Physical Activity, All-Cause Mortality, and Longevity of College Alumni." *New England Journal of Medicine* 314 (1986): 605–613.

Soman, V. R., V. A. Koivisto, D. Deibert, et al. "Increased Insulin Sensitivity and Insulin Binding to Monocytes after Physical Training." *New England Journal of Medicine* 301 (1979): 1200–1204.

Weintraub, M. S., Y. Rosen, R. Otto, et al. "Physical Exercise Conditioning in the Absence of Weight Loss Reduces Fasting and Postprandial Triglyceride-Rich Lipoprotein Levels." *Circulation* 79 (1989): 1007–1014.

47

Cardiac Rehabilitation Programs

OBJECTIVES FOR CHAPTER 47

After reading this chapter, the student should be able to:

1. Define cardiac rehabilitation.
2. Differentiate the four phases of a cardiac rehabilitation program according to setting, type, intensity, and duration of exercise at each phase.
3. Identify the different areas of instruction contributing to the holistic approach to cardiac rehabilitation.
4. Identify legal concerns and considerations associated with a cardiac rehabilitation program.

INTRODUCTION

Cardiovascular disease affects thousands of people each year. Many individuals who survive myocardial infarction or undergo coronary artery bypass grafting are faced with long-term treatment and care of their cardiac conditions. The prevalence of cardiovascular conditions, in particular coronary heart disease, led to the development and evolution of cardiac rehabilitation programs. Such programs have become a valuable component in the recovery process of the cardiac patient.

Chapter 47 begins with an overview of cardiac rehabilitation. The chapter then discusses the development of cardiac rehabilitation programs and the four phases of the programs generally in use today. The chapter concludes with a brief discussion of the guidelines for cardiac rehabilitation programs offered by various professional organizations and the legal aspects of these programs. ■

GENERAL OVERVIEW OF CARDIAC REHABILITATION

Cardiac rehabilitation can be defined as a program helping individuals faced with cardiovascular disease regain the most active, productive, and satisfying life possible within the boundaries of their disease. Generally, the programs are multiphasic and provide exercise therapy, as well as proper education and counseling for patients and their families. Emphasis is placed on the necessity of lifestyle changes with regard to diet, weight and stress reduction, termination of smoking, and exercise. Individuals are taught the importance of making a lifelong commitment to healthy lifestyle changes. Instruction is not limited to exercise therapy, but is expanded to include nutrition, relaxation skills, stress management, behavior modification, and group counseling.

Cardiac patients often experience emotional reactions such as depression, denial, and hostility while attempting to accept their condition. They are concerned and anxious about their future. The rehabilitation staff helps patients to cope with their feelings. Most programs provide peer group counseling, which aids in emotional recovery. The opportunity to exercise and converse with other cardiac patients in the peer group enhances emotional well-being and encourages participation. An important sense of camaraderie is nurtured within the cardiac rehabilitation program.

DEVELOPMENT OF CARDIAC REHABILITATION PROGRAMS

Cardiac rehabilitation programs were developed by cardiologists. Their theory was based on the need for controlled stress to cardiac muscle to aid it in developing its full potential following injury. As cardiac rehabilitation programs have evolved through the years, they have met obstacles and opposition from various groups.

Prior to the 1950s, opposition to cardiac rehabilitation—in particular, exercise therapy—was based on the idea that bed rest only was needed for cardiac recovery. Many believed physical activity would lead to severe complications such as cardiac rupture, congestive heart failure, or even sudden death.

Following the 1950s, opinions shifted as a result of continued research. It was demonstrated that physical activity actually prevents the adverse effects of prolonged bed rest. Cardiac rehabilitation programs emphasized the benefits of exercise and education in decreasing the risk of further disease. These programs also stressed the importance of helping individuals learn to manage their disease.

A major step forward in the evolution of cardiac rehabilitation was made in the 1970s with the introduction of a program design based on a graduated inpatient routine, followed by continued supervised exercise after discharge. These programs were further refined in the 1980s to incorporate a four-phase concept of cardiac rehabilitation that is generally accepted today.

FOUR PHASES OF THE CARDIAC REHABILITATION PROGRAM

The focus of the four-phase cardiac rehabilitation program is to provide care after the initial attack. Support and instruction are built into each progressive phase of the program (Table 47.1).

Phase I: Inpatient Phase

Phase I in cardiac rehabilitation is known as the *inpatient phase*. It is initiated as soon as the individual is considered stable and is concluded at the time of discharge.

Exercise Therapy

Individuals who have experienced a myocardial infarction (MI) usually begin low-level ambulation (walking) within 2 to 4 days following the attack. Patients who have undergone coronary artery bypass grafting are usually ambulated 1 to 2 days after surgery. Program initiation time differs from person to person. Range-of-motion exercises may be started prior to ambulation and then combined with the ambulation sessions. Exercise intensity in the inpatient phase is generally accepted as a heart rate of 20 to 30 beats per minute (bpm) over the standing resting heart rate. The program is performed twice a day, with a staff member supervising ambulation. All progress is recorded on the patient's chart. Prior to discharge, the individual may begin

TABLE 47.1. Summary of the Four-Phase Program

	Phase I	Phase II	Phase III	Phase IV
Location	Hospital (inpatient phase)	Hospital or clinic (outpatient phase following discharge)	Community "Y" or college facility (6–12 weeks post-discharge)	Community center or similar adult fitness program
Exercise	*Exercises:* Range of motion and ambulation *Frequency:* twice a day *Intensity:* 20–30 BPM over standing resting HR	*Exercise:* walking, jogging, stationary bike with ECG monitor *Frequency:* 3–4 times/week *Intensity:* started low and progressively increased based on GXT	*Exercise:* Phase II plus progression to recreational games *Intensity:* 60–85% max HR on GXT *Duration:* 20–60 minutes *Frequency:* 3 times/week	Maintenance program of patient's selection
Education	Individual and group: Dietary counseling Medical education Methods of coping	Exercise program, weight control, diet, discontinue smoking, importance of medication	Patient's own choice for further continuing education	Patient's own choice for further continuing education

to ambulate outside designated sessions utilizing guidelines taught by the staff.

Education

The Phase I program also provides education in combination with exercise therapy. Patients may receive instruction in individual and group sessions. Instruction includes dietary counseling, medical education, and information about cardiac disease, as well as methods of coping. Family members are often encouraged to participate in this process. Prior to discharge, a home exercise program and its components are outlined and explained to the patient and the family.

Phase II: Physical Rehabilitation

Phase II, a continuation of the inpatient program, begins immediately after discharge. The goal is to provide physical rehabilitation so the patient may resume everyday activities and promote healthy lifestyle changes. The program is conducted at a hospital or clinic and uses telemetry monitoring during exercise participation.

An individual is enrolled in an outpatient Phase II program for 6 to 12 weeks. Exercise intensity is kept low, and the duration of exercise is progressively increased. Typically, an initial exercise session lasts 10 to 15 minutes and progresses to 45 minutes.

Graded Exercise Test

An exercise prescription is developed for each individual, based on the results of a **graded exercise test (GXT)** administered prior to initiation into the program. This prescription sets a range for a target rate zone in which the individual maintains his or her heart rate during each exercise session. Individuals attend exercise sessions three to four times a week.

Recommended Activities

Patients in Phase II are encouraged to pursue activities such as walking, jogging, and stationary cycling. Range-of-motion exercises, as well as strength exercises (for example, rowing machines, wall cranks, wall pulleys, and the bench step), are also included. Weight lifting and static movements are discouraged because of the strain they place on the cardiovascular system.

Telemetry

All exercise during Phase II is done with electrocardiogram (ECG) continuous monitoring. During these sessions, the staff carefully observes any symptoms (such as fatigue, dyspnea, light-headedness, dizziness, claudication, nausea, or significant angina) or signs (greater than 2-millimeter ST-segment depression over baseline, significant arrhythmias, abnormal heart rate, or blood pressure responses).

Education

Education is an important component of Phase II. A portion of the instruction is conducted on a one-to-one level to assess each patient's understanding of the exercise prescription. Family members may also be included in this phase. Patients are instructed in the importance of regularly taking their medication. Medication side effects should be reviewed. Patients are also taught how important diet, weight control, and cessation of smoking are in improving their cardiac outlook. Peer group programs tend to reduce anxiety and depression levels while providing psychosocial support.

Individuals receive a summary of their results before discharge from the program, and each patient receives instruction and guidelines for an at-home exercise program. At this time the staff gives eligible and interested individuals information and recommendations for the Phase III outpatient program.

Phase III: Preparation for a Lifetime of Exercise

The primary focus of Phase III is to promote the need for lifelong adherence to exercise and to reinforce the behavior modification goals. Phase III is an outpatient program which is generally conducted in a community facility such as a YMCA or YWCA, or a college facility under the supervision of medical personnel. Emergency equipment (portable defibrillator with ECG recorder, emergency drugs and supplies, etc.) is maintained on-site at all times, and personnel are trained and certified to deal with cardiac emergencies. The ratio of staff to participants should be 1:10.

Patients are accepted into a Phase III program after discharge from Phase II; however, some patients may be accepted 6 to 12 weeks following discharge from the hospital. These are patients who have elected to exercise on a home program following discharge or those who do not have access to a Phase II program. Admittance into a Phase III program requires a physician referral, physical exam, completion of a medical history, and a recent GXT. Patients are encouraged to remain in Phase III for at least 3 to 6 months. Many individuals elect to remain in the program longer because of the need for a structured program.

Target Heart Rate

Phase III exercise sessions generally meet three times a week for 20 to 60 minutes. The duration of exercise tolerated varies among individuals. Exercise prescription and target heart rate are based on the results of the patient's GXT. The target heart rate may be determined by taking 60 to 85 percent of the maximum heart rate achieved on the GXT. Another, more individualized way of determining the heart rate is with the heart rate reserve formula: 60 to 85 percent (max $HR-RH$) + RH, where HR means heart rate and RH means resting heart rate. (This formula is particularly helpful if the patient is on beta-blocker medication, which slows the heart rate.) A lower percentage (60 percent) is used to determine the initial intensity (target heart rate); however, as an individual progresses in the program, the intensity and/or duration can be adjusted upward.

Vital Signs

Phase III programs do not utilize telemetry as seen in Phase II. Response to exercise is monitored by systematic checks of the heart rate and rhythm, and blood pressure prior to exercise, at the halfway point, at the termination of exercise, and before leaving the exercise area. These checkpoints may vary from program to program. The blood pressure is monitored before and after exercise; however, abnormal blood pressure readings indicate the need for more frequent monitoring and consultation with the physician. Patients are instructed in the technique of checking their heart rate by palpation of their pulse (see Chapter 11, Fig. 11.1); patients are also responsible for monitoring their heart rate in regard to the target zone.

Functional Activities

Individuals in Phase III are more medically and physically stable in comparison with patients in earlier phases. This enhanced functional status allows the participant in Phase III to engage in a wide variety of activities. Initially, the patient participates in walking, jogging, and stationary cycling, but may progress to recreational games and athletic activities. Individuals are encouraged to engage in different activities to maintain their interest and motivation to remain in the program and to encourage lifelong adherence to exercise (Table 47.2).

Phase IV: Maintaining Fitness

Patients who have participated in the Phase III outpatient program for at least 3 to 6 months without complications are generally considered to be at a maintenance level, or in Phase IV. These individuals exercise to maintain their level of fitness achieved through the previous levels of rehabilitation. Participants in Phase IV are unsupervised. As in the latter stage of Phase III, the individual is encouraged to participate in varied activities and exercise modalities to maintain interest and lifelong adherence to exercise.

TABLE 47.2. Approximate Energy Requirements of Selected Activities

Category	Self-Care or Home	Occupational	Recreational	Physical Conditioning
Very light	Washing, shaving, dressing Desk work, writing Washing dishes Driving auto	Sitting (clerical assembly) Standing (store clerk, bartender) Driving truck Operating crane	Shuffleboard Horseshoes Bait casting Billiards Archery Golf (cart)	Walking (2 mph) Stationary bicycling (very low resistance) Very light calisthenics
Light	Cleaning windows Raking leaves Weeding Power lawn mowing Waxing floors (slowly) Painting Carrying objects (15–30 lb)	Stocking shelves (light objects) Light welding Light carpentry Machine assembly Auto repair Paper hanging	Dancing (social and square) Golf (walking) Sailing Horseback riding Volleyball (6 man) Tennis (doubles)	Walking (3–4 mph) Level bicycling (6–8 mph) Light calisthenics
Moderate	Easy digging in garden Level hand lawn mowing Climbing stairs (slowly) Carrying objects (30–60 lb)	Carpentry (exterior home building) Shoveling dirt Using pneumatic tools	Badminton (competitive) Tennis (singles) Snow skiing (downhill) Light backpacking Basketball Football Skating (ice and roller) Horseback riding (gallop)	Walking (4.5–5 mph) Bicycling (9–10 mph) Swimming (breaststroke)
Heavy	Sawing wood Heavy shoveling Climbing stairs (moderate speed) Carrying objects (60–90 lb)	Tending furnace Digging ditches Pick and shovel	Canoeing Mountain climbing Fencing Paddleball Touch football	Jogging (5 mph) Swimming (crawl stroke) Rowing machine Heavy calisthenics Bicycling (12 mph)
Very heavy	Carrying loads upstairs Carrying objects (> 90 lb) Climbing stairs (quickly) Shoveling heavy snow Shoveling 10 min (16 lb)	Lumberjack Heavy laborer	Handball Squash Ski touring over hills Vigorous basketball	Running (≥ 6 mph) Bicycling (≥ 13 mph or up steep hill) Rope jumping

Source: Adapted from W. L., Haskell, "Design and Implementation of Cardiac Conditioning Programs," in Wenger, N. K., and Hellerstein, H. K., eds., *Rehabilitation of the Coronary Patient.* New York: Copyright © John Wiley & Sons, 1978. Reprinted by permission of John Wiley & Sons, Inc.

Individuals who have advanced to Phase IV may be placed in adult fitness programs. These programs mix adults who are considered asymptomatic with those who are at high risk of heart disease. The combination of both groups in these programs provides an atmosphere of motivation and enjoyment for all.

GUIDELINES OF VARIOUS PROFESSIONAL ORGANIZATIONS

While the four-phase program is considered "state of the art," it should be noted that several organizations have developed their own guidelines for specific programs. The

American College of Sports Medicine, for example, has published guidelines for its organization titled *Guidelines for Exercise Testing and Prescription*, now in its third edition. The American Heart Association also has developed guidelines for cardiac rehabilitation in *The Exercise Standards Book*. The American College of Cardiology defined a "Position Report on Cardiac Rehabilitation," which recommends cardiac rehabilitation strategies and services. And the American Association of Cardiovascular and Pulmonary Rehabilitation continually updates research and guidelines in its *Journal of Cardiopulmonary Rehabilitation*. While these and other groups have designated guidelines for cardiac rehabilitation, including the four-phase approach, the standards are not necessarily uniform or consistent.

LEGAL ASPECTS OF CARDIAC REHABILITATION

Program Documentation

The previously described four-phase, holistic approach to cardiac rehabilitation requires a wide variety of staff, ranging from board-certified physicians, psychologists, nurses, occupational and physical therapists, and athletic trainers to nutritionists and counselors. Because of the diversity of guidelines and personnel, it is imperative that written policies be developed and procedures specifically followed for the benefit of both patients and staff.

Documentation regarding which guidelines are being followed should be a part of the bylaws. State statutes should be examined carefully to determine if various providers are specifically prohibited in this type of setting. The scope of each team member's job description should be defined in detail, as should the program itself. Policies and procedures need to be originated and reviewed by medical, legal, and insurance staff.

Informed Consent

Cardiac rehabilitation patients should present a written prescription signed by their physician before being admitted to a program. Patients should be advised of the risks and benefits of a program prior to enrollment. Informed consent should be obtained by a physician to avoid unnecessary legal problems.

Negligence

Exercise testing raises specific legal concerns with respect to Phases I, II, and III. The American Heart Association and American Medical Association both stress the need for a physician to monitor this activity. In the absence of a physician, negligence may occur if the patient becomes ill or injured.

The patient's heart and/or pulse rate should be documented at each checkpoint daily. Along with routine daily statistics, any abnormalities should be noted carefully, along with specific instructions for referral, changes in program, or emergency treatment required. Protocols for emergency treatment should be clearly delineated and understood by all staff members.

Lack of Supervision in Phase IV

Phase IV of the four-phase program presents special legal consideration because of its lack of supervision. Patients should be carefully screened for participation in Phase IV, and once again, the risks and benefits of this phase should be reviewed and documentation obtained. As part of the program, family members should be instructed in cardiopulmonary resuscitation (CPR). (See Chapter 37 for details in administering CPR.)

IMPORTANT CONCEPTS

1. Cardiac rehabilitation involves lifestyle changes such as diet, weight and stress reduction, termination of smoking, and exercise.
2. Phase I of the four-phase rehabilitation program is an inpatient phase where ambulation and range-of-motion exercises are combined with education about diet, cardiac disease, and methods of coping with heart disease.
3. Phase II is a physical rehabilitation phase in which an exercise program of walking, jogging, and stationary cycling is set up, based on the results of GXT administered prior to initiation into Phase II of the program.
4. Phase III is outpatient preparation for lifelong adherence to exercise and behavior modification goals.
5. Phase IV is an unsupervised, maintenance level achieved by individuals who have spent at least 3 to 6 months in Phase III without complications.
6. The policies and procedures of a cardiac rehabilitation program must be written down and reviewed by medical, legal, and insurance staff, and the informed consent of participants should be obtained.

SUGGESTED READINGS

Franklin, B. A. "Safety of Outpatient Cardiac Exercise Therapy: Reducing the Incidence of Complications." *The Physician and Sportsmedicine* 14 (September 1986): 235–248.

Greenland, P., and J. S. Chu. "Efficacy of Cardiac Rehabilitation Services: With Emphasis on Patients after Myocardial Infarction." *Annals of Internal Medicine* 109 (1988): 650–663.

Herbert, W. G., and D. L. Herbert. "Legal Aspects of Cardiac Rehabilitation Exercise Programs." *The Physician and Sportsmedicine* 16 (October 1988): 105–111.

Thompson, P. "The Cardiovascular Risks of Cardiac Rehabilitation." *Journal of Cardiopulmonary Rehabilitation* 5 (July 1985): 321–324.

Wilson, P. K. "Cardiac Rehabilitation: Then and Now." *The Physician and Sportsmedicine* 16 (September 1988): 75–84.

48

Conditioning Programs for Senior Citizens

OBJECTIVES FOR CHAPTER 48

After reading this chapter, the student should be able to:
1. Identify physiological changes seen in the aging process.
2. Describe the important components of a pre-exercise assessment in this age group.
3. Identify considerations for writing an exercise prescription for the senior citizen.

INTRODUCTION

As time has progressed, our population is living longer than our forefathers of a century ago. Currently, almost 12 percent of U.S. citizens are 65 or older. While many senior citizens are truly enjoying their golden years, others are hampered by limited physical capabilities. Many individuals, inactive in their younger years, are afraid of becoming active as they grow older.

Chapter 48 begins with a discussion of the physiological changes observed with aging, including cardiovascular and respiratory changes, plasma lipoproteins and glucose tolerance changes, and musculoskeletal and nervous system changes. The chapter then describes what is involved in a pre-exercise assessment. The last section of Chapter 48 discusses an exercise prescription for the elderly individual. ■

PHYSIOLOGICAL CHANGES WITH AGING

To assist the elderly in an exercise program, one must examine the physiological changes observed in the aging. Some changes are not so dramatic in elderly individuals who have maintained a physically active lifestyle throughout their middle and advancing years. Although inactivity is not the only factor, it certainly has a dramatic effect on the physiologic changes in this group.

Cardiovascular Changes

Contraction

Actual changes in cardiac function are difficult to evaluate fully because of the prevalence of coronary heart disease and sedentary lifestyles in individuals 65 and older. In general, it is believed that myocardial contractility (the heart's capability to contract) is not altered with aging. However, duration of contraction increases with age.

Heart Rate, Stroke Volume, and Cardiac Output

Maximum stroke volume and cardiac output were previously thought to be reduced with age. However, more recent studies show that in the absence of coronary heart disease, these two factors are unchanged. Although heart rate and stroke volume rise with exercise, the increase in heart rate is significantly less in the elderly. To compensate, the elderly heart has an increased dependence on Starling's law of the heart, which states that within limits, an increase in the end-diastolic volume of the heart (increasing the length of the muscle fibers) increases the force of cardiac contraction during the following systole (Fig. 48.1). This often results in maximum cardiac output at a lower level. There is also a slower return to baseline heart rate, blood pressure, oxygen consumption, and carbon dioxide elimination after exercise.

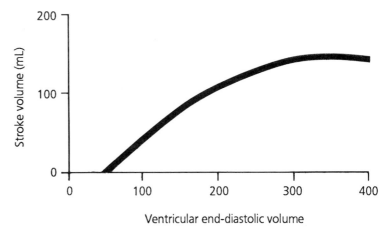

FIGURE 48.1. The relationship between ventricular end-diastolic volume and stroke volume (Starling's law of the heart). (From Vander et al., *Human Physiology: The Mechanisms of Body Function,* 3d ed. New York: McGraw-Hill, 1980. Reprinted by permission.)

Left Ventricular Volume and Filling Rates

Left ventricular volume does not differ with age, but left ventricular filling rates are affected. Several factors are believed responsible for this change, in the absence of coronary heart disease. Some of these factors include decreased closure rates of the mitral valve and an increase in chamber stiffness due to increased ventricular wall thickness and changes in viscoelastic properties. Thus, the amount of blood actually ejected from the left ventricle in relation to total cardiac output is also reduced.

Respiratory Changes

As one ages, lung compliance (the lung's ability to yield to pressure) increases while thoracic wall motility (the thoracic wall's ability to move spontaneously) decreases. Breathing usually becomes more frequent, which increases the work required to breathe during exercise. The athlete's cardiovascular status also affects respiratory function. Endurance training programs can improve the efficiency of breathing at submaximal (below normal) workloads.

In the sedentary individual, VO_2 max (the volume of maximally oxygenated blood) declines approximately 5 percent each decade after the age of 25 — a decline that can be halved with endurance training. While athletes may be spared some of the usual cardiovascular changes related to aging, even the previously sedentary individual should be encouraged to participate in some form of exercise, as recent studies reveal marked improvement in VO_2 max with gradually increasing training intensity in healthy senior citizens.

Plasma Lipoproteins

The average level of serum cholesterol of 200 mg/dl is a value considered low risk for coronary heart disease. Cholesterol levels increase with age and are thought to be related to increased low-density lipoprotein (LDL) production and decreased clearance of LDL. Since LDLs are increased, the total plasma cholesterol is increased. Total plasma cholesterol and LDLs are positively associated with coronary heart disease. While exercise does not affect total plasma cholesterol levels, it does decrease LDL levels. Also, high-density lipoproteins (HDLs), which are negatively associated with coronary heart disease, are higher in endurance athletes as compared with sedentary individuals.

Glucose Tolerance

Glucose tolerance decreases with age and may be related to hyperinsulinemia, which results from higher glucose concentrations or impaired clearance of insulin. The decrease in glucose tolerance in individuals past 40 puts the elderly individual at risk of developing **non-insulin-dependent diabetes mellitus** (**NIDDM**) (see Chapter 54). The treatment of choice for NIDDM is diet therapy, weight loss, and increased physical activity. Diet therapy alone reduces glucose production and improves hepatic sensitivity to insulin. Physical training not only enhances weight reduction, but also improves carbohydrate storage rates.

Musculoskeletal System Changes

Arthritis

Arthritis is perhaps the most consistent finding among the elderly population. Although the arthritis seen in an individual may result from systemic disease such as rheumatoid arthritis, pseudogout, hemophilia, or systemic lupus, the most common type of arthritis seen in the elderly is **degenerative joint disease** (**DJD**), or **osteoarthritis**. DJD is characterized by deterioration of the weight-bearing surface, which is distinguished by destruction of the hyaline cartilage, hardening of subchondral bone, narrowing of the joint space, and overgrowth of bone at the joint margins (Fig. 48.2).

The joint surfaces are often rough and produce an aching pain in the affected joints. Pain and overgrowth of bone at the

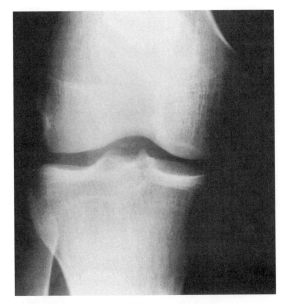 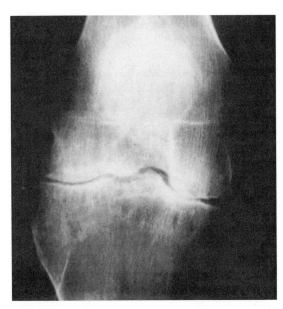

FIGURE 48.2.   (a) Normal knee. (b) Knee with degenerative joint disease.

joint margins often cause decreased range of motion. Pain, decreased range of motion, and associated inactivity often produce muscle weakness, which in turn often decreases metabolism, resulting in weight gain. The extra weight places more demand on the affected weight-bearing surface.

Exercise can have significant positive effects in the elderly. Regular exercise can help decrease or maintain weight; maintain existing range of motion; and improve overall functional status, conditioning, and per-

ceived joint discomfort. Exercise programs should be tailored according to the area affected. For instance, the individual with DJD of the knees should be encouraged to participate in activities that do not involve pounding, such as running or jogging. More appropriate for this individual are gliding sports, such as cross-country skiing or skiing machines. Swimming, water aerobics, or water running reduces stress on the knees because the water supports some of the person's weight (Table 48.1).

TABLE 48.1.   Exercise Devices Suitable for Patients with Arthritis*

	Joints Stressed				
	Hip	Knee	Ankle	Shoulder	Spine
Stationary bicycle	++	++	+	−	+
Arm-crank ergometer	−	−	−	++	++
Rowing machine	−	−	−	++	++
Cross-country skiing machine	+	+/−	+/−	+/−	+
Climbing machine	++	++	++	+	+
Water running with limited-buoyancy vest	−	−	−	+/−	+/−

*Explanation of symbols: ++, greatly stressed; +, stressed; +/−, somewhat stressed; −, not stressed.
Source: Reprinted from the February 1989 issue of *The Physician and Sportsmedicine* by special permission from McGraw-Hill, Inc. Copyright © 1990 by McGraw-Hill, Inc.

For individuals with arthritic changes in the cervical spine, swimming is not a recommended form of exercise. In fact, swimming may exacerbate their condition, and because of limited neck movement, these individuals may not be able to breathe comfortably while participating in this sport. Stationary bicycling may also strain the neck because most people tend to lean forward while pedaling and extend their neck so they are still looking up. Exercise bicycles should be evaluated carefully. Many of the newer bicycles are more upright for the rider and would not cause additional stress to this area. Brisk walking is a good alternative exercise program for individuals with arthritis in the cervical spine.

Osteoporosis

Osteopenia is the decrease of mineralized bone tissue in the body. **Osteoporosis** is actually irreversible osteopenia or decreased bone volume. With these problems, the bone is frail and often collapses without history of injury or fractures with minimal trauma. Vertebral collapse is considered the hallmark of the disease, although fractures of the proximal femur and distal radius are highly prevalent. On x-ray, the osteoporotic bone looks "washed out" as compared with normal bone (Fig. 48.3). Often, collapse or microfractures may be seen on x-ray.

Osteopenia and osteoporosis evolve as a result of intrinsic factors, such as age and inactivity, and extrinsic factors. Extrinsic factors include calcium homeostasis/estrogen disorders; gastrointestinal (malabsorption) problems; nutritional deficiencies (vitamin D, calcium, vitamin C); endocrine imbalances (sex hormones, thyroid, adrenals); renal diseases; hematologic and neoplastic disorders; and drug toxicity (alcohol, corticosteroids, etc.).

In general, the elderly are at higher risk for osteoporosis because they have a natural predisposition for this problem, although age itself is not the highest contributing factor. Inactivity, alcohol abuse, and nutri-

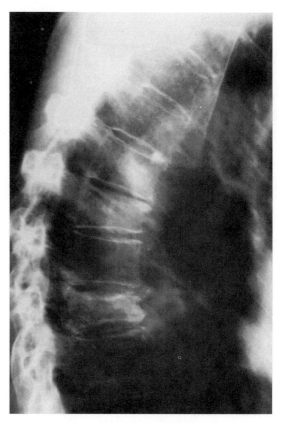

FIGURE 48.3. X-ray of osteoporotic bone with washed-out effect. Note the collapse of the thoracic vertebrae.

tional deficiency—problems frequently seen in the elderly—add to the risk. Osteoporosis affects approximately 30 percent of women over 65. This higher incidence among women is directly related to postmenopausal changes and a decrease in estrogen production.

Although treatment of osteoporosis is multifaceted and out of the realm of this chapter, studies do show that exercise has a positive effect on this problem in the elderly. Because the bone is at higher risk of compression with pounding, activities such as jogging should be excluded. Gliding sports such as cross-country skiing are at first glance advantageous, but the risk of falling is higher. Water activities or brisk walking on soft, even terrain are wiser choices for a conditioning program.

Nervous System Changes

Slowed nerve conduction velocities and lengthened reaction times affect many elderly individuals. They may become less sensitive to various stimuli and sensory deficits may increase. These changes are perceived as contributing to the greater number of falls in the elderly. While literature on this subject is not abundant, some studies suggest the benefits of exercise to include decreased perceptions of chronic pain and anxiety.

PRE-EXERCISE ASSESSMENT

The elderly individual requires a careful pre-exercise assessment prior to beginning participation in a safe, effective conditioning program.

Review of Medical History

The initial evaluation should include a thorough history to determine past and present medical problems that would affect the program. Past history of heart or respiratory disease would indicate the need for more meticulous screening of the problem and additional studies. Past history of trauma, degenerative changes, or surgery to a joint should alert the examiner to evaluate these areas more thoroughly for decreased range of motion and, strength, or pain with movement.

Review of Medication

Knowledge of medication taken is important to determine if alterations in dosage are indicated. Persons on insulin or oral diabetic medications may need adjustments. Diuretics may predispose the individual to arrhythmias, hypokalemia (abnormally low potassium level in the blood), or even fluid depletion. Some persons on heart medications may have reduced tolerance to exercise. Other medications may cause dizziness or syncope (fainting), or increase the individual's tolerance to heat or cold.

Review of Lifestyle

It is also important to evaluate lifestyle. Smoking, average alcohol intake, and dietary habits are important to know. Many senior citizens have poor dietary habits, and exercise programs may significantly affect their total caloric expenditure.

Review of Past and Present Exercise Habits

Reviewing what activities an individual has participated in previously may give the examiner some insight into activities of interest at this period of the person's life. This information may also help the examiner to designate an appropriate starting level for an activity.

Review of Symptoms

A review of symptoms would include such things as recent shortness of breath, dizziness, chest pain, heart palpitations, weakness, decreased range of motion, pain with movement, numbness or decreased sensation in the extremities, swelling of joints or extremities, and so forth. This information is important in targeting new problems that may need further investigation during the physical examination.

Thorough Physical Examination

A thorough physical examination looks more closely at prior existing medical conditions or new problems that were noted in the review. A graded exercise test is important for evaluation of cardiac and respiratory status. The test is often performed on a treadmill and should last long enough to ensure the individual is at a steady state for at least 2 to 3 minutes. Careful monitoring of pulse rate and blood pressure is necessary in all cases. Electrocardiogram (ECG) monitoring is suggested as well. Blood pressure should be measured before, during, and after testing.

The treadmill may not be an appropriate testing method for some individuals. The person with significant degenerative changes in the knees should be tested in an exercise mode with less stress to this area. Tests need to be modified for the senior citizen, as does the exercise prescription.

EXERCISE PRESCRIPTION

The exercise prescription should be tailored to the elderly individual's present physical condition, interests, accessibility of equipment, and mental and social needs. A well-defined swimming program is useless if the individual is afraid of the water. A conditioning program is only effective if it is applicable to one's way of life and if adherence is practiced.

Goals and expectations of the exercise program should be discussed and addressed early with the elderly individual. Goals can always be raised or reassessed, but goals set too high will produce early frustration and most likely lack of compliance with the exercise program.

Large Muscle Groups: Rhythmic Movements

Activities involving large muscle groups are best when they involve rhythmic movements, increasing the blood flow to the muscles and raising the heart rate. Strength and endurance are enhanced in a safe manner, and overstressing of the joints is avoided. Large muscle groups deserve particular attention in the previously sedentary individual.

Frequency of Activity

The individual should exercise at least twice a week when starting an exercise program. Eventually, frequency of activity should increase to three or four times per week. Duration of activity depends on the individual's pre-exercise status. Initially, the program may last only 5 or 10 minutes,

although 15- to 20-minute sessions are ultimately recommended. Once the individual's conditioning improves, duration and frequency may be increased.

Intensity

Intensity of exercise should be determined by monitoring the heart rate (HR). Elderly participants should be instructed in taking their own pulse early in the program. Blood pressures should be monitored regularly in the beginning stages and on a routine basis before and after exercise. Stress tests in the pre-exercise assessment provide important information for determining intensity levels. Once VO_2 max, HR max (maximal heart rate), and HR rest (resting heart rate) have been determined, the following equation can be utilized to determine training heart rate (THR):

$$THR = [(HR\ max - HR\ rest) \times \%\ VO_2\ max\ desired] + HR\ rest$$

Exercising at 50 to 70 percent VO_2 max is an average range for elderly individuals to achive cardiac fitness. The VO_2 max factor can be adjusted with tolerance to the training program. A slightly lower VO_2 percentage should be utilized in swimming exercise programs.

Program Sequence

The exercise program should consist of a gentle warm-up, followed by stretching of those muscle groups utilized during the actual exercise program, the aerobic activity, and the cool-down, which may also include another session of stretching. The aerobic activity should start slowly and gradually peak midway through the aerobic exercise phase. A typical exercise progression for a healthy but previously sedentary senior citizen begins with 10 minutes of exercise four times a week during week 1 and progresses to between 30 and 40 minutes five times a week during week 15 (Table 48.2).

Special Considerations

Many elderly do not tolerate extremes in heat or cold—a factor that should be considered when designing any exercise program. In colder environments, a longer warm-up time is necessary. Because of their less efficient sweating mechanism, elderly individuals have less tolerance to heat stress and heat exhaustion. Exercise in extreme heat is not suggested for the elderly.

Elderly individuals should also be advised on icing down sore joints and muscles after exercise. They should be aware that some soreness during exercise or the following day is not unusual. This discomfort usually diminishes as the day progresses and should be significantly decreased by the next exercise session. However, pain that persists for more than 1 hour after activity should be reassessed.

This age group should also be advised on proper footwear that will provide stability and cushioning during exercise. A Sorbothane insert often is recommended to reduce trauma to the joints of the lower extremities.

Benefits of an Exercise Program

The elderly can benefit significantly from physical conditioning programs. Although some physiological changes are inherent to this group, many of these changes are magnified by sedentary lifestyles. Exercise programs must be specifically tailored to the individual, considering such things as baseline physical condition, special restricting conditions, interests, accessibility of equipment, and cost. Such programs benefit the elderly because they provide them with strength and endurance to perform self-care and household activities, decrease their risk of health problems, provide them with social interaction, and enhance the quality of their daily living.

TABLE 48.2. A Typical Exercise Progression

Week	Sun	Mon	Tue	Wed	Thu	Fri	Sat	Total Min
1	10	off	10	off	10	off	10	40
2	10	off	12	off	10	off	15	47
3	10	off	15	off	10	off	15	50
4	10	off	10	10	10	off	15	55
5	10	off	12	10	12	off	15	59
6	10	off	15	10	15	off	15	65
7	12	off	15	12	15	off	15	69
8	12	off	20	12	15	off	15	74
9	15	off	20	15	20	off	15	85
10	20	off	20	15	20	off	15	90
11	25	off	20	20	20	off	20	105
12	30	off	20	25	20	off	25	120
13	30	off	25	30	25	off	25	135
14	35	off	30	30	30	off	30	150
15	40	off	30	35	30	off	35	165

(Important Concepts appear on next page.)

IMPORTANT CONCEPTS

1. In the absence of coronary heart disease, maximum stroke volume and cardiac output are not reduced with age.
2. In the sedentary individual, VO_2 max declines approximately 5 percent each decade after age 25, but that decline can be halved by endurance training.
3. Exercise does not affect total plasma cholesterol levels, but it does decrease LDL levels, which are positively associated with coronary heart disease.
4. Glucose tolerance decreases with age and puts those affected at risk of developing non-insulin-dependent diabetes.
5. For elderly individuals suffering from degenerative joint disease, a program of regular exercise can decrease or main tain weight; maintain existing range of motion; and improve overall functional status, conditioning, and perceived joint discomfort.
6. A pre-exercise assessment should include a review of the individual's past and present medical history, medications, lifestyle, past and present exercise habits, symptoms of new problems, and a thorough physical exam, including a graded exercise test.
7. An exercise prescription should involve large muscle groups and avoid overstressing of joints.
8. An exercise program for the elderly individual should include a gentle warm-up, stretching of the muscles used during activity, aerobic activity, and cool-down and stretching.

SUGGESTED READINGS

Balady, G., and D. Weiner. "Exercise Testing in Healthy Elderly Subjects and Elderly Patients with Cardiac Disease." *Journal of Cardiopulmonary Rehabilitation* 9 (1989): 35–39.

Fitzgerald, P. L. "Exercise for the Elderly." *Medical Clinics of North America* 69 (1985): 189–196.

Ike, R. W., R. M. Lampman, C. W. Castor. "Arthritis and Aerobic Exercise: A Review." *The Physician and Sportsmedicine* 17 (February 1989): 128–139.

Mahler, D. A., L. N. Cunningham, G. D. Curfman. "Aging and Exercise Performance." *Clinics in Geriatric Medicine* 2 (1986): 433–452.

Posner, J. D., K. M. Gorman, H. S. Klein. "Exercise Capacity in the Elderly." *American Journal of Cardiology* 57 (1986): 52C–58C.

Schulman, S., and G. Gerstenblith. "Cardiovascular Changes with Aging: The Response to Exercise." *Journal of Cardiopulmonary Rehabilitation* 9 (1989): 12–16.

Shephard, R. "Habitual Physical Activity Levels and Perception of Exertion in the Elderly." *Journal of Cardiopulmonary Rehabilitation* 9 (1989): 17–23.

Smith, E. L., P. E. Smith, and C. Gilligan. "Diet, Exercise, and Chronic Disease Patterns in Older Adults." *Nutrition Reviews* 46 (February 1988): 52–61.

Wenger, N. "Exercise for the Elderly: Highlights of Preventative and Therapeutic Aspects." *Journal of Cardiopulmonary Rehabilitation* 9 (1989): 9–11.

Wolfel, E., and K. Hossack. "Guidelines for the Exercise Training of Elderly Healthy Individuals and Elderly Patients with Cardiac Disease." *Journal of Cardiopulmonary Rehabilitation* 9 (1989): 40–45.

SIX

REHABILITATION TECHNIQUES

49

Basic Principles of Rehabilitation

CHAPTER OUTLINE

OBJECTIVES FOR CHAPTER 49

After reading this chapter, the student should be able to:

1. Identify the members of a rehabilitation team and define their roles.
2. Identify the components of a complete rehabilitation program.
3. Define and discuss the components of Phase I, the immediate care stage of rehabilitation.
4. Differentiate among the methods of increasing range of motion, strength, power, and endurance during Phase II of rehabilitation.
5. Discuss ways to return the athlete to activity, Phase III of rehabilitation.
6. Discuss the importance of documenting each phase of the rehabilitation process.
7. Identify the psychological concerns to be addressed when caring for an injured athlete.

INTRODUCTION

When discussing the basic principles of rehabilitation after injury, it is important to remember that everyone reacts to an injury differently, both physiologically and psychologically. Motivational levels, healing, and conditioning times must be individualized. Therefore, the time frames for rehabilitation provided in this chapter should be considered general guidelines. It is up to the athletic trainer and physician to select the methods they prefer to use.

Chapter 49 begins by describing how a rehabilitation plan is formulated for an injured athlete. The next three sections detail each of the three phases of rehabilitation: Phase I, immediate care; Phase II, restoring range of motion and strength; and Phase III, returning the athlete to play. The last two sections of Chapter 49 discuss the importance of documenting each phase of rehabilitation and the need to be sensitive during rehabilitation to the athlete's psychological response to injury. ■

THE REHABILITATION PLAN

Rehabilitation is defined as restoration. The process of rehabilitation for athletes must include not only restoration to a functional level for daily living, but also return to an appropriate level of competitive fitness.

A successful rehabilitation program requires the cooperation of everyone involved in the athletic program. The physician, athletic trainer, coach, teammates, and parents each have clearly defined roles, along with the injured athlete. The attending physician provides an appropriate diagnosis and recommends any necessary rehabilitation, including restrictions. The athletic trainer outlines a specific rehabilitation program for the athlete to follow and maintains daily contact with the athlete to ensure that adequate progress is being made. The coach keeps the athlete abreast of new team plays and strategies, makes sure the athlete stays as conditioned as possible considering the injury, and helps the athlete to share in the team camaraderie during the time the athlete is unable to participate in practice or competition. Teammates, friends, and parents provide the athlete with moral support and motivation, particularly if long-term rehabilitation is necessary.

After an acute injury occurs, a primary evaluation should be performed immediately (Fig. 49.1). It is important to stabilize the injured body part and prevent or control pain, ecchymosis, edema, and/or joint effusion. After these physiologic events are stabilized, rehabilitation of an injury can begin. Rehabilitation of acute injuries follows the same pattern as for chronic injuries. Reevaluation by the appropriate personnel provides a diagnosis and determines the extent of injury. An overall return-to-play plan is constructed for the athlete and properly communicated to the coach. The initial emphasis of this plan is on healing the injury. The other goals of the plan are to return the injured athlete to a functional level for daily living, and then completely recondition the athlete to allow a safe, full return to his or her sport.

In the construction of treatment and rehabilitation plans, consideration should be given to the athlete's level of play, the time frame within the competitive season when the injury occurs, and the athlete's desire to return to full competitive participation. The rehabilitation process can be divided into three phases: (1) immediate care, (2) restoration of motion and strength, and (3) return to competitive activity. Within each phase, goals for the athlete should be clearly outlined. These goals must be realistic and reachable for the injured player. In fact, several sets of goals may be needed within each phase, and goals may need to be reassessed as the athlete progresses. The pro-

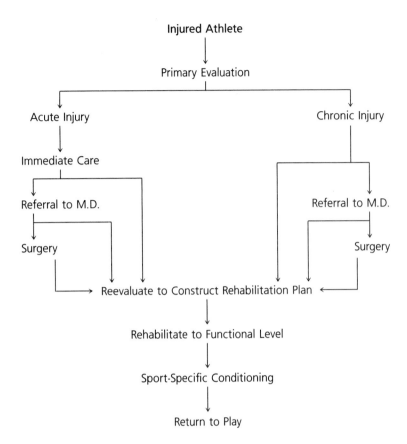

FIGURE 49.1.   Treatment protocol for an injured athlete.

gram should also permit the athlete to remain as active as possible to decrease deconditioning without interfering with the healing of the injury.

PHASE I: IMMEDIATE CARE

Immediate care encompasses those treatments rendered from the time when the athlete is first evaluated, either on the field or in the training room, up to completion of initial healing, when aggressive range-of-motion exercises can be initiated. In this immediate phase, control of pain, hemorrhage, and edema (tissue swelling) is of prime importance. An attempt should also be made to prevent loss of the athlete's present conditioned status, but the overall emphasis at this stage of rehabilitation is on healing (Fig. 49.2).

Control of Hemorrhage, Edema, and Pain

ICE Treatment

The three most commonly recognized means to control initial hemorrhage and edema following injury are *ice* directly on the affected site, a *compression* bandage over the ice, and *elevation* of the affected area. This treatment is commonly referred to as **ICE (ice, compression, and elevation) treatment**. The application of ice and compression produces a greater overall decrease in swelling than if ice alone is used. Ice with compression helps decrease further leakage of blood from injured vessels. Ice also slows the tissue metabolic rate, which diminishes

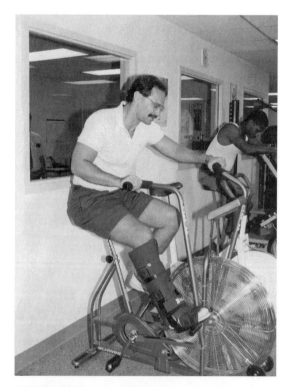

FIGURE 49.2. An athlete in a cast, riding a stationary bike to lessen deconditioning.

the inflammatory response. ICE treatment is usually continued for at least 24 hours, with a maximum duration determined by the severity of the injury. When ice is not available because of traveling, going to class, or for other reasons, an Ace bandage moistened in cold water can be applied as a compression wrap.

Ice should be left on the affected area for approximately 20 minutes of every hour, with appropriate protection given to the athlete's skin so that ice burns do not occur. Athletes should be warned to anticipate a burning or stinging sensation prior to feeling numb over the area receiving treatment. When the ice is removed, the injured area should remain compressed and elevated.

Compression is usually achieved by the use of an elastic bandage, wrapped toward the heart, with each circular application overlapping by one-half the width of the bandage. In some cases tape may be used for compression, particularly with ankle sprains, where an open basketweave taping technique can be applied and then left on by the athlete until the next treatment (see Chapter 43.) In applying compression, care should be taken not to apply the wrap too tightly. When compressive dressings are used, the symptom of increased pain or signs of increased swelling, decreased sensation, or decreased motor power indicate that the compressive wrap should be loosened, particularly in the acute phase. If the symptoms persist, despite loosening of the wrap, the athlete should seek further care immediately.

Adequate elevation involves keeping the extremity above the level of the heart whenever possible. Elevation is usually accomplished through the use of pillows. Rest and support for the injured area are important at this early stage to minimize further tissue injury.

Immobilization

In some injuries, complete immobilization in a cast may be required, particularly in

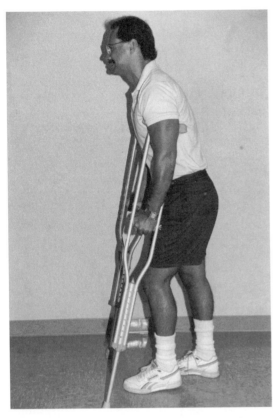

FIGURE 49.3a. Crutch walking using touchdown weight bearing with foot in plantigrade position. The crutches bear most of the athlete's weight.

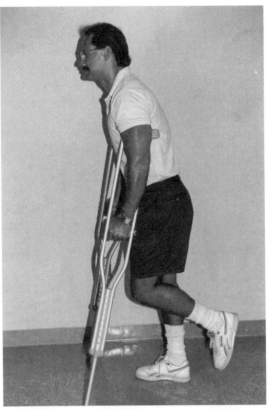

FIGURE 49.3b. Crutch walking with knee bent and foot plantar flexed. This total non-weight-bearing position can lead to Achilles tightening.

areas difficult to heal, such as the navicular of the wrist. Popular methods of immobilization include splints or cast braces that are easily removed so modalities may be used to decrease pain and swelling. Range-of-motion exercises can be initiated early in the treatment course to avoid stiffness and other complications of swelling from immobilization. When immobilization is used, the trainer should always be alert to side effects such as atrophy, decreased nutrition to the articular cartilage, and loss of range of motion. During the immediate treatment stage, the athlete may need to restrict use of the injured area. Crutches may be needed to decrease weight bearing in lower extremity injuries. An injured athlete should not bear full body weight until the swelling has dissipated, the joints above and below the area have almost full range of motion, and weight bearing does not produce pain. Limping indicates that the athlete is bearing weight too soon.

When crutches are used, it is frequently helpful to allow the foot of the injured extremity to contact the floor in a normal plantigrade position, even though most of the athlete's weight is being borne on the crutches (Fig. 49.3a). This position allows for normal "floor contact sensation" and prevents the athlete from holding the extremity with the knee bent and the foot plantar flexed, a position that promotes Achilles tightening (Fig. 49.3b). Partial or touch-down weight-bearing status should be approved by the physician.

Modalities and Medications

Modalities may be helpful in decreasing pain and swelling during the immediate care phase. Examples of these include ice, massage, electrogalvanic stimulation (EGS), and transcutaneous electrical nerve stimulation (TENS).

EGS is particularly useful in eliminating fluid accumulation because of its ability to alternate current, creating a pump effect which allows for vasoconstriction and vasodilation to occur. TENS may also be helpful not only in decreasing swelling (the mechanism for this is not clearly understood) but also in controlling pain by inhibiting spinal cord neurons, causing the release of endorphins and other natural pain relievers, and by blocking peripheral nerve fibers. (See Chapter 50 for additional discussion of these modalities.)

To control pain and swelling, the attending physician may prescribe nonsteroidal, anti-inflammatory drugs (NSAIDs), such as aspirin, ibuprofen (Advil, Nuprin, Motrin), naproxen (Naprosyn), diflunisal (Dolobid), diclofenac sodium (Voltaren), as well as numerous others (see Chapter 58). Acetaminophen (Tylenol) may relieve pain, but it does not have an anti-inflammatory function.

Healing Time

The amount of time needed for tissue repair is based on several factors, such as the degree and location of the injury, the presence of infection, and the age of the athlete. The determination of the degree of injury is based on physical findings such as edema, ecchymosis, effusion, joint laxity, and supplementary diagnostic studies (x-rays, scans, or arthroscopic evaluations). In general, the greater the disruption of the tissue, the longer the healing time. The location of the injury will also affect healing time. For instance, fractures occurring in an area with poor vascularity, such as a navicular fracture of the wrist, will heal more slowly than highly vascular bones.

Infection retards healing time. When an infection occurs, the body's defenses attempt to seclude the infection locally. Because of this targeting to the infected area, healing of bone or soft tissue will be delayed until the infection is well under control. The age of the athlete should also be considered when healing time is assessed. Fractures in an active adolescent athlete usually heal more quickly than those in an adult.

Other factors that may slow healing time significantly include the athlete's nutritional status, the presence of diabetes or other medical problems, medications the athlete may take on a regular basis because of concurrent medical problems, and the use of corticosteroids (not to be confused with anabolic steroids).

Close monitoring of the athlete's progress by the athletic trainer and the team physician during this initial phase of rehabilitation is needed to ensure that the athlete is progressing as successfully as expected. The physician should reevaluate the injury for healing and the need for immobilization. The athletic trainer, physical therapist, or sports therapist should advise the physician if the athlete is progressing more quickly or slowly than initially projected.

Limiting Deconditioning

Once pain is well under control, reconditioning should begin. For example, a soccer player whose ankle is in a cast will not be able to run to maintain cardiovascular conditioning. However, a stationary bicycle may provide an alternative conditioning program. Although not sport-specific in nature, these activities help to prevent the significant degree of cardiovascular retrogression one would see if the athlete waited until he or she was able to run again. Strength can be maintained through a weight-lifting program on an alternate-day schedule. This program should be as sport-specific as possible, although obviously it cannot involve the injured area. In the case of the soccer player with a short leg cast for an ankle fracture, the athlete could still work on strengthening the quadriceps, hamstrings, abductors, and adductors. A strengthening program for the opposite leg can be initiated to prevent deconditioning in the unaffected extremity. Moreover, such a program also benefits the injured extremity due to a crossover training effect. Isometric contractions can be beneficial in an immobilized limb, provided the athlete is able to isolate and contract the muscles. Of course, any maintenance conditioning programs should be reviewed and cleared by the treating physician.

Phase I Goals

Successful immediate care of an injury is important because decreased swelling and pain allow for earlier range of motion and use of the area, and will ensure a more rapid rehabilitation process. The goals of Phase I will vary depending on the type of injury and the athlete; however, they should resemble the following goals as much as possible:

- Keep swelling to a minimum.
- Decrease inflammation.
- Control pain with gradual decrease in the use of pain medications.
- Maintain strength of unaffected musculature.
- Maintain present level of cardiovascular endurance.

PHASE II: RESTORATION OF MOTION AND STRENGTH

Phase II of the rehabilitation process begins as soon as pain and swelling are controlled and complete immobilization is no longer necessary. The athlete may still be in an immobilizer part of the time or in a brace or splint that allows only limited motion. The athlete may also still be non–weight bearing.

Treatment programs are based on objective findings such as the physical exam. In many cases the physician and trainer have worked closely enough that although the parameters of the prescription are defined by the physician, the actual daily therapy routine is formulated by the trainer.

Progression in Phase II is based on subjective symptoms such as pain and on physical findings such as swelling. The goals of Phase II are to first regain range of motion of the affected part and then to work on regaining strength comparable to the unaffected extremity. Once substantial strength gains have been attained, power and endurance should be targeted. As in Phase I, maintenance of the strength of unaffected parts and cardiovascular endurance should not be neglected during this phase of the rehabilitation process.

Although general guidelines can be written for progression of therapy following a specific injury, the trainer must realize that every therapy prescription must be individualized for the athlete. The methods used, as well as the rate of progression of activities, depend not only on the particular injury, but also on the athlete's pain tolerance, motivation level, and rate of tissue healing.

Phase II of rehabilitation is similar for both acute and chronic injuries, and the emphasis is on restoring range of motion, strength, and endurance. Depending on the severity of an injury, varying amounts of time and emphasis will be spent on the components of this stage of the rehabilitation program.

Range of Motion

The targeted goal in a range-of-motion program is to attain full range of motion of an injured limb. A guideline for this goal can be easily obtained by measuring the range of motion on the unaffected, contralateral body part. Information on an appropriate range of motion may also be obtained from preseason physicals. With the exception of certain athletes like throwers who may require more external rotation in their throwing arm than in their nonthrowing arm, most athletes have equal range of motion when compared side to side.

Assessment

The easiest, most accurate way to assess full range of motion is by using a goniometer (see Chapter 10). In some cases full range of motion may be unattainable, such as after specific surgical procedures. (If this is the case, the physician and trainer should discuss this problem prior to goal setting.) Return of normal range of motion can be achieved through a combination of exercises that are performed passively or actively, or are actively assisted.

Achieving Motion

Passive range-of-motion exercises are those in which the stretching or range of motion is performed specifically by the trainer and not by the athlete. Passive range of motion is indicated in early rehabilitation programs to prevent degenerative changes in a joint and to promote healing. It is also indicated in situations where the athlete is stagnant in his or her range-of-motion program or is actually retrogressing. In these cases, as well as in situations in which the athlete has developed adhesions following an injury or more specifically a surgical procedure, passive range of motion may be vigorous but always controlled so that no damage of the healing tissue is incurred.

Passive range of motion should be performed with the athlete as relaxed as possible. The trainer must perform the exercise slowly and with great skill, thereby gaining the athlete's confidence and cooperation.

Active range-of-motion exercises allow the athlete to work on gaining full range of motion within the confines of pain. In the early stages, active range-of-motion exercises are usually most effective when performed in a position so that the athlete does not have to work against gravity. The support of water, such as in a whirlpool or swimming pool, also facilitates active range of motion. As the athlete's range of motion improves, he or she should work on exercis-

es against gravity to begin the strengthening phase.

Actively assisted range-of-motion exercises permit the athlete to go to the limits of his or her range of motion, and then the trainer assists to increase the range of motion slightly more. A technique frequently used is proprioceptive neuromuscular facilitation (PNF). This technique is described in Chapter 45.

During actively assisted or passive range-of-motion exercises, the athletic trainer must be careful not to apply more resistance than the athlete can tolerate. Resistance should be applied at a steady, continuous rate for approximately 10 seconds. This length of time is variable, depending on the nature of the injury and the personal preference of the trainer.

Modalities

Just as they did in Phase I of rehabilitation, modalities play an important role in Phase II. For example, warming up the tissues prior to attempting motion is beneficial. Moist heat, electrical stimulation, or diathermy can all be used effectively. Further, once the tissues are warm, massage therapy is extremely effective in breaking up scar tissue and adhesions and may precede range-of-motion exercises.

Cold, or cryotherapy, is applied (ice or cold whirlpool) after exercise to help prevent secondary swelling or effusion. In some situations, cold is applied prior to exercise. It decreases the amount of pain perceived and allows the athlete to work within a greater range of motion. An example is the application of ice to an injured muscle prior to working the muscle through its range of motion. While pain still sets the limits of motion, the discomfort level is less because the area is partially numb.

Exercise Equipment

On occasion, when difficulty is encountered in regaining an adequate pain-free range of motion, exercise equipment may be used to help the athlete meet the determined goals. Continuous passive motion (CPM) machines may be prescribed by a physician, particularly postoperatively to prevent adhesions. Isokinetic machines may be used to apply a static stretch to a lower extremity joint at an isometric setting at various degrees of allowable motion.

Strength

As the athlete progresses with his or her range of motion, strengthening exercises can be initiated. During the early stages of active exercise, training can occur every day. As the workload increases to about 25 percent of the noninjured muscle group, the frequency of exercise should be reduced to every other day. The 48 hours between sessions is necessary for cellular adjustments in the muscle tissue, which creates a climate for maximal strength gains. If the injury becomes inflamed again, usually the intensity or frequency of exercise is too great. Icing down after workouts helps to reduce inflammation.

Strength gains can be achieved through a combination of isometric, isotonic, and isokinetic exercises. Isometrics can be done early and when there is still a need to limit the range of motion in which strengthening exercises can be performed. They are even applicable when the athlete is immobilized because they help to decrease atrophy. In an isometric contraction, the muscle neither shortens nor lengthens, so the strengthening attained is specific to the joint angle. There is a 10-degree physiological overflow above and below a specific angle; therefore, working on isometric contractions at 20-degree intervals through a range of motion can, to some extent, strengthen the entire range.

Isotonic exercises involve strengthening muscle groups through a range of motion with fixed resistance. They can be incorporated into the athlete's program once a reasonable active range of motion has been achieved. Isotonic exercises are described in detail in Chapter 45. The progressive resist-

ance programs described in that chapter are appropriate for rehabilitation. However, the athlete should start with no weights and work against gravity before progressing to resistance exercises. When weights are applied, they should be increased in very small increments, making certain, in the early phases, that the athlete does not overstress his or her muscles. As the athlete is able to progress to larger weights, exercise machines can be incorporated into the therapy program. Isotonic exercises with free weights or machines should be performed in a very controlled fashion, using good form and including exercises which stress the muscles both concentrically and eccentrically.

Attention should be given to exercising all muscles of the injured extremity—not just those directly involved in the injury or those crossing the injured joint. For example, following a knee injury, the emphasis initially may be on the quadriceps and hamstrings but should rapidly move to include hip flexors, extensors, abductors, and so forth.

When working to regain strength in the injured area, the athlete should exercise one extremity at a time. In this way, the injured extremity will get the maximum benefit from the exercise without being carried through the exercise by the unaffected extremity.

The isokinetic exercises described in Chapter 45 have excellent application in rehabilitation programs. Isokinetics allow for slow strength work as well as high-speed endurance work at full and/or limited ranges of motion. One of the most beneficial types of isokinetic exercise is pool therapy. Running in waist-deep water, one form of pool therapy, has its advantages in that it is safer than running on land because the water accommodates resistance due to buoyancy. It also lightens the impact loads to the lower extremities. Exercising in this manner can often be sport-specific. Unfortunately, many schools do not have pools.

Most isokinetic exercises require specialized equipment (Cybex, Kincom, Biodex, etc.). The advantage of these exercise units is that they allow accommodations to pain and fatigue as the athlete works through a full range of motion with them.

Unlike free weights or nonisokinetic equipment (Nautilus), where the weight is set and the athlete accommodates his or her rate of exercise, isokinetic equipment is not limited in the weight the athlete can lift by the weakest point in his or her range, since the resistance is accommodating. This advantage enables the athlete to perform a strengthening program more efficiently. Caution must be used, however, in prescribing the use of isokinetic equipment too early in the rehabilitation program, especially for athletes who are used to the "no pain, no gain" philosophy of routine strength training. The equipment only allows the athletic trainer to set the rate; the athletic trainer cannot limit the resistance. The athlete who is overly aggressive on this equipment early in the rehabilitation course may develop secondary pain and swelling.

With both isotonic and isokinetic exercise, muscle strength during rehabilitation should be developed initially by using slow speed, low weights, and multiple repetitions. Unlike working normal muscle in strengthening programs which stress high weights and minimal to moderate repetitions in order to fatigue the muscle to encourage the further development of muscle fibers, injured muscle should not be worked to its maximal fatigue level, as secondary muscle spasm and edema will develop.

Power and Endurance

Having achieved muscle strength that is 80 percent of the unaffected limb, the athlete may begin working on muscle power and endurance. Regaining muscle power is achieved by lifting weights more quickly at faster contractile velocities. Muscle endurance is improved by lifting low weights through a range of motion at a faster contractile velocity of more than 60 degrees per second on an isokinetic machine.

Sport Specificity

In many cases a strengthening program can be designed to reproduce the motion that will actually be performed during the sport. An example would be the soccer player who practices running and kicking in waist-deep water. Another example would be the baseball pitcher who practices throwing with rubber stretch tubing.

Documenting Motion and Strength Gains

Range of motion is documented in the early phases through frequent goniometric measurements. Beginning levels of muscle strength, power, and endurance should be documented as each extremity is introduced into the program. Muscles above and below the injury site should be tested for weakness. The muscle strength test, whether it be isotonic, isometric, or isokinetic, should be precisely defined and reproducible. Once weakness has been documented, a specific program of exercise can be developed for that muscle group. Documentation of strength, power, and endurance gains should be made on a weekly basis, rather than with each session. When observing the athlete in a range-of-motion, strength, power, and endurance program, the trainer should make certain the athlete is not substituting alternative muscle groups to perform the particular exercise.

As in Phase I, the athlete in Phase II should continue to train and maintain any nonaffected body parts while receiving treatment for the injury. A program established to maintain conditioning should have both anaerobic and aerobic components. The program will need to be altered throughout the rehabilitation process as the athlete's injury permits engagement in a greater variety of activities.

Phase II Goals

As athletes work through Phase II of a rehabilitation program, they should be striving to attain the following goals:

- Reach full range of motion to the joint involved in the injury when compared to the unaffected side, unless the athlete's preseason examination documented a side-to-side variance. Joints above and below the injury should have full range of motion as well.
- Increase muscle strength in all muscle groups affected by the injury. Muscle strength is generally targeted to equal the athlete's unaffected side unless the athlete's preseason examination documented a side-to-side variance.
- Increase muscle power and endurance in all muscle groups affected by the injury. Power and endurance should be targeted to equal the athlete's unaffected side unless the athlete's preseason examination documented a side-to-side variance.
- Maintain cardiovascular endurance levels and pre-injury strength of all areas unaffected by the injury.

PHASE III: RETURN TO PLAY

The third phase of rehabilitation is a preparatory phase for returning the athlete to activity.

Biomechanics

Care is taken to make sure the athlete's normal biomechanical function has been restored. Analysis of sport technique is also extremely important, especially for the athlete who has sustained an overuse injury. Correction of any biomechanical imbalances or improper technique should be made at this time to prevent future recurrence.

Balance, Proprioception, and Kinesthetic Awareness

In the past, balance, proprioception, and kinesthetic awareness have been linked generally to lower extremity rehabilitation programs. However, as more information is gathered regarding successful rehabilita-

tion of shoulder and elbow injuries in throwing athletes, swimmers, and gymnasts, restoring these qualities in upper extremity injuries is now believed to be important also.

Lower Extremities

To restore balance, proprioception, and kinesthetic awareness following lower extremity injuries, the following routine is suggested. (Certainly, other programs exist that are equally as effective. Most programs employ the same principles; they merely differ somewhat in style.)

The athlete with an ankle or knee injury may begin balance and proprioception skill development with heel raises (Fig. 49.4) and single-leg stands. The athlete then progress-

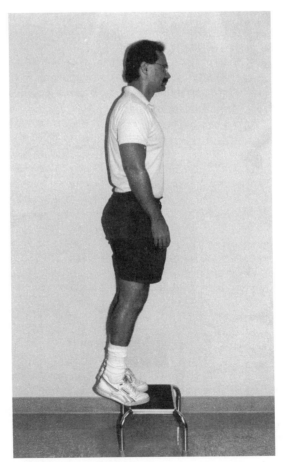

FIGURE 49.4. Heel raises are used to restore balance and proprioception.

es to the use of a balance board or circle (Fig. 49.5).

After the athlete is confident about sense of balance on the affected extremity, he or she progresses to jumping, starting with equal weight-bearing, two-legged jumps. These begin low and slowly increase in height. Gradually, weight is shifted to the affected foot alone. Once the athlete can jump ten times on the injured foot with equal weight, no pain or facial grimace, and no extra body movements, he or she is ready for the jog-to-run progression.

The jog-to-run progression is a step-by-step progression. Once the athlete completes a specific step without difficulty or limping, he or she is allowed to progress to the next step. The jog-to-run progression consists of the following ten steps:

1. Jog straight ahead on even ground; start with 1/4 mile and gradually progress to 1 mile.
2. Jog large figure eights, both directions.
3. Gradually increase the speed of jogging the figure eights.
4. Gradually decrease the size of the figure eights, jogging.
5. Increase the speed of Step 4 to full speed.

6. Jog, running straight ahead, then cut to the unaffected side; repeat, cutting to the affected side.
7. Progress to full speed in Step 6.
8. Progress to 25 yards of back pedaling.
9. Progress to 20 yards of a carioca step, both directions (moving sideways: step, cross over front, step, cross over back).
10. Add sport-specific activities in a non-competitive environment.

Upper Extremities

Restoring proprioception and kinesthetic awareness is equally important following injuries to the upper extremity, especially for athletes involved in throwing and racquet sports as well as swimming and gymnastics.

Redeveloping synchrony of motion of the upper extremity is the most important step in Phase III of rehabilitation. This is initially accomplished by performing the upper extremity motion specific to the sport in a slow and deliberate fashion. It is frequently helpful to perform this motion in front of a mirror. Emphasis should be given to stabilization of the scapula, especially during rehabilitation of shoulder injuries. When fluid motion is achieved, speed can gradually be increased. The next step is to perform the motion holding a ball (specific to the sport involved), racquet, or light weight (2 to 3 pounds) for gymnastics and swimming. When this exercise can be performed with a fluid motion at variable speeds without pain, the athlete progresses to sport-specific activities.

In the throwing athlete, an interval throwing program designed to increase gradually the amount and intensity of throwing is started. Such a program generally involves alternating intervals of "long toss" throwing (high arc lobs with fluid rainbow motion) and "short toss" throwing (shorter distances with less arc and more emphasis on cocking). The "long toss" is emphasized initially, and the "short toss" is gradually phased in. The number of throws and intensity are slowly increased. A similar interval program, leading to a

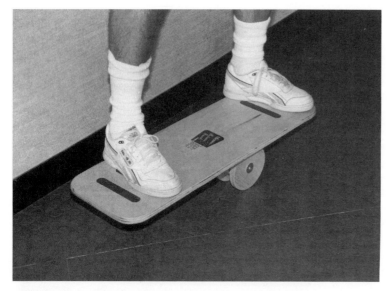

FIGURE 49.5. After doing heel raises, the athlete progresses to using a balance board to regain balance and proprioception.

gradual return to sport, can be developed for the racquet sports, swimming, and others.

Evaluation for Taping, Bracing, and Protective Devices

During Phase III, the athlete should be evaluated for the need for protective taping, bracing, padding, and the like. The athlete should understand that these protective devices do not take the place of a maintenance rehabilitation program. The athlete's present equipment, including footwear, should also be reevaluated prior to returning to activity.

Final Check

Prior to the athlete's return to full participation, there should be a final activity check. Note should be made of the athlete's range of motion, strength, endurance, power, balance, proprioceptive and kinesthetic awareness, and overall conditioned state, as well as the athlete's style of performance (techniques) and level of confidence. In an attempt to avoid reinjury, all of these parameters must be maximized before the player is released to full competition. A reinjury may not be physically more traumatic than the initial injury to an athlete, but generally it is psychologically more traumatic.

Phase III Goals

As athletes progress through Phase III of a rehabilitation program, they should be working to achieve the following goals:

- Attain normal biomechanical function.
- Increase balance, proprioception, and kinesthetic function.

- Wear the appropriate taping, bracing, or protective devices to ensure safe return to play.
- Return to practice and eventually to competitive play.

DOCUMENTATION

Record keeping is a necessary component of every athlete's rehabilitation program. Documentation allows everyone involved in the athlete's care to know that the proper procedures are being followed in a timely fashion and that the athlete is healing in a reasonable amount of time. If the athlete fails to progress as one would anticipate, reviewing the rehabilitation record may aid the trainer and physician in finding an alternative rehabilitation course so the athlete can progress more rapidly. The trainer should also review the rehabilitation progress reports with the injured athlete. Data on increased range of motion, strength, endurance, and power are frequently encouraging to the athlete and serve as a positive psychological motivational force.

PSYCHOLOGICAL CONSIDERATIONS

When dealing with an injured athlete, it is critical that the athletic trainer explain to the athlete the nature of the injury, the intent and overall anticipated progression of the rehabilitation program, and the prognosis for recovery. Expected goals should be clearly stated during each phase of the rehabilitation program. It is not uncommon for injured athletes to go through a period of denial, anger, and depression before they accept their injury (see Chapter 12). Therefore, it is critical that the trainer be sensitive to the psychological issues of injury and rehabilitation and address them with the athlete as rehabilitation progresses.

(Important Concepts appear on the next page.)

IMPORTANT CONCEPTS

1. Rehabilitation for the injured athlete includes restoration to a functional level for daily living and return to an appropriate level of competitive fitness.
2. Phase I of rehabilitation involves immediate care and healing of the injury.
3. Phase II involves restoring range of motion, strength, power, and endurance and returning the athlete to a functional level of daily living.
4. Phase III involves returning the athlete to competitive activity.
5. The ICE (ice, compression, elevation) treatment is used to control hemorrhage and edema.
6. Healing time is based on degree of the injury, location of the injury, presence of infection, age of the athlete, nutritional status, and presence of specific medical problems.
7. Passive range of motion is performed by the trainer; active range of motion is performed by the athlete; and actively assisted range of motion occurs when the athlete goes to the limits of his or her range of motion and is then assisted by the trainer to go a bit further.
8. During isometric strengthening, the muscle neither shortens nor lengthens during contraction.
9. In isotonic strengthening, muscle groups are strengthened through a range of motion with fixed resistance.
10. A final check before the athlete returns to full participation should include evaluation of range of motion, strength, endurance, power, balance, proprioceptive and kinesthetic awareness, overall conditioned state, and technique.
11. Documentation during the program of rehabilitation allows everyone involved to know that proper procedures are being followed in a timely fashion and that the athlete is healing in a reasonable amount of time.

SUGGESTED READINGS

Bernhardt, Donna B., ed. *Sports Physical Therapy.* New York: Churchill Livingstone, 1986, pp. 155–172.

Cruess, R. L. "Healing of Bone, Tendon, and Ligament." In *Fractures in Adults*, 2d ed., vol. 1, edited by Charles A. Rockwood, Jr. and David P. Green, pp. 147–167. Philadelphia: J. B. Lippincott, 1984.

Davies, G. J. "Isokinetic Approach to the Knee." In *Physical Therapy of the Knee*, edited by R. E. Mangine, pp. 221–243. New York: Churchill Livingstone, 1988.

Fisher, A. Craig., Mary A. Domm, and Deborah A. Wuest. "Adherence to Sports-Injury Rehabilitation Programs." *The Physician and Sportsmedicine* 16 (July 1988): 47–52.

Gould, James A., III, and George J. Davies, eds. *Orthopaedic and Sports Physical Therapy.* St. Louis: C. V. Mosby, 1985, pp. 181–198.

Harkess, J. W., W. C. Ramsey, and B. Ahmadi. "Principles of Fractures and Dislocations." In *Fractures in Adults*, 2d ed., vol. 1, edited by Charles A. Rockwood, Jr. and David P. Green, pp. 1–146. Philadelphia: J. B. Lippincott, 1984.

Kisner, Carolyn, and Lynn Allen Colby. *Therapeutic Exercise: Foundations and Techniques*. Philadelphia: F. A. Davis, 1985.

Kulund, D. N., ed. *The Injured Athlete*, 2d ed. Philadelphia: J. B. Lippincott, 1988.

Licht, Sidney, ed. *Rehabilitation and Medicine*. New Haven: Elizabeth Licht (Publisher), 1968.

Malone, Y. "Surgical Overview and Rehabilitation Process for Ligamentous Repair." In *Physical Therapy of the Knee*, edited by R. E. Mangine, pp. 163–189. New York: Churchill Livingstone, 1988.

Mangine, R. E., and S. Price. "Innovative Approaches to Surgery and Rehabilitation." In *Physical Therapy of the Knee*, edited by R. E. Mangine, pp. 191–220. New York: Churchill Livingstone, 1988.

Marino, M. "Current Concepts on Rehabilitation in Sports Medicine: Research and Clinical Interrelationships." In *The Lower Extremity and Spine in Sports Medicine*, vol. 1, edited by J. A. Nicholas and E. B. Hershman, pp. 117–194. St. Louis: C. V. Mosby, 1986.

O'Donoghue, D. H. *Treatment of Injuries to Athletes*, 3d ed. Philadelphia: W. B. Saunders, 1976.

Rusk, Howard A. *Rehabilitation Medicine*, 4th ed. St. Louis: C. V. Mosby, 1977, pp. 93–139.

Sloan, J. P., P. Giddings, and R. Hain. "Effects of Cold and Compression on Edema." *The Physician and Sportsmedicine* 16 (August 1988): 116–120.

50

Modalities

OBJECTIVES FOR CHAPTER 50

After reading this chapter, the student should be able to:

1. Understand the mechanism of inflammation in response to tissue injury.
2. Describe the therapeutic effects of cryotherapy and thermotherapy.
3. Identify the various cryotherapy and thermotherapy modalities, their indications, contraindications, and operational theories.
4. Understand the differences between superficial and penetrating thermotherapies.
5. Recognize the differences between diathermy and ultrasound.
6. Describe the use of ultrasound and phonophoresis.
7. Identify the differences between the categories of electrical stimulators.
8. Identify the mechanical therapies, along with their indications and their application techniques.

INTRODUCTION

The number of therapeutic modalities used in the athletic training environment is ever increasing. Unfortunately, however, they are too often applied in a very mechanized manner, without an understanding of the working principles relevant to that modality. An understanding of the capabilities of the modality—when it is indicated and contraindicated and how it is properly used—is essential if potentially harmful effects are to be avoided. Modalities should be used under the supervision of a physician.

Chapter 50 begins with a discussion of modality selection—the factors to be considered, the need to understand the inflammatory response, how intervention with modalities helps minimize the inflammatory response, and the types of modalities available. Then several modalities—specifically, cryotherapy, thermotherapy, electrical stimulation, and mechanical therapy—are discussed. ▪

MODALITY SELECTION

Selection Factors

Minimizing the time lost to injury is a major goal of the athletic training profession. Various **modalities**, or physical agents, available to the athletic trainer can create an optimum environment for injury healing, while reducing pain and discomfort. Modalities include forms of heat, cold, light, water, electricity, massage, and any mechanical means that will work to promote healing or rehabilitation. The selection of specific treatments or combinations of treatments is based on such factors as:

- Injury site, type, and severity.
- Modality indications and contraindications.

■ The physician's prescription.
■ The athlete's willingness to accept treatment.

A key point to remember is, "more is not better." Modalities are used to aid the athlete's tolerance to exercise, which is the ultimate modality. Misuse or overuse of modalities can often aggravate a condition, delaying rather than facilitating the athlete's return to play.

For legal reasons, therapeutic modalities must be administered in accordance with local physical therapy/athletic training regulations. Documentation of all treatments should be maintained to ensure continuity and to help assess the efficacy of the treatment.

The Inflammatory Response

A knowledge of the consequences of an injury to the body's tissues is a prerequisite to understanding how and why modalities can help create an optimum healing environment. **Inflammation** results when tissue is crushed, stretched, or torn. Vasodilation of local blood vessels, with formation of edema and pain, is the major element of the inflammatory response. Heat and redness are also signs of inflammation and result from increased blood flow to the injured area. Chemically, bradykinins and prostaglandins are synthesized, and histamines are released. These mediators increase local swelling and pain.

Hemorrhage from damaged, dilated blood vessels adds additional trauma to the injured area. Local circulation is disrupted, and the vessels are no longer able to meet the tissues' oxygen demands. Further cellular damage results from these secondary hypoxic conditions. Muscle spasm is induced in the body's effort to splint damaged tissues to prevent further trauma. In addition to the chemical mediators, pressure from swelling and spasm stimulates pain fibers and contributes to the pain-spasm cycle (pain causes spasm, which causes pain, etc.).

Intervention With Modalities

Early intervention with physical agents helps to limit the pain-spasm cycle by minimizing the inflammatory response. Success in this effort reduces the athlete's time lost to injury and allows better tolerance to rehabilitative exercise. As the injury matures, the progression of the modalities can augment circulation and nutrient transfer, which enhances the healing process.

The early utilization of exercise minimizes the degree of deconditioning. Therefore, rehabilitation can be accomplished more quickly, allowing the athlete to return to activity more expediently. The athletic trainer's goal, therefore, is to minimize the inflammatory response, augment the healing environment, and incorporate timely therapeutic exercise.

Types of Modalities

The following are basic types of modalities used in the athletic training setting:

■ Cryotherapy/cryokinetics: cold therapy, contrast therapy, cold therapy combined with exercise.
■ Superficial thermotherapy: whirlpool, hydrocollator packs, paraffin bath, Fluidotherapy.
■ Penetrating thermotherapy: diathermy, ultrasound.
■ Electrical stimulation: transcutaneous electrical nerve stimulation (TENS), high-voltage stimulation, low-voltage stimulation, interferential stimulation, point stimulation, portable TENS, neuromuscular stimulation.
■ Mechanical therapy: massage, manual therapy, traction, intermittent compression.

CRYOTHERAPY

Indications/Contraindications

Cryotherapy (cold therapy) cools tissue by transferring heat energy. Its indications include soft tissue injuries such as sprains, strains, contusions, and muscle spasms. Cryotherapy is also indicated for chronic inflammatory conditions such as tendinitis, tenosynovitis, and fasciitis. Contraindications include circulatory disturbances, hypersensitivity to cold, and prolonged application over superficial nerves.

Physiological Effects

The physiological effects of cryotherapy are the most effective means of reducing post-injury inflammation.

Decreased Tissue Temperature

Cryotherapy in the form of ice packs, ice massage, cold water immersion, and so forth decreases tissue temperature surrounding the injury site. In response to cold, nerve impulses and conduction velocities are diminished, and the athlete experiences an analgesic/anesthetic effect. Cold decreases muscle spindle firing, thus decreasing muscle activity, which diminishes the muscle spasm in the surrounding region. When spasm and pain sensations are decreased, the pain-spasm response also diminishes. To preserve core heat, superficial cutaneous vessels constrict, leading to decreased blood flow and lower capillary permeability in the injured area. Thus, hemorrhage and the release of metabolites into the injured tissues are lessened. Local tissue metabolism is decreased in response to cold, with a resultant decrease in the cells' oxygen demands. Therefore, fewer cells are destroyed from the inability of the damaged vessels to provide oxygen.

Hunting Reaction

The initial constriction of blood vessels following the application of cryotherapy is followed by a period of dilation as the body attempts to warm the cooled area. This process of cyclical vasodilation and vasoconstriction is called the **hunting reaction**, and its occurrence and effects on tissue temperature are controversial. The implication of this reflex vasodilation is believed to prevent the extreme lowering of tissue temperatures as the body attempts to protect itself from frostbite. The hunting reaction is most likely to occur in regions of high arteriovenous anastomoses, commonly found in the ears, hands, and feet.

Duration of Therapy

Cryotherapy is generally limited to 20 to 30 minutes, depending on the depth of the target tissues. Precautions are also necessary to prevent prolonged application of ice over areas with superficial nerves, such as the fibular head and the elbow. Cases of nerve palsy caused by excessive and unsupervised cold therapy at these sites have been reported.

ICE Principle

In acute conditions, cryotherapy is best combined with elevation and compression in the form of an elastic wrap. This treatment combination is known as the **ICE** (ice, compression, elevation) **principle**. ICE is standard treatment for most acute athletic injuries. Elevation of an injured extremity higher than the heart, as well as compression of the tissues with an elastic wrap applied distal to proximal, can minimize edema by decreasing blood flow and pressure to the area.

Cryotherapy Application

The physiologic effects of cryotherapy are similar, despite the various methods of delivery. The athlete will experience the sensations of cold, burning, aching, and finally numbness after the cold has been applied for a period of time. Care should always be taken to avoid freezing the skin and to limit ice pack and cold water immersion treatments to 20 to 30 minutes. Cold applications can be applied hourly, or at least several times a day during active inflammatory stages. Application techniques include ice massage, cold water immersion, ice packs, chemical cold packs, flexible gel cold packs, and vapocoolant sprays.

Ice Massage

A paper cup filled with water is frozen to form an ice cylinder that can be rubbed or massaged directly onto the skin surface. The ice is rubbed gently over the site of the injury until the skin becomes bright pink in color, usually 7 to 10 minutes for a 5-square-inch area. Ice massage is commonly used for its analgesic effect prior to cross-fiber (across tissues) friction massage.

Cold Water Immersion

A whirlpool tank, bucket, or other similar container is filled with a mixture of water and ice. The temperature should be maintained between 55 and 65 degrees F (13 and 18 degrees C); therefore, ice slurry mixtures are not advised. Immersion of the injured part lasts for 20 to 30 minutes. Cold water immersion is extremely effective in delivering cryotherapy to highly contoured areas such as the hands, feet, and ankles. The immersion technique offers excellent circumferential cooling; however, the extremity must be placed in a dependent position during the treatment. For this reason, alternative methods of cryotherapy may be utilized for athletes with moderate to severe edema.

Ice Packs

Plastic bags filled with flaked or crushed ice can be placed over the site of the injury. Crushed ice is more effective in conforming to the body's contours. The bag should not contain air, which acts to insulate the area. A single layer of wet elastic wrap can first be applied to provide pressure over the injured site, and the remainder of the wrap can be used to secure the ice pack in place. Treatment is 20 to 30 minutes in length. Elevation can be combined with the ice and compression for the injured extremity.

Chemical Cold Packs

Commercially manufactured chemical cold packs are expensive but convenient. Mixing the chemical contents produces the cold by creating an endothermic reaction. Temperatures are not always consistent; nor can the pack be reused. The length of time the pack stays cold also varies. Chemical burns can result from the alkaline contents if the pack ruptures.

Flexible Gel Cold Packs

Refreezable, flexible silica gel cold packs, encased in plastic, are a convenient means of applying cold therapy. A damp towel should be placed between the skin and the pack to guard against frostbite and for clinical hygiene. Treatment time is 20 to 30 minutes. Compression and elevation can be used in conjunction with this form of cryotherapy.

Vapocoolant Sprays

Cold sprays use rapid evaporation of chemicals, usually chloromethane or fluoromethane, sprayed on the surface of the skin to freeze it. The effects of such sprays are temporary and superficial. Cold sprays are used for the treatment of myofascial pain and trigger points, and are sometimes combined with stretching techniques to help break the pain-spasm cycle of soft tissue injuries—for example, hamstring or low back strains. The effect is primarily through a sensory response.

Cryokinetics

Cryokinetics is the use of cold and movement as treatment modalities (Fig. 50.1). Often, pain and spasm result in decreased range of motion in an injured body part. Cold therapy decreases pain sensation and allows range-of-motion activities to be incorporated with treatment. Cold therapy can also minimize temperature increases that occur from exercise, encouraging early motion while further reducing potential injury from activity. Active range of motion decreases dissociation, retards disuse atrophy, and prevents adhesions.

Simple, pain-free movement is done simultaneously or after the application of

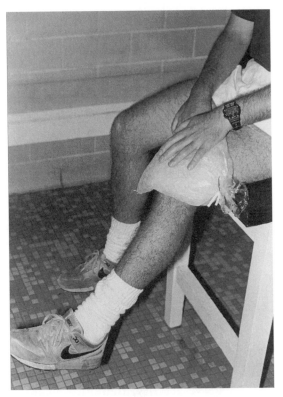

FIGURE 50.1. Cryokinetics is a treatment modality that combines cold and movement.

standard cold therapy. If active motion is painful, isometric exercises may be substituted. The athlete should never force movement or experience pain when performing exercise. Cryokinetics can be easily included in the athlete's home care and can be performed frequently throughout the day.

Contrast Therapy

Indications/Contraindications

Contrast therapy alternates cryotherapy and thermotherapy (heat therapy) in the postacute phase of injury. During the transition period between cold and heat application, contrast therapy is often incorporated into the treatment protocol. The efficacy of this treatment is largely empirical, but it has been found to be helpful in reducing pitting edema and in encouraging motion in the involved area.

Contrast therapy is initiated when an injury is not acutely painful, the swelling has stabilized, and progress with ice application is no longer being made. By applying cold to cause vasoconstriction, followed by heat to cause vasodilation, circulation and nutrition to the area are stimulated while minimizing the complications of increased swelling. Contraindications of contrast therapy include acute injuries and lesions with active hemorrhaging.

Technique of Application

The most common technique for contrast therapy uses two whirlpools or containers filled with water. One is filled with cold water at 55 to 65 degrees F (13 to 18 degrees C), and the other is filled with hot water at 100 to 110 degrees F (38 to 43 degrees C). The injured extremity is placed in the hot water for 2 to 4 minutes, followed by 1 to 3 minutes in the cold water. Generally, a 4:1 minute (hot to cold) cycle is assumed as the athlete's tolerance indicates. Hot and cold are alternated for four to five cycles, several times daily.

Generally all treatments should end with cold to provide an analgesic effect and decrease tissue temperature prior to rehabilitation exercises. Ending with cold immersion will also aid in the prevention of reactive swelling that the exercise might produce. Range-of-motion exercises can be performed while the extremity is in the water.

THERMOTHERAPY

Indications/Contraindications

Thermotherapy, or heat application, is a second major modality of athletic injury care. Heat has the opposite effect of cryotherapy in that it produces an immediate increase in circulation. Vasodilation occurs as the body attempts to shunt cooler blood to the warmed area to dissipate the heat. Because of the potential increase in interstitial fluid from the increased blood flow and dilated capillary beds, thermotherapy is

TABLE 50.1. Physiological Effects of Cryotherapy and Thermotherapy

Cold Applications	Short—30 minutes or less	Prolonged—more than 30 minutes
Skin capillaries	Constriction, then dilation	Constriction
Skin color	White, turning red	White
Skeletal muscle	Relaxed after shivering	Rigid voluntary and/or reflex contractions
Cell size	Little change	Slightly decreased
Tissue metabolism	Decreased	Decreased
Pain sensation	Decreased	Decreased
Deep circulation	Little change	Vasodilation

Heat Applications	Short—30 minutes or less	Prolonged—more than 30 minutes
Skin capillaries	Dilation	Continued dilation
Skin color	Pink, then red	Deep red
Skeletal muscle	Relaxed	Irritated
Cell size	Expanded	Less expanded but still larger than normal
Tissue metabolism	Increased	Levels off
Pain sensation	Decreased	Variable

Source: Donley, P.B. "The Uses of Therapeutic Modalities." Eastern Athletic Trainers Association Convention, Grossinger, NY. January 24, 1977.

contraindicated with acute inflammatory conditions.

A safe guideline for the progression to thermotherapy is to avoid heat until the active inflammatory process has ceased. The injured area should not be acutely painful, and show no increased signs of heat or swelling prior to thermotherapy application. If any of these signs are present, the injured part is not yet ready for heat treatments.

Physiological Effects

Despite its potential consequences, thermotherapy has the advantage of being a more comfortable modality than cryotherapy. Applied at the correct time during rehabilitation, heat can provide many beneficial effects. The therapeutic effects of heat include decreased pain, decreased muscle spasm, increased cell metabolism, and, when combined with stretching or movement, increased range of motion. The elevated blood flow encourages the removal of waste products and produces an influx of oxygen and nutrients to meet the metabolic demands of the injured area.

Heat reduces muscle spasm by inhibiting gamma nerve activity, therefore breaking the pain-spasm cycle (Table 50.1). Fluid congestion and pain in the injured area are diminished by reducing the viscosity of the edema and by augmenting lymphatic circulation. Higher temperatures cause the viscoelastic structure of connective tissue to become more pliable. The muscle, tendon, and/or joint capsule becomes elongated as a stretch is applied while the tissue is still warm.

Methods of Introduction

Heat, or thermotherapy, can be introduced to the body by four principal methods:

- *Conduction.* The transfer of heat through direct contact with its source (e.g., moist heat packs or paraffin bath).
- *Convection.* The transfer of heat via a medium such as the movement of air or water (e.g., whirlpool bath).
- *Radiation.* The transfer of heat or energy through space by electromagnetic waves (e.g., infrared lamp). (Rarely used.)

- *Conversion*: Heat developed by the passage of sound or electrical current through the tissues (e.g., ultrasound, diathermy).

The method used to deliver thermotherapy to the body varies with the athlete's specific injury, and depends on each modality's indications and contraindications.

Superficial and Penetrating Thermotherapies

Two categories of thermotherapies are used in sports medicine environments: **superficial thermotherapy** and **penetrating thermotherapy**. Superficial therapy, which includes whirlpools, moist heat packs, paraffin, and Fluidotherapy, has a maximal penetration of 0.4 inch (1 cm) into soft tissues. An example of penetrating thermotherapy is ultrasound, a deep heat modality which has varied penetration capabilities up to 2 inches (5 cm).

Superficial Thermotherapy

Whirlpool bath. The modality most commonly associated with athletic injury care is the whirlpool bath. While the whirlpool can be used in immediate injury care as a cryotherapy technique, it is most commonly a form of heat treatment. A turbine circulates the water in the tank, providing a hydromassage effect in addition to the thermal effects of the water. Range-of-motion activities can be performed in the water during treatment. Indications for whirlpool treatment include soft tissue trauma and postimmobilization conditions in need of increasing range of motion. Contraindications include active hemorrhaging or swelling, heat stress, or any acute condition.

Whirlpool baths increase superficial tissue temperatures, causing an analgesic action, a decrease in muscle spasm, production of relaxation, and the stimulation of circulation, thereby promoting healing. Table 50.2 contains the treatment times and temperatures for using the whirlpool bath.

A full body whirlpool treatment can produce dizziness and heat stress; therefore, it

TABLE 50.2. Whirlpool Treatment Times and Temperatures

Treatment	Temperature	Time (minutes)
Cold whirlpools	55–65°F (13–18°C)	20–30
Hot whirlpools		
Extremity	100–110°F (37.8–43.4°C)	20
Full body	94–100°F (34.4–37.8°C)	8–12

must be used cautiously. Only those body parts in need of treatment should be in the whirlpool bath. Electrical safety inspections and ground fault circuit interrupters are essential for the safe operation of whirlpool baths. Athletes receiving treatment should never be left unsupervised. To prevent the chance of electrical shock, athletes should never turn the unit off or on while they are in the water.

Whirlpool water and tanks must be kept clean. Frequent water changes and daily cleaning are essential. Antiseptics should be used regularly during wound care. Whirlpool management of open wounds or abrasions should be handled cautiously. Hydrotherapy environments that handle wound care must adhere to very stringent cleaning techniques to prevent contamination or spreading of infection to others.

Hydrocollator packs. Hydrocollator (moist heat) packs are an efficient and inexpensive means of applying moist heat to an injured body part (Fig. 50.2). Hydrocollator packs are indicated in postacute soft tissue injuries such as contusions, strains, and muscle spasms. As with any form of heat therapy, moist heat packs are contraindicated for acute injuries, over areas of impaired sensation, and over the eyes and genitals.

Moist heat packs are comprised of silicone gel encased in a canvas fabric which acts to absorb and hold moisture. Packs are stored in a hot water unit that keeps them at

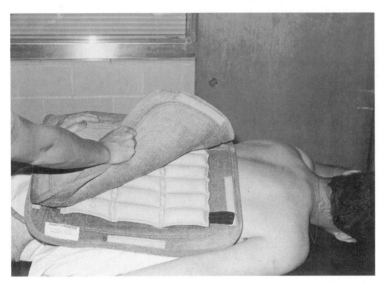

FIGURE 50.2. Hydrocollator packs are moist heat packs that work well in postacute soft tissue injuries such as contusions, strains, and muscle spasms.

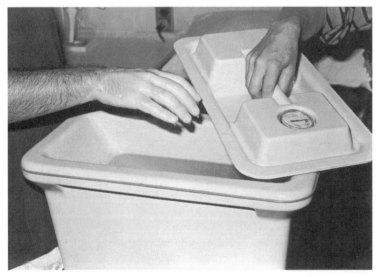

FIGURE 50.3. The dip-and-wrap technique for applying paraffin. After being dipped several times, the extremity is wrapped in a plastic bag and toweling.

150 to 170 degrees F (66 to 77 degrees C). A pack is removed from the unit, wrapped in six to eight layers of toweling, and applied to the injured area for 20 minutes. The athlete should be cautioned that hydrocollator packs can burn the skin, and adequate

toweling must be kept in between the pack and the skin. While receiving the treatment, the athlete should be in a comfortable, supported position, or in a comfortably stretched position if the goal of the treatment is to increase the range of motion. Athletes should not lie on the hot pack because the pressure from their body weight can impede the circulation necessary to dissipate the accumulated heat.

Paraffin baths. Paraffin baths are of particular use in providing superficial heat to angular, bony areas of the body (hands, feet, and wrists), while allowing the part to remain elevated. A mixture of paraffin and mineral oil (8:1 ratio) is kept at 125 to 130 degrees F (52 to 54 degrees C) in a thermostatically controlled unit. With its high melting point and low heat conductivity, paraffin can provide sustained heat, increasing circulation and decreasing pain in the affected area. The specific heat of the paraffin mixture is lower than that of water, so fewer calories are released to change its temperature; therefore, the body can tolerate the higher temperature without being burned. A paraffin bath is also useful in the hand care of gymnasts since the mineral oil helps to keep calluses soft and pliable. A disadvantage of paraffin is that active motion is not allowed during the heat application.

There are three techniques for applying paraffin:

- *Dip and soak.* Dip the extremity in and out of the paraffin several times to build up a layer of wax; soak in the wax for 15 to 20 minutes.
- *Dip and wrap.* Dip the extremity in the wax for several seconds, 6 to 12 times, and wrap the extremity in a plastic bag and toweling. The part is then elevated for 20 minutes, followed by massage and exercise (Fig. 50.3).
- *Painting.* Paint the extremity with 6 to 12 layers of paraffin; allow it to remain for 20 minutes.

Before paraffin is applied, the part should be cleaned and any jewelry removed; no open wounds should be present. Precautions include not allowing movement while dipping or soaking in the wax. Contraindications are the same as those with superficial heat applications.

Fluidotherapy. A more recent superficial heat modality is Fluidotherapy, which is a dry heat agent that transfers heat through convection. Small cellulose (corn husk) particles are suspended by forced air. The agitation can be controlled by adjusting the force with which the air is circulated through the particles. Although the unit has self-sterilizing capability, open wounds should be protected in a plastic bag as a precautionary measure. An extremity is placed in the unit and exercise is encouraged as tolerated. A back unit that allows the athlete to lie on a mesh hammock is also available; the particles circulate beneath it. The temperatures range from 100 to 125 degrees F (38 to 52 degrees C).

This modality has the same indications and contraindications as hydrotherapy applications. The contraindications include active hemorrhaging or swelling, a history of heat stress, or acute injuries. Precautions should be taken with vascular or sensory disorders.

Penetrating Thermotherapy

Of the penetrating therapies, diathermy and ultrasound are considered thermal agents. **Diathermy** uses high-frequency electromagnetic currents, and **ultrasound therapy** uses high-frequency acoustical energy to elicit thermal and mechanical responses. Of the electrical therapies used in physical medicine, diathermy is the only one that has a high enough current frequency to result in any significant thermal response when applied to an athlete.

Diathermy. Diathermy is the therapeutic application of high-frequency electrical current to heat the body's tissues. The effects of local heating by diathermy are the same as for any form of heat therapy: increased blood flow and tissue metabolism, decreased spasm, and so forth. In addition, internal tissue temperatures can be elevated as much as 9 degrees F.

The indications for diathermy are post-acute strains and inflammation of musculotendinous units, joints, bursae, and tendon sheaths. Contraindications include acute inflammation, nondraining infections, hemorrhage, limited circulation or sensation, peripheral vascular disease, epiphyseal growth plates, pregnancy, obesity, casts, dressings, and metal implants or screws. Metal and moisture will concentrate the current and can potentially cause burns. Only a sensation of mild warmth should be experienced during the treatment.

There are two forms of diathermy: shortwave and microwave. Shortwave diathermy uses an oscillating, high-frequency electrical current of 27 megacycles per second. The dosage is monitored by the athlete's subjective feeling of warmth, and treatment time is 20 to 30 minutes daily. One condenser plate is placed on either side of the injured part, or an induction coil is wrapped around the part. A condenser field places the athlete as a dielectric in the electrical circuit, while the induction field places the athlete in an electromagnetic field. A double layer of dry toweling should be placed between the athlete's skin and the plates or coil to absorb moisture and ensure proper spacing with the induction method (Fig. 50.4).

Microwave diathermy uses electrical current at a rate of 2,450 megacycles per second to heat tissues to 104 degrees F (40 degrees C) at a depth of 2 inches (5 cm) from the surface. Electromagnetic waves travel from the device's reflector head in a beamed or cylindrical heating pattern, depending on the type of director being used. Microwave energy is absorbed in tissues with high fluid content and has difficulty penetrating through thick layers of adipose (fatty tissue). The reflector head is placed approximately 2 inches (5 cm) above the bare skin, and treatment lasts 20 minutes. Any moisture that results during the treatment should be removed.

Microwave diathermy treats only one side of a joint at a time, but is a safer and

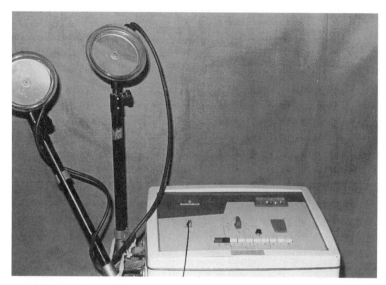

FIGURE 50.4. Shortwave diathermy. An oscillating, high-frequency electrical current generates heat in the injured part.

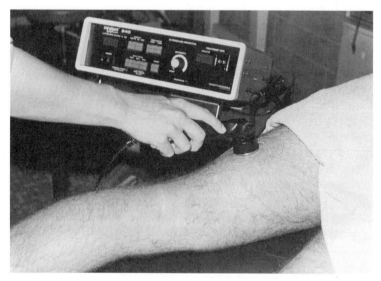

FIGURE 50.5. Ultrasound therapy. Electrical energy is converted into high-frequency sound energy to generate heat in the injured tissues.

easier modality than shortwave diathermy, due to less superficial heating.

Ultrasound. Ultrasound therapy involves the conversion of electrical energy into high-frequency sound energy beyond the audible range (Fig. 50.5) to generate heat in the tissues. Therapeutic ultrasound is generated most commonly at a frequency of 1 megahertz, but a 3.3-megahertz unit can be used. The higher-frequency unit provides a more superficial application of energy, which is beneficial when treating structures with minimal soft tissue coverage.

All energy applied to a system is either transmitted, absorbed, reflected, or refracted. Ideally, the energy is transmitted to the target area and absorbed where its therapeutic responses are desired. Absorption of ultrasound energy is highest in tissues with a high protein content. Reflection of the sound waves occurs at tissue interfaces, especially the bone-muscle interface where selective heating occurs.

As the sound waves penetrate the tissues, they produce thermal and mechanical effects which augment circulation and promote healing. Ultrasound is reported to raise tissue temperature 7 to 8 degrees F up to 2 inches (5 cm) below the skin's surface, with little or no change in skin temperature. Along with the thermal benefits, the energy also provides a micromassaging action on the cells, which provides the nonthermal effects. The nonthermal effects include an increase in cell permeability and an increased influx of ions across the cells.

Indications for ultrasound include postacute soft tissue trauma, bursitis, tendinitis, and fasciitis. Contraindications include treatment of acute inflammatory conditions with the continuous mode; treatment over areas of limited vascularity or sensation; and treatment over the ears, eyes, heart, reproductive organs, endocrine glands, central nervous system, or open epiphyses. Several of the deleterious effects of ultrasound over the above structures have occurred at dosages above the therapeutic levels, but due to the potential consequences that may occur, they are considered contraindications.

Ultrasound can be produced in a pulsed or continuous manner. Pulsed treatment produces primarily nonthermal effects due to interrupted flow and thus less total energy. It is used primarily in subacute conditions, with wound healing and over bony areas to avoid periosteal irritation. Continuous ultrasound provides both thermal and nonthermal responses.

Ultrasound at these frequencies is not transmitted through air, so a coupling medium such as lotion, gel, or water is necessary to transmit sound waves from the transducer (sound head) to the site of the injury. Treatment can also be given underwater when the treatment surface is highly contoured (Fig. 50.6). The transducer should be kept 1/2 to 1 inch (1.3 to 2.5 cm) from the skin surface and the intensity should be increased by .5 watts per square centimeter when applying ultrasound with the underwater method. Gas bubbles must be removed from the treatment surface and the transducer, as they will attenuate the energy transmission.

For all ultrasound treatments, the sound head should be kept moving in small circles or longitudinal strokes at a speed of 1 to 2 inches (2.5 to 5 cm) per second. The sound head should be perpendicular to the body, and steady pressure should be applied to help prevent cavitation (gas bubble formation) in the tissues. Treatment time is 5 minutes for an area three to four times the size of the sound head. The intensity of the treatment is determined by the stage of the injury, mode of transmission (pulsed or continuous), and the depth of the target tissues. The higher the intensity, the greater the thermal responses. Superficial tissues require lower intensities to prevent periosteal burns. Generally, the intensities range from .5 to 2.0 watts per square centimeter.

Phonophoresis. In **phonophoresis**, an application of ultrasound, whole molecules of a medication are driven through the skin to inflamed structures by ultrasound energy. The purpose of phonophoresis is to place anti-inflammatory medication into affected tissues as an alternative to injections. The most commonly used medication in phonophoresis is 10 percent hydrocortisone cream. Instead of mineral oil, lotion, or water, the hydrocortisone cream is the

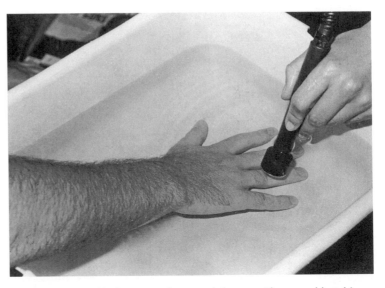

FIGURE 50.6.   Underwater ultrasound therapy. The sound head is kept moving 1/2 to 1 inch from the treatment surface.

coupling medium. Other medications such as 10 percent hydrocortisone with lidocaine (Xylocaine) ointment, or a combination of dexamethasone and 2 percent lidocaine gel, can be used for additional anesthetic benefits.

Phonophoresis is indicated in postacute soft tissue trauma such as tendinitis, strains, and contusions. Contraindications for phonophoresis are the same as for any ultrasound treatment. In addition, the contraindications for the medication administered with phonophoresis must also be considered. Phonophoresis treatment is generally of lower intensity but longer duration than standard ultrasound therapy—that is, 1 to 1.5 watts per square centimeter for 5 to 15 minutes.

Ultrasound combined with electrical muscle stimulation. Ultrasound therapy can also be combined with electrical muscle stimulation to treat postacute soft tissue trauma (e.g., sprains, muscle spasm, strains, and contusions). With combination therapy, the athlete receives both the deep heating effects of ultrasound and the benefits of muscular contractions via electrical muscle stimulation. Treatments generally last 5 to 7 minutes and can be given twice daily.

ELECTRICAL STIMULATION

Indications/Contraindications

In athletic injury care, the primary purposes of electrical stimulation are to control pain, exercise muscle tissue to decrease atrophy and its accompanying enzymatic and structural changes, encourage circulation, increase tissue temperature, encourage the breakdown of adhesions, reeducate muscles, and treat peripheral nerve lesions involving musculotendinous units. Contraindications for electrical stimulation include demand pacemakers, pregnancy, and positioning over the carotid sinuses. Muscular contractions are contraindicated where active motion is not wanted, such as with nonunited fractures or repaired tendons, thrombophlebitic conditions, areas of active bleeding, and near malignancies.

Physiological Effects

Electrical stimulation applied to the body with an intact peripheral nervous system is categorized as **transcutaneous electrical nerve stimulation (TENS)**. This modality can elicit either sensory or muscular responses by stimulating nerves when electrical current passes across the skin. Muscle membrane can be stimulated directly using direct electrical current, but muscle responses will be via the nerve if it is intact. By controlling current pulse width, frequency, and intensity, the desired responses can be obtained.

Pain Control

While the exact effects of TENS are subject to speculation, it has been shown to diminish pain in many conditions. Pain control is attained using electrical stimulation through several different mechanisms. The different methods of pain modulation are elicited by varying the type and intensity of the stimulation. The fastest pain relief is attained by a gating mechanism in the dorsal horn of the spinal cord. Stimulating large sensory fibers inhibits the transmission of pain impulses to higher recognition centers in the cortex. Applying a noxious stimulus or rhythmical muscle contractions is another method of targeting pain relief in higher levels of the central nervous system. These higher levels of pain relief are believed to include release of neurohumeral agents such as enkephalins and endorphins.

Methods of Application

There are numerous types of electrical stimulators, including high-voltage stimulators, low-voltage stimulators, interferential stimulators, point stimulators, portable TENS, and neuromuscular stimulators. Two forms of current are used with these electrical stimulators: (1) monophasic, in which galvanic or direct current flows in one direction; and (2) biphasic, in which current periodically reverses itself.

High-Voltage Stimulation

High-voltage stimulation uses a twin-peaked monophasic current and delivers between 0 and 500 volts (Fig. 50.7). High-voltage stimulation utilizes short pulse widths and long durations between pulses

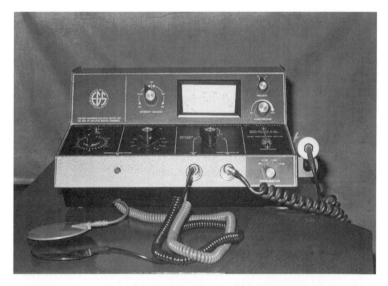

FIGURE 50.7. High-voltage stimulation. The high-peak current allows good penetration into affected tissues, and the short pulse widths minimize stimulation of nerve fibers that transmit pain.

to minimize any electrochemical responses associated with monophasic current. The high-peak current allows good penetration into the tissues, and the short pulse widths minimize stimulation of nerve fibers that transmit pain; thus a strong but comfortable stimulation can occur. The pulse widths with high-voltage stimulation are too short to stimulate denervated muscles or drive ions into the tissues (iontophoresis) effectively.

Low-Voltage Stimulation

Low-voltage stimulators frequently allow use of either biphasic or monophasic current, and typically deliver between 0 and 150 volts. The biphasic current, previously called faradic, most commonly delivers stimulation to motor nerves in a variety of ways, including pulsed, surged, or tetanizing contractions. This is typically called **electrical muscle stimulation** (**EMS**) and is used primarily to exercise muscles, reduce spasms, and enhance circulation through a mechanical massaging effect. The classic, low-voltage monophasic stimulators also deliver a true direct or galvanic current—a long, uninterrupted flow of current in one direction. The chemical responses that are associated with electrical current occur with this type of stimulation and depend on the polarity of the current. Effects at the positive and negative poles are as follows:

Positive	Negative
Vasoconstriction	Vasodilation
Hardens tissue	Softens tissue
Sedative	Stimulative
Local analgesic	Enhances venous and lymphatic return

Low-voltage monophasic current (direct current) is required to stimulate denervated muscle in areas where peripheral nerve lesions have occurred and is also necessary to perform iontophoresis (Fig. 50.8).

Iontophoresis

A specific application of low-voltage stimulation, **iontophoresis**, uses galvanic (D.C.) electrical current to drive ionized medications through the skin to injured tissues. Galvanic current causes ions in solution to travel according to their electrical charges. Current of identical polarity as the ions will act to repel the medication, obtaining the driving effect (Fig. 50.9). The most com-

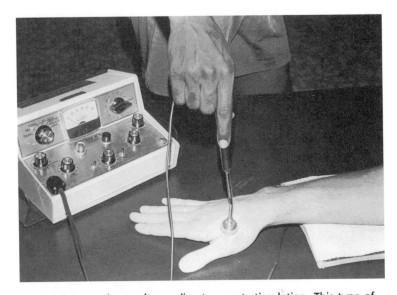

FIGURE 50.8. Low-voltage, direct current stimulation. This type of electrical stimulation is required to stimulate denervated muscle in areas where peripheral nerve lesions have occurred.

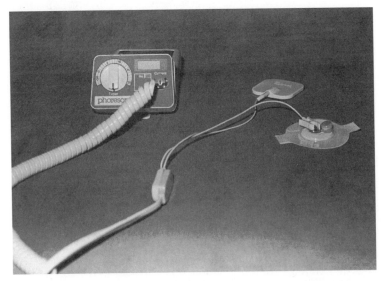

FIGURE 50.9. Iontophoresis. A galvanic (D.C.) electrical current drives ionized medications through the skin to injured tissues.

monly used medications for iontophoresis are hydrocortisone and salicylates. Hydrocortisone is a positively charged ion; therefore, the positive pole should be used as the active electrode, and the negative pole should be used for negative ions (salicylate). Low amperage (5 milliamperes maximum) and low concentration of ions (1 to 5 percent) have been found to be more effective than higher concentrations of ions in transferring ions into the tissues. The athlete should not experience discomfort or a burning sensation while receiving the treatment. Postacute soft tissue injuries—contusions, tendinitis, strains, bursitis, and so forth—can all be treated with iontophoresis. The contraindications for this procedure include those for the medications and for electrical muscle stimulation (demand pacemakers, pregnancy, and positioning over the carotid sinuses). Treatment times are 10 to 20 minutes, once a day.

Interferential Stimulation

Interferential stimulation uses two biphasic medium-frequency currents between 4,000 and 5,000 cycles per second simultaneously

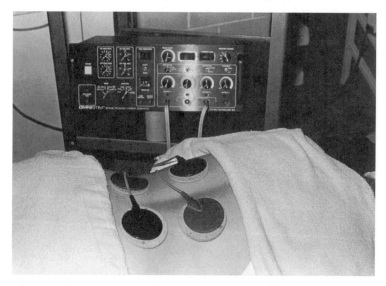

FIGURE 50.10. Interferential stimulation. Two biphasic, medium-frequency currents are superimposed on each other in the tissues, therefore eliciting a stronger response with less current intensity.

(Fig. 50.10). The higher frequencies are used to lower tissue resistance, therefore eliciting a stronger response with less current intensity. These frequencies also cause a decrease in sensory perception between the electrodes, so more current can be tolerated, allowing a stronger stimulation. The two currents will be superimposed in the tissues, causing a third current to result, with regions of increased and decreased intensities. The frequency of the third current can range from 1 to 100 beats per second by adjusting the frequency of one of the initial currents. The electrodes are placed diagonally across the treatment area, but will have to be adjusted so the perceived stimulation is concentrated in the target area. Treatment times are 20 to 30 minutes.

Point Stimulation

Point stimulators are used for hyperstimulation analgesia and are similar to acupuncture. This type of stimulation delivers a noxious stimulus to elicit a brain stem response. Regions in the brain stem activate a descending pathway that inhibits pain back at the dorsal horn of the spinal cord. In other words, eliciting a pain response triggers pain inhibition.

These stimulators use low-frequency currents of 1 to 4 pulses per second, with long pulse widths to enable stimulation of pain fibers. The intensity of the current should be the highest that the athlete can tolerate. Along with these stimulation parameters, the small size of the electrode further ensures the noxious response (Fig. 50.11).

Treatment sites include acupuncture, trigger, or motor points that are associated with the painful area. Point stimulators are frequently combined with resistance detection devices to help locate the optimal treatment sites. The current is applied for 30 seconds and can be repeated two to three times per point. It has been traditionally recommended to treat the points farthest away from the pain and work back toward it. Pain relief can be rapid and last for long durations.

Portable TENS

Portable TENS units are classically associated with sensory stimulation for pain reduction (Fig. 50.12). Numerous units that have been developed enable different modes of stimulation application. The different modes of application are named according to the parameter settings of current intensity, pulse frequency, and pulse widths. The clinical units described utilize the same parameter adjustments to elicit responses. The different modes of application include high-frequency TENs, low-frequency TENS, burst mode TENS, brief intense TENS, and neuromuscular stimulation.

Conventional, high-frequency TENS. This mode elicits a comfortable "pins and needles" sensation without any muscular response. It obtains the pain relief primarily from a gating control at the spinal cord level. It uses a high frequency between 40 to 100 pulses per second (pps) and short pulse widths. Pain relief is fast in onset, but tends to be short-lived.

Two to four electrodes can be placed in various locations, including over the pain site, dermatomes, myotomes, motor points, trigger points, peripheral nerve trunks, or nerve roots in the paraspinal region. Stimulation time can range from 30 minutes to 24 hours. A general rule is to apply the stimulation for the least amount of time that provides the maximum pain relief. The athlete accommodates quickly to this type of stimulation, so the intensity will have to be adjusted periodically.

Low-frequency TENS. This mode is referred to as acupuncturelike TENS, which elicits its pain response by indirectly stimulating the pituitary gland to release an endogenous opiate called endorphin. Current parameters include low frequencies of 1 to 4 pps and long pulse widths. The intensity must be high enough to elicit a muscular twitch response. The pain relief has a 20- to 30-minute latency, but can last for 4 hours or more. Electrode placement is recom-

mended over myotomes or appropriate acupuncture points, but can also be used over any of the other sites listed for high-frequency TENS. Stimulation is applied from 30 to 60 minutes at a time.

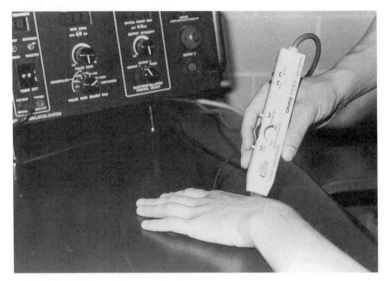

FIGURE 50.11. Point stimulation. This type of electrical stimulator uses low-frequency current to deliver a noxious stimulus to elicit a brain stem response that triggers pain inhibition.

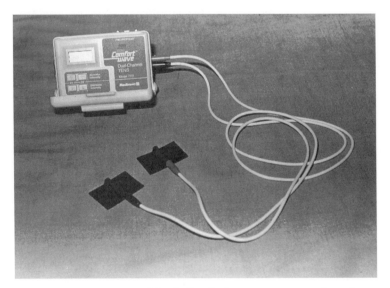

FIGURE 50.12. A portable TENS unit. Sensory responses for pain reduction are elicited when electrical current passes across the skin and stimulates nerves.

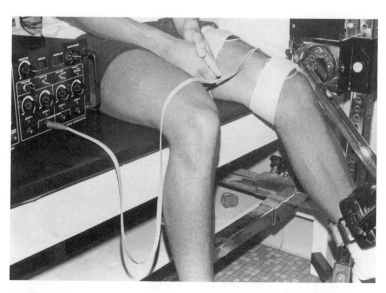

FIGURE 50.13. Neuromuscular stimulation. Electrodes, which are placed over the nerve trunk of the target muscle group and over the distal motor point, deliver electrical current to elicit controlled muscle contractions.

Burst mode TENS. This technique uses a combination of high- and low-frequency TENS parameters, but can only be applied if the unit is designed to do so. A high-frequency carrier current of 70 to 100 pps is packaged into 1 to 5 bursts per second. This will elicit the same responses as low-frequency TENS. This method was developed to allow a strong muscle contraction at a lower current intensity.

Brief intense TENS. This technique is similar to the point stimulation or hyperstimulation analgesic method, although the parameters will vary when using a portable TENS unit. The desired goal is to deliver a strong noxious stimulus that elicits the brain stem to activate a descending pathway that inhibits pain. The frequency is set at 150 pps, and the intensity is increased until a muscle twitching results. The treatment lasts for 15 minutes and can be repeated after several minutes of rest.

Neuromuscular Stimulation

Although neuromuscular stimulation is another mode of TENS, its principal purpose is to stimulate muscles with intact motor nerves for the intention of increasing force-generating capacity, reeducating muscles, maintaining range of motion, or retarding muscle atrophy. If the peripheral nerve has been damaged, then the muscle membrane has to be stimulated directly, and a direct current is required. Numerous units have the current parameters to elicit muscle contractions, but they lack an on-off cycle (duty cycle) that optimizes this effect.

The optimal parameters for neuromuscular stimulation include an intensity that can elicit maximal recruitment of the motor units; a frequency between 30 and 50 pps so a tetanic contraction will occur but not so high as to promote fatigue; a long pulse width; and a duty cycle with a 10-second contraction and a 50-second rest. Ten to 15 maximal contractions should be performed each session. Electrode placement should be over the nerve trunk of the target muscle group and over the distal motor points. A voluntary muscle contraction should be superimposed on the contraction generated by the stimulator. The distal part of the exercising limb should be secured to prevent it from exceeding normal joint ranges as normal inhibition that protects the joint is being overridden (Fig. 50.13).

MECHANICAL THERAPY

Mechanical therapies used in athletic injury care include massage, mobilization techniques, traction, and intermittent compression. Mechanical therapies are most often used in conjunction with, or as a supplement to, other methods of treatment.

Massage

Massage, one of the oldest modalities, is the systematic and scientific manipulation of the body's soft tissue. The therapeutic effects of massage include stimulating cell metabolism, increasing venous flow and lymphatic drainage, increasing circulation and nutrition, stretching superficial scar tissue, and relaxing muscle tissues. It is often used as an adjunct in treating postacute soft tissue trauma and strains. Conditions contraindicating the use of massage include areas of acute injuries, hemorrhaging, infection, thromboses, nerve damage, skin disease, and the possibility of calcification. Basic massage techniques include the following:

- Effleurage: superficial or deep stroking.
- Pétrissage: kneading.
- Tapotement: percussion or tapping.
- Vibration: trembling, forward and backward movement.
- Friction: pressure across muscles or tendons.

The effects of massage are both mechanical and reflexive. Mild stretching of scar and superficial tissue is its major mechanical effect. Reflexive effects include stimulation and relaxation of the tissues. Generally lubricants such as oil, lanolin, lotion, or powder should be used during massage therapy. Stroking toward the heart is also recommended to increase and promote venous return and to reduce swelling in the injured areas.

Manual Therapy

Manual therapy, also called **joint mobilization,** is the mobilization of joints and soft tissues to allow proper functioning of a body part. Joint mobilization is based on the concepts of joint play—the gliding and rolling of one joint surface on another that is necessary for normal joint function. For example, the humeral head must roll superiorly and glide inferiorly in the glenoid fossa to allow full abduction of the arm. All soft tissues in the body also have optimal resting positions. Normal joint play and the ability of the surrounding soft tissues to assume their optimal length may be lost secondary to an injury, perpetuating a painful condition.

Therapeutic Effects

Joint mobilization uses a combination of graded oscillations and traction to joint surfaces to restore normal joint function and reduce pain. The amount of force and amplitude used will vary, depending on whether the goal is to restore motion or relieve pain. Soft tissue spasms can result from direct injury or from a protective splinting mechanism to inhibit movement from an adjacent injury. The spasm itself may be painful, which can further perpetuate the spasms, resulting in the pain-spasm cycle. Passive restoration of soft tissues to their optimal length and maintaining the positioning for a certain duration allow the soft tissues to relax. The spasm accompanying joint dysfunction is treatable by conventional therapies, but joint mobilization often corrects the cause of the problem.

Manipulative Therapy

High-velocity, forceful mobilization techniques are referred to as **manipulative therapy**. Manipulation involves specific positioning of joint surfaces and applying a brief thrust at the end of the normal range of joint play. Manipulation is indicated to free a joint from a fixed pathological position—for example, a locked vertebral facet. Clinicians trained in manual therapy can use mobilization and positioning as an adjunct to the more conventional therapeutic modalities in the treatment of both acute and chronic athletic injuries.

Contraindications

No contraindications exist for the mild grades of mobilization. Contraindications for manipulative treatments include bone or joint disease or inflammation, healing ligament sprains or muscle strains, disc injuries, and vertebral fractures. The only contraindication for positioning of soft tissues is increased discomfort with passive movement.

Traction

Indications

Cervical and lumbar **traction** is used to treat noninflammatory musculoskeletal conditions, muscle spasm, nerve root impingement, facet sprains, and disc protrusion. Different effects can be achieved by altering the treatment variables, including mode of traction, positioning of the athlete, force of pull, and total treatment time. Traction can be applied in a continuous, static, intermittent, manual, positional, or gravitational method.

Types of Traction

Continuous traction is applied for several hours at a time and uses low poundages. This mode is considered to have minimal effects on spinal structures, but does impose the necessary rest to allow some back conditions to improve. Sustained or static traction applies traction from a few minutes to up to 30 minutes without a rest cycle. This mode is recommended if discogenic symptoms are present. Shorter treatment times of 8 to 10 minutes are recommended when using sustained traction for disc protrusions.

Intermittent traction involves traction that is applied and released periodically during the course of the treatment time.

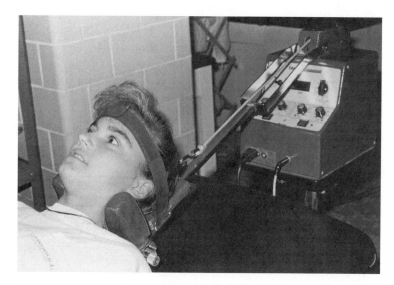

FIGURE 50.14. Cervical traction is applied with the athlete in the supine position to enhance relaxation and to allow the use of lower poundages.

This mode is most effective when treating joint hypomobility or degenerative joint disease. A 3:1 hold/release cycle—30 seconds hold, 10 seconds rest—is generally utilized. Manual traction is applied by the clinician for a few seconds, allowing time to assess the type of response an athlete may have to traction. Positional traction involves placing the athlete in various positions over pillows or blocks to impose a pull on spinal segments. Gravitational traction uses a portion of the athlete's body weight as the source of pull. This technique requires special straps and tables or boots.

Amount of Weight

Poundage necessary to obtain effective spinal separation is recommended to be at least 50 percent of the athlete's body weight when using lumbar traction. Cervical traction will incorporate poundages of 25 to 40 pounds, or 20 percent of the athlete's body weight. These poundages may have to be exceeded, but should be reached in a progressive manner. The traction poundage is ideally removed at the end of the treatment in a graduated regressive manner as well. Lower traction forces can be used for muscle spasms.

These forces are generalized and should be adjusted according to athlete's tolerance, as relaxation is essential to allow for the therapeutic effects of spinal traction. Traction units need to be as frictionless as possible. This state is attained by using either a sliding cervical unit or a "split" table, which enables the lower half of the body to slide essentially friction free with lumbar traction.

Position of Athlete

The athlete may either be placed prone or supine while receiving lumbar traction. Cervical traction should be applied in the supine position rather than sitting to enhance the athlete's relaxation and to allow lower poundages to be used (Fig. 50.14). The cervical spine is usually flexed 25 to 30 degrees while applying traction to help straighten the spinal curves. If traction is desired at the atlantoaxial joint, then 0 degrees of spinal flexion is recommended.

Traction With Other Modalities

As with all modalities, traction itself will rarely correct spinal dysfunction. Traction must be used in conjunction with proper flexibility and strengthening exercises and occasionally bracing. Instruction in proper body mechanics will help prevent further damage to the spine.

Contraindications

Contraindications for traction include subjective complaints of pain, increased radiating symptoms, hypermobility of the spine, structural disease, pregnancy, osteoporosis, and vascular compromise.

Intermittent Compression

Indications/Contraindications

In **intermittent compression**, an air-filled boot or sleeve applies pressure to an injured extremity to augment absorption of edema (Fig. 50.15). It is most effective when combined with elevation. The benefits of intermittent compression include decreasing blood flow and assisting venous return, ultimately decreasing edema.

Contraindications for this modality include infections or any conditions where a thrombosis may exist.

Usage

A layer of stockinette is applied to the extremity to absorb perspiration. The unit is adjusted to deliver inflation pressures between 40 and 100 mm Hg, lower pressures for the upper extremity. The athlete should not experience pain, paresthesia, or sense his or her pulse while the unit is

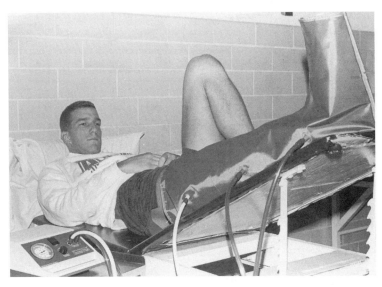

FIGURE 50.15. Intermittent compression. An air-filled boot or sleeve applies pressure to the injured extremity to augment absorption of edema.

inflated. The unit cycles at a 3:1 inflate-to-deflate ratio, most commonly 90 seconds on, 30 seconds off. The athlete should be encouraged to perform active range-of-motion exercises during the deflation cycle. Intermittent compression is frequently applied for 20 to 30 minutes, although longer treatment times may be used and it can be applied several times a day.

Use With Cryotherapy

Intermittent compression can also be combined with cryotherapy in which the boot or sleeve is filled with refrigerant fluid. This allows cold, pressure, and elevation to be applied simultaneously. By using a flexible gel cold pack, a standard intermittent compression device can be used to apply the ICE principle discussed earlier in this chapter. This is an effective initial and postacute therapy for joint sprains or injuries involving swelling.

IMPORTANT CONCEPTS

1. The selection of specific treatments or combinations of treatments is based on injury site, type, and severity; modality indications and contraindications; the physician's prescription; and the athlete's willingness to accept treatment.

2. The basic types of modalities used in the athletic training setting include cryotherapy/cryokinetics, thermotherapy, electrical stimulation, and mechanical therapy.

3. Cryotherapy/cryokinetics includes cold therapy, contrast therapy, and cold therapy combined with exercise.

4. Superficial thermotherapy includes whirlpool treatment, hydrocollator packs, paraffin baths, and Fluidotherapy.

5. Penetrating thermotherapy includes diathermy and ultrasound therapy.

6. Electrical stimulation includes TENS, high-voltage stimulation, low-voltage stimulation, interferential stimulation, point stimulation, portable TENS, and neuromuscular stimulation.

7. Mechanical therapy includes massage, manual therapy, traction, and intermittent compression.

SUGGESTED READINGS

Alon, G. *High Voltage Stimulation.* Chattanooga, Tenn.: Chattanooga Corporation, 1984.

Benton, L. A., L. L. Baker, B. R. Bowman, et al. *Functional Electrical Stimulation: A Practical Clinical Guide,* 2d ed. Downey, Calif.: Rancho Los Amigos Rehabilitation Engineering Center, 1981.

Bertolucci, L. E. "Introduction of Antiinflammatory Drugs by Iontophoresis: Double Blind Study." *The Journal of Orthopaedic and Sports Physical Therapy* 4 (1982): 103–108.

Castel, J. C. *Pain Management with Acupuncture and Transcutaneous Electrical Nerve Stimulation Techniques.* Lake Bluff, Ill.: Pain Control Services, Inc., 1979.

Dunn, F., and L. A. Frizzell. "Bioeffects of Ultrasound." In *Therapeutic Heat & Cold,* 3d ed., edited by J. F. Lehmann, pp. 386–403. Baltimore: Williams & Wilkins, 1982.

Gieck, J., M. Bamford, H. Stewart, and B. Ferguson. "Therapeutic Ultrasound: Technology, Performance Standards, Biological Effect, and Clinical Application." HHS Publication FOA 84–XXXX, August 1984.

Griffin, J. E. "Physiological Effects of Ultrasound as It Is Used Clinically." *Journal of American Physical Therapy Association* 46 (1966): 18.

Harris, P. R. "Iontophoresis: Clinical Research in Musculoskeletal Inflammatory Conditions." *The Journal of Orthopaedic and Sports Physical Therapy* 4 (1982): 109–112.

Hayes, K. W. *Manual for Physical Agents.* Chicago: Northwestern University, 1984.

Killian, C., T. Malone, and W. Carroll. *High Frequency and High Voltage Protocols.* Medtronic, Inc., 1984.

Kleinkort, J. A., and F. Wood. "Phonophoresis with 1 Percent versus 10 Percent Hydrocortisone." *Physical Therapy* 55 (1975): 1320–1324.

Kots, Y. M. "Notes from De Kot's (USSR) Lectures and Laboratory Periods." Canadian-Soviet Exchange Symposium on Electrostimulation of Skeletal Muscles, 1977.

Kramer, J. F. "Ultrasound: Evaluation of Its Mechanical and Thermal Effects." *Archives of Physical Medicine and Rehabilitation* 65 (1984): 223–227.

Kulund, D. N., ed. *The Injured Athlete*, 2d ed. Philadelphia: J. B. Lippincott, 1988.

Lehmann, J. F., and B. J. De Lateur. "Diathermy and Superficial Heat and Cold Therapy." In *Krusen's Handbook of Physical Medicine and Rehabilitation*, 3d ed., edited by F. J. Kottke, G. K. Stillwell, and J. F. Lehmann. Philadelphia: W. B. Saunders, 1982.

Mannheimer, J. S., and G. N. Lampe, eds. *Clinical Transcutaneous Electrical Nerve Stimulation*. Philadelphia: F. A. Davis, 1984.

Newton, R. A. *Electrotherapeutic Treatment: Selecting Appropriate Waveform Characteristics*. Clifton, N.J.: Preston Corp., 1981.

Nippel, F. J. *Interferential Current Therapy: An Advanced Method in the Management of Pain*. Nemectron Medical, Inc., 1979.

Stratton, S. A. "Role of Endorphins in Pain Modulation." *The Journal of Orthopaedic and Sports Physical Therapy* 3 (1982): 200–205.

Wolf, S. L., ed. *Clinics in Physical Therapy*, Vol. 2. *Electrotherapy*. New York: Churchill Livingstone, 1981.

Ziskin, M. C., and S. L. Michlovitz. "Therapeutic Ultrasound." In *Thermal Agents in Rehabilitation*, edited by S. L. Michlovitz. Philadelphia: F. A. Davis, 1986.

51

Injury-Specific Rehabilitation Programs

CHAPTER OUTLINE

INTRODUCTION

Chapter 51 discusses rehabilitation programs for a few of the commonly seen athletic injuries. The programs suggested are not all-inclusive and describe only one possible protocol for rehabilitating each injury. There are, in fact, many ways of treating each injury discussed here, and it is up to the athletic trainer to decide which exercises will work best for the athlete involved.

Chapter 51 presents exercises at the stages they should be attempted. The sports injuries covered are plantar fasciitis, ankle sprains, shin splints, calf strains, quadriceps muscle strains, groin strains, iliotibial band strains, hamstring muscle strains, low back strains and sprains, cervical strains and sprains, rotator cuff injuries, and epicondylitis of the elbow. The last section of Chapter 51 presents suggestions for pool exercises. ∎

OVERVIEW

Maintenance of present conditioning and rehabilitation of an injury should be as sport-specific as possible. However, when a rehabilitation program is devised, one should remember that injury healing is the primary consideration and that maintenance of the athlete's pre-injury physical condition may not be possible. Instead, the athlete must realize that even after an injury has healed, additional time may be required to regain the desired level of competitive fitness.

To ensure proper rehabilitation of the athlete, a thorough evaluation should be performed by the physician or trainer. Once the exercise prescription is designed, the athlete should be evaluated to make sure he or she understands the goals projected and performs the exercises correctly. Improper technique could result in unnecessary pain and a setback in rehabilitation.

This chapter does not include the use of cryotherapy, thermotherapies, or modalities prior to or after rehabilitation exercises. Modalities are discussed in Chapter 50 and are used according to the philosophy of the physician or trainer. Also, availability of these modalities would limit or extend the rehabilitation prescription. General sport-specific exercises have not been included either, as they are far beyond the scope of this chapter. The trainer should be flexible and creative enough to adapt the selected basic program to a specific sport.

Every injury cannot be covered in this chapter; therefore, selected areas frequently injured are discussed and exercises for their rehabilitation are presented. The trainer may wish to modify these exercises or add others that might be more appropriate for a particular athlete. Each athlete is an individual and should be treated as such; likewise rehabilitation exercises are not black and white or cut and dried.

Exercises in this chapter are broken down into different stage levels when appropriate. *Stage I* exercises are gentle exercises to work on stretching, regaining range of mo-

tion, and strengthening through the use of isometrics. *Stage II* exercises are more difficult and generally work on strengthening. They should be added to rather than replace Stage I exercises. Additional exercise stages increase in difficulty. The athlete should not progress to the next stage until he or she is able to perform the prior stage workouts comfortably.

PLANTAR FASCIITIS

Plantar fasciitis is an irritation or tear in the dense fibrous band that extends from the calcaneus to the toes on the plantar surface of the foot (Fig. 51.1). While the pain is not usually excruciating, it can be debilitating and difficult to control. Although an injury can lead to heel pain, there is rarely a clear cause-and-effect association. Heel pain can take the form of a sharp burning or aching sensation. In most cases, the pain occurs on only one heel, although both can be affect-

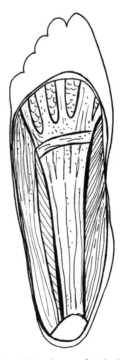

FIGURE 51.1. The plantar fascia is a dense, fibrous band of tissue extending from the calcaneus to the toes.

ed. Men and women seem to be equally vulnerable: most patients are middle-aged, and many tend to be overweight. Several other conditions can produce similar symptoms, so a physician should perform a thorough examination in order to rule out disorders such as neuritis, arthritis, and tendinitis.

Simple therapy usually gives relief. Sometimes, however, weeks or even months of therapy may be required for complete recovery. During this recovery period, the athlete should stay away from pounding activities such as running or basketball. Swimming or biking may be substituted to maintain aerobic conditioning.

The physician may suggest the following:

- Visco, Sorbathane, or Tulis heel cup with special shock-absorbing or shock-dispersing capacities.
- Nonsteroidal, anti-inflammatory medication.
- Ice massage to the affected area for 5 to 7 minutes before and after rehabilitation exercises.
- Specific, gentle rehabilitation exercises described in this chapter.

Most of the exercises that follow are shown in stages at which they should be attempted. If the exercise is continued from one stage to another, it is mentioned but not explained the second time.

Range-of-Motion Exercises

Exercise: Achilles tendon stretch. Stand about 2 feet away from an immovable object such as a wall. Lean into the wall, keeping your back straight and the affected foot pointing straight ahead. Bend the opposite knee toward the wall but keep the affected heel on the ground (Fig. 51.2). Hold the stretch for 20 counts; do 10 stretches a day.

Exercise: Stair toe raises. Stand on a stair with a railing or wall available for balance. Balance so the stair is under the ball of the foot and the midfoot and heels are over the edge. The feet should be pointing straight

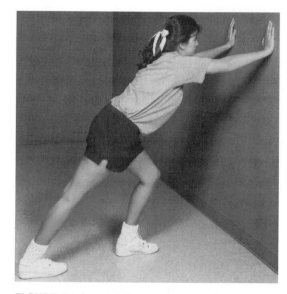

FIGURE 51.2. Achilles tendon stretch.

ahead. Slowly raise and lower yourself on your toes above and below the level of the step over a 10-count span (Fig. 51.3). Do 10 toe raises a day.

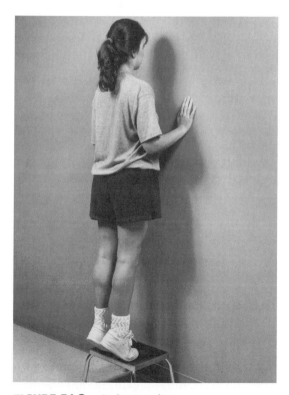

FIGURE 51.3. Stair toe raises.

Exercise: Plantar fascia stretch. With the ankle dorsiflexed, pull the toes back toward the ankle. The stretch should be felt in the plantar fascia (Fig. 51.4). Hold the stretch for 10 counts; do 10 stretches a day.

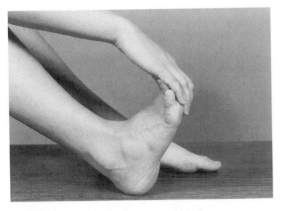

FIGURE 51.4. Plantar fascia stretch.

ANKLE SPRAINS

Ankle sprains most frequently occur to the lateral collateral ligaments as a result of an inversion injury of the ankle. The anterior talofibular ligament is most frequently the ligament that is completely ruptured. This injury shows up as a positive anterior drawer on physical exam or anterior drawer stress x-rays.

Another important mechanism of injury to the ankle is pronation with external rotation. This is rarely a true ligamentous injury, but when it does occur, the deltoid and anterior talofibular ligaments are torn. (Further discussion of these injuries can be found in Chapter 23.)

Rehabilitation following ankle sprains should emphasize strengthening those musculotendinous structures that surround the ligamentous injury. Rehabilitation may begin as soon as the physician allows. Ice massage contrast whirlpools or thermotherapies should be administered, based on the philosophy of the physician or trainer.

To regain normal function in an ankle that has experienced a sprain or a strain, it is important to combine strengthening, flexibility, and proprioceptive (balance) activities. The ankle positions shown in Figure 51.5 are considered normal and will be referred to in some of the exercises to follow:

- dorsiflexion
- plantar flexion
- eversion
- inversion

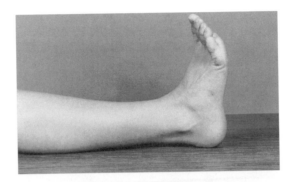

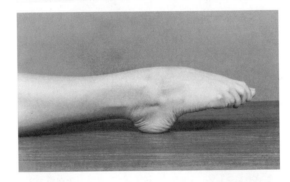

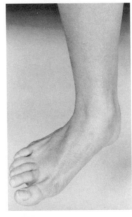 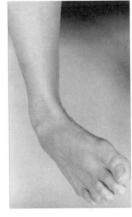

FIGURE 51.5. Normal ankle movements: (top) dorsiflexion; (middle) plantar flexion; (bottom left) eversion; (bottom right) inversion.

Stage I

Exercise: Alphabet writing. Write the alphabet, using the big toe as the pen. Create the letters by using ankle motion rather than lower-leg motion.

Exercise: Towel stretches. Place a towel under your foot. Holding the ends of the towel, perform the following movements:

1. Pull the foot up into dorsiflexion (Fig. 51.6).
2. Push the foot down into plantar flexion.
3. Pull the foot up and out into eversion.
4. Pull the foot up and into inversion.

Repeat for a set of 10. Do 3 sets of 10 for each movement. Perform the Achilles tendon stretch (see p. 814).

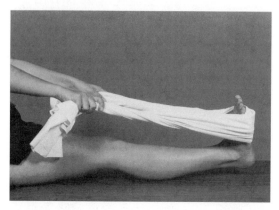

FIGURE 51.6. Using a towel stretch to pull the foot up into dorsiflexion.

Exercise: Functional balancing. Balance on one leg for 10 seconds with eyes open; repeat 10 times. Balance on one leg for 10 seconds with eyes closed; repeat 10 times. Walk heel to toe for 5 yards, 10 times with eyes open. Walk heel to toe for 5 yards, 10 times with eyes closed.

Strengthening Exercises

Exercise: Isometrics. Gentle strengthening can be accomplished through isometrics using the hand or uninjured foot to provide resistance. Make an isometric contraction by resisting the normal ankle movements of dorsiflexion, plantar flexion, eversion, and inversion (see Figs. 51.5a–d); hold each contraction for 10 seconds.

Stage II

Exercise: Isotonics. Isotonics can be performed with a variety of inexpensive equipment but only when isometrics are not painful. The following exercises (Figs. 51.7a–d) can be done with surgical tubing, Theraband, an old bicycle tube, or an elastic bandage. Use the elastic as resistance as you move in all directions of normal ankle movements. Work up to 3 sets of 10 repetitions. The tubing should be taut and the heel remains on the floor. The ankle is what moves—not the entire lower leg. The tubing should be placed as far down the foot as possible without having it slide off as the exercise is performed.

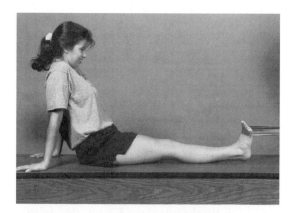

FIGURE 51.7a. Isotonics: dorsiflexion.

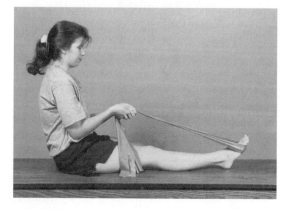

FIGURE 51.7b. Isotonics: plantar flexion.

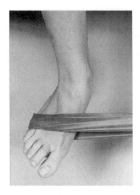

FIGURE 51.7c.
Isotonics: eversion.

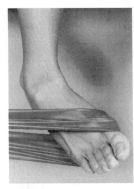

FIGURE 51.7d.
Isotonics: inversion.

Exercise: Calf raises without weight. Stand on a flat surface, with weight evenly distributed. Raise your heel off the floor as high as possible, using your own body weight as resistance. Work up to 3 sets of 10 repetitions. Gradually shift weight to the injured foot, performing the calf raises on this leg only (Fig. 51.8a).

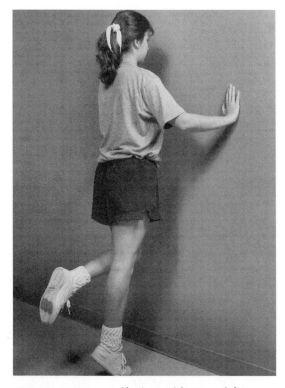

FIGURE 51.8a.   Calf raises without weight.

Exercise: Calf raises with weight. Perform the previous exercise with both legs, but this time, following the chart below, add weight to the shoulders as shown in Figure 51.8b.

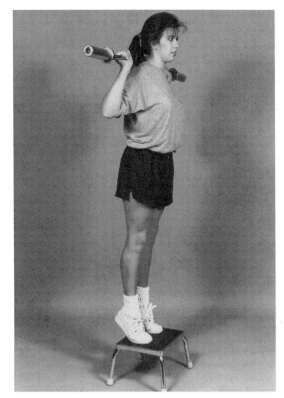

FIGURE 51.8b.   Calf raises with weight.

Step	Set I	Set II	Set III	Set IV
1		Barbell Only	Barbell Only	
2	5 lbs.	5 lbs.	5 lbs.	10 lbs.
3	10	10	10	15
4	15	15	15	20
5	20	20	20	25
6	25	25	25	30
7	30	30	30	35

Stage III

The athlete should gradually work back into normal functional activities. It may be necessary, especially during athletic activities, for the athlete to wear protective equipment (taping or bracing) on the ankle for several months after injury.

SHIN SPLINTS

For a runner, shin splints can be a devastating injury because this athlete's primary activity (running) is often completely restricted. Repetitive pounding may exacerbate the shin splints; resolving the problem requires rest. Runners, like many athletes, may find the concept of total rest unacceptable. Fortunately, activity modification may make it possible to maintain the conditioned state while the shin splints are healing. For example, a runner can wear a life jacket and walk or jog in chest-deep water in a swimming pool. Several commercial life jackets for this activity are available, as are special tanks with built-in treadmills for running in the water. A runner can also swim laps using an adaptive device such as a kickboard or buoy for resistance. If the athlete is not a good swimmer, a float aid may be used while swimming to maintain cardiovascular conditioning. Another alternative method of maintaining conditioning for a runner is cross-country skiing. By cross-country skiing or using an indoor Ski-master, the athlete may work on similar cardiovascular conditioning, providing the exercise is pain free.

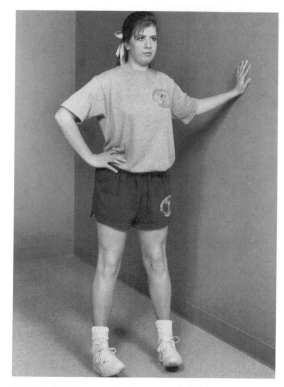

FIGURE 51.9a. Starting toe-in position.

Stage I

Range-of-Motion Exercises

Exercise: Toe raises. Perform stair toe raises as previously directed (see p. 814). This exercise should then be repeated in a toe-in position (Fig. 51.9a) and then in a toe-out position (Fig. 51.9b).

Perform the Achilles tendon stretch (see p. 814).

Stage II

Strengthening Exercises

Exercise: Towel pull. Sit in a chair, with a towel laid on the floor in front of you. Drag the towel toward you by curling the toes of the affected leg on the towel. It is important

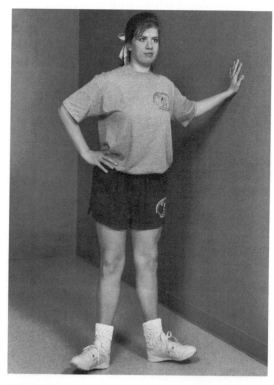

FIGURE 51.9b. Starting toe-out position.

to keep your heel on the ground during this exercise. As the exercise becomes easier to do, place a weight on the far end of the towel to increase the difficulty of the task. The exercise should be done for several minutes, with the time adjusted as weight is added. This exercise strengthens the muscles in the lower part of the leg and foot.

Perform the isotonic exercises (see pp. 816–817).

CALF STRAINS

The most commonly strained muscle in the leg is the medial head of the gastrocnemius. This injury is discussed in greater detail in Chapter 22.

Stage I

Range-of-Motion Exercises

Exercise: Towel stretch I. In a sitting position, with your legs extended all the way out, place a towel under your feet. Pull back on the towel, pulling your feet into dorsiflexion (up). Hold the feet in this position for 15 seconds. Repeat this maneuver three times. This exercise primarily works the gastrocnemius muscle (Fig. 51.10a).

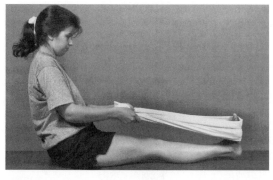

FIGURE 51.10a. Towel stretch I with leg in extension.

Exercise: Towel stretch II. Repeat towel stretch I with your knees partially bent. This position allows stretching of the soleus (Fig. 51.10b).

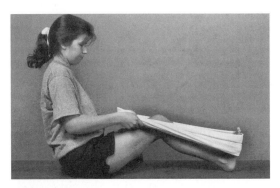

FIGURE 51.10b. Towel stretch II with knee partially bent.

Strengthening Exercises

Exercise: Towel push. Begin by performing towel stretches (see p. 816), dorsiflexing the ankle as far as it will go; then push down against the resistance of the towel as you hold it in your hands. Adjust the resistance according to how much your calf can tolerate (Fig. 51.11). Repeat this exercise until you have completed 3 sets of 10.

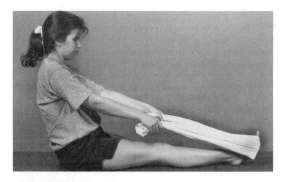

FIGURE 51.11. Towel push.

Stage II

Range-of-Motion Exercises

1. Continue to do towel stretches I and II.
2. Add the Achilles tendon stretch (see p. 814) to the towel stretches.

Strengthening Exercises

1. Continue to do towel stretches I and II.
2. Perform the isotonic exercises (see pp. 816–817).

3. Perform stair toe raises (see p. 814). Repeat in a toe-in and toe-out position (see Figs. 51.9a–b).

Stage III

Range-of-Motion Exercises

1. Discontinue the towel stretch.
2. Continue the Achilles tendon stretch (see p. 814), increasing the time to 30 seconds.

Strengthening Exercises

Continue with the isotonic exercises (see pp. 816–817), doing 3 sets of 10 repetitions.

Exercise: One-legged calf raise. From a standing position, with both feet flat on the floor, raise yourself up on your toes with one leg. Hold at the top for 5 seconds. Repeat until you have performed 3 sets of 10 repetitions, each with your foot in a neutral position, with your foot rotated inward, and with your foot rotated outward. Repeat the exercise with the other leg. When you can successfully perform 3 sets of 10 repetitions in each position for each leg, then perform the exercise over again, this time using a stair or raised object so that your toes are on the step and the rest of your foot is off the step. Lower your body slowly up and down off the step. Repeat for 3 sets of 10 repetitions in all three foot positions.

Stage IV

Range-of-Motion Exercises

Continue the Achilles tendon stretch (see p. 814).

Strengthening Exercises

1. Discontinue the isotonic exercises.
2. Perform calf raises with weight (see p. 817).

Stage V

Range-of-Motion Exercises

Continue the Achilles tendon stretch (see p. 814).

Strengthening Exercises

Continue performing the calf raises with weight (see p. 817).

QUADRICEPS MUSCLE STRAINS

Quadriceps strains occur to one or more combinations of muscles in the quadriceps mechanism. These are the rectus femoris, vastus intermedius, vastus lateralis, and vastus medialis. This injury is discussed in greater detail in Chapter 21.

Stage I

Range-of-Motion Exercises

Exercise: Active range of motion. Sit on the end of a bench or lay on your stomach on a table or bed. Place an ice bag on the injured area and begin extending and flexing the leg as far as possible. Continue for at least 10 minutes. Repeat this exercise twice a day.

Strengthening Exercises

Exercise: Quadriceps sets. Flex the ankle and contract the quadriceps by pulling the kneecap toward you, tightening the thigh muscles in an isometric contraction. Hold for 10 seconds. Repeat for 3 sets of 10 repetitions.

Stage II

Range-of-Motion Exercises

Exercise: Quadriceps stretch. Lean against a wall or immovable object with one hand. Use the other hand to pull your thigh straight back behind you. Make sure the leg you are pulling back remains straight. Hold the stretch for 10 to 15 seconds and repeat it three times (Fig. 51.12).

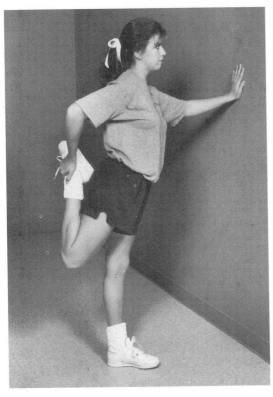

FIGURE 51.12.   Quadriceps stretch.

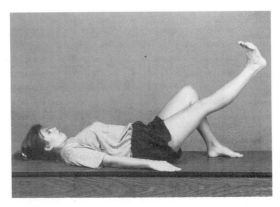

FIGURE 51.13.   Straight-leg raise.

ment but only the creation of tension in the muscle (contraction). Hold each contraction for 10 seconds and repeat over a variety of spots in the possible range of motion until you have performed at least 10 contractions (Fig. 51.14). Do 3 sets of 10 contractions.

Strengthening Exercises

Exercise: Straight-leg raises.   Begin by lying on your back with the injured leg straight and the foot dorsiflexed, and the other leg bent at the knee and hip to relax your back. First tighten your thigh. Raise the leg 6 to 10 inches off the ground and hold for 5 counts. Continue to perform repetitions until you have done 3 sets of 10 repetitions. When you can successfully perform 3 sets of 10, use ankle weights to add increments of 1 to 2 pounds. These can be hand made out of socks and sand if necessary. Continue to lift until you are able to lift 10 pounds successfully for 3 sets of 10 or 10 percent of your body weight, whichever comes first (Fig. 51.13).

Exercise: Isometric quadriceps exercise.   Begin by sitting on the edge of a table or chair that will allow you full range of motion. Using your uninjured leg as resistance, push up against the leg, allowing no move-

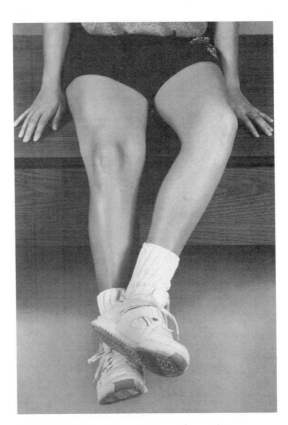

FIGURE 51.14.   Isometric quad exercise.

Stage III

Range-of-Motion Exercises

Continue the quadriceps stretch, increasing the hold time to 30 seconds.

Strengthening Exercises

Exercise: Short arc leg extensions. Begin by lying on your back with a pillow or other soft object under the injured leg. Place the pillow so that your knee is bent about 20 degrees (slight bend). From that position, extend your knee out as far as possible and hold for 5 seconds. Repeat this movement until you can do 3 sets of 10 repetitions. Then begin adding weight to your ankle in 1- to 2-pound increments until you can successfully lift 10 pounds or 10 percent of your body weight (Fig. 51.15).

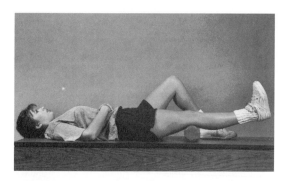

FIGURE 51.15. Short arc leg extension.

Stage IV

Range-of-Motion Exercises

Continue the quadriceps stretch if a partner is unavailable. If someone is available to help, begin doing the next exercise.

Exercise: Quadriceps stretch with a partner. Begin by lying on your stomach with the affected leg bent. Have a partner actively bend your knee, bringing the foot toward the buttock as far as possible, and hold for 30 seconds. The partner should gently push to assist in additional stretch (Fig. 51.16). Repeat three times.

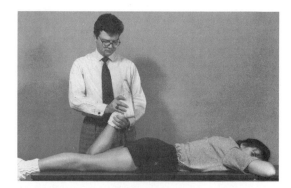

FIGURE 51.16. Quadriceps stretch with a partner.

Strengthening Exercises

Exercise: Leg extensions. Perform 4 sets of 10 repetitions by following the chart below. Continue adding 2.5 pounds to each set. Perform the exercise one leg at a time, three times per week.

Step	Set I	Set II	Set III	Set IV
1	5 lbs.	7.5 lbs.	10 lbs.	12.5 lbs.
2	7.5	10	12.5	15
3	10	12.5	15	17.5
4	12.5	15	17.5	20
5	15	17.5	20	22.5

The athlete can return to activity when both legs are equal in strength and normal flexibility has returned.

GROIN STRAINS

The adductor muscles of the anterior groin are frequently injured during athletics. Very mild to severe strains may occur during running, jumping, or twisting movements. This injury is discussed in greater detail in Chapter 20.

Stage I

Range-of-Motion Exercises

Exercise: Side straddle stretch. Stand with your legs spread in the position shown in Figure 51.17, with one leg straight with toes pointing straight ahead and the other

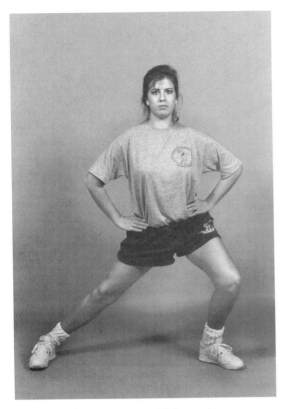

FIGURE 51.17.   Side straddle stretch.

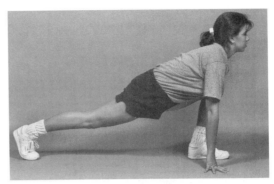

FIGURE 51.18.   Hip flexor stretch.

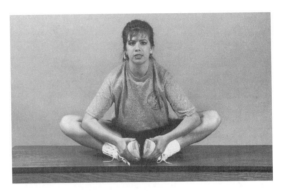

FIGURE 51.19.   Butterfly stretch.

leg bent at the knee with toes at a 45-degree angle. Lean forward on the knee that is bent and hold this position for 20 to 30 seconds. Repeat three times and reverse to include the other leg.

Exercise: Hip flexor stretch.   Start with one leg bent at the knee with toes pointing straight ahead and the injured leg straight behind you, with the toes of that foot pointed straight ahead as shown in Figure·51.18. Lean into the front knee, pressing your pelvis toward the floor. Bend the knee of the injured leg, bringing the heel toward the buttocks. Hold a comfortable stretch for 20 to 30 seconds and repeat three times.

Exercise: Butterfly stretch.   Sit on the floor. Bring heels together into the groin area and hold the toes of both feet. Lower knees until they are as far down as possible. Hold this position for 20 to 30 seconds (Fig. 51.19). Repeat three times.

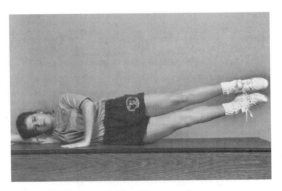

FIGURE 51.20.   Adduction exercise.

Strengthening Exercises

Exercise: Adduction exercise.   Lie on your side with your back arched slightly in and both legs together. Raise the top leg up 6 inches; then raise the other leg to meet it. Raise legs to a count of 2 seconds, hold the position for 3 seconds, and lower both legs to a count of 4 seconds. Work up to 3 sets of 10 (Fig. 51.20).

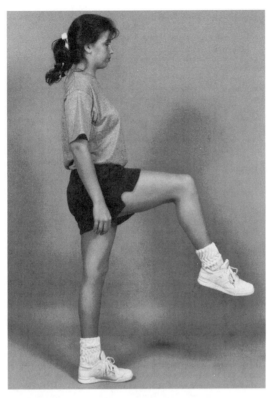

FIGURE 51.21. Hip flexion exercise.

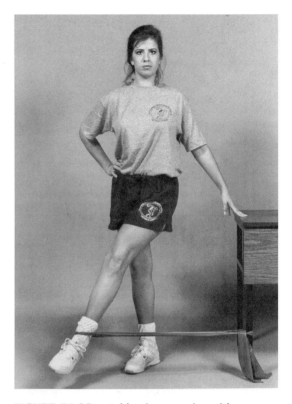

FIGURE 51.22. Adduction exercise with resistance.

Exercise: Hip flexion exercise. Stand with legs together. Raise one leg up in front by flexing at the hip (Fig.51.21) and lower. Repeat the hip flexion exercise until you have completed 3 sets of 10 repetitions.

Stage II

Range-of-Motion Exercises

1. Continue the side straddle stretch.
2. Continue the hip flexor stretch.
3. Continue the butterfly stretch.

Strengthening Exercises

Exercise: Adduction exercise with resistance. Continue with the adduction exercise, but begin adding resistance. Ankle weights are ideal. Start with 1 to 2 pounds and add 1 to 2 pounds each time 3 sets of 10 repetitions are completed. You can also use rubber tubing, an old bicycle tube, surgical tubing, or Theraband exercise tubing. If tubing of

any kind is substituted for ankle weights, the exercise should be performed standing, as shown in Figure 51.22.

Exercise: Hip flexion exercise with resistance. Continue to do the hip flexion exercise, but begin adding resistance. Ankle weights or sandbags can be worn on the thigh to provide resistance. Elastic tubing, an old bicycle tube, surgical tubing, or Theraband exercise tubing can be substituted for ankle weights and sandbags. If some type of tubing is substituted for ankle weights, the exercise should be performed as in Figure 51.23.

Stage III

Range-of-Motion Exercises

Continue the side straddle stretch.

Exercise: Hip flexor stretch with a partner. If a partner is available for stretching, per-

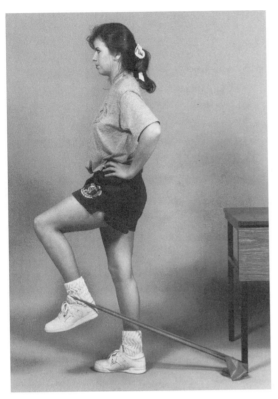

FIGURE 51.23. Hip flexion exercise with resistance.

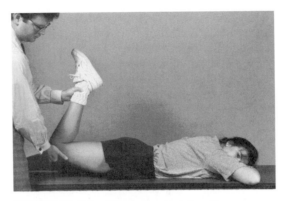

FIGURE 51.24. Hip flexor stretch with a partner.

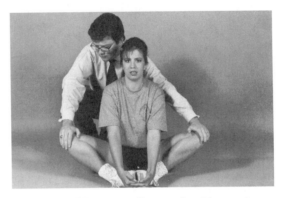

FIGURE 51.25. Butterfly stretch with a partner.

form this stretch instead of the hip flexor stretch. Start by lying on your stomach. Bend the knee of the leg to be stretched. Your partner should bring your heel down as close as it will come to the body. At the same time raise your knee up off the ground so the stretch is placed on the hip (Fig. 51.24). Hold this position for 20 to 30 seconds and repeat three times.

Exercise: Butterfly stretch with a partner. If a partner is available, substitute this stretch for the butterfly stretch. Start in the same position as in the butterfly stretch. Have your partner gently push your legs down until a comfortable stretch is felt. Hold this position for 5 seconds. Try to bring your knees together as your partner provides some resistance with his or her hands. The resistance should be enough to allow slow movement of the legs until the knees almost touch (Fig. 51.25). Repeat three times.

Strengthening Exercises

1. Continue the adduction exercise.
2. Continue the hip flexion exercise.

Stage IV

The athlete continues performing all stretching and strengthening exercises. If available to the athlete, hip flexion and adduction/abduction machines can be added to the program. Normal activities should be resumed under the direction of the athlete's physician.

ILIOTIBIAL BAND STRAINS

The iliotibial band is a thickening of the iliotibial tract that runs the length of the entire upper leg and inserts directly into the lateral tubercle of the tibia. The iliotibial band aids in both knee extension and flexion, as well as being the primary adductor at the hip (see Chapter 21). Strains can occur along the length of the iliotibial band. A program of stretching and strengthening the iliotibial band to withstand the forces of athletic activity will help prevent iliotibial band strains.

Stage I

Range-of-Motion Exercises

Exercise: Iliotibial band stretch. Start in a standing position. Use a wall or stationary object to lean against. Place the injured leg behind the other leg and lean into the wall as shown in Figure 51.26. Hold the stretch for 20 to 30 seconds. Repeat three times.

Strengthening Exercises

Exercise: Abduction exercise. Lie on unaffected side with both legs together. Raise the affected leg 6 to 8 inches off the ground and hold for 5 seconds (Fig. 51.27). Lower the leg and rest two counts.

Range-of-Motion Exercises

Continue the iliotibial band stretch.

Strengthening Exercises

Exercise: Abduction exercise with resistance. Continue the abduction exercise. Once 3 sets of 10 repetitions are successfully completed, begin adding resistance. Resistance can be provided by sandbags or ankle weights. Start with 1 to 2 pounds and add 1 to 2 pounds each time 3 sets of 10 are successfully completed. If ankle weights or sandbags are unavailable, elastic tubing or an old bicycle inner tube can be used. If elastic tubing is used, tie one end of the tube to the bottom leg and the other to the top leg, just below the knee. Pull up against the tube in the same motion one would use if using ankle weights (Fig. 51.28).

Exercise: Knee extension. Since the iliotibial band aids in the extension of the knee,

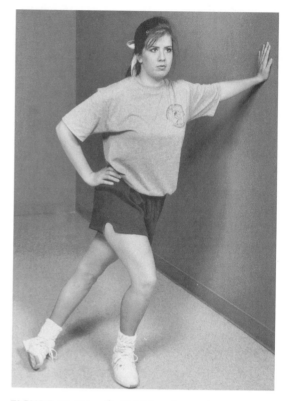

FIGURE 51.26. Iliotibial band stretch.

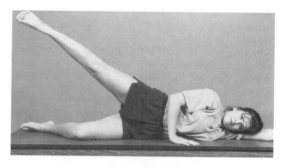

FIGURE 51.27. Abduction exercise.

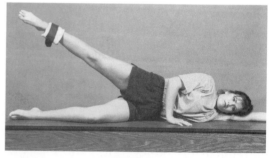

FIGURE 51.28. Adduction with resistance.

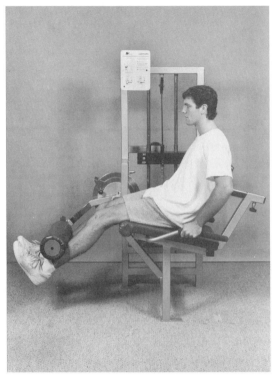

FIGURE 51.29.   Knee extension.

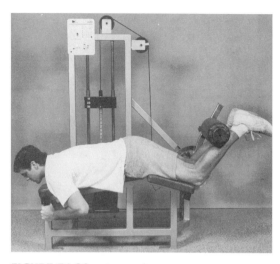

FIGURE 51.30.   Leg curls.

extension exercises are important to the total strength of the tissue. Perform 4 sets of 10, following the chart below. Continue adding 2.5 pounds to each set (Fig. 51.29). Perform the exercise one leg at a time, three times per week.

Step	Set I	Set II	Set III	Set IV
1	5 lbs.	7.5 lbs.	10 lbs.	12.5 lbs.
2	7.5	10	12.5	15
3	10	12.5	15	17.5
4	12.5	15	17.5	20
5	15	17.5	20	22.5

Exercise: Leg curls. The iliotibial band also contributes to knee flexion or bending of the knee. Following the chart above for knee extensions, perform 4 sets of 10 repetitions (Fig. 51.30).

Stage III

Range-of-Motion Exercises

Continue the iliotibial band stretch.

Strengthening Exercises

1. Continue to do the abduction exercise with resistance, and keep adding on weight.
2. Continue to do the knee extension exercises, and keep adding on weight.
3. Continue to do the leg curls exercise, and keep adding on weight.

HAMSTRING MUSCLE STRAINS

The hamstring muscles are strong flexors of the knee and major extensors of the hip. They are particularly vulnerable to strain because of the nature of their function (see Chapter 20). Hamstring injuries are among the most feared injuries to athletes because they tend to recur. They are more easily prevented through proper conditioning than treated once they have occurred. The following exercises are designed to stretch and strengthen the hamstrings.

Stage I

Range-of-Motion Exercises

Exercise: Active range of motion. Sit on the end of a bench or lie on your stomach on a table. Place an ice bag on the injured area. After about 5 minutes of icing, begin bending and extending the knee as far as possible. Continue moving the knee until the leg is numb (at least 10 to 15 minutes).

Strengthening Exercises

Exercise: Hamstring contractions. Tighten your hamstring muscles and hold in an isometric contraction for 10 seconds. Repeat until you have done 3 sets of 10 repetitions. Repeat this exercise two to three times per day.

Stage II

Range-of-Motion Exercises

Continue the active range-of-motion exercise.

Exercise: Modified hurdler stretch. Sit on the floor or table, extending the affected leg in front and bending the other so the heel is tucked into the groin area. Reach forward as if trying to dive. Pick a spot in front of you and extend your arms as far forward as possible. Remember to keep your back straight so the hamstrings are being stretched and not the low back muscles. Hold the stretch for 30 seconds; repeat three times. Placing both legs out in front can be substituted in situations where previous injuries do not allow the knee in front to be bent. The back must still remain straight and the arms should be up and out versus touching the toes (Fig. 51.31).

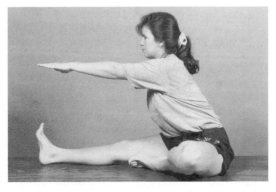

FIGURE 51.31. Modified hurdler stretch.

Strengthening Exercises

Combine the hamstring contractions with the straight-leg raises that follow.

Exercise: Straight-leg raises for hamstrings. Lie on your stomach. Extend the knee; then tighten the hamstrings of the affected leg. Raise your leg behind you as far as possible, holding the contraction for 5 counts (Fig. 51.32). Rest for 2 counts. Work up to 3 sets of 10 repetitions. When 3 sets of 10 can be successfully performed without pain during or after the exercise, then add 1- to 2-pound ankle weights to the ankle. Substitutions for ankle weights include socks filled with rolls of pennies or a pocketbook filled with weighted objects. Continue adding weight until either 10 pounds or 10 percent of your body weight is lifted for 3 sets of 10.

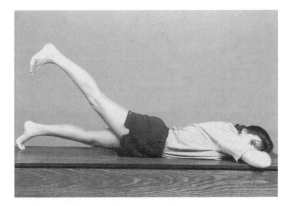

FIGURE 51.32. Straight-leg raises for hamstrings.

Exercise: Hip extension exercise. Repeat the straight-leg raises for hamstrings, but this time bend the knee 90 degrees and lift up from the hip. Lift up and back as far as possible. When adding weight, it can be added to either the ankle or back of the thigh, above the knee. Repeat until 3 sets of 10 repetitions are completed. Add 1- to 2-pound increments until 10 pounds or 10 percent of your body weight is lifted (Fig. 51.33).

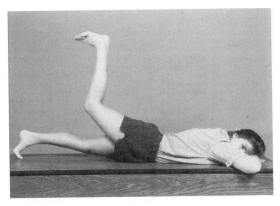

FIGURE 51.33. Hip extension exercise.

Exercise: Isometric hamstring exercise. Sit at the edge of a table and place the injured leg on top of the uninjured leg. Using the uninjured leg as resistance, push against the leg, trying to bend the knee. Apply enough resistance with the uninjured leg so there is no movement. Repeat the contraction 10 times at different spots in the normal range of movement. Repeat until you have done 3 sets of 10 repetitions.

Stage III

Range-of-Motion Exercises

1. Continue the active range-of-motion exercise.
2. Continue the modified hurdler stretch.

Strengthening Exercises

1. Discontinue the straight-leg raises for hamstrings when you are able to lift 10 pounds or 10 percent of your body weight. Continue to perform the hip extension exercise unless a hip extension machine is available.
2. Begin doing leg curls on a leg curl machine or by using ankle weights (see page 827). Perform 4 sets of 10 repetitions. Continue adding 2.5 pounds to each set after step 5. Perform the exercise one leg at a time, and do the exercise 3 days per week.

Stage IV

Range-of-Motion Exercises

Discontinue the active range-of-motion exercise. Continue to perform the modified hurdler stretch. If a partner is available, the modified hurdler stretch may be replaced by the next exercise.

Exercise: Modified hurdler stretch with a partner. Lying on your back with your knee locked into extension, have a partner lift your leg toward your head as far as it will go. Hold the stretch for 10 to 15 seconds (Fig. 51.34). Repeat three times, each time trying to stretch slightly farther.

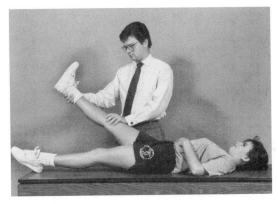

FIGURE 51.34. Modified hurdler stretch with a partner.

LOW BACK STRAINS AND SPRAINS

Back strains are injuries associated with the muscles that help support the spine, and sprains are injuries to the ligaments that connect one vertebrae to the next. Often, low back injuries are a combination of a sprain to the ligaments and a muscle strain (see Chapter 32). Rehabilitation of low back injuries is directed at regaining normal, pain-free motion through the use of flexibility exercises, selective strengthening exercises, corrections in posture, and adjustments in normal daily activities.

Stage I

Range-of-Motion Exercises

Exercise: Pelvic tilt. Lie on your back with knees bent and feet flat on the floor. Tighten your abdominal muscles and tilt the pelvis so that the small of your back flattens out against the floor. Hold this contraction for 5 seconds and repeat 10 times (Fig. 51.35).

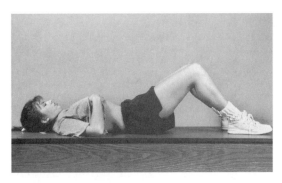

FIGURE 51.35. Pelvic tilt.

Exercise: Cat back stretch. Kneel on your hands and knees in a relaxed position. Raise your back up like a cat and hold for 5 seconds (Fig. 51.36). Repeat 10 times.

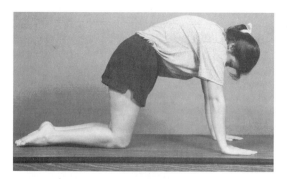

FIGURE 51.36. Cat back stretch.

Exercise: Williams flexion exercise. The position for this exercise is the same as for the pelvic tilt exercise. Begin the exercise with a pelvic tilt. Once your back is flattened, grasp one knee and bring it up to the chest as far as it will go. Lower your leg back to the starting position and grasp the other leg

in the same manner. Finally, grasp both legs and pull them up to your chest. Continue to alternate—first one leg, then the other, then both—until 10 of the rotations are completed (Fig. 51.37). Work up to 3 sets of 10.

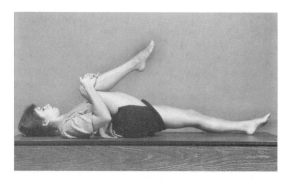

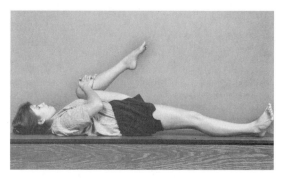

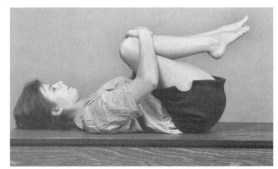

FIGURE 51.37. Williams flexion exercise: (top) one leg; (middle) other leg; (bottom) both legs.

Strengthening Exercises

Exercise: Card table exercise. Kneel on your hands and knees. Raise the left arm forward to shoulder height and hold it for 3 seconds; then lower it back to the starting position.

Raise the right arm and hold it for 3 seconds; now lower. Next, raise the left leg up with the knee straight and hold for 3 seconds; then lower. Raise the right leg in the same fashion and lower it. Finally, raise the right arm and left leg at the same time and hold for 3 seconds. Alternate and raise the left arm and right leg. Perform the entire sequence until a set of 10 repetitions is completed (Fig. 51.38). Build up to 3 sets of 10 repetitions.

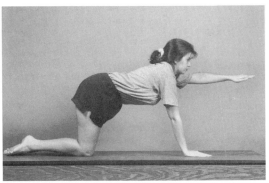

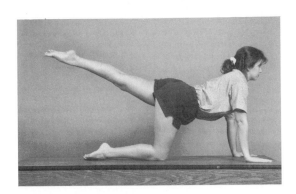

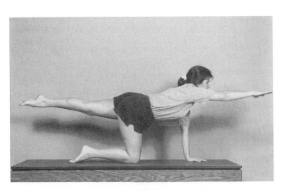

FIGURE 51.38. Card table exercise: (top) arm up; (middle) leg up; (bottom) arm and leg up.

Stage II

Range-of-Motion Exercises

1. Continue the pelvic tilt exercise.
2. Continue the cat back stretch.
3. Continue the Williams flexion exercise.

Exercise: Chair stretch. Sit in a chair and lean forward as far as possible, lowering your head to the ground as far as it will go. Hold the position for 5 seconds, coming up slowly, low back first, upper back and shoulders next, and head last. Repeat 10 times.

Exercise: Side stretch. Stand with feet shoulder-width apart. Place one hand on your hip and raise the other hand over your head, leaning to the opposite side. Hold this position for 15 seconds, repeating three times on each side (Fig. 51.39).

4. Perform the modified hurdler stretch (see p. 828).

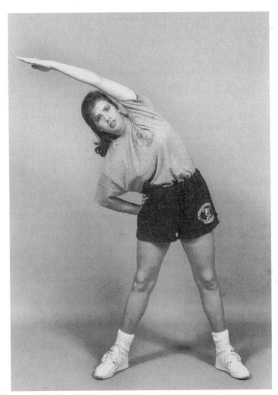

FIGURE 51.39. Side stretch.

Strengthening Exercises

Continue the card table exercise.

Exercise: Bent-leg, one-quarter sit-ups. Lie on your back, with knees bent. Place your hands across your chest and add a pelvic tilt. After doing the pelvic tilt, raise your upper body off the ground until one-quarter of the distance to your knees is reached. Return to the starting position (Fig. 51.40). Work up to 3 sets of 10 repetitions.

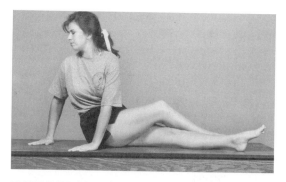

FIGURE 51.41. Sitting rotation stretch.

Strengthening Exercises

1. Continue the card table exercise.
2. Continue bent-leg, one-quarter sit-ups.

Exercise: Hip raises. Lie on your back with your knees bent, hands at your side. Raise your hips off the ground and hold this position for 5 seconds; then relax (Fig. 51.42). Repeat 3 sets of 10 repetitions.

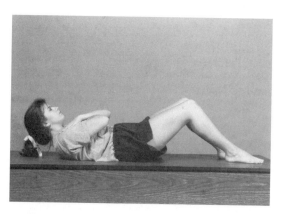

FIGURE 51.40. Bent-leg, one-quarter sit-ups.

Stage III

Range-of-Motion Exercises

1. Discontinue pelvic tilt exercise. Do pelvic tilts when doing bent-leg, one-quarter sit-ups.
2. Discontinue the cat back stretch and side stretch.
3. Continue the Williams flexion exercise.
4. Continue the chair stretch.
5. Continue the modified hurdler stretch.

Exercise: Sitting rotation stretch. Sitting in an upright position, cross one leg over the other and rotate your body toward the crossed leg and back in the other direction. Repeat in the opposite direction, switching crossed legs (Fig. 51.41). Hold each stretch for 30 seconds. Repeat three times in each direction for each leg.

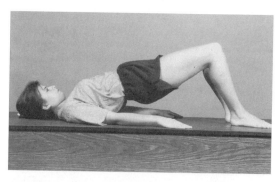

FIGURE 51.42. Hip raises.

Exercise: Prone-ups. Lie on your stomach. Raise yourself up on your hands and lean backward without lifting your hips off the floor. Hold this position for 5 seconds and relax. Continue until you have completed 3 sets of 10 repetitions.

Stage IV

Range-of-Motion Exercises

1. Continue the Williams flexion exercise.
2. Continue the chair stretch.

3. Continue the modified hurdler stretch.
4. Continue the sitting rotation stretch.

Strengthening Exercises

1. Continue the card table exercise.
2. Continue bent-leg, one-quarter sit-ups.
3. Continue the hip raises.
4. Continue the prone-ups.

Stage V

Range-of-Motion Exercises

Continue all flexibility exercises.

Strengthening Exercises

1. Add in any low back exercise machine.
2. You may discontinue other strengthening exercises; however, continue to do 3 sets of 10 repetitions of the bent-leg, one-quarter sit-ups (see p. 832).

CERVICAL STRAINS AND SPRAINS

A cervical strain is an injury to the musculotendinous unit, and a cervical sprain is a ligamentous injury. Both are common in athletes. They can occur at the extremes of motion, such as hyperflexion, hyperextension, or excessive rotation, or in association with violent muscle contraction (see Chapter 32). Generally, muscle strain symptoms subside within 3 to 7 days. If they persist, an underlying ligament injury may be prolonging the symptoms. As the injured connective tissue heals, resulting stiffness prohibits normal joint motion. Early range of motion done gently by the athlete may help prevent the stiffness. A flexibility and strengthening program will also help in the treatment of cervical strains and sprains.

Stage I

Range-of-Motion Exercises

Exercise: Active range, 10-position exercise. Move your neck to the farthest possible point in each of the following directions:

1. Straight back.
2. Straight forward.
3. Ear to shoulder on left.
4. Ear to shoulder on right.
5. On an angle back to the left.
6. On an angle forward to the right.
7. On an angle back to the right.
8. On an angle forward to the left.
9. Rotate head counterclockwise.
10. Rotate head clockwise.

Hold each position for 5 seconds. Perform this exercise at least two to three times daily.

Stage II

Range-of-Motion Exercises

Continue active range, 10-position exercise.

Strengthening Exercises

Exercise: 10-position strength exercise. Perform the 10 exercises described in the active range, 10-position exercise, but now push against hand resistance for an isometric contraction. Perform all 10 movements, holding each contraction for 10 seconds and repeat 3 times.

Stage III

Range-of-Motion Exercises

Continue the active range, 10-position exercise two to three times daily.

Strengthening Exercises

If no machines or weight-training equipment is available, continue with the active range, 10-position exercise. If training equipment is available, do the following exercises.

Exercise: Neck flexion, extension, lateral bending. On the appropriate machine (Universal, Nautilus, etc.) perform neck flexion (forward); neck extension (backward); and lateral bending to each side (to one shoulder and then the other). Start with a light weight (50 percent of max) and high repetitions (12 to 15). Decrease the repetitions and increase the weight as you feel comfortable. Make sure you can perform 3 sets of 12 to 15 repetitions of the chosen weight before advancing.

Helpful Daily Living Pointers for a Healthy Neck

- Avoid activities that place the neck in extremes of movement (bending far back when shaving, washing hair in a sink, looking up at the sky).
- Avoid maintaining any particular position for longer than 15 minutes (e.g., sitting at a desk, typing at a computer or typewriter, watching TV).
- Use a straw for drinking.
- Do all of your work at eye level.
- Avoid driving for prolonged amounts of time and support your neck with the headrest if possible.
- Avoid sleeping on your stomach because it forces the neck back into extension. Sleep on your side or on your back with a cervical pillow or a very flat pillow.
- Remember that posture is a key factor in how your neck and back feel during the day. Don't slouch or allow your shoulders to slump forward while sitting or standing.

ROTATOR CUFF INJURIES

The rotator cuff is a group of four shoulder muscles. All of the rotator cuff muscles are essential for effective abduction of the arm, as they must stabilize the humeral head in the glenoid during arm movement. Injuries to the rotator cuff muscles can occur through a variety of mechanisms. They are most often caused by a violent pull to the arm, an abnormal rotation, or a fall on the outstretched arm (see Chapter 16.) The throwing mechanism, swimming, and over-head tennis play can be major contributing factors. Rehabilitation of the rotator cuff after injury should include range of motion and flexibility exercises, as well as a comprehensive strengthening program designed specially to strengthen the rotator cuff muscles.

Stage I

Range-of-Motion Exercises

Exercise: Pendulum exercise I. Lean over a table, chair, or against a wall. Let the affected arm swing in a circular motion, starting with 25 small circles, then 25 medium circles, and finally 25 large circles in a clockwise direction. Wind down from the large circles with 25 large circles, 25 medium circles, and 25 small circles in a counterclockwise direction. The starting position is shown in Figure 51.43.

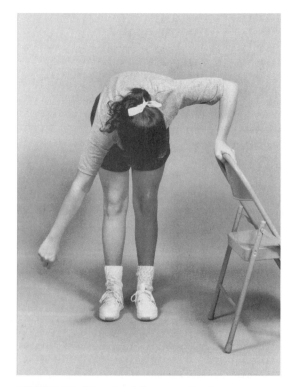

FIGURE 51.43. Pendulum exercise I.

Exercise: Pendulum exercise II. Let your arm swing from side to side, moving in each direction as far as your arm will allow (Fig. 51.44). Do 50 swings back and forth.

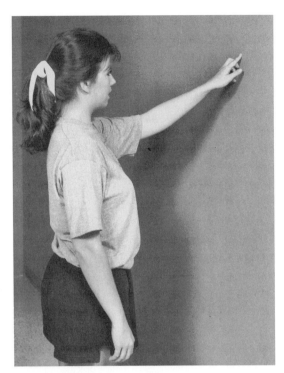

FIGURE 51.45.   Wall walking I.

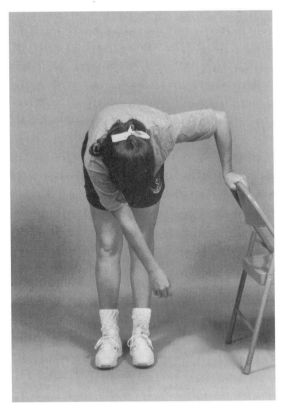

FIGURE 51.44.   Pendulum exercise II.

Exercise: Wall walking I. Face the wall at arm's length. Using your second and third fingers, "walk" up the wall as high as tolerable (Fig. 51.45). Repeat this exercise until you have successfully performed 10 climbs up the wall. Each time, try to go slightly higher than the time before.

Exercise: Wall walking II. Stand sideways next to the wall (Fig. 51.46) and climb the wall as you did in wall walking I. Repeat going up the wall until you have successfully managed 10 climbs up the wall.

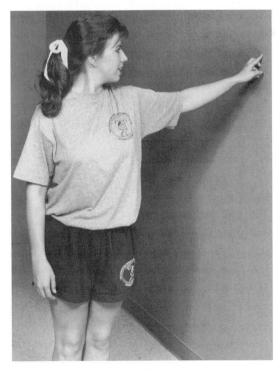

FIGURE 51.46.   Wall walking II.

Stage II

Range-of-Motion Exercises

Exercise: Wand exercises. Using a wand, stick, baseball bat, or broom handle (something as wide as your shoulders), grab the wand on the ends and move in the following directions:

1. Side to side (Fig. 51.47a).

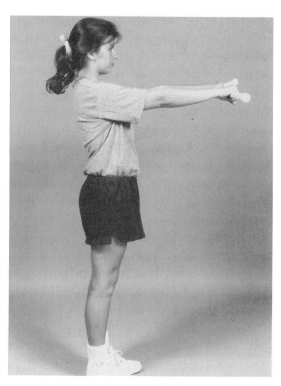

FIGURE 51.47b. Wand exercises, up in front to shoulder height.

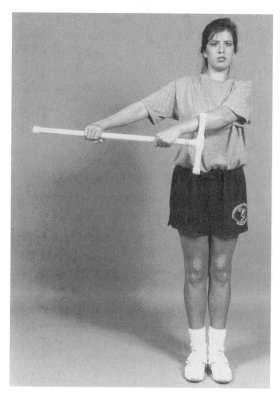

FIGURE 51.47a. Wand exercises, side to side.

2. Up in front to shoulder height (Fig. 51.47b).
3. In back and up as far as possible (Fig. 51.47c).

Perform 3 sets of 10 repetitions for each direction.

Exercise: Four-point shoulder movements. Move your arm in the following directions:

1. Flexion: thumb up and raise arm to shoulder level, no higher. Arm should be

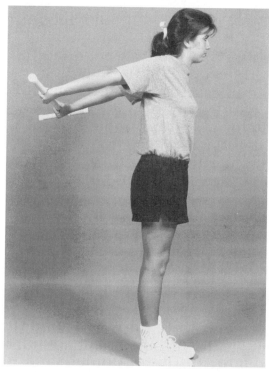

FIGURE 51.47c. Wand exercises, in back and up as far as possible.

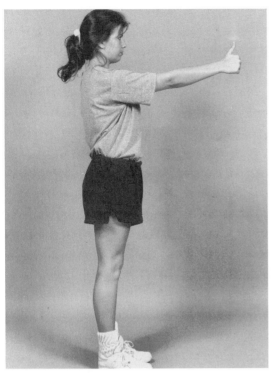

FIGURE 51.48a. Four-point shoulder exercise: flexion.

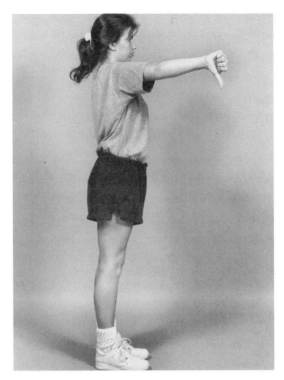

FIGURE 51.48b. Four-point shoulder exercise: rotator cuff position.

raised directly in shoulder flexion (Fig. 51.48a).

2. Rotator cuff position: move your arm up into flexion, but the position of your arm should be somewhere between directly in front of you and out to the side. The thumb should be pointing down as if you were going to empty a glass or can (Fig. 51.48b).
3. Abduction: raise your arm from the side to shoulder level (Fig. 51.48c).
4. Extension: raise your arm up to the back as far as you can (Fig. 51.48d).

Strengthening Exercises

Exercise: Isometric abduction. Stand next to a wall with the affected arm at your side and elbow bent. Push against the wall as if lifting your arm up from your side. Push for 10 seconds and relax. Repeat for 3 sets of 10, with 10-second holds for contraction (Fig. 51.49).

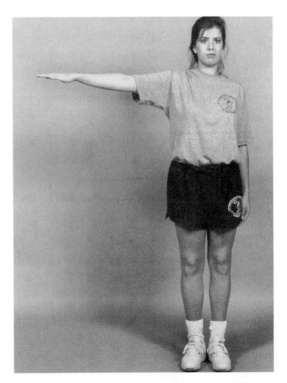

FIGURE 51.48c. Four-point shoulder exercise: abduction.

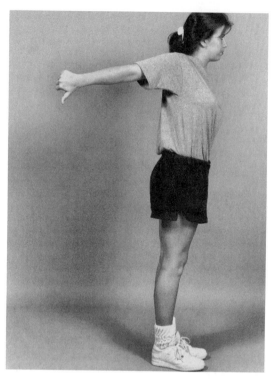

FIGURE 51.48d. Four-point shoulder exercise: extension.

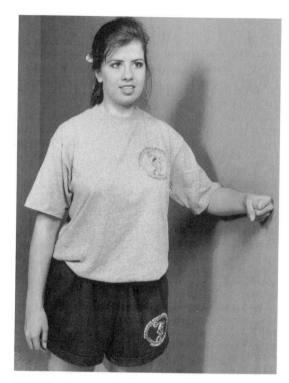

FIGURE 51.49. Isometric abduction.

Exercise: Isometric external rotation. Stand near a wall with the affected arm at your side and elbow bent. Rotate your arm outward against the wall and push for 10 seconds (Fig. 51.50). Repeat for 3 sets of 10, holding 10 seconds each.

Exercise: Isometric internal rotation. Using the opposite hand for resistance, place the affected arm at your side with your elbow bent. Rotate the arm inward against the other hand, pushing for 10 seconds. Repeat the exercise for 3 sets of 10 contractions, holding each contraction for 10 seconds.

Exercise: Isometric flexion. Stand facing a wall, 1 inch away. Push forward against the wall with your hand as if to raise your arm in front of you. Push for 10 seconds and repeat until you have performed 3 sets of 10 contractions.

Exercise: Isometric extension. Stand with your back 1 inch from a wall. Keeping your

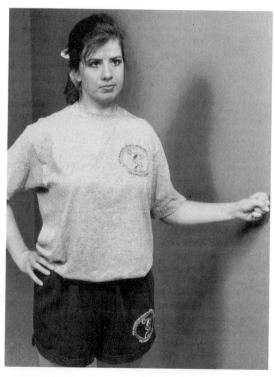

FIGURE 51.50. Isometric external rotation.

hand in a neutral position, push against the wall as if to bring your arm up and back. Hold the push for 10 seconds. Repeat, working up to 3 sets of 10 contractions.

Stage III

Range-of-Motion Exercises

1. Discontinue wand exercises.
2. Continue with four-point shoulder movements.

Strengthening Exercises

Discontinue isometric exercises.

Exercise: 4-point shoulder movements with weight. Repeat four-point shoulder movements, but this time add weight. Begin with a light weight (1 to 2 pounds) and increase 1 to 2 pounds when you can successfully complete 3 sets of 10 repetitions. Continue until you can successfully lift 10 percent of your body weight or 10 pounds, whichever comes first. When you can successfully do these repetitions with the appropriate weight, proceed to Stage IV strengthening exercises.

Exercise: Shoulder pulley, internal rotation. Stand with the affected shoulder perpendicular to the pulley, with the shoulder adducted and elbow flexed to 90 degrees. Start with the arm in external rotation and pull to an internally rotated position (Fig. 51.51). Shoulder pulleys can be substituted with elastic surgical tubing, bicycle tubing, or Theraband exercise tubing. Do 3 sets of 10 repetitions.

Exercise: Shoulder pulley, external rotation. Turn 180 degrees from the last exercise position so the affected arm is away from the pulley system. With the shoulder in adduction and elbow flexed to 90 degrees, pull the weight from an internally rotated to an externally rotated position (Fig. 51.52). Do 3 sets of 10 repetitions.

If no pulley system or elastic tubing material is available for the last two exercises, do internal and external rotation by lying

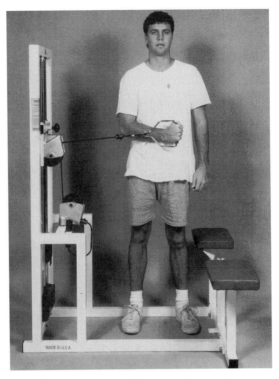

FIGURE 51.51.   Shoulder pulley, internal rotation.

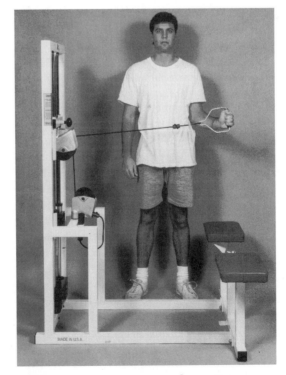

FIGURE 51.52.   Shoulder pulley, external rotation.

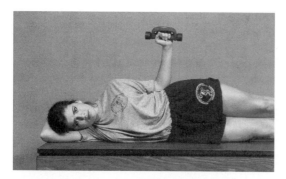

FIGURE 51.53. Internal and external rotation with weight.

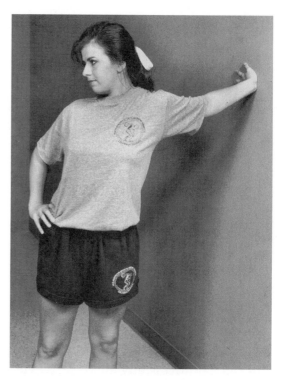

FIGURE 51.54. Chest stretch.

on your side and using dumbbells or ankle weights for resistance (Fig. 51.53).

Stage IV

Range-of-Motion Exercises

Discontinue four-point shoulder movements.

Exercise: Chest stretch. With an extended arm, place your palm against a wall and turn your upper body in the opposite direction. Hold each stretch for 30 seconds (Fig. 51.54). Repeat three times.

Exercise: Posterior shoulder stretch. Place the affected arm across your chest and use the other arm to pull in adduction. Hold each stretch for 30 seconds (Fig. 51.55). Repeat three times.

Exercise: Wand stretch I. Perform this stretch in a supine position on a table or bench. For the first stretch, the shoulder is adducted with the elbow flexed to 90 degrees and supported by the table or bench. Use a wand, dowel, broomstick, baseball bat, or even a hammer. Using your other hand, with the wand pushing into the arm to stretch, push the hand down until you feel a good but comfortable stretch (Fig. 51.56). Hold the stretch for 30 seconds.

Exercise: Wand stretch II. Perform this stretch in a supine position. Begin with the

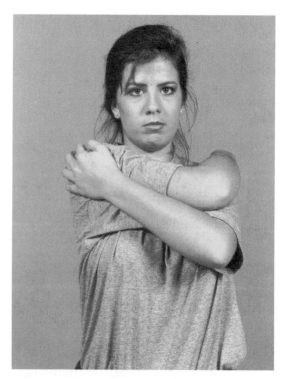

FIGURE 51.55. Posterior shoulder stretch.

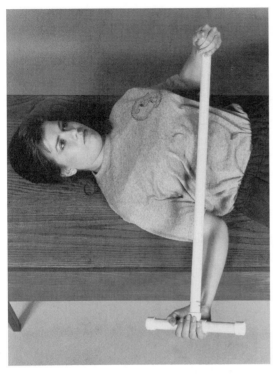

FIGURE 51.56.   Wand stretch I.

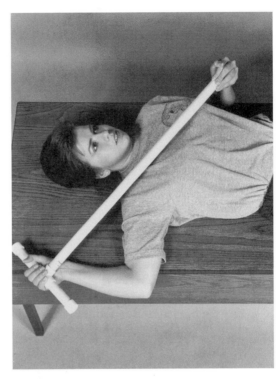

FIGURE 51.57.   Wand stretch II.

shoulder and the elbow bent to 90 degrees, with the shoulder supported by the table or bench. Using a wand or related object, push down until a good but comfortable stretch is felt (Fig. 51.57). Hold the stretch for 30 seconds.

Exercise: Wand stretch III.   Perform this stretch in a supine position. Begin with the affected arm against your ear on the same side of your head. Support the scapula with the table and allow the rest of your arm to hang off the end. Push with a wand or stick until a good but comfortable stretch is felt (Fig. 51.58). Hold the stretch for 30 seconds.

Strengthening Exercises

1. Continue the four-point shoulder movements (see pp. 836–838).
2. Continue internal and external rotation exercises, using a pulley, elastic tubing, or weight.

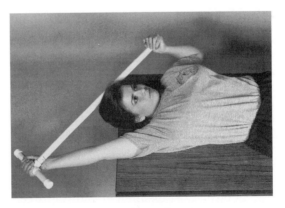

FIGURE 51.58.   Wand stretch III.

Exercise: Prone empty-can exercise.   Start by lying prone, with the affected arm in the empty-can position midway between straight out in front of you and straight out to your side. Bring your arm from the leg of the table or ground to shoulder level as shown in Figure 51.59. Perform this exercise for 3 sets of 10 repetitions.

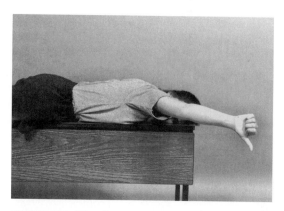

FIGURE 51.59. Prone empty-can exercise.

Stage V

Range-of-Motion Exercises

1. Continue all stretching from Stage IV.
2. Continue all strengthening from Stage IV.
3. Return to functional activity.

EPICONDYLITIS OF THE ELBOW

Epicondylitis is an inflammatory response to overuse of either a flexor or an extensor muscle group attaching into the medial and lateral epicondyle of the humerus, respectively (see Chapter 17). Tennis elbow, or lateral epicondylitis, is perhaps the most common of these inflammatory injuries. Medial epicondylitis is a frequent occurrence in athletes participating in the throwing sports. Factors that contribute to epicondylitis are muscle weakness, overuse, poor playing technique, and improper equipment. A program of stretching and strengthening over several months is required in order for the athlete to regain strength and range of motion.

Stage I

Range-of-Motion Exercises

Exercise: Active flexion/extension. Sit with the affected forearm resting on your thigh with the wrist extending past the knee. First, flex the wrist, holding it in this posi-

tion for 5 seconds; then extend and hold for the same amount of time. Work up to 3 sets of 10.

Exercise: Active supination/pronation. Begin in the same position as for active flexion/extension. Rotate your hand and forearm to extreme supination and hold 5 seconds; then turn to extreme pronation and hold for the same period of time. Work up to 3 sets of 10 repetitions.

Stage II

Range-of-Motion Exercises

1. Continue active flexion/extension exercise.
2. Continue active supination/pronation exercise.

Strengthening Exercises

Exercise: Grip-strengthener exercise. Grasp a ball, gripping it with all of your fingers. Hold the grip as tightly as possible for 10 seconds. Work up to 3 sets of 10 repetitions. Start with a Nerf or sponge ball; work up to a racquetball and finally to a tennis ball or the manufactured grip strengtheners that can be found in local sporting goods stores.

Exercise: Towel-wringing exercise. Grab a towel with both hands as if one was wringing water out of the towel. Perform this motion using both hands and alternate wringing directions. Wring the towel so that one downward wring and one upward wring is one repetition. Work up to 3 sets of 10 repetitions.

Stage III

Range-of-Motion Exercises

1. Discontinue active flexion/extension.
2. Continue active supination/pronation exercise.

Exercise: Wrist flexion stretch. Extend your arm and hand out as if signaling someone to "stop." Place the opposite hand across the palm and push the hand back gently into extension as far as it will go and hold the wrist there for 10 to 15 seconds (Fig. 51.60). Repeat three times.

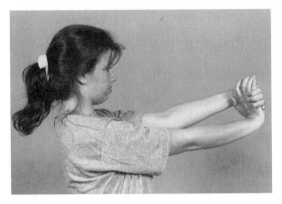

FIGURE 51.60.   Wrist flexion stretch.

Exercise: Wrist extension stretch.   Begin with your arm extended and the wrist in full flexion. Use the opposite hand to apply gentle pressure to the back of the hand, forcing the hand into flexion as far as it will go. Hold this position for 10 to 15 seconds and then release (Fig. 51.61). Repeat three times.

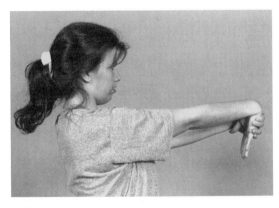

FIGURE 51.61.   Wrist extension stretch.

Strengthening Exercises

1. Continue grip-strengthener exercise.
2. Continue towel-wringing exercise.

Exercise: Wrist flexion curls.   Perform active flexion/extension exercise with the palm up, using a 1/2-pound weight. Work up to 3 sets of 10; then increase weight in 1/2-pound increments (Fig. 51.62).

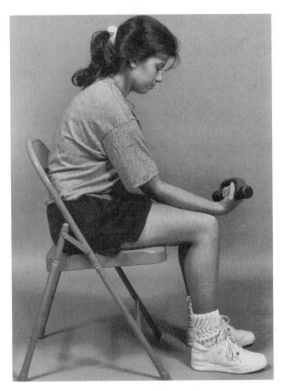

FIGURE 51.62.   Wrist flexion curls.

Exercise: Wrist extension curls.   Repeat wrist flexion curls with palm down (Fig. 51.63).

Stage IV

Range-of-Motion Exercises

1. Continue active supination/pronation exercise (see p. 842).
2. Continue wrist flexion stretch.
3. Continue wrist extension stretch.

Strengthening Exercises

1. Discontinue grip-strengthener exercise.
2. Discontinue towel-wringing exercise.
3. Discontinue wrist flexion and wrist extension curls.

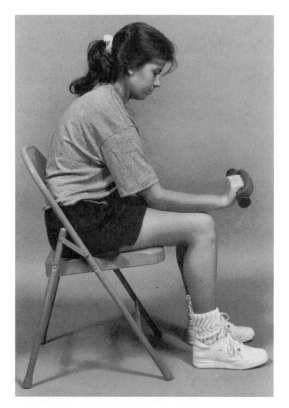

FIGURE 51.63. Wrist extension curls.

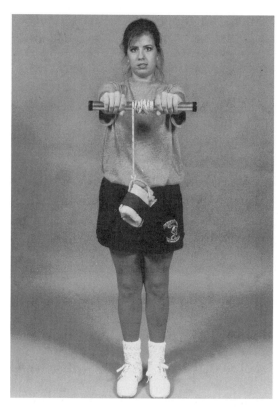

FIGURE 51.64. Broom handle flexion curls.

Exercise: Broom handle flexion curls. Tie one end of a rope about 3 feet long to a broom handle. Place a plate weight or something that will act as a weight on the other end of the rope. Grab the broom handle with both hands, palms down. Roll the rope up around the broom handle until it cannot be rolled up anymore. Unroll the rope and start again. Repeat until you have completed 3 sets of 10 repetitions (Fig. 51.64).

Exercise 2: Broom handle extension curls. Repeat the broom handle flexion curls but with both palms up as you grip the broom handle. Repeat this exercise until you have done 3 sets of 10 repetitions.

Substitutions for Broom Handle Exercises

Exercise: Elastic tubing flexion exercises. Hold elastic tubing, surgical tubing, or an old bicycle inner tube in one hand and make a loop in the other end. Grab the looped end with your hand palm up. Pull the affected elbow's hand into extension as far as it will go, add resistance as tolerable, and pull your wrist into flexion against the resistance of the tubing. Complete 3 sets of 10 repetitions.

Exercise: Elastic tubing extension exercises. Repeat the previous exercise but start the affected hand palm down and in extreme flexion. Pull the hand up into extension. Repeat until you have completed 3 sets of 10 repetitions.

Stage V

Range-of-Motion Exercises

1. Discontinue active supination/pronation exercise.
2. Continue wrist flexion stretch and wrist extension stretch.

Strengthening Exercises

Continue with broom handle flexion curls and broom handle extension curls, or elastic tubing flexion exercises and elastic tubing extension exercises.

Return to Activity Tips

If you are returning to tennis:

- Use a lighter racquet.
- Grip the racquet higher.
- Start back slowly and build up time and amount of strokes gradually.
- At first avoid hitting backhands since this is one of the major injury-causing strokes in tennis. Or substitute a two-handed backhand for a one-handed backhand when you first return to sport.
- Reduce your string tension.
- Change grip size.
- Consult a professional at a club to improve your technique and discuss your equipment choices.

For other sports the principles are the same: start slowly and build endurance by increasing amounts of activity *gradually*.

SUGGESTIONS FOR POOL EXERCISES

Water is an excellent medium for exercise. Buoyancy and the relative density of a body in water contribute to the fact that most human beings have a tendency to float. This allows exercise with decreased gravitational and weight-bearing pressure on the lower limbs. Water also provides resistance equal to the force applied. This makes it easy for the athlete to gauge how much resistance is possible.

Stage I

Water Level: Waist to Neck

Exercise: Balancing. Try balancing on one foot for 5 seconds. Relax for 5 seconds and repeat until you have balanced 30 times.

Exercise: Walking. Walk from the beginning of the low end to water that is neck deep and return. It should be about 10 yards. Begin doing 10 walks up and back.

Water Level: 8 Feet or More

Exercise: Running with a flotation device. With a life vest or flotation device of some kind, kick your legs in as normal a jogging style as possible. Do 5 minutes of running in deep enough water so you are not touching when fully extended.

Stage II

Water Level: Waist to Neck

Continue to balance, holding each balance for 5 seconds and repeating until you have completed 30 balances.

Exercise: Walk/jog. Begin walking about 10 yards in the pool from the beginning of the low end to water that is neck deep. After 10 walks back and forth, begin jogging with as natural a motion as possible. Repeat until you have completed 10 jogs or as many as possible up to 10 jogs.

Water Level: 8 Feet or More

Exercise: Running with a flotation device. Begin increasing amount of time running by 1 minute each session until you have reached 10 minutes.

Stage III

Water Level: Waist to Neck

Discontinue balancing activity.

Exercise: Walk/jog/run. Begin walking 10 yards in the pool from the beginning of the low end to water neck deep. After 5 walks back and forth, begin jogging with as natural a motion as possible. After 5 jogs begin running. Repeat until you have completed 10 runs or as many as you possibly can up to 10 runs back and forth.

Water Level: 8 Feet or More

Discontinue running with a flotation device if you can swim and begin the second exercise, treading water. If you cannot swim, continue using the flotation device and add 1 minute to the 10 minutes each day until 15 minutes of running is reached.

Exercise: Water tread. If you can swim, start treading water without a flotation device. Begin with 3 minutes and progress 1/2 minute each day, up to 10 minutes.

Stage IV

Water Level: Waist to Neck

Exercise: Walk/jog/run. Begin with 5 walks and 5 jogs. Add one run onto the 10 runs that you were doing in the previous stage until you have reached 20 runs.

Exercise: High steps. Begin running by high stepping through the water. Work on speed and power. Begin with 5 high steps.

Water Level: 8 Feet or More

Continue treading water or running with a flotation device.

Exercise: Flutter kicking with kickboard or flotation device. Begin flutter kicking with a kickboard the full length of the pool. Start with 5 laps back and forth. Add one full lap each day until you have reached 10 laps.

Exercise: Scissor kicking with a kickboard. Begin scissor kicking with a kickboard or

flotation device. Do as many as possible up to 5 laps.

Stage V

Water Level: Waist to Neck

1. Continue walk/jog/run program.
2. Continue high steps.

Water Level: 8 Feet or More

1. Continue treading water.
2. Continue flutter kicking with a kickboard.
3. Continue scissor kicking with a kickboard.

Exercise: Begin swimming crawl stroke. Start with 5 laps of the crawl with a small break in between each lap. Add one lap or try to swim an increasing amount more at one time each time you attempt the exercise. Your final workout should look like this:

1. Walk 5 laps back and forth.
2. Jog 5 laps back and forth.
3. Run up to 20 laps back and forth.
4. High stepping: up to 5 laps.
5. Lunges: up to 5 laps.
6. Tread water: up to 10 minutes.
7. Kickboard work: flutter kick for up to 10 laps.
8. Scissor kick: up to 5 laps.
9. Swim crawl stroke: up to 10 laps.

Build each day but do not exceed the recommended amounts suggested above. Do what time allows and the accommodations can provide.

SUGGESTED READINGS

Kulund, D. N. *The Injured Athlete,* 2d ed. Philadelphia: J. B. Lippincott Co., 1988.

Peterson, L., and P. Renstrom. *Sports Injuries: Their Prevention and Treatment.* Chicago: Year Book Medical Publishers, 1986.

Roy, S., and R. Irvin. *Sports Medicine: Prevention, Evaluation, Management, and Rehabilitation..* Englewood Cliffs, N.J.: Prentice-Hall, 1983.

Torg, J. S., J. J. Vegso, and E. Torg. *Rehabilitation of Athletic Injuries: An Atlas of Therapeutic Exercise.* Chicago: Year Book Medical Publishers, 1987.

SECTION

SEVEN

OTHER MEDICAL ISSUES

52

Environmental Problems

849

OBJECTIVES FOR CHAPTER 52

After reading this chapter, the student should be able to:
1. Discuss the physiology of thermal regulation and the three classifications of heat exposure syndromes.
2. Describe the physiologic response of the human body to cold exposure and various types of cold exposure injury.
3. Understand the pathologic conditions which may result from high-altitude exposure.
4. Discuss the types of diving disorders the underwater diver may encounter.

INTRODUCTION

The injuries and conditions to which the athletic trainer must respond are sometimes related to the environment in which the sport is taking place. The athlete may suffer from heat exhaustion in a hot climate, frostnip in a cold climate, mountain sickness in a high altitude, or decompression sickness while scuba diving.

Chapter 52 reviews the pertinent information concerning the causes, recognition, treatment, and prevention of injuries and conditions unique to certain environments. These areas include excessive heat and humidity, cold, altitude, and underwater environments. The chapter also stresses the prevention of these conditions and the immediate medical care given to people who develop them. ▪

HEAT DISORDERS

Physiology of Thermal Regulation

The main center for thermal regulation in the body is in the hypothalamus, where thermal receptors sense the local temperature of the heated or cooled blood to this area. Autonomic impulses to increased body sweating and peripheral vasodilation result from hypothalamic temperature elevations.

Normal body temperature is maintained by precise balance between heat production and heat loss. Body heat is produced by basic metabolic processes, by food intake (specific dynamic action), and by muscular activity. Heat loss occurs in five ways.

- **Conduction**: When the body comes in contact with an object—for example, a cold, wet shirt—heat is directly transferred from the warmer body to the cooler object.
- **Convection**: When cool air moves across the body surface, heat is transferred to the cooler air, warming it and cooling the body.
- **Evaporation**: When water on the body surface is transformed from a liquid to a vapor, the body loses heat. Vapor-

ization of approximately 1 gm of water removes about 0.6 kcal of heat by perspiration.

- **Respiration**: When inspired, cooler air is raised to the body temperature in the lungs, and heat is lost through respiration.
- **Radiation**: Heat can be radiated by the body to the environment.

Most of these mechanisms of heat loss depend on the fact that the environmental temperature is lower than the body temperature. If the external temperature is higher than the body temperature, the primary source of heat loss is vaporization of sweat, assuming the humidity is low enough to accept the vaporization.

Mechanisms of Heat Regulation

When the body is challenged by an elevated environmental temperature, mechanisms to increase heat loss, including cutaneous vasodilation, sweating, and increased respiratory rate, are activated. Extreme heat produces both an immediate and a delayed effect on body physiology. The immediate response is vasodilation of the vessels in the skin, with increased blood flow to the skin and increased sweat production, maximizing losses through radiation and convection. With moderate heat exposure, the increased blood flow to the skin is achieved at the expense of flow to other organs. Greater heat stress increases the pulse rate to maintain cardiac output. Respiratory rate also increases to aid cooling when air temperature is less than body temperature.

There are approximately 2 million eccrine (sweat) glands in the body. Sweat production increases sharply with increasing temperature and may result in the loss of 2 to 8 liters of water in a 24-hour period. The average person loses about 2 gm of sodium chloride in each liter of sweat at the beginning of warm weather. With acclimatization, the body conserves sodium chloride. Sweating is an efficient means of cooling when the humidity is low, with up to 600 kcal dissipated for each liter of sweat

that evaporates. When the humidity rises, evaporation of sweat decreases. No heat loss results from sweat that drips off or remains in clothing. When the environmental temperature is less than skin temperature, 87 degrees F (30.6 degrees C), heat is transferred out of the body. At rest, with the temperature below 87 degrees F (30.6 degrees C), about two-thirds of the body's normal heat loss occurs due to radiation and convection of heat. The rest of the heat is lost through evaporation from the skin and the lungs, and a small amount is lost through the urine and feces. As the ambient temperature approaches skin temperature and exceeds 87 degrees F (30.6 degrees C), loss of body heat through radiation and convection is sharply curtailed. As heat transfer is reversed, heat loss is mostly achieved by evaporation.

There are five principal mechanisms of human thermal regulation:

- Excitation of sweating by the central heat receptors.
- Vasodilation elicited by central heat receptors.
- Inhibition of sweating by cold receptors of the skin.
- Excitation of metabolic heat production by cold receptors of the skin.
- Inhibition of thermal regulatory heat centers.

The rate of water loss can be substantially increased by sweating. Evaporation over most of the body surface directly cools the blood that runs through the capillaries in the skin. The rate of cooling by evaporation depends on the amount of body surface exposed, the condition and nature of the covering material, the degree of humidity in the air in contact with the skin, and the rate of air circulation over the surface.

Electrolyte Losses

For years controversy has existed as to whether or not athletes who perspire heavily consume more salt in the summer than in the winter, or more than the average population. An adequate consumption of salt is rarely a problem in the typical American diet. In fact, most Americans consume an excessive amount of sodium, averaging 5 to 10 gm of sodium per day, although we probably require only 1 to 3 gm. Sodium is widely used as a flavoring agent and a preservative in packaged foods, and most Americans use table salt on food. One "Big Mac" supplies the sodium needs for 1 day.

Several key electrolytes are lost in sweat —namely, sodium, chloride, potassium, and magnesium. The quantity of electrolytes varies from day to day and from individual to individual, depending in part on the person's degree of conditioning or acclimatization. The well-conditioned athlete loses fewer electrolytes than his or her poorly conditioned counterpart. The electrolyte concentrations in sweat vary greatly: .3 to 2.7 gm of sodium, .3 to 2.8 gm of chloride, and .2 to 1.2 gm of potassium per liter. Since a typical mixed diet furnishes 3 to 10 gm of sodium, 2.5 to 8 gm of chloride, and 2 to 6 gm of potassium, net deficiencies of these electrolytes are highly unlikely, even with profuse sweating.

Most electrolyte losses can be made up at meals following athletic events. Rarely, an athlete may lose 5 to 6 liters of sweat per athletic event, manifested by weight loss of 2 to 10 pounds, and probably requires electrolyte replacement. Water is most important to replace electrolytes during and immediately after the event. Then, a diet including potassium-rich foods such as potatoes, tomatoes, tomato juice, citrus fruits, vegetables, meat, peas, fish, and beans is recommended. Whenever athletes add extra sodium to their diets, they should drink liberal amounts of water simultaneously. Otherwise, excessive sodium can draw water out of the body cells, accentuating the dehydration.

Water Loss

Water loss in a sweating athlete exceeds sodium loss and is generally of greater concern. Adequate fluid intake is essential to maintain the hydrated state and prevent an abnormal rise in body temperature. An average adult exercising in a neutral environment requires approximately 2.5 liters of water a day. This water comes from all fluids consumed, as well as from food. The average runner requires an additional 1.5 to 2 liters of water per hour of active sweating and 2 to 4 liters of water per hour when competing in endurance events. An athlete should conscientiously consume fluids before, during, and after an event to ensure hydration.

Thirst alone is not an adequate indicator of fluid needs, as thirst does not occur until the athlete has lost 2 percent of his or her body weight. In addition, satisfying thirst only replaces about 50 percent of the needed fluid. The athlete should be weighed before and after the event to determine the amount of fluid that needs to be replaced. Players who lose over 3 percent of their body weight in vigorous practice should be encouraged to take water frequently during practice and to rehydrate adequately prior to the next practice.

While maintaining hydration, the athlete should avoid excessive protein, caffeine, alcoholic beverages, and foods that increase urine output, which might result in further dehydration. Beverages containing large amounts of salt and/or sugar should be avoided because they tend to delay gastric emptying. Most authorities agree that plain water is the best replacement fluid. Salt-containing hypertonic beverages probably should be avoided because their sodium content aggravates dehydration. (For more on fluid replacement, see Chapter 42.)

Heat Exposure Syndromes

Aside from skin disorders such as prickly heat and sunburn, basically three types of syndromes result from exposure to heat: heat cramps, heat exhaustion, and heatstroke.

Heat Cramps

Normal muscle contractions or relaxations require a strict balance of salt and water within the muscle. With excessive perspiration, both water and salt are lost. Some physicians believe **heat cramps** are due to excessive fluid loss in the muscles; others believe electrolyte imbalance causes the muscle spasm. Blood volume is usually well preserved, and the individual is alert and otherwise in good condition. Heat cramps occur in persons who sweat profusely and, like all disorders due to heat, usually take place at the beginning of the warm weather season before acclimatization. These cramps may involve the legs, abdominal muscles, or arms. Heat cramps differ from cramps resulting from overexertion, and there is no history of injury, such as a pulled muscle. The diagnosis is largely by exclusion to rule out an acute muscle injury. Often, athletes with heat cramps have a history of these cramps.

Once heat cramps have developed, treatment consists of rest from the exertional stress and passive stretching. Drinking water or a hypotonic saline solution (made by mixing 1 teaspoon of table salt to 1 quart of water) may help reverse the cramps. Prevention involves ensuring adequate fluid intake and a normal salt diet during times of excessive sweating. Conditioning and acclimatization also help reduce the incidence of cramps.

Heat Exhaustion

Heat exhaustion is a more severe heat syndrome caused by inadequate cardiovascular responsiveness to circulatory stresses induced by heat. Vasoconstriction in other parts of the body or volume expansion normally compensates for initial diversion of blood flow to the skin. Otherwise fit individuals involved in extreme physical exertion in a hot environment can develop heat exhaustion. Under these conditions, the muscle mass of the body and the brain require increased blood flow. At the same time the skin needs an increased blood flow to radiate heat from the skin in the form of sweat. Because the vascular system is inadequate to meet the simultaneous demands placed on it by the skin, muscle, and viscera, heat exhaustion results. It is an insidious, slowly progressive, peripheral vascular collapse, or "shock" syndrome.

Heat exhaustion, also called **heat prostration**, is characterized principally by the signs of peripheral vascular collapse or shock—that is, weakness, dizziness, headache, loss of appetite, nausea, pallor, diffuse sweating, vomiting, an urge to defecate, and postural syncope (fainting). Heat exhaustion is known to be of two types: salt depletion (excessive salt loss) and water depletion (excessive water loss). The latter type of heat exhaustion is experienced more often by athletes.

The symptoms of heat exhaustion develop because of reduced blood volume from fluid loss. The athlete may appear ashen and gray. In salt depletion heat exhaustion, the skin is cold and clammy; with water depletion heat exhaustion, the skin is hot and dry, a symptom that may indicate the more serious condition of heatstroke. With both types, vital signs are normal, and body temperature may even be below normal. A hypertonic state is caused by a relative increase in electrolytes. The athlete may become unconscious if not treated. Heat exhaustion due to excessive water loss is also seen in people who take salt tablets. While water and salt depletion heat exhaustion may coexist, again, water depletion heat exhaustion is by far the most serious, as it can lead to heatstroke.

The treatment for heat exhaustion, in addition to replenishing electrolytes and fluids, is to treat the accompanying mild state of hypovolemic shock by having the athlete lie down in a cool room. Rest diminishes the demands on the circulatory system. The athlete may or may not need intravenous fluids. Heat exhaustion is common and is ordinarily promptly reversed. Preexisting conditions such as cardiovascular disease, vomiting, and diarrhea, however, can aggravate it.

All athletes should be closely monitored during activity. The trainer should be alert for poorly conditioned athletes who are more susceptible to heat exposure syndromes and for overeager athletes who may ignore the symptoms of heat illness in their desire to participate. Athletes who have previously experienced any form of heat exposure syndrome should also be watched closely. An athlete who has suffered from heat illness should be permitted to participate only after he or she has been rehydrated and all symptoms have abated.

Heatstroke

Heatstroke is the third and most serious heat syndrome. In heatstroke all of the mechanisms for body cooling have failed to the extent that severe **hyperpyrexia** (body temperature above 105 degrees F [40 to 41 degrees C]) ensues. It may develop suddenly or progress from water depletion heat exhaustion. Although heatstroke is the least common of the heat disorders, it is often a problem for distance runners in hot environments. In football, it is second only to head injury as the most frequent cause of fatalities. Wrestlers dehydrated through weight loss are also particularly susceptible to heatstroke.

Heatstroke is a true emergency with a very high mortality rate. Untreated victims of heatstroke die because of damage to the cells of the central nervous system. Because some survivors may have permanent nerve damage because of hyperpyrexia, rapid and vigorous treatment is essential for full recovery. Heatstroke in the athlete is almost always precipitated by prolonged, strenuous physical exercise, either when the athlete is poorly acclimatized or in situations that do not allow evaporation of sweat. Strenuous muscular work contributes to the development of heatstroke by increasing the production of body heat.

Under conditions of maximum heat stress, when the ambient temperature approaches the skin temperature and the humidity increases, evaporation of sweat efficiently removes heat from the body. However, the initially high rates of sweat production cannot be maintained indefinitely. When the rate of sweat production falls, the body temperature rises abruptly.

This failure of perspiration is known as **sweat fatigue** or **anhidrosis**. The maximum amount of sweat that can be produced upon exposure to heat is related to the humidity. The absence of sweating and the presence of moderate dehydration in the exercising athlete intensify hyperpyrexia. For every rise of 1 degree F in core temperature, metabolism increases 7 percent, creating a vicious cycle. Heatstroke usually occurs when the ambient temperature is over 95 degrees F (35 degrees C) for a day or two and the relative humidity is in the range of 50 to 75 percent, as heat illness is cumulative.

With fluid loss from exercise, the heat regulatory mechanism fails, and the central sweating mechanism shuts off to avoid further dehydration. As the heat generated by metabolic activity builds up, body temperature rises yet the skin remains dry. The rising temperature increases cell metabolism, especially in the central nervous system where damage occurs.

Premonitory symptoms are irritability, aggressiveness, emotional instability, and hysteria, progressing to apathy, failure to respond to questions, and disorientation. The athlete may have an unsteady gait and glassy stare. Hot, dry skin accompanies the final signs of collapse and unconsciousness. Early in the course of the disorder, the pulse is rapid and full. As the changes of heatstroke become established and tissue is damaged by body heat, vasomotor collapse occurs, blood pressure falls, and the pulse becomes rapid and weak.

Treatment must begin as soon as heatstroke is diagnosed. Emergency care is designed to rid the body of excessive heat as rapidly as possible, reducing temperature below 100 degrees F (37.7 degrees C). The athlete should be immersed in a bathtub of water cooled with ice, if available; or, wet sheets or compresses and fans can be used while transporting the athlete to the hospital. Any form of cooling available should be initiated immediately. Treatment for shock may require intravenous fluids, but cooling is the priority and must be continued during transportation to the hospital. Medica-

TABLE 52.1.   Heat Stress Syndromes

Disorder	Cause	Clinical Signs and Symptoms	Treatment
Heat cramps	Excessive fluid loss in muscles Electrolyte imbalance Athlete is not acclimated to local climate	Profuse sweating Cramps involving abdominal muscles or extremities	Rest in cool environment Passive stretching Ingestion of H_2O or hypotonic solution
Heat exhaustion (excessive salt loss)	Profuse sweating; with inadequate replacement of body salts; vomiting or diarrhea	Weakness, faintness, dizziness, headache, loss of appetite, nausea, pallor, profuse sweating, urge to defecate Skin is gray and ashen, cold, and clammy	Rest in a cool room in recumbent position Fluids or IV if unconscious, increase fluid and salt intake in normal diet Discontinue activity until well under control
Heat exhaustion (excessive H_2O loss)	Profuse sweating; with inadequate replacement of body fluids; vomiting or diarrhea	Skin is hot and dry, small urine volume, excessive thirst, weakness, headache, unconsciousness	Rest in cool room in recumbent position Sponge with cool H_2O Increase intake of fluids Keep record of body weight Discontinue activity until well under control
Heatstroke	Progress from H_2O depletion Failure of all mechanisms for body cooling This is a true medical emergency	Irritability, aggressiveness, emotional instability, hysteria, progression to apathy, disorientation, unsteady gait, glassy stare Skin is hot and dry, pulse is rapid and full, blood pressure falls	Immerse athlete in bathtub cooled with ice or wet compresses with fan blowing Transport to hospital immediately, treat for shock Cooling is top priority

tion may be required to prevent shivering during body cooling.

Air-conditioned room cooling is effective only for minor hyperpyrexia. Antipyretic drugs, such as aspirin, do not help, because they require an intact heat-losing mechanism. Although external cooling should be carried out until the athlete's temperature falls below 100 degrees F (37.7 degrees C), the athlete should be observed for secondary rises in temperature.

Preventing Heat Stress Syndromes

Heat stress syndromes are obviously related to climate, determined by temperature and humidity. Since climate and humidity cannot be controlled, other factors must be,

especially the athlete's condition and acclimatization. Coaching techniques, color and type of uniforms, the time of day, and the intensity of training all contribute to heat injuries. Table 52.1 lists the causes, clinical signs and symptoms, and treatments for heat stress syndromes.

Acclimatization

Acclimatization is the body's adaptation to heat stress and increased capacity to work at high environmental temperatures. Acclimatization was first studied when military personnel were exposed to tropical climates. Unable to work for the first few days, they gradually became able to tolerate high temperatures without becoming exhausted. Acclimatization involves modification in neural, hormonal, and cardiovascular physiology. The changes in cardiovascular physiology are very similar to those observed during general physical training. After acclimatization, there is less subjective discomfort during heat exposure, with less increases in pulse and respiratory rates under the same conditions of heat and stress. Cardiovascular stability with postural changes and activity is also greater. Skin and rectal temperatures remain close to normal, and sweat production increases after acclimatization. Sweating begins sooner after exposure to heat and work, or at a lower environmental temperature, than before acclimatization.

There is a diversity of opinion as to how long full acclimatization takes. Many say that in 4 to 7 days and as little as 90 minutes of exposure to heat per day, the body can fully adapt to the stress of heat, whereas others say that full acclimatization may take 2 months. Previous physical conditioning and exercise enhance the ability to adapt to heat. Once achieved, acclimatization is maintained for several weeks with short periods of reexposure. After 6 weeks of heat exposure, the body may be able to produce two and a half times the person's normal volume of sweat.

Preseason Conditioning

The body's heat-regulating mechanism becomes accustomed to the elevation of internal temperature that accompanies vigorous exercise, often as high as 103 degrees F (39.4 degrees C) in the trained athlete. When tested under conditions of high heat and high humidity, physically fit athletes require much less acclimatization to heat than those out of condition. Because the long-distance runner characteristically can produce elevated internal temperatures, running is a good preseason conditioning exercise. At least 4 weeks of long-distance running should be done in the preseason.

Environmental Conditions

The trainer can test the air a short time prior to any practice or game using a wet

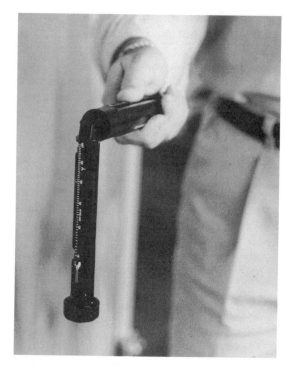

FIGURE 52.1.   A sling psychrometer.

bulb globe temperature index (WBGT index), which is based on the combined effects of air temperature, relative humidity, radiant heat, and air movement. The military has established standards when training is allowed to continue. A sling psychrometer can be used to correlate the dry bulb temperature with relative humidity (Fig. 52.1). Again, when to allow, modify, or prohibit training when the humidity is high should be based on existing standards (Table 52.2). In the event of severe thunderstorms with lightning, all outdoor athletic activities, practices, and games should be suspended.

Coaching Techniques

Equipment and uniforms should be lightweight, porous, and light in color. Sleeves should be short and socks should be low. The athlete should have the opportunity to change perspiration-soaked uniforms during the practice session. As much skin as possible should be exposed to the air.

Practices during hot, humid weather should be held early in the morning or late in the afternoon to avoid the worst heat. Early in the season, night games should be scheduled when possible. However, if games must be played during the late morning or early afternoon in hot, humid climates, the players must be acclimatized to those conditions.

Practice sessions during high-temperature and high-humidity conditions to acclimatize athletes should be shorter and less intense, with less clothing or uniforms and more frequent rest and water breaks than a normal practice session held during the cool part of the day. Frequent rest breaks (10 minutes every half hour) should be allowed during practice. The trainer should consider canceling practice in extreme temperature and humidity. Athletes should weigh out and in after practice daily. Those who have lost 3 percent of their body weight should be excluded from practice. Those who have symptoms of heat illness should also be excluded from practice for 24 hours.

Fluid Replacement

Free intake of fluid during games and practice sessions should be encouraged, but large amounts at any one time should be avoided. The rate of water replacement should be about 1 pint for each pound lost, or 10 ounces every half hour. In ideal situations, the rate of dehydration is controlled by weighing athletes and rehydrating them between practice sessions. Weight should be checked daily and recorded. Research shows that a well-hydrated athlete achieves a state of physical conditioning more rapidly than a poorly hydrated athlete.

Electrolyte Replacement

Electrolyte solutions are unnecessary for individuals with a normal diet unless they are in an event lasting more than 1 hour. No more than 2.5 mg/100 ml of sugar should be contained in fluids available to athletes. Athletes participating in events lasting

TABLE 52.2. Training Standards for High Humidity

Temperature (°F)	Humidity	Procedure
80°–90°	Under 70%	Watch those athletes who tend toward obesity.
80°–90° 90°–100°	Over 70% Under 70%	Athletes should take a 10-minute rest every half hour and tee shirts should be changed when wet. All athletes should be under constant and careful supervision.
90°–100° Over 100°	Over 70%	Under these conditions it would be well to suspend practice. A shortened program conducted in shorts and tee shirts could be established.

longer than 1 hour may benefit from a 5 to 8 percent carbohydrate drink for the prevention of exhaustion.

COLD INJURIES

Pathophysiological Effects of Cold

The human body is a heat-generating mechanism. Its temperature must remain within a narrow range simply for survival—that is, 75 to 112 degrees F (23.9 to 44.4 degrees C). For proper bodily function, the range is even narrower: 98.6 degrees F (37 degrees C), plus or minus a few degrees. In addition to the warmth and heat the body produces, it also gains heat from external sources such as sun, fire, and ingestion of warm foods.

For the purpose of heat regulation, the body consists of a *core* (the brain, heart, lungs, and major abdominal organs) and a *shell* (the skin, muscles, and extremities). When exposed to cold, the body attempts to increase internal heat production by increasing muscular activity, such as shivering, and by increasing the basal metabolic rate at which food stored within the body is burned. Heat loss is decreased by reducing the circulation of blood in the shell.

Cold injury occurs in two ways. In the first way, the core temperature is maintained but the shell temperature decreases, resulting in local injuries that include frostnip, superficial frostbite, deep frostbite, chilblain, trench foot, or immersion foot. In the second way, both the core temperature and the shell temperature fall, systemic hypothermia occurs, all body processes slow down, and the athlete may die if not treated.

Body parts freeze when not enough heat is available to counteract external cold resulting in local injury. Predisposing factors include:

- Inadequate insulation from cold and wind.
- Restricted circulation because of arterial disease or tight clothing, especially footwear.
- Fatigue.
- Poor nutrition.
- The use of alcohol.
- The body's normal effort to maintain its core temperature by shunting the flow of blood away from the shell.

The most commonly affected body parts are hands, feet, ears, and exposed parts of the face. All of these areas are located far from the heart and are normally subjected to rapid heat loss because of a large surface area to volume ratio.

Freezing temperatures affect the cells in the body in a predictable fashion. A cell is mostly water, which becomes cool and eventually freezes and is no longer able to function. The ice crystals that result then destroy the cell. Local cold injuries are the result of injuries of the capillary blood vessels and to other tissue components of the skin and the subcutaneous cells. Cell injuries are all essentially the same, varying only in degree and depth. Duration of the exposure, the temperature to which the skin has been exposed, and wind velocity are the three most important factors to consider when determining the severity of a local injury.

Local Injuries

Frostnip

Frostnip usually affects the tips of the ears, nose, cheeks, chin, fingertips, and toes, usually in conditions of high wind, extreme cold, or both. It is manifested as a sudden blanching or whiteness of the skin. Frostnip comes on slowly and painlessly. The afflicted person often does not notice it, and frequently a companion first perceives it. There may be no permanent tissue damage, and it can be treated effectively by the firm, steady pressure of a warm hand, by blowing warm breath, or by holding the nipped fingers motionless in the armpit. The skin should not be rubbed with snow. As warmth and color return, tingling may occur. After thawing, the skin may turn red and may flake for several days.

Superficial Frostbite

Superficial frostbite usually involves the skin and the underlying superficial tissue. The skin appears white and waxy and is firm to the touch, but the tissue beneath it is soft and resilient. The person should be taken indoors, protected from the cold, and subjected to the same, steady, careful rewarming as for frostnip. Again, the affected area should not be rubbed with snow or by the hand. When the injured area thaws, it is first numb; then it turns mottled blue or purple. Capillary damage and plasma leaks into the tissue cause swelling. If the frostbite is severe, the tissue beneath the outer layers of skin is involved, and blisters may form. Throbbing, aching, and burning may last for weeks. The skin may remain permanently red, tender, and sensitive to reexposure to cold, so these susceptible areas should receive extra protection.

Deep Frostbite

Deep frostbite is extremely serious and usually involves the hands and feet. The tissues are cold, pale, and solid. The tissues deep to the skin and subcutaneous layers are usually injured and may be completely destroyed. Emergency treatment must be rendered as quickly as possible to keep the athlete dry and provide external warming. The injured area turns purplish blue and becomes extremely painful after thawing. Large blisters or gangrene may develop in the first day or two. Permanent tissue damage depends on the temperature and the duration of freezing.

The treatment of the above three conditions calls for early and rapid rewarming by whatever means possible, including warm water baths. If a prolonged delay is anticipated before a medical facility can be reached, rapid rewarming with warm water should be instituted. The temperature of the water should be between 100 to 105 degrees F (37.7 to 40.6 degrees C) with thermometer control, making sure it does not become too hot; the temperature should be kept 6 to 7 degrees F warmer than normal body temperature. The temperature must be checked continually, because immersing the cold extremity causes loss of heat. The container should be large enough so that neither the extremity nor the athlete touches the sides. Rewarming should continue until the frozen area is deep red or bluish in color. The athlete's body temperature can be maintained with warm drinks. Analgesic medication may be needed. When treating frostbite, the trainer must always guard against infection by applying bandages loosely under sterile conditions, being careful not to rupture blisters, and inserting pads between the toes.

Chilblain

Chilblain results from repeated exposure of bare skin to low temperatures for prolonged periods. The injury results in red, swollen, hot, tender, itching areas, usually on the fingers or toes, and the lesions tend to recur in the same areas during cold weather each season. There may be permanent skin changes between the periods of recurrence. This injury represents a chronic injury of the skin and the peripheral capillary circulation. There is no treatment once the skin injury has been established except to prevent recurrence and to protect the area from further exposure to cold.

Trench or Immersion Foot

Trench or **immersion foot** results from the wet cooling of an extremity over hours or days at temperatures slightly above freezing. The lesion represents primary damage to the capillary circulation of the skin, which may progress to necrosis or gangrene of the skin, muscle, and nerves. The involved extremity is cold, swollen, waxy, mottled, and numb. After it is warmed, it becomes red, swollen, and hot, and blisters as well as gangrene may develop. The treatment is to remove the wet, cold footgear and gently rewarm the extremity, maintaining good local hygiene and applying a warm, dry covering.

Treatment of Local Injuries

Only frostnip and superficial frostbite should be treated in the field, with direct application of body heat. Athletes with more serious cold injuries should be taken to a hospital as soon as possible. En route, the damaged area should be protected from further injury, especially from rubbing, chafing, and contusion. If absolutely necessary, an athlete may be allowed to walk on a frostbitten extremity, providing that no thawing has occurred. Walking even a long distance on a frostbitten limb does not lessen the chance of successful treatment if the limb has not thawed. However, once the frozen limb has thawed, the athlete should not be allowed to walk. Walking on a thawed limb with the resulting chance of refreezing is extremely painful and dangerous. Blisters are usually a good prognostic sign, indicating that only a partial thickness of skin has been damaged.

Systemic Hypothermia

General, severe body cooling, or **hypothermia**, can occur at temperatures well above freezing. It is usually caused by exposure to low or rapidly dropping temperatures, cold moisture, snow, or ice. It is aggravated by hunger, fatigue, and exertion and may be associated with other local cold injuries. Documentation of the extent of hypothermia requires a clinical thermometer that can reach a low temperature.

Generalized body cooling progresses through the following five states:

1. Shivering, which is the body's attempt to generate heat.
2. Apathy, sleeplessness, listlessness, and indifference, which may accompany rapid cooling of the body.
3. Unconsciousness, with a glassy stare, a very slow pulse rate, and slow respiratory rate.
4. Freezing of the extremities.
5. Death.

Shivering usually begins at a rectal temperature of 95 degrees F (35 degrees C) and, as the cooling proceeds, clumsiness, fumbling, stumbling, falling, slow reactions, mental confusion, and difficulty in speaking follow. Death may occur within 2 hours of the onset of the first symptoms.

Systemic hypothermia is an acute, first-priority medical emergency and requires the rapid transfer of the athlete to an emergency facility. The basic principles of emergency care are to prevent further heat loss, rewarm the athlete as rapidly and safely as possible, and be alert for complications.

Mild to moderate hypothermia (rectal temperature of 81 to 95 degrees F [27.2 to 35 degrees C] with the athlete conscious) is treated by preventing further heat loss by removing the athlete from the wind, replacing wet clothing, adding appropriate insulating material, and providing external heat in any way possible (hot water bottles, electric blankets, camp fires, or body heat from rescuers). If the athlete is conscious, hot liquids may be given. An effective way of rewarming someone with systemic hypothermia is to immerse the person in a tub of warm water kept between 105 to 110 degrees F (40.6 to 43.3 degrees C). Severe

hypothermia (rectal temperature below 81 degrees F [27.2 degrees C] with unconsciousness) carries serious dangers from cardiac arrhythmias and rewarming shock. While the above procedures are carried out, facilities to diagnose and treat cardiac arrhythmias, especially ventricular fibrillation, should be available. Rewarming shock occurs as the circulatory system of the body warms and veins dilate before the heart becomes able to support the expanded circulation within a dilated system. Vital signs must be monitored and this athlete must be evacuated to a medical facility. Athletes with severe hypothermia should not be warmed in the field. These persons may appear dead yet may still be revived.

Contributing Factors in Cold Injuries

Lack of Preparation

Local cold injuries obviously occur in colder climates when the ambient temperature is closer to freezing and the skin is exposed. Systemic hypothermia, however, can occur during all months of the year, depending on the activities and the altitude. Hunters, hikers, skiers, and climbers exposed to unusually severe weather for which they have not been prepared are in danger of hypothermia. The alcoholic or other ill person whose normal defenses from cold are insufficient can also experience hypothermia in mild conditions.

Inability to Acclimatize

Athletes cannot acclimatize to cold as they can to heat. They therefore must prepare for cold by anticipating weather changes; by having the right clothing available in layers; by having dry clothing available if possible; and, above all, by recognizing the ever-present possibility of hypothermia, regardless of the season. At the same time, the athlete should avoid overdressing, especially with synthetic materials that promote sweating and prevent evaporation.

TABLE 52.3. Wind-chill Factor

						Equivalent Temperature (°F)								
Calm*	35	30	25	20	15	10	5	0	−5	−10	−15	−20	−25	−30
		COLD												
5	32	27	22	16	11	6	0	−5	−10	−15	−21	−26	−31	−36
		VERY COLD												
10	22	16	10	3	−3	−9	−15	−22	−27	−34	−40	−46	−52	−58
		BITTER COLD												
15	16	9	2	−5	−11	−18	−25	−31	−38	−45	−51	−58	−65	−72
20	12	4	−3	−10	−17	−24	−31	−39	−46	−53	−60	−67	−74	−81
25	8	1	−7	−15	−22	−29	−36	−44	−51	−59	−66	−74	−81	−88
		EXTREME COLD												
30	6	−2	−10	−18	−25	−33	−41	−49	−56	−64	−71	−79	−86	−93
35	4	−4	−12	−20	−27	−35	−43	−52	−58	−67	−74	−82	−89	−97
40	3	−5	−13	−21	−29	−37	−45	−53	−60	−69	−76	−84	−92	−100

Wind Speed (miles per hour) is the vertical axis label for the leftmost column.

*"Calm-air" as used in wind-chill determinations actually refers to the conditions created by a person walking briskly (at 4 miles-per-hour) under calm wind conditions.
Source: National Oceanic and Atmospheric Administration.

All people subjected to a cold environment are susceptible to cold injuries. They should be aware of the effect not only of cold but also of windchill (Table 52.3) and understand the value of insulating materials and the layering principle in clothing.

ALTITUDE DISORDERS

Altitude sickness is a maladjustment of the individual to the hypoxia (lack of oxygen) of a high altitude and is generally divided into three syndromes: acute mountain sickness, high-altitude pulmonary edema, and high-altitude cerebral edema. These three forms may appear separately or simultaneously. They are not clear-cut entities and probably represent a common, underlying physiologic response to hypoxia. Almost everyone gets acute mountain sickness when exposed to high altitudes, but few develop the advanced stages. High-altitude pulmonary edema and cerebral edema are serious and potentially fatal.

Altitude sickness is becoming more common as more people are hiking, skiing, and participating in recreational activities at higher altitudes than ever before. Inadequate time on weekend trips to acclimatize to high altitudes is definitely a factor in this condition. Symptoms may appear at 7,500 to 8,000 feet, and death has occurred at altitudes of 8,000 to 9,000 feet. In addition to the problems of hypoxia, people at higher altitudes face insidious temperature changes and increased exposure to ultraviolet rays and radiation.

The basic cause of mountain sickness has not been proved. The severity of symptoms and rapidity of onset vary from person to person. Some people are inherently more susceptible than others, especially young people who have made a rapid ascent.

The symptoms are directly proportional to the rapidity of the ascent, the duration, and the degree of exertion; they are inversely proportional to acclimatization and physical conditioning. The initial signs and symptoms of altitude sickness are from oxygen lack or hypoxia. They are thought to be secondary changes since there may be a lag period before symptoms develop.

Acute Mountain Sickness

Acute mountain sickness is the mildest form of altitude sickness, and most people will experience it when ascending to high altitudes. There is no direct relationship between the altitude and the severity of the illness. Mild to moderate cases occur at all altitudes.

There is a time lag of 6 to 96 hours between arrival and the onset of symptoms, which include headache, difficulty sleeping, early morning arousal, dyspnea on exertion, loss of appetite, light-headedness, fatigue, confusion, weakness, alteration of heart rate, and edema.

Acute mountain sickness is usually self-limited, lasting 2 to 5 days. Headaches usually respond to aspirin. Activities during the early days in high altitude should be reduced, since most people adapt to higher altitudes in a few days. Avoiding fatty foods and eating a high-carbohydrate diet will help control nausea.

High-Altitude Pulmonary Edema

High-altitude pulmonary edema is a more dramatic form of altitude illness and an unusual form of noncardiac pulmonary edema. It may develop on the first exposure to high altitude, but frequently is seen after descent and reascent.

The symptoms of high-altitude pulmonary edema vary in severity. After the symptoms of acute mountain sickness subside, shortness of breath, increased rate of respiration, an irritating cough progressing to hemoptysis (coughing up bright, red blood), and substernal chest pain may develop. The cough produces bloody, frothy sputum. The diagnosis is suspected when rales (the sounds of air bubbling through fluid) are heard in the chest. It is imperative that these people return to a lower altitude as quickly as possible and that they be given oxygen whenever available. They must be thoroughly reevaluated before allowing reascent.

High-Altitude Cerebral Edema

High-altitude cerebral edema is a less common but very dangerous form of altitude sickness. Death has occurred as low as 8,000 feet but is rare below 12,000 feet. Its relationship to high-altitude pulmonary edema is unclear.

The symptoms are initially those of acute mountain sickness but with increasingly severe headaches followed by mental confusion, aggressiveness and emotional instability, hallucinations, and, finally, localized motor weakness and reflex changes. The condition may progress to coma and death. Bradycardia (unusually slow but regular beating of the heart) is an initial finding and may be related to increased cerebral pressure. Judgment and coordination are impaired due to direct local swelling of the brain, especially the cerebellum. Ocular signs and symptoms such as blurring of vision, papilledema (edema of the optic nerve as it enters the eyeball), and retinal and vitreous hemorrhage may develop.

High-altitude pulmonary edema and cerebral edema are emergencies and when suspected, persons should descend. Oxygen should be used when available, and the athlete should be carried down as exercise aggravates both conditions. Corticosteroids, such as dexamethasone or betamethasone, may be used to treat high-altitude cerebral edema, but all of these measures are secondary to descent. A diuretic such as acetazolamide may stabilize breathing.

Preventing Altitude Illness

Preparation for high-altitude activities should include months of cardiovascular and strength training and aerobic conditioning. An aerobically fit person has a higher altitude threshold than an unfit person.

The symptoms of altitude illness are proportional to altitude and duration and degree of exertion divided by acclimatization and physical conditioning. Acclimatization involves a long, slow ascent, going up higher during the day and coming down lower to sleep and rest. Those with coronary vascular disease or chronic obstructive pulmonary disease should avoid areas of low oxygen tension.

UNDERWATER DIVING DISORDERS

The effects of absolute pressure on compressed air/gas exchange may be categorized in three ways. The first way is the direct effects of pressure; second, the indirect effects of pressure; and third, are the interaction of the direct and indirect effects of pressure on the diver. It should also be noted that the diver may have a combination of diving disorders simultaneously.

Direct Effects of Pressure: Squeeze Injuries

Pressure-related problems may occur on descent when the diver is unable to equalize pressure in internal anatomical rigid air spaces or equipment air spaces. Human body natural air spaces have vents which normally allow internal and external pressure to equalize. The lungs are vented by breathing; the middle ear and sinuses are connected by passageways at the back of the throat. If these passageways are blocked due to congestion or a head cold, air trapped in these spaces cannot be equalized on descent. This situation can be painful, and if the pressure imbalance is great enough, can result in ruptured blood vessels or other tissue damage. In diving, the term applied to this problem is **barotrauma**, or **squeeze injury**.

Uncomplicated squeeze injuries of these areas are not medical emergencies and frequently do not require medical treatment. Sinus squeezes and mask area squeezes can be treated by cold packs. Ear squeeze can be complicated by rupture of the eardrum, and immediate treatment is indicated to minimize the chances of middle ear infection, with subsequent hearing loss and balance disturbances. A person with a suspected ruptured eardrum should be transported to an emergency department immediately. A diver who sustains a perforated eardrum must avoid diving until the injury heals, usually in several weeks.

If cold water enters the middle ear, the diver may suddenly experience vertigo, panic, and rapidly ascend to the surface while holding his or her breath. The rapid ascent may cause an air embolism, a problem discussed later in the chapter. Vertigo can cause mental confusion and lead to drowning.

An exceedingly rare descent condition is lung compression, or thoracic squeeze, which occurs when the diver descends deeply and rapidly while holding his or her breath. The prominent symptom is severe chest pain. Emergency treatment consists of resuscitation and life support during transportation to a medical facility. This condition is primarily seen in breath-hold diving and is rare due to the depth of the free dive required to create the disorder.

Indirect Effects of Pressure

Physiologic problems may arise due to increased partial pressure of the breathing mixture while diving. This increased partial pressure of oxygen, nitrogen, and other gases is the culprit in the onset of nitrogen narcosis, oxygen toxicity, carbon dioxide toxicity, carbon monoxide poisoning, and air embolism.

Nitrogen Narcosis

If a diver descends too deeply, increasing partial pressure of nitrogen in the body creates a euphoric effect on the central nervous system—**nitrogen narcosis**, or "rapture of the deep." Divers at or below 100 feet have impaired judgment, even though they do not think so. It is immediately corrected by rising to shallower water. Divers who fail to ascend may become so narcotized that they disregard their own safety and remove their breathing equipment while in the water. Most sports diving instructors limit dives to 130 feet because of the insidious danger of nitrogen narcosis. Susceptibility varies greatly from person to person.

Oxygen Toxicity

Oxygen toxicity may occur in two different ways. The first way is if the diver executes a dive deep enough to increase the partial pressure of the oxygen component in the air mixture to 0.6 atmosphere, 1.6 atmosphere exposure depth, depending on the individual's oxygen tolerance. It should also be noted that the development of toxicity symptoms requires long exposure. Oxygen toxicity will also result if the diver breathes 90 percent pure oxygen at a depth of 33 feet or 2 atmosphere exposure depth. Symptoms include muscle twitching, confusion, nausea, and convulsions.

Treatment of oxygen toxicity is ascension to the surface and breathing normally without the aid of diving equipment. The diver should be watched for evidence of lung irritation or shock and transported to an emergency department for care. Oxygen toxicity is not usually a problem for the sport diver due to time and air restrictions.

Carbon Dioxide Toxicity

The primary concern for the sport diver regarding carbon dioxide toxicity is the buildup of carbon dioxide through improper breathing patterns. This carbon dioxide buildup is due to poor respiratory exchange and may be magnified due to increased partial pressure of carbon dioxide in blood gases. Symptoms may include air hunger (deep labored breathing at an abnormally high or low respiratory rate), shortness of breath, headaches, panic, confusion, and unconsciousness. Primary contributory factors are excessive work or swimming efforts, inadequate respiratory exchange (diver initiated or equipment malfunction), and excessive resistance to breathing for a variety of reasons, both psychological and physical.

Treatment of carbon dioxide toxicity is ascension to the surface and breathing of fresh air. Administration of oxygen is gen-

erally not necessary. Vital signs should be closely monitored, and the athlete should be transported to the emergency department. Carbon dioxide toxicity occurs rarely, but the athletic trainer should be able to recognize the symptoms and provide supportive care prior to transport.

Carbon Monoxide Poisoning

Carbon monoxide poisoning results from filling tanks with air contaminated with carbon monoxide. The symptoms are similar to those seen on the surface: headaches, shortness of breath, and, ultimately, unconsciousness. Carbon monoxide combines with hemoglobin, thus decreasing the oxygen going to the brain. Carbon monoxide poisoning is treated by the immediate breathing of oxygen, which forces the carbon monoxide from the hemoglobin molecule. It can be prevented by careful inspection of all facilities selling compressed air. Unconsciousness may result on ascent due to decreased partial pressure of oxygen, which reduces the amount of available oxygen and creates the hypoxic condition.

Air Embolism

Air embolism, or **arterial gas embolism**, is a condition that occurs in the body when air or other gas bubbles are forced into the arterial system, causing obstruction of blood flow and leading to local hypoxia and tissue death. This condition is the most serious for the compressed air diver and usually affects the central nervous system and the pulmonary system.

Air embolism can occur in dives as shallow as 4 feet if the diver holds his or her breath during a rapid ascent. When water pressure on the chest is rapidly reduced, air within the lungs expands. Rapid expansion of air can rupture alveoli within the lung and damage the adjacent blood vessels. The air can then be forced from the lungs into the blood vessels to travel as emboli in the vascular system to any part of the body. Air bubbles act as obstructions, preventing body tissue from receiving its normal supply of blood and oxygen. Brain damage is obviously the most serious result of air embolisms. Additionally, air can be forced from the lungs into the pleural space or into the mediastinum to create a pneumothorax, mediastinal emphysema, or subcutaneous emphysema.

The following are signs and symptoms of air embolism:

- Mottling or blotching of the skin.
- Frothy or bloody fluid at the nose and mouth.
- Pain in muscles, joints, tendons, or abdomen.
- Difficult breathing and chest pain.
- Dizziness, vomiting, and convulsions.
- Difficulty in speaking and seeing.
- Paralysis and coma.

Immediate treatment for air embolism is to rescue the diver from the water, keep the person calm and quiet, and arrange immediate transport to an emergency department while giving basic life support, including oxygen administration. The person must be kept flat and will require immediate recompression in a hyperbaric chamber.

Direct *and* Indirect Effects of Pressure: Decompression Sickness

Decompression sickness, also known as the **bends**, or **Caisson's disease**, is primarily caused by violating established time/depth limits and exceeding prescribed rates of ascent. The average human body at sea level contains about 1 liter of dissolved nitrogen. All of the body tissues are saturated with nitrogen at a partial pressure equal to the nitrogen partial pressure in the alveoli. When the partial pressure of nitrogen changes in the air mixture during a dive, the body strives to reach equilibrium at the new depth pressure.

The process of taking on more nitrogen gas is called *absorption* or *saturation*, and correspondingly, the process of giving up gas is called *elimination* or *desaturation*. Although the processes of nitrogen uptake and elimination occur in the same way, desaturation occurs much more slowly than saturation, and this is why the diver's as-

cent rate is so critical. Ascending too quickly will not allow the excess nitrogen gained at depth to vent off naturally through respiration. If the diver is over the prescribed time limits at a given depth and returns to the surface without making the required decompression stops, this excess nitrogen will come out of solution in the body in the form of venous gas emboli. As previously mentioned, even the diver who does not exceed time limits at depth, but merely is near time limits and ascends too quickly (faster than 30 to 60 feet/minute), might experience symptoms of decompression sickness.

The pathophysiology of decompression sickness is venous gas emboli forming on the low-pressure side, the venous side, of circulation. These bubbles cause mechanical distortions in the tissues, resulting in pain, edema, hypoxia, and impairment.

There are two types of decompression sickness: Type I (musculoskeletal bends) and Type II (central nervous system bends). Often what determines the type and severity of decompression sickness is the time/depth exposure aggravated by a rapid ascent. It should be noted that decompression sickness is a very complex physiologic event, which is further complicated by individual factors predisposing people to the disorder. Some of these factors are fatigue, age, alcohol, smoking, respiratory/circulatory efficiency, previous surgery or injury, diving in cold water, and strenuous diving.

Symptoms of decompression sickness will vary, depending on whether it is Type I or Type II bends. Symptoms include joint pain, chest pain, back and abdominal pain, shortness of breath, confusion, tingling and numbness in the extremities, loss of bladder control, and paralysis. Unlike the symptoms of air embolism, which are usually immediate, the symptoms of decompression sickness may not occur until some hours after a dive is concluded.

The only treatment for decompression sickness is recompression. The individual is placed in a pressure chamber and subjected to high pressure once again. The nitrogen that was released into the blood is forced back into the tissues, the bubbles are reduced in size, and the symptoms subside. The athlete is then gradually decompressed to allow for the slow and steady release of excess nitrogen.

Damage from the bends is usually temporary. However, if a major cerebral or spinal vessel is blocked, tissue damage may produce permanent effects, including paralysis. To minimize brain damage, oxygen should be given while the person is being transported to a recompression chamber.

Preventing Diving Disorders

To prevent these potentially serious injuries, divers must understand the physiology of gas exchange and the need to use proper breathing techniques while ascending and descending. They must plan the duration and depth of their dives based on the available charts and tables and their level of experience. Finally, their equipment must be checked regularly to ensure it is functioning properly.

IMPORTANT CONCEPTS

1. Body heat is produced by basic metabolic processes, by food intake, and by muscular activity.
2. Heat loss occurs from conduction, convection, evaporation, respiration, and radiation.
3. Heat exhaustion can occur from salt depletion (cold and clammy skin) or excessive water loss (hot and dry skin).
4. Heatstroke is a serious emergency in which tissue is damaged by body heat, vasomotor collapse occurs, blood pressure falls, the pulse becomes rapid and weak, and death ensues if the athlete is not cooled rapidly.
5. Cold injuries occur when either the shell temperature falls or both the core and shell temperatures fall.
6. Deep frostbite is a serious condition because tissues deep to the skin and subcutaneous layers are injured and may be completely destroyed.
7. Dangers of severe hypothermia include cardiac arrhythmias and rewarming shock, which occurs as the circulatory system of the body warms and veins dilate before the heart becomes able to support the expanded circulation within a dilated system.
8. "Squeeze injuries," which can occur underwater during descent when the diver is unable to equalize pressure in the air spaces of the body or the diving equipment, can result in ruptured blood vessels or other tissue damage.
9. Air embolism is a condition that occurs in the body when air or other gas bubbles are forced into the arterial system, causing obstruction of blood flow and leading to local hypoxia and tissue death.

SUGGESTED READINGS

Aamon, H. V. *Principles Governing the Absorption of Water, Electrolytes, and Other Nutrients.* Washington, D.C.: Food and Nutrition Board, National Research Council, 1982.

Adolph, E. F. *Physiology of Man in the Desert.* New York: Interscience Publishers, 1947.

Armstrong, L. E., R. W. Hubbard, P. C. Szlyk, I. V. Sils, et al. "Heat Intolerance, Heat Exhaustion Monitored: A Case Report." *Aviation Space and Environmental Medicine* 59 (1988): 262–266.

Costill, D. L., and J. M. Miller. "Nutrition for Endurance Sport: Carbohydrate and Fluid Balance." *International Journal of Sports Medicine* 1 (1980): 2–14.

Fox, E., ed. *Nutrient Utilization during Exercise.* Columbus, Ohio: Ross Laboratories, 1983, pp. 1–138.

Graver, D., ed. *Advanced Diving Technology and Techniques.* Montclair, Calif.: National Association of Underwater Instructors, 1989.

Leithead, C. S., and A. R. Lind. *Heart Stress and Heat Disorders.* Philadelphia: F. A. Davis, 1964.

Mitchell, J. B., D. L. Costill, J. A. Houmard, et al. "Effects of Carbohydrate Ingestion of Gastric Emptying and Exercise Performance." *Medicine and Science in Sports and Exercise* 20 (1988): 110–115.

Murray, R. "The Effects of Consuming Carbohydrate-Electrolyte Beverages on Gastric Emptying and Fluid Absorption during and following Exercise." *Sports Medicine* 4 (1987): 322–351.

Nielsen, B., G. Sjφgaard, J. Ugelvig, et al. "Fluid Balance in Exercise Dehydration and Rehydration with Different Glucose-Electrolyte Drinks." *European Journal of Applied Physiology and Occupational Physiology* 55 (1986): 318–325.

Thomas, B., and B. McKenzie. *The Diver's Medical Companion.* Brisbane, Australia: Diving Medical Services, 1981.

Additional Information on Scuba Diving

Divers Alert Network
Duke University Medical Center
Durham, NC 27710

The National Association of Underwater Instructors
P.O. Box 14650
Montclair, CA 91763-1150

The Professional Association of Diving Instructors
1243 East Warner Avenue
Santa Ana, CA 92705

The Young Men's Christian Association
6083A Oakbrook Parkway
Norcross, GA 30093

53

Asthma

OBJECTIVES FOR CHAPTER 53

After reading this chapter, the student should be able to:

1. Understand the pathogenesis of asthma and its clinical manifestations.
2. Identify which medications are commonly used to treat asthma and which of these medications are permitted by the International Olympic Committee for use by competitive athletes with asthma.
3. Understand the cause and treatment of exercise-induced asthma.

INTRODUCTION

Asthma is a condition with profound medical and economic consequences. Almost 10.5 percent of the U.S. population is estimated to have asthma, and since 1977, mortality from asthma has been slowly increasing. In 1984, mortality reached 3,600. Some researchers theorize that environmental factors such as air pollution and increased bronchodilator use may be causative factors in the increasing mortality rate. The annual cost of asthma therapy in the United States is estimated at $11 billion.

Chapter 53 begins with an explanation of the symptoms and causes of asthma. The chapter next discusses the pharmacologic treatment of asthma and describes the major drugs that are delivered by inhalation, orally, and intravenously. The last section focuses on exercise-induced asthma, a type of asthma that athletic trainers and coaches commonly see. ▪

PATHOGENESIS

Asthma is a Greek word for panting or shortness of breath. It is defined as a clinical syndrome characterized by increased responsiveness of the tracheobronchial tree to a variety of stimuli. The major symptoms of asthma are paroxysms of dyspnea, wheezing, and coughing, which may vary from being mild and almost undetectable to severe and unremitting. The primary physiological manifestation of this hyperresponsiveness is variable airway obstruction.

In asthma, the airways narrow as a result of a combination of events, including spasm in the smooth muscle layers of the airways (which may be caused by cooling of the airways), edema in the airway lining cells, and changes in the quantity and character of mucus secreted.

The narrowed airways affect conduction of air to the alveoli, which disrupts the normal relationship between ventilation and perfusion. Inadequate oxygen may thus be supplied by ventilation, and a waste product, carbon dioxide, may not be sufficiently cleared. The work of breathing is increased as a result of airway narrowing, in turn increasing resistance to airflow.

CLINICAL MANIFESTATIONS

Diagnosis

The asthmatic athlete has difficulty in breathing as a consequence of the aforementioned increase in the work of breathing. Auscultation of the chest (listening to sounds inside the chest) reveals continuous whistling noises called **wheezes**, which are most commonly heard during expiration. Expiration is markedly prolonged, and inspiration may be either normal or prolonged. Expiratory effort is increased and, therefore, is often tiring and frightening for the athlete. Repetitive coughing usually accompanies wheezing, although occasionally coughing is the only presenting sign of asthma.

In contrast, partial upper airway obstruction, which usually occurs at the level of the larynx, results in the athlete's experiencing difficulty with inspiration. In **hyperventilation**, which can occur without any obvious cause, the athlete feels unable to inhale a deep enough breath but can exhale easily.

Precipitating Factors

Allergy has been found to be an important precipitating factor in both childhood-onset and adult-onset asthma. However, asthma often occurs in those with no allergies. Respiratory infections (particularly viral infections), occupational agents, environmental factors, medications, and exercise are among stimuli that can provoke an asthma attack in susceptible individuals.

TREATMENT

Avoidance of Known Stimuli

Although asthma can occur or subside at any age, treatment should be initiated based on the assumption that the condition is chronic. Avoidance of stimuli known to precipitate an attack in an individual is desirable whenever possible and can be aided by use of devices such as air conditioners and electrostatic cleaners.

Pharmacologic Therapy

Pharmacologic therapy is the mainstay of treatment for asthma. Several categories of medications are used to treat asthma, and the drugs within each category can often be delivered by more than one route. In general, inhaled medications have fewer side effects but a shorter duration of action. They are also more time-consuming to administer than their oral counterparts. Parenteral (intravenous) medication is reserved for emergency situations and hospital treatment. The proper combination of oral and inhaled therapy will permit optimal control of a potentially debilitating condition. A description of the major classes of medications, which may be used singly or in combination in asthma treatment, depending on the severity of the athlete's asthma, follows.

Beta Adrenergic Drugs

Beta adrenergic drugs such as albuterol, terbutaline, and metaproterenol cause dilation of bronchial smooth muscle, alter airway responsiveness, and inhibit release of chemicals from mast cells (connective tissue cells that contain histamine and heparin) which result in airway inflammation. These medications can be administered in inhaled, oral, or parenteral form and are very effective in the treatment of exercise-induced asthma. A 12-hour sustained release form of albuterol is available. Side effects include skeletal muscle tremors and vasodilation.

Theophylline

Theophylline, a methylxanthine, appears to exert a direct relaxing effect on the smooth and skeletal muscle, perhaps through calcium ion exchange. It may also reduce mucous tenacity. It has recently been downgraded in importance in the treatment of asthma because of its narrow therapeutic range, interactions with other medications, adverse side effects such as vomiting and diarrhea when the drug is given in therapeutic doses, and potentially toxic effects such as arrythmias and convulsions. However, its prolonged duration of action in sustained release form, as well as its beneficial effect in exercise-induced asthma, makes it a valuable medication in the proper setting. It is available as a continuous intravenous medication or in oral form.

Cromolyn Sodium

Cromolyn sodium, or disodium cromoglycate, is an inhaled medication that stabilizes mast cells against attack by both specific antigens and nonspecific stimuli such as exercise and ozone. Mast cells release mediators that induce or exacerbate asthma attacks. Cromolyn helps prevent mediator release. It also appears to blunt some immunological challenges that do not involve mast cells and reduces bronchial hyperreactivity when used long term in allergic asthmatic individuals. It seems to be more useful in children than adults and is not as effective as inhaled beta adrenergic agents in treating exercise-induced asthma.

Corticosteroids

Corticosteroids are available in oral, parenteral, and inhaled forms. They exert an anti-inflammatory effect which is delayed in onset. They also enhance the responsiveness of airways to beta adrenergic drugs. The latter effect is much more rapid in onset. Prolonged use of any but the inhaled form of this class of medications should be avoided if possible because of potentially serious side effects, for example, fluid and electrolyte disturbances, peptic ulcer, and convulsions.

Ipratropium Bromide

Ipratropium bromide is an anticholinergic drug available in inhaled form only. Stimulation of cholinergic receptors in the lung causes bronchospasm. Anticholinergic drugs relieve bronchospasm, but they are not direct bronchodilators. This medication is not as effective in treating asthma as beta adrenergic agents.

EXERCISE-INDUCED ASTHMA

Exercise-induced asthma (exercise-induced bronchospasm) is not an uncommon problem in athletes. This condition is an acute, reversible, self-limited episode of airway obstruction that occurs in both small and large airways either during or after physical activity.

Frequency

Exercise-induced asthma occurs in individuals with a previous history of asthma, as well as those who have never had an attack. Three percent of the U.S. population are asthmatic, and 90 percent of these people will get exercise-induced asthma. Of the 12 percent of the population who suffer from allergies, 30 percent will develop exercise-induced asthma. Three to 4 percent of the population without allergies will develop exercise-induced asthma.

At the 1984 Olympic Games, 67 athletes had exercise-induced asthma. Forty-one of these athletes won medals. Several medal winners have had exercise-induced asthma, including Rick Demont, who was disqualified from the 1972 Olympics because he used Marax for asthma control. Marax contains ephedrine and hydroxyzine in addition to theophylline. Ephedrine and hydroxyzine are banned by the International Olympic Committee. Theophylline is a permitted medication as long as athletes notify their own national Olympic committee that they are on such medication.

Cause

Why does exercise-induced asthma occur? No one really knows. At one time, it was thought that exercise-induced asthma was related to arterial-alveolar oxygen difference, but that link has not been proven. Others believe that it is caused by a loss of heat or water from the respiratory tract through breathing cold, dry air during exercise. This school of thought believes that swimming is not as inducive to developing asthma as is running. In keeping with this theory, athletes with a tendency to develop exercise-induced asthma have been encouraged to breathe through their noses so the air will be better humidified and warmed, and hence, their risk of developing exercise-induced asthma will decrease.

Others believe that the development of exercise-induced asthma is related to histamine release with exercise. Cooling of the mast cells in the respiratory tree is thought to cause them to release histamine. There is, however, no proof that this activation occurs. Among other proposed causes is the fact that physical stress and increased intensity of exercise can increase the reactivity of smooth muscle in the airways.

Prevention and Treatment

As mentioned earlier in this chapter, medications that are particularly effective in the treatment of exercise-induced asthma include the beta adrenergic drugs and theophylline. Among the anti-asthmatic medications that are approved by the International Olympic Committee for use dur-

ing competition are the various types of beta adrenergic drugs (inhalant form only), theophylline, cromolyn sodium, and ipratropium bromide.

IMPORTANT CONCEPTS

1. Asthmatics have difficulty with expiration; inspiration may be normal or prolonged.
2. Precipitating factors for asthma include allergies, respiratory infections, occupational agents, environmental factors, medications, and exercise.
3. Medications used in the treatment of asthma include beta adrenergic drugs, theophyl-line, cromolyn sodium, corticosteroids, and ipratropium bromide.
4. Asthma medications permitted by the International Olympic Committee for use in competitive athletes include the beta adrenergic drugs (inhalant form only), theophylline, cromolyn sodium, and ipratropium bromide.

SUGGESTED READINGS

Bailey, W. C., ed. *Clinics in Chest Medicine*, vol. 5, no. 4. Philadelphia: W. B. Saunders, 1984.
Journal of Respiratory Diseases (June 1989), Supplement.
Journal of Respiratory Diseases (August 1989), Supplement.
Standards for the Diagnosis and Care of Patients with Chronic Obstructive Pulmonary Disease (COPD) and Asthma. New York: American Lung Association, 1987.

54

Diabetes

OBJECTIVES FOR CHAPTER 54

After reading this chapter, the student should be able to:

1. Understand how diabetes mellitus affects carbohydrate metabolism.
2. Discuss the ways in which diet, exercise, and hypoglycemic agents may be used to regulate diabetes mellitus.
3. Recognize the signs and symptoms of insulin shock and diabetic coma, and be able to provide emergency treatment for each situation.
4. Describe the steps to take in order to prevent insulin shock in athletes.

INTRODUCTION

Diabetes, a disorder of carbohydrate metabolism caused by a deficiency of available insulin, can usually be controlled by careful regulation of factors such as diet, exercise, and hypoglycemic agents such as insulin. When these factors are in dysequilibrium, problems develop, and some of them can be life-threatening. The athletic trainer and coach should understand the importance of maintaining proper blood sugar levels and how to respond when the diabetic athlete requires medical assistance.

Chapter 54 describes the disorder of diabetes mellitus and how it is classified into insulin-dependent and non-insulin-dependent diabetes. The chapter then focuses on the effects of too much or too little insulin—insulin shock and diabetic coma, respectively. The last section of Chapter 54 presents procedures to be followed in the prevention of insulin shock in athletes. ■

PATHOGENESIS

Diabetes mellitus is a disorder of carbohydrate metabolism caused by a deficiency of available insulin. **Insulin**, a hormone secreted by the pancreas, is essential in the metabolism of glucose. It promotes storage of glucose in the muscles and liver in the form of glycogen. Insulin is also needed for the efficient transfer of glucose from the bloodstream into skeletal and cardiac muscles.

Carbohydrate Metabolism

When carbohydrates are eaten, they are digested into monosaccharides and then changed into glucose. Glucose is absorbed from the small intestine into the bloodstream. As the glucose level rises, the beta cells of the islets of Langerhans in the pancreas are stimulated to secrete insulin. As the glucose level drops, the secretion of insulin decreases.

Other hormones in the body such as epinephrine, glucagon, growth hormone, cortisol, and catecholamines raise the blood glucose level. The interaction of these substances with insulin, in addition to diet and exercise, regulates the blood sugar level. Normal blood sugar levels are between 70 and 120 mg/dl.

In diabetes mellitus, because of a deficiency or total lack of insulin, the blood sugar level rises above normal levels, a condition called **hyperglycemia**. Hyperglycemia leads to the excretion of glucose in the urine (**glycosuria**). When glucose is excreted, it draws with it a large amount of water. The excretion of excessive urine is called **polyuria** and leads to excessive thirst (**polydypsia**).

Ketoacidosis

Without insulin, the body cannot metabolize glucose, and the primary source of energy is then derived from burning fats. The end products of fat metabolism are **ketone bodies**. These ketone bodies alter the acid-base relationship, resulting in a decrease in the body's pH, a condition called **ketoacidosis**. In an attempt to diminish the acidosis and bring the pH of the body back to normal (7.35 to 7.45), the respiratory system tries to increase its elimination of carbon dioxide by deep respirations. The deep sighing respirations seen in diabetic ketoacidosis or coma are called **Kussmaul breathing**.

Ketoacidosis, plus dehydration, depresses the nervous system, and the person becomes confused and somnolent and may lapse into diabetic coma. In diabetic coma, acetones are expired from the lungs and give the breath a fruity odor.

CLASSIFICATION OF DIABETES MELLITUS

Diabetes mellitus for clinical purposes is classified into two main types: **insulin-dependent diabetes mellitus (IDDM)** and **non-insulin-dependent diabetes mellitus (NIDDM)**.

Insulin-Dependent Diabetes Mellitus (IDDM)

As the name implies, IDDM (also known as **Type I** or **juvenile-onset diabetes**) can be regulated only by the daily use of insulin. The onset of IDDM is usually quite sudden and is most commonly found in individuals less than 30 years of age. IDDM, often termed "brittle diabetes," is sometimes difficult to regulate. In these insulin-sensitive individuals, swings in blood sugar levels from hyperglycemic (high blood sugar) to hypoglycemic (low blood sugar) can be quite rapid. Insulin must be injected, because when taken orally, it is broken down by digestive enzymes in the stomach before its effects are realized.

Non-Insulin-Dependent Diabetes Mellitus (NIDDM)

NIDDM (also known as **Type II** or **adult-onset diabetes**) can usually be controlled by diet and exercise alone, or by the addition of medications (oral hypoglycemics) which lower blood glucose levels. The onset of NIDDM is usually much slower. It is usually found in obese individuals over the age of 40 and is generally not associated with the development of ketoacidosis.

EFFECTS OF TOO MUCH OR TOO LITTLE INSULIN

Insulin Shock

The three factors that can stabilize or control diabetes mellitus are diet, exercise, and hypoglycemic agents such as insulin or the oral hypoglycemics. In well-controlled diabetes, these three factors are in equilibrium. Since exercise lowers the blood sugar, any increase in the level of exercise must be compensated for by increasing food intake or by lowering the amount of hypoglycemic agent given. If compensatory changes are not made, the blood sugar will drop below normal levels (**hypoglycemia**) and the athlete will go into **hypoglycemic shock**, also called **insulin shock.**

Symptoms

Severe hypoglycemia or insulin shock is life-threatening. Symptoms of hypoglycemia are variable and nonspecific. They include irritability, trembling, hunger, sweating, apprehension, confusion, convulsions, and coma. All diabetic athletes should be watched closely, especially during the first weeks of exercise until the diet, insulin, and exercise levels are stabilized and constant. Since exercise lowers the blood sugar, the level of training should be increased slowly, and frequent adjustments in diet and/or the amount of insulin given must be made.

Treatment

Many diabetic athletes require sugar about every 30 minutes during the exercising session and a carbohydrate snack before the exercise session begins. At the first signs or symptoms of hypoglycemia, all exercise should cease, and sugar should be given immediately. Sugar can be given in the form of such foods as sweetened orange juice, candy bars, fruit, sugar-sweetened soft drinks, or sugar cubes. Many diabetic athletes carry commercial glucose tablets and gels for "low-sugar" emergencies. They can be used if the athlete is responsive enough to swallow. Prompt recovery should follow their administration.

If the onset of hypoglycemia is so abrupt that the athlete is unable to swallow, he or she should be immediately transported to a medical facility where intravenous glucose can be given. The trainer should never try to put sugared fluid into the mouth of an unconscious individual, as aspiration of this material into the lungs may occur. Failure to respond promptly to insulin shock may result in brain damage or death.

Diabetic Coma

Hyperglycemia may progress to **hyperglycemic shock,** also called **diabetic coma.** Contrary to the rapid onset of hypoglycemic shock, diabetic coma from hyperglycemia usually develops quite slowly, usually over a period of several days. Precipitating factors can be severe infections, dietary indiscretions, and failure to take insulin or hypoglycemic agents.

Symptoms

As sugar levels rise, the athlete becomes dull and somnolent. Polyuria results in dehydration. Kussmaul breathing is usually apparent, as is the fruity odor of acetone on the breath. Diabetic coma is rarely seen in an actively exercising diabetic athlete.

Treatment

The symptoms of hyperglycemia are somewhat similar to those of hypoglycemia, and the trainer may not be certain which condition the athlete has. For this reason, *all* stuporous or lethargic diabetic athletes should be assumed to have hypoglycemic shock and be given sugar immediately as described previously in the treatment of hypoglycemia. The amount of sugar ingested could be lifesaving for the hypoglycemic athlete and generally results in immediate improvement in medical status. In the unlikely event that the athlete is suffering shock from hyperglycemia, this sugar dose would not improve mental status, but neither would it cause additional harm. Therefore, sugar should be given as an emergency measure to any diabetic athlete who is lethargic or stuporous, followed by prompt transport to the hospital if recovery is not immediately apparent.

PREVENTION OF HYPOGLYCEMIA IN ATHLETES

Since exercise reduces the blood sugar level, to prevent hypoglycemia reactions the following procedures should be followed:

■ An athlete's diabetes should be well controlled before he or she is permitted to play.

■ Exercise sessions should be consistent, at the same time every day, and of approximately the same intensity and duration.

■ Exercise during the peak of insulin activity should be avoided, or if this is not possible, the athlete should eat a high-carbohydrate snack like juice and crackers or milk and cookies about 30 minutes before exercise begins.

■ Since exercise enhances circulation to the muscles of the legs and arms and, hence, would enhance the absorption of insulin, insulin should be given in the abdomen, not the arms or legs.

■ During prolonged activity, about 10 gm of carbohydrates should be ingested every 30 minutes (a piece of fruit, 4 ounces of juice, or a soft drink). Sugar cubes, candy bars, fruit, and soft drinks containing sugar should be available at all times, and the athlete should be told to stop all activities and to ingest some sugar at the first sign or symptom of hypoglycemia.

■ Adequate replacement of fluid is essential.

Since hypoglycemia may occur at anytime, sports such as mountain climbing, in which falls may be catastrophic, should probably be discouraged.

Any diabetic athlete who becomes confused, dizzy, apprehensive, and sweaty should be treated for insulin shock and transported to the nearest medical facility immediately if he or she does not respond to sugar within 2 or 3 minutes. Diabetic coma is extremely rare in active athletes, and the amount of sugar given will not significantly aggravate hyperglycemia.

Most diabetic athletes are well versed in controlling their blood glucose levels. As a part of the medical history taken in conjunction with the preseason physical evaluation, the diabetic athlete should detail his or her normal management plan—how he or she best balances food intake, insulin requirements, and activity levels—so that this information is available to those providing medical coverage for the team. Sports medicine professionals covering an unfamiliar team should be alerted to any diabetic athletes who may require assistance.

Blood glucose monitoring devices that analyze blood sugar levels through fingertip puncture blood samples have given the diabetic athlete even more control over adjusting the insulin dosage to meet the glucose fluctuations that result from exercise and other vigorous activities. Those caring for the diabetic athlete should be familiar with the use of these monitoring devices.

IMPORTANT CONCEPTS

1. Insulin is a hormone released by the pancreas that promotes the storage of glucose in the muscles and liver.
2. In diabetes mellitus, because of a deficiency or total lack of insulin, the blood sugar level rises above normal levels, a condition called hyperglycemia.
3. Insulin-dependent diabetics need daily doses of injected insulin; non-insulin-dependent diabetics can usually be controlled by diet and exercise alone, or by taking medications that lower blood glucose levels.
4. When blood sugar levels drop below normal, the athlete develops hypoglycemia, which can progress to insulin shock.
5. At the first signs of insulin shock, the conscious athlete must be given sugar in the form of orange juice, candy bars, sugar-sweetened soft drinks, or sugar cubes.
6. Any time a diabetic athlete is lethargic or stuporous, he or she should be treated for insulin shock because sugar is life-saving if the athlete is hypoglycemic and not harmful if the athlete is hyperglycemic.
7. Any diabetic athlete who does not recover within 2 or 3 minutes of receiving sugar should be transported immediately to the hospital.

SUGGESTED READINGS

Koivisto, V., and P. Felig. *Exercise in Diabetes: Clinical Implications in Diabetes Mellitus*, vol. 5, edited by H. Rifkin and P. Raskin. Bowie, Md.: Robert J. Brady Co., 1981, pp. 137–144.
LaPorte, R. E., J. S. Dorman, N. Tajima, et al. "Pittsburgh Insulin-Dependent Diabetes Mellitus Morbidity and Mortality Study: Physical Activity and Diabetic Complications." *Pediatrics* 78 (1986): 1027–1033.
Ruderman, N. B., O. P. Ganda, and K. Johansen. "The Effect of Physical Training on Glucose Tolerance and Plasma Lipids in Maturity-Onset Diabetes." *Diabetes* (Supplement 1) 28 (1979): 89–92.

55
Epilepsy

OBJECTIVES FOR CHAPTER 55

After reading this chapter, the student should be able to:

1. Understand the diagnosis of epilepsy and its manifestations.
2. Know how to manage the athlete experiencing a seizure.
3. Recognize the medical considerations involved in permitting epileptics to participate in sports.

878

INTRODUCTION

An athlete who is suddenly stricken with a seizure may or may not be a diagnosed epileptic. It could be the athlete's first epileptic seizure, or the seizure could be related to other problems or disorders. What is important for the athletic trainer to know is what kind of seizures are possible and how to manage them when they do occur.

Chapter 55 begins by describing epilepsy and the seizures that accompany this disorder. The chapter then discusses two types of seizures, generalized and partial, and their management. The last section of Chapter 55 discusses the somewhat controversial issue concerning sports participation by epileptics. ■

A SEIZURE DISORDER

Epilepsy refers to any of the disorders caused by an abnormal focus of electrical activity in the brain that produces seizures. A **seizure**, or **convulsion**, is characterized by generalized, uncoordinated muscular activity and changes in the level of consciousness which last for variable periods of time. Seizures can vary in form from severe convulsions to simply "blacking out" for a few seconds. A state of sleepiness or unconsciousness follows the seizure.

Not all seizures are caused by epilepsy; they may also occur as a result of a recent or old brain injury, a brain tumor, a cerebral embolus causing an acute block of blood flow within the brain (stroke), infection, fever, diabetes, or simply a genetic predisposition.

CLASSIFICATION OF SEIZURES

Seizures are generally classified according to the degree and location of abnormal electrical activity in the brain. Seizure episodes are classified into two categories: generalized seizures and partial seizures.

Generalized Seizure

In a **generalized seizure** (convulsive or **tonic-clonic**), most of the brain is affected. There are usually three phases of a generalized seizure: the aura, the convulsion, and the postictal state.

Aura

The **aura** is a sensation that something is about to happen; it precedes the convulsion in many persons with epilepsy. It can take many forms (a sound, a twitch, dizziness, a feeling of anxiety, or a characteristic smell), but for the epileptic the aura is usually the same and is a warning that a seizure is about to begin. The aura lasts only a few seconds and is followed by the convulsion.

Convulsion

During the convulsion, the jaw muscles contract, which may lead to biting the tongue or lips. Loss of bowel or bladder control is common, and involuntary urination or defecation often occurs. Sustained, *tonic* (rigid) muscular contractions, which can cause abnormal posturing of the body, may last several minutes. *Clonic* (repetitive) muscular activity, or spasms, may be superimposed on the rigid muscular contractions.

Postictal State

After one to several minutes, the convulsive phase is followed by the **postictal state**. The postictal state is a period of exhaustion and recovery following the convulsion. During this phase, which may last for 10 to 30 minutes, the athlete's level of consciousness is depressed; the airway may become obstructed by mucus, vomitus, or the relaxed pharyngeal muscles; and respirations may be slowed.

Partial Seizure

Simple partial seizures involve less extensive areas of the brain. The seizure activity may be limited to one or more extremities or one side of the body, in which case it is called a simple partial seizure.

In a **complex partial seizure**, consciousness may be clouded, or the individual may display automatic behavior such as chewing, fumbling with clothes, walking aimlessly, muttering, or unresponsiveness.

MANAGEMENT OF SEIZURES

Management of a Generalized Seizure

The first important step in the management of a generalized seizure is to protect the athlete from inflicting self-injury. When an epileptic athlete says that a seizure is about to occur (the aura is present), the trainer should immediately help the athlete to lie down on the ground away from danger, to minimize chance of injury during the seizure. The athlete's head, arms, and legs should be protected, but not rigidly restrained. Clothing should be loosened.

Nothing should be forced into the athlete's mouth, especially if the teeth are clenched or if the person is convulsing. Padded "bite sticks" made by taping tongue depressors together have been popular to prevent an epileptic from biting his or her lips, cheeks, or tongue. In some cases, however, the person has bitten the stick in two, or it has become lodged in the pharynx and obstructed the airway. The athletic trainer's fingers should never be put into the athlete's mouth.

Contraction of the chest muscles may cause the convulsing athlete to appear to have an airway obstruction and to become cyanotic. Normal respiration almost always follows a seizure. Lack of respiration during the seizure rarely presents a problem unless

several convulsions follow one another in quick succession. The trainer can help keep the airway open by placing the athlete on one side, head down, so that gravity will help keep the tongue out of the pharynx and prevent aspiration of vomitus.

During the postictal state, the athletic trainer should assess the athlete's airway, clear any mucus or vomitus, and maintain the airway adequately until the athlete is fully awake. Once vital signs are assessed and recorded, a secondary survey of the person should be performed. The trainer should look for any injuries that may have occurred during the seizure.

The athlete who has a history of epilepsy and who has frequent, recurring seizures usually achieves complete recovery of function soon after the seizure, and transportation to the hospital is not necessary. However, the athlete should consult his or her physician to determine whether an alteration in the seizure medication is needed. Athletes without a history of previous seizures should have a thorough medical evaluation to discover the cause of the seizure and receive treatment for prevention of further seizures.

Some people with epilepsy experience **status epilepticus**, in which one seizure closely follows another, with no return of full consciousness between them. This situation is potentially serious, since the person does not have time to breathe well and recover from the stress of the initial seizure. Respiratory distress and fatigue also may occur if a single seizure is prolonged, lasting longer than 10 minutes. The athlete who experiences either status epilepticus or prolonged convulsion should be transported promptly to the hospital for emergency medical assistance.

Management of a Partial Seizure

In managing a partial seizure, the same general rules apply as for managing a generalized seizure. It may be difficult to diagnose a complex partial seizure, which may be mistaken for intoxication, drug abuse, insulin shock, or another medical condition causing abnormal behavior.

A cardinal rule concerning the management of anyone with aberrant behavior is that the person should not be physically restrained unless it is essential for safety. The person may react violently to restraint.

During a complex partial seizure, which may last 15 minutes or longer, the person is in a confused state but is usually amenable to suggestions and comments given in a friendly manner. It is usually possible to control the person for the duration of the seizure. The trainer must stay with the athlete, provide reassurance, and observe the athlete carefully until the abnormal behavior ceases. The athlete with a history of such seizures should consult his or her physician to determine if a change in medication is required. A thorough medical evaluation is needed to evaluate and diagnose the cause of this type of seizure.

Role of the Athletic Trainer

Seizures may be generalized or partial, but in all cases the role of the athletic trainer is to protect the athlete from injury when possible; keep the airway open; determine the extent of injuries, if any, incurred during the seizure; and transport the athlete to the emergency department when necessary. The athletic trainer should provide a calm, reassuring presence at all times, not only for the benefit of the athlete, who may be disoriented following the seizure, but also for the benefit of the athlete's teammates, who may not be familiar with epilepsy.

SPORTS PARTICIPATION

Epileptics' participation in sports has recently received increased publicity as several prominent professional football and baseball athletes with epilepsy have spoken publicly on the ability of epileptics to pursue athletics. Two issues on this subject merit discussion. Is there a risk of precipitating seizures with exercise? Is there a risk of serious injury if the seizure occurs during exercise?

Some authorities believe that people with epilepsy should not participate in exercise, because stress or exhaustion secondary to exercise would increase the risk of seizures. However, this is not presently a commonly held belief. Other authorities believe that hyperventilation during swimming would precipitate a seizure. This issue is currently being debated, with no known answer.

Some authorities still believe that seizure-prone athletes should not participate in sports in which a high risk of injury is possible if a seizure occurred, such as gymnastics, diving, mountain climbing, hang gliding, and biking. However, most experts do not believe epileptics should be restricted from participating in all physical exercise. When epileptics do participate in sports, proper seizure control is mandatory, as is supervision during sports participation. The American Academy of Pediatrics in its position statement in 1983 concluded that the responsibility of determining whether an epileptic child can participate in sports is a "joint responsibility of parent, physician, and child."

(Important Concepts appear on next page.)

IMPORTANT CONCEPTS

1. Epilepsy refers to any of the disorders caused by abnormal electrical activity in the brain and is characterized by convulsions or seizures.
2. Seizures are classified into generalized (most of the brain is affected) and partial (less extensive areas of the brain are involved).
3. Three phases of a generalized seizure are the aura (feeling that an attack is about to occur), convulsion, and postictal state (period of exhaustion and recovery, following a seizure).
4. Status epilepticus, or when one seizure follows another with no return to full consciousness between them, constitutes a medical emergency.

SUGGESTED READINGS

American Academy of Pediatrics: Committee on Children with Handicaps and Committee on Sports Medicine. "Sports and the Child with Epilepsy." *Pediatrics* 72 (1983): 884–885.

Jeavons, P. M., and A. Aspinall. *The Epilepsy Reference Book: Direct and Clear Answers to Everyone's Questions.* London: Harper & Row, 1985.

Porter, R. J. *Epilepsy: 100 Elementary Principles.* London: W. B. Saunders, 1984.

Solomon, G. E., H. Kutt, and F. Plum. *Clinical Management of Seizures: A Guide for the Physician,* 2d ed. Philadelphia: W. B. Saunders, 1983.

56

Communicable Diseases

CHAPTER OUTLINE

Terms and Definitions
Modes of Transmission
Precautions against Contamination

OBJECTIVES FOR CHAPTER 56

After reading this chapter, the student should be able to:

1. Understand what a communicable disease is and how it is transmitted.
2. Recognize the signs and symptoms of the various communicable diseases.
3. Take precautions to reduce the risk of self-contamination and contamination of other personnel from communicable diseases.

INTRODUCTION

Communicable diseases can range in severity from mild to life-threatening. Athletic trainers and coaches should understand the nature of a communicable disease and be able to recognize the signs and symptoms of the most frequently encountered communicable diseases. They should also know how to reduce the risk of contamination to themselves and others. Chapter 56 defines the terms that are routinely used to describe communicable diseases, describes the major modes of transmission, and stresses the importance of taking precautionary measures to protect against contamination from infectious agents. ▪

TERMS AND DEFINITIONS

Infection: The disease state produced in a host by the invasion of an infecting organism such as a virus, bacterium, or parasite.

Contamination: The presence of an infectious agent on body surfaces, in water or food, or on objects such as wound dressings. All surfaces, unless sterilized, should be considered contaminated.

Host: The organism or person in whom an infectious agent resides. A host is infected.

Carrier: A person or animal that may transmit an infectious disease while having no clinical evidence of the disease.

Reservoir: The place where the infecting organisms live and multiply.

Source of infection: The thing, person, or substance from which an infectious agent passes to a host. Sometimes the reservoir is also the source of the infection.

Communicable period: The time during which an infectious agent may be transferred from one host to another.

Incubation period: The time between infection of the host and the first appearance of signs of the disease.

Communicable disease: A contagious disease—that is, a disease that can be transmitted from one person to another person.

MODES OF TRANSMISSION

The term *communicable (infectious) disease* refers to an illness that can be transmitted from one person to another. The method of transfer is called the **mode of transmission**; it can take place in one of four ways:

1. **Contact transmission.** There are two methods of contact: direct and indirect. Direct physical contact takes place between an individual and the infected person. Indirect physical contact takes place between an individual and inanimate objects that may have infectious organisms on them—for example, locker room surfaces, dressings, athletic equipment, or linens.
2. **Airborne transmission.** The infective organism is introduced into the air by an athlete who is coughing or sneezing. Droplets of mucus that carry bacteria or other organisms can then be inhaled by another individual.
3. **Vehicle transmission.** The infective organism is introduced directly into the body through the ingestion of contaminated food, or water, or by the infusion of contaminated drugs, fluid, or blood.
4. **Vector transmission.** The infective organism is transmitted to an individual by animals; for example, mosquitoes transmit malarial parasites, and ticks

transmit Rocky Mountain spotted fever. Vector-borne diseases rarely present a great risk to prehospital care providers.

The greater opportunity for acquiring an infectious or communicable disease is through direct or indirect contact. When rendering care, athletic trainers often do not take the time to wash their hands thoroughly following contact with an athlete or contaminated materials. When this simple procedure is omitted, the opportunity for infection increases, especially if the care provider engages in hand-to-nose or hand-to-mouth activity.

Airborne transmission can present a risk of infection; but it is less likely than with direct or indirect contact. The method of organism transfer and the duration of expo-sure to the athlete play major roles. In general, there must be contact with a coughing or sneezing athlete, direct contact with sputum produced, or prolonged exposure to the person.

PRECAUTIONS AGAINST CONTAMINATION

Depending on the disease, trainers can take precautions to protect themselves and others from contamination. Risks do exist in managing athletes with communicable diseases, but proper care can minimize them.

Table 56.1 reviews the types of infectious diseases and their characteristics, source, transmission, incubation, communicability, and precautions.

TABLE 56.1.   Infectious Diseases

Disease	Characteristics	Source	Mode of Transmission	Incuba-tion Period	Period of Communi-cability	Care of Personnel
Acquired immune deficiency syndrome (AIDS)*	Unexplained weight loss; fever of unknown origin; night sweats over several weeks; dry, hacking cough not associated with upper respiratory infection; persistent, unexplained diarrhea; enlarged lymph nodes in the neck, armpits, and groin; small painless, purple papules or nodules on the skin or mucous membranes that gradually enlarge	Human immuno-deficiency virus (HIV)	Sexual contact with, blood donations from, and sharing of or contact with needles used by HIV carriers	Unknown	Unknown	Wash hands. Use precautions when disposing of needles or instruments used for AIDS patients
Chickenpox	Acute febrile viral disease; itchy red rash that leaves scabs; more common in children	Respiratory tract secretions (scabs do not carry infection)	Direct contact; droplet contact	2–3 weeks	1 day before skin lesions appear to 6 days after skin lesions appear	Wash hands; shower; change clothing

*Individuals at risk with suggestive symptoms should seek immediate medical evaluation. The Centers for Disease Control has an AIDS task force (800) 342-AIDS.

TABLE 56.1. (continued)

Disease	Characteristics	Source	Mode of Transmission	Incubation Period	Period of Communicability	Care of Personnel
Diphtheria	Acute bacterial infection of throat, tonsils, nose, and sometimes skin with local pain and swelling	Discharge from nose and throat	Direct or indirect contact	2–5 days	2–4 weeks	Immunization; wear mask if not immune
German measles (rubella)	Feverish viral illness with rash; more common in children; danger of birth defects if contracted during first 3 months of pregnancy	Discharge from nose and throat	Direct contact; indirect contact; droplet contact	14–21 days	1 week before rash appears to 4 days after rash appears	None
Gonorrhea	Bacterial venereal disease characterized by thick yellow urethral discharge in males; more difficult to detect in females and may lead to chronic infection	Exudate from mucous membrane	Sexual intercourse	3–4 days	Months or years unless treated	None
Herpes I[†] (labialis)	Vesiculo-ulcerative lesions of the mucous membrane of the oral cavity; irritability and local lymphadenopathy	Viral	Direct contact (saliva, stools); indirectly from utensils contaminated with saliva of a virus carrier	3–5 days	Usually self-limiting, 1–2 weeks	Wash hands
(gladiatorum)	Commonly found on arms and face of wrestlers					
Herpes II[‡]	Multiple vesicles surrounded by diffuse inflammation and edema; intense itching and burning along vulva, vagina, and cervix or penis (often preceding vesicles and associated with hemophilus vaginitis or trichomonas vaginitis); fever, malaise, and inguinal lymphadenopathy; with cervical or vaginal involvement, may be asymptomatic	Viral	Sexual intercourse	3–5 days; occasionally less than 24 hours	Recurrent, with or without systemic reactions, probably due to reactivation of latent viral infection	Wash hands

[†]Treatment is symptomatic. Protect athlete from sources of infection at the lesion site.
[‡]Diagnosis easily made from cultures of suspected lesions. Serologic tests are also available. Symptomatic treatment includes topical acyclovir ointment in initial management, and then topical anesthetic agents as well as drying, antipruritic agents.

TABLE 56.1.   (continued)

Disease	Characteristics	Source	Mode of Transmission	Incubation Period	Period of Communicability	Care of Personnel
Herpes zoster[§]	Inflammation of posterior nerve roots and ganglia, with crops and vesicles over skin supplied by affected sensory nerves; fever and malaise soon followed by severe pain in skin or mucosa along affected nerve route	Viral	Response of partially immune host to reactivation of latent varicella virus	7–21 days	Varies	Wash hands
Infectious hepatitis	Acute viral infection with fever; loss of appetite; jaundice; fatigue	Feces, urine, blood from infected person; dishes, clothing, or bed linen used by infected person; injuries from needles used by or for infected person	Fecal-oral contamination through handling clothes and linen; contaminated water, food, syringes; transfusion from infected person	15–30 days	Unknown	Wash hands, use precautions when disposing of needles or instruments used for these athletes
Lyme disease	Fever, chills, malaise, enlarging red rash on trunk, buttocks, and thighs initially	Spirochete (*Borrelia burgdorferi*) carried by the tick *Ixodes*	Tick bite	3–30 days	May be transmitted in pregnancy to fetus	Take precautions against tick bites: wear long pants tucked inside socks and long-sleeved shirt tucked into pants when in wooded areas and fields; wear shoes; use a product such as permethrin to kill ticks
Measles	Acute viral disease; fever; bronchitis; red blotchy rash; common in childhood	Nose and throat secretions	Direct contact; indirect contact; droplet contact	10 days	4 days before rash appears to 5 days after	None
Meningitis	Acute bacterial disease with fever; severe headache; nausea; vomiting; coma	Nose and throat secretions	Direct contact; droplet contact	2–10 days	Varies	If close contact has occurred, see physician
Mononucleosis	Acute viral disease with fever; sore throat; lymph node swelling	Respiratory tract secretions	Unknown; possibly person-to-person oral route	2–6 weeks	Unknown	None

[§]With severe symptoms, massive IV doses of Cytarabine inhibits further dissemination of lesions. Other IV drugs have had varying success. Topical anesthetic and drying antipruritic agents are helpful in mild cases. Protect athlete from irritation and infection.

TABLE 56.1.   (continued)

Disease	Characteristics	Source	Mode of Transmission	Incubation Period	Period of Communicability	Care of Personnel
Mumps	Acute viral disease with fever; swelling and tenderness of the salivary glands	Saliva of infected person	Direct contact; indirect contact; droplet contact	12–26 days	7 days before swelling appears to 9 days after	None
Pneumonia	Acute viral or bacterial disease; fever; chills; cough; chest pain	Respiratory tract secretions	Direct contact; indirect contact; droplet contact	Varies	Varies	None
Poliomyelitis	Acute viral disease with fever; headache; gastro-intestinal symptoms; stiff neck; paralysis	Nose and throat secretions; feces	Direct contact	7–12 days	6 weeks	None
Rocky Mountain spotted fever	Acute bacterial disease with fever; headache; rash over the body including palms and soles	Infected tick; reservoirs are rodents and dogs	Tick bite	3–10 days	Tick's life span	Remove ticks without crushing, protecting hands with gloves if possible
Smallpox	Acute viral disease with fever; headache; abdominal pain; rash with scabbing and eruptions; still present in many countries but has been eradicated from the U.S. through prevention by vaccination programs	Respiratory discharge; scabs	Direct contact; indirect contact; droplet contact	7–16 days	From first symptoms to disappearance of symptoms	Revaccinate
Scarlet fever	Acute bacterial disease with headache; fever; nausea; vomiting; sore throat	Respiratory discharge	Direct contact; indirect contact; droplet contact; carriers exist	2–5 days	Unknown	Wear mask; change; shower; boil clothes
Syphilis	Acute bacterial venereal disease; primary lesion seen at 3 weeks as a hard sore that erodes; secondary skin eruptions appear during next 4–6 weeks; late disabling complications of heart and brain	Saliva; semen; blood; vaginal discharge during the infectious period	Direct contact through mucosal surface or open wounds; sexual intercourse	10 days–10 weeks	Variable	If scratched or bitten, contact physician
Tuberculosis	Chronic bacterial disease; cough; fatigue; weight loss; chest pain; coughing up of blood	Respiratory secretions; occasionally milk	Direct contact; indirect contact; droplet contact; carriers exist	4–6 weeks	As long as live tubercle bacilli are excreted	Wear mask; chest x-ray yearly; skin test periodically

TABLE 56.1.   (continued)

Disease	Characteristics	Source	Mode of Transmission	Incubation Period	Period of Communicability	Care of Personnel
Typhoid fever	Fever; loss of appetite; diarrhea	Feces and urine	Direct contact; indirect contact; raw fruits; vegetables; milk; carriers exist	2 weeks	As long as typhoid bacilli are excreted	Wash hands
Whooping cough	Acute bacterial disease with violent attacks of coughing; a high-pitched whooping; common among children	Respiratory discharge	Direct contact; indirect contact; droplet contact	7 days–3 weeks	7 days–3 weeks	Change; shower; boil clothes

SUGGESTED READINGS

Hoeprich, P. D., ed. *Infectious Diseases: A Modern Treatise of Infectious Processes*, 3d ed. Philadelphia: Harper & Row, 1983.

Kass, E. H., and R. Platt. *Current Therapy in Infectious Disease*, vol. 2. Toronto: B. C. Decker, 1986.

Mandell, G. L., R. G. Douglas, Jr., and J. E. Bennett, eds. *Principles and Practice of Infectious Diseases*, 3d ed. New York: Churchill Livingstone, 1990.

57

Poisons, Stings, and Bites

CHAPTER OUTLINE

OBJECTIVES FOR CHAPTER 57

After reading this chapter, the student should be able to:

1. Define a poison, describe the common symptoms of poisoning, and discuss general treatment guidelines.
2. Identify the most frequently encountered insect stings and bites and institute the emergency treatment necessary.
3. Describe the symptoms of a snakebite and know how to provide emergency care.
4. Administer first-aid care for dog bites and human bites.
5. Discuss the various types of injuries from marine animals and identify how they are treated.

INTRODUCTION

Accidental poisoning is not an uncommon event, especially food poisoning and plant poisoning. Poisoning from the bites and stings of insects and animals is less common but requires emergency treatment when it occurs. The athletic trainer should be familiar with the various types of poisonings, stings, and bites that can occur on or off the playing field and be prepared to administer first aid.

Chapter 57 discusses ingested, surface contact, inhaled, and injected poisons and offers treatment guidelines. Bites from spiders, snakes, dogs, and humans, as well as stings and injuries from marine animals, are described. Treatment protocols are also presented for these injuries. ■

POISONS

Each year approximately 1 million children and thousands of adults accidentally swallow poisons. From 5,000 to 10,000 people in the United States die annually from accidental or intentional poisoning. Of all poisonings, 80 percent occur in children under the age of 6. Approximately 20 percent of all poisonings require some sort of emergency treatment at a hospital. Most athletic trainers will never need to administer first aid to a poisoning victim; nevertheless, all should be prepared to handle such an emergency if it arises.

A **poison** is any substance that can produce a harmful effect on the body process-es. Poisons may act by modifying normal metabolism of cells or by actually destroying the cells. Poisoning can result from ingestion, inhalation, injection, surface contact, or absorption through the skin and mucous membranes of substances in toxic amounts.

The first decision to make when faced with a possible poisoning victim is whether a poisoning has actually occurred. Some substances are harmless and require no treatment. Others require nothing more than drinking a glass of milk or water to offset an upset stomach. However, if there is the slightest doubt, the poison control center should be contacted and treatment should be started as needed.

Some of the more common symptoms of poisoning are nausea, vomiting, abdominal pain, diarrhea, dilation or constriction of the pupils, excessive salivation or sweating, difficulty in breathing, unconsciousness, or even convulsions. If respiration is inadequate, cyanosis occurs. Chemical burns or surface irritants cause inflammation of the skin or mucous membranes with blisters or even third-degree burns.

When responding to a poisoning, the athletic trainer should try to determine the nature of the poison. Objects at the scene, such as overturned bottles, pills lying around, or toxic fumes from spilled chemicals or gases might provide clues. The remains of any food or drink at the scene may also be important. All suspicious material should be collected, put into a plastic bag, and taken to the hospital with the individual. If the person vomits, some or all of the vomitus should be collected in a plastic bag and brought to the hospital for chemical analysis. Again, the most important response, in addition to resuscitating the individual, is to identify and bring along any suspicious medicines, drugs, or substances that may have caused the poisoning, along with the bottle or can that contained the material. The ingredients of many substances are often listed on the label, which can be of great help to the poison control center. In addition, knowing how much material is left in the container can give the physician some idea of how much was ingested. If the brand name of the material is known, sometimes the manufacturer can be contacted for a specific description of the material in the container. By bringing the container with the person, proper treatment may be hastened and a life saved.

Several hundred poison control centers throughout the United States are located in large hospitals, medical schools, or pharmacy schools. The telephone numbers of these poison control centers are readily available. Medical personnel who staff the poison control centers have access to information on virtually all of the commonly used drugs, chemicals, and substances that could possibly be poisonous. They should also be able to supply information on how to administer first aid to an athlete following a sting or bite from a potentially poisonous insect or snake. The poison control centers are usually staffed 24 hours a day, and they should be contacted for help whenever a poisoning occurs.

Most poisons do not have a specific antidote or remedy. Support for the individual may range from reassuring an anxious athlete to instituting cardiopulmonary resuscitation. In general, the most important treatment for poisons involves physical removal of the agent. Removal can be accomplished by surface flooding and washing of the skin, inducing vomiting for ingested poisons, or administering oxygen for inhaled noxious agents. Certain poisons may require a specific antidote. Injected poisons pose urgent problems since they are difficult to remove or dilute.

Ingested Poisons

Poisonous substances most likely to be ingested include drugs, drinks, household products, contaminated food, or plants. Children are often victims of accidental household poisonings (Fig. 57.1). With the exception of contaminated food, adults usually ingest poisonous agents as a method of committing suicide or as unsuspecting victims of murder. While drug ingestions are common sources of poisonings, approximately 60 percent of all poisonings are caused by other liquid or solid agents, cleaners, soaps, acids, or alkalis. Plant poisonings are also prominent among children who like to explore and often bite the leaves of various bushes or shrubs. (Food poisoning, even though technically an ingested poison, and plant poisoning are discussed later in this section.)

Treatment

Dilute the poison. The first step after determining that a poisoning with an ingested

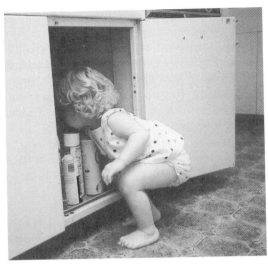

FIGURE 57.1. A curious child will try to taste or swallow almost any substance. A common victim of accidental ingestion of dangerous compounds is the unwatched toddler.

agent has occurred is to attempt to dilute the agent in the stomach if the poison is acting as a gastric irritant. A glass of water or milk may be given to drink.

Induce vomiting. The next step is to remove the poison physically by inducing vomiting in the person. Vomiting may be stimulated only if the person is conscious and alert, and, especially, if the poison control center has so instructed. Vomiting is most easily induced by the oral administration of **syrup of ipecac**, an over-the-counter medication available at most drugstores. The dosage is 1 to 2 teaspoonsful for children under 1 year and 3 teaspoonsful for older children and adults, followed by a glass of water. The athlete should be transported promptly after swallowing the dose of ipecac. Vomiting will usually occur in about 15 to 20 minutes. The vomitus should be saved. If vomiting has not occurred after 20 minutes, the dose should be repeated, but only once. Transport should not be delayed to administer a second dose.

When not to induce vomiting. Vomiting should *not* be induced under the following circumstances:

- If the individual is unconscious, semiconscious, or having a convulsion.
- If the poison is corrosive, such as a strong acid, lye, or drain cleaner, or has caused obvious burns on the lips or mouth.
- If the poison contains any petroleum product such as kerosene, gasoline, lighter fluid, or clear furniture polish. These agents cause a serious chemical pneumonia if aspirated into the lungs.

Use of activated charcoal. Some substances are best neutralized by local absorption onto **activated charcoal**, which is most commonly available as a solution. The usual first dose is 4 ml/kg of solution or 25 to 30 gm/120 ml. This medication is given at the direction of the poison control center after the center has been provided with information as to the nature of the agent taken. Activated charcoal inhibits the action of ipecac; therefore, it should not be given after a dose of this medication. Many children are afraid to swallow this dirty, inky, messy substance. Often some coaxing is required to get them to do so. The athletic trainer should never force it into anyone's mouth, however.

Ventilatory support. In cases of ingested drugs such as opiates, sedatives, or barbiturates, expect central nervous system depression and especially respiratory depression. These athletes may require aggressive ventilatory support and even cardiopulmonary resuscitation, since absorption of some agents from the gastrointestinal tract is quite rapid. Prompt transportation of the athlete to the emergency department is mandatory.

Food Poisoning

The term *ptomaine poisoning* was coined in 1870 and is used frequently in news accounts of episodes of food poisoning. Unfortunately, it is nonspecific and indicates little about the problem. Food poisoning is caused by the ingestion of contaminated food, or food that is carrying bacteria. There are two types: one type occurs when the bacteria themselves cause disease, and the other type occurs when the bacteria have produced toxins (poisons) that cause disease.

An example of the former is typhoid fever, which represents the ingestion of the bacterium *Salmonella typhosa*. It produces characteristic gastrointestinal problems that develop up to 72 hours after ingestion. Only ingested living bacteria can produce the disease. A variety of other organisms can also produce milder intestinal complaints. Usually, proper cooking will kill bacteria, and proper cleanliness in the kitchen will prevent the contamination of noncooked foods.

The ingestion of preformed bacterial toxins is probably the most common cause of food poisoning. Far and away, the most frequent offender is food contaminated with staphylococcus; some strains can produce a potent toxin. This agent is responsible for the occasional episodes of food poisoning reported at large gatherings. It results from the early preparation of food which has been kept warm for many hours so that contaminating bacteria have a chance to grow and produce toxins. Usually, staphyloccal food poisoning results in the onset of violent gastrointestinal problems (nausea, vomiting, and diarrhea) within 1 to 3 hours after ingestion. In general, the episode is over in 6 to 8 hours.

The most severe form of toxin ingestion is **botulism**. Frequently fatal, this disease usually results from eating improperly canned food in which the spore of the bacterium has grown and developed its toxin. Symptoms of botulism develop as long as 24 hours after ingestion and may take weeks to subside.

In general, the athletic trainer should not try to separate specific causes of acute gastrointestinal problems from one another. Transport to the emergency department is warranted for diagnosis. In obvious instances in which two or more individuals in one group have the same problem, it is wise to bring along the suspected food.

Plant Poisoning

Several hundred thousand cases of poisoning from plants occur each year; some are severe. Many household plants are poisonous if they are accidentally ingested, especially by children who like to nibble strange-looking leaves. Some poisonous plants cause local irritation of the skin; others can affect the circulatory system, the gastrointestinal tract, or the central nervous system.

Thirty to 50 minutes after ingesting a poisonous plant that affects circulation, the person may show the classic signs of circulatory collapse: tachycardia (a rapid heart rate); falling blood pressure; sweating; weakness; and cold, moist, clammy skin. The treatment is the same as for shock. The trainer positions the person lying down with the legs elevated; if available, oxygen should be administered; and the person should be transported promptly to the hospital. The plant, or at least several loose leaves, should also be brought along for positive identification.

Small amounts of many plants can produce severe gastrointestinal disturbances. The usual symptoms of gastrointestinal disturbance from plant ingestion are the same as those caused by any other toxic substance: vomiting, diarrhea, and cramps. Symptoms can occur within 20 to 30 minutes after ingestion. If the athlete does vomit, the vomitus should be collected. Vomiting may be induced at the direction of the poison control center if the plant has been positively identified. The athletic trainer should arrange transport of the athlete to the hospital.

Some agents in plants are locally irritating to oral and throat mucosa. In these instances, it is unwise to increase the irritation. If gastrointestinal symptoms occur very soon after the ingestion, vomiting may help rid the individual of the substance; if symptoms are late, vomiting is unlikely to do much good. Again, bringing leaves or the whole plant to the emergency department may help identify the toxin.

Poisonous plants sometimes affect the central nervous system. Signs of such problems include depression, hyperactivity, excitement, stupor, mental confusion, or coma. The treatment for this type of poisoning is basic life support. Vomiting should not be induced in a person who shows any signs of stupor or coma. The individual should be brought promptly to the hospital, along with a sample of the plant or its leaves, if possible.

Skin irritation certainly is the most common form of plant poisoning. Problems include itching, burning, and local blister formation. One of the most common plants to produce such reactions is poison ivy (Fig. 57.2, color insert). In general, skin irritation occurs after direct contact with the plant and from a spreading onto the skin of the plant's sap or juice. Contact with these plants rarely produces systemic symptoms such as tachycardia, hypotension, or respiratory distress. The emergency treatment of skin irritants is thorough cleansing with soap and water. This treatment is most effective if done within 30 to 60 minutes of exposure to the poison. Athletes occasionally need medical attention for prolonged symptoms.

A specific problem of skin or mucous membrane irritation occurs with dieffenbachia, a common houseplant (Fig. 57.3, color insert). If a leaf of this plant is chewed, a severe irritation of the oral mucous membrane and the lining of the upper airway can occur. This irritation is enough to cause difficulty in swallowing, breathing, and speaking. Partial, and once in a while complete, airway obstruction can occur. For this reason the plant has been given the conversational name "dumb cane." The emergency medical treatment involves maintaining an open airway, giving oxygen if available, and transporting the person as promptly as possible to the hospital.

Surface Contact Poisons

Many corrosive substances cause damage of the skin, mucous membranes, or eyes by direct contact. Acids, alkalis, and some petroleum or benzene products are very destructive. Contact with these agents will cause inflammation, chemical burns, or specific rashes or lesions in affected areas.

The emergency treatment for contact poisoning is to remove the irritating or corrosive substance as rapidly as possible. Dry materials are dusted off thoroughly; then the affected area is washed with soap and water or flooded under a shower. When a large amount of material has been spilled, flooding may be the most rapidly effective treatment. All clothing that has been contaminated with poisons or irritating substances should be removed as rapidly as possible so the skin may be cleaned with running water.

Chemical agents that have come in contact with the eyes must be flushed by rapid and copious irrigation for several minutes. At least 15 minutes of irrigation are needed for acid substances and 15 to 20 minutes for alkalis.

Substances should not be neutralized on the skin. Rather, they should be washed off immediately with water. This procedure is safer and more effective than attempting to neutralize a substance chemically. The one exception to flooding the contact area with water is if the agent is known to react violently with water. For example, phosphorus and elemental sodium are dry, solid chemicals that ignite when they contact water. The incidence of exposure to these elements is rare. As with other dry chemicals, they should be dusted off and the athlete's clothing removed while awaiting or during transport to a medical facility.

Inhaled Poisons

For inhaled poisons such as natural gas, carbon monoxide, chlorine, or other gases, the emergency treatment is to move the person into fresh air. An individual exposed to prolonged inhalation may require supplementary oxygen and basic life support. Because it is easy to inhale noxious fumes in an emergency situation, athletic trainers

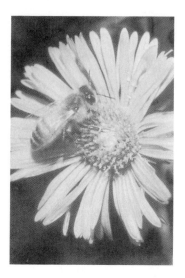
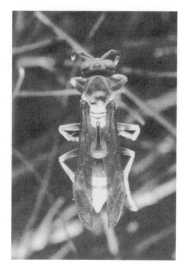
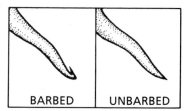

FIGURE 57.4. Most stinging insects inject venom through a small hollow spine that projects from the abdomen. The stinger of the honeybee (left) is barbed and so cannot be withdrawn. Wasps (right) have unbarbed stingers and can sting repeatedly.

BARBED   UNBARBED

must be careful to protect themselves as well as their athletes.

Some inhaled poisons such as carbon monoxide are odorless and produce profound hypoxia (an oxygen deficiency in the tissues) without much damage to the lungs. Some such as chlorine are very irritating and induce pulmonary edema (fluid in the lungs) and airway obstruction. Oxygen is needed whenever hypoxia, pulmonary edema, or airway obstruction results from inhaled poisons. Affected persons should be transported as quickly as possible to a medical facility because some inhaled agents cause progressive lung damage.

Injected Poisons

Poisoning by injection is usually the result of deliberate drug overdose. Other sources of injected poisons are the stings and bites of insects or animals. These will be considered in more detail in the next sections of this chapter.

Most injected poisons are impossible to dilute or remove. Usually they are absorbed quickly into the body or cause intense local tissue destruction. Thus, prompt transport to the emergency department is mandatory. If the area around the site of an injection starts to swell, all rings, watches, or bracelets should be removed.

STINGS

Many different kinds of insects can inflict pain from stings or bites. Some of these injuries are potentially dangerous. They are associated with stings or bites from bees, wasps, yellow jackets, hornets, certain ants, scorpions, and some spiders.

Stinging Insects

There are over 100,000 species of hymenopteran, including bees, wasps, and hornets. Fatalities from stinging insects outnumber those from snakebites; 60 percent are related to bee, wasp, and hornet stings. The stinging organ of most bees, wasps, and hornets is a small hollow spine that projects from the abdomen. **Venom** can be injected through this spine directly into the skin. The stinger of the honeybee is barbed so that it cannot be withdrawn. The bee must disembowel itself after stinging to fly away. Wasps or hornets with their unbarbed stingers can sting repeatedly (Fig. 57.4). Identification of the stinging insect is often impossible because it tends to fly away immediately after the injury.

Some species of ant, especially the fire ant, can bite repeatedly and often inject a particularly irritating toxin at the bite site. These bites usually occur on the feet and legs. It is not uncommon for the athlete to sustain multiple bites within a short period of time (Fig. 57.5, color insert). Typically, fire ant bites produce an acute inflammation and ulcerations that are slow to heal.

Symptoms

Symptoms associated with insect stings or bites usually occur at the site of injury. Local symptoms of stings and bites are sudden pain, swelling, heat, and redness about the affected area. Sometimes a whitish, firm elevation of the skin called a **wheal** may occur, with itching (Fig. 57.6, color insert). While there is no specific treatment for these injuries, sometimes the application of ice may make the athlete more comfortable. The swelling accompanying insect stings and bites may be considerable and sometimes frightens athletes. However, the local manifestations of these stings are not serious.

Treatment

The stinging organ of a honeybee with its attached muscle can continue to inject venom for up to 20 minutes after the bee has flown away because the stinger has remained in the wound. Anyone assisting a person who has been stung by a honeybee should gently attempt to remove the stinger and that portion of the abdomen of the bee by scraping it off the skin. Tweezers or forceps should not be used, as squeezing the stinger may only inject more venom into the athlete.

Some insect bites are not noticed by the individual for some hours until a **cellulitis**, or spreading redness and swelling of the skin, has developed. This person requires transport to the emergency department with immobilization of the injured area. Warm, moist packs may produce some comfort.

Anaphylactic Reaction and Allergic Reaction

Approximately 5 percent of all people are allergic to the venom of the honeybee, hornet, yellow jacket, or wasp. This allergy accounts for approximately 200 deaths per year. More than two-thirds of those who die do so within the first hour after the sting.

Honeybee venom is commonly associated with allergy and very severe reactions. In an allergic person, the sting of such an insect will usually result in a hypersensitivity reaction called **anaphylaxis**. Anaphylactic reactions occur in minutes or even seconds after contact with the substance to which the person is allergic.

Signs of an Anaphylactic Reaction

Anaphylaxis can also occur from injection (from drugs such as penicillin), ingestion (eating certain foods such as shellfish or the use of some medications or drugs), or inhalation (dusts, pollens, or other materials to which the person is sensitive). The following signs are characteristic of an anaphylactic reaction:

- Generalized itching and burning.
- **Urticaria** (hives) (Fig. 57.7, color insert).
- Swelling about the lips and tongue.
- Bronchospasm and wheezing.
- Chest tightness and cough.
- Dyspnea.
- Anxiety.
- Abdominal cramps.
- Occasionally, respiratory failure.

Such a reaction can proceed to **anaphylactic shock** and, if untreated, to death from respiratory obstruction. As fluid pours into the bronchi in reaction to the sensitizing agent, the individual tries to cough up this fluid. The smaller bronchi constrict, and the passage of air into the lungs becomes increasingly difficult. Expiration, normally the passive part of the breathing cycle, becomes forced. The fluid in the air passages and the constricted small bronchi cause the development of a characteristic wheeze as the person works hard to exhale. With anaphylactic shock, there is no loss of blood, no cardiac or vascular damage, and no vascular dilation. The body is, however, rapidly deprived of needed oxygen.

Treatment for an Allergic Reaction

The athlete with skin wheals, hives, and wheezing respiration should be immediately transported to the hospital with first-priority status. Oxygen should be given if it is available, and preparations should be made to maintain an airway or give full cardiopulmonary resuscitation. An attempt should be made to remove the stinger from the wound by gently scraping it off with the edge of a knife blade. An ice bag placed over the injury site may help to slow the rate of absorption of the toxin.

Athletes who have a history of severe allergic reactions to stings may carry bee sting kits (Fig. 57.8, color insert). Commercially manufactured, they are usually prescribed specifically for the hypersensitive person by a physician. The kits usually contain the medication epinephrine prepared in a syringe and ready for injection.

Epinephrine is a rapidly acting agent which produces bronchodilation to reverse the effects of the allergen on the airway. It has a short period of action and produces acute relief. Most kits also contain some oral or intravenous **antihistamine**. These agents, of which a variety are available, are specific to counter the production of histamine, which is believed to be responsible for the attack. Usually, they are slower in onset of action and effective over a longer period than epinephrine is. The athlete who is able to do so should be assisted in administering these lifesaving medications by the athletic trainer where local laws permit. Specific instructions for the use of epinephrine are in the kit.

The athlete who is injected with epinephrine will experience tachycardia and, on occasion, increased anxiety or nervousness. The emergency care outlined earlier for support for this athlete should be completed and the athlete transported promptly to the hospital.

An athlete's medical history taken prior to sports participation should indicate any allergies to bee, wasp, and ant stings, as well as to other bites and stings. The athletic trainer can then discuss with the athlete and the athlete's physician an individualized treatment plan for use in the event of an allergic reaction.

Scorpion Stings

Scorpions and spiders are related, in that both are eight-legged insects from the same biological group (Arachnida). Scorpions are rare; they are found primarily in the Southwest and in deserts. Scorpions have a venom gland and a stinger at the end of their tail. Except for the sting of a specific scorpion in the desert of the Southwest, the Arizona scorpion, scorpion injuries are ordinarily very painful but not dangerous. Only 4 percent of fatalities related to insect stings are associated with scorpions.

Localized swelling, pain, and discoloration result from a scorpion sting. Arizona scorpion venom may produce a severe systemic reaction that brings about circulatory collapse, severe muscle contractions, excessive salivation, hypertension, convulsions, and cardiac failure.

The emergency treatment for a scorpion sting is basic life support. **Antivenin**, a serum that contains antibodies that counteract the venom, is available but must be administered by a physician.

SPIDER BITES

Many of the fatalities associated with insect stings and bites are related to spiders. Spiders are numerous and widespread in the United States. Two species, the black widow spider and the brown recluse spider, are able to deliver serious, and sometimes even life-threatening, bites. Most other spiders will bite, but these injuries do not produce complications.

Black Widow Spider Bites

The black widow spider is approximately 1 inch long with its legs extended; it is not particularly large. It is glossy black and has a distinctive, bright red-orange marking in the shape of an hourglass on its belly. Black widow spiders are found in every state except Alaska. They prefer dry, dim places around buildings, in woodpiles, and among debris.

Symptoms

Commonly, a black widow spider bite is overlooked. The individual may not recall the bite itself, since the area may become numb after the bite. The venom is **neurotoxic** (poisonous to nerve tissue) and directly attacks spinal nerve centers. Thus, the major problem with these bites lies in their systemic manifestations. Severe cramps, with boardlike rigidity of the abdominal muscles, tightness in the chest, and difficulty in breathing occur over 24 hours. Abdominal symptoms are more commonly seen with bites in the lower half of the body. Chest symptoms tend to accompany bites on the upper extremities and the upper part of the body. Other complaints include dizziness, sweating, vomiting, nausea, and skin rashes. Generally, the signs and symptoms subside over 48 hours, but the muscle cramps and ensuing pain can be agonizing.

Although the complaints following the bites are severe, death is not common (12 deaths were reported in 1986). A specific antivenin is available, although its use is reserved for very severe bites, the aged or very feeble, and some infants. It will be administered, if necessary, by a physician.

Treatment

In general, emergency treatment for a black widow spider bite is basic life support if the athlete is in respiratory distress. Much more commonly, the athlete will require relief from pain. The individual often is unaware of having been bitten or where the bite is located. If the site can be identified, putting ice against it may slow the absorption of toxin. The athlete should be transported to the emergency department as soon as possible for treatment of the symptoms of pain and muscle rigidity. It is also important, if possible, to identify the spider and bring it with the athlete to the hospital.

Brown Recluse Spider Bites

Dull brown in color, the brown recluse spider is somewhat smaller than the black widow. It has a dark violin-shaped mark on its back, which can be easily seen from above. Although the brown recluse spider is found mostly in the southern and central United States, it is currently moving to other areas. The spider takes its name from the fact that it tends to live in dark areas, in corners, in old unused buildings, under rocks, and in woodpiles. It has moved indoors in cooler areas and inhabits closets, drawers, cellars, and old piles of clothing.

Symptoms

The bite from the brown recluse, in contrast to the black widow, produces local rather than systemic problems. The venom of the brown recluse spider causes severe local tissue damage, which will result in local gangrene and a large, nonhealing ulcer if not treated promptly (Fig. 57.9, color insert). Typically, the bite is not painful initially but becomes so within hours. The area becomes red, swollen, and tender, and it develops a pale, mottled cyanotic center. A small blister may form. Over the next several days, a large scab of dead skin, fat, and debris will develop and deepen to produce a large ulcer.

Treatment

Systemic symptoms and signs from brown recluse spider bites rarely occur. When they do, the emergency treatment is basic life support and transport to the emergency department. No specific antivenin exists for this toxin, but use of dapsone, a drug which reduces the immune reaction to the toxin, seems promising. Thus, emergency treatment for a suspected brown recluse spider bite without symptoms is also prompt transportation to the emergency department. Again, it is helpful if the spider can be identified and brought to the hospital along with the athlete.

SNAKEBITES

Snakebite is a worldwide problem of some significance. More than 300,000 injuries from snakebites occur annually; 30,000 to 40,000 deaths result. The greatest number of the fatalities from snakebites occur in Southeast Asia and India (25,000 to 30,000), and in South America (3,000 to 4,000). Snakebites are fairly common in the United States: 40,000 to 50,000 are reported annually. Approximately 7,000 of them are caused by poisonous snakes. However, fatalities in the United States from snakebites are extremely rare: about 15 a year for the entire country.

Of the approximately 150 different species of snakes in the United States, only four are poisonous: the rattlesnake, the copperhead, the cottonmouth (water) moccasin, and the coral snake. Only Alaska, Hawaii, and Maine do not have at least one species of venomous reptile. As a general rule, these creatures are retiring and timid. They usually do not bite unless provoked, angered, or accidentally injured (as when one steps on them). There are a few exceptions to these rules. Moccasins are often rather aggressive snakes, and certainly very little provocation is needed to annoy a rattlesnake. Coral snakes, on the other hand, are very shy and retiring and usually bite only when being handled.

Most snakebites occur between April and October when the reptiles are active. Most involve young male snakes, and most occur within a very few states. Texas reports the largest number of bites. Other states with a major concentration of snakebites are Alabama, Louisiana, Georgia, Oklahoma, North Carolina, Arkansas, West Virginia, and Mississippi.

Envenomation

When responding to a snakebite, it is extremely important to identify whether envenomation (deposit of venom into the wound) has occurred. In one classification of all snakebites throughout the United States, 27 percent were found to have had no envenomation and an additional 37 percent were rated as minimal. Thus, only one-third of snakebites in general result in severe local or systemic problems. There are several reasons why envenomation does not occur. Most commonly, the snake recently has struck another animal and has exhausted its supply of venom.

Nonpoisonous snakes can also cause bites, which usually leave a horseshoe shape of tooth marks. With the exception of the coral snake, poisonous vipers in the United States all have hollow fangs in the roof of the mouth, which inject the poison from two sacs at the back of the head. The characteristic appearance of the poisonous snakebite, therefore, is two small puncture wounds, usually about a half-inch apart, with surrounding discoloration, swelling, and pain (Fig. 57.10, color insert). Some poisonous snakes have teeth as well as fangs. The mere presence of tooth marks does not necessarily mean that a poisonous snake attack has occurred. Fang marks, on the other hand, are a clear indication of a bite by a poisonous snake.

Pit Viper Bites

Rattlesnakes, copperheads, and cottonmouth (water) moccasins are all pit vipers (Fig. 57.11). The head of the pit viper is triangular and flat; there is a small pit located just behind the nostril and in front of each eye. The pupil of the eye is vertical and slitlike. The pit is a heat-sensing organ that allows the snake to strike accurately at any warm target, especially in the dark when it cannot see. Localization by the pit is much more accurate than that provided by the eye.

The fangs of the pit viper normally lie flat against the roof of the mouth. When the snake is striking, the mouth opens wide and the fangs extend, so that if the mouth strikes an object, the fangs will penetrate. The fangs are hollow adapted teeth that act

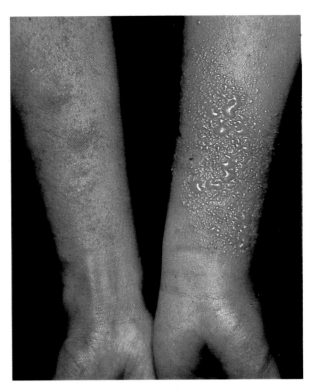

FIGURE 57.2. The sap or juice from poison ivy can cause itching, burning, and blister formation. Severe cases can become infected and require medical treatment.

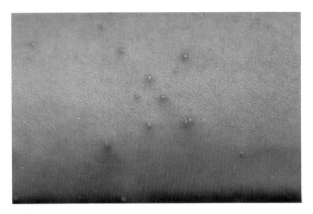

FIGURE 57.5. Fire ants, imported from Brazil, have become a serious problem in several southern states. They inject a particularly irritating toxin. They can bite repeatedly, and some persons sustain multiple bites within a short time.

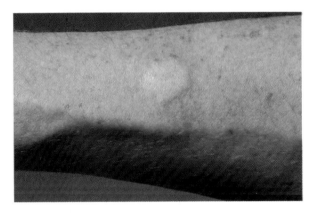

FIGURE 57.6. A wheal is a whitish, firm elevation of the skin that occurs after an insect sting or bite.

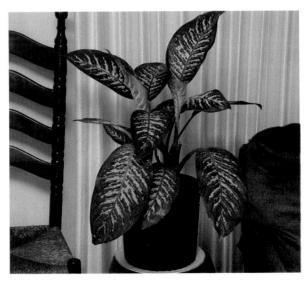

FIGURE 57.3. Dieffenbachia, also called "dumb cane," is a common houseplant that can cause severe irritation and swelling of the mouth and throat if ingested.

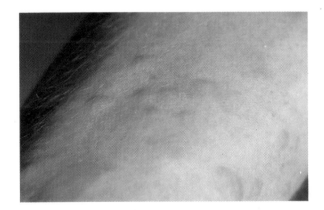

FIGURE 57.7. Hives that appear following a bee, hornet, or wasp sting are one of the warning signs of an impending anaphylactic reaction.

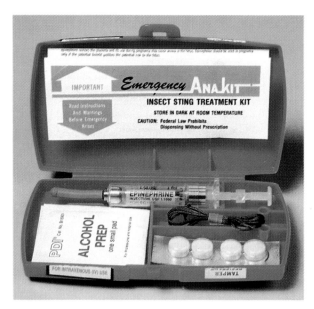

FIGURE 57.8. A typical prescription bee sting kit. The syringe is loaded with two premeasured doses of epinephrine solution. Instructions for proper administration, including self-examination, are attached to the kit.

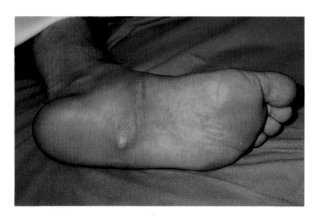

FIGURE 57.9. The venom from the bite of a brown recluse spider causes severe local tissue damage, which, if not treated promptly, can result in gangrene and a large, nonhealing ulcer.

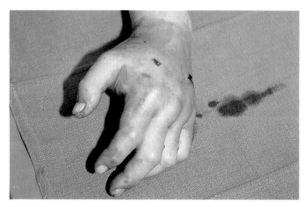

FIGURE 57.10. The presence of fang marks signals a poisonous snakebite. Swelling and discoloration of the hand indicate envenomation.

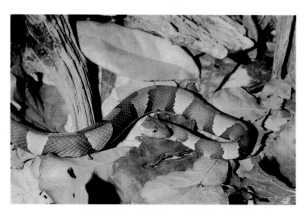

FIGURE 57.13. The copperhead is a reddish, copper-colored pit viper that accounts for most of the venomous snakebites in the eastern United States.

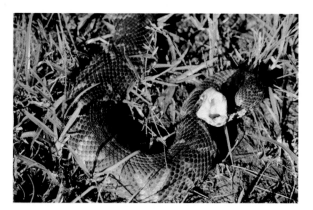

FIGURE 57.14. Cottonmouth (water) moccasins are pit vipers that live in the water. They are aggressive snakes whose bites cause serious tissue destruction.

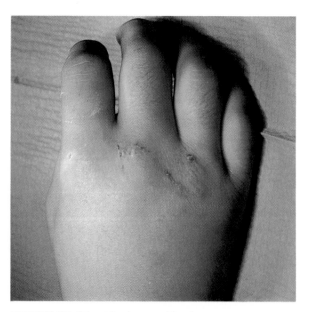

FIGURE 57.15. The human bite is a very serious injury because if left untreated, it will become the source of significant spreading infection.

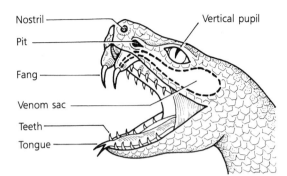

FIGURE 57.11. Rattlesnakes, copperheads, and cottonmouth (water) moccasins all have hollow fangs in the roof of the mouth, which inject poison from two sacs at the back of the head. These snakes are called *pit vipers* because they have small, heat-sensing organs (pits) located in front of their eyes that allow them to strike at warm targets, even in the dark.

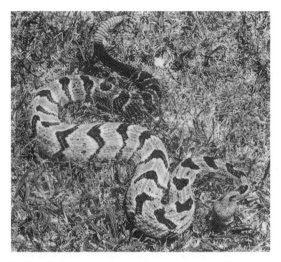

FIGURE 57.12. The rattlesnake is the commonest of the pit vipers. The "rattle" is actually layers of shed skin that lie against a small nubbin on the end of the tail.

much like hypodermic needles. They are hinged to swing back and forth as the mouth opens. They are connected to a sac containing a reservoir of venom, which in turn is attached to a poison gland. The gland itself is an adapted salivary gland that produces powerful enzymes which digest and destroy tissue. The purpose of the venom is to kill the small animal the snake attacked and also to start the digestive process prior to the animal's being eaten by the snake.

Rattlesnake

Among the pit vipers, the most common is the rattlesnake (Fig. 57.12). Several different species of rattlesnake exist. Apart from the features of the pit vipers in general, rattlesnakes can usually be identified by the rattle on the tail. The rattle is actually numerous layers of shed skin which come to lie against a small nubbin on the end of the tail. Each year the skin is not completely shed; a small piece remains. As the snake sheds annually, the dried skin remnants that do not come off completely form the characteristic rattle. Generally, rattlesnakes have many patterns of color, often with a diamond pattern. They can develop to 6 feet or more in length.

Copperhead

Copperheads are smaller than rattlesnakes. They are usually 2 to 3 feet long and have a characteristic reddish coppery color with brown or red cross-bands (Fig. 57.13, color insert). Shier than rattlesnakes, they inhabit woodpiles and abandoned dwellings, often close to areas of habitation. They account for most of the venomous snakebites in the eastern United States. Fatalities are rare following these injuries.

Cottonmouth Moccasin

Cottonmouth moccasins grow to about 4 feet. Also called water moccasins, these snakes are olive or brown, with black cross-bands and a yellow undersurface (Fig. 57.14, color insert). They are water snakes with a particularly aggressive pattern of behavior. Although fatalities from these snakebites are rare, tissue destruction from the venom may be severe.

Symptoms of Pit Viper Bites

The sign of envenomation by a pit viper is severe burning pain at the site of the injury, followed by swelling and discoloration. These signs are evident within 5 to 10 minutes after the bite has occurred and spread slowly over the next 8 to 36 hours. Bleeding under the skin (ecchymosis) causes bluish discoloration. An envenomated bite is painful and ecchymotic. Systemic signs, which may or may not occur, include weakness, sweating, fainting, and shock.

Occasionally, the athlete bitten by a snake will faint. Usually this situation is corrected promptly when the athlete is supine (lying flat). Consciousness returns, and the episode, triggered by fright, is temporary. A fainting spell should not be confused with shock, which ordinarily develops much later after the bite has occurred.

The venom of the pit viper causes localized destruction of all tissues: protein, fat, and entire cells. It can also interfere significantly with the body's clotting mechanism and cause bleeding at various distant sites. Tissue destruction locally starts from the moment of envenomation.

Treatment for Pit Viper Bites

The emergency treatment of snakebites from pit vipers is directed primarily at local containment of venom and then at the systemic effects. The trainer should carry out the following steps when treating an athlete with a bite from a pit viper.

1. Calm and reassure the athlete. Place the athlete supine and explain that staying quiet will decrease the spread of any venom through the system.
2. Locate the bite area; clean it gently with soap and water or a mild antiseptic.
3. Immobilize the extremity with a splint.
4. Monitor the vital signs: blood pressure, pulse, and respiration.
5. If any signs of shock are present, elevate the lower extremities about 12 inches, and give supplemental oxygen, if it is available.
6. Transport the athlete promptly to the hospital. Notify the hospital that you are bringing in a snakebite victim and, if possible, describe the snake.
7. If the snake has been killed, as is often the case, bring it along to the hospital.

Identification of the offending snake is extremely important in administering the correct antivenin. Be aware, however, that "dead" snakes can still bite by reflex for several hours after death. It is, therefore, very important to be careful when handling the killed snake.

8. Be alert for vomiting. Athletes may often vomit from anxiety rather than from the effects of the toxin itself.
9. Do not give the athlete anything by mouth, especially alcohol.

If the athlete shows no sign of envenomation, basic life support should be provided as needed, a sterile dressing should be placed over the suspected bite area, and the athlete should be immobilized. The same procedure applies for the athlete who shows early signs of envenomation but who can be delivered to the hospital in less than 30 minutes.

All suspected snakebite victims should be brought to the emergency department whether they show signs of immediate envenomation or not. Whether or not envenomation has occurred, these wounds are treated like all other deep puncture wounds to prevent infection. Athletic trainers who work in an area where poisonous snakes are known to live should always keep a snakebite kit available.

Coral Snakebites

The coral snake is a small, very colorful reptile with a series of bright red, yellow, and black bands that completely encircle its body. Many harmless snakes are colored in a fashion similar to the coral snake. The difference is that the red and yellow bands of the coral snake are next to one another, completely encircling the body. There is a rhyme for remembering this fact: "Red on yellow will kill a fellow; red on black, venom will lack."

The coral snake lives primarily in Florida and in the desert Southwest. It is not found in the northern regions of the United States. In fact, it is only rarely found at all, since it is shy and will only bite when provoked or handled. The coral snake is not a pit viper; the head is not triangular, there are no pits, and there are no projecting fangs. A relative of the cobra, the coral snake has tiny fangs and injects the venom with its teeth by a chewing motion, not an injection. Because of its small mouth and teeth and limited jaw expansion, the coral snake usually bites its victim on a small part of the body, especially a finger or toe. Following the bite of a coral snake, one puncture or more scratchlike wounds can be found in the area.

Symptoms

The danger of this particular snake is that its venom is a powerful toxin that causes paralysis of the nervous system. Usually, there are minimal or no local manifestations of a coral snake bite. However, within a few hours bizarre behavior may occur, followed by progressive paralysis of eye movements and respiration as a result of the toxic effects on the nervous system.

Treatment

Treatment, either emergency or long-term, depends on positive identification of the snake. Antivenin is available, but most hospitals or doctors must order it from a central supply area, often in another city. Therefore, the need for it should be made known as soon as possible. The steps for emergency care of a coral snakebite are very similar to a pit viper snakebite except that the area of the bite should be flushed with 1 to 2 quarts of warm, soapy water to wash away any poison left on the skin surface.

In the case of a coral snakebite, the danger is to the nervous system from an absorbed neurotoxin. Antivenin is the most effective means of control.

DOG BITES

The exact incidence of dog bites is unknown because most people who are bitten do not report the bite. Dog bites, however, are potentially serious problems. The animal's mouth is contaminated with bacteria, and infection may result. All of the wounds are punctures which require **tetanus prophylaxis** (treatment to prevent tetanus, a potentially fatal infectious disease characterized by extreme body rigidity and muscle spasms). All dog bites should be considered as potentially infected wounds.

People who have been bitten by a dog are often extremely upset and frightened. Calm reassurance is extremely important. A dry, sterile dressing should be placed over the wound and the person transported to the emergency department as promptly as possible for local wound care and antibiotics.

A major concern with dog bites is the spread of rabies. **Rabies** is an acute viral infection of the central nervous system. Ordinarily, the virus is present in saliva of the infected carrier or host and is transmitted by biting or by licking an open wound. All warm-blooded animals can be affected. Once contracted and well developed in humans or animals, rabies is almost always fatal. Prevention of the disease in a bitten person is possible but requires treatment with antibiotics and vaccine. Although rabies is extremely rare today, particularly with widespread inoculation of pets, it still exists. There are still stray dogs that have not been inoculated and that could be carriers of the disease. Certain other animals— squirrels, bats, foxes, skunks, and raccoons —may also carry rabies.

A rabid animal (one with rabies) may act perfectly normal, may appear vicious, may salivate excessively, or may act in an abnormal way. One cannot tell for certain if an animal is rabid by its behavior. If the animal has been inoculated against rabies, it ordinarily will have a tag so stating on its collar. It is, therefore, very important to determine if the animal can be located. Usually, in the case of dog bites, the dog is a pet and can be identified. If it does not have a rabies tag, it should be captured (not killed) by an animal control officer and turned over to the health department for observation. If the animal is then suspected of having rabies, it is killed and the brain is studied. Results (positive or negative) of this study for rabies are needed to diagnose the presence of the disease in the bitten athlete.

When the animal cannot be found or identified, then the individual bitten usually must undergo a series of rabies inoculations, using a new vaccine introduced in 1980. If started early enough, these inoculations will prevent rabies from developing. They are painful and expensive, and are administered over a 2-week period. The trainer should know locations of the local rabies control center and the closest institution that has human rabies vaccine.

HUMAN BITES

A somewhat neglected area of emergency medical treatment is the human bite. It is relatively uncommon but potentially one of the most severe injuries seen today. The human mouth contains an exceptionally wide range of bacteria, some of which live best without oxygen (anaerobic). The variety of germs contained in the human mouth is greater than that in dogs or many other animals. For this reason, any human bite or laceration from a human tooth that has penetrated the skin must be regarded as a very serious injury, as it can result in a severe infection if not properly treated (Fig. 57.15, color insert).

All bites and tooth wounds should be evaluated. If only minimal skin disruption is noted, proper cleansing, with the wound left open, is recommended. If the wound penetrates deeply or is extensive, surgical débridement (removal of devitalized tissue and foreign matter from a wound) may be needed. Antibiotic coverage is recommended for most human bite wounds.

The emergency treatment for human bites is prompt immobilization of the area with a splint or bandage; application of a dry, sterile dressing; and transport to the emergency department for surgical cleansing of the wound and antibiotic therapy.

INJURIES FROM MARINE ANIMALS

Shark Bites

In recent years there has been a good deal of publicity concerning shark bites. They remain extremely rare. The emergency treatment of a large marine animal bite is the same as for any other major open wound. The athlete should be removed from the water, hemorrhage controlled, dressings and splints applied, shock treated, and the athlete transported to the emergency department promptly (Table 57.1).

Many other injuries may result from marine animals, but none of them is as dramatic or as potentially life-threatening as the large marine animal bite. With the exception of the shark and barracuda, most marine creatures are not aggressive and will not deliberately attack. Injuries from these animals occur when they are disrupted or provoked—for example, if a scuba diver accidentally steps on a shark on the ocean floor.

Stinging Injuries

The most frequent injuries from marine animals occur from swimming into the tentacles of a jellyfish, stepping on the back of a stingray, or falling on a sea urchin. Athletic trainers should be familiar with marine life in their locality. Stings from the tentacles of a jellyfish, a Portuguese man-of-war, various anemones, corals, or hydras can be treated by removing the athlete from the water and gently irrigating the area with salt water to remove loose tentacles.

For Portuguese man-o-war exposures, household vinegar should be poured gently over the affected area to inhibit any further toxin release and provide pain relief. Emergency medical care should be immediately sought if the athlete's symptoms appear to be potentially life-threatening. If not, the athletic trainer, using a gloved hand, should pick off individually any remaining tentacles. The area should *not* be rubbed. The affected area should again be irrigated gently with salt water followed by vinegar. At this point, if symptoms persist, the athlete should be transported for further medical care (see Table 57.1).

For jellyfish envenomations, a baking soda slurry should be applied to the affect-ed area after the initial irrigation with salt water. If emergency medical care is not needed for potentially life-threatening symptoms, any remaining tentacles should be individually picked off by the athletic trainer using a gloved hand. A repeat application of baking soda slurry should be performed. At this point, if symptoms persist,

TABLE 57.1.   Guide to Diagnosis and Emergency Treatment of Injuries from Marine Animals

Type of Injury	Marine Animal Involved	Emergency Treatment	Possible Complications

Trauma (bites and lacerations)	Major wounds by
	    Shark
	    Barracuda
	    Alligator
		Control bleeding
		Prevent shock
		Give basic life support
		Splint the injury
		Secure prompt medical care
			Shock
			Infections

	Minor wounds by
	    Moray eel
	    Turtle
	    Corals
		Cleanse wound
		Splint the injury	

Sting (by tentacles)	Jellyfish Portuguese man-of-war Anemones Corals Hydras	Baking soda slurry Vinegar and salt water Salt water	Allergic reactions Respiratory arrest
Puncture (by spines)	Urchins Cone shells Stingrays Spiny fish (catfish, toad, or oyster fish)	Inactivate with hot water[1]	Allergic reactions Collapse Infections Tetanus Granuloma formation

Poisoning (by ingestion)[2]	Puffer fish
	Scromboids (tuna species)
	Ciguatera (large colored
	    fish)
	Paralytic shellfish
		Give basic life support;
		    prevent self-injury from
		    convulsions
			Allergic reactions
			Asthmatic reactions
			Paresthesia, numbness
			Temperature reversal
			    phenomena
			Respiratory arrest and
			    circulatory collapse

Miscellaneous:
    Shocks
    Skin rashes
	Electric fish
	Marine parasites
		No treatment required;
		    injuries usually
		    self-limiting
			Electric fish or electric eel
			    may precipitate a panic
			    reaction

[1] A toxin is introduced with some of the puncture wounds from this group. In any case, the wounds are excruciatingly painful. It appears that the foreign material or poison introduced into the wound is heat-sensitive. Dramatic treatment results occur with soaking in quite hot water for 30 to 60 minutes. Be careful, however, not to scald the athlete with water that is too hot, as the pain of the wound will mask the normal reaction to heat.

[2] Should ingestion of a poisonous fish be suspected, reference to Halstead's *Poisoning and Venomous Marine Animals of the World* or seeking immediate assistance from poison control centers is suggested.

the athlete should be transported for further medical care.

On very rare occasions, a systemic allergic reaction may result from the sting of one of these animals. The athlete should be treated for anaphylactic shock; basic life support must be given and the athlete transported promptly to the hospital.

Puncture Wounds

Punctures from the spines of urchins, stingrays, or certain spiny fish such as a catfish can best be treated by immobilizing the affected area and soaking it in hot water for 30 minutes. The water should be as hot as the athlete can stand without risking a burn. Toxins from these animals are heat-sensitive, and dramatic relief from local pain often occurs just from the application of hot water. Also, allergic reactions may occur with injections from these animals. There is always the possibility that tetanus and other infections could develop. These athletes should be taken to the emergency department for appropriate treatment for these problems (see Table 57.1).

Shocks and Skin Rashes

Other rare conditions include shocks from electric eels or skin rashes from marine parasites (see Table 57.1). In general, these injuries are mild. Panic from contact with electric eels can be the most impressive part of this particular injury.

IMPORTANT CONCEPTS

1. A poison is any substance that can produce a harmful effect on the body processes.
2. Common symptoms of poisoning are nausea, vomiting, abdominal pain, diarrhea, dilation or constriction of the pupils, excessive salivation or sweating, difficulty in breathing, unconsciousness, convulsions, cyanosis, and skin or mucous membrane inflammation.
3. Symptoms of an anaphylactic reaction to an insect sting or bite include generalized itching, hives, swelling about the lips and tongue, bronchospasm and wheezing, chest tightness and cough, dyspnea, anxiety, abdominal cramps, and anaphylactic shock.
4. Anaphylactic shock is a life-threatening emergency that may require full cardiopulmonary resuscitation.
5. The two species of spiders that can deliver serious, sometimes life-threatening, bites are the black widow and brown recluse.
6. The four species of poisonous snakes in the United States are the rattlesnake, the copperhead, the cottonmouth (water) moccasin, and the coral snake.
7. Rabies, usually fatal once it is contracted and well developed by humans, is carried by uninoculated dogs, as well as squirrels, bats, foxes, skunks, and raccoons.
8. The variety of germs contained in the human mouth is greater than the types found in the mouths of dogs or many other animals, thus making any injuries from human bites and lacerations by human teeth subject to serious infection.

SUGGESTED READINGS

Ellenhorn, M. J., and D. G. Barceloux. *Medical Toxicology: Diagnosis and Treatment of Human Poisoning.* New York: Elsevier, 1988.

Goldfrank, L. R., N. E. Flomenbaum, N. A. Lewin, et al., eds. *Goldfrank's Toxicologic Emergencies,* 3d ed. Norwalk, Conn.: Appleton-Century-Crofts, 1986.

Haddad, L. M., and J. F. Winchester, eds. *Clinical Management of Poisoning and Drug Overdose.* Philadelphia: W. B. Saunders, 1983.

Litovitz, T. L., B. F. Schmitz, N. Matyunas, et al. "1987 Annual Report of the American Association of Poison Control Centers National Data Collection System." *American Journal of Emergency Medicine* 6 (1988): 479–515.

58

Drugs in Sports

OBJECTIVES FOR CHAPTER 58

After reading this chapter, the student should be able to:

1. Describe the various types of anti-inflammatory medications available to treat athletic injuries.
2. Discuss the use of analgesics and anesthetics in the control of pain.
3. Be familiar with other medications athletes may use to treat conditions such as infections, allergies, and gastrointestinal and respiratory ailments.
4. Identify the categories of drugs banned by the National Collegiate Athletic Association (NCAA).
5. Understand the considerations involved in establishing a drug-testing program.

INTRODUCTION

Many drugs are used in the sports setting for the control of pain and the treatment of medical ailments. In recent years, certain drugs have been found to enhance performance, and their use has sparked much controversy. The athletic trainer must be knowledgeable about the drugs used to treat athletes, drugs that are banned, and the problems of drug abuse that unfortunately affect athletes as well as other individuals.

Chapter 58 describes medications used to control pain and inflammation from sports-induced acute or overuse injuries, as well as medications used to treat common medical conditions such as infections, allergies, and respiratory and gastrointestinal disturbances. Issues of drug misuse and drug testing are also discussed. ■

MEDICATIONS USED TO TREAT ATHLETES

As a result of the physical demands placed on them, all athletes can expect to experience an injury during the scope of their endeavor. Unfortunately, some athletes must endure painful chronic inflammatory injuries in addition to acute injuries. Medications that are used to control pain and inflammation include anti-inflammatory agents, analgesics, and anesthetics.

Anti-inflammatory medications are effective in controlling the production of prostaglandin, a chemical that is released at the site of injury and contributes to the body's inflammatory response to the injury. Anti-inflammatory agents are available in nonprescription and prescription formulas (Fig. 58.1). The most widely used anti-inflammatory is aspirin. Aspirin has analgesic effects (controls pain) as well as antipyretic effects (reduces body temperature).

Athletic trauma will produce varying degrees of pain and tissue insult, depending on the severity of the injury. Analgesics such as aspirin and acetaminophen are used to manage pain of nonvisceral origin, such as headaches and mild to moderate joint or muscle injuries. If the injury is severe, such as a glenohumeral dislocation or a wound that requires suturing, the physician will use an anesthetic such as lidocaine to control the athlete's pain.

Anti-inflammatory Agents

Systemic Anti-inflammatory Agents

Aspirin. Aspirin is a nonsteroidal, anti-inflammatory drug (NSAID). Aspirin has analgesic, anti-inflammatory, and antipyretic qualities. The analgesic and anti-inflammatory effects of aspirin on the body

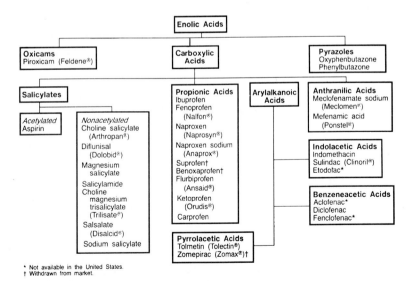

* Not available in the United States.
† Withdrawn from market.

FIGURE 58.1. Nonsteroidal anti-inflammatory drugs. (From *Nonsteroidal Anti-inflammatory Therapy—Some Questions and Answers.* Reprinted with permission of The Upjohn Company, Kalamazoo, Michigan.)

TABLE 58.1 Prescription NSAID

Medication	Dosage
Diclofenac (Voltaren)	50–75 mg twice a day
Diflunisal (Dolobid)	Initial dose of 500–1000 mg, followed by 250–500 mg 2–3 times a day
Fenoprofen (Nalfon)	400–800 mg 3–4 times a day
Flurbiprofen (Ansaid)	100 mg twice a day
Ibuprofen (Motrin)	400–800 mg 3–4 times a day
Indomethacin (Indocin)	75–100 mg a day in 3 or 4 divided doses
Ketoprofen (Orudis)	75 mg 3 times a day
Meclofenamate (Meclomen)	200–400 mg 4 times a day
Naproxen (Naprosyn, Anaprox)	250–500 mg twice a day
Phenylbutazone (Butazolidin)	300–600 mg 3–4 times a day (Serious side effects include aplastic anemia and agranulocytosis)
Piroxicam (Feldene)	20 mg a day
Sulindac (Clinoril)	200 mg twice a day
Tolmetin (Tolectin)	400 mg 4 times a day

result from its ability to inhibit the synthesis of prostaglandins. The recommended dosage of aspirin used in treating pain and inflammation is 650 mg, three to four times daily. Because aspirin can cause gastrointestinal disturbances, a buffered or enteric-coated form of aspirin can be taken to alleviate this discomfort. Aspirin, like most anti-inflammatory medications, should preferably be taken with food or a large quantity (240 ml) of water to minimize gastric irritation.

Ibuprofen. Ibuprofen, another NSAID, acts similarly to aspirin, phenylbutazone, and indomethacin. Ibuprofen is available in nonprescription as well as prescription strengths. A physician's prescription is needed for a dosage strength that is greater than 200 mg.

Higher doses of ibuprofen are required for anti-inflammatory effects than for analgesic effects. The usual adult dosage of ibuprofen in the symptomatic treatment of acute and chronic inflammation is 400 to 800 mg, three or four times daily. Dosage should be adjusted according to the ath-

lete's response and tolerance and should not exceed 3.2 grams daily. Therapeutic response usually occurs within 2 weeks of beginning ibuprofen. For relief of mild to moderate pain, the usual adult doses of ibuprofen are less than those used for treatment of inflammation.

Commonly prescribed NSAIDs. At times, a stronger anti-inflammatory medication may be indicated for the athlete. The stronger prescription anti-inflammatory agents act similarly to other NSAIDs. Table 58.1 lists the commonly used prescription-strength NSAIDs in sports medicine, along with suggested dosage strengths.

Local Anti-inflammatory Agents

Local corticosteroids, such as cortisone or cortisone-like derivatives, may occasionally be indicated in the treatment of an inflammatory condition. However, their use in athletics is controversial. Undoubtedly, local steroids can markedly decrease intra-articular inflammatory conditions, but they also can inhibit normal cartilage metabolism. Although local steroids can reduce periarticular or peritendinous inflammatory conditions, when they are injected into collagenous tissues such as tendons or ligaments, they can cause microscopic disorganization and subsequent weakening of these tissues. Repeated injections often lead to pathologic rupture. Therefore, steroids should be injected carefully, adjacent to ligaments and tendons—not into them. If local steroid injection therapy is used to treat tendinitis, particularly in the lower extremity, the part should be rested for 7 to 12 days following injection to minimize the risk of rupture.

Dimethyl Sulfoxide

Dimethyl sulfoxide (DMSO), a solvent derived from wood, aroused great interest because of claims of significant anti-inflammatory action. No studies to date have documented the efficacy of DMSO in managing inflammatory conditions related to athletics. Its use remains restricted by the Food and Drug Administration to the treatment of interstitial cystitis.

Several side effects from DMSO may occur from possible impurities in commercially available preparations. High doses of the drug have been shown to induce cataracts in experimental animal studies. Because DMSO is quickly absorbed through the skin after application, athletes who elect to use DMSO should be advised to thoroughly wash off chemicals or other substances from the area where the drug will be used to avoid absorption of these materials along with the DMSO. Also, DMSO will cause a strong garlic taste and breath after use.

Analgesics

Acetaminophen

One of the most common analgesics in use today is acetaminophen. It is used extensively to reduce mild to moderate pain and lower fever. Acetaminophen has been used in the treatment of pain in various combinations with aspirin, caffeine, and salicylamide. These combinations have not been clearly shown to have a greater analgesic effect than an optimal dose of acetaminophen alone. For relief of mild to moderate pain, the suggested daily dosage is 325 to 650 mg, every 4 to 6 hours.

Codeine

Codeine is a mild prescription analgesic used in the relief of mild to moderate pain which is not relieved by a nonopiate, analgesiclike acetaminophen. The usual oral dosage for relief of mild to moderate pain is 30 mg, every 4 hours. Codeine, at times, is prescribed in combination with aspirin or acetaminophen.

Morphine and Meperidine

Two other prescription analgesics that are available to the physician to control pain are morphine and meperidine. Morphine is dangerous to use because it can suppress respiration and is habit-forming. Meperidine is used to manage severe muscular pain and is habit-forming.

Anesthetics

When needed, local anesthetic agents are a valuable asset in controlling acute traumatic pain. The three common types of local anesthetics are lidocaine 1 percent (Xylocaine 1 percent) for common use; lidocaine 2 percent (Xylocaine 2 percent) with epinephrine for longer action; and bupivacaine 0.5 percent (Marcaine 0.5 percent) for use when prolonged action is needed. Not only are these agents useful in minor surgery (e.g., wound suturing), but also they can be used when a fracture or dislocation requires reduction.

Other Medications

Antibiotics

In addition to topical antibiotics for localized infections, athletes may occasionally require systemic antibiotics. Oral tetracycline, usually coupled with an expectorant, is often used to treat athletes with chronic bronchitis. A chest film can confirm the absence of alveolar disease. Tetracycline, or its relative minocycline, is also used to treat acne, a common problem among teenage athletes. Dosages used for acne treatment are low, typically 250 mg per day. Infected skin lesions (postoperative wounds, blisters, and abrasions), although treated with local antibiotic preparations following sterile cleansing, occasionally require systemic antibiotics. A common causative agent in infected skin wounds is penicillinase-resistant Staphylococcus aureus. This bacterium is susceptible to many of the cephalosporins as well as dicloxacillin. Therapy with one of these medications can begin before the culture results and sensitivity study are known.

"Strep" throat is occasionally seen in athletes, especially when resistance is decreased by long, strenuous workouts and little sleep. Athletes whose throats appear infected should have a culture, especially if exudate (thick fluid that has oozed out through the capillary walls) is present. If the culture is positive for beta streptococci, oral penicillin is the treatment of choice. If the athlete is allergic to penicillin, erythromycin may be substituted.

TABLE 58.2 NCAA Banned Drug Classes, 1990–1991 (Bylaw 31.2.3.1)

Psychomotor and central nervous system stimulants:

amiphenazole	dimethylamphetamine	pemoline
amphetamine	doxapram	pentetrazol
bemigride	ethamivan	phendimetrazine
benzphetamine	ethylamphetamine	phenmetrazine
caffeine	fencamfamine	phentermine
chlorphentermine	meclofenoxate	picrotoxine
cocaine	methamphetamine	pipradol
cropropamide	methylphenidate	prolintane
crothetamide	nikethamide	strychnine
diethylpropion		*and related compounds*

Anabolic steroids:

boldenone	methenolone	oxymesterone
clostebol	methandienone	oxymetholone
dehydrochlormethyl-testosterone	methyltestosterone	stanozolol
fluoxymesterone	nandrolone	testosterone
mesterolone	norethandrolone	*and related compounds*
	oxandrolone	

Substances banned for specific sports:

Rifle:

alcohol	metoprolol	propranolol
atenolol	nadolol	timolol
	pindolol	*and related compounds*

Diuretics:

acetazolamide	flumethiazide	quinethazone
bendroflumethiazide	furosemide	spironolactone
benzthiazide	hydrochlorothiazide	triamterene
bumetanide	hydroflumethiazide	trichlormethiazide
chlorothiazide	methyclothiazide	*and related compounds*
chlorthalidone	metolazone	
ethacrynic acid	polythiazide	

Street drugs:

heroin	THC (tetrahydrocannabinol)
marijuana	

Source: 1990/91 NCAA® Drug Testing/Education Programs, September 1990. Reprinted with permission of the National Collegiate Athletic Association.

Allergy Medications

Antihistamines are effective in treating allergic rhinitis, conjunctivitis, and hives. They will also control pruritus (itching) in contact dermatitis. However, their potential side effects of drowsiness and slow reaction time may be unacceptable to the competing athlete. Newer drugs, like terfenadine and astemizole, help control symptoms in the athlete with allergies without promoting drowsiness. In allergic rhinitis, decongestants may be as effective as antihistamines in alleviating upper airway obstruction and offer symptomatic relief without drowsiness. If antihistamines are indicated, the team physician and/or athletic trainer should make certain that the medication is not on the NCAA's banned substances list (Table 58.2).

Asthmatic athletes may find their symptoms are decreased if they remain well hydrated. Cromolyn sodium (Intal), theophylline, and beta adrenergics (epinephrine, isoproterenol, metaproterenol sulfate, and terbutaline sulfate) can also be used to control bronchospasms in the asthmatic. Again, any medications must be checked to make sure they are not on the NCAA's banned substances list. Beclomethasone dipropionate (Vanceril), a synthetic steroid, is available as an inhalant to treat allergic athletes. Many physicians feel steroids (oral or inhalant), though effective, should not be used in the daily management of the asthmatic athlete and should be employed only briefly to manage a severe allergic reaction. **Exercise-induced asthma** is bronchospasm precipitated by exercise. It frequently occurs in previously nonallergic persons. Similar to the treatment of the asthmatic athlete, treatment of exercise-induced asthma focuses on hydration and the use of bronchodilators prior to exercise.

Exercise-induced anaphylaxis is another medical emergency. Like any anaphylactic reaction, the symptoms are sweating, high blood pressure, fever, and a feeling of "impending doom." Immediate treatment with fluids, subcutaneous epinephrine, and intravenous diphenhydramine (25 to 50 mg) is needed while transporting the athlete to the nearest emergency department. The etiology of exercise-induced anaphylaxis is not known, but it is probably multifactorial. As in exercise-induced asthma, the athlete may have no allergic history. One episode of exercise-induced anaphylaxis does not necessarily predispose the athlete to future attacks (see Chapter 53).

Gastrointestinal Medications

Occasionally, the nervous or agitated athlete will have gastric upsets and problems of hyperacidity for which magnesium and aluminum hydroxide preparations (Maalox, Amphojel, Gelusil, etc.) are useful. An effective drug for nausea is prochlorperazine (Compazine) or promethazine hydrochloride (Phenergan) in oral doses of 5 to 15 mg. These medications are also available in injectable and suppository forms.

Diarrhea, of either functional or organic origin, may be a problem on road trips, particularly with indiscriminate or irregular eating. In most conditions, diphenoxylate with atropine (Lomotil) has replaced other antidiarrheal agents because of its convenience, low toxicity, and effectiveness. It is given in doses of 1 to 2 tablets, 4 to 6 hours apart.

Medications for the Common Cold

The symptoms of the common cold are difficult to treat, at best. With the athlete's high level of exertion and resulting fatigue, cold symptoms can be particularly troublesome. Decongestants open up nasal passages, and because of their drying effect can secondarily reduce cough. The combination of decongestants and antihistamines is even more effective in relieving congestion. As in the treatment of allergic rhinitis, the secondary effects of decreased reaction time and drowsiness of the antihistamines must be balanced against their increased effectiveness over decongestants alone. Timing may be an important factor in choosing a medication. Prescribing a decon-

gestant during the day and an antihistamine at night (when drowsiness may be beneficial and not detrimental) is often a good treatment plan.

BANNED DRUGS AND PRACTICES

Unfortunately, illegal use of drugs has become part of the athletic arena. Recent episodes of athletes caught using banned substances such as steroids and cocaine during and after competition have resulted in drug-testing regulations and drug awareness programs. The NCAA has issued strict guidelines about drugs and procedures that are subject to restrictions (see appendix on p. 918). Even athletes who are taking prescription medicine for treatment of illness or injury have to be careful that the medication does not contain ingredients that are on the NCAA's list of banned substances (see Table 58.2).

Athletes are first members of society; therefore, managing the demands and pressures of their athletic endeavors comes on top of managing the stresses of their everyday lives. Most athletes find coping with these dual stresses comes as naturally as their athletic ability. For some athletes, however, drugs and alcohol offer an escape and a potentially deadly outlet from unmanageable stress or seemingly unsolvable problems.

Athletic trainers and others involved with athletes must learn to recognize the symptoms and dangers of drug and substance abuse. Even more important is learning how to direct an athlete with symptoms of substance abuse into a treatment or counseling program.

Psychomotor Drugs

Stimulants

The primary effect of psychomotor stimulants is on the brain and central nervous system. They increase motor activity and delay the onset of the subjective feeling of fatigue. Because stimulants cause excessive energy expenditure, they probably do not improve muscular performance. Depending on the dosage, the individual's sensitivity, and other factors, stimulants may be toxic and often create psychological dependency problems.

Caffeine, considered one of the least dangerous of the psychomotor stimulants, is one of the most common. Found in tea, coffee, cocoa, and colas, caffeine not only acts as a psychomotor stimulant, but also stimulates cardiac muscle. Recently, it was shown that 330 mg of caffeine (equivalent to about 2½ cups of coffee) increases plasma fatty acids by enhancing lipolysis. This effect spares glycogen depletion and, hence, may aid performance in endurance exercise.

Depressants

Psychomotor depressants include narcotic analgesics, antihistamines, sedatives, antidepressants, hypnotics, and alcohol. These drugs decrease activity of the central nervous system and have been used to increase physical and psychological tolerance of pain in an attempt to improve athletic performance. Because many psychomotor depressants are used legitimately to lessen pain or relieve muscle spasms following an injury, they highlight the major problem that drug regulation committees for organized sports must face: where does therapy end and "doping" begin?

Alcohol is the most widely used and abused drug among both teenagers and adults. Alcohol is a powerful, central nervous system depressant. As is the case with all other drugs, the user builds up a certain tolerance to alcohol; individuals addicted to alcohol require larger amounts to get the same effect. Alcoholics can be young, middle-aged, elderly, males, females, executives, blue-collar workers, students, athletes, or "bums." More than 50 percent of all traffic fatalities or injuries involve at least one drunken driver. Chronic alcoholics are often suicidal.

Why athletes abuse alcohol is a complex topic that cannot be addressed here. One misguided belief is that alcohol will decrease nervous tremors and, therefore, will increase precision in marksmanship sports —riflery, archery, etc. Another myth is that alcohol decreases anxiety and, therefore, improves concentration and serves as a readily available source of carbohydrates for endurance events. Actually, alcohol's benefit in a carbohydrate-loading diet is far below that of other high-carbohydrate sources such as pastas and sweetened juices. Moreover, alcohol provokes dehydration by blocking antidiuretic hormones produced by the pituitary to prevent water loss from the kidneys. Alcohol decreases alertness, slows reaction time, and impairs coordination and judgment. It causes fat to accumulate in the liver and can lead to fatty degeneration of this organ.

Performance-Enhancing Practices and Abuses

Blood Doping

Blood doping refers to withdrawing a unit of blood from the athlete and storing it for several weeks prior to competition. Normal homeostatic mechanisms then begin synthesizing red blood cells to return the red blood cell count to the "predraw" level. Prior to the event, the athlete is transfused with the previously drawn unit of blood. These added cells raise the red blood cell count to greater than normal levels. The theory, of course, is that additional red blood cells will increase oxygen-carrying capacity and, hence, improve aerobic endurance. Data substantiating this conclusion are controversial. One risk of blood doping is the **hyperviscosity syndrome**, in which the hematocrit is greater than 60 percent. Intravascular clotting, heart failure, and death may occur. Blood doping is not advised.

Anabolic Steroids

Anabolic steroids are synthetic modifications of testosterone developed to increase the anabolic action of this compound relative to its androgenic effects. Athletes combine anabolic steroids with an intense progressive resistance exercise program and a high-protein diet during their training periods in an attempt to increase body weight and muscle mass. Although there is general agreement that anabolic steroids increase muscle mass if taken in combination with adequate weight-training programs and protein-rich diets, this increase in muscle bulk does not appear to provide gains in endurance. The risks of taking anabolic steroids are significant, including sterility, premature epiphyseal closure in the adolescent, salt and water retention, testicular atrophy, oligospermia, prostatic hypertrophy, hypercalcemia, cholestatic jaundice, and hepatocellular carcinoma (liver cancer). In females, male-patterned baldness, clitoral hypertrophy, facial hair, and a deepening of the voice may also occur.

Contemporary research indicates that anabolic steroids have not only a physiological effect, but also a psychological effect. Athletes taking steroids usually have noticeable personality changes. They may become aggressive, in some cases even to the extreme of borderline sociopathic. Additionally, research indicates that like any abused drug, anabolic steroids can cause future psychological disorders. Since some athletes inject these substances into their bodies, concern must be also directed to the passive transmission of the AIDS virus through contaminated needles.

Substance Abuse

Overdose Signs and Symptoms

Frequently abused stimulant drugs include amphetamines ("speed," "bennies") and cocaine ("coke," "crack," "snow"). Caffeine, found in coffee and cola drinks, is a mild stimulant, as are certain anti-asthmatic drugs such as epinephrine (Adrenalin) and aminophylline. Certain drugs commonly used as nasal decongestants, such as ephedrine and isoproterenol, are also mild stimulants. These drugs are taken orally with the exception of cocaine, which is frequently sniffed.

The sale of certain equipment, particularly that used to prepare cocaine, is legal in many states. The presence of such drug paraphernalia as spoons, lamps, and pipes should alert the trainer to the possibility of drug abuse. Physical findings that suggest addiction to depressants and stimulants include small, nonreactive pupils and multiple needle marks on the skin of the forearms and hands.

All of these stimulants can cause a profound reactive depression when they are stopped or if they are suddenly taken in large amounts. The usual manifestation of overdose of a stimulant drug is an obviously excited, agitated athlete with rapid pulse and respirations, and even convulsions. An overdosed athlete is seriously ill.

An athlete who has taken a hallucinogenic drug such as LSD or marijuana usually is in an altered state of awareness. These athletes rarely take a large enough overdose to cause coma or unconsciousness, but occasionally the hallucinatory effect may be extremely unpleasant and result in a panic state—the "bad trip." In the case of an overdose, the trainer should establish and maintain an adequate airway. Then the emergency care of these athletes is the same as for any other emotionally ill athlete: emotional support; a calm, professional, straightforward manner; and prompt transportation to the hospital. These athletes should not be restrained unless they are physically dangerous, and they should never be left alone.

A depressant such as alcohol dulls the sense of awareness, slows reflexes, and decreases reaction time. Athletes under the influence of alcohol may show the same signs as athletes with physical illnesses or injuries, specifically head injuries, toxic reactions, or uncontrolled diabetes. Always bear in mind that an athlete suffering from the effects of alcohol could have a physical illness as well. If there is the slightest question a person may have some illness other than alcoholic overdose, bring the athlete to the hospital. Often the family or acquaintances can provide a good history of the athlete's drinking pattern.

Intoxicated athletes may show aggressive and inappropriate behavior, fall easily, and be combative. Steps must be taken to protect them from self-injury. Occasionally, an athlete consumes so much alcohol that signs of central nervous system depression appear, and respiratory support may be necessary. These athletes must be transported promptly to the hospital.

Overdose Management

In cases of drug overdose, as with any illness or injury, an overall assessment of the athlete is necessary, and treatment priorities must be established. In general, airway maintenance is the first priority. Preventing self-injury, maintaining level of consciousness, and evaluating the athlete for other injuries are the other crucial parts of the initial assessment.

Athletes who have overdosed have an altered sense of consciousness and are often depressed. Vomiting in any athlete who is not fully conscious and fully alert should not be induced due to the danger of aspiration of the vomited material into the tracheobronchial tree. Convulsions are frequently seen in athletes who have overdosed. The trainer should protect the athlete from falls or biting the tongue by the usual techniques for managing athletes with convulsions (see Chapter 55).

The athletic trainer should try to maintain the athlete's level of consciousness by constant stimulation such as gentle shaking, conversation, or light pinching. If the athlete becomes unconscious, severe respiratory depression may follow rapidly. If respirations are severely depressed, the trainer will need to establish and maintain an adequate airway.

Athletes who are under the influence of hallucinogenic or stimulant drugs must be approached in a calm, professional, sympathetic manner. Often it is possible to "talk the athlete down,"—that is, to calm and reorient the athlete. The trainer should try to gain the athlete's confidence and avoid the use of restraints if possible.

Athletes in severely depressed states often injure themselves unknowingly. The athletic trainer should quickly check the athlete for suspected fractures or other injuries. Sometimes the athlete has a head injury as well as a drug overdose, and it is difficult, if not impossible, to separate the effects of the two. These athletes should be taken to the hospital promptly and treated as though they had sustained a serious head injury.

Athletes who abuse injectable drugs may have fever from deep infections of the brain, heart, or other organs resulting from the use of contaminated equipment and unsterile drugs. The source of these infections may not be apparent. The incidence of hepatitis is particularly high in these athletes, and they may be jaundiced. Jaundice can be detected by a yellow coloring of the sclera (white portion of the eye) or the skin. Always remember that hepatitis is extremely contagious and precautions should be taken to avoid infection. Additionally, it is a documented fact that HIV can be transmitted through contaminated needles and blood. Extreme caution must be used when handling needles or treating wounds of a known drug user.

DRUG TESTING

Drug testing is a controversial issue in contemporary athletics. While most of the discussion about drug testing has centered on its legal ramifications, drug testing is now standard practice in national and international competitions. Reviewing the legal ramifications of drug testing is beyond the scope of this chapter, so discussion is limited to specific components of a drug-testing program that must be in place before an athlete is tested for using a banned substance. The NCAA has established the following guidelines for colleges and universities that are considering implementing a drug-testing program:

1. The college's or university's legal counsel must be kept informed at every stage,

particularly in regard to right-to-privacy statutes.

2. Before initiating drug-testing activity, a specific written policy on drug testing should be developed, distributed, and publicized. The policy should include such information as (a) a clear explanation of the purposes of the program; (b) the drugs to be tested, how often, and under what conditions; and (c) actions to be taken, if any, against an athlete who tests positive.

3. An appropriate waiver form should be developed wherein the athlete agrees to submit to the drug-testing program. (This is the one facet of drug testing that has faced most of the legal challenge.)

4. Agree on the list and/or types of drugs to be tested. The NCAA provides a listing to schools of its banned substances (see Table 58.2). The NCAA and International Olympic Committee have similar banned substances lists and update their lists annually. It is advisable that all athletes be made aware of these lists so that they, along with their physicians and athletic trainers, be assured that any medication they are presently using is not now banned.

Logistical aspects of a drug-testing program must also be in place before an athlete is tested. These administrative components include:

1. When, from whom, and how will urine samples be collected, secured, and transported to the laboratory?

2. Who will select the laboratory that will analyze the urine samples? Questions concerning the laboratory staff's qualifications and experience with drug testing need to be addressed. Does the laboratory have the necessary equipment to test the types of drugs to be analyzed?

3. How will urine samples be stored and how soon will analysis be initiated?

4. What type of analytical procedures will be conducted—radioimmunologic assay or gas chromatography? Is the laboratory capable of performing mass spectrometry analysis as well?

5. What are the laboratory's false-positive and false-negative rates?

6. How will false-positives be identified and processed?

7. Who will receive the test results and how will the results be used?

It is important throughout the entire process to protect the athlete's right to privacy and to make available to the athlete educational materials and resources on drug education and related topics and matters.

IMPORTANT CONCEPTS

1. Nonsteroidal, anti-inflammatory agents are used to treat pain and inflammation.

2. Local anesthetics are used for controlling acute pain, minor surgery, and reducing a fracture or dislocation.

3. Psychomotor depressants are controversial because they increase physical and psychological tolerance of pain in an attempt to improve performance.

4. Alcohol decreases alertness, slows reaction time, and impairs coordination.

5. Anabolic steroids increase muscle mass but are controversial because of the physiological and psychological risks attached to their use.

6. Amphetamines and cocaine can cause a profound depression when they are stopped or if they are suddenly taken in large doses.

SUGGESTED READINGS

The 1988–89 NCAA Banned Substance Listing Book. Mission, Kans.: NCAA Publishing, 1988.

The 1990–91 NCAA Drug-Testing Educational Program. Mission, Kans.: NCAA Publishing, 1991.

Physicians' Desk Reference for Nonprescription Drugs, 11th ed. (annual). Oradell, N.J.: Medical Economics Company, 1990.

Physicians' Desk Reference, PDR, 44th ed. (annual). Oradell, N.J.: Medical Economics Company, 1990.

APPENDIX: NCAA BYLAW 31.2.3.1.1

Drugs and Procedures Subject to Restrictions

The use of the following drugs and/or procedures is subject to certain restrictions and may not be permissible, depending on limitations expressed in these guidelines and/or quantities of these substances used:

(a) *Blood Doping.* The practice of blood doping (the intravenous injection of whole blood, packed red blood cells or blood substitutes), as well as the use of erythropoietin (red blood cell producing hormone), is prohibited and any evidence confirming use will be cause for action consistent with that taken for a positive drug test.

(b) *Growth Hormone.* The use of growth hormone (human, animal or synthetic) or human chorionic gonadotropin (HCG) is prohibited and any evidence confirming use will be cause for action consistent with that taken for a positive drug test.

(c) *Local Anesthetics.* The Executive Committee will permit the limited use of local anesthetics under the following conditions:

(i) That procaine, xylocaine, carbocaine without epinephrine or any other vaso-constrictor may be used, but not cocaine;

(ii) That only local or topical injections can be used (i.e., intravenous injections are not permitted);

(iii) That use is medically justified only when permitting the athlete to continue the competition without potential risk to his or her health, and

(iv) That the Association's crew chief in charge of testing must be advised in writing by the team physician if the anesthetic has been administered within 24 hours of the competition. He or she also must be advised of time, route and dose of administration.

(d) *Manipulation of Urine Samples.* The Executive Committee bans the use of substances and methods that alter the integrity and/or validity of urine samples provided during NCAA drug testing. Examples of banned methods are catheterization, urine substitution, and/or tampering or modification of renal excretion by the use of diuretics, probenecid or related compounds.

(e) *Additional Analysis.* Drug screening for select nonbanned substances may be conducted at NCAA championships and certified postseason football contests for nonpunitive purposes.

EIGHT

SELECTED ATHLETIC GROUPS

59

Female Athletes

OBJECTIVES FOR CHAPTER 59

After reading this chapter, the student should be able to:

1. Describe the anatomic and physiologic factors in women that affect their sports performance.
2. Describe the psychological adjustments that female athletes must make.
3. Discuss how proper conditioning, including a weight-training program, is as important for preventing injuries in female athletes as it is for preventing injuries in male athletes.
4. Discuss the diagnosis and treatment of common orthopedic problems seen in female athletes.
5. Identify the most common medical problems of female athletes.

INTRODUCTION

In the last several years, more and more women have been competing in athletic events. With this increase in participation has come the realization that female athletes benefit just as much as their male counterparts from conditioning and weight-training programs. They also suffer the same kinds of injuries as male athletes. However, anatomic and physiologic differences do exist between male and female athletes, giving each sex certain advantages. The trainer who understands the inherent genetic strengths and weaknesses of both sexes will be able to help female athletes maximize their athletic performance.

Chapter 59 begins with an explanation of the anatomic and physiologic differences that exist between the sexes and addresses the psychological factors that influence the participation and performance of female athletes. The chapter then discusses the relationship between conditioning and injury rates and the effects of weight training in female athletes. The last two sections of Chapter 59 discuss common orthopedic and medical problems of female athletes. ■

MALE AND FEMALE ATHLETES: COMPARISONS

"A Range of Normal"

The anatomic and physiologic differences between men and women explain the uniqueness of each sex in athletics. Despite the data on the "typical" man and the "typical" woman, the spectrum of these differences overlaps. In reality, these differences are not as definitive as they may seem in the following discussion, nor do they absolutely define male and female sports dominions. They do, however, provide each sex with "an edge" in certain areas of sports performance.

Training diminishes absolute genetic advantages and disadvantages. These differences are not explained to catalogue the abilities of each sex, but rather to assist the athletic trainer with the conditioning, treatment, and rehabilitation of athletes. By recognizing inherent genetic strengths and weaknesses of individuals, trainers will be able to help athletes maximize their performance.

Anatomic Comparisons

Size and Weight Variations

In general, females have smaller bones and correspondingly smaller areas of articular surface than males. Males have longer legs, comprising 56 percent of their height, as compared to 51 percent in women. Males' heavier, larger, more rugged structure gives them a mechanical and structural advantage in athletic activities. The longer bones of males are greater levers, producing more force in sports that require striking, hitting, and kicking.

Overall Form

Females have narrower shoulders, a wider pelvis, and a greater valgus angle of their legs at the knee than their male counterparts. In female athletes, the greater varus of the hips and valgus of the knees are sometimes blamed for the increased number of overuse syndromes seen in these areas, particularly in the unconditioned state (Fig. 59.1).

The wider pelvis and shorter lower extremities of females give them a lower center of gravity than males. The location of females' center of gravity is 56.1 percent of their height compared to 56.7 percent in males. Females, therefore, have a distinct advantage in balance sports such as gymnastics. Males must widen their stance to obtain the same degree of balance. Hence, the balance beam is one of four major events in women's gymnastics competition, but not in men's gymnastics competition.

Physiologic Comparisons

Aerobic Capacity

For the same body weight, females have smaller hearts, lower diastolic and systolic blood pressures, and smaller lungs and thoracic capacities than equally trained males. These differences decrease female athletes' effectiveness in both anaerobic (burst) and aerobic (endurance) activities. Aerobic capacity depends on one's genetic ability to maximally consume oxygen. Training can and does enhance **maximal oxygen consumption** (VO_2 max), but the baseline is genetically determined. VO_2 max reflects the body's ability to maximally extract and use oxygen for aerobic metabolism. VO_2 max also measures the lung's ability to extract oxygen, the heart's ability to deliver oxygen to the muscle, and the muscle's ability to maximally assimilate oxygen in energy pathways.

Because of her smaller heart, stroke volume, and lung and muscle mass, a female with the same weight and conditioned state as a male has a lower baseline VO_2 max upon which to build aerobic capacity. However, these physiologic parameters have a continuum for each sex. Some females on the upper spectrum of the VO_2 max capacity have a greater genetic baseline than some males on the lower end of the masculine profile (Fig. 59.2).

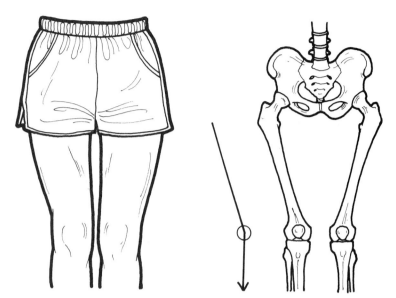

FIGURE 59.1. Females have a greater varus of the hips and a greater valgus angle of the legs at the knee than their male counterparts.

Body Composition

With regard to body composition, normal college-age females have approximately 25 percent fat per body weight versus 15 percent fat for college-age males. Conditioned athletes vary significantly according to sport. For track athletes, the average conditioned female has about 10 to 15 percent body fat, while the conditioned male has generally less than 7 percent.

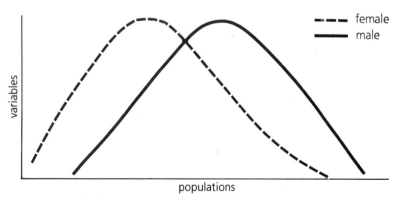

Note: Overlap between sexes

FIGURE 59.2. Spectrum of anatomic and physiologic variables between the sexes.

TABLE 59.1. Male and Female Body Composition

	% Fat*	% Muscle Mass*
Conditioned female	10–15	23
Unconditioned female	25	
Conditioned male	<7	40
Unconditioned male	15	

*Percent per total body weight

The muscle mass of females is approximately 23 percent of body weight, whereas equally trained males have approximately 40 percent muscle mass. Because a female has less muscle per body weight, it is more difficult for her to achieve the same power and speed as an equally trained male of the same body weight. The greater percentage of fat per body weight in the female adds to her power and her speed disadvantages (Table 59.1).

The increased percentage of body fat per body weight in females is a disadvantage when matched with males of equal muscle mass, since females must use the same muscle mass to "energize" their extra body fat. If a male performs in a weighted vest equal to a woman's excess body fat, his VO_2 max lowers to the female's range.

Female athletes have been compared with race horses carrying a heavier handicap. Their extra load of fat reduces their work capacity and stamina. But fat does insulate and give buoyancy—an advantage for swimmers, especially in natural waters. It is a female who holds the record for swimming the English Channel; in 1978, Penny Dean achieved the best one-way time of 7 hours, 40 minutes.

Fat also provides energy when glycogen is depleted. Females may be able to convert to fatty acid metabolism more readily than their male counterparts, an advantage in marathons and ultramarathons.

Sudorific Response

Previously, it was thought females were more prone to heat exhaustion than males and needed higher core body temperatures to increase their sudorific (sweating) response. However, recent evidence demonstrates that training influences thermal regulation, and early reports of females' poor sweating response merely reflected a lack of proper conditioning.

Basal Metabolic Rate

Basal metabolic rate is lower in females, meaning that the female athlete burns fewer calories than a male performing the same activity. This difference is important to remember when planning training tables and pre-game meals for female athletes. Women need nutritionally balanced meals with fewer total calories than men. This fact, although seemingly obvious, can be easily overlooked.

When women first entered the military academies, the diet of the cadets was not altered. The women gained weight from eating the same high-calorie foods (gravy, potatoes, bread, sauces, etc.) that were provided for male cadets to ensure them of adequate caloric intake to maintain basal body weights during a time of intense physical effort. The academies learned they had to provide nutritional meals with fewer total calories (lean meats, fewer sauces, more fruits, and vegetables) for their female cadets.

Coordination and Dexterity

Coordination and dexterity are difficult parameters to measure, but there appears to be no gender-related superiority.

Effect of Puberty

Anatomic and physiologic variations occur in hormonally mature men and women. The prepubertal female is fairly equal to the prepubertal male in strength, aerobic power, oxygen, pulse, heart size, and weight. In the male, puberty is a time of maturation of fitness, but in the female it is a period of great alteration of physical characteristics and abilities, making her no longer equal to the male in size or strength.

A female must adjust timing and performance techniques to accommodate increases in weight and height without the help of a parallel increase in muscle mass. Recall the prepubertal Nadia Comaneci of the 1976 Olympics, the talented gymnast who won everyone's heart during her outstanding performance (Fig. 59.3). Four years later, puberty had taken its toll. Comaneci's percentage of body fat had increased, curves had replaced her previously straight lines, and her center of gravity had changed. She was never able to regain her prepubertal performance level.

PSYCHOLOGICAL ADJUSTMENT

Puberty is not the only problem requiring psychological adjustments on the part of the female athlete. Since ancient Greek times, independence, fortitude, aggressiveness, achievement, and the desire to win or conquer have been classified as masculine or "nonfeminine" qualities. Yet, these are the important characteristics in successful athletes. Traditionally, the winning male athlete has proven his masculinity, whereas the winning female athlete often finds she must justify her femininity. This attitude is slowly changing, but it will be years before prejudices arbitrarily qualifying masculinity and femininity disappear.

Female athletes may face depression because they feel they are not living up to the image expectations of their sex. Those involved in the care of female athletes should be aware that these feelings may develop, and they should be prepared to help female athletes cope with them.

Injury can be precipitated by lack of confidence, and sometimes both female and male athletes may appear for sick call for many minor "hurts." Physically they are fine, but they may be reaching out for psychological reassurance. The athletic trainer must be sensitive to this need and respond accordingly.

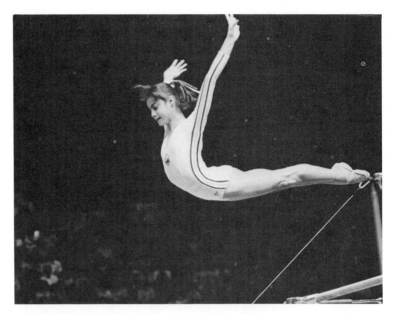

FIGURE 59.3. Nadia Comaneci scoring a perfect 10 at the 1976 Olympic women's gymnastic competition.   (From AP/Wide World Photos.)

CONDITIONING AND REHABILITATION

Relationship of Conditioning and Injury Rates

Prior to the 1980s, authorities blocked the participation of women in long-distance running events because they believed women were not physically strong enough to sustain such an activity and would harm themselves. The performance of the first women to run the 800-meter race only reinforced this theory. The majority of the participants, untrained and uncoached, tried to sprint the entire distance, and many collapsed along the way.

Lack of conditioning was probably also responsible for early reports demonstrating an increased rate of injuries in female athletes compared with males. Similarly, studies of the first female cadets admitted to the military academies found that women had an increase in minor injuries and a greater time loss from duty.

The early conclusion from these studies was that women were physiologically inferior to men. In reality, these studies merely reflected the fact that females entering the military academy had not been subjected during their high school years to physical training programs as rigorous as those of males. After several months at the academy, the number of minor injuries and days lost from duty decreased significantly for female cadets.

Recently, several studies have demonstrated greater differences in the number and types of injuries sustained by athletes in different sports than by males and females in the same sport. As in male athletes, most injuries seen in female athletes are sprains, strains, and contusions, especially of the lower extremities. Injury studies done on female athletes show that conditioning programs, including properly structured weight-training programs, are as important for women as they are for men. Conditioning increases endurance, strength, and flexibility, and therefore decreases the number of injuries.

Weight Training, Hormones, and Muscle Mass

Weight training increases strength but will not necessarily result in increased muscle bulk in females. A female can increase her strength by 44 percent without any significant increase in muscle mass. Muscle size is hormonally regulated. Within a sex, the secretion of testosterone, androgen, and estrogen (the sex hormones) varies considerably and accounts for marked variations in terms of muscularity and general morphology among males and females.

COMMON ORTHOPEDIC PROBLEMS

Some common orthopedic problems seen in female athletes more frequently than in male athletes include retropatellar pain, shoulder pain, spondylolysis, stress fractures, and bunions. These problems have been discussed more fully in the chapters on musculoskeletal injuries (Section Three).

Only a brief summary of each will be presented here.

Retropatellar Pain

Women commonly complain of **retropatellar pain**, also known as **patellofemoral stress syndrome (PFSS)** or pain behind the kneecap. Pain may develop from direct trauma to the patella or from repetitive knee flexion-extension activities.

Decreasing retropatellar pain is frequently difficult. Hamstring-stretching and quadriceps-strengthening exercises are the basis of any therapy program. As in most acute inflammatory processes, icing following activity may be helpful.

Physicians may also prescribe various braces, shoe orthoses, or nonsteroidal anti-

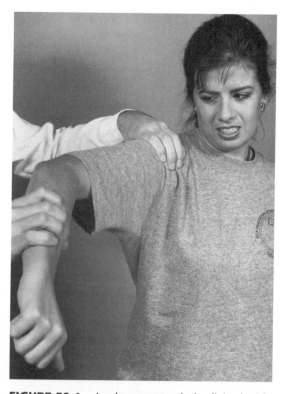

FIGURE 59.4. Impingement pain is elicited with the examiner's hand exerting downward pressure on the acromion while the athlete's arm is internally rotated and elevated into forward flexion.

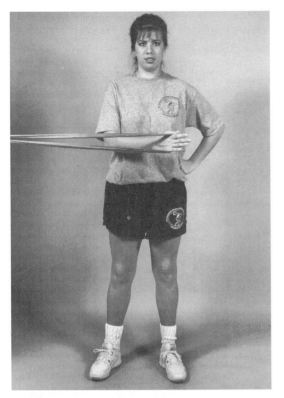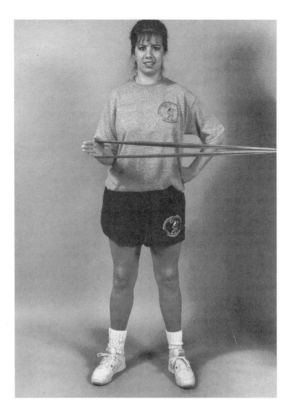

FIGURE 59.5. Shoulder rotator cuff exercises can be done by attaching a small piece of surgical or rubber tubing onto a door: (left) sustained internal rotation against the tubing; (right) sustained external rotation against the tubing.

inflammatory medications. Muscle-stimulating units to strengthen the vastus medialis have also met with some success. Stair climbing and deep squats should be eliminated from the conditioning program.

Shoulder Pain

Shoulder pain in female athletes, particularly in swimmers and softball players, is usually due to either subluxation or impingement. The female with shoulder **subluxation** complains of pain in the anterior region of her shoulder when her shoulder is placed in external rotation, abduction, and extension. In this position, the humeral head subluxes against the anterior shoulder capsule, stretching the capsular tissue and thereby causing pain in this area.

In the female athlete with **impingement**, a weakened rotator cuff (weakened secondary to repetitive use or other trauma) allows the humeral head to migrate superiorly, rather than staying centrally located in the glenoid fossa. With a weak rotator cuff, deltoid contraction, such as occurs with overhead motions like throwing and tennis serves, results in tissue (the supraspinatus) being impinged between the acromion and the upwardly migrated humeral head. Inflammation and pain result. Downward pressure on the acromion while elevating the humerus in a forward-flexed manner reproduces the pain (Fig. 59.4).

Both shoulder subluxation and shoulder impingement can be managed by strengthening programs for the rotator cuff and shoulder muscles. Rubber tubing provides an excellent way to perform exercises in a "pseudo" isokinetic fashion (Fig. 59.5).

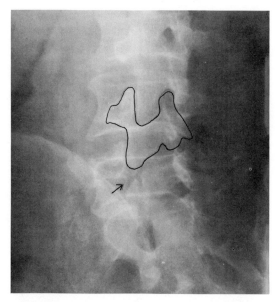

FIGURE 59.6. Spondylolysis shown at the level of L3. Note the Scotty dog configuration at L4 and L3. The disruption at the dog's neck in L5 is spondylolysis.

Spondylolysis

Low back pain in female athletes may be associated with defects in the posterior elements of the spine, a condition called **spondylolysis** (Fig. 59.6). This defect occurs four times more often in the female gymnast than in the general population.

The team physician must determine whether a symptomatic athlete's radiologic defect is an acute stress fracture or an aggravation from chronic spondylolysis. If symptoms are secondary to an acute stress fracture, prolonged rest is recommended. In cases of aggravating chronic pain from spondylolysis, rest during the acute phase, with gradual return to activity, is usually prescribed. Anti-inflammatories, muscle relaxants, ice massage, and other physical therapy modalities may be helpful. A regular exercise program for abdominal and back muscles should be instituted.

Stress Fractures

Stress fractures occur when the rate of bone breakdown from activity (a normal process) is greater than the rate of bone formation (repair). Slow and sensible conditioning for sport is necessary to give bone time to increase in cortical thickness to meet the mechanical demands of exercise. The pain of a stress fracture is typically restricted to a specific area, becomes worse with activity, and is often relieved with rest.

Initially, radiographs may not demonstrate the area of fracture, since many stress fractures are "microfractures" of bone. X-rays can be helpful, however, at about 2 weeks, when healing (increased bony reaction around the stress fracture) becomes apparent. A bone scan is more sensitive than routine radiographs and is positive in the early phases of bone healing. (See Chapter 15 for a more complete discussion of stress fractures.) The greater incidence of stress fractures in female athletes probably represents a lack of conditioning and proper training techniques, rather than true predisposition to injury.

Some physicians have expressed concern over the possibility of a greater incidence of stress fractures in female athletes with **amenorrhea** (lack of regular menstrual periods). Amenorrhea may be associated with low levels of estrogen. Estrogen has a protective effect on preserving bone calcium. In postmenopausal women, estrogen-protective effects are absent and bone minerals may be lost, resulting in **osteoporosis**, which predisposes these women to fractures. Some argue that the low estrogen levels associated with amenorrhea may also result in loss of normal bone minerals and increase the incidence of stress fractures. Much is still to be learned on this issue.

Healing will usually occur if the stress on the bone is reduced. If the lower extremity is involved, a cane or crutch may be helpful until the athlete can bear weight on the extremity without pain. When the athlete can walk long distances unaided and pain-free, she may attempt to run.

In the interim, non–weight-bearing activities such as biking and swimming will maintain cardiovascular endurance and muscle tone without stressing the injured area. Ongoing participation in an exercise program will benefit the athlete psychologically and hasten her return to her desired sport.

Bunions

Perhaps because of shoe styles, **bunions** of the first toes (inflammation of the bursa over the medial side of the metatarsophalangeal joint of the great toe) are more common in females than in males. The inflamed bursa is generally associated with a deformity of the toe at this level. Bony hypertrophy of the metatarsal head often underlies the inflamed bursa.

All conservative modalities should be used to treat bunions, since surgery may alter foot mechanics and precipitate other problems for the athlete. Treatment for painful bunions is directed to decreasing pressure over the inflamed medial metatarsal area. Shoe alterations (wider toe box), orthoses, and protective pads may be successful in diminishing symptoms.

COMMON MEDICAL PROBLEMS

Common medical problems unique to female athletes include iron deficiency, with or without anemia; amenorrhea; dysmenorrhea; and vaginitis.

Iron Deficiency

The mineral iron, present in the hemoglobin molecules within red blood cells, is necessary for oxygen transport. A normal iron level, then, is especially important for athletes who need maximal oxygen-carrying capacity for maximal energy output. Iron deficiency in women is more common than in men because a woman can lose up to 1.2 to 2 mg of iron per day during menstruation. Menstruating females have a higher incidence of iron deficiency than the general population.

Iron may also participate as a catalyst in removing the lactate formed during aerobic exercise. Women who are iron deficient but not anemic have increased lactate levels with submaximal exercise when compared with women with normal levels of iron.

Strenuous exercise during early conditioning programs has been reported to lower plasma iron levels in both sexes, perhaps because of increased destruction of red cells with vigorous activity, but the exact cause is not known.

Iron supplementation in women is advised unless sufficient quantities are part of the athlete's diet. The recommended daily allowance of iron for menstruating women is 18 mg per day. Only 10 percent of all ingested iron is absorbed through the gastrointestinal system. Foods high in iron include liver, oysters, beef, turkey, dried apricots, and prune juice. Ferrous sulfate, taken as a 300-gm tablet each day, may be used to supplement dietary iron sources. A multivitamin plus iron generally has only 12 mg of iron.

Too much iron is as harmful as too little. Megadoses of iron will not make blood "iron rich" or improve oxygen-carrying capacity. Iron overdose can be toxic.

The Menstrual Cycle

Normal ovulation and menstruation depend on proper hormonal secretion by the hypothalamus, the pituitary, and the ovaries. A delicate balance of positive and negative feedback channels exists within this system. Basically, the hypothalamus, which is located at the base of the brain, secretes releasing and inhibiting factors that act on the pituitary to cause it to release two pituitary hormones: follicle stimulating hormone (FSH) and luteinizing hormone (LH). These hormones travel to the ovaries, where they promote the development of ovarian follicles and the production of estrogen and progesterone (the ovarian hormones).

Ovarian follicles have two basic stages: a follicular stage prior to ovulation, and a luteal phase that follows ovulation (Fig. 59.7). FSH causes follicles within the ovary to mature and produce estrogen. This increased estrogen causes the pituitary to respond by producing a surge of LH. This

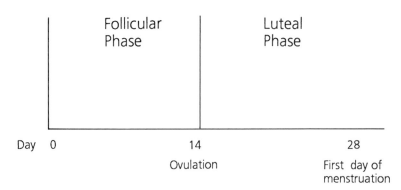

FIGURE 59.7. The normal menstrual cycle.

surge of LH, combined with the FSH produced by the pituitary, acts on the ovary to stimulate ovulation in the ovarian follicle that is most mature at this time.

Following ovulation, the follicle that produced the ovum involutes, forming the corpus luteum that secretes progesterone as well as estrogen, beginning the luteal or second phase of the monthly menstrual cycle. The normal menstrual cycle is 28 days, with a range of 25 to 32 days. The length of the follicular and luteal phases of the cycle are equal, approximately 14 days each.

Amenorrhea

In female athletes, the onset of menstruation (**menarche**) is typically later than that of the nonathletic female (Table 59.2). Most female athletes, however, do begin menstruating by age 16. Delay of the onset of menstruation beyond this age is termed **primary amenorrhea**. An athlete with primary amenorrhea should be referred to her physician for further evaluation to make certain this delay is not due to some pathologic abnormality of the hypothalamic-pituitary-ovarian axis.

TABLE 59.2. Average Age of Beginning Menses

Nonathletic U.S. girls	12.5–12.8 years
Runners	15.1 years
Ballerinas	14.3 years

Secondary amenorrhea is the cessation of normal menstrual periods for greater than 3 months in a previously menstruating female. This phenomenon is not uncommon in female athletes and has been related to physical and emotional stresses, as well as to the low percentage of body fat in conditioned athletes with high energy demands. Stress or increased energy demands may play a major role in causing secondary amenorrhea and, in fact, may be more important than a low percentage of body fat. This stress-related secondary amenorrhea is thought to be due to the absence of the LH surge necessary for proper ovulation and menstruation.

Those who argue that secondary amenorrhea is due to a low percentage of body fat suggest that the pituitary realizes the body lacks sufficient fat to support pregnancy and therefore "turns off" the pituitary axis. This mechanism is proposed for the amenorrhea commonly seen in **anorexia nervosa**, a psychological disturbance resulting in the lack of food intake (see Chapter 42).

Much is still to be learned about secondary amenorrhea in the female athlete. It seems fairly certain that the condition is reversible and does not result in long-term fertility problems. Usually, if the athlete diminishes her training or gains a little weight, normal menstrual cycles return.

Since a female athlete with secondary amenorrhea may begin ovulating at any time and start a normal cycle, she is always at a risk of becoming pregnant if she has unprotected intercourse. Female athletes with secondary amenorrhea should be advised of this possibility, as many of them believe that the lack of regular periods protects against pregnancy. Because secondary amenorrhea is relatively common in female athletes, most gynecologists believe that evaluation is necessary only if the amenorrhea persists for longer than a year.

Dysmenorrhea

Dysmenorrhea, or painful menstruation, is far less common in athletic females than in nonathletic females. The pain appears to be caused by the release of prostaglandins (another hormonal-type substance) by the lining of the uterus. Prostaglandin inhibitors such as ibuprofen, aspirin, and naproxen may help control dysmenorrhea.

Contraception

Birth control pills, intrauterine devices, diaphragms, foams, spermicidal jellies, and suppositories all can be used by the female athlete for birth control. Some women find that oral contraceptives cause increased water retention and a feeling of premenstrual sluggishness. For others, intrauterine devices cause heavy menstrual flow and pelvic pain that can negatively influence athletic activity. Diaphragms, if worn during training episodes, have been reported to cause cramping and abdominal pain. No methods of contraception seem universally accepted, but neither are any contraindicated in the female athlete.

Women should be warned against the practice of using birth control pills to alter their normal menstrual cycle so they will be at a given point in the cycle at the time of competition. A study done during the 1972 Olympics found gold medalists in all phases of their menstrual cycles. There is no scientifically proven advantage or disadvantage to competition in any phase of the menstrual cycle despite some women's testimonials regarding premenstrual "bloating" and decreased performance.

Vaginitis

Vaginitis is common in women and typically results in a pruritic discharge. Yeast and Trichomonas infections are the two most frequent causes of vaginitis. These infections can be differentiated by examining a vaginal smear; following identification, proper treatment should be instituted. Vaginal suppositories for yeast infections and oral medications for Trichomonas infections are extremely effective.

PROTECTIVE EQUIPMENT FOR WOMEN

At one time there was much discussion regarding protective equipment for the external female genitalia, even though injuries to this area are extremely rare. Protective pelvic girdles and protective bras with molded plastic cups were offered; today, they are no longer marketed.

Sport bras with few, if any, metal fasteners and broad straps designed not to slide off easily or cut into the shoulder are available. For maximal comfort, these bras are generally made of a lightweight material that "breathes" and is easy to launder. However, bras manufactured as sport bras are expensive, and a conventional bra style may have all of the same characteristics and be less expensive.

The amount of breast support needed during exercise depends on the individual's preference and should be determined by comfort rather than by any arbitrary standard. Some women prefer very supportive bras, and others prefer to wear no bra—a preference not always determined by breast size. The type of sport does not seem to influence the degree of support preferred by the female athlete. Surveys indicate that women generally want the same type of bra for all sports.

Nipple chafing and excoriation occur in both men and women, especially in women who wear no bras. Long-distance runners are particularly susceptible to nipple irritation from shirts rubbing over the nipple area. Vaseline smeared on the nipples, with or without bandage coverage, may decrease symptoms.

(Important Concepts appear on next page.)

IMPORTANT CONCEPTS

1. Knowing the genetic strengths and weaknesses of the female athlete helps the athletic trainer adjust training and conditioning techniques to maximize performance.
2. Anatomically, females have a lower center of gravity; shorter legs, arms, and overall height; a wider pelvis; and narrower shoulders than males.
3. Physiologically, females have a smaller heart, lower blood pressure, smaller lung mass, and a lower basal metabolic rate than males.
4. Prepubertal males and females are very similar in strength, aerobic power, oxygen, pulse, heart size, and weight.
5. Most injuries seen in female athletes are sprains, strains, and contusions—the same types of injuries seen in male athletes.
6. Common orthopedic problems in female athletes include retropatellar pain, shoulder pain, spondylolysis, stress fractures, and bunions.
7. Common medical problems in women athletes include amenorrhea, dysmenorrhea, iron deficiency, and vaginitis.

SUGGESTED READINGS

Albohm, M. "Equal but Separate: Insuring Safety in Athletics." *Journal of the National Athletic Trainers Association* 13 (1978): 131.

Clarke, K. S., and W. E. Buckley. "Women's Injuries in Collegiate Sports: A Preliminary Comparative Overview of Three Seasons." *American Journal of Sports Medicine* 8 (1980): 187–191.

Haycock, C. E., ed. *Sports Medicine for the Athletic Female.* Oradell, N.J.: Medical Economics Company, Book Division, 1980.

Lutter, J. M. "Mixed Messages about Osteoporosis in Female Athletes." *The Physician and Sportsmedicine* 11 (September 1983): 154–165.

Puhl, J. L., C. H. Brown, and R. O. Voy, eds. *Sport Science Perspectives for Women: Proceedings From the Women and Sports Science Conference.* Champaign, Ill.: Human Kinetics Books, 1988.

Shangold, M. M., and G. Mirkin, eds. *Women and Exercise: Physiology and Sports Medicine.* Philadelphia: F. A. Davis, 1988.

Wells, C. L. *Women, Sport and Performance: A Physiological Perspective.* Champaign, Ill.: Human Kinetics Publishers, 1985.

Whiteside, P. A. "Men's and Women's Injuries in Comparable Sports." *The Physician and Sportsmedicine* 8 (March 1980): 130–140.

Pediatric and Adolescent Athletes

OBJECTIVES FOR CHAPTER 60

After reading this chapter, the student should be able to:

1. List the anatomic and biomechanical differences in the child and adolescent that make their injuries in sporting activities different from an adult's injury.
2. Identify special considerations when performing a thorough history and physical on an adolescent.
3. Identify the frequent locations of fractures and dislocations unique to growing children, the common mechanisms of injury, and the signs and symptoms seen on physical examination.
4. Describe the common overuse injuries that occur in children and adolescents.
5. Discuss common congenital and developmental disorders that impact on the sports performance of adolescents.

INTRODUCTION

With the increasing participation of children and adolescents in recreational and competitive sports, it is not surprising that many musculoskeletal disorders are appearing in the skeletally immature athlete. Those involved with young athletes must recognize that children are not merely small adults. In children, the special properties of growing bones, cartilage, and soft tissue can result in healing rates and potential for long-term disability from injury that are different from those of adult athletes.

Chapter 60 begins with the anatomy and biomechanics of growing bone, cartilage, and soft tissue. The chapter then stresses the importance of obtaining a thorough history, conducting a careful physical examination, and allowing enough time for treatment and rehabilitation of young injured athletes. The next two sections of Chapter 60 address macrotrauma that causes fractures and dislocations and microtrauma that produces overuse injuries. Other musculoskeletal disorders, including joint instability, myositis ossificans, and osteochondroses are discussed next. The final section of Chapter 60 describes congenital disorders. ■

ANATOMY AND BIOMECHANICS

Unique Fracture Patterns

The biomechanics of growing bone can result in fracture patterns that are unique to children. **Bowing deformities** occur in young children when the bone is stressed beyond its elastic recoil limits into a state of permanent plastic deformation. Also, in young children, greenstick and torus frac-

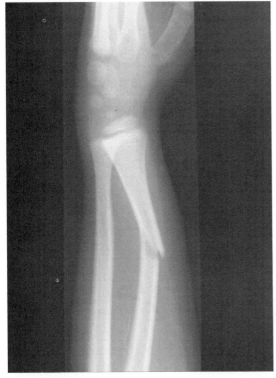 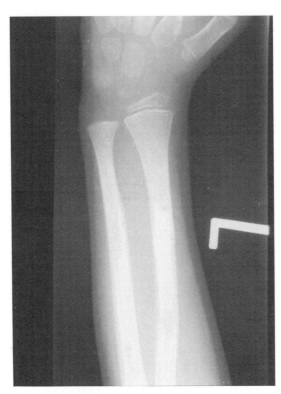

FIGURE 60.1.   (left) Anteroposterior view of a greenstick fracture of the distal third of the forearm. (right) Note the remodeling that has occurred since the original angulation.

tures are common. In a **greenstick fracture,** the bone is incompletely broken, with a portion of the cortex and periosteum remaining intact on the compression side (Fig. 60.1). In a **torus fracture,** an impaction fracture occurs in the metaphyseal bone of the child (Fig. 60.2).

Rapid Bone Healing

In all pediatric fractures, because of an abundant blood supply in the developing bone and the extremely thick osteogenic periosteum, bone healing is relatively rapid. The dynamic nature of the growing bone allows for remodeling of healed fractures, so mildly angulated fractures or overriding fracture fragments will "straighten" as the bone matures (see Fig. 60.1). This remodeling potential is greatest in younger athletes and in fractures that occur close to the growth plate.

Cartilage

The structure and the location of cartilage are why special consideration must be given to athletic injuries in the child and adolescent. **Cartilage,** a form of connective tissue containing a tough, elastic substance, is found in joints and at the developing ends of bones. Three areas of cartilage that are of particular importance in the growing child are cartilage of the growth plate, cartilage of the apophysis, and articular cartilage (Fig. 60.3).

Growth Plate (Physis)

Cartilage of the growth plate, also known as the **physis,** is responsible for the rapid longitudinal growth of bones and also somewhat for their increase in width. The plate is subdivided into zones, with differences in cellular architecture and arrangement of the intercellular matrix. The zone between

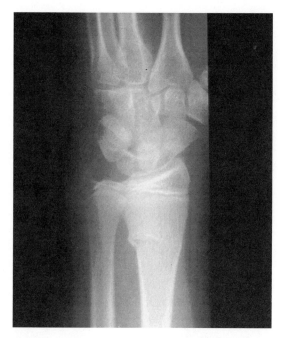

FIGURE 60.2. Anteroposterior view of a torus fracture of the distal radius. Note the buckling of the medial cortex.

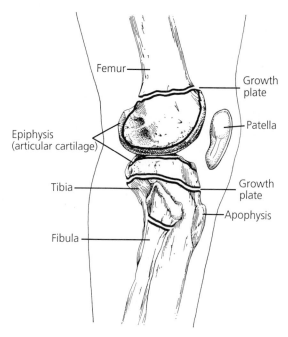

FIGURE 60.3. Areas of cartilage in a child's knee. Note apophysis, epiphysis, and growth plate.

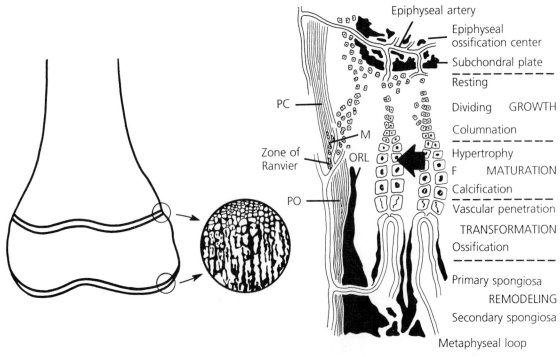

FIGURE 60.4. A schematic showing potential area of fracture at the zone between the hypertrophic cells and the region of calcification.

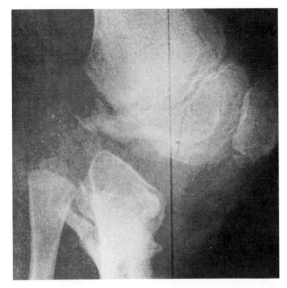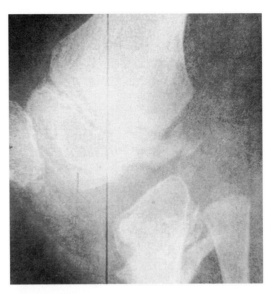

FIGURE 60.5.   (left) A physeal fracture with complete closure of the injured physis. Note marked growth disturbance of distal femur and proximal tibia secondary to severe knee trauma. (right) Note the abnormality shown in the sagittal section of bone from the proximal tibia and its growth plate. (From John A. Ogden, *Skeletal Injury in the Child,* 2d ed. Philadelphia: W. B. Saunders Company, 1990. Reprinted by permission.)

the hypertrophic cells and the region of calcification is thought to be the weakest part of the physis, and it is through this zone that most fractures are believed to occur (Fig. 60.4). **Physeal fractures** are common injuries and are of great concern because of the potential for later growth disturbance, with either complete closure of the injured physis, or formation of a localized area of closure known as a physeal bridge (Fig. 60.5).

Apophysis

An **apophysis** is a cartilaginous structure near the end of a long bone, which is subjected primarily to tensile forces, as opposed to an **epiphysis**, which is subjected mostly to compressive forces. Tensile forces are most often produced through a musculotendinous insertion, such as the insertion of the patellar tendon on the tibial tubercle apophysis. An apophysis is thus susceptible to overuse syndromes in the pediatric athlete. Whereas tendinitis is commonly seen in the adult athlete with an overuse syndrome, in the child, the apophysis will usually become symptomatic before the muscle-tendon unit itself is affected.

Articular Cartilage

Articular cartilage, the layer of cartilage that covers the ends of bones to form the joint surface, may be affected by macrotrauma or microtrauma in the growing child. Some evidence suggests that the child's articular cartilage is more susceptible to shear forces than the adult's. Repetitive trauma may be responsible for osteochondritis dissecans, which is seen in the knee, the ankle, and the elbow. It remains to be seen if more subtle changes in the articular cartilage of young athletes will occur, possibly resulting in as yet unknown, long-term effects.

Biomechanical Properties of Soft Tissues

The biomechanical properties of the soft tissues of the growing child and their con-

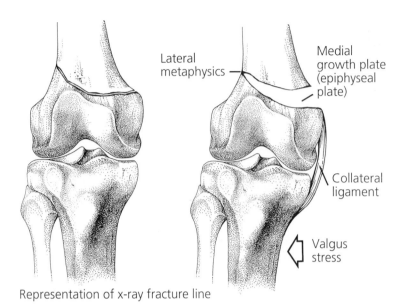

Representation of x-ray fracture line

FIGURE 60.6. Fracture line through the medial growth plate and extending through the lateral metaphysis of a femur that was injured when valgus stress was applied to the knee.

tribution to the unique injuries of children must also be considered.

Ligaments and Tendons

In children, ligaments and tendons insert into the fibrous and fibrocartilaginous periosteal and perichondrial regions of the metaphysis, instead of directly into osseous tissue as they would in adults. This produces a more uniform gradation of tissue elasticity, protecting the soft tissue–bone interface from injury. As a result, traumatic lesions in children will tend to be intra-osseous. For example, an injury that produces a rupture of the anterior cruciate ligament in the adult will, when it occurs in the child, more commonly produce an avulsion of this ligament still attached to an underlying piece of tibial eminence. Any time instability about a joint is suspected, the possibility of growth plate injury must be considered (Fig. 60.6). Ligamentous injuries in children are quite a rare occurrence. Ligaments are stronger than the growth plate and apophysis. Plain radiographs are mandatory if any instability is present.

Mismatches Between Bone and Soft Tissue Growth

Another aspect of soft tissue growth which may contribute to childhood injuries is the potential for mismatches between bone and soft tissue growth. It has been suggested that during periods of rapid growth, such as the adolescent growth spurt, longitudinal bone growth occurs more rapidly than the growth of the surrounding soft tissues, which elongate only in response to this bone growth. Therefore, an increase in muscle-tendon unit tightness and a loss of flexibility are seen during these growth periods, perhaps putting the adolescent at greater risk for overuse injuries.

TREATING YOUNG INJURED ATHLETES

Importance of Thorough History

Certain general principles apply to all physical complaints seen in growing children. The most important step in treating injured pediatric and adolescent athletes and returning them to play is to make the correct diagnosis. There is no substitute for obtaining an adequate history. Even in the situation of an observed acute traumatic event, it is imperative to rule out any preexisting disease or antecedent trauma. Since children, especially younger children, are often poor historians, it is important to elicit information from parents, coaches, athletic trainers, and other family members, as well as from the child. Recent training history, participation in sports other than the one in which the injury occurred, the type of playing surface involved, and the presence of concurrent disease are all relevant points of information to gather for the medical history.

Careful Physical Examination

Once an adequate history has been obtained, a careful physical examination is mandatory. In the case of acute trauma during a sporting event, the presence of an obvious deformity and the inability to bear weight or use an upper extremity are indications for referral to a physician and radiographic evaluation. With all complaints, the pain may be caused by an abnormality in an adjacent joint, a possibility that should not be overlooked. A phenomenon known as **referred pain** occurs when there is no pathology in the painful region, but the pain is referred from elsewhere. The child should be examined thoroughly, with careful attention paid to the site of the complaint and to the joints above and below the injury. In the child and teenager, knee symptoms often result not only from abnormal knee architecture, but also from abnormal foot and ankle mechanics. A classic example of referred pain in the growing child is the presence of anterior thigh or knee pain that actually reflects hip pathology (Fig. 60.7). Radiographic evaluation is usually indicated to rule out fractures, dislocations, or deformity secondary to growth plate abnormalities. One must remember that there are other fairly uncommon causes of pain, including congenital anomalies, tumors, and infection. The occurrence of minor trauma in the child may simply call attention to these underlying disorders.

Duration of Treatment

Although the diagnosis may have been established and treatment initiated, the care of the athlete is not complete until the youngster has returned to his or her previous activity level. Parents, coaches, trainers, and the athletes themselves should not be misled by the seemingly rapid healing process which occurs following most pediatric injuries, especially fracture healing. As with adults, deconditioning occurs during injury and recovery from injury. It is critical that range of motion and flexibility be restored to the affected extremity, followed by restoration of strength, speed, and coordination before the child is allowed to return to competition.

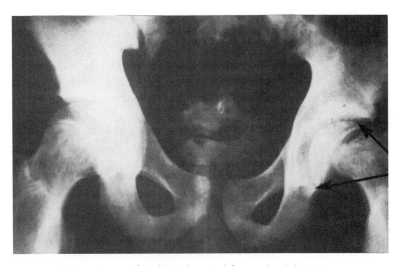

FIGURE 60.7. X-ray of a slipped capital femoral epiphysis (see arrow). This adolescent football player presented with anterior thigh and knee pain but not hip discomfort.

MACROTRAUMA: FRACTURES AND DISLOCATIONS

Osseous Injuries

Osseous injuries (those involving the bones) are more common than ligamentous injuries in pediatric and adolescent athletes. Most osseous injuries result from single, acute traumatic events—either direct or indirect trauma—incurred during participation in contact sports. However, as previously discussed, due to the inherent strength of the ligamentous insertions in children and adolescents, noncontact injuries will often result in osseous injuries. These may include growth plate fractures and avulsion fractures. Intraligamentous injuries, although rare, do occasionally occur. Muscle tears are also seldom seen in the growing child. Again, it should be stressed that radiographic evaluation of these injuries is usually indicated. If a fracture does occur after seemingly minor trauma, the presence of an underlying pathologic lesion of the bone must be ruled out. A child who has suffered multiple fractures should be carefully evaluated for underlying endocrine or metabolic disorders.

A description of all the fractures and dislocations commonly occurring during sports participation in both adults and children is beyond the scope of this chapter. Some of the more common injuries include fractures of the wrist, radius and ulna, clavicle, tibia, and fibula, as well as dislocations of the shoulder, elbow, and interphalangeal joints. The treatment of most of these injuries is generally the same for the child as for the adult. (See Chapters 13–24 for a description of treatment protocols.) Exceptions to this rule include certain forearm fractures or tibial fractures that would be treated with operative fixation in the adult, but for which cast immobilization is usually appropriate in the immature athlete.

Fractures unique to the growing child include plastic deformation and the incomplete (greenstick) fractures seen in younger children due to the biomechanics of the growing diaphysis and metaphysis. Most of these fractures are successfully treated with cast immobilization.

In the older child and adolescent, fractures involving the growth plate are not uncommon. Since these injuries often occur at the wrist and ankle, it is important to obtain x-rays when even a simple sprain is suspected.

Due to the unique properties of ligamentous attachments in the child, osseous injuries, including growth plate injuries, are often sustained through the traumatic pull of these ligaments. Common examples are valgus or varus stress injuries to the knee. On clinical examination, these injuries present with laxity. The laxity, however, will show as a fracture to the growth plate of the distal femur or proximal tibia on x-ray. Another example is the bony mallet finger, which is usually a fracture of the growth plate in a young child or adolescent. Unlike adult ligamentous injuries, these osseous injuries will heal rapidly through fracture healing mechanisms. Most of these fractures can be treated with casting alone. Restoration of the growth plate or articular surface deformity may require operative intervention. These children must be fol-

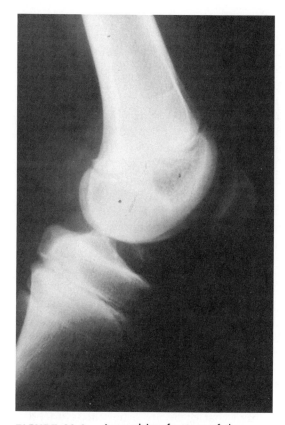

FIGURE 60.8.　An avulsion fracture of the anterior intercondylar eminence of the tibia, which represents an avulsion of the attached anterior cruciate ligament. Note the small fragment of bone within the knee joint.

lowed for long-term disability due to partial or complete growth arrest from physeal plate disruption.

Avulsion Fractures

Avulsion fractures are a result of the unique properties of the muscle-tendon unit attachment to bone in the growing child. Acute muscular contractions or ligamentous sprains will result in avulsion of an osseous origin or insertion.

Two of the most common of these fractures occur around the knee. First is the fracture of the anterior intercondylar eminence of the tibia, which represents an avulsion of the attached anterior cruciate ligament (Fig. 60.8). This fracture is often

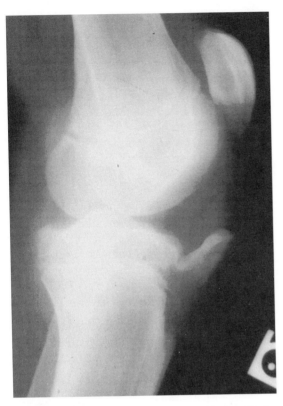

FIGURE 60.9. An avulsion fracture of the tibial tubercle by the patellar tendon.

(usually requiring operative fixation). Often, a hemarthrosis is present, and loss of active knee extension is seen with displaced fractures. Again, the diagnosis is confirmed on x-ray.

Also of concern are avulsion fractures of the pelvis. These represent avulsions of the apophyses by the muscle-tendon units which originate there (Fig. 60.10). Apophysitis in these areas may be seen as a result of overuse injuries. However, acute separations of the apophyses do occur with sudden contractions or stretching of the hamstrings, adductors, or other muscles that

seen in children after falls from bicycles. It may also occur during any athletic trauma known to produce anterior cruciate ligament tears in adults, such as twisting injuries while playing football or skiing. Usually, a large hemarthrosis (a collection of blood within a joint) is present in addition to anterior laxity on clinical exam. The diagnosis is confirmed on x-ray.

The second common avulsion fracture around the knee is an avulsion of the tibial tubercle by the patellar tendon (Fig. 60.9). This fracture results from jumping activities, as in basketball or track. The severity of these injuries varies from a simple avulsion of the tibial tubercle apophysis (which can usually be reduced nonoperatively and treated in a cast) to a fracture which propagates across the primary ossification center of the proximal tibia into the knee joint

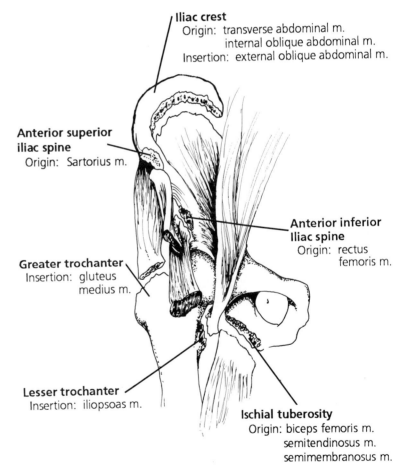

FIGURE 60.10. Origins and insertions of muscles about the pelvis and proximal femur, where avulsions of the apophysis frequently occur. (From *Orthopedic Clinics of North America*, October 1987, vol. 18, no. 4, p. 700. Reprinted with permission of W. B. Saunders, Philadelphia.)

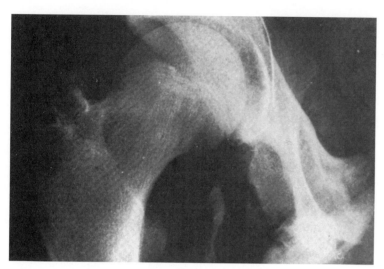

FIGURE 60.11. Repeat x-ray shows avulsion injury of ischium. Note displacement where muscle originates. (From John A. Ogden. *Skeletal Injury in the Child,* 2d ed. Philadelphia: W. B. Saunders Company, 1990. Reprinted by permission.)

originate from or insert on the pelvis and proximal femur. Most of these separations are successfully treated conservatively. Rarely, open reduction and internal fixation are indicated for significantly separated fragments. If symptoms persist beyond the usual time for recovery (about 6 weeks), reevaluation with repeated x-rays is indicated (Fig. 60.11). Occasionally, a symptomatic nonunion may occur, necessitating surgical excision of the fragment and repair of the musculotendinous origin or insertion.

MICROTRAUMA: OVERUSE INJURIES

Overuse injuries include disorders resulting from repetitive microtrauma (see Chapter 15). Overuse injuries have been described for nearly every bone and joint in the body. As with adult injuries, incorrect training is often the major cause. The following discussion highlights those overuse injuries unique to the growing athlete.

Apophysitis

This group of common disorders represents fatigue fractures of the growing apophyses.

Seen in the growing athlete, these disorders result from repetitive microtrauma at musculotendinous origins or insertions. They would present as tendinitis in adults, but due to the mechanical properties of these attachments in the growing child, younger athletes may have an osseous injury.

As discussed under "Avulsion Fractures," overuse injuries around the pelvis and proximal femur can result in apophysitis clinically similar to acute traumatic avulsions except by history. These disorders similarly respond to conservative therapy. Two well-known examples of apophysitis that occur around the knee, in the extensor mechanism, are Osgood-Schlatter's disease and Sinding-Larsen-Johansson syndrome.

Osgood-Schlatter's Disease

Osgood-Schlatter's disease affects the secondary ossification center of the tibial tubercle (Fig. 60.12). The injury occurs because

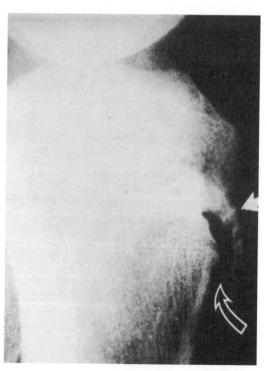

FIGURE 60.12. Osgood-Schlatter's disease. Note elevation and fragmentation of tibial tubercle at patellar ligament insertion.

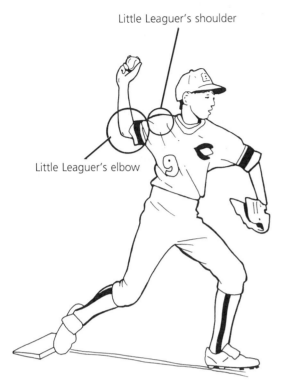

Little Leaguer's shoulder

Little Leaguer's elbow

FIGURE 60.13. Little Leaguer's elbow results from repetitive valgus stress on the elbow during overhead throwing.

the tubercle is subjected to traction forces by the patellar tendon insertion. Osgood-Schlatter's is usually seen during the adolescent growth spurt, more commonly in males than in females. It is frequently associated with sports that require repetitive jumping, such as basketball, track, and gymnastics. **Jumper's knee**, another disorder of the extensor mechanism, is not truly an apophysitis but does represent a repetitive traction injury to the patella that occurs when the distal pole of the patella is injured by the insertion of the quadriceps mechanism.

Sinding-Larsen-Johansson Syndrome

When the lower pole of the patella is injured by the pull of the patellar tendon, it is referred to as **Sinding-Larsen-Johansson syndrome**. All of these overuse disorders of the extensor mechanism are diagnosed by

clinical examination, supported by a history of repetitive jumping activity. Radiographs may show fragmentation of the tibial tubercle or small bony avulsions at either pole of the patella. The majority of these athletes respond to a period of rest and avoidance of pain-producing activities for about 6 to 8 weeks, sometimes supplemented by nonsteroidal anti-inflammatory medication. As with all overuse injuries, a proper regimen of stretching and reconditioning must be established before the child is allowed to return to competitive activity.

Little Leaguer's Elbow

An overuse syndrome seen in the elbows of adolescent pitchers is called **Little Leaguer's elbow**. It is the result of a repetitive valgus stress during overhead throwing (Fig. 60.13). The valgus stress results in lateral compression and medial traction on the elbow (Fig. 60.14). The resultant injuries are variable and include osteochondral injuries of the capitellum (with or without the presence of loose bodies), injury to the proximal radial epiphysis and physeal plate (with early closure and overgrowth of the radial head), and inflammatory changes or avulsion of the medial epicondyle. The extent of injury determines its management. The throwing child who complains of elbow pain should be evaluated carefully. Early institution of rest, followed by appropriate stretching, strengthening, and refinement of the throwing technique, may prevent progression and long-term sequelae of this disorder. These effects may include the formation of loose bodies in the joint, abnormal growth of the bones of the elbow, and/or permanent flexion contractures.

Little Leaguer's Shoulder

The syndrome known as **Little Leaguer's shoulder** is also an overuse injury noted in overhead throwing activities. In this case a stress fracture of the proximal humeral physis occurs. It should be differentiated from other complaints of shoulder pain seen in

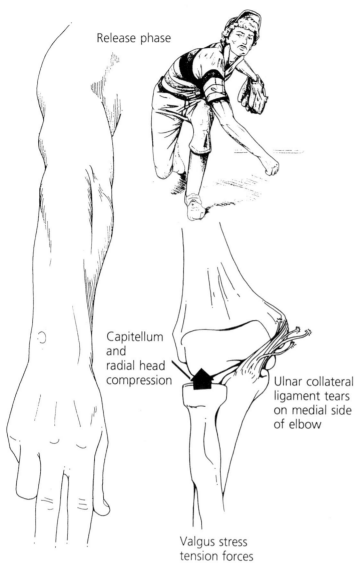

Release phase

Capitellum
and
radial head
compression

Ulnar collateral
ligament tears
on medial side
of elbow

Valgus stress
tension forces

FIGURE 60.14. Throwing places compression forces on the radius and capitellum and tension forces on the medial side of the elbow.

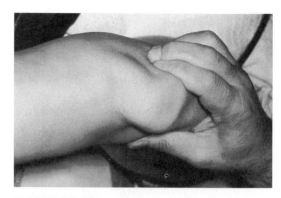

FIGURE 60.15. Patellar instability may result from many factors, including patella alta, a shallow trochlear groove, or laxity of the static retinacular restraints.

young pitchers and swimmers which result from an impingement syndrome or instability. X-rays or a bone scan may be useful in the diagnosis.

OTHER MUSCULOSKELETAL DISORDERS

Joint Instability

Joint instability is a common problem in pediatric and adolescent athletes. The two most symptomatic joints are the patellofemoral and the glenohumeral joints.

Patellofemoral Joint Instability

The patellofemoral joint is dependent on dynamic restraints (especially the vastus medialis portion of the quadriceps), static restraints, and limb alignment for stability. Acute injuries can result in medial restraint ruptures that cause traumatic subluxation or dislocation, occasionally with an associated chondral or osteochondral fracture. All children with acute dislocations of the patella should be evaluated for associated fractures. Recurrent subluxation can occur in the young athlete (Fig. 60.15). Conservative treatment is directed at strengthening the dynamic restraints and may include use of patellar bracing during activity.

The patellofemoral joint may be affected by tightness in the lateral restraints, resulting in patellar compression and pain rather than subluxation. This pain syndrome is known as **excessive lateral pressure syndrome**, **patellofemoral pain syndrome**, or **patellofemoral stress syndrome**. It manifests as peripatellar or retropatellar pain and is especially noted after overuse situations such as long training sessions and hill running. The syndrome may correlate with the pathologic condition known as **chondromalacia**, which affects the patella and/or the articulating femoral cartilage.

The treatment of this syndrome begins with cessation of the offending activity. An exercise program is begun to strengthen the medial restraints (i.e., the vastus medialis muscle) and stretch the lateral restraints. A surgical procedure, such as a lateral retinacular release, or a realignment procedure may be indicated in symptomatic athletes who have not responded to at least 6 months of exercise therapy.

Glenohumeral Joint Instability

The shoulder may also be a source of painful instability in young athletes. Frank dislocation of the glenohumeral joint is uncommon in the young child, but may be seen in the adolescent athlete. Of more importance are the painful shoulder syndromes in children associated with repetitive swimming or throwing activities. These conditions are commonly referred to as **swimmer's shoulder** but actually represent impingement, laxity, and overuse occurring separately or concurrently.

There is much discussion in the orthopedic literature as to the true relationship between subtle anterior laxity and rotator cuff or biceps tendon impingement. The impingement lesion in these young athletes is usually a reversible inflammatory process which responds to conservative therapy. The presence of associated instability can usually be established with a careful history and physical exam. The shoulder should be examined for subluxation and the presence of an apprehension sign in abduction and external rotation (Fig. 60.16). The presence of generalized physiologic laxity is common in these young competitors. Athletes with generalized physiologic laxity should also respond to conservative therapy, with an exercise program aimed at maintaining a full range of motion, strengthening the shoulder musculature, and stretching of the posterior capsule.

Myositis Ossificans

Myositis ossificans is the formation of heterotopic bone within muscle. This condi-

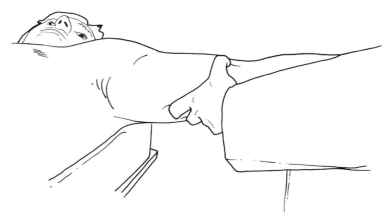

FIGURE 60.16. The athlete will often be apprehensive when his or her shoulder is placed in abduction and external rotation, suggesting subluxation.

tion may be seen as a complication of blunt trauma, which frequently occurs in athletic activities, especially contact sports. The most common sites of occurrence are the quadriceps, deltoid, and brachial muscles (Fig. 60.17).

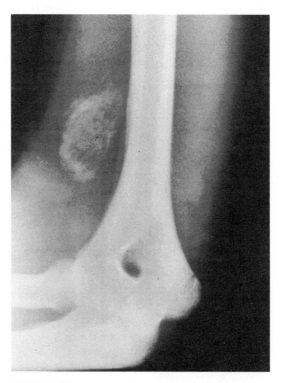

FIGURE 60.17. Myositis ossificans in the brachialis muscle.

The etiology of heterotopic bone formation is unclear, but it is believed to result from an inflammatory process initiated in bleeding muscle after a contusion. The diagnosis of myositis ossificans should be suspected if a child presents 2 to 4 weeks after injury, with restricted range of motion (such as restricted knee flexion after an anterior thigh contusion) and a palpable hard mass in the affected muscle. The diagnosis is confirmed radiographically. The x-ray appearance may suggest an osteogenic sarcoma or other malignant tumors; thus, the history of a significant soft tissue injury should be obtained. The converse, however, is that history of trauma does not exclude a tumor. All severe soft tissue contusions should be treated as if the potential for the development of myositis ossificans exists.

These injuries should be treated with initial compression, ice, rest, and anti-inflammatory medication; passive stretch, massage, and any activity causing pain should be avoided. Established myositis ossificans should be treated with rest and avoidance of any treatment modality that causes pain or swelling. The heterotopic bone will mature in 3 to 6 months. In the child, this bone will frequently resorb by 12 months after the injury. Uncommonly, surgical excision of the new bone mass is considered if symptoms persist after complete maturation of the bone.

Osteochondroses

Juvenile osteochondroses, also known as **osteochondritis,** are a group of clinical entities thought at one time to have a similar pathogenesis. Although this may not be the case, they do have a similar radiographic appearance, and all occur in the pediatric age group. These conditions are not specifically sports-related, but they may be the underlying cause of local pain in a young athlete and therefore should be discussed. Each of these regional conditions is more commonly known by an eponym. There are thought to be two subgroups of osteochondroses: true localized osteonecrosis and variations of normal ossification.

True Localized Osteonecrosis

The first group are those disorders due to a true localized osteonecrosis in an epiphysis or apophysis. The relationship to either acute or repetitive trauma is unclear. This group includes **Freiberg's disease,** a painful affliction of the second metatarsal head, seen in young adolescents. This condition sometimes requires the use of protective shoe wear during revascularization. **Panner's disease,** an osteonecrosis of the capitellum, also occurs in young teenagers. It is usually self-limited and heals rapidly.

An important condition in this first group is **Legg-Calvé-Perthes disease,** or avascular necrosis of the proximal femoral epiphysis. This condition is seen in young children, especially males between the ages of 3 to 8 years. Legg-Calvé-Perthes must be considered in the differential diagnosis of any young athlete noted to have a painless limp, and then found to have decreased range of motion and a hip flexion contracture on clinical exam.

One more form of osteochondrosis is **osteochondritis dissecans.** This localized area of avascular necrosis results in separation of a fragment of subchondral bone, with or without injury to the overlying cartilage (Fig. 60.18). A relationship to acute trauma is suspected but not definite in all cases. In the knee, the child presents with pain, possibly intermittent locking, and swelling, associated with localized tenderness. The lateral aspect of the medial femoral condyle is the most common site of osteochondritis dissecans in the knee. Unlike adults, children under 15 usually show spontaneous healing and resolution of symptoms within a year or so. Osteochondritis dissecans is also seen in the ankle, and less commonly in the hip.

Variations of Normal Ossification

The other subgroup of osteochondroses is thought to be variations of normal ossification, or derangement of endochondral ossification, as opposed to true avascular necrosis. Again, the radiographic appearance of localized sclerosis and fragmenta-

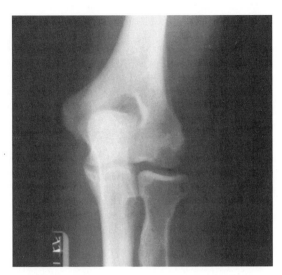

FIGURE 60.18. Osteochondritis dissecans of the capitellum in an adolescent tennis player. Note radiolucency.

tion on the epiphysis or apophysis is seen. The relationship between these disorders and trauma is also unclear.

Osgood-Schlatter's disease is actually considered to be an osteochondrosis. Other conditions in this group are **Köhler's disease** of the tarsal navicular and **Scheuermann's disease**, which affects the ring apophyses of the spine. Scheuermann's disease results in increased thoracic kyphosis in the preteen and early adolescent years.

Sever's disease, which affects the calcaneal apophysis, is seen in children 6 to 10 and may mimic Achilles tendinitis. It is treated similarly with rest and elevation in the heel of the shoe.

CONGENITAL AND DEVELOPMENTAL DISORDERS

Congenital and developmental disorders include a wide array of conditions that are thoroughly addressed in any textbook of pediatric orthopedics. If a young athlete refuses to participate because of pain, or is noted to have a deformity, the presence of some underlying disorder should always be considered in the differential diagnosis.

Three important conditions discussed in the following sections are discoid meniscus, slipped capital femoral epiphysis, and tarsal coalition.

Discoid Meniscus

A **discoid meniscus** is a congenital abnormality in which the meniscus is discoid in shape instead of its usual semilunar shape. This abnormality more commonly occurs on the lateral side of the knee. It should be considered in the differential diagnosis of a "clicking" sensation in the lateral aspect of the knee with or without associated lateral knee pain. The pain may be aggravated by activity, suggesting this condition in the athletic child. The diagnosis may be confirmed by arthrography, magnetic resonance imaging, or arthroscopy. Symptomatic discoid menisci may be converted into a semilunar shape by operative arthroscopy. It should be stressed that a discoid meniscus is inherently different from a normal meniscus; restoring a semilunar shape will not convert this fibrocartilage into a "normal" functioning meniscus.

Slipped Capital Femoral Epiphysis

An entity known as **slipped capital femoral epiphysis** is the most common hip disorder occurring during adolescence (see Fig. 60.7). As a result of a growth disturbance in the proximal femoral growth plate, displacement of the femoral head on the femoral neck occurs. These athletes usually present with a painful limp. Groin pain is frequently reported, but referred pain to the anterior thigh or knee is also common. Therefore, it is imperative that a slipped capital femoral epiphysis be considered in the differential diagnosis of any preadolescent or early adolescent athlete who complains of hip or knee pain.

On clinical examination, there will be pain on hip motion and limitation of abduction and external rotation. As the thigh of the affected limb is flexed, the hip will roll into external rotation and abduction. The diagnosis is confirmed on anteroposterior and lateral radiographs of the hip. The treatment is surgical.

Tarsal Coalition

Tarsal coalition is a congenital synostosis or failure of segmentation between two or more tarsal bones (Fig. 60.19). This condition is also referred to as **peroneal spastic flatfoot**. Most affected athletes present with a painful foot, usually occurring after activity or injury, and resulting in the inability to participate. Symptoms of tarsal coalition are not usually manifested until the early teenage years.

On examination, the foot shows pes planus (flatfoot) and limited or absent subtalar motion. There may be associated spasticity in the peroneal or anterior tibial muscles. The diagnosis can sometimes be confirmed on oblique x-rays of the foot, but

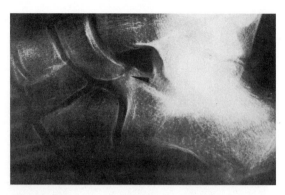

FIGURE 60.19. Tarsal coalition is seen in this oblique radiograph of the foot showing bony bar between the navicular bone and the calcaneous.

more often plain tomography or computed tomography scanning is necessary. The treatment varies with the location and nature of the coalition as well as the athlete's symptoms.

IMPORTANT CONCEPTS

1. Pediatric bone fractures undergo rapid bone healing because of an abundant blood supply in developing bone and extremely thick osteogenic periosteum.

2. Three areas of cartilage that are of particular importance in athletic injuries of children are cartilage of the growth plate, cartilage of the apophysis, and articular cartilage.

3. Ligament injuries in children occur infrequently because the ligaments are stronger than the growth plate and apophysis.

4. The three most important principles involved in treating injured children are taking a thorough history, conducting a careful examination, and planning adequate duration of treatment before return to play.

5. Osseous injuries are common in the growing child and are often sustained through the traumatic pull of ligamentous attachments.

6. Overuse injuries in the growing child often involve fatigue fractures of the growing apophysis.

7. Patellofemoral and glenohumeral joint instability are common problems in adolescent athletes.

8. A discoid meniscus is a congenital abnormality in which the meniscus is discoid instead of its usual semilunar shape.

9. Myositis ossificans is the formation of heterotopic bone within muscle that is believed to result from an inflammatory process initiated in bleeding muscle after a contusion.

10. Osteochondrosis, a disease of the growth or ossification centers in children, begins as a degeneration or necrosis followed by regeneration or recalcification.

11. Slipped capital femoral epiphysis (SCFE) is a common hip disorder in which growth disturbance in the proximal femoral growth plate causes displacement of the femoral head on the femoral neck.

12. Tarsal coalition is a congenital synostosis or failure of segmentation between two or more tarsal bones.

SUGGESTED READINGS

Hensinger, R. N., ed. *The Orthopedic Clinics of North America*, vol. 18, no. 4. Philadelphia: W. B. Saunders, 1987.

Micheli, Lyle J., ed. *Pediatric and Adolescent Sports Medicine*. Boston: Little, Brown, 1984.

Ogden, John A. *Skeletal Injury in the Child*. Philadelphia: Lea & Febiger, 1982.

Sullivan, J. A. and W. A. Grana, eds. *The Pediatric Athlete*. Park Ridge, Ill.: American Academy of Orthopaedic Surgeons, 1990.

The Physically Impaired Athlete

OBJECTIVES FOR CHAPTER 61

After reading this chapter, the student should be able to:

1. Recognize the growth in sports participation among the physically impaired and the demand for sporting and recreational programs to serve this population.
2. Identify the special considerations that must be addressed when establishing sporting and recreational events for physically impaired athletes.
3. Establish injury prevention programs based on special medical problems noted in specific groups of physically disabled athletes.
4. Describe the national classification system for wheelchair competition.

INTRODUCTION

Physically impaired athletes have participated in sporting activities on an individual basis for years, but not until recently did formal competition among these athletes come into being. As sports participation has increased among this group, so, too, has the need for programs to serve these athletes.

Chapter 61 begins with a brief account of the growth in sports participation by the physically impaired, followed by the criteria needed to set up a successful program for these athletes. The chapter then discusses injury prevention for athletes with amputations, arthritic athletes, athletes with cerebral palsy, seizure-prone athletes, athletes with spinal cord defects or injuries, and wheelchair athletes. The last section of Chapter 61 presents the national classification system for wheelchair competition. ■

GROWTH OF SPORTS PARTICIPATION BY THE PHYSICALLY IMPAIRED

The first national wheelchair basketball tournament was held in the late 1940s, but not until wheelchair racer Bob Hall finished the 1975 Boston Marathon in less than 3 hours did people begin to recognize the physically disabled as serious, competitive athletes. The Amateur Sports Act of 1978 expanded the job of the U.S. Olympic Committee to coordinate, promote, and support amateur competition for physically impaired athletes. Individual and team sports participation by this group of athletes has skyrocketed over the last 15 years. Now, physically impaired individuals can participate in almost any sport which their impairment will allow.

Today, most schools offer adaptive physical education programs, but few have enough similarly disabled students to foster a competitive atmosphere for these individuals. Nor do school programs meet the needs of disabled individuals after they graduate from high school. These programs do, however, provide an avenue in which developmental and individual skills can be taught to help physically impaired children become stronger and more capable of dealing independently with obstacles of daily living. Some programs also provide the basis for a structured competitive program.

Sports medicine team members have an excellent opportunity to set up and develop sporting and recreational programs for physically impaired individuals. Many physicians and physical therapists have worked with these potential participants as patients in the hospital or clinical setting. Thus, a pool of physically impaired athletes may be available to start such a program.

DEVELOPING A SPORTING/ RECREATIONAL PROGRAM

Developing a safe and enjoyable sporting or recreational program for the physically disabled requires the establishment of several criteria, including proper assessment of the disabling condition, identification of areas of particular concern and special considerations in children, realistic goal setting, physical conditioning, and special instructor training.

Assessing the Disabling Condition

To provide an overview of the person's physical abilities, the trainer must assess the following factors:

- Range of motion and flexibility of the extremities and trunk.
- Strength.
- Balance and equilibrium skills.

- Postural discrepancies.
- Associated reactions produced by increased activity (of particular importance with central nervous system involvement).
- Sensory discrimination and circulation problems.
- Rhythmic and coordination skills.
- Leg length and other discrepancies of bone growth or size.
- Visual and/or auditory accuracy.
- Orthopedic or other special appliances worn.

An accurate assessment of these factors will be valuable in establishing realistic goals for each individual. Assessment of these factors will also help to determine guidelines for exercise prescription and sport adaptation.

Identifying Areas of Particular Concern

The initial assessment should include identification of any areas of concern or contraindications to participation in a particular sport. These areas of concern include the following:

- Seizure activity (especially if the athlete's seizures are not totally controlled by medication).
- Osteoporosis.
- Cardiac and respiratory conditions.
- Unstable orthopedic conditions (such as dislocated hips, instability of major weight-bearing joints, scoliosis).
- Recent trauma and surgery.
- Bleeding diatheses.

Identifying Special Considerations in Children

Adults are capable of understanding the risks involved in an activity and can usually make a judgment regarding the appropriateness of the activity for themselves. Children, on the other hand, often do not realize the full implications of their condition. Proper guidance from medical personnel is both valuable and necessary. Another special problem that children present is that many conditions that are stable in the adult are greatly affected by the child's growth and development. Because of this problem, periodic reassessment is necessary during participation.

Establishing Realistic Goals

It is important to establish realistic goals that are attainable within a reasonable length of time. The primary goal should be easily obtained, with minimal dependence on physical equipment, geographic location, and the involvement of others. Higher goals can always be established later. Sporting activities should be fun and enjoyable! If goals cannot be reached, the physical limitations can become an unnecessary emotional handicap. The overall goal of the physically impaired athlete should be an easily pursued lifetime activity.

Ensuring Proper Conditioning

Proper conditioning is essential for all athletes; physically disabled athletes are no exception. Good strength and flexibility help reduce the possibility of injury. Cardiovascular endurance is another concern. Balance and coordination activities may be necessary aspects of specific conditioning programs. Using assessment data, the proper conditioning program can be easily established.

Selecting Program Instructors

Instructors who work with the disabled require special training, as well as knowledge of disabling conditions and their implications. Without this knowledge, their intervention could be detrimental to athletes' health. With proper training and guidelines, instructors can provide a tremendously positive and safe experience for physically impaired athletes.

The creativity of the instructor is often the key to success. Having the ability to improvise and adapt special equipment for an individual (either as an aid or for safety) is essential.

INJURY PREVENTION FOR SPECIFIC PHYSICAL PROBLEMS

Injury prevention is as important for the physically impaired athlete as it is for the able-bodied athlete. For those establishing injury prevention programs, having an awareness of specific physical problems permits targeting of conditioning programs and special precautionary measures to diminish the risk of injury for participants. The specific physical problems addressed here are those related to amputees, arthritic athletes, athletes with cerebral palsy, seizure-prone athletes, athletes with spinal cord defects or injuries, and wheelchair athletes.

Amputees

Conditioning programs for the athlete with an amputation are the same as those for the unimpaired athlete. Just as able-bodied athletes must be cognizant of problems that relate to the toes and bottoms of their feet, amputees must be particularly aware of pressure, friction, and moisture at the end of their stumps. Thus, stump care should be an integral part of the amputee's athletic routine.

Special sport prostheses have been developed for amputees to allow them to be more competitive than is possible with routine artificial limbs. However, in some sports such as Alpine skiing, a prosthesis may not be used. In this case, the single-legged skier uses adapted ski poles and needs to concentrate on balance and coordination skills in the conditioning program.

Arthritic Athletes

Most arthritic individuals who participate in an athletic program are suffering from osteoarthritis (degenerative joint disease) as opposed to the more crippling types of arthritis such as rheumatoid arthritis. Because their joints are often irregular and mechanically unsound, arthritic individuals have to be taught to warm up very slowly and increase their activity level gradually within the confines of comfort. As range of motion of specific joints is often compromised, special attention has to be paid to maintaining the present range of motion and, if possible, gradually and gently increasing range of motion to a more normal level. Water sports and activities are often excellent for arthritic individuals. Because the water supports some of their weight, they are able to work on range of motion and even strengthening without the ill effects of full weight bearing. Weight control is particularly important for this group to help preserve joint structures and also to allow them to be more active.

Athletes With Cerebral Palsy

Cerebral palsy is a disorder of movement and posture caused by an irreparable lesion of the central nervous system. Individuals with cerebral palsy may have musculoskeletal problems, mental retardation, speech and hearing difficulties, eye problems, and seizures. Musculoskeletal evaluations should include the individual's ability to sit, stand (with or without assistance), and/or walk (with or without assistance or equipment). Multiple musculoskeletal abnormalities may or may not be present and can include scoliosis, kyphosis, lordosis, or combinations of the aforementioned; deformity of bones; and subluxation or even dislocation at the joints because of overwhelming spasticity of muscle groups.

Range of motion of the individual with cerebral palsy should be actively and passively evaluated. In the spastic athlete, an exaggerated stretch reflex may come into play, in which the muscle actually contracts more forcefully, displaying an apparent lack of motion.

It should also be remembered there are many types of cerebral palsy. While the majority of individuals suffer from a spastic component, athetoid cerebral palsy may present with continuous slow motions and bizarre positions.

Mentally, athletes with cerebral palsy vary significantly. Some are particularly bright, but because of speech abnormalities, intelligence may be difficult to assess by casual observation. Trainers must take the time to listen carefully to what these individuals are trying to say.

In many cases, individuals with cerebral palsy are able to participate in the large number of activities, clinics, and competitions offered at the local, state, national, and international levels of the Special Olympics (see Chapter 62).

The sports medicine team member who is planning to work closely with athletes with cerebral palsy needs to seek further training in this area and maintain close contact with the primary care and orthopedic physicians of these individuals.

Seizure-Prone Athletes

Medication taken by seizure-prone athletes may reduce their awareness and reflex responses. If the athlete has a seizure, it is important to protect the person from harm and embarrassment. Following the seizure, the athlete should rest before attempting to resume activity. Seizure-prone athletes should not be allowed to participate in sports without physician clearance (see Chapter 55).

Athletes With Spinal Cord Defects or Injuries

The sports participation of individuals born with spina bifida, a defect of the spinal cord, may be similar to that of people who have had a spinal cord injury. The majority of spina bifida individuals are paraplegic, whereas a spinal cord injury may cause either quadriplegia or paraplegia. Individuals with spinal cord injury can participate in a number of activities when wheelchair bound. These individuals are rated into

classes for purposes of participation (see pp. 954–955). Athletes with neurological impairment may have bowel and bladder incontinence. Most individuals with spinal cord injury know their own care routines but need privacy to perform these vital functions.

Sensation is lost below the level of the spinal cord lesion; thus, sitting in a wheelchair may become a problem for those with sensitive skin. Appropriate cushions are necessary to protect pressure areas over the ischium, sacrum, and possibly the greater trochanter. Presently, there are several excellent cushions for wheelchair athletes.

The loss of sensation also creates problems with excessive exposure to heat or cold. Many of these athletes also sustained damage to their internal "thermostat" and need to take extra precautions concerning overheating or excessive exposure to cold.

Wheelchair Athletes

The rapid growth of wheelchair athletics has prompted improvement in competition chairs. In accordance with the National Wheelchair Athletic Association (NWAA), these chairs must have no gears, levers, or chains to help limit speed. Improvements have also been made in maneuverability.

The injuries most frequently sustained by wheelchair athletes are blisters and lacerations of the hands and arms, tendinitis or bursitis at the shoulders, and, not surprisingly, carpal tunnel syndrome because of constant impact of the heel of the hand on the racing wheel. Wheelchair racers should protect themselves with specially designed gloves.

CLASSIFICATION OF WHEELCHAIR COMPETITION

Wheelchair competition is regulated by classification to maintain fair competition for all degrees of disability, in both men's and women's divisions. Archery is open competition, meaning that no classification is necessary. Weight lifting is open competition for men. The following is the national system for classification:

- *Class IA.* All cervical lesions with complete or incomplete quadriplegia; involvement of both hands; weakness of triceps (up to and including grade 3 on testing scale); and severe weakness of the trunk and lower extremities, interfering significantly with trunk balance and ability to walk.
- *Class IB.* All cervical lesions with complete or incomplete quadriplegia; involvement of upper extremities but less than Class IA; preservation of normal or good triceps (grade 4 or 5 on testing scale); and generalized weakness of the trunk and lower extremities, interfering significantly with trunk balance and ability to walk.
- *Class IC.* All cervical lesions with complete or incomplete quadriplegia; involvement of upper extremities but less than Class IB; preservation of normal or "good" finger flexion and extension (grasp and release) but no intrinsic hand function; and generalized weakness of the trunk and lower extremities, interfering significantly with trunk balance and ability to walk.
- *Class II.* Complete or incomplete paraplegia below T1 down to and including T5 or comparable disability; total abdominal paralysis or poor abdominal muscle strength (0–2 on testing scale); and no useful trunk sitting balance.
- *Class III.* Complete or incomplete paraplegia or comparable disability below T5 down to and including T10, and upper abdominal and spinal extensor musculature sufficient to provide some element of trunk sitting balance but not normal.
- *Class IV.* Complete or incomplete paraplegia or comparable disability below T10 down to and including L2; no quadriceps or very weak quadriceps (a value up to and including 2 on the testing scale); and gluteal paralysis.
- *Class V.* Complete or incomplete paraplegia or comparable disability below L2 down to and including S5, and quadriceps in grades 3 to 5.

For Swimming Events Only

- *Class V.* Complete or incomplete paraplegia or comparable disability below L2 down to and including L4, and quadriceps in grades 3 to 5 (up to and including 39 points on the points scale).
- *Class VI.* Complete or incomplete paraplegia or comparable disability below L4 down to and including S5 (40 points and above).

(Important Concepts appear on next page.)

IMPORTANT CONCEPTS

1. Individual and team sports participation by the physically impaired has skyrocketed over the past 15 years, creating an opportunity for sports medicine teams to set up sporting and recreational programs for this population.
2. The criteria for developing a safe and enjoyable sporting or recreational program for the physically impaired include proper assessment of the disabling condition, identification of areas of concern and special considerations in children, realistic goal setting, physical conditioning, and special instructor training.
3. Focusing on injury prevention is important in the disabled athlete, and requires knowledge of special considerations required by specific physical disabilities, such as amputations, arthritis, cerebral palsy, seizures, spinal cord problems, and wheelchair confinement.

SUGGESTED READINGS

Curtis, K. A., S. McClanahan, K. M. Hall, et al. "Health, Vocational, and Functional Status in Spinal Cord Injured Athletes and Nonathletes." *Archives of Physical Medicine and Rehabilitation* 67 (1986): 862–865.

Madorsky, J. G., and K. A. Curtis. "Wheelchair Sports Medicine." *American Journal of Sports Medicine* 12 (1984): 128–132.

McCormick, D. P., F. M. Ivey, Jr., D. M. Gold, et al. "The Preparticipation Sports Examination in Special Olympics Athletes." *Texas Medicine* 84 (1988): 39–43.

Shephard, R. J. "Sports Medicine and the Wheelchair Athlete." *Sports Medicine* 5 (1988): 226–247.

Stewart, M. J. "The Handicapped in Sports." *Clinics in Sports Medicine* 2 (1983): 183–190.

Valliant, P. M., I. Bezzubyk, L. Daley, et al. "Psychological Impact of Sport on Disabled Athletes." *Psychological Reports* 56 (1985): 923–929.

ORGANIZATIONS FOR THE PHYSICALLY IMPAIRED ATHLETE

Amputees

Amputee Service Association
Suite 1504
520 North Michigan Avenue
Chicago, IL 60611

Amputee Sports Association
11705 Mercy Boulevard
Savannah, GA 31406

National Amputee Golf Association
5711 Yearling Court
Bonita, CA 92002

The National Amputation Association, Inc.
12-45 150th Street
Whitestone, NY 11357

United States Amputee Association
Route #2
County Line
Fairview, TN 37062

Arthritis

The Arthritis Foundation
3400 Peachtree Road, N.E.
Atlanta, GA 30326

Cerebral Palsy
United Cerebral Palsy Association, Inc.
66 East 34th Street
New York, NY 10010

Epilepsy
Epilepsy Foundation of America
1828 L Street, N.W.
Washington, DC 20036

Hearing Impairment
American Athletic Association of the
Deaf
3916 Lantern Drive
Silver Spring, MD 20902

National Association of the Deaf
814 Thayer Avenue
Silver Spring, MD 20910

Multiple Sclerosis
Association to Overcome Multiple
Sclerosis
79 Milk Street
Boston, MA 02109

National Multiple Sclerosis Society
205 East 42nd Street
New York, NY 10017

Spina Bifida
Spina Bifida Association
c/o The Texas Medical Center
2333 Moursund
Houston, TX 77025

Spina Bifida Association of America
104 Festone Avenue
New Castle, DE 19720

Spinal Cord Injury
American Spinal Injury Association
250 East Superior Street
Room 619
Chicago, IL 60611

National Paraplegia Foundation
333 North Michigan Avenue
Chicago, IL 60601

Paralyzed Veterans of America
7315 Wisconsin Avenue, N.W.
Washington, DC 20014

Visual Impairment
American Blind Bowlers Association
150 North Bellaire
Louisville, KY 40206

American Foundation for the Blind
15 West 16th Street
New York, NY 10011

Blind Outdoor Leisure Development, Inc.
(BOLD)
533 East Main Street
Aspen, CO 81611

Braille Sports Foundation
Room 301
730 Hennepin Avenue
Minneapolis, MN 55402

National Association for Visually
Handicapped
3201 Balboa Street
San Francisco, CA 94121

Wheelchair
American Wheelchair Bowling Association
6718 Pinehurst Drive
Evansville, IN 47711

American Wheelchair Pilots Association
P.O. Box 1181
Mesa, AZ 85201

Canadian Wheelchair Sports Association
333 River Road
Ottawa, Ontario K1L 8B9
Canada

International Foundation for Wheelchair
Tennis
1909 Ala Wai Boulevard
Suite 1507
Honolulu, HI 96815

International Wheelchair Road Racers
Club, Inc.
165 78th Avenue, East
St. Petersburg, FL 33702

National Foundation for Wheelchair
Tennis
3855 Birch Street
Newport Beach, CA 92660

National Wheelchair Athletic Association
2107 Templeton Gap Road
Colorado Springs, CO 80901

National Wheelchair Marathon
380 Diamond Hill Road
Warwick, RI 02886

Sports 'n Spokes (Magazine for
Wheelchair Sports)
5201 North 19th Avenue
Suite 111
Phoenix, AZ 85015

Wheelchair Pilots Association
11018 102nd Avenue, North
Largo, FL 33540

General
Disabled Sportsmen of America, Inc.
P.O. Box 26
Vinton, VA 24179

Handicapped Scuba Association
1104 El Prado
San Clemente, CA 92672

International Council on Therapeutic Ice
Skating
P.O. Box 13
State College, PA 16801

International Sports Organization for the
Disabled
International Stoke-Mandeville Games
Federation
Stoke-Mandeville Spinal Injury Center
Aylesbury, England

National Handicapped Sports and
Recreation Association
Ferragut Station
P.O. Box 33141
Washington, DC 20033

62

The Special Olympics

OBJECTIVES FOR CHAPTER 62

After reading this chapter, the student should be able to:

1. Explain how the Special Olympics began.
2. Be aware of common orthopedic and medical problems seen in Special Olympic athletes.
3. Understand special organizational and logistical problems at Special Olympic competitions at the local, state, national, and international levels.

INTRODUCTION

In the last several years, opportunities have increased for those with mental and physical disabilities to improve their motor skills and compete at the local, state, national, and international Special Olympics. The Special Olympics provides a unique and rewarding experience to mentally and physically impaired athletes and the sports medicine team. Injuries to the Special Olympian are similar to those of other athletes. However, because these athletes typically have underlying medical problems, special considerations must be made for documenting these problems prior to the event and for organizing the event so that the athlete's prior history is easily accessible. Moreover, the athletic trainer should be knowledgeable about the special needs of these athletes to ensure that the games run as smoothly and as safely as possible.

Chapter 62 discusses the history of the Special Olympics, reviews the common medical problems associated with mentally and physically impaired athletes, and examines the particular considerations to be taken into account when organizing a Special Olympics event. ■

HISTORY OF THE SPECIAL OLYMPICS

The Special Olympics, founded by Eunice Kennedy Shriver in the late 1960s, is an international sports program for the mentally disabled. The first international competition was held in Chicago in 1968 and brought together approximately 1,000 mentally disabled children and adults. Today, Special Olympic competitions are held all over the United States.

Months of organization and preparation go into the 1- to 3-day Special Olympic events, which rely heavily on volunteers to implement the programs. Athletic trainers, physicians, physical therapists, nurses, emergency medical technicians (EMTs), and other paraprofessionals are frequently asked to help. Most medical volunteers are glad to assist in the games, but they often find themselves poorly prepared.

Motto

The Special Olympic motto sums up the goal of the competition: "Let me win, but if I cannot win, let me be brave in the attempt." While winning a Special Olympic event provides a boost in self-esteem and offers a moment of pride, the benefits of improvement in motor skills, social interaction, and perhaps conditioning, to some extent, are not to be overlooked.

Scheduled Events

Special Olympic events include track and field, bowling, swimming, diving, wheelchair races, softball, gymnastics, tennis, soccer, basketball, floor hockey, ice skating, skiing, and individual skill events. Most events are divided into summer and winter competitions. Athletes who participate in these events gain skill and experience by attending clinics, workshops, and schools for their training. Because exposure and availability of the activities, as well as innate individual ability, differ, skill and performance vary widely at the Special Olympics.

PREPARTICIPATION PHYSICAL EVALUATION

Each Special Olympic athlete is required to have a current preparticipation physical evaluation prior to attending any local, state, national, or international event. Areas of special consideration in this population include heart abnormalities, sickle cell trait, musculoskeletal abnormalities, and potential for seizures.

Congenital Heart Defects

Although Down's syndrome is not the only cause of mental retardation, it is probably the most widespread and easily recognized form. Approximately 50 percent of the Down's population has a congenital heart defect. The more common congenital findings are tetralogy of Fallot, atrioventricularis communis, and Cushing septal defect. Individuals with tetralogy of Fallot are generally impaired in their physical capacity and occasionally die of arrhythmias, even after surgery. Cardiac abnormalities should be evaluated on an individual basis.

Sickle Cell Trait

Sickle cell trait is frequently found in this population. Although it is thought that these athletes may have more difficulty with anoxia at high altitudes and with strenuous exercise, they are believed to have the same capacity for exercise as normal athletes.

Seizure Disorders

Seizure disorders are frequently seen among participants in the Special Olympics. (Management of an acute seizure is discussed in Chapter 55.) It is important to note the type and dosage of medication taken by these athletes. A multitude of physical problems underlying the seizure disorder may be associated with the athlete's health status. These must be considered on an individual basis.

General Orthopedic Problems

Orthopedic problems are commonly related to poor muscle tone and general joint laxity. One orthopedic problem frequently seen in Down's syndrome is atlantoaxial subluxation (AAS). AAS poses a significant risk to athletes participating in Special Olympic events involving bodily contact. In AAS, the C1 vertebra slips forward as a result of joint looseness, ligamentous laxity, or malformation of the vertebrae or surrounding structures. In this situation, the spinal cord can be compressed, particularly when the neck is in flexion or extension. In the Down's athlete with juvenile rheumatoid arthritis, the potential for AAS increases. This population is often unable to provide a thorough history, and AAS in this population often occurs without a prior history of trauma. Clinical findings may be difficult to assess. Nor is neck pain necessarily a consistent finding. In addition, congenital motor abnormalities may mask neurologic dysfunction.

Because of the risk of AAS and its association with the Special Olympic population, flexion/extension x-rays are mandatory for all developmentally disabled participants who are planning to participate in any sport potentially involving collision (Fig. 62.1).

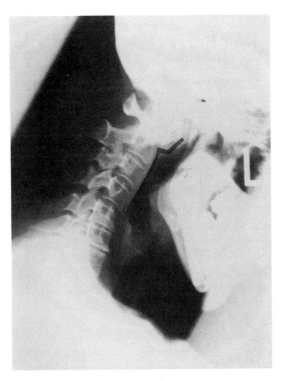

FIGURE 62.1. X-ray of ligamentous laxity, with C1 slipping forward on C2.

Other orthopedic problems common to Special Olympic athletes have been discussed in previous chapters. These problems include subluxating and dislocating patella (see Chapter 21); pes planus (flat foot), hallux valgus, and metatarsus primus varus (see Chapter 24); and thoracolumbar scoliosis (see Chapter 32).

EVENT ORGANIZATION

Organizational preparation is particularly essential for Special Olympic events, as rarely does one elsewhere encounter a large number of participants with multiple medical problems at one gathering.

Game Site

Events may be held in several geographic locations, and each game site should be inspected prior to the event. It is important to determine how many first-aid stations will be needed and, depending on the schedule of events, the number of medical volunteers needed.

Preparticipation History and Physical Evaluation Forms

Physical forms are sent to the participants and coaches prior to the event. The importance of making sure these forms are complete must be stressed.

Medications

Particular note should be made of the dosage and frequency of all medications an athlete is currently taking or has recently taken. Medications should remain in the container in which they were bought and should be appropriately labeled. Special arrangements should be made prior to the Special Olympics for medications requiring refrigeration, special mixing, or administration instructions. This is particularly true for overnight stays or multiple-day events. A responsible person such as a parent, trainer, or coach should be assigned to monitor medications, because often the athlete is not able to assume this responsibility.

Wrist Bands

Once the physical forms are collected, wrist bands containing the athlete's name, age, pertinent medical problems (e.g., asthma, diabetes, epilepsy), medications, and allergies should be compiled. Often these bands are color coded according to the general location of the athlete's hometown. These bands should be worn by the athletes at all times. Frequently, an athlete who is injured is unable to communicate or becomes flustered when surrounded by unfamiliar faces. A wrist band will provide important medical information immediately, and the athlete's coach can be summoned to provide a full history. Also, the athlete's physical evaluation form can be pulled.

Central Operations and Communications

Physical evaluation forms are best kept in one central location rather than at each site because frequently athletes will participate in events at more than one site. It is difficult to separate and duplicate these forms so they will be at the appropriate place. The athletes themselves cannot be responsible for these documents.

Many Special Olympic events have short-wave operators covering the events. This provides good communication for all organizational crews working the event. Medical personnel should be on a separate frequency, with an operator available at each first-aid station.

Emergency Services

The services of a volunteer ambulance squad should be secured well in advance of the event. If the ambulance is present for the entire event, it can provide a multitude of services, decreasing the equipment needed at each site. The hospital to be utilized should also be contacted in advance.

Insurance Forms

Each ambulance and first-aid station should have Special Olympic insurance forms available should an emergency injury occur. In such a situation, the ambulance should be alerted of the location of the emergency, and the athlete's physical evaluation and associated waiver form should be pulled at the central operation center. This information must go with the athlete to the hospital.

First-Aid Stations

First-aid stations should be well marked and stocked prior to the event. Individuals working the medical stations should have identifying clothing (T-shirts, for example) that will make them easy to locate when an injury occurs. Each station should have an adequate supply of ice for injuries. Arrangements should be made for ample fluids for the participants.

A central first-aid station should be available in the general area where the participants are staying in the case of multiple-day events. A central station should also be designated for special events, such as a dance following closing ceremonies. Surprisingly, just as many injuries occur at these events as in the actual games.

Injuries

The most common injuries seen at the Special Olympics are abrasions, contusions, sprains, and strains. Environmental conditions should also be considered. Athletes can be affected by sunburn, heat cramps, fatigue, and exhaustion. During the winter Olympics, hypothermia, frostbite, and circulatory impairment can occur.

Special Considerations

Age of the Athlete

Special Olympic athletes vary widely in age, from adolescents to athletes in their 50s. Often their age is difficult to determine from their appearance or actions. The ath-

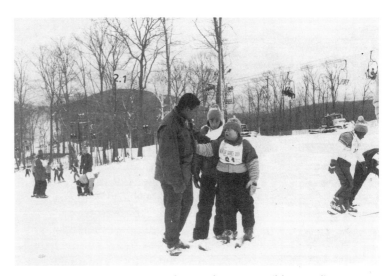

FIGURE 62.2. A parent, coach, or other responsible guardian may be able to provide additional information about the athlete.

lete's age can be found on the wrist band and physical evaluation form and is important to know when evaluating complaints. For example, a 12-year-old boy complaining of chest pain the night before an event is most likely suffering from anxiety about the upcoming event or is anxious because this is one of his first nights away from home; consulting his evaluation form will be of value in making certain he does not have a history of prior cardiac abnormalities. A 48-year-old athlete with chest pain is more likely to have medical rather than psychological reasons for pain.

Prior Medical History

The Special Olympic athlete will often be a poor historian, making the job of evaluation more difficult. Unless the problem is an emergency, a parent, coach, or other responsible guardian should be summoned to give additional information about the athlete (Fig. 62.2). Parents may be hard to locate in any type of outdoor event. Prior to an event, arrangements should be made with parents to secure their easy accessibility in an emergency. In most cases, spectators are not allowed in the competition area. In an emergency, the coach will be extremely valuable in finding the parents.

IMPORTANT CONCEPTS

1. Special Olympics events include track and field, bowling, swimming, diving, wheelchair races, softball, gymnastics, tennis, soccer, basketball, floor hockey, ice skating, skiing, and individual skill events.
2. Fifty percent of the Down's population has a congenital heart defect.
3. Orthopedic problems, particularly atlantoaxial subluxation, are related to poor muscle tone and joint laxity.
4. Medications of the participants should list dosage, frequency, and conditions (e.g., with food, etc.), and they should be under the supervision of a responsible person such as a parent, trainer, or coach.
5. Participants should wear wrist bands that contain the athlete's name, age, allergies, medications, and significant medical problems, and that are color coded for general location of the athlete's hometown.
6. First-aid stations should be well marked, stocked with ample ice and plenty of fluids, and staffed by easily identifiable medical personnel.

SUGGESTED READINGS

Cope, R., and S. Olson. "Abnormalities of the Cervical Spine in Down's Syndrome: Diagnosis, Risks, and Review of the Literature, with Particular Reference to the Special Olympics." *Southern Medical Journal* 80 (1987): 33–36.

Diamond, L. S., D. Lynne, and B. Sigman. "Orthopedic Disorders in Patients with Down's Syndrome." *Orthopedic Clinics of North America* 12 (1981): 57–71.

Magnus, B., and R. French. "Wanted: Athletic Trainers for Special Olympic Athletes." *Athletic Training* (Fall 1985): 204–205.

Maxwell, B. M. "The Nursing Role in the Special Olympic Program." *Journal of School Health* 54 (1984): 131–133.

Starek, P. J. K. "Athletic Performance in Children with Cardiovascular Problems." *The Physician and Sportsmedicine* 10 (February 1982): 78–89.

GLOSSARY

abdomen the more inferior of the two major body cavities, lying between the thorax and the pelvis.

abdominal catastrophe most severe form of acute abdomen.

abdominal cavity cavity between the diaphragm and the pelvis that contains all the abdominal organs.

abdominal thrust series of manual thrusts to the upper abdomen to relieve upper airway obstruction.

abrasion rubbing off or scraping off of the skin or a mucous membrane.

acclimatization body's adaptation to a new environment.

acetabulum the socket of the hip joint into which the femoral head fits.

Achilles tendinitis inflammation of the Achilles tendon.

Achilles tendon tendon joining the gastrocnemius and soleus muscles in the calf of the leg to the bone of the heel.

acidosis pathologic condition caused by accumulation of acid or loss of base in the body.

acinar cells cells in the pancreas that secrete many enzymes that digest fat, starch, and protein.

acne vulgaris chronic inflammatory disease (often hereditary) of the oil glands and hair follicles, presenting as blackheads, inflammatory papules, pustules, or cysts.

acromioclavicular joint joint at the top of the shoulder, formed by bony articulations of the scapula and clavicle.

acromioclavicular separation injury to the acromioclavicular joint, in which some of the supporting ligaments are either stretched or torn; shoulder separation; *sprain.*

activated charcoal powdered charcoal that has been treated to increase its powers of adsorption; used as a general-purpose antidote for ingested toxins.

active team individuals who play a vital role in the health, safety, and welfare of the athlete in an intercollegiate sports program.

acute of abrupt onset.

acute abdomen an abdominal condition causing acute irritation or inflammation of the peritoneum (peritonitis), which causes severe pain.

acute cervical intervertebral disc herniation protrusion of cervical intervertebral disc, resulting in nerve root impingement.

acute injury injury characterized by a rapid onset and resulting from a traumatic event.

acute mountain sickness mildest form of altitude sickness.

acute myocardial infarction (AMI) death of heart muscle caused by lack of oxygen to the muscle; "heart attack."

acute peroneal compartment syndrome increased soft tissue pressure in the peroneal compartment of the lower leg, resulting in localized pain and numbness in the distribution of the peroneal nerve.

acute tenosynovitis inflammation of the tendon sheath.

Adam's apple the firm prominence (more prominent in men than in women) in the upper part of the larynx formed by the thyroid cartilage.

adductor muscles muscles which draw toward the midline of the body.

adenosine triphosphate (ATP) adenosine compound containing three phosphoric acid groups; stored form of muscle energy.

adhesive capsulitis self-limiting condition resulting from any inflammatory process about the shoulder in which capsular scar tissue is produced, resulting in pain and limited range of motion; frozen shoulder.

adult-onset (Type II) diabetes milder form of diabetes mellitus that affects primarily adults, in which insulin is still produced but at a lower, insufficient level.

advanced life support the use of adjunctive equipment, cardiac monitoring, defibrillation, intravenous lifeline, and drug infusion to treat respiratory and/or cardiac failure.

aerobic exercise exercise which utilizes oxidative metabolic pathways to provide energy.

aerobic metabolism state in which the body's oxygen needs are being met during activity.

afterload impedance of forward flow of blood from the ventricle; a measure of arterial system resistance.

airborne transmission a method of disease transmission in which the infective organism is introduced into the air by coughing or sneezing; droplets of mucus that carry bacteria or other organisms are then inhaled by another person.

air embolism bubbles of air released into the blood, as from rupture of lung alveoli during ascent from the water or flying too high in an unpressurized plane.

air pressure splint double-walled plastic tube that immobilizes a limb when the space between the walls is inflated.

air splint a precontoured, inflatable plastic type of soft splint.

alkalosis pathologic condition resulting from accumulation of base or loss of acid in the body.

altitude sickness maladjustment to the hypoxia (lack of oxygen) of a high altitude.

alveoli the air sacs of the lungs where the exchange of oxygen and carbon dioxide takes place.

amenorrhea lack of regular menstrual periods.

anabolic steroid testosterone, or a steroid hormone resembling testosterone, that stimulates anabolism in the body.

anabolism conversion of simple substances into complex compounds by cells.

anaerobic exercise exercise of short duration, not requiring the body's utilization of oxygen to make fuel available.

anaerobic metabolism oxygen debt; when the cardiovascular system is unable to meet the needs of the working muscles, the anaerobic metabolism is activated.

anaphylactic shock shock caused by an allergic reaction.

anaphylaxis the most severe form of an allergic reaction, resulting in shock.

anemia condition in which there is a reduction in the number of circulating red blood cells or hemoglobin or in the volume of red cells.

aneurysm weakened and bulging area of a blood vessel.

angina suffocating, choking pain; usually refers to angina pectoris.

angina pectoris attacks of chest pain with squeezing or tightness in the chest and difficulty breathing; caused by insufficient oxygen supply to the heart.

angle of Louis a bony prominence on the breastbone, just inferior to the junction of the clavicle and sternum and just opposite the second intercostal space.

anhidrosis inadequate perspiration which causes the body temperature to rise.

anisotropic when the biological properties are specific to the direction of force application.

anorexia nervosa a condition, common in young females, in which the patient takes in less and less food and may become seriously emaciated and malnourished; a manifestation of a severe underlying psychological disorder.

anterior chamber space between the iris and the cornea.

anterior compartment syndrome increased soft tissue pressure in the anterior compartment of the lower leg, resulting in pain, decreased sensation, and muscle paralysis.

anterior cruciate ligament ligament that passes from the lateral intercondylar notch of the femur to attach anteriorly on the articular surface of the tibia.

anterior glenohumeral dislocation displacement of the humeral head and stretching or tearing of the anterior capsule within its substance or at its attachment to the anterior glenoid.

anterior sternoclavicular dislocation tear of the sternoclavicular joint; the most common type of sternoclavicular dislocation capsule recognized clinically by the anterior prominence of the proximal clavicle on the involved side.

anterior superior iliac spines blunt bony projection on the anterior border of the ilium, forming the anterior end of the iliac crest.

anterior surface surface at the front of the body, facing the examiner.

anterior talofibular ligament one of the three lateral ligaments of the ankle; arises from the anterior border of the lateral malleolus to attach to the neck of the talus.

anterior tibial tendon structure from which comes the extrinsic support; arises in the anterior crucial compartment of the leg and passes downward and medially to insert on the first cuneiform and the base of the first metatarsal.

anterior tibiofibular ligament part of the tibiofibular syndesmosis; it arises from the anterior calculi on the lateral side of the tibia and blends into the interosseous membrane above the ankle joint.

anterolateral rotatory instability anterior internal rotational subluxation of the lateral tibial condyle on the femur, reflecting damage to the anterior cruciate ligament and lateral structures.

anteromedial rotatory instability when the medial plateau of the tibia rotates anteriorly and medial joint opening occurs, indicating disruption of the superficial tibia collateral ligament, medial and posteromedial capsular structures, and anterior cruciate ligament.

anteroposterior drawer test test for anterior and posterior laxity in which the examiner holds the knee in 30 degrees of flexion, stabilizes the thigh, and carries out an anteroposterior drawer motion with the proximal tibia; the test is positive if changes in anteroposterior displacement of the tibia are noted.

antihistamine drug that counteracts the effects of histamine; one use is to relieve the symptoms of an allergic reaction.

antivenin antitoxin (remedy) for a venom.

anus distal or terminal ending of the alimentary canal.

aorta major artery leaving the left side of the heart that carries freshly oxygenated blood to the body.

Apley compression test test for a meniscal tear; the examiner places the athlete in a prone position with the knee flexed to 90 degrees and rotates the knee joint; the result is positive if the test produces pain.

aponeurosis broad fibrous sheet attaching a muscle to another muscle.

apophysis a projection from a bone, such as a tubercle tuberosity or process.

apophysitis inflammation of an apophysis.

appendicitis inflammation of the appendix.

appendix small, closed end tube that opens into the cecum in the lower right quadrant of the abdomen.

apprehension test test for patellar laxity; examiner attempts to subluxate the patella laterally to see whether apprehension or pain is elicited.

aqueous humor fluid located in the anterior chamber of the eye.

arachnoid the middle of the three layers of tissue that envelop the brain and spinal cord; lies between the dura mater and the pia mater.

arcuate ligament posterior third of the lateral capsule, which together with the popliteus attachments, provides considerable stability to the posterolateral corner of the knee.

arrhythmia disturbance in heartbeat rhythm.

arterial gas embolism *see* air embolism.

arterial hypotension low blood pressure in the arteries that produces decreased carotid sinus stretch, triggering the sympathetic nervous system to increase blood pressure.

arterial pressure point point where an artery passes over a bony prominence or lies close to the skin; allows an artery to be palpated and the arterial pulse taken.

arteriole small branch of arteries.

arteriosclerotic heart disease condition characterized by thickening and loss of elasticity of the arterial walls.

artery tubular vessel that carries oxygenated blood from the heart to the body tissues.

arthrogram imaging of a joint by x-ray after injection of a radiopaque contrast medium into the joint space.

arthroscopic surgery surgery in which the interior of a joint is visualized through a scope attached to a camera.

articular cartilage cartilage covering the joint surfaces.

artificial circulation a means of providing circulation by external chest compression in one who has sustained a cardiac arrest.

artificial ventilation opening the airway and restoring breathing, in one who has sustained a respiratory arrest, by mouth-to-mouth ventilation, mouth-to-nose ventilation, or by the use of mechanical devices.

ascending colon part of the colon that lies in the vertical position on the right side of the abdomen and extends to the lower border of the liver from the cecum.

aspiration inhalation; taking foreign matter into the respiratory tract during inhalation.

assistive team individuals who play important but secondary roles in the care of athletes in an intercollegiate setting.

assumption of risk when an individual who participates in an activity is injured as a result of the ordinary risk associated with the activity and thus has no action for negligence.

asthma a disorder characterized by responsiveness of the trachea and bronchi to various stimuli, resulting in narrowing of the airways.

asystole lack of heartbeat.

atlas the ring-shaped first cervical vertebra beneath the skull.

atrium either of the heart's two upper chambers.

atrophy wasting of a tissue or organ.

auditory ossicles with the tympanic membrane, forms the middle ear.

aura the first phase of a generalized epileptic seizure.

auricle with the external acoustic meatus, forms the external ear.

auscultation listening with a stethoscope to sounds within the organs to aid in diagnosis and treatment.

automatic (involuntary) nervous system portion of the nervous system regulating involuntary functions, such as digestion and sweating.

avascular necrosis a condition in which cells die as a result of inadequate blood supply.

avulsion injury in which a piece of skin, with varying portions of subcutaneous tissue or muscle, is torn loose.

axis the second cervical vertebra beneath the skull.

Baker's cyst localized fluid accumulation in the posterior fossa of the knee.

ballistic stretch use of body momentum to bounce at the end range of a stretch, causing activation of the muscle fibers; not recommended due to risk of injury.

Bankart lesion injury to the anterior capsule of the shoulder which involves separation (tear) of the labrum from the glenoid.

barium enema an enema of barium sulfate used as contrast material for x-ray examination of the colon; for this test to be useful, the gastrointestinal tract must be completely free of contents.

barium swallow an x-ray examination of the esophagus during and just after the swallowing of a barium sulfate.

barotrauma ruptured blood vessels or other tissue damage mainly affecting the middle ear and facial sinuses due to a head cold, trapped air, change in atmospheric pressure; common among air travelers and divers.

basal ganglia demarcated masses of gray matter in the interior of the cerebral hemispheres.

basal skull fracture fracture of the base of the skull; bleeding from the ear or leakage of cerebrospinal fluid may be among the presenting symptoms.

baseball (mallet) finger rupture of the extendor tendon at its insertion on the terminal phalanx caused by a sudden flexion force on the DIP joint while the finger is actively extended.

basic life support emergency lifesaving procedure used to resuscitate a person who has sustained respiratory or cardiovascular system failure.

basilar skull fracture *see* basal skull fracture.

bends *see* decompression sickness.

biceps brachii deep anterior muscle of the shoulder with two heads of origin, both of which insert on the radial tuberosity .

biceps muscle large muscle that covers the front of the humerus; functions include forearm flexion and hand supination.

bicipital tendinitis inflammation of the biceps tendon in its subacromial location.

bile duct one of the ducts conveying bile from the liver to the intestines.

bladder musculomembranous sac where urine is collected and stored.

blister fluid under the outer layer of the skin that forms when the skin rubs against a hard or rough surface, causing the epidermis to separate from the dermis.

blood doping withdrawing a unit of blood from an athlete and storing it for several weeks prior to competition, and reinfusing it prior to the event; controversial practice banned by the International Olympic Committee.

blood pressure pressure of the blood circulating against the walls of the arteries.

blunt (closed) injury injury caused by a blunt object such as a steering wheel; the skin remains intact.

body the trunk; also the principal part of a structure.

body rehearsal mental rehearsal technique in which the athlete is given a detailed explanation of his or her injury and the healing process and is asked to repeatedly visualize the latter to influence healing.

bone osseous connective tissue that makes up the skeleton.

bone marrow the central portion of all bones that produces the cellular components of the blood.

bone scan an imaging technique in which a radioactive substance is injected into a vein and absorbed by bone; a few hours later a scanner is used to detect abnormal amounts of radioactive uptake in the bone.

botulism the most severe form of food poisoning; usually results from eating improperly canned food that contains bacterial toxins.

boutonnière deformity rupture of the central slip of the extensor tendon of the middle phalanx caused by rapid, forceful flexion at the PIP joint; characterized by flexion of the PIP joint and hyperextension of the DIP joint.

bowing deformity a state of permanent plastic deformation occurring in young children when the bone is stressed beyond its elastic recoil limits.

brachial artery artery on the inside of the arm

between the elbow and the shoulder; used in taking blood pressure and for checking pulse in infants.

brachial muscle originates on the humerus, extends anteriorly across the elbow joint, and attaches into the ulna; functions in forearm flexion.

brachial plexus network of nerves that pass from the lower part of the cervical spine and upper part of the thoracic spine down the arm.

bradycardia slow heartbeat; a sinus rhythm with a rate below 60 in an adult or below 70 in a child.

brain stem area of the brain between the spinal cord and cerebrum, surrounded by the cerebellum; controls functions necessary for life, such as respiration.

bridge the proximal one-third of the nose that is formed by bone (the rest of the nose is made of cartilage).

bronchi the two main branches of the trachea that lead into the right and left lungs; bronchus (singular).

bronchiolitis inflammation of the bronchioles.

bronchitis inflammation of the mucous membrane of the bronchi.

bucket-handle tear complete longitudinal tear of the central segment of the meniscus.

bulimia a psychological disorder manifested by significant overeating followed by induced vomiting and ingestion of laxatives or diuretics, in an effort not to gain weight from the extra food.

bunion prominence of the first metatarsal head often associated with lateral shift of the great toe (hallux valgus deformity).

bunionette *see* Tailor's bunion.

bursa synovial sac generally located over bony prominences throughout the body.

bursitis inflammation of a bursa.

bursitis of the shoulder inflammation of the subacromial bursa.

Caisson's disease *see* decompression sickness.

calcaneal tendon *see* Achilles tendon.

calcaneofibular ligament the longest of the three lateral ligaments of the ankle; inserts on the lateral surface of the calcaneus.

calcaneus heelbone.

callosity area of thickened skin overlying a bony prominence.

callus *see* callosity

cancellous bone less dense and more trabecular layer of bone; predominates in the epiphyseal regions.

capillary small vessel that connects the arterioles and venules and permits the interchange of various substances between the blood and tissue fluid.

capsulorrhaphy *see* lateral retinacular release.

carbohydrate loading dietary program which, when combined with depletion exercise, can increase storage of glycogen in the muscle and thus improve athletic performance.

cardiac arrest sudden ceasing of heart function.

cardiac compression external heart massage to restore circulation and the pumping action of the heart in the event of cardiac arrest.

cardiac cycle electromechanical sequence of events that occurs with one contraction and relaxation of the heart muscle.

cardiac ischemia inadequate blood supply to the heart.

cardiac muscle specialized form of striated muscle that makes up the walls of the heart.

cardiac output effective volume of blood expelled by either ventricle per unit of time; the product of stroke volume and heart rate.

cardiac rehabilitation multiphasic program involving exercise, therapy, education, and counseling; designed to help individuals with cardiovascular disease regain the most active and satisfying life possible within the boundaries of their disease.

cardiogenic shock shock resulting from inadequate functioning of the heart as a pump.

cardiopulmonary resuscitation (CPR) artificial establishment of circulation of the blood and movement of air into and out of the lungs in a pulseless, nonbreathing patient.

cardiorespiratory endurance the ability of the heart, blood vessels, and lungs to deliver oxygen to the tissues while removing unnecessary materials and wastes.

cardiovascular fitness ability of the cardiovascular system to meet the oxygen delivery and carbon dioxide removal demands of high workloads and maintain efficiency for long periods of time.

carotid artery one of the principal arteries of the neck running upward and dividing into the external and internal carotid arteries to supply the face and head and brain, respectively; can be palpated on either side of the neck.

carotid sinus hypotension low blood pressure detected by the stretch receptors in the carotid sinus; produces arterial vaso constriction which increases peripheral vascular resistance and aortic impedance, thus increasing blood pressure.

carpal bones bones of the wrist.

carpal tunnel syndrome pressure on the median nerve where it passes through the carpal tunnel of the wrist, causing soreness, numbness, and weakness of the thumb muscles.

carrier person or animal capable of transmitting an infectious disease but does not display any symptoms of the disease.

cartilage connective tissue containing a tough, elastic substance; found in joints, at the developing ends of bones, and in specific areas such as the nose and ear.

cauda equina roots of the upper sacral nerves which have not exited the spinal canal; located below the second lumbar vertebra.

cavus foot a foot with an excessively high and rigid longitudinal arch; if the deformity is significant, a varus heel and clawing of the toes may also be present.

cecum first part of the large intestine into which the ileum opens.

cellulitis inflammation of soft or connective tissue.

central nervous system brain and spinal cord and their nerves and end organs.

cerebellum brain area located posteriorly and attached to the brain stem; works in concert with the brain stem and cerebral cortex to coordinate movement.

cerebral contusion bruising of the brain tissue from a blow to the head; bleeding, swelling, and brain damage may occur.

cerebral concussion jarring injury of the brain resulting in disturbance of brain function.

cerebral cortex outer part of the hemispheres, controls speech, motor, and sensory functions.

cerebral hemispheres the two cerebral hemispheres forming the bulk of the brain.

cerebrospinal fluid fluid contained in the four ventricles of the brain and in the subarachnoid space about the brain and spinal cord.

cerebrovascular accident stroke; a sudden lessening or loss of consciousness, sensation, or voluntary movement caused by rupture or obstruction of an artery in the brain.

cerebrum main brain area with two hemispheres controlling movement, hearing, speech, balance, and visual perception.

cervical spine upper seven bones of the back, found in the neck.

cervical sprain injury to the ligaments of the cervical spine.

cervical strain injury to the musculotendinous unit of the cervical spine.

cervix the lower and narrow end of the uterus.

chance (slice) fracture spinal fracture with a horizontal disruption of the vertebral body and ligamentous structures.

charitable immunity doctrine based on the notion that a person who is carrying out a charitable function should not be held accountable for negligent acts.

chemistry profile a basic chemistry profile generally consists of testing for blood levels of sodium, potassium, chloride, CO_2, and sometimes glucose, urea nitrogen, and creatinine; a more comprehensive profile may include proteins, fats, and enzymes.

chilblain a mild form of cold exposure affecting the fingers, toes, or ears.

chin-lift maneuver a procedure used to open the airway in preparation for CPR by tilting the athlete's head backward and lifting the chin.

chondromalacia pathologic condition involving softening of the patella and/or articular femoral cartilage.

choroid plexus vascular portion of the pia mater which secrets the cerebrospinal fluid.

chronic bronchitis long-standing form of bronchitis characterized by attacks of coughing and changes in the lung tissue.

chronic injury injury characterized by a slow, insidious onset, implying a gradual development of structural damage.

chronic obstructive lung disease slow process of disruption of the airways, alveoli, and pulmonary blood vessels caused by chronic bronchial obstruction, in which lung function is increasingly compromised.

chronic rotator cuff tear tear of the rotator cuff of the shoulder resulting from degeneration within the rotator cuff tendon.

circumferential compression a type of injury to the chest; in extreme instances of circumferential compression, the upper part of the body may be bluish and swollen, the neck veins distended, and the eyes bulging.

clavicle collarbone.

clavicular epiphyseal fracture fracture of the growth plate of the clavicle; may appear clinically as a dislocation, especially if some displacement is present.

clavicular fracture fracture of the clavicle.

claw toe deformity involving hyperextension of the MP joint and a hyperflexion of the interphalangeal joint; can be congenital or result from muscle imbalances or neurological disorders.

closed (blunt) injury soft tissue damage that occurs beneath the skin with no break in the surface.

closed chest injury injury to the chest in which the skin has not been broken.

closed fracture a fracture in which the bone ends have not penetrated the skin and no wound exists near the fracture site.

closed wound soft tissue damage that occurs beneath the skin but with no break in the surface of the skin.

coach's finger a painful, stiff finger with a fixed flexion deformity of the joint resulting from a hyperextension injury.

coccygodynia pain in the coccygeal area.

coccyx the tailbone; the small bone below the sacrum formed by the final three to four vertebrae.

coffee grounds vomitus vomitus consisting of dark-colored matter, usually digested blood.

colic intermittent painful spasm in an organ.

collagen family of 13 stiff, helical, insoluble protein macromolecules, providing the scaffold for tensile strength in fibrous tissue for rigidity in bone.

Colles' fracture fracture of the distal radius, with dorsal displacement of the fragments; often caused by a fall on an outstretched arm with the hand extended.

colon part of the large intestine that extends from the ileocecal valve to the rectum.

comminuted fracture a fracture in which the bone is broken into more than two fragments.

comminuted skull fracture fracture of the skull consisting of multiple fragments.

common peroneal nerve nerve lying below the head of the fibula that controls movement at the ankle and supplies sensation to the top of the foot.

communicable disease a disease that can be transmitted from one person to another.

communicable period time during which an infectious agent may be transferred from one host to another.

comparative negligence doctrine that compares the negligence of two parties.

complete blood cell count commonly performed test used to evaluate white and red blood cell populations in a sample of blood; complete blood count (CBC).

complex partial seizure partial epileptic seizure in which consciousness may be clouded or the athlete may display automatic behavior.

compound fracture any fracture in which the over-

lying skin has been penetrated.

computerized axial tomography (CAT) scan a computer assisted x-ray tomogram providing detailed images of tissue based on their relative density; only axial and not sagittal or transverse images can be obtained by this technique.

concentric muscle contraction contraction in which tension is developed when the actin filaments slide over the myosin filaments, causing the muscle to shorten in length.

conduction loss of heat from a body by direct contact with a cold object; also the transfer of electrical or nervous impulses or sound waves.

condyle rounded prominence at one or both ends of a bone.

congestive heart failure (CHF) condition in which the damaged heart muscle is unable to pump enough blood to meet the demand of the body; difficulty breathing due to pulmonary edema and swelling of the feet and ankles.

connective tissue tissue which connects and supports the structures of the body.

contact allergy allergic response of the skin that produces inflammation to an external agent.

contact irritant dermatitis inflammatory, nonallergic reaction of the skin to exposure to irritating or caustic substances or to a physical agent that damages the skin.

contact transmission a method of transmitting a communicable disease from direct physical contact between an individual and the infected person, from indirect physical contact between a person and contaminated inanimate objects, or from inhalation of infected droplets or dust.

contamination soiling, staining, or infecting by contact with bacteria or other infectious agents.

contractility overall capacity of the muscle fibers of the ventricles to shorten and do useful work; cannot be measured directly.

contrast therapy alternating cryotherapy and thermotherapy in the post-acute phase of injury to reduce swelling and pain and improve range of motion.

contributory negligence when the plaintiff commits an act that causes his or her own injury and the defendant thus bears no liability.

contusion bruise; injury to soft tissue without a break in the skin.

convection loss of heat from a body to a moving current of air.

coping rehearsal mentally practicing solutions to difficult situations with an emphasis on effective responses.

coracoacromial ligament ligament lying anteromedially and superior to the glenohumeral joint; defines the subacromial space.

coracoclavicular ligaments strong stabilizers of the acromioclavicular joint, consisting of the conoid and trapezial ligaments.

cornea transparent tissue layer in front of the pupil and the iris of the eye.

coronal plane frontal section of the body.

cortical bone dense outer layer of bone; the bone's cortex.

costal arch fused costal cartilages of the sixth to tenth ribs forming the upper border of the abdomen.

costovertebral angle angle that is formed by the spine and the tenth rib; the kidneys lie beneath the back muscles in the costovertebral angle.

crab louse *see* pediculosis pubis.

cranial nerves twelve pairs of peripheral nerves associated with the brain.

cranium area of the head above the ears and eyes; the bones forming the vault that lodges the brain.

crepitus a grating or grinding sound.

cricoid cartilage a firm ridge of cartilage that forms the lower part of the larynx.

cricothyroid membrane a thin sheet of connective tissue (fascia) that connects the thyroid and cricoid cartilages that make up the larynx.

crimp regular, wavy undulation of cells and matrix that is seen under a microscope.

cross-finger technique method of using crossed fingers to open the athlete's mouth and probe for foreign bodies.

cryokinetics use of cold and movement as treatment modalities.

cryotherapy cold therapy; cools tissue by transferring heat energy.

cuboid bone bone on the lateral side of the foot that articulates with the foot.

cuneiform one of the three bones of the midfoot that are stable joints and produce little movement.

curvature abnormal curve.

cyanosis blue color of the skin and mucous membranes, resulting from poor oxygenation of the circulating blood.

dead arm syndrome condition that occurs in throwing athletes whereby after ball release their arm goes numb and is extremely weak and they are unable to throw.

decompression sickness bubbles of nitrogen released in the blood stream during rapid ascent from deep water which causes blockage in the vessels.

deep frostbite severe cold injury usually involving the hands and feet, in which the skin and subcutaneous tissues are damaged.

deep medial collateral ligament *see* medial capsular ligament.

deformation state of mechanical strain in the body.

degeneration destruction of normal, healthy tissue from disease.

degenerative joint disease (DJD) deterioration of the weight-bearing surface, distinguished by destruction of the hyaline cartilage and narrowing at the joint space; osteoarthritis.

deltoid muscle in the most superficial layer in the shoulder found anteriorly.

deltoid ligament one of the major support ligaments of the ankle; originates on the medial malleolus and spreads to attach to the medial border of the talus.

depressed skull fracture fracture of the skull in which a fragment or fragments of bone are pushed inward against the brain.

dermis the deeper layer of the skin, containing hair follicles, sweat glands, sebaceous glands, nerve endings, and blood vessels.

descending colon part of the colon that lies on the left side of the abdomen, extending from below the stomach to the level of the iliac crest.

diabetes mellitus a disorder of carbohydrate metabolism caused by a deficiency of available insulin.

diabetic coma *see* hyperglycemic shock.

diabetic ketoacidosis condition caused by build-up in the blood stream of acid metabolic products (ketones) as a result of the body's use of substances other than sugar for energy.

diaphragm flat, circular sheet of muscle separating the thoracic and abdominal cavities.

diaphysis shaft or middle part of a long cylindrical bone.

diarrhea condition of abnormally frequent and liquid bowel movements.

diastolic pressure the blood pressure noted during ventricular relaxation as the heart fills with blood.

diathermy therapeutic application of high frequency electrical current to heat the body's tissues.

diencephalon portion of the brain between the cerebral hemispheres forming the upper part of the brain stem.

diffusion spread of a substance in fluid from an area of high concentration to one of lower concentration, until the concentration is equal throughout.

direct bone healing method of fracture treatment in which the broken bone ends are immobilized and are in contact, allowing direct deposit of woven bone.

discoid meniscus congenital variation of the normal semilunar meniscus, in which the meniscus is discoid in shape.

dislocation disruption of a joint so that the bone ends are no longer in contact.

displaced fracture a fracture that produces deformity of the limb.

distal location in an extremity nearer the free end; location on the trunk farther from the midline or from the point of reference.

distention the state of being stretched or inflated.

dorsalis pedis artery the continuation of the anterior tibial artery on the anterior surface of the foot.

duodenum first or most proximal portion of the small intestine, connecting the stomach to the jejunum.

drawer test *see* anteroposterior drawer test.

dura mater outermost of the three layers of tissue that envelop the brain and spinal cord.

duration time necessary to do something, as in the time necessary to complete the desired exercise.

dynamic exercise exercise involving the rhythmical contraction of flexor and extensor muscle groups, such as in walking and jogging.

dysmenorrhea painful menstruation, less common in athletic females than in nonathletic females.

dysphagia sensation of sticking or discomfort when swallowing.

dyspnea difficulty or pain with breathing.

dysuria sensation of pain, burning, or itching that occurs during urination.

eburnation in osteoarthritis, the loss of the articular cartilage, exposing the underlying subchondral bone.

eccentric muscle contraction development of tension through actin and myosin interaction and muscle lengthening.

ecchymosis bruise; dislocation of the skin due to subcutaneous and intracutaneous bleeding.

edema condition in which fluid escapes into the tissues from vascular or lymphatic spaces and causes local or generalized swelling.

electrical muscle stimulation (EMS) treatment in which the biphasic current delivers stimulation

to muscles in a variety of ways, including pulse, surged, or tetanizing contractions.

electrocardiogram (ECG or EKG) recording of the electrical current which flows through the heart.

emergency cardiac care (ECC) cardiopulmonary resuscitation.

emotive imagery visualization technique in which the athlete imagines scenes that produce positive self-enhancing feelings.

emphysema disease of the lung in which there is extreme dilation of pulmonary air sacs and poor exchange of oxygen and carbon dioxide.

enchondral bone healing process in which capillaries grow among mesenchymal cells, forming a fibrovascular tissue known as callus that bridges the gap between bone ends.

enchondral ossification process of bone formation whereby a cartilage model is replaced by bone.

endometrium the lining of the uterus.

endosteum tissue which forms the inner layer of long bones.

enthesopathy injury in which tendon fibers are torn directly off their insertion.

envenomation the deposit of venom into a victim via a poisonous bite.

epicondylitis inflammatory response to overuse of either a flexor or an extensor muscle group attaching into the medial and lateral epicondyle of the humerus, respectively.

epidermis the outer layer of skin which is made up of cells that are sealed together to form a watertight protective covering for the body.

epididymis cordlike structure along the posterior border of the testis where sperm is stored.

epididymitis inflammation of the epididymis.

epidural hematoma hematoma outside the dura mater and under the skull.

epiglottis a thin, leaf-shaped valve that allows air to pass into the trachea but prevents food or liquid from entering.

epilepsy a disorder caused by an abnormal focus of electrical activity in the brain that produces seizures.

epinephrine hormone that stimulates the heart and the sympathetic nervous system.

epiphyseal fracture injury to the growth plate of a long bone in children; may lead to arrested bone growth.

epiphyseal plate transverse cartilage plate near the end of a child's bone responsible for growth in length of the bone.

epiphysis end of a long bone.

epistaxis nosebleed.

erectile tissue tissue containing large vascular

spaces that fill with blood on stimulation (a process called erection) as in the penis and clitoris.

erythrocyte sedimentation rate indicator of both the pressure of infection and inflammation; performed by watching red cells "sediment out" from whole blood; also called "sed rate."

esophageal varices large dilated veins in the wall of the esophagus in patients with cirrhosis secondary to long-term alcohol abuse; shorting of blood flow from the GI tract around (instead of through) the liver results in the development of these veins.

esophagus passage leading from the pharynx to the stomach.

evaporation loss of heat from the body by conversion of moisture or perspiration on the body's surface to a vapor.

eversion turning outward.

evisceration the protrusion of viscera or internal organs through an abdominal wound.

excessive lateral pressure syndrome pain produced by excessive pressure on the lateral facet and lateral structures about the patellofemoral joint.

exercise-induced anaphylaxis an allergic response to exercise; symptoms include sweating, high-blood pressure, fever, and a feeling of "impending doom."

exercise-induced asthma acute, reversible, self-limited episode of airway obstruction that occurs in both small and large airways during and after physical activity; exercise-induced bronchospasm.

expiration exhaling, breathing out, or expelling air from the lungs.

expiratory reserve volume the maximum volume which can be expired at the end of a normal expiration.

extensor digitorum brevis short toe extensor on the dorsum of the foot.

extensor digitorum longus muscle in the anterior compartment of the muscles of the leg; divides and inserts on the dorsum of the small toes.

extensor hallucis longus muscle in the anterior compartment of the leg which inserts on the dorsum of the great toe.

extensor mechanism complex interaction of muscles, ligaments, and tendons that stabilizes the patellofemoral joint and acts to extend the knee.

extensor supinator muscle group muscle group originating on the lateral epicondyle and extending down the forearm dorsally into the wrist and hand.

external acoustic meatus with the auricle, forms the external ear.

external chest compression technique to produce artificial circulation by applying rhythmic pressure and relaxation to the lower half of the sternum; has the effect of compressing the heart between the sternum and the spine.

external hemorrhage bleeding that can be seen coming from a wound.

external maxillary arteries artery anterior to the angle of the mandible on the inner surface of the lower jaw that contributes much of the blood supply to the face.

external rotation-recurvatum test test for postero-lateral rotatory instability of the knee in which the athletic trainer lifts the affected extremity by the foot and evaluates the external rotation of the lateral tibial on the femur.

eyeball the ball of the eye sphere approximately 1 inch in diameter.

eyelid a protective fold covering the front of the eye; contains the eyelashes and the conjunctiva.

fabella sesamoid bone that is sometimes found in the lateral gastrocnemius muscle tendon.

fabellofibular ligament *see* short collateral ligament.

fallopian tubes: long, slender tubes that extend from the uterus to the region of the ovary on the same side, and through which the ovum passes from ovary to uterus.

fascia sheet or band of tough fibrous connective tissue; lies deep under the skin and forms an outer layer for the muscles.

fascia lata originates from the lateral crest region and continues over the lateral aspect of the knee, enveloping the lateral aspect of the thigh; iliotibial tract.

fascicles bundles covered by a tough outer layer which form axons or groupings of nerve fibers.

fast twitch muscle fibers Type I muscle fibers adapted for anaerobic activity.

fatigue fracture microfracture that occurs when the bone is subjected to frequent, repeated stresses, such as in running or marching long distances, and the rate of bone breakdown exceeds the rate of bone repair.

fat pad specialized soft tissue structure for weight bearing and absorbing impact.

felon purulent infection of the pulp of the distal phalanx of the finger.

female genitalia the uterus, ovaries, fallopian tubes, and vagina.

femoral artery principal artery of the thigh, a

continuation of the external iliac artery; supplies blood to the lower abdominal wall, external genitalia, and legs.

femoral condyles two surfaces at the distal end of the femur that articulate with the superior surfaces of the tibia.

femoral head proximal end of the femur, articulating with the acetabulum.

femoral neck heavy column of bone connecting the head and the shaft of the femur.

femur the thigh bone; extends from the pelvis to the knee and is the longest and largest bone in the body.

fibrillation continuous, uncoordinated quivering of the muscle fibers of the heart; causes uncontrolled and ineffective beating of the heart.

fibrocartilaginous discs spacers and shock absorbers between each vertebral body.

fibrositis diffuse, multiple-site inflammation associated with pain and stiffness.

fibula outer and smaller of the two bones of the leg, extending from just below the knee to form the lateral portion of the ankle joint.

fibular collateral ligament ligament that inserts from the femoral condyle to the fibular head.

finger sweep procedure used to remove foreign bodies from the mouth; care should be taken when using the finger sweep not to push the dislodged foreign body farther back into the airway.

first-degree concussion the least severe brain injury; involves no loss of consciousness; slight mental confusion, memory loss, dizziness, and ringing of the ears may occur.

flail chest condition that occurs when three or more ribs are broken each in two places and the chest wall lying between the fractures moves in a direction opposite the rest of the chest wall during respiration.

flail segment segment of the chest wall in a flail chest injury that lies between the rib fractures and moves paradoxically as the patient breathes.

flat foot *see* pes planus.

flexibility range of motion at a specific joint; the capacity of a muscle to lengthen or stretch.

flexion-rotation drawer test a modification of the pivot shift test and the Lachman test, the test is positive if anterolateral subluxation of the lateral femorotibial articulation occurs; test for anterolateral rotatory instability of the knee in which the leg is held in neutral rotation at 20 degrees of the knee flexion.

flexor digitorum longus muscle one of the medial stabilizers of the ankle, located in the posterior compartment of the muscles of the leg, that flexes the lateral four toes.

flexor hallucis longus muscle one of the three muscles of the deep portion of the posterior compartment that flexes the great toe.

flexor pronator muscle group muscle group originating on the medial epicondyle and then extending along the epicondylar ridge.

floating ribs eleventh and twelfth ribs, which do not connect to the sternum.

folic acid deficiency lack of adequate folic acid in the body; cause of megaloblastic anemia.

fontanelles area in a baby's head where the skull bones have not yet completely grown together.

foot strike hemolysis a cause of anemia in long-distance runners, which results from multiple foot strikes on hard pavement, bursting red blood cells in the bloodstream.

foramen magnum large opening in the base of the skull through which the brain connects to the spinal cord.

foramina openings in the arches allowing paired branches of nerves to exit the spinal cord at each vertebral level.

force action that changes the state or motion of a body to which it is applied.

forced expiratory volume (FEV) volume of air expired during the first second of the forced vital capacity maneuver.

forced lateral deviation of the neck an injury in which the neck is driven laterally, stretching the nerve trunks of the upper portion of the brachial plexus.

fracture any break in the continuity of a bone.

fracture-dislocation two-fold injury in which the joint is dislocated and a part of the bone near the join is fractured.

Freiberg's disease specific avascular necrosis that occurs in the head of the second metatarsal in some adolescents.

frequency the number of occurrences of a process per unit of time.

frontal bone bone forming the skeleton of the forehead.

frostnip *see* chilblains.

frozen shoulder *see* adhesive capsulitis.

functional residual capacity volume of air remaining in the lung at the end of expiration, during normal breathing.

funnelization process whereby the bone grows in width by apposition of new bone on the periosteal surface and remodeling of the metaphysis.

furuncle tender inflammation around the hair follicle that becomes a fluctuant mass; caused predominantly by a staphylococcal organism.

Galeazzi fracture   dislocated ulna with a fractured radius.

gallbladder   pear-shaped sac on the undersurface of the liver that collects bile from the liver and discharges it into the duodenum through the common bile duct.

galvanic stimulation   treatment modality that provides an external electrical stimulation of more than 100 volts with a pulsatile waveform that is between 5 and 100 microseconds in duration.

gamekeeper's thumb   rupture of the ulnar collateral ligament.

ganglion   a mass of nerve cell bodies usually found lying outside the central nervous system.

gastric distention   inflation of the stomach.

gastritis   inflammation or irritation of the lining of the stomach.

gastrocnemius muscle   muscle located in the posterior compartment of the leg; the medial and lateral heads of this muscle arise from the capsule of the knee and form the inferior boundary of the popliteal fossa; helps to extend the foot and flex the knee.

gastrocnemius-soleus group   muscle group located in the superficial part of the posterior compartment of the leg; leads to the calcaneal tendon and inserts on the posterior aspect of the calcaneus; acts to extend and rotate the foot.

gastroenteritis   viral or bacterial infection of the lining of the stomach and/or the intestines.

generalized seizure   an epileptic seizure involving most of the brain; also called a convulsive or tonic-clonic seizure.

genital system   the male and female reproductive systems.

genitourinary system   organs of reproduction together with the organs concerned in the production and excretion of urine.

genu recurvatum   tendency of the knee to hyperextend.

germinal layer   layer of skin cells that constantly reproduce to replace outer cells that are being shed or rubbed off.

glenohumeral dislocation   injury in which the humeral head may displace from the joint; the majority of these dislocations are anterior and inferior to the glenoid rim.

glenohumeral joint   true shoulder joint.

glenoid labrum   fibrocartilaginous rim around the glenoid that slightly widens and deepens the socket.

glenoid labrum tear   tear of the glenoid labrum; can result from acute trauma or overuse.

glycosuria   excretion of glucose in the urine as a result of hyperglycemia.

gout   hereditary form of arthritis, resulting from excessive uric acid in the blood and characterized by recurrent painful attacks of arthritis in one joint.

gracilis muscle   one of the three pes anserinus muscles of the knee that help protect the knee against rotatory and valgus stress (the other ones are the sartorius and semitendinosus).

graded exercise test (GXT)   exercise prescription administered prior to initiation into a cardiac rehabilitation program; sets a range for the target rate zone in which the athlete maintains his or her heart rate during each exercise session.

granulocytes   any cell containing granules, especially a leukocyte.

gravity drawer test   test for posterior laxity of the knee in which the athlete lies supine and the hip and knee are flexed to 90 degrees.

gravity external rotation test   test for determining posterolateral rotatory instability; the knee, as well as the hip joint, is flexed to 90 degrees; the trainer rotates the tibia and foot externally and notes the excursion of the fibular head and tibial tubercle.

greater trochanter   broad, flat process at the upper end of the lateral surface of the femur to which several muscles are attached.

greenstick fracture   incomplete fracture that passes only partway through the shaft of a bone; occurs only in children.

guarding   refusal to use an injured part because motion causes pain; involuntary abdominal muscular contraction reflecting inflammation and pain within the peritoneal cavity.

hair follicles   the small organs that produce hair.

hallux valgus deformity   *see* bunion.

hamate hook fracture   fracture of the hook of the hamate; usually occurs with a strong, twisting force or from a direct blow.

hammertoe   flexion deformity of the DIP joint of the foot.

hamstring   one of the large muscle groups at the back of the thigh that flex the knee.

hamstring muscles   *see* hamstring.

hamstring strain (tear)   tear of the hamstring; can be recurrent and disabling.

hangman's fracture   fracture of the pedicles of C2.

HDL cholesterol (high-density lipoprotein)   one of the two types of cholesterol; HDL-chol produced only by the body, and is thought to play a preventive role in heart disease.

head   the upper or proximal portion of a structure;

the head of a bone is the rounded end that allows joint rotation.

head-tilt/chin-lift maneuver opening the airway by tilting the athlete's head backward and lifting the chin forward, bringing the entire lower jaw with it.

head-tilt maneuver opening the airway by tilting the athlete's head backward as far as possible.

heart hollow muscular organ that receives blood from the veins and propels it into the arteries.

heart rate frequency of heart muscle contraction.

heat cramps painful muscle spasms of arms and legs caused by excessive body heat and depletion of fluids and electrolytes.

heat exhaustion *see* heat prostration.

heat prostration form of shock that occurs when the body loses water and electrolytes through very heavy sweating after exposure to heat; symptoms include weakness, dizziness, nausea and vomiting, and pallor; also called heat exhaustion.

heatstroke most serious form of heat injury in which rapidly rising internal body temperature overwhelms the body's mechanisms for release of heat; symptoms include hot, dry skin, lack of sweating, emotional irritability, and disorientation.

heel spur a bony spur on the calcaneus.

Heimlich maneuver a series of six to ten manual thrusts to the upper abdomen, just above the umbilicus and well below the xiphoid, to relieve upper airway obstruction; the abdominal thrust maneuver.

hemarthrosis collection of blood within a joint.

hematemesis vomiting of bright red blood.

hematochezia passage of bright red blood from the rectum.

hematocrit ratio of the volume of packed red blood cells to the total volume of blood.

hematoma a pool of blood collecting within the damaged tissue.

hematuria the passage of blood in the urine.

hemopneumothorax blood and air within the pleural space, but outside the lung.

hemoptysis coughing up of bright red blood.

hemorrhage bleeding; blood escaping from arteries or veins.

hemorrhagic shock shock resulting from blood loss.

hemothorax presence of blood in the chest cavity within the pleural space outside the lung.

hernia protrusion of a loop of an organ or tissue through an abnormal opening.

herniated disc rupture of the nucleus pulposus or annulus fibrosis of the intervertebral disc; presentation may include pain radiating into the extremities and altered motor and sensory function of the extremities with diminished reflexes.

herpes infection highly contagious, recurrent skin eruption caused by infection from the herpes virus.

high-altitude cerebral edema very dangerous form of altitude sickness, whose symptoms include headache, confusion, hallucination, and coma.

high-altitude pulmonary edema form of altitude illness and unusual form of noncardiac pulmonary edema, characterized by shortness of breath, increased respiratory rate, cough, hemoptysis, and chest pain.

Hill-Sachs lesion indentation or compression fracture of the articular surface of the humeral head created by the sharp edge of the anterior glenoid as the humeral head dislocates over it.

hip joint joint where the femur articulates with the innominate bone.

hip pointer painful injury caused by irritation or avulsion of the attachments of the abdominal and thigh muscles at the iliac crest.

HLA-B27 seriologic antibody-antigen test used to detect certain arthritic disorders, especially ankylosing spondylitis.

hollow organs tubes through which materials pass, such as the stomach, intestines, ureters, and bladder.

horizontal cleavage tears meniscal injuries usually due to cartilage degeneration; horizontal meniscal tears.

horizontal meniscal tears *see* horizontal cleavage tears.

host organism or individual attacked by an infecting agent.

Hughston jerk test a test for anterolateral rotatory instability of the knee in which the athlete lies supine, with the knee flexed approximately to a right angle and the hip at about 45 degrees of flexion; while the knee is extended, an internal rotational force is placed on the tibia and a valgus stress applied; a positive test produces a snap and a pop.

humerus bone of the arm articulating with the scapula to form the shoulder joint and with the ulna and radius to form the elbow joint.

humoral response centers on the activation of Hageman factor (clotting factor XII) in the plasma, resulting in four subsystems of mediator production.

hunting reaction the initial constriction of blood vessels following the application of cryotherapy after which vasodilation occurs.

hydroceles a collection of fluid in the scrotal sac.

hyperglycemia abnormally increased content of sugar in the blood.

hyperglycemic shock (diabetic coma) stuporous or unconscious state in the diabetic athlete caused by hyperglycemia; symptoms include polyuria, dehydration, Kussmaul breathing and the odor of acetone on the breath.

hyperplasia condition in which the muscle fibers split and increase in number.

hyperpyrexia body temperature above 40 to 41 degrees C (105 degrees F).

hypertrophy of muscle increase in the cross-sectional area of individual muscle fibers caused by resistance training.

hyperventilation overbreathing to the extent that the level of carbon dioxide in the blood falls way below normal.

hyperviscosity syndrome condition in which the hematocrit is greater than 60 percent; this is one risk of blood doping.

hyphema bleeding into the anterior chamber of the eye, obscuring the iris.

hypoglycemia insufficient sugar in the blood.

hypoglycemic (insulin) shock insulin shock resulting from an abnormally low sugar content in the blood.

hypokalemia potassium deficiency; may result from chronic vomiting or laxative/diuretic abuse.

hypothermia a body temperature below 33.3 C (95 F).

hypovolemic shock shock resulting from loss of body fluid or blood.

hypoxia deficiency of oxygen reaching the tissues of the body.

ICE principle treatment combination in acute conditions, in which cryotherapy is combined with elevation and compression in the form of an elastic wrap.

ICES ice, compression, elevation, and splinting.

ICE treatment ice, compression, and elevation, used to decrease hemorrhage and edema after an injury.

ileum more distal portion of the small intestine, between the jejunum and the colon.

ileus obstruction of the bowel.

iliac crest the upper border of the pelvic bone.

iliac spines blunt, bony projections on the borders of the ilium which form the posterior iliac crest.

iliocecal valve valve at the junction of the ilium and the cecum allowing passage of bowel contents in only one direction, into the colon of the large intestine.

iliofemoral one of the three extremely strong ligaments surrounding the hip joint anteriorly and posteriorly and reinforcing the capsule; the other two ligaments are the ischiofemoral and the pubofemoral.

iliopsoas bursa one of the two most important bursae (the other being the trochanteric bursa) about the hip joint; located between the capsule and the iliopsoas muscle anteriorly.

iliotibial band thickening of the iliotibial tract that inserts directly into the lateral tubercle of the tibia.

iliotibial band friction syndrome acute inflammatory condition occurring when the iliotibial band repeatedly rubs against the bony prominence of the lateral femoral epicondyle.

iliotibial tract *see* fascia lata.

ilium one of the three bones (ilium, ischium, and pubis) that fuse to form the pelvic bones.

immersion (trench) foot a form of cold exposure that occurs when the feet suffer prolonged exposure to cold but not freezing water.

impaled foreign object object such as a knife, splinter of wood, or piece of glass that penetrates the skin and remains in the body.

impetigo bacterial infection of the skin caused by streptococcus and staphylococcus.

impingement condition in which the rotator cuff impinges on the acromion and coracoacromial ligament; the weakened rotator cuff allows the humeral head to migrate superiorly, rather than staying centrally located in the glenoid fossa.

incontinence inability to control the bowels or bladder.

incubation period time between exposure of the host to the infectious agent and the appearance of symptoms of that infection.

infection invasion of a host or host tissue by organisms such as bacteria, viruses, or parasites.

infectious mononucleosis mildly contagious viral disease primarily affecting the respiratory system.

inferior portion portion of the body or body part that lies nearer the feet than the head.

inferior vena cava one of the two largest veins in the body that carries blood from the lower extremities and the pelvic and abdominal organs into the heart.

inflammation heat, redness, swelling, and pain that accompany musculoskeletal injuries; occurs when tissue is crushed, stretched, or torn.

inflammation repair process a three-phase response to bone injury (acute vascular inflammation response, repair regeneration, and remodeling maturation).

influenza specific viral bronchitis due to influenza viruses A or B.

informed consent consent given by a person who understands the nature and extent of any procedure before agreeing to it and who has sufficient mental and physical capacity to make such a judgment.

infrapatellar fat pad dynamic shock absorber and source of nutrition for the tendon; extends from the lower pole of the patella to the level of the tibia.

infraspinatus muscle of the rotator cuff that arises from the dorsal surface of the scapula and inserts on the greater tuberosity.

inguinal ligament fibrous band running from the anterior superior spine of the ilium to the tubercle of the pubis.

innominate bone bone forming one half of the pelvic girdle and arising from a fusion of the ilium, ischium, and pubis.

insertion site of attachment of a muscle.

inspiration inhaling; breathing in, drawing air into the lungs.

inspiratory reserve volume maximum volume of gas which can be inspired at the end of a normal inspiration.

instability looseness; unsteadiness.

insulin hormone produced by the pancreas that enables glucose to be converted to glycogen and stored until needed; used in treatment and control of diabetes mellitus.

insulin-dependent diabetes mellitus (IDDM) a form of diabetes mellitus that can be regulated only by the daily use of insulin.

insulin (hypoglycemic) shock shock caused by an overdose of insulin or failure to eat enough food to balance the insulin, resulting in a sudden drop in the blood sugar level; chief symptoms are sweating, tremor, anxiety, vertigo, and double vision, followed by delirium, convulsions, and collapse.

intensity amount of effort extended to perform a task.

intercondylar eminence proximal tibial process; anterior and posterior to the intercondylar eminence are attachment sites for the cruciate ligaments' menisci.

intercondylar notch bony notch that separates posteriorly the condyles of the femur.

intercondylar tubercles a lateral spur projecting upward from the intercondylar eminence.

interferential stimulation method of electrical stimulation that uses simultaneously two biphasic medium-frequency currents between 4000 and 5000 cycles per second.

intermittent compression air-filled boot or sleeve that applies intermittent pressure to the injured extremity to augment absorption of edema.

internal hemorrhage bleeding not visible to the eye.

interosseous membrane (ligament) a fibrous sheet that connects the radius to the ulna and the tibia to the fibula.

interval throwing program a program for shoulder rehabilitation that allows the athlete to get a light workout several times a day at a submaximal level without fatiguing the arm.

intervertebral disc fibrocartilaginous shock-absorbing disc located between vertebrae composed of the annulus fibrosis and the nucleus pulposus.

intramembranous ossification formation of bone within a preexisting cartilage.

intravenous pyelogram (IVP) scan performed by injecting contrast medium into a vein and allowing it to pass through excretion into the kidneys and ureters and bladder.

inversion injury ankle injury in which the athlete lands on the lateral aspect of the foot; bony stability is greater laterally than medially, predisposing the ankle to inversion.

involuntary muscles muscles that continue to contract rhythmically regardless of conscious control.

iontophoresis therapeutic modality that uses galvanic electrical current to drive ionized medications through the skin to injured tissues.

iris muscle behind the cornea that dilates and constricts the pupil, regulating the amount of light that enters the eye.

iron deficiency anemia anemia resulting from lack of iron; treated by increasing the amount of iron in the diet and by correcting any underlying medical problems.

ischial tuberosity the bony prominence felt in the middle of each buttock; the major attachment site for the hamstrings; the major weight-bearing structure for sitting.

ischiofemoral one of the three extremely strong ligaments surrounding the joint anteriorly and posteriorly and reinforcing the capsule; the other two ligaments are the iliofemoral and the pubofemoral.

ischium one of the three bones (ilium, ischium, and pubis) that fuse to form the pelvic bones.

islets of Langerhans cells in the pancreas, which produce insulin and other regulatory hormones.

isokinetic exercise develops tension in the muscle as it shortens; performed on specialized machines or underwater.

isometric exercise contraction of muscles without shortening or lengthening of the muscle fibers.

isometric muscle contraction *see* isometric exercise.

isotonic exercise contraction of muscles concentrically or eccentrically against resistance with movement of the part.

jaundice yellow color of the skin seen in liver disease.

jaw-thrust maneuver opening the airway by bringing the athlete's jaw forward and pulling the lower lip down.

Jefferson fracture burst fracture that occurs when the condyles of the occiput are driven down against the ring of the atlas.

jejunum portion of the small intestine that extends from the duodenum to the ileum.

jersey finger rupture of the insertion of the flexor digitorum longus tendon by forced extension of the flexed finger.

joint articulation, place of union, or junction between two or more bones of the skeleton.

joint arthritis *see* degenerative joint disease.

joint articulation the juncture where two bones come in contact.

joint fluid analysis a gross and microscopic chemical analysis of fluid removed from a joint to differentiate viral, bacterial, chemical, degenerative, and other inflammatory conditions.

joint mobilization *see* manual therapy.

Jones fracture stress fracture of the proximal shaft of the fifth metatarsal.

jugular notch superior border of the sternum.

jumper's knee overuse injury of the extensor mechanism; occurs when the proximal pole of the patella is injured by repetitive traction of the insertion of the quadriceps mechanism.

juvenile-onset (Type I) diabetes insulin-dependent type of diabetes mellitus found usually in children.

juvenile osteochondrosis inflammation of an epiphysis in children and adolescents.

ketoacidosis acidosis seen in diabetic patients and associated with an enhanced production of ketone bodies from incomplete metabolism of fats.

ketone bodies metabolic end products of the use of fat for routine energy needs.

kidneys the two retroperitoneal organs that excrete the end products of metabolism as urine and regulate the body's salt and water content.

kidney stones stones formed in the kidney from calcium and oxalate crystals or uric acid.

kinetic energy (KE) energy in action that produces motion.

Kohler's disease osteochondrosis of the tarsal navicular.

Kussmaul breathing air hunger, manifested by deep sighing respirations, associated with diabetic acidosis.

kyphosis excessive backward curvature of the spine.

labrum acetabulare fibrocartilaginous rim reinforcing the acetabulum or socket of the joint; acetabular labrum.

labyrinth complicated, fluid-filled spaces in the inner ear that sense balance.

laceration cut that may leave a smooth or jagged wound through the skin, subcutaneous tissues, muscles, and associated nerves and blood vessels.

Lachman test test for instability of anterior cruciate ligament of the knee in which the examiner stabilizes the thigh while performing an anteroposterior drawer motion with the hand holding the proximal tibia to direct tibial displacement.

large bowel portion of the digestive tube extending from the ileocecal valve to the anus; made up of the cecum, colon, and rectum.

large intestine *see* large bowel.

laryngitis inflammation of the larynx usually caused by infection and resulting in hoarseness.

larynx voice box; a structure composed of thyroid cartilage on the top and cricoid cartilage on the bottom.

lateral lying away from the midline.

lateral collateral ligament ligament in the elbow; consists of a capsular thickening, extending from the lateral epicondyle to the annular ligament; also the fibular collateral ligament of the knee, the lateral collateral ligament of the ankle.

lateral condyle forms the lateral border of the upper surface of a joint.

lateral ligament structure the three pairs of the lateral collateral ligament of the ankle: the posterior talofibular ligament, the calcaneofibular ligament, and the anterior talofibular ligament.

lateral malleoli projects down to the level of the subtalar joint much farther than the medial malleoli, providing bony stability for the lateral side of the ankle joint.

lateral malleolus bony prominence at the end of the fibula that, together with the medial malleolus, forms the socket of the ankle joint.

lateral meniscus the lateral C-shaped fibrocartilaginous structure of the knee; *see* menisci.

lateral patellar compression syndrome *see* retropatellar pain.

lateral patellar retinacula expansion on both sides of the patella, made up of extensions of the vastus lateralis that help extend the knee joint.

lateral pivot shift test test for anterolateral rotatory instability of the knee in which the tibia is internally rotated on the femur and pushed anteriorly to note subluxation of the lateral tibial plateau.

lateral retinacular release the lateral retinaculum is weakened by surgical release to allow the patella to move more centrally in the groove; also known as capsulorrhaphy.

latissimus dorsi one of the muscles of the trunk that help to stabilize and maneuver the shoulder girdle.

law of valgus any stabilizing deficiency in the extensor mechanism leads to patellar malposition manifested by lateral patellar subluxation or dislocation.

laxity gross ligamentous instability.

LDL cholesterol (low-density lipoprotein) lipoprotein found in foods and produced by the body; contributes to high circulating levels of blood cholesterol.

left lower quadrant abdominal quadrant containing the stomach, the spleen, a portion of the transverse and descending colon, and a small portion of the liver.

left upper quadrant abdominal quadrant containing the liver, gallbladder, and a portion of the colon.

Legg-Calvé-Perthes disease avascular necrosis of the proximal femoral epiphysis.

lesser trochanter medial large prominence distal to the neck of the femur.

levator ani broad shelf of muscle which forms the entire pelvic floor.

levator scapulae muscle of the trunk which helps to stabilize and maneuver the shoulder girdle; *see* latissimus dorsi.

ligament band of the fibrous tissue that connects bones to bones and supports and strengthens joints.

ligamentum nuchae a band of tissue extending from the skull to the seventh cervical vertebra.

linear acceleration change in an object's speed in a straight direction.

linear and nondepressed skull fracture skull fracture involving minimal indentation of the skull toward the brain.

Lisfranc fracture rare but severe fracture-dislocation in the midfoot.

Little Leaguer's elbow overuse syndrome in the elbows of young athletes; the result of repetitive valgus stress during overhead throwing, resulting in lateral compression and medial traction on the elbow.

Little Leaguer's shoulder overuse injury consisting of a stress fracture of the proximal humeral physis; seen in young athletes who perform overhead throwing activities.

liver large solid organ that lies in the upper right quadrant of the abdomen; produces bile, stores sugar for immediate use by the body, and chemically treats all products of absorption in the gastrointestinal tract.

load any force or combination of forces applied to the outside of a structure and therefore sustained or carried by the matter in the structure.

load-deformation curve mathematical relationship of the load applied to a structure.

longitudinal arch arch formed by the bones of the foot; starts at the weight-bearing surface of the calcaneus and ends at the metatarsal heads; supports the head of the talus.

longitudinal meniscal tear meniscal tear caused by the displacement to some extent of the posterior medial segment of the meniscus; can be partial or complete.

lordosis accentuation of the normal curve, which is normally present to a minor degree in the lower back.

lumbar spine lower part of the back formed by the lowest five nonfused vertebrae.

lung parenchyma the alveoli in which oxygen is transferred to the blood and carbon dioxide is transferred from the blood.

lungs organs that aerate the blood, occupying the lateral cavities of the chest and separated from each other by the heart and mediastinal structures.

lymphocyte type of leukocyte; mainly responsible

for the specific defenses of the body against foreign invaders.

McMurray test meniscal test used to detect a posterior horn tear; the examiner, with the athlete's knee in full flexion, externally rotates the leg and extends the knee; a click indicates a medial meniscal tear. To test for a lateral meniscal tear, the leg is internally rotated.

magnetic resonance imaging (MRI) diagnostic technique using magnetism to provide high-quality cross-sectional images of organs and structures within the body without x-rays or other radiation.

main stem bronchi one of the two main branches of the trachea that lead into the left lung and the right lung.

male genitalia testicles, vasa deferentia, seminal vesicles, prostate gland urethra, and penis.

mallet (baseball) finger avulsion of the insertion of the tendon of the exterior digitorum communis into the distal phalanx of the finger caused by forced flexion of the extended joint.

mandible bone of the lower jaw.

manipulative therapy high-velocity, forceful mobilization technique to free a joint from a fixed pathological position.

manual therapy (joint mobilization) mobilization of joints and soft tissue to allow proper functioning of the body.

massage systematic and scientific manipulation of the body's tissue, usually using hands; one of the oldest modalities.

mastery rehearsal mentally practicing a desired outcome in an enthusiastic and positive way.

mastoid process prominent, hard, bony mass at the base of the skull behind the ear.

matrix intercellular substance of a tissue.

maxilla bone forming the upper jaw on either side of the face; contains the upper teeth, orbit of the eye, nasal cavity, and palate.

maximal oxygen consumption (VO$_2$ max) reflects the body's ability to maximally extract and use oxygen for aerobic metabolism; measures the lung's ability to extract oxygen.

medial lying toward the midline.

medial capsular ligament midthird of the true capsule of the knee joint; ligament extending from the femur to the midportion of the meniscus and then to the tibia.

medial collateral ligament ligament on the medial aspect of the knee consisting of anterior, posterior, and oblique components and extending from the femur to the tibia.

medial condyle forms the medial border of the upper surface of a joint.

medial malleoli *see* medial malleolus.

medial malleolus the bony prominence at the end of the tibia that, together with the lateral malleolus, forms the socket of the ankle joint.

medial meniscus the medial C-shaped fibrocartilaginous structure of the knee; *see* menisci.

medial patellar retinacula extension of the vastus medialis that helps extend the knee joint.

medial retinaculum structure composed of the aponeurosis of the vastus medial muscle itself; attaching along the medial border of the patella, its primary function is to hold the patella medially.

median nerve nerve that controls sensation of the central palm, the thumb, and the first three fingers, as well as the ability to oppose the thumb to the little finger.

mediators protein messengers that allow cell-to-cell self-regulation.

medullary (canal) cavity central open area of the bone.

melena passage of dark black stools with the consistency of tar.

menarche the onset of menstruation.

meninges the three layers of tissue that envelop the brain and spinal cord: the dura mater, pia mater, and arachnoid.

menisci fibrocartilaginous structures that lie between the hyaline cartilage surface of the femur and tibia.

meniscofemoral ligament with the meniscotibial ligament, it attaches the midportion of the medial meniscus peripherally to the tibia and the femur.

meniscotibial (coronary) ligament with meniscofemoral ligament, attaches the midportion of the medial meniscus peripherally to the tibia and femur.

meniscus cushion of cartilage that fills up a space between bones and aids in the gliding motion and stability of the joint.

menstrual period regular shedding of the endometrial lining occurring when the released ovum is not fertilized; menstrual periods usually begin at puberty and continue until menopause.

mesenchymal syndrome group at risk for connective tissue breakdown in the face of relatively benign load or use.

mesentery delicate tissue formed by peritoneum that suspends the organs within the abdomen from the body walls and carries blood vessels and nerves to all these organs.

metabolic shock shock caused by loss of body fluid.

metacarpal bones the five bones of the hand that extend from the wrist to the fingers.

metacarpals *see* metacarpal bones.

metaphysis portion of long bone in the wide part of the extremity containing the growth zone in children.

metatarsal bones five long bones of the foot between the instep and the toes.

metatarsals *see* metatarsal bones.

metatarsus abductus *see* metatarsus varus.

metatarsus adductus *see* metatarsus valgus.

metatarsus valgus congenital deformity of the forefoot in which the forefoot is rotated laterally in relation to the hindfoot.

metatarsus varus congenital deformity of the forefoot in which the forefoot is rotated medially in relation to the hindfoot.

microtrauma destruction of a small number of cells caused by additive effects of repetitive forces.

midline imaginary straight vertical line drawn from midforehead through the nose and the umbilicus to the floor.

modalities physical agents that can create an optimum environment for injury healing, while reducing pain and discomfort.

mode of transmission the manner by which an infection is spread: by contact, airborne, by vehicles, or by vectors.

modulus of elasticity value for stiffness obtained by dividing the stress at any point in the elastic portion of the curve by the strain at that point.

molluscum contagiosum a viral disorder characterized by flesh-colored pink papules, with a central dimpling, on the skin surface.

moment of inertia a measure of resistance to change.

moment of torque force that acts through a distance.

mono spot a blood test used to assist in the diagnosis of infectious mononucleosis, and where the antibodies to the virus that produces mononucleosis are tested for in the athlete's serum.

Monteggia fracture dislocation of the radial head in association with an ulnar fracture.

morphostasis process by which tissues renew their cell populations and their matrix content.

Morton's foot congenital abnormality characterized by a short first metatarsal, which throws weight-bearing stresses to the second metatarsal head, often resulting in pain.

Morton's neuroma an interdigital neuroma of the foot.

motor nerves nerves that transmit impulses to muscles, causing them to move.

motor unit a motor neuron and all the muscle fibers it innervates.

mouth-to-mouth ventilation artificial ventilation performed by the resuscitator's mouth making a seal around the athlete's mouth as he or she exhales into the athlete's mouth.

mouth-to-nose ventilation artificial ventilation in which the resuscitator's lips make a seal around the athlete's nose.

muco-ciliary escalator the protective function of the cilia and mucus of the lungs in sweeping particulate matter and cellular debris up to the pharynx where it can be swallowed.

mucoid degeneration loss of normal crimped, wavy collagen fiber array and normal cellularity noted under a microscope.

mucous membranes mucous-secreting lining of body cavities and passages that communicate directly or indirectly with environment outside body.

mucus opaque, sticky secretion of the mucous membranes that lubricates the body openings.

muscle endurance repetitive muscle contractions carried out over time without undue fatigue.

muscle power the speed movement or the rate at which a resistance can be moved per unit of time.

muscles tissue composed of bundles of specialized cells that have the ability to contract and relax, thus producing movement or force.

muscle strength force or tension that a muscle or muscle group can exert against a resistance.

myelogram x-ray study of the spine carried out after injection of a contrast material into the spinal cord sheath; helpful in diagnosing ruptured or bulging discs.

myocardial contusion bruise of the heart muscle.

myocardial infarction damage or death of an area of the heart muscle; heart attack.

myocardium heart muscle.

myofascial pain syndrome a painful musculoskeletal response that can follow muscle trauma.

myositis ossificans the formation of heterotopic bone within muscle, often as a result of blunt trauma; most commonly occurs in the quadriceps, deltoid, and brachialis muscles.

navicular bone bone with which the head of the talus articulates on the medial side of the foot; also a bone in the wrist that articulates with the trapezium, trapezoid, and other carpal bones.

neck portion of the body between the head and shoulders; also, the constricted portion of a structure (e.g., femoral neck).

negligence unintentionally harmful conduct of an individual.

neural arch *see* vertebral arch.

neuralgia pain along the course of a nerve.

neuritis inflammation or irritation of a nerve.

neuroma a tumor composed of nerve cells.

neuromuscular system a group of interrelated parts that work together to perform certain functions.

neurotmesis total disruption of a nerve.

neurotoxic a substance poisonous to nerve tissue.

nitrogen narcosis state of euphoria caused by increased blood nitrogen during a too rapid diving descent.

nitroglycerin medicine used in treating angina pectoris; relaxes vascular smooth muscle and increases blood flow and oxygen supply to the heart muscle.

nocturia excessive passage of urine at night.

nondisplaced fracture fracture in which there is no deformity of the limb.

non-insulin-dependent diabetes mellitus (NIDDM) form of diabetes mellitus usually found in individuals over 40 that can be controlled by diet and exercise or by oral hypoglycemics; *see* adult-onset (Type II) diabetes.

nonlamellar (woven) bone immature bone.

occiput back part of the head.

occlusive dressings dressing or bandage that closes a wound and protects it from the air.

olecranon bursa bursa in the elbow that separates the skin from the underlying ulna; allows the soft tissue to glide smoothly over the olecranon process.

olecranon process bony process of the proximal ulna preventing hyperextension of the elbow.

open chest injury injury in which the chest wall has been penetrated.

open fracture *see* compound fracture.

open injury injury caused by a penetrating object that breaks the skin or the mucous membrane that lines the mouth, nose, anus, or vagina.

open (penetrating) injury injury occurring when a foreign body enters the abdomen, opening the peritoneum-lined cavity to the external environment.

open wound *see* open injury.

orbit eye socket.

orifices the openings to the body (mouth, nose, anus, vagina).

origin the more fixed end or attachment of a muscle.

os calcis *see* calcaneus.

Osgood-Schlatter disease partial avulsion of the tibial tubercle because the tubercle is subjected to traction forces by the patellar tendon insertion, causing painful swelling in the knee of the adolescent.

osteitis pubis arthritic condition from continued stress placed on the pubic symphysis; characterized by localized pain and difficulty running.

osteoarthritis *see* degenerative joint disease.

osteoblasts cells which lay down new bone.

osteochondral fracture intra-articular fracture in which part of the articular surface is separated from the remainder of the epiphysis by a fracture through the subchondral bone.

osteochondritis inflammation of bone and cartilage.

osteochondritis dissecans localized area of avascular necrosis resulting in separation of a fragment of subchondral bone with or without injury to the underlying cartilage under a joint surface.

osteoclast large multinuclear bone cell associated with absorption and removal of bone.

osteocytes osteoblasts imbedded within bone.

osteoporosis irreversible decrease in mineralized bony tissue.

osteosynthesis fixation that fixes and reduces the fracture fragments with wire, screws, and pins, to obtain bony union.

os trigonum syndrome a congenital variant consisting of a bony ossicle posterior to the talus; usually asymptomatic, but can become inflamed with repetitive plantar flexion activities as in dancing, skating, and kicking.

ovaries glands found in females that produce sex hormones and ova (eggs).

overload principle states that strength, power, endurance, and hypertrophy of muscle can only increase when a muscle performs workloads greater than those previously encountered.

overuse injury any injury that has been caused by repetitive movement of part of the body.

ovum female reproductive cell which, when fertilized by the sperm, develops a new member of the same species.

palpation the last portion of the abdominal examination; using the hands to feel for masses and muscle resistance and to determine the size and shape of abdominal organs.

pancreas large, elongated gland situated transversely behind the stomach, between the spleen and the duodenum; major source of digestive enzymes and producer of insulin.

Panner's disease osteonecrosis of the capitellum seen in teenagers.

paradoxical motion in flail chest, the motion of the chest wall segment between the rib fractures is opposite the motion of the rest of the chest wall during respiration.

paralysis complete or partial loss of the ability to move.

parasympathetic (craniosacral) nervous system a part of the autonomic nervous system that causes blood vessels to dilate, slows the heart rate, and relaxes muscle sphincters.

parasympathetic stimulation type of stimulation that has the opposite effect of sympathetic stimulation; predominates to maintain the usual resting heart rate of about 65 to 75 beats per minute.

parietal pleura portion of the pleura lining the inside of the chest cavity.

parietal regions more lateral portions of the cranium.

paronychia inflammation of folds of tissue surrounding the fingernail.

parrot-beak tear traumatic meniscal tear of youth, mainly located in the middle segment of the lateral meniscus and usually a combination of tears associated with previous pathology; radial tear.

pars interarticularis part of the vertebra posteriorly between the spinal arch and the pedicle.

patella kneecap.

patellar crepitus grating, grinding sensation that is noted during movement of the patellofemoral joint.

patellar dislocation displacement of the patella; usually the patella reduces, leaving a painful, swollen, and tender knee.

patellar ligament see patellar tendon.

patellar plicae a synovial fold which may persist into adult life and cause medial knee pain in the absence of trauma.

patellar subluxation syndrome the patella repetitively subluxates laterally, placing strain on the medial restraints and excessive stress on the patellofemoral joint.

patellar tendinitis pain and inflammation of the patella tendon; causes pain over the tendon and difficulty jumping or running.

patellar tendon the extension of the quadriceps mechanism from the patella to the tibia; also called patellar ligament.

patellectomy surgical excision of the patella.

patellofemoral groove groove that runs anteriorly between the condyles of the femur and accepts the patella.

patellofemoral joint joint between the patella and the femur.

patellofemoral pain syndrome the lateral retinaculum is tight or the muscles are imbalanced so that the patella is pulled laterally; excessive pressure develops on the lateral facet and the lateral tissues about the patellofemoral joint, causing pain.

patellofemoral stress syndrome (PFSS) see retropatellar pain.

pathologic fracture fracture that occurs from minimal force because the bone is weak or diseased.

pectoralis major large, fan-shaped muscle that covers much of the upper part of the front of the chest.

pediculosis pubis oftenly referred to as "crabs"; infestation caused by small, wingless insect that lives in the pubic hair and feeds on blood; is contracted through intimate contact with affected individuals; the lice cause extreme itching of the involved sites.

pelvic cavity space between the pelvis walls.

pelvic inflammatory disease infection in the fallopian tubes and the surrounding tissue of the pelvis.

pelvic ring see pelvis.

pelvis a bony ring, consisting of the sacrum, coccyx, and innominate bones, that connects the trunk to the lower extremities, supports the abdominal contents, and allows passage of the excretory canals.

penetrating injury see open injury.

penetrating thermotherapy deep-heat modality which has varied penetration capabilities up to 2 inches and uses high-frequency electromagnetic currents or acoustic energy to elicit thermal and mechanical responses.

penile urethral discharge any material other than urine or semen passed out of the male urethra.

penis male organ of urinary excretion and copulation.

peptic ulcer ulcers in the stomach or duodenum caused by the action of pepsin.

perceptual alternatives viewing and interpreting the same situation in many different ways.

percussion part of the abdominal inspection; performed by placing one's nondominant hand lightly on the athlete's abdomen to determine the presence and location of hollow versus solid organs or masses.

perfusion process of blood entering an organ or a tissue through its arteries and leaving through the veins, providing tissue nourishment.

pericardial tamponade condition in which blood or other fluid is present in the pericardial sac outside the heart, exerting an unusual pressure on the heart.

periodization concept of dividing the annual training plan into smaller segments, phases, or cycles.

periosteum specialized connective tissue covering all bones of the body.

peripheral nervous system portion of the nervous system that consists of the nerves and ganglia outside the brain and spinal cord.

peristalsis wormlike movement caused by contraction of the muscles in the walls of the gastrointestinal tract that propels food through the digestive tract.

peritendinitis inflammation of the tendon sheath, marked by pain, swelling, and, occasionally, local crepitus.

peritoneum membrane lining the abdominal cavity (parietal peritoneum) and reflected inward over the abdominal organs (visceral peritoneum).

peritonitis inflammation of the lining of the abdomen.

peritonsillar abscess bacterial infection of the peritonsillar and tonsillar areas characterized by pain and inability to open the mouth fully.

pernicious anemia anemia caused by deficiency of vitamin B12, which is essential for normal red blood cell production in the bone marrow.

peroneal spastic flatfoot peroneal muscle spasm that usually occurs after activity or injury, resulting in pes planus (flatfoot) or absent subtalar motion.

peroneus brevis muscle muscle in the peroneal compartment on the lateral aspect of the leg, averting the ankle; passes distal and inferior to the lateral malleolus and inserts on the base of the fifth metatarsal; acts to extend and abduct the foot.

peroneus longus muscle muscle in the peroneal compartment on the lateral aspect of the leg, averting the ankle; it passes under the cuboid bone and inserts on the inferior surface of the medial cuneiform and base of the first metatarsal; it acts to extend, abduct, and evert the foot.

peroneus longus tendon one of the structures that creates a dynamic sling supporting the longitudinal arch, from which comes the extrinsic support.

peroneus tertius muscle that extends from the distal fibula to the fifth metatarsal and acts to flex the foot.

pes anserinus conjoined tendon, composed of the sartorius, gracilis, and semitendinosus muscles, which inserts onto the upper medial aspect of the tibia.

pes planus a pronated foot with a flattened longitudinal arch.

phalanges bones making up the skeleton of the fingers or toes.

pharyngitis inflammation of the pharynx.

pharynx cavity at the back of nose and mouth; the throat.

phonophoresis an application of ultrasound in which molecules or a medication are driven through the skin to inflamed structures.

physeal fractures fractures of the physis which, with complete closure of the injured physis or formation of a localized area of closure known as a physeal bridge, may cause later growth disturbance.

physis growth plate or epiphyseal plate; separates the metaphysis from the epiphysis and is responsible for the rapid longitudinal growth of bones.

pia mater innermost of the three layers of tissue that envelop the brain and spinal cord.

pillow splints a soft splint; *see* splint.

pinna the external ear.

plantar calcaneonavicular ligament sling ligament supporting the longitudinal arch.

plantar fascia fibrous tissue band that runs from the calcaneal tuberosity to the phalanges and supports the talus.

plantar fasciitis irritation of the plantar fascia, usually from overuse; the pain is most severe at the calcaneal tuberosity.

plantar flexion extension of the foot.

plantar warts skin-growth on the sole of the foot caused by a localized viral infection; virus called papillomavirus.

plasma sticky, yellow component of blood that carries the blood cells and nutrients and transports cellular waste material to the organs of excretion.

platelets tiny disc-shaped elements that are a component of blood clot formation; primary function is to seal the holes in blood vessels.

pleura layer of smooth, glistening tissue that covers the lungs.

pleural cavity potential space between the pleural layers, the visceral pleural and the parietal pleura.

plyometric exercises variety of exercises that utilize explosive movements to increase athletic power.

pneumonia infection of the lung.

pneumothorax presence of air within the chest cavity in the pleural space but outside the lung.

point stimulators treatment modality used to produce hyperstimulation analgesia; similar to acupuncture.

point tenderness tenderness at the site of injury or disease, which can be located by gently pressing with one finger.

Poiseuille's law formula indicating that volume flow in a tube is directly proportional to the pressure drop along the length of the tube and to the radius of that tube to the fourth power, and inversely proportional to the length of the tube and to the viscosity of the fluid.

poison substance producing a harmful effect on body process.

polydipsia excessive thirst for long periods of time, as in diabetes.

polyuria frequent and copious urination.

popliteal artery continuation of the superficial femoral artery in the popliteal space (posterior surface of the knee); supplies the knee and the calf.

popliteal cyst *see* Baker's cyst.

popliteal fossa the hollow area that appears on the posterior surface of the knee; popliteal space.

popliteal space *see* popliteal fossa.

popliteus muscle muscle deep to the popliteal artery with three proximal insertions on the tibia; its primary function is internal rotation of the tibia on the femur.

posterior cruciate ligament ligament extending from the intercondylar area of the posterior tibia to the lateral surface of the medial femoral condyle; functions with the anterior cruciate ligament in anteroposterior and rotatory stability of the knee; shorter, thicker, stronger, and less oblique than the anterior cruciate ligament.

posterior glenohumeral dislocation disruption of the glenohumeral joint in a posterior direction; the athlete holds the shoulder in internal rotation and the humeral head may be prominent posteriorly in the shoulder.

posterior interosseous nerve the major terminal branch of the radial nerve that winds around the radius to the dorsal side of the forearm to provide motor and sensory function to the dorsal forearm and wrist.

posterior process that part of each vertebra which can be palpated as it lies just under the skin in the midline of the back.

posterior sternoclavicular dislocation disruption of the sternoclavicular joint posterior; while it is less common than the anterior dislocation of the sternoclavicular joint, it has higher morbidity, with potential injury to the great vessels.

posterior surface surface at the back of the body.

posterior talofibular ligament one of the three lateral ligaments of the ankle; the strongest of the three, it helps to resist forward dislocation of the leg on the foot.

posterior tibial artery artery that is just posterior to the medial malleolus; supplies blood to the foot.

posterior tibial syndrome pain along the medial border of the tibia; associated with running.

posterior tibial tendon one of the structures that creates a dynamic sling supporting the longitudinal arch; attaches directly on the tuberosity of the navicular bone and indirectly on the plantar surface of the navicular and middle cuneiform bones.

posterior tibiofibular ligament part of the talofibular syndesmosis, arises from the posterior calculi on the lateral side of the tibia; helps to hold the fibula snug in its tibial groove.

posterolateral rotatory instability the lateral tibial plateau rotates posteriorly in relationship to the femur.

posteromedial rotatory instability the medial tibial plateau rotates posteriorly on the femur, with associated medial opening.

postictal state third and final phase of a generalized seizure—the period of exhaustion and recovery following a convulsion.

potential energy (PE) energy stored in a body by virtue of its position in space and equal to the mass times the vertical height.

preload reflection of cardiac muscle quality; an elastic distensible ventricle propels more blood more rapidly than a stiffer, less distensible ventricle.

pressure dressing pressure applied to a wound through a dressing to control bleeding.

priapism permanent and painful erection caused by certain spinal injuries, some diseases, and certain drugs.

primary amenorrhea delay of the onset of menstruation beyond the age of 16.

primary survey process of finding and treating the most life-threatening emergencies first.

principle of transition states that sports injury is most likely to occur when the athlete experiences any change in load or use of the involved part.

progressive resistance exercise (PRE) overloading the muscle in a progressive, gradual manner so overtraining and fatigue are avoided.

prominence projection, protrusion.

prominence of the cheek formed by the zygomatic bone.

proprioceptive neuromuscular facilitation (PNF) stretching techniques designed to enhance the neuromuscular response.

prostate gland small gland that surrounds the male urethra where it emerges from the urinary bladder; it secretes a fluid that is part of the ejaculatory fluid.

proteoglycans group of matrix macromolecules that possess great water-binding capacity.

proximal describing structures that are closer to the trunk.

proximal realignment proximal soft tissue reconstruction designed to align the muscle pull on the patella to enhance the action of the vastus medialis obliquus and to tighten the medial capsule.

pseudoanemia *see* sports anemia.

pubic symphysis firm fibrocartilaginous joint anteriorly between the two innominate bones.

pubis one of the three bones (ilium, ischium, and pubis) that fuse to form the pelvic bones.

pubofemoral one of the three extremely strong ligaments surrounding the joint anteriorly and posteriorly and reinforcing the capsule; the other two ligaments are the iliofemoral and the ischiofemoral.

pulmonary circulation the circulation, sometimes called the lesser circulation, that carries unoxygenated blood from the right ventricle through the lungs and back to the left atrium.

pulmonary contusion bruise of the lung.

pulse the wave of pressure that is created by the heart contracting and forcing blood out the left ventricle and into the major arteries.

puncture wound wound resulting from a stab with a knife, ice pick, splinter, or any other pointed object or from a bullet.

pupil the circular opening in the middle of the iris of the eye.

P wave the wave on an electrocardiogram that represents depolarization of the atria.

pyarthrosis pus in a joint cavity.

Q angle the angle made by the rectus femoris and patellar tendon as it attaches to the tibial tuberosity.

QRS complex the wave of an electrocardiogram that represents depolarization of the ventricles.

quadriceps *see* quadriceps muscle.

quadriceps femoris tendon located at the patella, or kneecap.

quadriceps muscle extensor muscle situated at the front of the thigh; composed of four components: the vastus medialis, vastus lateralis, vastus intermedius, and rectus femoris.

quadriceps tendon convergence of the rectus femoris, vastus intermedius, vastus medialis, and vastus lateralis; inserts in the superior pole of the patella.

rabies acute viral infection of the central nervous system that is transmitted by the bite of a rabid animal.

radial artery one of the major arteries of the arm; it can be palpated at the base of the thumb.

radial humeral bursa bursa anteriorly between the radial head and the lateral epicondyle.

radial nerve nerve carrying sensation to the greater portion of the back of the hand and controlling extension of the hand at the wrist.

radial styloid bony prominence felt on the lateral (thumb) side of the wrist.

radial tear *see* parrot-beak tear.

radiation sending forth of radiant energy.

radius bone on the thumb side of the forearm.

rales sound of air bubbling through fluid in the alveoli and bronchi; may sound like sand falling on an empty tin can or be musical or whistling.

rebound tenderness pain elicited upon withdrawal of both the examiner's hands from the abdomen after putting deep pressure on the abdomen; reflects the presence of intra-articular pathology.

rectosigmoid colon lower part of the large intestine that joins the rectum.

rectum the lowermost end of the large intestine.

rectus femoris anterior thigh muscle of the quadriceps group.

rectus femoris muscle *see* rectus femoris.

red blood cells cells in the blood stream that contain hemoglobin to transport oxygen; erythrocytes.

referred pain pain felt on a distant body surface associated with the same area of the spinal cord as the organ causing the pain.

reflex fairly fixed pattern of response or behavior similar for any given stimulus; does not involve a conscious action.

reflex pathway consists of sensory fibers bringing impulse into the spinal cord and motor fibers capable of effecting a response, plus all the interconnections between the two.

regeneration process whereby new matrices and cells, identical in structure and function to those they replace, are formed.

regurgitation a backflow of fluid as a result of the stomach's being too full.

rehabilitation restoration of the injured athlete to self-sufficiency and an appropriate level of competitive fitness.

renal pelvis cone-shaped collecting area that connects the ureter and the kidney.

renal stone *see* kidney stones.

repair process where damaged or lost cells and matrices are replaced by new cells and matrices.

reservoir place where infectious organisms live and multiply, such as in stagnant water or a sewer.

residual volume air remaining in the lungs after maximal expiration.

resorption first step in bone remodeling or taking away bone.

respiration breathing.

respiratory zone generations of branching in the airway system beyond the terminal bronchiole.

respondeat superior doctrine stating that the principal or employer must respond for the tortious conduct of the agent or employee; vicarious liability.

retina a layer of cells at the back of the eye which are carried by the optic nerve to the brain and change the light image into electrical impulses.

retropatellar pain pain behind the kneecap caused by direct trauma to the patella or repetitive knee flexion-extension activities.

retroperitoneal space space between the posterior parietal peritoneum and the posterior abdominal wall, containing the kidneys, adrenal glands, ureters, duodenum, ascending and descending colons, pancreas, and large vessels and nerves.

reversibility an important training concern; basically states that "if you don't use it, you lose it."

rheumatoid arthritis type of joint inflammation (arthritis) mostly affecting the smaller peripheral joints, which become swollen, red, painful, and stiff; also termed rheumatoid disease.

rheumatoid factor a test done to identify proteins found in 50 to 95 percent of individuals with rheumatoid arthritis (RA).

rhomboid muscle of the trunk that helps to stabilize and maneuver the shoulder girdle.

ribs paired arches of bone, twelve on either side, that extend from the thoracic vertebrae toward the anterior midline of the trunk.

right lower quadrant abdominal quadrant which has as principal organs two portions of the large intestine (the cecum and the ascending colon).

rigid splint splint made from firm material and applied to sides, front, and/or back of an injured extremity to prevent motion at the injury site.

ringworm infection, caused by a variety of different fungi, characterized by well-defined, slightly reddened patches with peripheral scaling; commonly found on the feet, groin, scalp, nails, or trunk.

rotator cuff musculotendinous cuff that reinforces the structure around the shoulder joint.

rotator cuff impingement impingement of the rotator cuff on the acromion and the coracoacromial ligament; causes microtrauma to the cuff, resulting in local inflammation, edema, cuff softening, pain, and poor function of the cuff.

sacroiliac joint the joint formed by the articulation of the sacrum and ilium.

sacrum one of the three bones (sacrum and two pelvic bones) that make up the pelvic ring.

sagittal plane vertical section of the body.

saliva secretion of water, protein, and salts into the mouth by salivary glands; makes food easier to chew and begins breaking down starch for digestion.

salivary glands glands that produce saliva to keep the mouth and pharynx moist.

sarcomere the basic unit of structure and function in skeletal muscle, composed of actin and myosin.

sartorius muscle one of the pes anserinus muscles that help protect the knee against rotatory and valgus stress (the other pes anserinus muscles are the gracilis and semitendinosus).

scabies skin infestation caused by a mite, characterized by itching and elevated burrows on the skin surface.

scapula the shoulder blade.

scapular fractures fractures of the scapula.

scapulothoracic joint articulation in which the scapula is suspended from the posterior thoracic wall through muscular attachments to the ribs and spine.

Scheuermann's disease osteochondrosis of the vertebral epiphysis resulting in increased thoracic kyphosis in the preteen and early adolescent years.

sciatic nerve nerve arising from the sacral plexus that carries major motor and sensory innervation to the foot and leg.

sclera white portion of the eye; the tough outer coat of the eye that protects the delicate, light-sensitive inner layer.

scoliosis lateral curvature of the spine to the left or right.

screw-home mechanism medial rotation; final motion of the femur before full extension.

sebaceous glands glands producing an oily substance called sebum which is discharged along the shafts of the hairs on the head and body.

sebum oily substance secreted by the sebaceous glands which seals the epidermal cells and keeps the skin supple.

secondary amenorrhea cessation of normal menstrual periods for greater than three months in a previously menstruating female.

secondary survey the final step in the assessment process in which the athletic trainer carefully examines the patient from head to toe, looking for wounds and deformities and observing whether the patient feels pain or sensation.

second-degree concussion moderate brain injury involving momentary loss of consciousness that may last from several seconds up to 5 minutes, transient confusion, mild retrograde amnesia, moderate dizziness and tinnitus, and possible loss of coordination.

sed rate *see* erythrocyte sedimentation rate.

seizure (convulsion) episode characterized by generalized uncoordinated muscular activity and changes in the level of consciousness which lasts for variable periods of time.

semen seminal fluid ejaculated from the penis and containing sperm.

semimembranosus muscle muscle extending from the ischial tuberosity to the tibia which acts to flex the leg and extend the thigh; important stabilizing structure to the posterior aspect of the knee.

seminal vesicles storage sacs for sperm and seminal fluid, which empty into the urethra at the prostate.

semitendinosus muscle one of the pes anserinus muscles that help protect the knee against rotatory and valgus stress (the other pes anserinus muscles are the gracilis and sartorius).

sensory dermatome scheme pattern of sensory innervation of the skin by one posterior or spinal nerve root.

sensory nerves nerves that carry sensations of touch, taste, heat, cold, pain, or other modalities to the spinal cord or brain.

septum dividing wall or membrane between body spaces or masses of soft tissue.

serosa peritoneum that covers organs.

serratus anterior muscle of the trunk that helps to stabilize and maneuver the shoulder girdle.

sesamoid bones two small bones located beneath the first metatarsal head that function as extra weight-bearing structures and leverage points for the mechanics of the great toe.

sesamoiditis inflammation of the sesamoid bones of the great toe.

Sever's disease osteochondrosis of the calcaneal apophysis seen in children aged 6 to 10 years.

shaft the long, straight, cylindrical midportion of a bone.

shin splints anterior or posterior tibial tendinitis.

shock state of collapse of the cardiovascular system; inability of the cardiovascular system to provide sufficient circulation to the entire body.

short collateral ligament ligament running parallel to the fibular collateral ligament and attaching to the fibular head posterior to the biceps tendon; also called fabellofibular ligament when it is attached to the fabella; reinforces the posterior capsule and contributes to the lateral stability of the knee.

shoulder dislocation *see* glenohumeral dislocation.

signs readily apparent manifestations of changes in body functions.

simple partial seizures partial epileptic seizures in which the seizure activity is limited to one or more extremities or one side of the body.

Sinding-Larsen-Johansson syndrome overuse injury of the extensor mechanism in which the lower pole of the patella is injured by the pull of the patellar tendon; seen in the growing athlete.

skeletal (voluntary) muscle striated muscles that are attached to bones and usually cross at least one joint.

skeleton the skeletal system; the supporting framework of the human body, composed of 206 bones.

sling and swathe triangular bandage that is tied around the neck to support the weight of the injured upper extremity (sling) and is used in conjunction with a bandage that passes around the chest, securing the injured extremity to the chest (swathe).

slipped capital femoral epiphysis displacement of the femoral head on the femoral neck as a result of a growth disturbance in the proximal femoral growth plate; the most common hip disorder occurring during adolescence.

Slocum anterolateral rotatory instability test modification of the lateral pivot shift test in which the athlete lies on his or her side with the uninvolved leg flexed at the hip, the examiner applies an internal rotation force to the proximal tibia and a valgus stress to the joint; at 20 degrees of flexion the knee visibly, palpably, and audibly reduces.

Slocum external rotation test one of the tests for anteromedial-rotatory instability conducted with the hip flexed to approximately 45 degrees and the knee to approximately 80 degrees; a forward motion is applied to the thigh and the degree of anterior drawer is assessed.

slow twitch muscle fibers Type II muscle fibers that are adapted for more efficient aerobic or endurance activities.

small bowel the portion of the digestive tube between the stomach and the cecum, consisting of the duodenum, jejunum, and ileum.

small intestine *see* small bowel.

smooth muscle nonstriated, involuntary muscle which constitutes the bulk of the gastrointestinal tract and is present in nearly every organ to regulate automatic activity.

soleus muscle muscle, extending from the proximal fibula to the calcaneus, that acts to extend and rotate the foot.

somatization a condition in which the individual complains over several years of various physical problems for which no physical cause can be found.

source of infection origin of the infection or infectious agent; it may be a person, object, or any substance carrying bacteria, viruses, or parasites.

sovereign immunity doctrine in English common law whereby individuals were deprived of a remedy when their injury or damage was caused by the negligence of the king or other governmental entity.

Spanish windlass tourniquet consisting of a bandage tied around a body part and twisted by a stick passed under it.

specificity important training concept that states that training must be relevant to the demands of the sport.

sphincters circular muscles that encircle a duct or opening in such a way that their contraction constricts the opening.

spinal column central supporting bony structure of the body; vertebral column.

spinal cord extension of the brain, composed of virtually all the nerves carrying messages between the brain and the rest of the body. It lies inside of and is protected by the vertebrae and the spinal column.

spine column of 33 vertebrae extending from the base of the skull to the tip of the coccyx.

spinous processes palpable prominences in the vertebrae.

spleen large, solid organ in the upper left quadrant of the abdomen; its major function is the production and destruction of blood cells.

splint device used to immobilize part of the body.

spondylolisthesis displacement of one vertebra on another through the spondylitic defect of the pars interarticularis; usually occurs between the fourth and fifth lumbar vertebrae.

spondylolysis defect in the pars interarticularis; may be congenital or traumatic.

spontaneous pneumothorax presence of air in the chest cavity caused by the rupture of a congenitally weak area on the surface of the lungs.

sports anemia false anemia or pseudoanemia caused by extensive aerobic training, which increases the plasma volume, producing a relative decrease in hematocrit.

sprain injury to a ligament sprain.

spur a pointed bony projection.

squeeze injury *see* barotrauma.

stabilizing dressing dressing used to keep bandages in place during transport—i.e., soft roller bandages, rolls of gauze, triangular bandages, or adhesive tape.

standard of care recognized manner in which the individual is expected to act or behave when giving care.

static exercise occurs with isometric contraction to the point of fatigue, such as in weight lifting.

static stretch stretching muscle tissue to a comfortable position, then holding this position for a period of time.

status epilepticus condition in which one epileptic seizure succeeds another with little or no intermission.

sternoclavicular dislocation disruption of the articulation which lies between the clavicle and the sternum.

sternoclavicular joint articulation between the sternum and the clavicle.

sternocleidomastoid cervical muscle that produces rotation of the head.

sternum breastbone.

stomach expansion of the alimentary canal between the esophagus and the duodenum; receives food, stores it, and provides for its movement into the small bowel.

stone bruise injury as a result of direct trauma to the heel pad.

straight anterior laxity true anterior instability of the knee; straightforward motion of the tibia on the femur, which indicates damage to the anterior cruciate ligament.

straight lateral laxity abnormal motion with lateral opening of the joint, or varus laxity; demonstrating injury to the fibular collateral ligament and lateral capsular structures.

straight medial laxity abnormal motion with medial opening of the joint, or valgus laxity, reflecting damage to the tibial collateral ligament.

straight posterior laxity the tibia can be displaced posteriorly in a neutral position, without any rotation, indicating damage to the posterior cruciate ligament.

strain stretching or tearing of a muscle; also, the deformation at a point in a structure under loading.

stress load per unit area which develops on a plane surface within a structure in response to externally applied loads.

stress fracture *see* fatigue fracture.

stress-strain curve curve reflecting the mathematical relationship of stress to strain of a structure.

striated muscle muscle with characteristic stripes, or striations, under the microscope; voluntary, skeletal muscle.

stroke sudden lessening or loss of consciousness, sensation, and voluntary movement resulting from rupture or obstruction of an artery in the brain.

stroke volume amount of blood ejected per beat of the heart.

styloid processes bony prominences at the ends of the radius and ulna that form the socket for the wrist joint.

subacromial bursa bursa that lies in the subacromial space and acts as the "protective" tissue between the cuff and the bony acromion.

subacute stage time period between acute and chronic injury.

subcutaneous emphysema presence of air in soft tissues of the body, causing a very characteristic crackling sensation on palpation.

subcutaneous tissue tissue, largely fat, that lies directly under the dermis and insulates the body.

subdiaphragmatic thrust a series of six to ten manual thrusts to the upper abdomen just above the umbilicus and well below the xiphoid to relieve upper airway obstruction; also called the abdominal thrust maneuver.

subdural hematoma hematoma, or collection of blood, beneath the dura mater and outside the brain.

subluxation partial dislocation.

subscapularis muscle that arises from the ventral surface of the scapula and inserts on the lesser tuberosity; part of the rotator cuff.

subungual hematoma hematoma beneath a finger or toe nail.

sucking chest wound wounds of the chest wall through which air passes into and out of the pleural space with each respiration.

superficial frostbite cold injury involving the skin and the superficial tissue.

superficial temporal arteries arteries supplying the scalp, palpable just anterior to the ear at the temporomandibular joints.

superficial thermotherapy therapeutic heat modalities including whirlpools, moist heat packs, paraffin, and fluidotherapy.

superior and inferior articular processes form the small joints of the posterior elements of the vertebra.

superior portion portion of the body or body part that lies nearer the head than the feet.

superior vena cava one of the two largest veins in the body that carries blood from the upper extremities, head, neck, and chest into the heart.

supraspinatus the most superior muscle that arises from the dorsal surface of the scapula and inserts on the greater tuberosity; part of the rotator cuff.

sustained and dynamic exercise exercise that creates a mixed response, such as when a person walks rapidly while carrying a heavy object.

sweat fatigue *see* anhidrosis.

sweat glands glands that secrete sweat.

swimmer's shoulder partial rotator cuff tear associated with repetitive swimming or throwing activities.

sympathetic stimulation the "fight or flight" response; release of adrenaline increases heart rate, constricts blood vessels, and relaxes bronchioles.

sympathetic (thoracolumbar) nervous system part of the autonomic nervous system that causes blood vessels to constrict, stimulates sweating, increases the heart rate, causes the sphincter muscles to constrict, and prepares the body to respond to stress.

symphysis pubis *see* pubic symphysis.

symptom evidence of change in body functions apparent to the patient and expressed to the examiner on questioning.

synovial fluid fluid produced by the synovium that nourishes and lubricates the articular cartilage of a joint.

synovitis nonspecific inflammation of the lining of a joint.

synovium the inner surface of the joint capsule.

syrup of ipecac preparation of the dried root of a shrub found in Brazil and other parts of South America that is used therapeutically to induce vomiting when a toxic substance has been ingested.

systematic desensitization technique used to rehabilitate injured athletes psychologically; helps athletes handle anxiety by combining relaxation training and visual imagery.

systemic circulation circulation, often called the greater circulation, that carries oxygenated blood from the left ventricle of the heart throughout the body and back to the right atrium.

systemic hypothermia systemic lowering of the body temperature below 95 degrees F.

systolic pressure the blood pressure noted at the moment of ventricular contraction of the heart.

tachycardia rapid but regular beating of the heart; high pulse rate.

tackler's exostosis *see* myositis ossificans.

tailor's bunion enlargement of the lateral aspect of the fifth metatarsal.

talus the ankle bone.

tarsal bones seven bones that make up the rear portion of the foot.

tarsal coalition congenital synostosis or failure of segmentation between two or more tarsal bones.

tarsal tunnel syndrome a neuritis of the posterior tibial nerve resulting in pain and/or numbness along the course of the nerve.

temples lateral portions of the cranium.

temporal regions *see* temples.

temporomandibular joint joint formed by the articulation between the mandible and the cranium, just in front of the ear.

tendinitis inflammation of a tendon, usually caused by injury.

tendinosis lesion asymptomatic tendon degeneration caused either by aging or by cumulative microtrauma without inflammation.

tendon tough, ropelike cord of fibrous tissue that attaches skeletal muscles to bones.

tenesmus straining of the anal sphincter with an urge to defecate that cannot be satisfied.

tennis elbow inflammation of the lateral epicondyle.

tenosynovitis inflammation of the thin inner lining of a tendon sheath.

tension pneumothorax condition in which air continuously leaks out of the lung into the pleural space, increasing pressure within the space at every breath; occurs when a spontaneous pneumothorax fails to seal with the collapse of the lung.

teres minor the most inferior muscle that arises from the dorsal surface of the scapula and inserts on the greater tuberosity; part of the rotator cuff.

terminal bronchiole last subdivision of the bronchi which terminates in the alveoli, beyond which is the respiratory zone.

testicle male genital gland containing specialized cells that produce hormones and sperm.

testis *see* testicle.

tetanus prophylaxis treatment to prevent tetanus, a potentially fatal infectious disease characterized by extreme body rigidity and muscle spasms.

thermotherapy heat application; physical modality that reduces muscle spasm and stiffness and eases motion at joints and between fascial planes.

third-degree concussion severe brain injury resulting in prolonged loss of consciousness beyond 5 minutes; neurovascular coordination is markedly compromised, with severe mental confusion.

Thompson test simple test to determine whether the gastrocnemius-soleus group is intact; the athlete kneels in a chair with the feet hanging free while the examiner squeezes the calf muscle; a lack of plantar flexion indicates disruption of the gastrocnemius-soleus-Achilles tendon complex.

thoracic spine the 12 vertebrae that attach to the 12 ribs; the upper part of the back.

thorax the chest; the upper part of the trunk between the neck and the abdomen.

thought stoppage psychological technique whereby the athlete, upon recognizing faulty thinking, says "stop."

throat culture a test to determine whether a bacterium (most frequently strep, group A) is causing symptoms of sore throat; a throat swab is obtained, and the bacteria are inoculated on culture medium and evaluated in 24 to 48 hours.

thrombus a blood clot within a vessel.

thyroid cartilage largest cartilage of the larynx; forms the Adam's apple.

thyroid gland ductless gland lying on the upper part of the trachea; it produces thyroid hormone.

tibia shinbone; the larger of the two leg bones.

tibial collateral ligament one of the major ligamentous support structures of the knee; extends from the medial condyle of the femur to the medial condyle of the tibia and its shaft.

tibialis anterior muscle muscle located in the anterior compartment of the lower leg; inserts on the medial cuneiform and acts to flex and elevate the foot.

tibialis posterior muscle one of the three muscles of the deep portion of the posterior compartment of the muscles of the leg; one of the medial stabilizers of the ankle, it acts to invert the foot and extend the ankle.

tibial nerve provides motor and sensory function to the lower leg; disappears from view as it courses deep to the gastrocnemius muscle.

tibial plateaus the expanded upper ends of the tibia; form the interior surface of the knee joint and articulate with the femoral condyles.

tibial tubercle the bony prominence of the proximal tibia.

tibiofemoral joint polycentric hinge joint that bears the body's weight during locomotion; joints between each tibial and femoral condyle.

tibiofibular syndesmosis one of the three groups of ankle ligaments; arrangement of dense fibrous tissues between the osseous structures just above the ankle joint that maintains the relationship of the distal tibia and fibula.

tidal volume amount of air breathed in and out during one respiratory cycle.

tidemark thin line that lies between the radial zone and the calcified zone of the articular cartilage.

tinea versicolor ringworm infection of the skin caused by a yeast fungus; produces patches of white or brown finely flaking skin over the trunk and neck.

tomograms cross-sectional image (slice) of an organ or part of the body at various depths of field produced by an x-ray technique.

tongue-jaw lift maneuver method of opening the athlete's mouth by grasping the tongue and lower jaw between the thumb and fingers and lifting forward to probe for foreign bodies.

tonic-clonic a generalized seizure involving rigid (tonic) muscular contractions and repetitive (clonic) muscular spasms.

tonsillitis inflammation of the tonsils due to infection; *see* pharyngitis.

topographic anatomy superficial landmarks of the body.

topography external features of the body.

torus fracture impaction fracture that occurs in the metaphyseal bone of the child.

total lung capacity volume of gas contained in the lungs at the end of full inspiration.

trachea windpipe; main trunk for air passing to and from the lungs.

traction action of drawing or pulling on an object.

traction splint splint that holds a lower-extremity fracture or dislocation immobile; allows steady longitudinal pull on the extremity.

tragus small, rounded, fleshy protuberance immediately at the front of the ear canal.

transcutaneous electrical nerve stimulation (TENS) therapeutic modality in which electrical stimulation is applied to the body with an intact peripheral nervous system; can elicit either sensory or muscular responses by stimulating nerves when electrical current passes across the skin.

transverse arch arch formed by the metatarsal bones when the foot is non-weight bearing and at rest.

transverse colon part of the colon that runs transversely across the upper part of the abdomen.

transverse plane horizontal section of the body.

transverse processes together with the posterior process, allow the attachment of strong intervertebral ligaments that support the spine and also provide anchors for muscles attached to the spinal column.

trapezius large diamond-shaped muscle of the most superficial layer of the shoulder girdle lying posteriorly.

traumatic spondylolysis the affected vertebra slips anterior to the one below it when both the right and left pars interarticularis of a vertebra are defective.

trench foot *see* immersion foot.

triage sorting or selection of patients to determine priority of care.

triceps the muscle in the back of the upper arm that acts to extend the arm and forearm.

triglyceride major storage for fats, consists of a glycerol and three fatty acids.

trochanter prominence on a bone where tendons insert; specifically, two protuberances, greater and lesser, on the femur.

trochanteric bursa one of the two most important bursae about the hip joint located just behind the greater trochanter and deep to the gluteus maximus and tensor fascia lata muscle.

trochlea a structure shaped like a pulley; for example, the patellofemoral groove.

tuberosity prominence on a bone where tendons insert.

turf toe sprain of the metatarsophalangeal joint of the great toe.

T wave wave of an electrocardiogram that represents repolarization of the ventricles.

tympanic membrane eardrum.

Type I diabetes *see* juvenile-onset diabetes.

Type II diabetes *see* adult-onset diabetes.

Type I muscle fibers fast twitch muscle fibers adapted for anaerobic activity.

Type II muscle fibers slow twitch muscle fibers adapted for aerobic (endurance) activity.

ulna inner and larger bone of the forearm, on the side opposite the thumb.

ulnar artery artery originating from the brachial artery and supplying the forearm, wrist, and hand.

ulnar nerve nerve originating from the brachial plexus that controls sensation over the fifth and fourth fingers; controls most of the muscular function of the hand.

ulnar styloid bony prominence of the ulna felt on the medial (little finger) side of the wrist.

ulna shaft the long cylindrical portion of the ulna.

ultrasound thermal agent which uses high-frequency acoustical energy to elicit thermal and mechanical responses; has long been used to treat inflammatory conditions.

ultrasound therapy therapeutic modality using high-frequency acoustical energy to elicit thermal and mechanical responses; *see* ultrasound.

umbilicus the navel; a small depression in the abdominal wall marking the point where the fetus was attached to the umbilical cord.

universal dressing a dressing made of thick, absorbent material, measuring 9 by 36 inches and folded into a compact size; can also be used as a cervical collar or as padding for splints.

upper gastrointestinal (UGI) series x-rays taken of the esophagus, stomach, and upper small intestine after the athlete swallows a mixture of water and barium sulfate, an oil-based nonabsorbable radiodense material.

upper right quadrant abdominal quadrant which has as its major organs the liver, the gallbladder, and a portion of the colon.

uremia toxic condition caused by waste products of metabolism accumulating in the blood as a result of a failure of kidney function.

ureters fibromuscular tubes that convey urine from the kidney to the bladder.

urethra membranous canal conveying urine from the bladder to outside the body.

urinalysis one of the oldest known clinical laboratory tests, used to determine kidney function.

urinary bladder musculomembranous sac for collecting and storing urine.

urinary frequency abnormally high number of voiding episodes during a 24-hour period.

urinary system organs for production and excretion of urine.

urticaria hives; allergic reaction characterized by bumps on the skin.

use accumulation of load over time; load and use are the primary mechanisms by which connective tissue change occurs in response to sport activity.

uterus muscular organ of the female reproductive system that opens into the vagina through the cervix; holds and nourishes the fetus.

vacuum splints splint using a vacuum created by suction to expand synthetic beads creating a rigid splint; splints that are not temperature sensitive and form around deformities.

vagina muscular, distensible tube connecting the uterus with the external female genitalia; receives the penis during intercourse.

vaginitis inflammation of the vagina.

valgus extension overload injury to the medial flexor mass and medial elbow joint ligaments in a throwing athlete.

valgus laxity *see* straight medial laxity.

varicoceles abnormally distended veins of the spermatic cord in the scrotum.

varus laxity *see* straight lateral laxity.

vas deferens spermatic duct of testicles.

vastus intermedius a component of the quadriceps muscle.

vastus lateralis a component of the quadriceps muscle.

vastus medialis a component of the quadriceps muscle.

vastus medialis obliquus (VMO) a smaller component of the vastus medialis muscle.

vector transmission method of disease transmission in which the infective organism is transmitted to an individual by animals.

vehicle transmission method of disease transmission in which the infective organism is introduced directly into the body through the ingestion of contaminated food or water or by the infusion of contaminated drugs, fluid, or blood.

vein tubular vessel that carries blood from the capillaries toward the heart.

venom poison secreted by animals and transmitted via bite wounds or stings.

ventricle either of the two lower chambers of the heart.

venules small veins into which blood passes from the capillaries.

vertebrae *see* vertebral column.

vertebral arch part of the vertebra composed of the right and left pedicles and the right and left laminae.

vertebral body compression compression fracture of the vertebral body without damage to the ligamentous structures; the most common thoracic fracture; also called wedge fracture.

vertebral column segmented spinal column composed of 24 movable vertebrae, 5 fixed sacral vertebrae and 4 fixed coccygeal vertebrae.

vertebrochondral ribs ribs that articulate directly with the sternum via their costal cartilages.

vertebrosternal ribs ribs that connect the first 10 thoracic vertebrae to the sternum.

vicarious liability *see* respondeat superior.

visceral peritoneum continuation of the parietal peritoneum that covers the stomach, spleen, liver, intestines, bladder, and female reproductive organs.

visceral pleura smooth, glistening tissue that covers the outer surface of the lungs.

viscoelastic time-dependent deformation behavior of biological materials.

vital capacity maximum volume of gas that can be expired after a maximum inspiration.

vitreous humor fluid behind the lens of the eye.

Volkmann's contracture ischemic necrosis of the forearm muscles.

voluntary (skeletal) muscle muscle, under direct voluntary control of the brain, which can be contracted or relaxed at will.

vomiting disgorging of the stomach contents through the mouth.

vulva the external female genitalia.

warts viral infection of the skin or mucous membranes, caused by a papillomavirus found within the skin of the body.

wedge fracture *see* vertebral body compression.

wheal raised area on the skin resulting from an allergic reaction.

wheezes whistling sounds resulting from respiratory airway narrowing.

white blood cells leukocytes.

Wolff's law phenomenon where the bone is deposited on areas subjected to stress and reabsorbed from areas where little stress is present.

work energy (WE) energy stored in a structure under deformation.

woven (nonlamellar) bone immature bone.

xiphoid process the pointed process of cartilage supported by a core of bone connected with the lower end of the body of the sternum.

x-rays radiant energy produced by exposing tungsten to a beam of electrons; useful in imaging many body parts.

zone of primary injury extent of the initial hematoma and the area of devitalized tissue.

zone of secondary injury zone created by the intense chemical activity and exudation of the acute inflammatory response.

zygomatic arch process from the temporal bone to which is connected the prominence of the cheek.

zygomatic bone cheekbone.

Index